Textbook of Palliative Care Communication

Textbook of Palliative Care Communication

Edited by

Elaine Wittenberg, PhD

Betty R. Ferrell, RN, PHD, MA, FAAN, FPCN, CHPN

Joy Goldsmith, PhD

Thomas Smith, MD

Sandra L. Ragan, PhD

Myra Glajchen, BSW, MSW, DSW

The Rev. George F. Handzo, MA, BCC

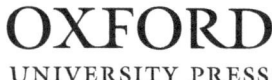

OXFORD
UNIVERSITY PRESS

Oxford University Press is a department of the University of
Oxford. It furthers the University's objective of excellence in research,
scholarship, and education by publishing worldwide.

Oxford   New York
Auckland   Cape Town   Dar es Salaam   Hong Kong   Karachi
Kuala Lumpur   Madrid   Melbourne   Mexico City   Nairobi
New Delhi   Shanghai   Taipei   Toronto

With offices in
Argentina   Austria   Brazil   Chile   Czech Republic   France   Greece
Guatemala   Hungary   Italy   Japan   Poland   Portugal   Singapore
South Korea   Switzerland   Thailand   Turkey   Ukraine   Vietnam

Oxford is a registered trademark of Oxford University Press
in the UK and certain other countries.

Published in the United States of America by
Oxford University Press
198 Madison Avenue, New York, NY 10016

© Oxford University Press 2016

All rights reserved. No part of this publication may be reproduced, stored in
a retrieval system, or transmitted, in any form or by any means, without the prior
permission in writing of Oxford University Press, or as expressly permitted by law,
by license, or under terms agreed with the appropriate reproduction rights organization.
Inquiries concerning reproduction outside the scope of the above should be sent to the
Rights Department, Oxford University Press, at the address above.

You must not circulate this work in any other form
and you must impose this same condition on any acquirer.

This material is not intended to be, and should not be considered, a substitute for medical or other
professional advice. Treatment for the conditions described in this material is highly dependent on
the individual circumstances. And, while this material is designed to offer accurate information
with respect to the subject matter covered and to be current as of the time it was written, research
and knowledge about medical and health issues is constantly evolving and dose schedules for
medications are being revised continually, with new side effects recognized and accounted for
regularly. Readers must therefore always check the product information and clinical procedures
with the most up-to-date published product information and data sheets provided by the
manufacturers and the most recent codes of conduct and safety regulation. The publisher and the
authors make no representations or warranties to readers, express or implied, as to the accuracy or
completeness of this material. Without limiting the foregoing, the publisher and the authors make
no representations or warranties as to the accuracy or efficacy of the drug dosages mentioned in the
material. The authors and the publisher do not accept, and expressly disclaim, any responsibility
for any liability, loss or risk that may be claimed or incurred as a consequence of the use and/or
application of any of the contents of this material.

Library of Congress Cataloging-in-Publication Data
Textbook of palliative care communication / edited by Elaine Wittenberg.
   p. ; cm.
Includes bibliographical references and index.
ISBN 978–0–19–020170–8 (alk. paper)
I. Witten berg, Elaine, editor.
[DNLM: 1. Palliative Care. 2. Advance Care Planning. 3. Communication. 4. Decision
Making. 5. Patient-Centered Care. 6. Professional-Patient Relations. WB 310]
R726.8
616.02′9—dc23
2015011427

9 8 7 6 5 4 3 2
Printed in the United States of America
on acid-free paper

Disclosures

Chapter 7: Sponsored by the Donald W. Reynolds Foundation Consortium for Faculty Development to Advance Geriatric Education.

Chapter 20: Support was provided by a grant from the National Institutes of Health/National Cancer Institute.

Chapter 30: Matthew Loscalzo is the co-inventor of the SupportScreen and receives royalties from the City of Hope for licensees external to the City of Hope.

Preface

Communication has long been recognized as a core component of quality palliative care. Historically, the field of palliative care has privileged communication as central to clinical practice by emphasizing the communication of bad news with patients and families. As a result, palliative care providers are among the best communicators in healthcare, as well as the most well practiced. However, the relatively brief history of communication in palliative care has been shaped by tools and protocols that are not inclusive of evidence and science that is representative of communication scholarship. Communication tools and protocols have been informed by books written by one person, from one discipline, about his or her own communication experiences with patients and families. We truly believe that advancement in the field will take place only by working collectively across disciplines and bridging an interest in communication across professional boundaries, methodological expertise, and care settings.

We are committed to quality care for seriously ill patients and their families and are steadfast in the belief that quality care requires excellent communication about palliative care topics, enables shared decision-making, includes family, and empowers patient preferences. While we have become proficient at explaining the physical aspects of care, we must now focus on ways to address other quality of life dimensions (social, psychological, and spiritual), begin to define and articulate the role and nature of other palliative care team members, extend the scope of issues within palliative care (such as with non-oncology patient populations and in other settings of care), and learn about the variety of approaches and research methods that can be used to study communication. This textbook is designed to meet all of these needs, and our goal is that it will serve as the essential communication training resource for clinicians and researchers across all disciplines involved in palliative care.

Uniquely, we have gathered prominent communication scholars, clinicians, and researchers all dedicated to palliative care in order to supply readers with one comprehensive book that symbolizes the power of interdisciplinary scholarship and defines the field of palliative care communication. We set out to find the best in the field of communication and palliative care; to include the busiest, most productive authors already forging new territory in communication research in palliative care; and to explore the most challenging palliative topics. We are grateful that they recognized the value of this first *Textbook of Palliative Care Communication* and the importance of providing an interdisciplinary text devoted to the topic. We recognize the major commitment and that they took time from their work to share their expertise.

Identified by Oxford University Press as a distinct field, this dedicated textbook establishes communication as a focal area within palliative care practice, defining the scope and breadth of palliative care communication, and naming it as an essential clinical feature that spans across all disciplines and conditions. The textbook legitimates the field of palliative care communication by providing frameworks and tools grounded in communication theory, research, and education. It represents a movement from "good" communication to evidence-based communication practice by changing the ways that we think about and approach communication in palliative settings. This state-of-the-art resource gives evidence to the knowledge, expertise, and practice of palliative care communication. The Palliative Care Communication Institute website (www.pccinstitute.com) serves as an additional resource and companion for this textbook, providing lectures, teaching activities, and audio and video examples of communication tools presented here. It is our hope that this comprehensive, evidence-based text will provide background as well as direction for future scholarship in palliative care communication.

Acknowledgment

The concept and execution of this volume was championed by our editor, Andrea Knobloch, at Oxford University Press, who shrewdly recognized its value and sagely navigated the project through the Oxford system. The book would not have been possible without the tireless efforts of Ellen Friedmann, who provided stellar editorial labors, and Lisa Vallecorsa, who gracefully stewarded the entire editorial process. We dedicate this book to the many patients, families, providers, and students of palliative care who willingly shared their experiences and have shaped the practice of palliative care communication as we know it today.

Contents

Contributors *xiii*	**12 Health Literacy and Communication in Palliative Care** 90
1 Overview of Communication *1* Sandra L. Ragan	Wen-ying Sylvia Chou, Anna Gaysynsky, and Alexander Persoskie
2 A Historical Perspective of Palliative Care Communication *10* Betty Ferrell, Elaine Wittenberg, and Tammy Neiman	**13 Patient- and Family-Centered Written Communication in the Palliative Care Setting** 102 Antoinette Mary Fage-Butler and Matilde Nisbeth Jensen
3 Transactional Communication *14* Athena du Pré and Elissa Foster	**14 Health Disparities** 111 Susan Eggly, Lauren M. Hamel, Louis A. Penner, and Terrance L. Albrecht
4 Consumer Communication and Public Messaging About Palliative Care *22* Rebecca A. Kirch	**15 The Role of Communication and Information in Symptom Management** 119 Gary L. Kreps and Mollie Rose Canzona
5 Communication Ethics *27* Timothy W. Kirk, Nessa Coyle, and Matthew Doolittle	**16 Patient Experience of Illness** 127 Terry Altilio and Meagan Lyon Leimena
6 Communication in Palliative Social Work *35* Myra Glajchen and Susan B. Gerbino	**17 Family Member Experience of Caregiving** 135 Maryjo Prince-Paul and Karen S. Vrtunski
7 Communication in Palliative Medicine *44* Jennifer Gabbard and Thomas Smith	**18 Family Caregiver Communication Goals and Messages** 144 Joy Goldsmith
8 Communication in Palliative Nursing *54* Constance M. Dahlin	**19 Cultural Considerations in Palliative Care and Serious Illness** 153 Guadalupe R. Palos
9 Communication in Palliative Care Chaplaincy *63* George F. Handzo	**20 Family Conversations About In-Home and Hospice Care** 161 Wayne A. Beach, Kyle Gutzmer, and David M. Dozier
10 Communication in Clinical Psychology *71* Sunita K. Patel, Stephanie Davidson, and Jeanelle Folbrecht	**21 Chronic Obstructive Pulmonary Disease and Heart Disease** 173 Niharika Ganta and Laura P. Gelfman
11 Cultural Humility *79* Kathryn Neubauer, William Dixon, Rosalie Corona, and Joann Bodurtha	

xii CONTENTS

22 **Oncology Across the Trajectory** 183
Lillie D. Shockney

23 **Transplantation and Organ Donation** 189
James D. Robinson and Teresa Thompson

24 **Communication Challenges in Providing Advance Care Planning for People Living With HIV/AIDS** 197
Maureen E. Lyon, Blaire Schembari, Brittney Lee, and Peter Selwyn

25 **Homeless, Mentally Ill, and Drug-Addicted Patients** 205
John D. Chovan

26 **Seriously Ill Veterans** 214
VJ Periyakoil

27 **Neonatal and Pediatrics** 220
Barbara L. Jones and Kendra D. Koch

28 **Lesbian, Gay, Bisexual, and Transgender Communication** 229
Carey Candrian and Hillary Lum

29 **Patient-Centered Communication** 238
Marleah Dean and Richard L. Street Jr.

30 **Care Coordination and Transitions in Care** 246
Finly Zachariah, Brenda Thomson, Matthew Loscalzo, and Laura Crocitto

31 **Trust, Hope, and Miracles** 255
Rhonda S. Cooper, Louise Knight, and Anna Ferguson

32 **Physical Pain and Symptoms** 263
Danielle Noreika, Barton Bobb, and Patrick Coyne

33 **Complementary and Alternative Medicine** 271
Paul Posadzki and Fiona Poland

34 **Redefining Comfort Measures: Communicating About Life Support, Artificial Hydration, and Nutrition** 276
Dawn M. Gross, Nancy Clifton-Hawkins, and Mariela Gallo

35 **Advance Care Planning** 285
Jeanine Blackford and Annette F. Street

36 **Palliative Care Communication and Sexuality** 294
Les Gallo-Silver

37 **Spiritual Communication** 301
Shane Sinclair

38 **Grief Reactions** 311
E. Alessandra Strada

39 **Team Communication in the Acute Care Setting** 321
Andrew Thurston, Lyle Fettig, and Robert Arnold

40 **Team Communication in the Outpatient Care Setting** 330
Jennifer Philip, Jenny Hynson, and Jennifer Weil

41 **Team Communication in the Hospice Setting** 340
Anne Arber

42 **Team Communication in the Nursing Home Setting** 346
Carol O. Long

43 **Communication Education for Physicians** 355
Jillian Gustin, Katie H. Stowers, and Charles F. von Gunten

44 **Communication Education for Nurses** 366
Pam Malloy

45 **Communication Education for Social Workers** 375
John G. Cagle and Kaila Williams

46 **Communication Education for Chaplains** 382
Angelika A. Zollfrank and Catherine F. Garlid

47 **Interprofessional Education** 390
Barbara Anderson Head and Tara J. Schapmire

48 **Qualitative Communication Research** 399
Patrick J. Dillon and Lori A. Roscoe

49 **Quantitative Communication Research** 408
Melinda M. Villagran and Brenda L. MacArthur

50 **The State of the Science on Palliative Care Communication** 417
Elaine Wittenberg

Index 425

Contributors

Terrance L. Albrecht, PhD
Professor of Family Medicine and Public Health
Associate Center Director, Population Sciences
Leader, Population Studies and Disparities Research Program
Wayne State University School of Medicine/Karmanos Cancer Institute
Detroit, Michigan

Terry Altilio, LCSW, ACSW
Social Work Coordinator
Department of Pain Medicine and Palliative Care
Beth Israel Medical Center
New York, New York

Anne Arber, PhD, MSc, RN
Senior Lecturer, Faculty of Health and Medical Sciences
University of Surrey
Guildford, Surrey, United Kingdom

Robert Arnold, MD
Professor of Medicine
Chief, Section of Palliative Care and Medical Ethics
Director, Institute for Doctor-Patient Communication
University of Pittsburgh
Medical Director, UPMC Palliative and Supportive Institute
Pittsburgh, Pennsylvania

Wayne A. Beach, PhD
Professor, School of Communication
San Diego State University
San Diego, California

Jeanine Blackford, PhD, RN
Senior Lecturer
School of Nursing & Midwifery
La Trobe University
Melbourne, Victoria, Australia

Barton T. Bobb, MSN, FNP-BC, ACHPN
Palliative Care and Pain Consult Team
VCU Medical Center
Richmond, Virginia

Joann Bodurtha, MD, MPH, FAAP, FACMG
Professor of Pediatrics and Oncology
McKusick-Nathans Institute of Genetic Medicine
The Johns Hopkins University
Baltimore, Maryland

John Cagle, PhD, MSW
Assistant Professor
University of Maryland, School of Social Work
Baltimore, Maryland

Carey Candrian, PhD
Assistant Professor
University of Colorado School of Medicine,
Division of General Internal Medicine Palliative Care Research Cooperative Group (PCRC)
Aurora, Colorado

Mollie Rose Canzona, PhD
Department of Communication
Wake Forest University
Winston-Salem, North Carolina

Wen-ying Sylvia Chou, PhD, MPH
Program Director
Health Communication and Informatics Research Branch
Division of Cancer Control and Population Sciences
National Cancer Institute
Rockville, Maryland

John D. Chovan, PhD, DNP, RN, CNP, CNS, PMHNP-BC, PMHCNS-BC, ACHPN, AHN-BC
Assistant Professor & Director, DNP Program
Otterbein University
Westerville, Ohio
Palliative Care Nurse Practitioner
Mount Carmel Hospice & Palliative Care
Columbus, Ohio

Nancy Clifton-Hawkins, MPH, MCHES
Community Benefits Manager
City of Hope
Duarte, California

Rhonda S. Cooper, MDiv, BCC
Chaplain
The Johns Hopkins Kimmel Cancer Center
Baltimore, Maryland

Rosalie Corona, PhD
Associate Professor
Director, Latino Mental Health Clinic
Virginia Commonwealth University
Richmond, Virginia

Nessa Coyle, PhD, RN, FAAN
Consultant
Palliative Care and Clinical Ethics in Oncology
New York, New York

Patrick Coyne, MSN, ACHPN, ACNS-BC, FAAN, FPCN
Director of Palliative Care
Medical University of South Carolina
Charleston, South Carolina

Laura Crocitto, MD, MHA
Clinical Associate Professor of Urology
  and Urologic Oncology
Medical Director of Enterprise Quality
  and Safety
City of Hope
Duarte, California

Constance M. Dahlin, ANP-BC, ACHPN, FPCN, FAAN
Director of Professional Practice
Hospice and Palliative Nurses Association
Pittsburgh, Pennsylvania
Palliative Nurse Practitioner
North Shore Medical Center
Salem, Massachusetts
Palliative Care Consultant
Beverly, Massachusetts

Stephanie Davidson, Psy.D
Clinical Psychologist
Department of Supportive Care Medicine
City of Hope
Duarte, California

Marleah Dean, PhD
Assistant Professor
Department of Communication
University of South Florida
Tampa, Florida

Patrick J. Dillon, PhD
Assistant Professor, Department
  of Communication
University of Memphis
Memphis, Tennessee

William K. Dixon, DMin, MDiv
Staff Chaplain
Burn Unit, Neuro ICU and ENT Oncology
James Comprehensive Cancer Hospital
The Ohio State University Wexner Medical Center
Columbus, Ohio

Matthew Doolittle, MD
Assistant Attending
Department of Psychiatry and Behavioral Sciences
Memorial Sloan Kettering Cancer Center
New York, New York

David M. Dozier, PhD
Professor, SDSU School of Journalism and Media Studies
San Diego State University
San Diego, California

Athena du Pré, PhD
Professor and Graduate Program Director
Communication Arts
University of West Florida
Pensacola, Florida

Susan Eggly, PhD
Associate Professor
Population Studies and Disparities Program, Department
  of Oncology
Wayne State University School of Medicine/Karmanos
  Cancer Institute
Detroit, Michigan

Antoinette Mary Fage-Butler, PhD
Associate Professor
School of Business and Social Sciences
Department of Business Communication
Aarhus University
Aarhus C, Denmark

Anna Ferguson, RN, BSN
Research Nurse
The Johns Hopkins Kimmel Cancer Center
Baltimore, Maryland

Betty Ferrell, PhD, RN, MA, FAAN, FPCN, CHPN
Director and Professor
Division of Nursing Research and Education
City of Hope
Duarte, California

Lyle Fettig, MD
Director, Hospice and Palliative Medicine Fellowship Program
Assistant Professor of Clinical Medicine
Indiana University School of Medicine
Eskenazi Health Palliative Care
Indianapolis, Indiana

Jeanelle Folbrecht, PhD
Associate Clinical Professor, Director of Psychology
Department of Supportive Care Medicine
City of Hope
Duarte, California

Elissa Foster, PhD
Associate Professor, Director of M.A. Health
    Communication Program
College of Communication
DePaul University
Chicago, Illinois

Jennifer Gabbard, MD
Assistant Professor, Geriatrics and Palliative Medicine
Section of Geriatrics, Gerontology, Palliative Medicine
Wake Forest University
Winston-Salem, North Carolina

Mariela Gallo, MPH, CHES
Senior Health Education Specialist
Sheri & Les Biller Resource Center, Department
    of Supportive Care Medicine
City of Hope
Duarte, California

Les Gallo-Silver, LCSW-R
Associate Professor
Program Director, Human Services Program
Health Sciences Department
LaGuardia Community College
The City University of New York
Long Island City, New York

Niharika Ganta, MD, MPH
Assistant Professor
Perelman School of Medicine
University of Pennsylvania
Philadelphia, Pennsylvania

Catherine F. Garlid, MDiv, BCC, ACPE
Director, Spiritual Care
Maine Medical Center
Portland, ME

Anna Gaysynsky, MPH
Health Communications Intern
Health Communication and Informatics Research Branch
Division of Cancer Control and Population Sciences
National Cancer Institute
Rockville, Maryland

Laura P. Gelfman, MD, MPH
Assistant Professor
Brookdale Department of Geriatrics and Palliative Medicine
Icahn School of Medicine at Mount Sinai
New York, New York

Susan B. Gerbino, PhD, LCSW
Clinical Professor
Director, Zelda Foster Studies Program in Palliative and
    End-of-Life Care
Silver School of Social Work
New York University
New York, New York

Myra Glajchen, DSW
Director of Medical Education
Associate Program Director, Fellowship Training Program
MJHS Institute for Innovation in Palliative Care
New York, New York
Assistant Professor
Department of Family and Social Medicine
Albert Einstein College of Medicine
Bronx, New York

Joy Goldsmith, PhD
Associate Professor
Department of Communication
University of Memphis
Memphis, Tennessee

Dawn M. Gross, MD, PhD
Arthur M. Coppola Family Chair, Department of Supportive
    Care Medicine
Professor of Supportive Care and Palliative Medicine
City of Hope
Duarte, California

Jillian Gustin, MD
Program Director, Hospice and Palliative Medicine
    Fellowship
Division of Palliative Medicine, Department of Internal
    Medicine
The Ohio State University Wexner Medical Center
Columbus, Ohio

Kyle Gutzmer, PhD
Student-SDSU/UCSD Joint Doctoral Program in Public Health
San Diego State University
University of California
San Diego, California

Lauren M. Hamel, PhD
Assistant Professor
Population Studies and Disparities Program, Department of
    Oncology
Wayne State University School of Medicine/Karmanos Cancer
    Institute
Detroit, Michigan

George F. Handzo, BCC, CSSBB
Director, Health Services Research & Quality
HealthCare Chaplaincy Network: *Caring For The Human
    Spirit*TM
New York, New York

Barbara Head, PhD, CHPN, ACSW, FPCN
Associate Professor
Interdisciplinary Program for Palliative Care
    & Chronic Illness
University of Louisville School of Medicine
Affiliated Associate Professor
University of Louisville Kent School of Social Work
Louisville, Kentucky

Jenny Hynson, PhD
Medical Director
Victorian Paediatric Palliative Care Program
The Royal Children's Hospital
Melbourne, Victoria, Australia

Barbara L. Jones, PhD, MSW
Assistant Dean for Health Affairs & Professor
Co-Director, The Institute for Palliative
  Care Family Survival
UT Austin School of Social Work
Austin, Texas

Rebecca A. Kirch, JD
Director, Quality of Life and Survivorship,
  Cancer Control
American Cancer Society
Washington, DC

Timothy W. Kirk, PhD
Associate Professor of Philosophy
City University of New York, York College
New York, New York

Louise Knight, MSW, LCSW-C, OSW-C
Director
Harry J. Duffey Family Patient
  and Family Services Program
The Johns Hopkins Kimmel Cancer Center
Baltimore, Maryland

Kendra D. Koch, MA
PhD Student
University of Texas at Austin, School
  of Social Work
Research Scientist
Children's Comprehensive Care Clinic
  Seton Healthcare Family
Austin, Texas

Gary L. Kreps, PhD, FAAHB
University Distinguished Professor, Department of
  Communication
Director, Center for Health and Risk Communication
George Mason University
Fairfax, Virginia

Brittney Lee, MPH
Clinical Research Coordinator II
FAmily CEntered Advance Care Planning (FACE) Team
Center for Translational Science
Children's National Health System
Washington, DC

Carol O. Long, PhD, RN, FPCN, FAAN
Principal, Capstone Healthcare & Founder, Palliative Care
  Essentials
Adjunct Faculty
Arizona State University College of Nursing and Health
  Innovation
Phoenix, Arizona

Matthew Loscalzo, LCSW
Liliane Elkins Professor in Supportive Care Programs
Administrative Director, Sheri & Les Biller Patient and Family
  Resource Center
Executive Director, Department of Supportive Care Medicine
Professor, Department of Population Sciences
City of Hope
Duarte, California

Hillary Lum, MD, PhD
Assistant Professor
Division of Geriatric Medicine
University of Colorado School of Medicine
VA Eastern Colorado Health Care System
Aurora, Colorado

Maureen E. Lyon, PhD, ABPP
Clinical Health Psychologist
Research Professor in Pediatrics
George Washington University School of Medicine and Health
  Sciences
Center for Translational Science/Children's Research Institute
Children's National
Washington, DC

Meagan Lyon Leimena, LMSW, MPH
Palliative Care Social Work Consultant
Asheville, North Carolina

Brenda L. MacArthur, MA
Doctoral Candidate
Department of Communication
George Mason University
Fairfax, Virginia

Pam Malloy, RN, MN, FPCN
Director and Co-Investigator of the ELNEC Project
American Association of Colleges of Nursing (AACN)
Washington, DC

Tammy Neiman, MS, RN-BS
PhD Student, College of Nursing
Jonas Nurse Leader Scholar, 2014-2016
University of Wisconsin
Milwaukee, Wisconsin

Kathryn Neubauer, MD
Department of Pediatrics
The Johns Hopkins Hospital
Baltimore, Maryland

Matilde Nisbeth Jensen, PhD
Assistant Professor
School of Business and Social Sciences
Department of Business Communication
Aarhus University
Aarhus C, Denmark

Danielle Noreika, MD
Physician
VCU Massey Cancer Center
Richmond, Virginia

Guadalupe R. Palos, DrPH, LMSW, RN
Clinical Trials Administration Manager
Office of Cancer Survivorship, Department
 of Medical Affairs
M.D. Anderson Cancer Center
Houston, Texas

Sunita K. Patel, PhD
Assistant Professor
Population Sciences and Supportive Care Medicine
City of Hope
Duarte, California

Louis A. Penner, PhD
Professor
Population Studies and Disparities Program,
 Department of Oncology
Wayne State University School of Medicine/Karmanos Cancer
 Institute
Detroit, Michigan

VJ Periyakoil, MD
Director, Palliative Care Education & Training,
Stanford University School of Medicine
Stanford, California

Jennifer Philip, PhD, FAChPM, MMed, MBBS
Associate Professor, Deputy Director
Palliative Medicine & Centre for Palliative Care
St Vincent's Hospital
University of Melbourne
Melbourne, Victoria, Australia

Fiona Poland, PhD
Professor of Social Research Methodology
School of Health Sciences
University of East Anglia
Norwich, United Kingdom

Paul Posadzki, PhD, MSc, BSc
Research Fellow
Lee Kong Chian School of Medicine, Nanyang Technological
 University and Imperial College
London, United Kingdom

Maryjo Prince-Paul, PhD, APRN, ACHPN, FPCN
Assistant Professor
Case Western Reserve University
Frances Payne Bolton School of Nursing
Cleveland, Ohio

Sandra L. Ragan, PhD
Professor Emerita, University of Oklahoma
Norman, Oklahoma

James D. Robinson, PhD
Professor, Communication
University of Dayton
Dayton, Ohio

Lori Roscoe, PhD
Associate Professor, Department of Communication
University of South Florida
Tampa, Florida

Tara J. Schapmire, PhD, MSSW, CSW, CCM, OSW-C
Assistant Professor
Interdisciplinary Program for Palliative Care & Chronic Illness
University of Louisville School of Medicine
Affiliated Assistant Professor
University of Louisville Kent School of Social Work
Louisville, Kentucky

Blaire Schembari, MA
Clinical Research Assistant
Children's National Health System
Center for Translational Science
Washington, DC

Peter Selwyn, MD, MPH
Chair, Department of Family
 and Social Medicine
Professor of Family Medicine, Internal Medicine, and
 Epidemiology & Population Health
Director, Palliative Care Program
Montefiore Medical Center
Albert Einstein College of Medicine
Bronx, New York

Lillie D. Shockney, RN, BS, MAS
University Distinguished Service Associate Professor of
 Breast Cancer
Departments of Surgery and Oncology
Administrative Director, the Johns Hopkins Breast Center
Director, Cancer Survivorship Programs at the Sidney Kimmel
 Cancer Center at Johns Hopkins
Associate Professor, JHU School of Medicine, Departments of
 Surgery, Oncology & Gynecology and Obstetrics
Associate Professor, JHU School of Nursing
Baltimore, Maryland

Shane Sinclair, PhD
Assistant Professor & Cancer Care Research Professor
Faculty of Nursing
University of Calgary
Clinician Scientist, Person Centred Care
Cancer Control, Alberta Health Services
Adjunct Assistant Professor, Cumming School of Medicine,
 Department of Oncology
Division of Palliative Medicine
University of Calgary
Calgary, Canada

Thomas J. Smith, MD, FACP, FASCO, FAAHPM
Professor of Palliative Medicine and Oncology
Johns Hopkins Medicine
Baltimore, Maryland

Katie H. Stowers, DO
University of Texas Health Science Center San Antonio
Division of Geriatrics, Gerontology, Palliative Medicine
San Antonio, Texas

E. Alessandra Strada, PhD, MSCP, FT
Director of Integrative Medicine and Bereavement Services
MJHS Institute for Innovation in Palliative Care
MJHS Hospice and Palliative Care
Clinical Assistant Professor
Department of Family and Social Medicine
Albert Einstein College of Medicine, New York
Adjunct Associate Professor of East-West Psychology
California Institute of Integral Studies, San Francisco

Annette F. Street, PhD
Emeritus Professor
La Trobe University
Bundoora, Melbourne, Victoria, Australia

Richard L. Street Jr., PhD
Chief, Health Decision-Making & Communication Program
Center for Innovations in Quality, Effectiveness and Safety
Michael E. DeBakey VA Medical Center
Professor of Medicine, Department of Medicine, Section of Health Services Research, Baylor College of Medicine
Professor, Department of Communication
Texas A&M University
College Station, Texas

Brenda Thomson, RN, BSN, PHN, MSN
Director of Case Management
City of Hope
Duarte, California

Teresa Thompson, PhD
Professor, Communication
University of Dayton
Dayton, Ohio

Andrew Thurston, MD
Medical Director of Palliative Care, UPMC-Mercy
UPMC Section of Palliative Care and Medical Ethics
UPMC Palliative and Supportive Institute
Pittsburgh, Pennsylvania

Melinda Villagran, PhD
Professor and Chair
Department of Communication Studies
Texas State University
San Marcos, Texas

Charles F. von Gunten, MD, PhD
Vice President, Medical Affairs, Hospice & Palliative Care
Ohiohealth Kobacker House
Columbus, Ohio

Karen S. Vrtunski, MSSA, LISW-S, ACHP
Clinical Resource Education Counselor
Hospice of the Western Reserve, Inc
Cleveland, Ohio

Jennifer Weil, FAChPM, FRACP, MBBS
Center for Palliative Care
St Vincent's Hospital
Melbourne, Victoria, Australia

Kaila Williams, MSW
Southeast Florida Regional Development Manager
The ALS Association Florida Chapter
Broward/Miami-Dade and Palm Beach, Florida

Elaine Wittenberg, PhD
Associate Professor
Division of Nursing Research and Education
City of Hope
Duarte, California

Finly Zachariah, MD
Assistant Clinical Professor
Division of Supportive Medicine
Department of Supportive Care Medicine
City of Hope
Duarte, California

Angelika A. Zollfrank, MDiv, BCC, ACPE
Coordinator, Pastoral Education
Yale-New Haven Hospital
New Haven, Connecticut

CHAPTER 1

Overview of Communication

Sandra L. Ragan

Introduction

In *New Yorker* cartoonist Roz Chast's[1] brilliant new book on the aging and deaths of her elderly parents, *Can't We Talk About Something More Pleasant?*, she presents in one series of cartoon frames a commonly held perception of the process of dying (see Figure 1.1). "Here's what I used to think happened at 'the end,'" she writes:

Chast concludes by saying: "What I was starting to understand was that the middle panel was a lot more painful, humiliating, long-lasting, complicated, and hideously expensive."[1(p148)]

While the editors of this text on the communication of palliative care would *not* choose those adjectives that Chast used to describe end of life (i.e., painful, humiliating, long-lasting, complicated, and hideously expensive), we do discuss, in particular, the "complicated" nature of communication in the context of serious illness and death. Yet, we advocate that palliative care brings comfort, compassion, and expense-saving measures to the care of the acutely ill and dying. Unlike Chast's experience with her dying parents, the end of life can be a peaceful, pain-free, and sacred time for patients and families.

Our volume covers seven overarching themes as we navigate the role and practice of communication throughout the illness trajectory: communication principles; health literacy; patients and families; specific populations; clinical communication topics; team communication; and research and education. We are concerned throughout with presenting the most recent research findings and the best practices in that nexus between communication and palliative care.

This chapter discusses how and why effective palliative care is predicated on communication; elucidates our concept of interpersonal communication in the health context; delineates the differences between our approach to palliative care communication and those limited only to physician-derived approaches; and reviews, in brief, the contributions of communication scholars to the context of serious illness and dying. We end by focusing on a model of palliative care communication at the heart of this volume, the COMFORT™ SM model.[2]

The Preeminence of Communication in Palliative Care

With three of this volume's seven co-editors schooled in the communication discipline, it is no wonder that we are squarely rooted in the concept that communication is the *sine qua non* of palliative care. In fact, from the inception of hospice[3] to the present, palliative care practitioners have viewed communication as the vehicle for the practice of palliative care. From Dame Cicely Saunders' reliance on the stories her dying patients told her to the current National Consensus Project Clinical Practice Guidelines[4] for hospice and palliative care professionals, effective palliative care is inextricably bound with and dependent upon effective communication.

A major proponent of the palliative care movement in the United States, Dr. Diane Meier, director of the Center to Advance Palliative Care at the Icahn School of Medicine at Mt. Sinai, recently wrote of the myriad needs for skilled communication, as she related the story of a dying patient whose oncologist is reluctant to give up treatment.[5] The case involved Jenny, a middle-aged, married, clinical psychologist who had lived six years with stage 4 non-small-cell lung cancer and who had contacted Meier because her oncologist had refused to engage the "what-if" questions about the efficacy of her cancer treatments. Jenny wished to know what her quality of life might become if the next treatment did not work. In other words, she came to Meier in hopes of getting straight answers. Her well-meaning oncologist, unable to give his patient those answers, persisted in giving her further treatment until questioned by Meier about a proposed new round of chemotherapy. At that point, he acknowledged that the treatment would be futile but that he did not want Jenny to think that he was abandoning her.

Meier explains that the oncologist's honesty about his motivation to prolong treatment as a way of expressing his care and commitment to his patient changed her perspective about why many of her colleagues persisted in futile treatment: many doctors are untrained about caring for patients at end of life. Says Meier,

> Physicians are trained to make diagnoses and to treat disease. Untrained in skills such as pain and symptom management, expert communication about what to expect in the future, and achievable goals for care, physicians do what we have been trained to do: order more tests, more procedures, more treatments, even when these things no longer help. Even when they no longer make sense.[5(p897)]

Meier adds that a remedy to this dilemma is a change in physicians' education and training as well as change in their professional and clinical culture, including the management of pain and symptoms and "intensive training on doctor-patient communication: how to relay bad news, how to stand with patients and their

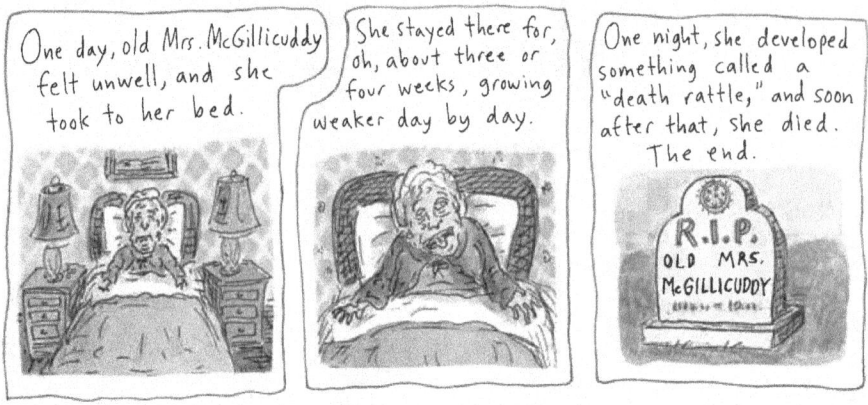

Figure 1.1
© Chast, R., May 2014, *Can't We Talk About Something More Pleasant? A Memoir*, New York: Bloomsbury Publishing; 2014:148. Reprinted with permission.

families until death, and how to help patients and families make the best use of their remaining time together."[5(p897)]

Jenny's case is fraught with communication crises and the lack of communication skills to resolve them. Nearly every communication topic we address in the present volume is suggested by this case: for example, communication as a transaction between mutually influencing participants; relational communication (Jenny's oncologist's care for her and fear of abandonment); communication ethics (how much should be disclosed to patients about their medical situation); health literacy (vis-à-vis Jenny's understanding of the proposed treatment); patient experience of illness; family conversations regarding serious illness; patient-centered communication; trust, hope, and miracles in critical illness; advance care planning; palliative care team communication; and communication training for physicians and other members of the palliative care team.

Bakitas and colleagues[6] also acknowledge the paramount need for quality communication in shared decision-making between the patient, family, and palliative care team in serious illness. Identified by Epstein and Street[7] as a communication deficit in a patient-centered approach to cancer care, the needs for decision-making include discussion of alternative options such as foregoing cancer treatment, surrogate decision-making, and decision-making at the end of life. Bakitas et al.[6] propose broadening the collaboration between the fields of palliative medicine and decision science, in order to address these topics and guide best practices for patients and families. They outline four decision junctures in the serious illness/end of life trajectory: (a) selecting a surrogate and other advance care planning decisions; (b) treatment choices when cure is not possible; (c) whether or not to be admitted to an ICU and receive life-prolonging treatments or to focus on comfort care; and (d) where to receive end-of-life care. Each of these decision junctures involves advanced communication strategies for palliative care team members that will facilitate optimal decision-making for patient and family. Decision-coaching, specialized and individualized clinician assistance that is designed to assist patients to make more informed, optimal decisions at these junctures, is also recommended.[6]

Palliative care physician Jessica Zitter[8] presented a case that exemplifies both the critical nature of decision-making and the concomitant need for patient-centered medicine. In treating an ICU patient with an unrecoverable brain injury, Zitter relied on the advice of the patient's sister (the only visitor seen) who wanted everything done to keep the patient alive. When she later relayed this information to the social worker, Zitter learned that she had completely missed the fact that the patient had a wife whom the patient's sister had deprived of information about him. Knowing that her husband did not want to be kept alive in such a debilitated state, the wife brought him home immediately with hospice support. Zitter remarked that she had followed Gawande's[9] "checklists" for medical care systematically, but despite her checks and balances, she had almost allowed the wrong person to make crucial decisions for the patient. She realized she needed a checklist that puts patients, not just their organs, at the center of their care. Such a checklist,

> would account for the human needs that we weren't always taught to prioritize, ones that didn't seem fatal if overlooked—clearly identifying the patient's next of kin, communicating with the family and identifying the goals of care, asking about symptoms like pain, delirium, shortness of breath. My critical oversight would not have happened had I sought out the social worker on the first day to confirm the true next of kin.[8]

Since putting her patient-centered checklist into practice, Zitter has never misidentified a surrogate decision-maker.[8]

In addition to Bakitas et al.'s[6] and Zitter's[8] emphasis on communication at key decision-making points, the evolution of palliative care from end of life to early initiation illustrates the critical need for effective communication throughout the disease course. Several physician contributors to the handbook edited by Kissane et al.[10] discuss the "transition from curative to palliative" (e.g., Baile and Parker, Clayton and Kissane) and "transitioning patients to palliative care"[10(p101)] as one of the most difficult tasks for cancer clinicians; Clayton and Kissane reference palliative care as "the goal of care changes from curative to palliative at some point along the disease trajectory"[11(p203)]; yet they also acknowledge that cancer patients may receive palliative care at diagnosis, and they recognize the relational benefits to patients of early referral to palliative care.[11] More recently, clinicians' widespread acceptance of the benefits of early palliative care[12] has shifted historical views of palliative care as tantamount to end-of-life or hospice care. Many healthcare providers now see palliative care as optimally beginning at the onset of a critical or life-limiting illness, at diagnosis rather than at a transition from curative to comfort care. This enlarged view of palliative care enhances the need for effective communication interventions, making them critical junctures along the trajectory of disease, from diagnosis until end of life.

The preeminence of communication as it undergirds the practice of palliative care is further illustrated by the experience of one of our co-editors, Dr. Betty Ferrell, who recently served as a grant reviewer for the Cambia Health Foundation (a foundation that focuses on advancing healthcare transformation). The Cambia Foundation had issued a call to nurses and physicians for proposals for a new Sojourner Award in palliative care—identifying 8 to 10 individuals who would be supported in their development as leaders to advance the field of palliative care. The award would provide two years of funding for salary and project costs with the goal of enticing early-career scholars who would continue to champion palliative care. In addition to a written proposal, finalist applicants met with the review panel in a face-to-face interview that included a presentation of their projects. Ferrell noted that all of the finalists, the future palliative care leaders in the trenches, presented projects involving communication in the service of palliative care.

Ferrell concludes that these providers recognize communication as a defining feature of palliative care; further, they realize that more evidence-based research is required to further legitimize the integral role of communication in the palliative care context. That is one of the overarching goals of the current text.

Our Concept of Communication

A major problem in attempting to teach communication skills—both to undergraduate communication majors and to health professionals alike—is the assumption that everyone already knows how to communicate. Many of us believe that the ability to communicate is like language, hard-wired in the human brain. Decades of communication research, however, has revealed that effective communication is a learned skill rather than an innate predisposition. Another misconception about human communication skills is that only public-speaking skills matter; interpersonal communication—including impression management, persuasion, forming and ending relationships, and listening—must be learned through trial and error or through life experience. Again, interpersonal communication research tells us that interpersonal skills can be improved through communication training undergirded by communication theory.

Traditional models of communication, even in the discipline itself, were based on a sender–receiver concept. Effective communication was seen as the skillful crafting of a message by a sender, such that the receiver accurately perceived the content of the message. Such a model—one that justified the widespread teaching of public speaking in communication departments with no emphasis on listening or relationship skills—now can be viewed as mechanistic, reductionist, and information-driven and as largely ignoring the context of the message, the listening process, and the importance of the receiver to the communication process.

We adopt a transactional model (see chapter 3, this volume) in which both parties contribute to and negotiate the meaning of messages, both verbally and nonverbally. In this model, listening is as important as speaking for effective communication, and both participants are mutually and reciprocally influencing the design and reception of and the attachment of meaning to messages. This notion of communication has vast implications for the practice of communication in the palliative care context, as shown in an example of a conversation between a nurse and dying patient:

RN: How is your family doing with all of this?
PT: None of them are talking to me.
RN: They might be afraid. You might need to bring it up.
PT: Yes, they are.
(LONG PAUSE)
RN: You might need to bring it up.
PT: I have a niece and nephew. I haven't seen them in two years, and they live right here in town. They said they were coming yesterday, and they didn't. But maybe I was sleeping. I feel like they are using it as an excuse, but I don't care. They have an excuse now. I was not the most popular person in my family. I'm the oldest, and I've always had to do the most, and sometimes it put me in an unpopular position. I was the tattle-tale. Mommy and Daddy expected me to report everything.[13(pp69–70)]

This example illustrates the mutual influence of communicators, as they shape and reshape the other's responses, attending both to verbal and nonverbal cues. Note that the patient gives a truncated response to the nurse's utterance of "They might be afraid.

You might need to bring it up." This utterance, along with the long silence that follows, affects the nurse's repeated advice, "You might need to bring it up." The patient follows with an elaborated response to the nurse's initial question: "How is your family doing with all of this?" The patient has modified her original response, perhaps in part due to the nurse's repeated advice that she might need "to bring it up." The elaborated response gives the nurse valuable information about the patient and the social/relational world surrounding her illness, information that might aid the nurse in eliciting the support of a palliative care team social worker.

Our transactional model of communication is built on several basic principles or axioms[14] of communication, the most essential of which are (a) one cannot *not* communicate and (b) all messages have at least two levels of meaning—the task or informational level and the relationship level, which cues interactants on how to interpret and process the message itself, as well as how to view the relational context of the message. In the previous conversational example, the first axiom is illustrated by the communicative value of silence: the long pause following the patient's brief second utterance signifies to the nurse that she might need to repeat her former suggestion to the patient that she communicate with her family about her dying. Silence is pregnant—it is assigned meaning by communicators. Likewise, nonverbal behaviors, including facial expressions, tone of voice, physical proximity, and touch, will communicate loudly without the use of words or in concert with words. In fact, we know that communicators interpret and construct meaning based on nonverbal behavior with much more assuredness than they rely on what is said.

The second axiom—that multiple levels of meaning are carried by every message—also notes the preeminence of nonverbal channels, since it is generally nonverbal communication that manifests the relational import of a message. While the conversation in the example does not include the nonverbal communication of the nurse or patient, we can speculate that tone of voice, eye contact, proximity, gesture, and other nonverbal messages are being encoded and decoded by each participant as she listens to one utterance and shapes the next. These nonverbal behaviors also help participants define their relationship as caring nurse and concerned patient and their conversational exchange as one in which the nurse sincerely wishes to assist the patient in dealing with familial issues around her dying.

Our communication model is one in which the relationship between the interactants (the palliative care professional and the patient/family member) is attended to and prized. It is a model consonant with patient-centered care,[7] in which both verbal and nonverbal behaviors manifest concern for patient participation and patient understanding.

Approaches to Palliative Care Communication

Fortunately, because of our belief that palliative care offers optimal care during life-limiting illness and at end of life, researchers from many disciplines are writing about palliative care and the preeminence of communication therein. Physicians, nurses, and communication scholars have offered several notable texts in recent years.[2,10,15–17]

While each discipline contributes meaningfully to the conversation about how best to communicate with patients, family, and team members in the palliative care context, we note throughout this volume some of the differences in approaches. Such differences seem particularly apparent between texts focused only on physician communication and this text, which features an interdisciplinary focus. The present text also deals with the gamut of life-threatening/life-limiting diseases rather than being limited to one disease, such as cancer.

The largest and overarching difference between our approach and common approaches resides in a basic definition of communication, one explicated in the previous section of this chapter. In short, we view the communication interaction as transactional, relational, and mutual. We question the terms "sender," "receiver," and "information" that mark former conceptualizations of communication by our discipline and that frequently characterize the approach to communication by physicians and others outside the discipline. We do not see the outcome of accurately sent "information" as the measure of effective communication, even when that "information" has been adapted to the "receiver." Other approaches to the communication of palliative care appear information-centered at the expense of privileging both parties (the traditional "sender" and "receiver") in the interaction. While we would not disagree that, for example, "message framing requires information to be customized both in style and content in a patient-centered manner,"[10(pix)] we would further add that "both physician and patient co-construct the meaning of the message." For example, a patient with end-stage heart disease might collaborate with his or her physician in deciding that further ICU admissions would be futile.

The difference is not a trivial one: if we view communication as being mutually influenced by both parties in an interaction, then information cannot be the *sine qua non* of communication, no matter how expertly it is delivered. For example, what an MD believes is "bad news" that must be communicated accurately may be interpreted very differently by a patient[18] who brings his or her own experiences and filters to the situation. Occasionally, patients and family members inject their own hopeful interpretations into a physician's message: for example, an MD might tell a late-stage dementia patient's family that her pneumonia is better, yet he is fully aware that the patient is still dying. The family, on the other hand, might view the good news about their loved one's pneumonia as an indication that she is getting better overall, thus misinterpreting the MD's message. Kissane et al. acknowledge "the seminal role of communication in information delivery, decision-making, competent treatment, compassionate support and healing."[10(px)] We would add a focus on the shaping of "information delivery" by patients and their families. Our own approach to communication in the palliative care context is relationship-driven rather than information-driven and sender-based. Rather than focusing on medical knowledge that must be communicated to patients and families, we see those patients and families not as mere receivers of this knowledge but as co-creators in constructing its meaning. In short, viewing communication as simply sending information emphasizes the performance of the provider; viewing communication as mutually negotiated meaning is about the outcome of the relationship between the provider and the patient/family.

Communication scholars who write about palliative care undergird their work with communication theory: for example, narrative theory, problematic integration theory, family communication patterns theory, relational dialectics theory, and communication privacy management theory are employed as frameworks for effective palliative care communication.[19-21] As Babrow and Mattson acknowledge in their seminal piece on health communication theories in the 21st century, "we are motivated by the belief that theoretically informed/informing work is of the greatest importance in this late—or postmodern age."[22(p18)] We do not see palliative care communication as merely assembling a set of skills that can be taught and then applied to patients and families. Much of the communication advice offered by physicians is experiential and anecdotal, despite claims of being evidence-based. Further, skills-based approaches are frequently atheoretical; effective communication can be reduced to formulaic recipes and algorithms. The reason we teach undergraduate communication majors communication theory is to provide them with an understanding of and conceptual richness for their communication behaviors; we would argue that healthcare professionals also need rudimentary training in social science theory, not just in rote verbal and nonverbal communication practices that help to ensure effective information delivery. To be sure, physicians, nurses, social workers, and chaplains must necessarily focus on communication skills, training, and assessment. Yet an exclusive preoccupation with the practice of the skills of communication limits an understanding of its complexities and nuances—inherently the hallmarks of palliative care communication.

An additional difference between approaches to communication is our insistence that qualitative inquiry and research methods be incorporated into the study and practice of communication in palliative care. We believe that many approaches largely dismiss the contributions to communication made by narrative inquiry, ethnographic methods, and conversation analysis. While some social scientists (including communication researchers) also eschew qualitative methods in the pursuit of advancing communication as a rigorous science with measurable, valid, and reliable results, many others herald qualitative inquiry for its illumination of clinician–patient interaction.[23-29] Whereas Lipkin and colleagues[30] believe that Roter's Interactional Analysis System[31] is the gold standard for analyzing communication empirically, Robinson[32] states that "traditional coding is not itself a method for describing and explaining the social organization of interaction; that is the modus operandi of CA [Conversation Analysis],"[32(p501)] a method concerned with how people create, maintain, and negotiate meaning. Robinson goes on to describe how conversation analysis and traditional coding methods (e.g., Bales; Roter) share a symbiotic and "social-scientifically pragmatic" relationship, "the former qualitatively bringing validity to the latter, and the latter quantitatively empowering the former."[32 (p501)]

In simpler terms, the writers of this volume embrace both quantitative and qualitative inquiry; like Robinson, we believe that these methods can be complementary. Further, we posit that qualitative methods such as narrative inquiry hold rich promise both for investigating discourse in palliative care interactions and for teaching clinicians how to engage optimally in conversation with patients and their families.[2] Eliciting, attending to, and incorporating patients' and family members' stories of illness transforms the communication and the resulting climate of care in the context of palliative medicine.

Contributions by Communication Scholars to the Literature on Death/Dying and Palliative Care

Given the rich theoretical work of communication scholars in the healthcare context,[7,22,33-41] in addition to their specific research contributions to describing, coding, and assessing the MD–patient interaction,[26-29,32,42-44] (see also chapter 20, this volume), the dearth of communication research devoted to end of life is lamentable. Few communication scholars have contributed to the scholarly literature on death and dying in general and on palliative care specifically. Brown and Bylund[42] introduce the Comskil model for oncology settings, one of the few communication models for skills training that appears theoretically grounded on sociolinguistic theory and on goals, plans, and action theories. They critique former models of MD–patient communication as being good for initial visits but not suited for continuing care or for palliative and end-of-life care. Hauser and Makoul[44] offer the SEGUE framework (**S**et the stage; **E**licit information; **G**ive information; **U**nderstand patient perspective; **E**nd the counter) for teaching and assessing MD communication skills; Cegala and Eisenberg[43] are two of the few communication researchers intent on discovering which patient communication skills interventions are effective in MD–patient interactions. Albrecht, Eggly, and Ruckdeschel[45] posit the convergence model in discussing the importance of communicating with families and companions in oncological interactions. Other communication researchers are interested in areas of research and teaching on oncology and palliative care that are not focused on communication skills per se. For example, Siminoff[46] is well known for her work in the communication ethics of end-of-life issues such as informed consent, decision-making, and persuasion.

Lest it appear that we have been overly critical of previous communication approaches by some that we assess as mechanistic, reductionist, and skills and information driven, we are disappointed that scholars in the communication discipline largely have failed to illuminate our understanding of conversations surrounding end of life and, specifically, palliative care. This is a sad irony given our discipline's solid theorists in the area[22,33-41] (also see chapter 29, this volume). Either communication researchers have not broached the context of medical interaction with very ill patients or we have not been engaged in the sort of translational research that would "go the extra mile and translate health communication research into practice."[47(p595)]

What *is* the best hope for parlaying communication theory/research into practice that would benefit healthcare professionals and patients in the palliative care context? We pose three interdisciplinary lines of research that appear most promising: narrative inquiry and narrative medicine;[41,48-50,53] the micro-analysis of interaction details, particularly the work of conversation analysts Beach[26,27] (see also chapter 20, this volume) and Robinson[28-29,32] and their colleagues in sociology Heritage[24,25] and Maynard;[24] and research generated by a model grounded in interdisciplinary theory and undergirded by the relational, mutual influence concept of communication—the COMFORT™ SM model.[2]

Theoretical Contributors

Problematic integration theory,[22,33-35] in its explanation of how we attempt to manage uncertainty, offers an excellent theoretical base for understanding end-of-life conversations and the inherent decision-making therein. Hines et al.[51] investigated how the seriously ill elderly coped with uncertainty in their transition from wellness to death. Babrow and Mattson[22,35] also discuss the dialectic of scientific and humanistic assumptions and values in shaping our attitudes and practices related to death and dying. Petronio's[36-37] work in privacy management theory illuminates family communication at end of life: when private information is self-disclosed to another, that individual assumes co-ownership of the information, creating privacy rules and boundary conditions: "Terminally ill patients and their family members must ultimately manage collective boundaries in the uncertainty of illness."[2(p80)] Street's[7,38-40] (also see chapter 29, this volume) work in the health context, especially in his delineation of the verbal and nonverbal communication correlates of patient-centered care, has also guided communication research in clinician–patient interaction.

While our own theoretical approach has been shaped by Babrow and colleagues,[22,33-35,51] Petronio,[36,37] and particularly Street,[7,38-40] (see also chapter 29, this volume), we are most indebted to the theory of narrative inquiry and to narrative medicine. Borrowing from Fisher's[52] elucidation of the narrative paradigm, Wittenberg-Lyles et al. state: "The narrative paradigm assumes that all forms of human communication can be seen fundamentally as stories, as interpretations of aspects of the world occurring in time and shaped by history, culture, and character."[2(p56)] Family illness narratives both shape and reshape the context of illness. They reveal ongoing interpretations of illness, co-constructed by patient, family member, and palliative care team members alike. Sharf and Vanderford[41] wrote about the five actions of narratives in the social construction of health, and Harter, Japp, and Beck[48] explored this notion more fully in their volume on the role of narratives on health and healing. All of these researchers would concur that "narration is a way to organize, understand, make meaning, and reduce uncertainty in the course of an illness; it is a communicative vehicle to perform these tasks."[2(p57)] The narrative medicine movement[49-50,53] manifests that physicians, as well as communication scholars, understand the value of story in assessing and treating patients. It is not surprising, then, that narrative is at the heart of our research approach: in fact, the founder of the modern hospice movement, Dame Cicely Saunders[3] heard and collected the stories of more than 1,000 of her dying patients in formulating her expansive notion of pain.

The COMFORT™ SM Model

Building upon the concepts of patient-centered care and narrative clinical practice and on the notion of communication as transactional, relational, and co-constructed by both parties to an interaction, Wittenberg-Lyles and colleagues developed an evidence-based communication model that elaborates seven principles of communication.[2,13,18-19,21,54] The model is elucidated here, followed by brief explanations of each of its seven components. (Box 1.1)

Box 1.1 Overview of the COMFORT™ SM Model

C—*Communication (clinical narrative practice)*

3Rs

Reflection on the patient before illness (ask)

Remember the patient as an individual (listen)

Re-author the story (use story in conversation)

- explicit recognition of life
- elaboration in context
- acknowledgment of loss/change

O—*Orientation and Options (O & O)*

Questions to ask to determine family orientation

Use plain language planner for palliative care

Questions to ask to understand patient/family culture

M—*Mindful Communication*

Awareness of emotions

Avoiding judgment

Adaptability

   Notice signs of stress
   Identify positives for patient/family
   Silence as a strategy

F—*Family Caregivers*

Caregiver communication tool

Patient and family information needs

Concern/response: Pain

Prompt/response: Assessment

O—*Openings*

Address the topic

Comment on topic

Incorporating quality of life

Spiritual review

R—*Relating*

   Uncertainty checklist
   AMEN protocol
   Goal questions

T—*Team Communication*

Interprofessional collaboration

Groupthink (risk and solutions)

Discipline-specific communication in team meetings

C—COMMUNICATE

This principle grounds the COMFORT™ SM communication model in the theory of narrative clinical practice,[2] which elicits and privileges the illness stories of patients and their families. It approaches communication between palliative care professional and patient/family as transactional and relational, with equal attention given to task (information) and relational meanings of a message. Messages are patient-centered[7] and person-centered.

O—ORIENTATION AND OPTIONS

The second principle of the COMFORT™ SM model involves determining the patient's/family's level of understanding of the illness, enumerating and discussing care options, assessing the health literacy of both patient and family, and orienting patient/family to both medical and lifeworld aspects of the illness. It also involves the palliative care team's assessment of the patient's/family's culture and ensuing cultural constraints.

M—MINDFUL COMMUNICATION

This principle involves the practice of mindful presence: those psychological attributes of refusing to judge patients, staying in the moment, and being able to adapt to rapid change in an interaction with a patient/family. Being mindful involves nonverbal mindfulness as well as verbal—it sometimes means being silent or communicating with a simple touch on the shoulder. Mindful communication is that which avoids talk about self and predetermined scripts; it is instead patient-driven and aware of the moment-by-moment details of interaction.

F—FAMILY

This principle recognizes that both patient and family form the unit of care in palliative care communication. The complexity of multiparty communication is also recognized. Family communication patterns are seen as affecting the nature of the communication, as are caregiver types and caregiver communication patterns.

Seeing families as a conduit to the patient in implementing care and thus honoring family members is a primary goal of communication. Family meetings are encouraged to elicit feelings and to clarify goals of care.

O—OPENINGS

The fifth principle of the COMFORT™ SM model views critical transitions in patient care as opportunities for intervention by the palliative care team. This is when skilled, strategic communication can create the possibility for positive change. These opportunities frequently occur at painful transitions on the disease trajectory (e.g., diagnosis, treatment options, disease recurrence, transition to hospice, etc.). Palliative care team members can help patients reframe these transitions and tensions as opportunities for resilience and coping. Quality-of-life considerations are paramount in these reframings.

R—RELATING

This principle means that the palliative care team is aware of the patient's/family members' understanding of the disease and its probable course and is willing to meet patients and families where they are in accepting the change brought by serious illness. It recognizes that prognosis and treatment options may need to be repeated numerous times in order for patients/families to reach an acceptable level of awareness and understanding. Relating also acknowledges that uncertainty and multiple goals affect patients'/families' treatment decisions. It champions relationship, both between palliative care team member and patient/family and between patient and family.

T—TEAM

The last principle in the COMFORT™ SM model centers on the concept of a multidisciplinary approach to palliative care, such that each of the disciplines of medicine, nursing, social work, chaplaincy, and clinical psychology is recognized for the positive contribution it makes to effective care. Team communication is emphasized, and strategies for improving communication are sought and implemented.

The COMFORT™ SM concept "is driven by narrative practice in nursing, the prioritization of family, early intervention of palliative care, and radically adaptive communication between and among patient/family/team members/clinicians."[13(p291)] With the primary goals of ensuring patient-centered care and assuring patients' quality of life, the COMFORT™ SM model acknowledges the complex, multiparty, nonlinear, and repetitive nature of communication in the palliative care context.[2] We believe that it also promises a more effective approach to communicating with patient/families and palliative care teams than do physician-derived models. The seven principles of communication that comprise the COMFORT™ SM model are designed to be used concurrently and in tandem rather than sequentially, as we do not believe them to be mutually exclusive. Used collectively, these principles offer patients and families the kind of patient-centered care that we find most effective in the palliative care context.

The following chapters focus on communication principles, and discuss the historical development of palliative care communication (chapter 2); the notion of communication as a transactional process (chapter 3); the communication of palliative care to the public (chapter 4); ethical issues in palliative care communication (chapter 5); and communication in specific palliative care disciplines: social work (chapter 6); medicine (chapter 7); nursing (chapter 8); chaplaincy (chapter 9); and clinical psychology (chapter 10).

References

1. Chast R. *Can't We Talk about Something More Pleasant? A Memoir.* 1st ed. New York, NY: Bloomsbury USA; 2014.
2. Wittenberg-Lyles E, Goldsmith J, Ferrell B, Ragan S. *Communication in Palliative Nursing.* New York, NY: Oxford University Press; 2013.
3. Saunders C. *The Management of Terminal Illness.* London: Hospital Medicine Publications; 1967: 1–29.
4. National Consensus Project for Quality Palliative Care. *Clinical Practice Guidelines.* 3rd ed. Pittsburgh, PA: National Consensus Project for Quality Palliative Care; 2013. http://www.nationalconsensusproject.org/NCP_Clinical_Practice_Guidelines_3rd_Edition.pdf. Accessed September 8, 2014.
5. Meier DE. "I don't want Jenny to think I'm abandoning her": Views on overtreatment. *Health Aff.* May 2014;33(5):895–898.

6. Bakitas M, Kryworuchko J, Matlock DD, Volandes AE. Palliative medicine and decision science: The critical need for a shared agenda to foster informed patient choice in serious illness. *J Palliat Med.* 2011;14(10):1109–1116.
7. Epstein RM, Street RL, Jr. Patient-centered communication in cancer care: Promoting healing and reducing suffering. In: Epstein RM, Street RL Jr, eds. *Patient-Centered Communication in Cancer Care: Promoting Healing and Reducing Suffering*, NIH Publication No. 07-6225. Bethesda, MD: National Cancer Institute; 2007.
8. Zitter JN. Who can speak for the patient? *The New York Times.* June 2014. http://well.blogs.nytimes.com/2014/06/19/who-can-speak-for-the-patient/?_php=true&_type=blogs&_r=0. Accessed September 8, 2014.
9. Gawande A. *The Checklist Manifesto: How to Get Things Right.* New York, NY: Picador; 2009.
10. Kissane DW, Bultz BD, Buttow PM, Finlay IG, eds. *Handbook of Communication in Oncology and Palliative Care.* New York, NY: Oxford University Press; 2011.
11. Clayton JM, Kissane DW. Communication about transitioning patients to palliative care. In: Kissane D, Bultz B, Butow P, Finlay I, eds. *Handbook of Communication in Oncology and Palliative Care.* New York, NY: Oxford University Press; 2011:203–214.
12. Rhondali W, Burt S, Wittenberg-Lyles E, Bruera E, Dalal S. Medical oncologists' perception of palliative care programs and the impact of name change to supportive care on communication with patients during the referral process: A qualitative study. *Palliat Support Care.* 2013;11(5):397–404.
13. Wittenberg-Lyles E, Goldsmith J, Ragan, S, Sanchez-Reilly, S. *Dying with Comfort: Family Illness Narratives and Early Palliative Care.* Creskill, NJ: Hampton Press; 2010.
14. Watzlawick P, Beavin Bavelas J, Jackson DD. *Pragmatics of Human Communication: A Study of Interactional Patterns, Pathologies and Paradoxes.* New York, NY: W.W. Norton; 1967.
15. Back A, Arnold R, Tulsky J. *Mastering Communication with Seriously Ill Patients: Balancing Honesty with Empathy and Hope.* New York, NY: Cambridge University Press; 2009.
16. Ferrell BR, Coyle N, eds. *Oxford Textbook of Palliative Nursing.* 3rd ed. New York, NY: Oxford University Press; 2010.
17. Matzo M, Sherman DW, eds. *Palliative Care Nursing: Quality Care to the End of Life.* 3rd ed. New York, NY: Springer; 2009.
18. Wittenberg-Lyles EM, Goldsmith J, Sanchez-Reilly S, Ragan SL. Communicating a terminal prognosis in a palliative care setting: Deficiencies in current communication training protocols. *Soc Sci Med.* 2008;66(11):2356–2365.
19. Ragan SL, Wittenberg-Lyles EM, Goldsmith J, Sanchez-Reilly S. *Communication as Comfort: Multiple Voices in Palliative Care.* New York, NY: Routledge/Taylor & Francis; 2008.
20. Wittenberg-Lyles E, Parker Oliver D, Demiris G, Baldwin P. The ACTive intervention in hospice interdisciplinary team meetings: Exploring family caregiver and hospice team communication. *J Comput Mediat Commun.* 2010;15(3):465–481.
21. Wittenberg-Lyles E, Goldsmith J, Richardson B, Hallett JS, Clark R. The practical nurse: A case for COMFORT communication training. *Am J Hosp Palliat Care.* 2013;30(2):162–166.
22. Babrow A, Mattson M. Building health communication theories in the 21st century. In: Thompson TL, Parrott R, Nussbaum JF, eds. *The Routledge Handbook of Health Communication.* 2nd ed. New York, NY: Routledge; 2011:18–35.
23. Glaser B, Strauss A. *Awareness of Dying.* San Francisco, CA: Aldine; 1965.
24. Heritage J, Maynard D. Problems and prospects in the study of doctor-patient interaction: 30 years of research in primary care. *Annu Rev Sociol.* 2006;32:351–374.
25. Heritage J, Robinson JD. The structure of patients' presenting concerns 1: Physicians' opening questions. *Health Commun.* 2006;19:89–102.
26. Beach WA. Preserving and constraining options: "Okays" and "official" priorities in medical interviews. In: Morris B, Chenail R, eds. *Talk of the Clinic: Explorations in the Analysis of Medical and Therapeutic Discourse.* Hillsdale, NJ: Lawrence Erlbaum; 1995:259–290.
27. Beach WA, Mandelbaum, J. "My mom had a stroke": Understanding how patients raise and providers respond to psychosocial concerns. In Harter LH, Japp PM, Beck CM, eds. *Narratives, Health, and Healing: Communication Theory and Research.* Mahwah, NJ: Lawrence Erlbaum; 2005:343–364.
28. Robinson JD. Getting down to business: Talk, gaze, and body orientation during openings of doctor-patient consultations. *Human Commun Res.* 1998;25:97–123.
29. Robinson JD. Soliciting patients' presenting concerns. In: Heritage J, Maynard D, eds. *Communication in Medical Care: Interaction Between Primary Care Physicians and Patients.* Cambridge, UK: Cambridge University Press; 2006:22–47.
30. Lipkin M. The history of communication skills knowledge and training. In: Kissane D, Bultz B, Butow P, Finlay I, eds. *Handbook of Communication in Oncology and Palliative Care.* New York, NY: Oxford University Press; 2010:3–12.
31. Roter D, Larson S. The Roter Interaction Analysis System (RIAS). Utility and flexibility for analysis of medical interactions. *Patient Educ Couns.* 2002;46:243–251.
32. Robinson JD. Conversation analysis and health communication. In: Thompson TL, Parrott R, Nussbaum JF, eds. *The Routledge Handbook of Health Communication.* 2nd ed. New York, NY: Routledge; 2011:501–518.
33. Babrow AS. Communication and problematic integration: Understanding diverging probability and value, ambiguity, ambivalence, and impossibility. *Commun Theory.* 1992;2(2):95–130.
34. Babrow AS. Uncertainty, value, communication, and problematic integration. *J Commun.* 2001;51(3):553–573.
35. Babrow AS, Mattson M. Theorizing about health communication. In: Thompson TL, Dorsey A, Parrott R, Miller K, eds. *The Handbook of Health Communication.* New York, NY: Routledge; 2003:35–62.
36. Petronio S. *Boundaries of Privacy: Dialectics of Disclosure.* Albany, NY: SUNY Press; 2002.
37. Petronio S. Translational research endeavors and the practices of communication privacy management. *J Appl Commun Res.* August 2007;35(3):218–222.
38. Street RL, Jr., Makoul G, Arora NK, Epstein RM. How does communication heal? Pathways linking clinician-patient communication to health outcomes. *Patient Educ Couns.* 2009;74(3):295–301.
39. Street RL Jr. Communication in medical encounters: An ecological perspective. In: Thompson TL, Dorsey A, Miller KL, Parrott R, eds. *Handbook of Health Communication.* New York, NY: Routledge; 2003:63–93.
40. Street RL Jr. Interpersonal communication skills in healthcare contexts. In: Greene JO, Burleson BR, eds. *Handbook of Communication and Social Interaction Skills.* Mahwah, NJ: Lawrence Erlbaum; 2003:909–933.
41. Sharf BF, Vanderford ML. Illness narratives and the social construction of health. In: Thompson TL, Dorsey A, Parrott R, Miller K, eds. *The Routledge Handbook of Health Communication.* New York, NY: Routledge; 2003:9–34.
42. Brown R, Bylund CL. Theoretical models of communication skills training. In: Kissane DW, Bultz BD, Butow PM, Finlay IG, eds. *Handbook of Communication in Oncology and Palliative Care.* New York, NY: Oxford University Press; 2010:28–40.
43. Cegala DJ, Eisenberg D. Enhancing cancer patients' participation in medical consultations. In: Kissane DW, Bultz BD, Butow PM, Finlay IG, eds. *Handbook of Communication in Oncology and Palliative Care.* New York, NY: Oxford University Press; 2010:87–97.

44. Hauser J, Makoul, G. Medical student training in communication skills. In: Kissane DW, Bultz BD, Butow PM, Finlay IG, eds. *Handbook of Communication in Oncology and Palliative Care*. New York, NY: Oxford University Press; 2010:75–85.
45. Albrecht TL, Eggly SS, Ruckdeschel JC. Communicating with relatives/companions about cancer care. In: Kissane DW, Bultz BD, Butow PM, Finlay IG, eds. *Handbook of Communication in Oncology and Palliative Care*. New York, NY: Oxford University Press; 2010:157–164.
46. Siminoff LA. The ethics of communication in cancer and palliative care. In: Kissane DW, Bultz BD, Butow PM, Finlay IG, eds. *Handbook of Communication in Oncology and Palliative Care*. New York, NY: Oxford University Press; 2010:51–61.
47. Kreps GL. Translating health communication research into practice: The influence of health communication scholarship on health policy, practice, and outcomes. In: Thompson TL, Parrott R, Nussbaum JF, eds. *The Routledge Handbook of Health Communication*. 2nd ed. New York, NY: Routledge; 2011:595–609.
48. Harter LM, Japp PM, Beck CS, eds. *Narratives, Health, and Healing: Communication Theory, Research, and Practice*. New York, NY: Taylor & Francis; 2005.
49. Charon R. Narrative medicine: A model for empathy, reflection, profession, and trust. *JAMA*. 2001;286(15):1897–1902.
50. DasGupta S, Charon R. Personal illness narratives: Using reflective writing to teach empathy. *Acad Med*. 2004;79(4):351–356.
51. Hines SC, Babrow AS, Badzek L, Moss A. From coping with life to coping with death: Problematic integration for the seriously ill elderly. *Health Commun*. 2001;13(3):327–342.
52. Fisher WR. *Human Communication as Narration: Toward a Philosophy of Reason, Value and Action*. Columbia: University of South Carolina Press; 1987.
53. Charon R. Narrative medicine as witness for the self-telling body. *J Appl Commun Res*. 2009;37(2):118–131.
54. Wittenberg-Lyles E, Goldsmith J, Ragan SL. The COMFORT Initiative: Palliative nursing and the centrality of communication. *J Hosp Palliat Nurs*. 2010;12(5):282–292.

CHAPTER 2

A Historical Perspective of Palliative Care Communication

Betty Ferrell, Elaine Wittenberg, and Tammy Neiman

Introduction

Although palliative care emerged in the United States in the mid-1990s, it was built on a foundation initiated 20 years prior by the hospice movement. This important history included communication as an essential element in care philosophy and delivery models. During this time, the role of communication in the field of palliative care has evolved in significant ways. This chapter provides a historical perspective on the role of communication in palliative care, identifies key communication concepts in the palliative care literature, and highlights future directions for palliative care communication research, education, and policy development.

Evolving Focus on Communication

Hospice began in the mid-1970s as an alternative form of care and was largely a social movement challenging the traditional paradigm of care in a death-denying society. Pioneers such as Elizabeth Kubler Ross emphasized the "silences" of communication surrounding seriously ill patients and the desperate, unmet needs of these patients within a society that did not publically recognize death and dying.[1] Early discussions about communication at the end of life centered on whether or not patients understood their terminal condition. Protecting the patient from distress by avoiding communication about diagnosis and prognosis was seen as beneficent care.

This early era of end-of-life care in the context of hospice was vital in identifying the lack of communication to the overall experience of dying.[2] Hospice providers were staunch supporters of open communication with dying patients and their families. They advocated for breaking the silence and encouraged communication to allow patients to complete life tasks and focus their remaining time on relationships. Hospice providers were also the first to advocate that meaningful communication could be nonverbal, suggesting that presence during the patient's passing was an important component of the dying process.[3] The initial concept of interdisciplinary care, and attention to the concept of team communication, was also introduced by the hospice movement. With a focus on treating the whole person, including physical, psychological, social, and spiritual well-being, it was recognized early on that the quality of communication among providers was an important aspect of care delivery.

Expanding the ideas of hospice, palliative care emerged in healthcare as an approach to "upstream" care for the seriously ill much earlier in the course of disease than hospice care. Monumental work initiated by support from the Robert Wood Johnson Foundation and the Open Society Institute in the late 1990s sparked the introduction of palliative care teams within acute care settings. This was a broad leap, to incorporate a culture of hospice that was largely highly personalized care at home into the chaotic, cure-focused, and physician-dominant hospital culture. In 2004, a major advance in palliative care was the development of clinical practice guidelines by a consortium of the leading palliative care organizations, the National Consensus Project for Quality Palliative Care.[4] These guidelines specified domains of care, and each domain revealed strong reliance on quality communication. Table 2.1 identifies the eight domains of the guidelines and related aspects of communication.

Given that palliative care has always been patient-focused and compassionate, with an emphasis on whole-person care, it has perhaps been assumed that communication in these settings is of high quality in this developing field. Unfortunately, there is extensive literature that indicates communication is a weak skill for healthcare providers across virtually all settings. This is particularly concerning in palliative care, where healthcare providers are charged with discussing serious diagnosis, prognosis, treatment options, and quality of life decisions with patients and families. The field of palliative care is relatively new, and thus the concept of palliative care communication is also new. Some key communication concepts in the palliative care literature include honest and open communication, communicating hope, barriers to communication, pediatric palliative care communication, and the use of technology to improve communication.

Table 2.1 National Consensus Project Clinical Practice Guidelines and Palliative Care Communication

Domain	Communication Aspects
1 Structure and Processes Of Care	Service model is dependent upon interdisciplinary team and patient communication.
2 Physical Aspects of Care	Effective assessment and management of symptoms are contingent upon effective communication between patients and healthcare professionals.
3 Psychological and Psychiatric Aspects of Care	Routine attention to emotional responses to illness requires active listening, assessment of psychological symptoms, and therapeutic communication to address issues such as anxiety, depression, hopelessness, and uncertainty.
4 Social Aspects of Care	Family focus requires communication with patients about social/relationship concerns. Equally important is communication with family members including family conferencing.
5 Spiritual, Religious, and Existential Aspects of Care	Spiritual, religious, and existential concerns are addressed through communication to assess needs, respond, and link community resources.
6 Cultural Aspects of Care	Culturally respectful care begins with communication to assess culturally based values, beliefs, and practices.
7 Care of the Patient at the End of Life	Communication to address signs of approaching death and respond to emotions in the final hours.
8 Ethical and Legal Aspects of Care	Address intensely complex issues such as withdrawal of life support, proxy decision-making, and conflicting values and beliefs. Attention to ethical and legal concerns is facilitated by mediated communication.

Honest and Open Communication

Palliative patients and family members describe poor communication skills among healthcare providers, with many professionals lacking the skills to engage in difficult conversations or the ability to deliver bad news to patients and families.[5] Overwhelmingly, patients want their healthcare providers to be honest and open with them in discussing their health or illness.[6-10] Barriers to open, honest communication include the provider's concern about the patient's hope, difficulty in deciding the right moment to discuss end-of-life issues, not knowing what the patient wants to discuss, not carefully listening to patients, and relying on the patient to initiate a conversation topic.[9] There are also patient-related barriers such as unwillingness to hear prognostic information even if provided, dependence on the provider to make decisions, shame in not understanding the information, and difficulty forming expectations.[9]

One key way to create open and honest communication with patients is to assess patient preference for information.[6-8,10,14-15] The most common assessment question asked by providers is: "How much information do you want and how much detail do you prefer?" Studies have indicated that providing patients with a list of questions to ask informs healthcare providers about pertinent patient information as well as empowers the patient to ask questions and obtain needed information.[8,16] Ongoing, continual assessment of patient preference and understanding of the illness has been identified as a key communication role of the palliative care team.[8,14]

While it is important for patients and families to understand their disease to make informed decisions, healthcare providers need to recognize there is no standard for how patients and families process information. Information-giving needs to be shaped to enhance the patients' and families' unique preferences. Jackson et al.[14] discussed the natural pattern of patients moving between a form of denial and awareness that aids the patient with coping. Prognosis awareness is the "capacity to understand his or her prognosis and the likely illness trajectory."[14]

Communicating Hope

Many patients have described needing hope from their healthcare providers.[6-10,14,15,17] Hope in palliative care and end-of-life care may sound contradictory to the situation, but hope during this time in a person's life does not necessarily mean the person is hoping to be cured. Hope can be related to many aspects of care, including hope for improved symptom management, hope for reconciled relationships, and hope for making meaning out of life.[7] Healthcare providers primarily help to maintain hope through their communication efforts. Being open to discussing difficult topics, exploring emotional and spiritual needs, and maintaining a focus on goals of care are a few ways that healthcare providers can maintain the hope of their patients.[9]

Barriers to Palliative Care Communication

Barriers to communication between healthcare providers and patients and families include prognosis uncertainty, physician hesitation and lack of skill, use of unfamiliar medical terminology, and the complex environment of care. Healthcare providers find it difficult to determine the timing of death or decide when to refer a patient to palliative or hospice care. This has been called "grayness" or "fence sitting."[5-6,9-10,14,17] Avoidance or hesitancy to talk about prognosis by the healthcare provider or patient can lead to uninformed or delayed decisions about care.[5] In Jackson et al.'s[14] guide to early palliative care interventions, step zero is the providers' preparation in describing accurate information regarding life expectancy and illness progression. Healthcare providers fear that bad news will cause psychological harm to patients and families, including a loss of hope.[7] It is understandable that healthcare providers need accurate information before discussing a prognosis with the patient and family; however, patients in Coad et al. described healthcare provider behaviors as "delay, denial and evasion," while they waited for test results.[6(p303)]

Another barrier to palliative care communication is the physician's hesitation or lack of skill to introduce palliative care. Physicians have described the act of telling patients about diagnosis and prognosis as emotional, drawn out, dreaded, and difficult.[17] Besides difficulty in communicating this information because of emotional challenges, physicians describe difficulty in accurately describing palliative care.[17] Strategies for telling a patient about prognosis vary, including pushing hard to make patients recognize the situation, easing patients toward palliative care, and presenting information with a "positive spin."[17] Broom et al. acknowledged that many times patients need to come to the realization of the severity of their disease on their own before accepting palliative care or foregoing life-prolonging treatments.[17]

The provider's use of medical terminology has also been frequently cited as confusing to patients and creating a barrier to understanding.[5,7,9] Not only do patients report difficulty in understanding the language used during clinical interactions, but they also report not understanding statistical information surrounding prognosis. In some cases, misunderstanding has resulted in the families' perception that the patient's death was sudden and could not have been anticipated.[5]

Last, environmental factors can be a barrier to communication between healthcare providers and patients and families. Busy hospital settings limit patients and families from receiving information they want and need.[5] There is an abundance of research demonstrating that patient and family dissatisfaction with care is linked to the lack of time and communication with providers.[6-10] Providing adequate time with patients and families demonstrates commitment to patient care and allows patients and families to discuss important information at their own pace. In the hospital setting, there is a lack of privacy, and often patients and families feel uncomfortable expressing emotions in such a public space, especially when discussions involve end-of-life care.[5]

Pediatric Palliative Care Communication

Researchers often focus on the communication needs of specific populations when exploring end-of-life or palliative care. According to the literature on adults, infants, and children, many of the communication concerns are similar across these populations. Parents of ill children desire honest and hopeful communication from their healthcare providers.[6,15] Medical terminology and challenges in understanding the statistical odds of survival are barriers to communication in pediatric palliative care populations. Assessing patient preference for information is key to palliative care communication, especially in pediatric populations; however, unique to this population is consideration of how parents want their children to be told about diagnosis and prognosis. Some parents want healthcare providers to deliver prognostic information, while other parents prefer to act as information gatekeepers.[6] Providers need options for training on communication for pediatric palliative care,[6] as physicians report difficulty discussing prognosis when the patient is young.[17]

Technology in Palliative Care Communication

In the early 2000s, the telephone was the primary communication tool used in palliative care to facilitate provider accessibility and relationship-building with patients and families.[10] Communication that took place over the phone primarily involved reassuring patients and family members with medication dosages and administration, resulting in decreased hospital admissions, emergency department visits, and number of hospital bed days.[18] Although telephones allowed quick assess to providers, the absence of empathetic contact and the inability to observe nonverbal cues were a disadvantage to establishing quality communication.[10] Skype, a video-conferencing Internet software program, is being used facilitate communication between long-distance family members and patients[19] and between family caregivers and hospice providers,[20] and to deliver cognitive behavioral interventions to family caregivers.[21] While there are benefits to using technology to facilitate communication between patients, families, and providers, personal presence is still considered a key component in palliative care communication.

Looking Forward

Communication is one of the most crucial aspects of palliative care. Patients and families request open and honest communication while being able to maintain some degree of hope in the illness progression. Professionals find it emotionally difficult to discuss diagnosis, prognosis, and treatment options, especially when the patient is young or has children to care for. Some guidelines and intervention tools, such as quality of life self-assessments and consult-question prompt sheets, have been found to aid the communication of prognosis and diagnosis between healthcare providers and patients and families.[8,16] In addition to these tools, healthcare providers need improved or repeated communication education, especially regarding breaking bad news, discussing treatment options, and considering referral of a patient and family to a palliative care team. Assessment of patient preferences, coping mechanisms, and the importance of maintaining hope should be included in communication education.

Similar to the hospice movement, palliative care has by its nature of interdisciplinary, holistic care supported communication as a key aspect of care. However, there have been several limitations to the literature, research, and clinical practice of communication for the field of palliative care thus far. For example, while the interdisciplinary team (IDT) approach may have been novel in bringing multiple disciplines together, little attention has been given to the patterns or quality of IDT communication. Limited research has been done in this area, but available evidence suggests that IDT meetings, while well intended, are often physician-dominated, with many members providing limited input and communication focused only on physical aspects of care.[3] The general concepts of listening and presence have also been cornerstones of palliative care, but there has been very little specific discussion of communication processes in the literature and a significant void of theoretical contributions from the field of communication. As the field moves forward, key limitations for palliative care communication need to be addressed. Table 2.2 summarizes these limitations and identifies needs for future research, education, and practice.

The field of palliative care is now affirming the importance of communication and the need for major improvement in this essential skill. Communication education is urgently needed to develop healthcare providers' skills and improve the palliative care experiences for seriously ill patients and their families. Key

Table 2.2 Limitations and Future Directions for Communication as a Key Aspect of Palliative Care

Limitation	Potential Future Direction
Communication has been largely focused only on physician–patient interactions	All members of the interdisciplinary team are vitally involved in communication, thus communication training must be greatly expanded.
Communication has focused predominantly on "breaking bad news"	There are many issues beyond initial breaking bad news requiring skilled communication across all domains.
Much of the education to improve communication in palliative care has been protocol driven or "step" approaches	Communication education should include a relational approach that recognizes the unique relationship issues, including those of patients, family members, and healthcare professionals
Communication training has often been limited to lectures	Advancing communication skills requires experiential learning through techniques such as role play, standardized patients and simulations

elements of communication skills building need to involve all members of the interdisciplinary team, expand beyond "breaking bad news" skills, focus on relationship-building with patients and families, and include experiential learning methods.[12,13]

Addressing the needs of patients and families during serious, chronic, or terminal illness is emotionally challenging work,[7] and healthcare providers require advanced communication skills to deliver quality palliative care and to facilitate their own self-care in these settings.

References

1. Kubler-Ross E. *On Death and Dying*. New York, NY: Routledge; 1969.
2. Milone-Nuzzo P, Ercolano E, McCorkle R. Home care and hospice home care. In: Ferrell B, Coyle N, Paice J. ed. *Oxford Textbook of Palliative Nursing*. 4th ed. New York, NY: Oxford University Press; 2015:727–739.
3. Ragan S, Wittenberg-Lyles E, Goldsmith J, Sanchez-Reilly S. *Communication as Comfort: Multiple Voices in Palliative Care*. New York, NY: Routledge; 2008.
4. National Consensus Project for Quality Palliative Care Website. www.nationalconsensusproject.org. Accessed June 15, 2015.
5. Robinson J, Gott M, Ingleton C. Patient and family experiences of palliative care in hospital: What do we know? An integrative review. *Palliat Med*. 2014;28(1):18–33.
6. Coad J, Patel R, Murray S. Disclosing terminal diagnosis to children and their families: Palliative professionals' communication barriers. *Death Stud*. 2014;38(5):302–307.
7. Dea Moore C, Reynolds A. Clinical update: Communication issues and advanced care planning. *Semin Oncol Nurs*. 2013;29(4);e1–e12.
8. Rodin G, Mackay J, Zimmerman C, Mayer C, Howell D, Katz M, Sussman J, Brouwers M. Clinician-patient communication: A systematic review. *Support Care Cancer*. 2009;17:627–644.
9. Slort W, Schweitzer B, Blankenstein A, Abarshi E, Riphagen I, Echteld M, Aaronson N, Van der Horst H, Deliens L. Perceived barriers and facilitators for general practitioner-patents communication in palliative care: A systematic review. *Palliat Med*. 2011;25(6):613–629.
10. Van Gurp J, Hasselaar J, van Leeuwen E, Hoek P, Vissers K, van Selm M. Connection with patients and instilling realism in an era of emerging communication possibilities: A review on palliative care communication heading to telecare practice. *Patient Educ Couns*. 2013;93:504–514.
11. Eggenberger E, Heimerl K, Bennett M. Communication skills training in dementia care: A systematic review of effectiveness, training content, and didactic methods in different care settings. *Int Psychogeriatr*. 2013;25(3):345–358.
12. Johnson L, Gorman C, Morse R, Firth M, Rushbrooke S. Does communication skills training make a difference to patients' experiences of consultations in oncology and palliative care services? *Eur J Cancer Care*. 2013;22:202–209.
13. Shaw E, Marshall D, Howard M, Taniguchi A, Winemaker S, Burns S. A systematic review of postgraduate palliative care curricula. *J Palliat Med*. 2010;13(9):1091–1108.
14. Jackson V, Jacobsen J, Greer J, Pirl W, Temel J, Back A. The cultivation of prognostic awareness through the provision of early palliative care in the ambulatory setting: A communication guide. *J Palliat Med*. 2013;16(8):894–900.
15. Wool C. State of the science on perinatal palliative care. *J Obstet Gynecol Neonatal Nurs*. 2013;42:372–382.
16. Fawole O, Dy S, Wilson R, Lau B, Martinez K, Apostol C, Vollenweider D, Bass E, Aslakson R. A systematic review of communication quality improvement interventions for patients with advanced and serious illness. *J Gen Intern Med*. 2012;28(4):570–577.
17. Broom A, Kirby E, Good P, Wootton, J, Adams J. The troubles of telling: Managing communication about the end of life. *Qual Health Res*. 2014;24(2):151–162.
18. Capurro D, Ganzinger M, Perez-Lu J, Knaup P. Effectiveness of e-health interventions and information needs in palliative care: A systematic literature review. *J Med Internet Res*. 2014;16(3):1–14.
19. Jones J. Using Skype to support palliative care surveillance. *Nurs Older People*. 2014;26(1):16–19.
20. Demiris G, Parker Oliver D, Kruse RL, Wittenberg-Lyles E. Telehealth group interactions in the hospice setting: Assessing technical quality across platforms. *Telemed J E Health*. 2013;19(4):235–240.
21. Demiris G, Parker Oliver D, Wittenberg-Lyles E, et al. A noninferiority trial of a problem-solving intervention for hospice caregivers: In person versus videophone. *J Palliat Med*. 2012;15(6):653–660.

CHAPTER 3

Transactional Communication

Athena du Pré and Elissa Foster

Introduction

> He told me he had had only a "wash and a brush up" that morning as he had felt too exhausted to be moved to the bathroom. A fastidious man, this seemed to concern him. Then he looked at me intently and asked, "Do you know the origin of the phrase, 'A wash and a brush up?' I didn't, and he, the librarian to the end, took delight in explaining it to me. Those were the last words he said to me: not profound, in fact, quite pedestrian. But I felt they symbolized the long walk we had begun together a year previously and which ended with his perfect death shortly after that conversation.[1(p125)]

With these words, social worker and palliative care provider Lois Pollock remembers a special relationship with Graham, a 57-year-old man with colon cancer.[1] Their relationship, and others like it, illustrates the deeply personal aspect of care meant to optimize one's quality of life and to prevent suffering during a time of serious illness.[2] In Pollock's words, palliative care is a "shared journey" without a clear roadmap.[1(p125)]

Because palliative care experiences are co-created by the people engaged in them, a transmission model of communication that emphasizes one-way or asymmetrical communication is inadequate. Such a model treats information as a commodity to be provided (transmitted) by one person and received by another.[3] It is easy to imagine the power differential that such a model supports, particularly if one person does most of the talking, as has been the tradition in healthcare encounters. Physicians in one study interrupted three out of four patients' opening statements of concerns within 16.5 seconds.[4] Other research points to a similar pattern.[5-7] Many argue that this is not an effective model for healthcare in general,[8] but, as we will discuss, it is particularly ill suited for palliative care. A more promising alternative is the transactional model of communication, which emphasizes feedback and mutual influence.[9]

In this chapter we briefly explore the shortfalls of sender-oriented communication in palliative care. Then we focus on communication approaches designed to enhance relationships and facilitate teamwork.

Communication Models

The transmission and transactional models of communication differ in terms of the power and autonomy granted to participants, the assumed purpose of communication, and the factors considered relevant to a communication episode.

Transmission Model of Communication

The transmission model of communication (also called a sender approach) proposes that people are alternately senders and receivers.[3] Senders transmit messages to receivers either face to face or through channels such as the telephone or computer. In terms of this model, physical noise (such as static, music, other voices, or loud machinery) may distort the message or how it is understood.

As mentioned, one shortfall of this approach is that it tends to support an uneven balance of power. The person assumed to have the most valuable information is often given license to set the tone and terms of an interaction.[10] Part of the reason physicians have dominated medical conversations is that patients have typically been nonassertive and quick to yield the floor in their presence.[11] Information and expertise are valuable. However, palliative care is not based solely or even primarily on the type of expertise that people typically seek from healthcare professionals. Palliative care providers are called upon, in extraordinary measure, to provide what nursing scholar Philip Larkin calls the "intangibles"—compassion, presence, hope, intuition, and understanding.[12] These require more than medical knowledge. As Larkin expresses it, "bereavement care takes the nurse beyond the 'safe' zone of technical expertise to relationship based in mutuality."[12(pp337-338)] This mutuality relies on give and take rather than a power differential.

Another limitation of the transmission model is that it depicts communication as the product of relatively detached and discrete components. Information, senders, and receivers are portrayed as distinct and separate entities, and the channel is assumed to be a neutral conduit for information (albeit one that is subject to the effects of noise). A common metaphor of the transmission model is tossing a ball back and forth. For the most part, we expect a ball to arrive at the receiver in the same form it left the sender, not to morph during the process. By the same token, senders and receivers are treated as independent agents. We may blame or congratulate one party or another for a "wild pitch" or a "great catch." In healthcare, this may translate into blaming the patient for failing to understand or comply with the information provided. It may mean that we consider someone a great communicator because he or she maintains eye contact, speaks clearly, or has a large vocabulary. It may also mean that we deliver information over the phone or via letter that would be more compassionately delivered through a different channel, such as face-to-face communication. As we discuss later, which communication behaviors and channels are the most effective depends a great deal on the people, culture, and circumstances involved.

In sum, the greatest weakness of the transmission model for palliative care is that it presents an overly simplistic, sender-oriented perspective on communication. Based on this, we might expect that the best healthcare providers are good at crafting messages they can use as reliable scripts in nearly any circumstance. In reality, that expectation misses the mark in palliative care—a context in which patients and their loved ones benefit more from two-way communication and emotional support,[13] which we discuss next.

Transactional Model of Communication

An alternative to the simple sender/receiver model is the transactional model of communication, which proposes that people are simultaneously senders and receivers in an ongoing process of reciprocal influence.[7] What one person says and does influences other people and vice versa. Because the emphasis is on shared meaning rather than simply transmitting information, the focus is on what happens "between people."

One benefit of the transactional perspective is that it encourages people to share power relatively equitably. In palliative care, this means minimizing status differences. For example, a patient's spouse may be considered as important and influential as his or her physician to the illness experience. This is not only good communication; indications are that it is good medicine. People with serious health concerns typically experience less stress and greater well-being when loved ones are actively involved in their care and communicate openly with them about it.[14,15]

A transactional perspective also reminds people to be attentive to cues (both verbal and nonverbal) about how others are interpreting a transaction. For example, women with breast cancer say they appreciate being fully informed, but they feel overwhelmed when healthcare professionals give them more information than they can process and adapt to at one time.[16] Respecting this, the best communicators do not toss messages around as if they are playing ball. They weigh their words and actions in light of how they are received by other people. They ask for feedback, observe feedback cues, and listen as much as they talk.

Another contribution of the transactional model is recognition that environmental, social, and personal factors influence how messages are interpreted. For example, members of some Native American cultures find silence comforting. To them, having others present without the obligation to make conversation is deeply appreciated.[17] Members of other cultures may consider silence awkward and wonder what they are "supposed to say" at a difficult time. Around the world and in any one community, cultures also differ in terms of how and if they talk about death, how they define family, how they regard spiritualism, what information they share with others, and much more.[18] In addition to culture, differences arise in terms of past experiences, emotions, pain, physical distractions, difficulties hearing or seeing, personality, family structure, age group, and so on.[19] The transactional model includes as "noise" any factor—including internal thoughts and feelings and external stimuli—that may interfere with shared meaning.[9] However, the model does not prescribe that communicators eradicate or minimize components of noise that are natural expressions of who people are. Instead, participants are encouraged to recognize the potential for misunderstanding and find mutually rewarding ways to honor diversity.

The transactional model calls attention to the idea that communication is a collaborative and unique accomplishment embedded in an ongoing process in which everyone involved shapes the meaning that emerges from a transaction. In the next section, we explore how these ideas translate into communication techniques and perspectives essential to palliative care.

Transactional Approach to Person-Centered Care

Consider the following comments by clients of a hospice in England that provides palliative, during-the-day care for people with multiple sclerosis:

> It's like being at home but with friends because you know you haven't got to explain what's wrong with you. I don't have to explain it here. Everybody knows. You actually feel good because you are part of a group.[20(p404)]
>
> ...
>
> It gives me a more confident frame of mind I think. Puts me in control.[16(p405)]
>
> ...
>
> I would miss it so much. I look forward to coming ... and it's just a nice relaxing day out.[16(p405)]
>
> ...
>
> Me coming here for the day takes a hell of a lot of pressure off my wife, who knows full well that I am fed and watered and looked after and couldn't be better.[16(p405)]

Contrary to the idea that palliative care is only for people who are dying (people do not usually die of multiple sclerosis), it also includes people whose conditions are not terminal or end stage but who benefit from the symptom management, social support, counseling, knowledge, spiritual connectedness, and overall comfort and caring that palliative care can offer them and their loved ones as they cope with serious health concerns.[21] As palliative physician Jacob Strand and colleagues put it, palliative care is increasingly being implemented "upstream," when serious illness is first detected, rather than only "downstream," at life's end.[22]

Even with diverse goals, however, palliative care in all its form shares an emphasis on relational and person-centered care. This section explores the role of transactional communication in accomplishing four key aspects of palliative care alluded to in the hospice clients' comments: (a) a focus on relationships, (b) the importance of emotions, (c) the need for empathy, and (d) the value of being present with each other.

The relational approach to understanding human interaction originated in one of the earliest publications devoted to communication as a distinct field of research. In *The Pragmatics of Human Communication*,[23] Paul Watzlawick, Janet Beavin, and Don Jackson proposed several axioms, one of which is particularly relevant to the relational approach. The axiom posits that all communication exists at two levels: the content level, which conveys the information of the message, and the relational level, which constitutes the relationship between the communicators. A relational approach to communication differs from an interpersonal approach, which focuses on individual acts, because it emphasizes the interdependency of relational members and their behaviors.[24] As the comments by hospice participants with multiple sclerosis illustrate, relationships are central to their experience, as much because of what is not said (such as explaining the illness to others) as what is.

The relational approach is aligned with the transactional model in that it focuses on what emerges between people rather than on the actions and responses of individual actors. Thus relational communication recognizes that relationships are not defined by the sender or receiver in isolation but rather are mutually and simultaneously co-constructed.

Instead of focusing primarily on message content, a relational approach is concerned primarily with the quality of the relationship that is generated through communication. The emergent nature of relational communication involves messages that are often conveyed implicitly rather than explicitly and through nonverbal cues. These messages convey emotions, attitudes, power and status, norms of interaction, expectations, cues about how to interpret the experience, and inferences.

The relational approach is also consistent with person- or patient-centered care, which involves respect for people's unique needs, values, and preferences.[25] Note that we use the term "person-centered" synonymously with "patient-centered" but prefer the former term as a means to recognize that palliative care (a) typically involves all aspects of a person's life, not just his or her role as a patient, and (b) includes loved ones and others who are not themselves the "patient." Rita Charon, an advocate of honoring patients' narratives, proposes that listening intently to people's stories and concerns bridges the "chasms" and "discontinuities" that often separate people who are ill from those who are not.[26(p197)] This bridging of that gap is particularly vital to palliative care.

Engaging in relational, person-centered communication requires that communicators be attuned to individual preferences and the myriad, complex elements that make each person unique. The capacity to recognize and respond appropriately at a relational level was long framed as intuitive and unteachable.[27] However, that position was refuted by the now well-established relationship-centered care paradigm.[28-30] This approach emphasizes values and practices related principally to emotions, empathy, and presence. The following is a brief overview of communication perspectives relevant to each of these.

Focus on Emotions

Emotions are not clearly represented in the transmission model of communication, which focuses mostly on intentional message delivery. By contrast, the relational, patient-centered approach emphasizes the emergent and unintentional features of relationships.[22]

Despite the "invisible" nature of relational dynamics such as emotions, reciprocal influence, authenticity, and respect, their impact is highly consequential to the meaning derived from any given interaction,[20] particularly in palliative care. For example, imagine a situation in which a patient has just received news of a terminal prognosis. The patient responds by becoming very still and quiet. Even in the context of this apparent absence of cues, the response of the healthcare provider who delivered the prognosis may be influenced by a wide variety of factors, including (but not limited to) prior training in how to deliver bad news, memories of being in this situation with other patients, an involuntary impulse to compare the patient to his or her aging parent, a sense of his or her own sorrow or anxiety, or a desire to better understand what the patient is thinking and feeling. If, in the next few moments, the patient's eyes begin to well with tears (an external cue), a new cascade of internal responses might guide the healthcare provider down a different path of communicative choices.

Paying attention and responding to cues, both internal and external, is key to communicating effectively when the stakes are high. Understanding the relational dimension of communication is essential if communicators hope to be mindful of the relationships that they are constructing in the moment and over time.

This experience reminds us that the focus should not only be on patients' emotions but on healthcare providers' as well. Relational theorists emphasize the importance of self-reflection for providers.[22] Robert Wicks, author of *The Resilient Clinician*,[31] encourages care providers to take daily stock of their emotions, to seek out people and activities that replenish them, and to be mindful of what makes them happy.

The Role of Empathy

One essential capacity/competency of healthcare providers in the palliative care context is empathy for others. Because this requires attending to both content and relational dimensions, empathy is appropriately framed within a transactional or relationship-centered approach. At its core, empathy involves three dimensions: attending to the emotions of another person (relational), understanding those emotions (cognitive), and responding to those emotions (communicative).[19,32]

Researchers often find that physicians avoid responding relationally to the emotional cues of patients and focus instead on cognitive, clinically oriented questions and treatment plans.[19] This may be because relational communication requires a sophisticated set of talents and sensitivities. However, a number of heuristics are available to help healthcare providers and others when it comes to communicating empathy.

Suchman and colleagues[23] present a framework that encourages care providers to become attuned to empathic opportunities and to consider how they might react to them. In the model, the three main reactions are characterized as *empathic responses, empathic opportunity continuers* (invitations to extend the conversation into the realm of feelings), and *empathic opportunity terminators* (comments or gestures that steer the conversation away from expressions of emotion). In the previous example of a patient reacting to a terminal prognosis, the patient's initial silence presents an *empathic opportunity* for the care provider to offer an explicit expression of emotion, perhaps by saying, "I can sense that this is a lot for you to take in, and I'm wondering how you are feeling about what I've just told you." The appearance of tears also represents an *empathic opportunity* because it is clear that the patient is feeling a strong emotion, although the provider should not assume to know what it is. One *empathic response* option would be to say, "I can see that this news has triggered some strong emotions for you, and that's perfectly understandable" and include an *empathic opportunity continuer* such as, "Would you like to share with me what you are thinking and feeling right now?" or even simply reaching out a hand to offer comfort. Conversely, an *empathic opportunity terminator* is any response that ignores the emotions in the room, perhaps by disconfirming the feelings of the patient—"You shouldn't be worried about that; just focus on taking your medication"—or changing the topic, as in, "I see. Well, we need to get the results of your bloodwork and schedule your biopsy."

Another technique designed to support empathic responses is represented by the acronym BATHE, which offers a five-part guide for responding in situations to where a patient or loved one is experiencing strong emotions and may feel overwhelmed by current circumstances.[33,34] The process includes (a) asking the patient for B—*background* information ("Briefly, what has been going on?"); (b) exploring A—*affect* (both affect as in emotion and affect as in "How has this affected you emotionally?"); (c) inviting talk about a particular aspect of the problem or T—*trouble* ("What troubles you the most about this situation?"); (d) considering how the patient is H—*handling* things emotionally and practically ("How have you been handling this situation?"); (e) and offering E—*empathy* without trying to change or fix the situation or change the emotional response of the patient ("It sounds like you've been working hard to keep things going" or "This seems like a very stressful time for you").

Underlying both the framework of empathic opportunities and responses[23] and the BATHE model[25] is a relational commitment that gives patients and their loved ones ample space and encouragement to pay mindful attention to their emotions and to experience the support of people around them. Empathic responses and encouragement, combined with the relational quality of presence, which we discuss next, are conducive to a supportive communication environment.

The Importance of Presence and "Being There"

The stigma surrounding incurable conditions and death was so great in the mid-20th century that patients were often abandoned to cope mostly alone, with little comfort or compassion.[35,36] Healthcare professionals often considered dying and death experiences to be "medical embarrassments" that belittled the supposed omnipotence of their expertise and technology.[37(p24)] In recent decades, however, the hospice and palliative care movement has made great strides in overcoming the fear and failure people used to associate with incurable conditions.

A new paradigm has emerged that honors the unique set of skills (many of which are related directly to communication) involved in palliative care. Talk is a valued component within the paradigm, which invites participants to co-construct a "good death" or "quality of life" during a serious illness. At the same time, researchers have posed a pertinent critique to the role that talk plays.[28,38]

To illustrate, an influential and popular book, *Tuesdays with Morrie*,[39] takes readers through the story of Morrie Schwartz's final months, as relayed by his friend and former student Mitch Albom. The book's popularity did a great deal to support a national conversation about death and dying. It also promoted a vision of the end-of-life journey as being accomplished through open, articulate, and insightful reflections offered by the person who is dying. A similar vision is offered in the Pulitzer Prize-winning play *Wit*,[40] in which the audience experiences the final months in the life of an English professor, Vivian Bearing, as she battles metastatic ovarian cancer, initially with biting humor and intelligence and eventually with vulnerability and humanity.

While such depictions help readers and viewers to vicariously experience important end-of-life challenges and emotions, they also lead us to overlook bodily experiences. As Foster puts it in the book *Communicating at the End of Life*,[41] focusing on cognition, thoughts, and words can be helpful, but it can also overshadow instinctive and emotional responses in palliative care situations. The desire to support persons who are dying or very ill primarily through conversation is not feasible when the person has advanced dementia, is aphasic or heavily medicated, or is simply unable or unwilling to talk explicitly about his or her experiences.

A different kind of end-of-life narrative is offered in *Derek*, a television production starring, written by, and directed by Ricky Gervais.[42] The series is set in a 26-bed nursing home in England and revolves around the quiet lives of the manager (Hannah), the caretaker (Dougie), and the title character (Derek), who is a care worker. What is remarkable about the program is the way it highlights both the relative social isolation of the nursing home's residents and the extraordinary connections that are built through very simple acts of kindness—listening, sitting and holding hands, reading a celebrity magazine, or offering a cup of tea. Although illness and death are ever-present, the dignity and humanity of the residents and workers is made evident through the quality of their interactions (relationships) with one another, so that the overarching message is a positive one.

Perhaps because words are relatively easy to observe and control, the emphasis of much palliative care communication training (including models described in this chapter and others) rests on how to prepare and enact conversations. An equally important emphasis, however, is on how to be fully present in the care of patients and their loved ones, even in the absence of talk. An example of this is the following story from a hospice volunteer, Tom, who was visiting a patient dying from cancer. The patient was not cognitively impaired, but she was not able to engage in conversation and, at first, this was very challenging for the volunteer.

> At first I felt the need to keep the conversation going, and with her not contributing the only thing I could really talk about was me ... but I remembered Patrice [volunteer coordinator] saying that it's fine to sit there and not say a word. So I said, "Do you want me to leave? Because you look really tired." And she said, "No, I'm just tired, but I want you to stay." So I just sat there looking at her and every now and then she would open her eyes to see if I was still there.[32(p137)]

In this example, Tom began by doing what made him feel comfortable—specifically, keeping up a one-sided conversation—until he realized that this did not constitute the kind of supportive relationship he wanted to have with this patient. In that instant, Tom's consciousness moved from himself to the patient and, most important, to the present moment. He was able to check his perceptions with the patient by sharing his observation that she looked tired and then ask what she wanted. When she indicated that she wanted him to stay, he was able to relax and simply be there for her.

Another aspect of "being there" with someone may also involve participating in conversations or interactions that have nothing explicitly to do with healthcare but can contribute dramatically to maintaining a humane and supportive relationship. Hospice or palliative care patients exist in what anthropologist Turner[43] calls a liminal space (literally, a threshold) between the time of their terminal diagnosis and death. This time constitutes a crisis both physically and socially because there is a process of *social dying*[32] that accompanies the bodily changes, shifts in consciousness, and pain of the dying process that are often the focus of palliative care. The social dying process has its own associated pain and often culminates in a social death[29,44] that precedes physical death if a patient has lost meaningful social or relational contacts and is attended only by healthcare professionals responding to physical contingencies. An antidote to the pain of social dying lies in reconnecting patients to the fabric of social life by recognizing their uniqueness and allowing their presence to generate a sense of immediacy and "being there."

Communicators within the palliative care context have the best chance of communicating effectively if they recognize that communication does not consist solely of content (words, gestures) but also includes a relational dimension through which attitudes, feeling, intentions, and care are conveyed. Ordinary gestures, such as rubbing patients' hands with lotion, reading articles to them about their favorite soap operas or sports stars, remembering a special anniversary, or introducing them by something other than their diagnosis can all serve to help reconnect them to the social fabric that we otherwise tend to take for granted.

Transactional Approach To Teamwork

Imagine a scenario in which a patient's oncologist (or other specialist) wishes to advocate for further treatment, but the palliative care team believes the time has come for comfort measures. On the surface, this is a difference of opinion at a content level. They may disagree about the "facts" of the case as they affect the prognosis. However, a transactional approach encourages us to think the matter through more thoroughly and examine it at multiple levels.

Returning to the communication axiom presented earlier,[17] the idea that communication occurs simultaneously at two levels is also reflected in theories of group communication, which recognize that groups function at both a task (content) and a social (relational) level. To be fully effective, group members must address both tasks to be accomplished (productivity) and relationships among the members (cohesion).

In keeping with this principle, the Relationship-Centered Care Model (RCCM) advanced by Dana Safran and colleagues[29] argues that attention must be paid to how relationships are enacted across the constellation of healthcare providers responsible for providing care (a transactional approach)—and not merely to the exchange of information (a sender-oriented approach). The Safran team has identified seven interdependent relational qualities that are essential to a "relationship-centered" team approach. In the following sections, we explore five that are most relevant to the current discussion.

Mindful Communication

"Mindfulness" refers to participants' awareness of self, of others, of relationships, and of what is happening in the larger scheme of things. It also involves being open to new ideas and different perspectives.[21(pS12)]

In the opening example involving a difference of opinion, being mindful may involve a conversation in which every member of the team (including the patient, if possible) is open to hearing the others' perspectives and why they feel as they do. The goal of mindfulness is not to debate the issue or reach a decision (that may come later) but to exercise sincere curiosity and consider multiple perspectives.

Diversity of Mental Models

An important dynamic that should be included in any consideration of a relationship-centered approach is how to manage diversity within the context of care. Within the RCCM, diversity of mental models refers to the degree to which members value multiple ways of thinking and capitalize on them to enhance group problem-solving and creativity.[21]

Diversity may include culture, race, gender, age, education, and many other individual characteristics that contribute to different standpoints. It may also include people's training and background. The best palliative care teams are made up of people with diverse expertise and ideas, including medical specialists, nurses, dieticians, therapists, clergy, social workers, volunteers, family members, pharmacists, and many others. The significant principle to remember is not simply to incorporate diversity into a group but to actually realize the benefits by nurturing positive and productive relationships among people with diverse ideas.[21]

Mindfulness is key to truly respecting diversity, but skillful conflict management is required as well. Particularly when the consequences are serious and emotions run high, divergent perspectives often lead to conflict. Those are most visible at the content level, but it is likely that relational issues are also involved. The oncologist advocating for continued treatment may feel that a transition to palliative care represents a vote of no confidence regarding his or her ability to serve the patient well. Conversely, members of the palliative care team may feel that the specialist is being domineering and insensitive by refusing to consider the contributions they might make.

People skilled at a relational, transactional approach are in the best position to understand and address conflict at multiple levels. They may realize, first of all, that part of the emotional intensity on both sides stems from underlying, relational factors. In other words, the issue is not only a decision to be made but a commentary on their identity and validity as care providers. When diverse participants are mindful of that, it may be easier to surface those issues and respect them. For example, members of the palliative care team may say to a physician, "This can't be easy for you. We know you have a long-standing relationship with this patient and have helped her immensely through the years. We'd like to work together with you."

Mutual Respect

Mutual respect is demonstrated when team members display honesty, tactfulness, and respect for every person's contributions.[21] It is imperative that diverse healthcare providers have mutual respect for each other, but it is just as important that patients and their loved ones be included. They should rightfully be treated as members of the care team rather than only as care recipients or bystanders.

Echoing the reciprocity principle of the transactional model, even as palliative care emphasizes the importance of focusing on the patient's and family's needs, patients and family members may express concern for their healthcare providers' well-being. They may wish to share small gifts or give advice or in some other way reciprocate the care that is being shown to them. One of the particularly challenging yet important ways that patients connect to the social world is caring for those around them, including health professionals. To deny patients and family members the opportunity to express their own sense of relationship to healthcare providers is to take a condescending or patronizing stand that forestalls the potential for connection through mutuality or reciprocity.[41] The challenge is to keep the reciprocation in balance so that neither patients and family members nor professionals become burdened with obligations. As described by Beach et al.,[20(pS4)] "While achievement of the patient's goals and the maintenance of health are the more obvious focus of any encounter, allowing a patient to have an impact on the clinician is a way to honor that patient and his or her experience."

Mix of Social and Task-Related Interactions

The RCCM reminds us that conversations should include both relationship-focused and function-oriented communication.[21] The goal is to involve team members in the right mix of these communication goals. In her extensive ethnography of an interdisciplinary oncology team, Ellingson[45,46] points out the dynamic of frontstage and backstage communication among clinical team members. The concepts of frontstage and backstage do not neatly align with task (content) and social (relational) communication but rather describe the shifting dynamic for the team when they are in front of a patient and family (frontstage) versus in the clinic spaces out of sight of patients and family members (backstage). A good deal of work occurs in the clinical backstage. This includes formal reporting but also informal information exchanges, sharing of impressions, and relationship-building among team members.[36] Ellingson[36,37] argues for what she calls an embedded model of understanding that recognizes team members as interdependent, inseparable, and mutually productive based on the quality of both their frontstage and backstage communication. Effective teamwork always incorporates both.

Ellingson[36] points out that healthcare providers may have good intentions when they exclude patients from the messy and sometimes contentious work that goes on backstage. And certainly, patients need not be part of all backstage communication. But she cautions that excluding patients unduly puts them at a disadvantage. In the difference-of-opinion scenario, a good deal of the work in resolving whose recommendation will hold sway—the oncologist's or the palliative care team's—is likely to be carried out backstage, away from the patient. Once the care team has reached some form of resolution (or at least an agreeable set of options), they are likely to convene a family meeting to discuss them. This seems reasonable on the surface, but Ellingson[36] points out that it puts patients and their loved ones at a distinct rhetorical disadvantage. By this time, the professionals have already spent significant time discussing the situation, hearing each others' viewpoints, and shaping how thinking about it evolves and emerges. Patients, on the other hand, are more likely to be caught off guard by what emerges and to feel that they must make decisions with limited information and minimal opportunity to engage in a collaborative thinking through of the issues. In short, being asked to make a decision at the end is not the same as being involved in the process.

Mindfulness

Mindfulness (what researchers sometimes call heedful interrelating) occurs when team members' interactions are rooted in ongoing awareness of how their work and others' contribute to practice goals.[21] Interrelating is not a simple process. It involves a great deal of give and take and a commitment to achieving balance between changing and contradictory goals.

The concept of relational dialectics[47] offers a framework for understanding dilemmas such as reciprocity within caregiving relationships. Relational dialectics is not a theory as much as it is a metatheoretical construct that emphasizes the fluid and changing nature of relationships and the tendency for multiple opposing forces (dialectic tensions) to be operating at any given time. The overarching dynamic in relational dialectics is the movement of coming together (centripetal force) and coming apart (centrifugal force).[38(p44)] In the palliative care context, a primary dialectic exists between recognizing and sustaining quality of life (coming together) and preparing for death (coming apart). At any given moment in palliative care, one may feel the influence of one of these forces more strongly than the other.

Dialectics are not only negotiated internally but between people who depend on each other. For example, during a family meeting to discuss vent removal, the patient's willingness to undergo extubation may indicate a readiness to "let go," while a family member argues strongly for continuing the patient on respiratory support, continuing to "hold on." All the while, healthcare providers' feelings may fall somewhere in the middle on this continuum.

A relational dialectics perspective also reminds us that roles are truly interrelated. There will be moments of role reversal when the patient reaches out to care for the healthcare provider and the provider feels more like a care recipient than a caregiver. The concept of mindful communication reminds us that this is natural and acceptable in the ongoing flow of teamwork. Such moments are not to be feared or avoided but rather embraced as transient and precious artifacts of human expression.

Conclusion

Collaborative communication is essential to creating the unique roadmap of every palliative care experience. In contrast to the transmission model, which depicts communication partners as relatively distinct and separate from one another, the transactional perspective represents people as interdependent members of communities connected by authenticity, mutual concerns, emotions, social activity, and more. The focus is on the uniqueness of every person and relationship.

A key principle of the transactional model is that messages are considered valuable to the extent that they enhance shared understanding. In palliative care, this provides the opportunity for participants to co-create the experience of a "good death" or "quality of life" in the context of a serious illness. Relational communication requires that people pay attention to both content and relational messages. This is consistent with a person- and patient-centered approach that places a premium on relationships, emotions, empathy, and the value of presence.

Palliative care is intrinsically team oriented, typically involving an array of professionals as well as volunteers and loved ones. The potential for collaborative sense making is extraordinary, but only if participants truly honor the diversity among them and are skillful at handling the inevitable conflict that arises from multiple perspectives. The RCCM suggests that palliative care teams are most helpful when members exercise and encourage mindfulness, embrace a diversity of mental models, show mutual respect, pay attention to both social and task goals, and interrelate in a manner that honors competing and contradictory inclinations among dialectic continua such as "holding on" and "letting go."

The focus in palliative care is not so much on communication as an information commodity as on communication as a means of sharing and relating. One last example, posted by a loved one on the National Hospice Foundation website, calls to mind the extraordinary and varied contributions of palliative healthcare providers who provide both tangible assistance and the intangibles of comfort, compassion, and presence. In this posting, Sue Hazelton remembers treasured time with Cathy, her 34-year-old sister and mother of three boys, who was dying of a rare cancer.[48] "The call was made to hospice and things quickly changed for the best," Hazelton recalls, describing what happened first:

> A knock on the door brought a hospital bed, toilet help, and a wheelchair. Another knock and in came a charge nurse, a counselor for the boys, and even someone to help with shopping and household chores. I felt like a weight was lifted off my shoulders. Better pain management brought her spirits up; she was more talkative, like her old self; and could visit more with everyone for a couple of weeks.

Later, on Cathy's last day of life, hospice was present in a different way. Hazelton describes the experience:

> The boys and my Dad came in to say goodbye ... I played [Cathy's] favorite CD as her breathing changed. The hospice nurse would give us updates until she said "Sue, I think it will be in the next hour or so." She was an amazing nurse that was quietly checking her, rubbing her legs, keeping her free of pain and just being there telling us what an honor it was for her to be there. I was honored along with my brother to hold each of Cathy's frail hands as she passed, whispering our goodbyes and I love you.

References

1. Pollock L. Accompanying the dying: The spiritual perspective. In: Mason C, ed. *Journeys Into Palliative Care: Roots and Reflections*. Philadelphia, PA: Jessica Kinglsey; 2002:119–134.
2. Department of Health and Human Services. Federal Register. Medicare and Medicaid programs: Hospice conditions and participation. http://www.gpo.gov/fdsys/pkg/FR-2008-06-05/pdf/08-1305.pdf. Published June 5, 2008. Accessed June 24, 2014.
3. Shannon C, Weaver W. *The Mathematical Theory of Communication*. Urbana: University of Illinois Press; 1949.
4. Dyche L, Swiderski D. The effect of physician solicitation approaches on ability to identify patient concerns. *J Gen Intern Med*. March 2005;20(3):267–270.
5. Nelson M, Hamilton HE. Improving in-office discussion of chronic obstructive pulmonary disease: Results and recommendations from an in-office linguistic study in chronic obstructive pulmonary disease. *Am J Med*. 2007;120(8 Suppl 1):S28–S32.
6. Mazor K, Gaglio B, Arora N, et al. Assessing patient-centered communication in cancer care: Stakeholder perspectives. *J Oncol Pract*. September 2013;9(5):e186–e193.
7. Lipton R, Hahn S, Nelson M, et al. In-office discussions of migraine: Results from the American Migraine Communication Study. *J Gen Intern Med*. 2008;(8):1145–1151.
8. Boykins D. Core communication competencies in patient-centered care. *ABNF J*. April 2014;25(2):40–45.
9. Barnlund D. A transactional model of communication. In: Sereno, KK, Mortensen, CD, eds. *Foundations of Communication Theory*. New York, NY: Harper; 1970:83–102.
10. Merkelsen H. Risk communication and citizen engagement: What to expect from dialogue. *J Risk Res*. 2011;14(5):631–645.
11. Delmar C. The interplay between autonomy and dignity: Summarizing patients' voices. *Med Health Care Philos*. 2013;16(4):975–981.
12. Larkin P. Listening to the still small voice: The role of palliative care nurses in addressing psychosocial issues at end of life. *Prog Palliat Care*. December 2010;18(6):335–340.
13. Gallagher R, Krawczyk M. Family members' perceptions of end-of-life care across diverse locations of care. *BMC Pall Care*. January 2013;12(1):25–33.
14. Li Q, Loke A. A literature review on the mutual impact of the spousal caregiver–cancer patients dyads: "Communication," "reciprocal influence," and "caregiver-patient congruence." *Eur J Oncol Nurs*. February 1, 2014;18:58–65.
15. Fletcher B, Miaskowski C, Given B, Schumacher K. The cancer family caregiving experience: An updated and expanded conceptual model. *Eur J Oncol Nurs*. September 1, 2012;16:387–398.
16. van Vliet L, Francke A, Tomson S, Plum N, van der Wall E, Bensing J. When cure is no option: How explicit and hopeful can information be given? A qualitative study in breast cancer. *Patient Educ Couns*. March 1, 2013;90:315–322.
17. Basso K. "To give up on words": Silence in Western Apache culture. In: Monogahn L, Goodman JE, Robinson JM, eds. *A Cultural Approach to Interpersonal Communication: Essential Readings*. 2nd ed. Malden, MA: Blackwell; 2012:73–83.
18. Chaturvedi S, Loiselle C, Chandra P. Communication with relatives and collusion in palliative care: A cross-cultural perspective. *Indian J Paliatl Care*. January–June 2009;15(1):2–9.
19. Eggly, SS, Albrecht, TL, Kelly, K, Prigerson, HG, Sheldon, L, Studts, J. The role of the clinician in cancer clinical communication. *J Health Commun*. 2009;14:66–75.
20. Embrey N. Exploring the lived experience of palliative care for people with MS, 3: Views of group support. *British J of Neuro Nurs*. September 2009;5(9):402.
21. Greer J, Jackson V, Meier D, Temel J. Early integration of palliative care services with standard oncology care for patients with advanced cancer. *Cancer J Clin*. September 2013;63(5):349–363.
22. Strand J, Kamdar M, Carey E. Concise review for clinicians: Top 10 things palliative care clinicians wished everyone knew about palliative care. *Mayo Clin Proc*. 2013;88:859–865.
23. Watzlawick P, Beavin JH, Jackson, DD. *The Pragmatics of Human Communication*. New York, NY: Norton; 1967.
24. Rogers LE, Escudero V. Theoretical foundations. In Rogers LE, Escudero V, eds. *Relational Communication: An Interactional Perspective to the Study of Process and Form*. Mahwah, NJ: Lawrence Erlbaum; 2004:3–21.
25. A physician's practical guide to culturally competent care. U.S. Department of Health & Human Services, Office of Minority Health. https://cccm.thinkculturalhealth.hhs.gov/. Published December 6, 2004. Accessed June 25, 2014.
26. Charon R. The polis of a discursive narrative medicine. *J Appl Commun Res*. 2009;37:196–201.
27. Buckman R, Tulsky JD, Rodin G. Empathic responses in clinical practice: Intuition or tuition? *CMAJ*. 2011;183(5):569–571.
28. Beach MC, Inui T, Relationship-Centered Care Research Network. Relationship-centered care: A constructive reframing. *J Gen Intern Med*. 2006;21:S3–S8.
29. Safran DG, Miller W, Beckman H. Organizational dimensions of relationship-centered practice: Theory, evidence, and practice. *J Gen Intern Med*. 2006;21:S9–S15.
30. Suchman AL. A new theoretical foundation for relationship-centered care: Complex responsive processes of relating. *J Gen Intern Med*. 2006;21:S40–S44.
31. Wicks RJ. *The Resilient Clinician*. Oxford: Oxford University Press; 2008.
32. Suchman AL, Markakis K, Beckman HB, Frankel R. A model of empathic communication in the medical interview. *JAMA*. 1997;277 678–682.
33. Miller W. The clinical hand: A curricular map for relationship-centered care. *Fam Med*. 2004;36:330–335.
34. Stuart MR, Lieberman JA III. *The Fifteen-Minute Hour: Practical Therapeutic Interventions in Primary Care*. 3rd ed. Philadelphia, PA: Saunders; 2002.

35. Connor SR. *Hospice: Practice, Pitfalls, and Promise.* Washington, DC: Taylor & Francis; 1998.
36. Morris DB. *Illness and Culture in the Postmodern Age.* Berkeley: University of California Press; 1998.
37. Walter T. *The Revival of Death.* London: Routledge; 1994.
38. Seale C. *Constructing Death: The Sociology of Dying and Bereavement.* Cambridge, UK: Cambridge University Press; 1996.
39. Albom M. *Tuesdays with Morrie: An Old Man, A Young Man, and Life's Greatest Lesson.* New York, NY: Doubleday; 1996.
40. Edson M. *Wit: A Play.* New York, NY: Faber & Faber; 1999.
41. Foster E. *Communicating at the End of Life: Finding Magic in the Mundane.* Mahwah, NJ: Lawrence Erlbaum; 2007.
42. Hanson C, prod. *Derek* [television series]. London, UK: Channel 4; 2013.
43. Turner V. *The Ritual Process: Structure and Anti-Structure.* Hawthorne, NY: Aldine DeGruyter; 1995.
44. Lawton J. *The Dying Process: Patients' Experiences of Palliative Care.* London: Routledge; 2000.
45. Ellingson L. Interdisciplinary health care: Teamwork in the clinic backstage. *J Appl Comm Res.* 2003;31:93–117.
46. Ellingson L. *Communicating in the Clinic: Negotiating Frontstage and Backstage Teamwork.* Cresskill, NJ: Hampton Press; 2005.
47. Baxter LA, Montgomery BM. *Relating: Dialogues and Dialectics.* New York, NY: Guilford Press; 1996.
48. Hazelton S. Lessons from my sister Cathy, Disney and hospice. National Hospice Foundation. http://www.nationalhospicefoundation.org/i4a/pages/index.cfm?pageID=507. Accessed June 28, 2014.

CHAPTER 4

Consumer Communication and Public Messaging About Palliative Care

Rebecca A. Kirch

Introduction

For seriously ill adults and children of any age and at any illness stage, treating the pain, symptoms, and stress that interfere with their quality of life is as important as treating their disease. Patients and their families place a premium on maintaining good quality of life and functioning for as long as possible so they can continue to pursue what matters most to them and participate in aspects of daily life that give them joy and make them feel their lives are worth living. Yet in today's disease-centric delivery system, quality of life priorities within this personal choice and value construct are not typically identified or discussed early enough to ensure they are considered, and they are rarely documented in medical records to help guide the course of therapeutic treatment and follow-up care. In a national poll conducted by the American Cancer Society Cancer Action Network (ACS CAN) in 2010 among 1,011 adults with cancer or a history of it, fewer than one-third (29%) reported that their physician or other health team member asked what was important to them in terms of quality of life before starting treatment.[1] Similarly, only about one-third (32%) said that they were asked regularly about stress, depression, anxiety, or other emotional concerns during and after cancer treatment, and fewer than half (47%) stated that they were provided any information or referral for treatment even after identifying their emotional concerns.[1]

Findings such as these underscore the need for action to make personalized medicine that treats the person beyond the disease a prioritized part of quality clinical practice. This means supporting and encouraging all providers to ask patients about what is important to them so they make quality of life concerns a routine part of the clinical conversation and course of care. At the same time, patients and families need help to feel more knowledgeable, skillful, and confident in their ability to cope with the challenges of serious illness diagnosis, treatment, and aftermath—including feeling that they would be supported in raising these quality of life matters as clinical concerns important to them alongside their disease-directed treatment.

Patients/families consistently report that they want to be involved in understanding their disease prognosis and treatment options and making decisions about their care. In a recent Institute of Medicine national survey of 1,068 US adults who had seen at least one healthcare provider in the previous year,[2] the majority of people responding confirmed that they want their healthcare provider to listen, tell the full truth about diagnosis (even though it may be uncomfortable or unpleasant), give the risks associated with each option, and explain how options impact quality of life, and they want to understand their goals and concerns regarding options of care.

These are important aspects of person-centered and goal-directed care that treats the whole person by focusing on what is important to a particular patient and his or her loved ones. Identifying and tending to these personal choices to ensure goal-concordant care is also the cornerstone of palliative care and the communication strategies that constitute its foundation.

Because patients and families often do not know what they do not know, they must be equipped and empowered with the right words to obtain the care they need. Adults and children with serious illness and their families require practical assistance to help them ask questions and articulate their healthcare concerns, needs, and wishes. They also require clear information and skilled professional communication to help them understand their diagnosis, prognosis and treatment options, and the implications of treatment in terms of their survival, functioning, and quality of life so that they can make informed decisions during and after disease-directed treatment that align with their personal values and goals. Providers in all disciplines and at every point in care serve as an essential gateway to ensuring that these quality of life needs are discussed, valued, and continuously addressed across the care continuum.

Quality of Life and Quality of Living

Currently, if personal preferences are addressed in clinical settings, poor prognosis is the typical trigger. Resulting conversations tend to focus on advanced care planning in the context of terminal illness and the end of life, relying on completing advance directives, DNR orders, and other such tools. Those are important discussions, but they are not designed to meet quality of life needs from the onset of serious illness and across what can be a long-term trajectory of ongoing chronic care. Moreover, this prevailing end-of-life focus may actually shortchange the survival and quality of life benefits that can be derived from earlier integration of palliative care.[3]

To meet the needs of patients and families, particularly as the United States faces unprecedented and rising numbers of adults and children living longer lives with complex chronic conditions, the focus must shift to prioritize earlier and continuous attention on personal choices about *how these patients want to be living*—right up until the time they die. This focus on quality of life and quality of living—optimally initiated at diagnosis—is a central tenet of palliative care. As described in more detail in this chapter, it is also the foundation of a growing national movement to raise awareness of palliative care so that it can extend to every seriously ill adult and child and their families and to every care setting—whether inpatient, outpatient, in the community, or at home.

Clinical conversations should identify early and document often what is important to patients and families and what are they hoping for—before, during, and after disease-directed treatment. Triggers for these conversations should occur routinely as part of care transitions throughout long-term chronic disease management and at the end of life. This upstream and ongoing person-centered focus enables and empowers adults, children, and families to articulate their own quality of living formula during treatment, follow-up, and in the weeks, years, or decades of life they have ahead. Those documented and accessible quality of life goals can then guide informed treatment decisions, long-term chronic care planning, and advanced care planning preferences and directives as these seriously ill adults or children approach the end of life.

What's in a Name?

Using consistent and clear messages about palliative care as a lifeline to quality of life really matters. A 2011 national poll commissioned by the Center to Advance Palliative Care, the American Cancer Society, and ACS CAN revealed that 7 in 10 Americans are "not at all knowledgeable" about palliative care.[4] While palliative care is a relative unknown among consumers, most providers associate palliative care with terminal prognosis and believe it becomes useful only near the very end of life.[4] These misconceptions conflating palliative care with "giving up hope" or hospice, particularly among disease specialties, remain one of the biggest barriers to patients and families accessing palliative care's benefits.

Consumer research findings confirm this language barrier can be effectively addressed using the public's own words to describe palliative care. An overwhelming majority of people (92%) in the Center to Advance Palliative Care/American Cancer Society poll confirmed that they would be likely to consider palliative care for themselves or their loved ones and believe it should be accessible in hospitals when it was explained using these key messages[4]:

- Palliative care helps to provide the best possible quality of life for patients and their families.
- Palliative care helps patients and families manage the pain, symptoms, and stress of serious illness.
- Palliative care is a partnership of patient, medical specialists, and family.
- Palliative care provides an extra layer of support for families and patients with serious illness.
- Palliative care is appropriate at any age and at any stage of a serious illness and can be provided along with curative treatment.

Additional detailed findings from this consumer research, which involved extensive in-depth interviews, focus groups, and a national poll, are provided in Box 4.1.

Despite evidence demonstrating the benefits of concurrent palliative care, many disease specialists still believe palliative care is done only when there is nothing left to do. Some studies, particularly in oncology, have suggested that changing the name to "supportive care" might help encourage earlier palliative care referrals.[5,6] But with the more recent consumer research findings and messaging

---

Box 4.1 Palliative Care Consumer Market Research Findings

The Center to Advance Palliative Care 2011 Public Opinion Research on Palliative Care can be found at https://www.capc.org/media/filer_public/18/ab/18ab708c-f835-4380-921d-fbf729702e36/2011-public-opinion-research-on-palliative-care.pdf

Most significant concerns for patients with serious illness:

- Doctors might not provide all of the treatment options or choices available
- Doctors might not talk and share information with each other
- Doctors might not choose the best treatment option for a seriously ill patient's medical condition
- Patients with serious illness and their families leave a doctor's office or hospital feeling unsure about what they are supposed to do when they get home
- Patients with serious illness and their families do not have enough control over their treatment options
- Doctors do not spend enough time talking with and listening to patients and their families

Palliative care definition (developed through the Center to Advance Palliative Care, www.capc.org):

Palliative care is specialized medical care for people with serious illnesses. This type of care is focused on providing patients with relief from the symptoms, pain, and stress of a serious illness—whatever the diagnosis. The goal is to improve quality of life for both the patient and the family.

Palliative care is provided by a team of doctors, nurses, and other specialists who work with a patient's other doctors to provide an extra layer of support. Palliative care is appropriate at any age and at any stage in a serious illness and can be provided together with curative treatment.

Key takeaways from the consumer research findings:

Once informed about palliative care using this definition and its key messages:

- 95% of poll respondents agree that it is important that patients with serious illness and their families be educated about palliative care.
- 92% of poll respondents say they would be likely to consider palliative care for a loved one if they had a serious illness.
- 92% of poll respondents say it is important that palliative care services be made available at all hospitals for patients with serious illness and their families.

now available, multiple thought leaders have cautioned against any such name change because it risks adding to the ambiguity and confusion rather than resolving it. Emphasizing that improved communication is essential to appropriate and timely engagement with palliative care services, the Institute of Medicine and several professional organizations have now recommended using the consumer-derived messages provided previously to describe palliative care, and they have used the term "palliative care" consistently in their own reports[2,7] and quality care guidance documents.[8,9]

If healthcare providers, professional and patient organizations, and others use this terminology consistently to talk about palliative care and tap the quality of life communication resources already available, great gains can be achieved in raising palliative care awareness among the public, professionals, and policymakers—important initial strategies for improving quality of care through advancing the US quality of life agenda. Communication skills training programs and resources for professionals are available in multiple formats, including an innovative new Vital talk platform that offers online talking and teaching maps, a smartphone app, and in-person advanced communication skills courses and faculty training programs built to nurture healthier connections between patients and healthcare providers.[10] Another palliative care communication mobile resource for healthcare providers, "Health Communication," is available for free at iTunes. Developed through the Palliative Care Communication Institute,[11] which is dedicated to advancing palliative care by fostering clinical communication practices for healthcare professionals, this smartphone app provides a handy mobile toolkit that is theory-driven and evidence-based to help address hard questions and challenging topics, guiding practitioners to provide compassionate and culturally sensitive care to seriously ill patients and their families. Similarly, multiple resources for consumers are available to help guide their quality of life focused conversations and decisions, including a novel "PREPARE" website that helps patients and families build skills needed for communication and in-the-moment decision making.[12] Table 4.1 lists these and other

Table 4.1 Resources for Communicating With Patients and Families

Organization	Description	Website
American Academy of Hospice and Palliative Medicine	Mobile-friendly site for patients and families seeking information on hospice and palliative care, including pages with patient stories, frequently asked questions, and links to important resources	http://palliativedoctors.org/
American Cancer Society and American Cancer Society Cancer Action Network	Consumer brochure and links to additional information and videos about palliative care and pediatric palliative care	http://www.cancer.org/treatment/treatmentsandsideeffects/palliativecare/index www.acscan.org/qualityoflife
Center to Advance Palliative Care	Consumer resources explaining palliative care and pediatric palliative care, including videos, podcasts, blog, and links	http://getpalliativecare.org/
University of California San Francisco	**PREPARE** interactive, easy-to-use communication-focused website designed to provide a quality of life-focused framework for assisting consumers in identifying and discussing their healthcare priorities	https://www.prepareforyourcare.org/
Courageous Parents Network	Pediatric palliative care information, videos, and network for parents and families of seriously ill children	www.courageousparentsnetwork.org
National Institutes of Health—National Institute Nursing Research	Palliative Care: Conversations Matter™ campaign materials for consumers and professionals explaining pediatric palliative care	http://www.ninr.nih.gov/newsandinformation/conversationsmatter#.U73k2vldXQo
American Childhood Cancer Organization	Pediatric palliative care handbook for families of children with cancer	http://acco.org/
Center to Advance Palliative Care	Full range of palliative care resources for professionals including e-learning communication curricula	http://www.capc.org/
Vitaltalk	Advanced communication skills resources and courses for professionals focused on balancing honesty with empathy when discussing serious illness	www.vitaltalk.org
Palliative Care Communication Institute	Free teaching materials to advance the COMFORT™ SM patient-centered training program that offers healthcare professionals extensive materials—PowerPoint presentations, knowledge assessments, example cases, and standardized patient assessment forms—designed to teach communication strategies for patient-centered palliative care	www.pccinstitute.com
American Society Clinical Oncology	Palliative care in oncology resource center provides a central location for a range of reference materials for physicians and patients	www.asco.org/practice-research/palliative-care-oncology

helpful, readily available communication resources that use quality of life and palliative care language and approaches that are consistent with the consumer research findings.

Advancing the National Quality of Life Movement

The number of hospital palliative care teams in the United States has grown dramatically over the past decade, with the prevalence of palliative care in hospitals having 50 beds or more nearly tripling since 2000, reaching 61% of all hospitals of this size.[13] This translates to 1,734 out of 2,844 hospitals with 50 beds or more reporting a team as of 2012. While these palliative care teams are serving an estimated 6 million Americans,[13] it remains difficult for the majority of seriously ill patients, such as those living at home, to access palliative care outside the hospice or hospital setting. Significant variation also exists in pediatric palliative care services availability among US children's hospitals.[14] With the US hospital uptake soaring, efforts now must also focus on making palliative care services universally available in outpatient clinics and other community care settings.

Coordinated and strategic action is essential to stretch palliative care's reach so that all seriously ill adults and children and their families can benefit from it. To begin, the public needs to understand what palliative care actually is and the benefits it brings to improve the quality of care so they can be empowered to ask for it and expect it. At the same time, we need to expand training opportunities that will boost generalist palliative care skills among physicians, nurses, social workers, and other healthcare providers so the workforce is equipped to meet the rising public demand for this level of person-centered and comprehensive care. Finally, health systems and policymakers need to prioritize and support these awareness, training, and professional practice activities so that palliative care can be available and integrated into quality medical care in every healthcare setting.

To advance these goals, multiple stakeholders representing many different diseases and disciplines have spearheaded the development of a new Patient Quality of Life Coalition[15] with an associated advocacy campaign[16] to promote person-centered care for all seriously ill adults and children and their families that focuses on what is important to them. This initiative is gaining steam. The campaign involves federal and state legislation and regulatory initiatives that are creating an echo chamber across the nation to build better understanding about palliative care and its role in promoting quality of life while also continuing to advocate for balanced pain care and prescribing public policies.

A key message of the quality of life advocacy campaign emphasizes palliative care's role in treating the person beyond the disease—a core component of ACS CAN's ad campaign promoting this platform among policymakers. Figures 4.1 and 4.2 show the ads used to launch this online and print campaign. ACS CAN also publishes an annual *How Do You Measure Up* report,[17] released every summer at the National Conference of State Legislators, that includes quality of life content-evaluating states' palliative care and pain public policy landscape, offering a handy reference tool for stakeholders interested in targeting coordinated action.

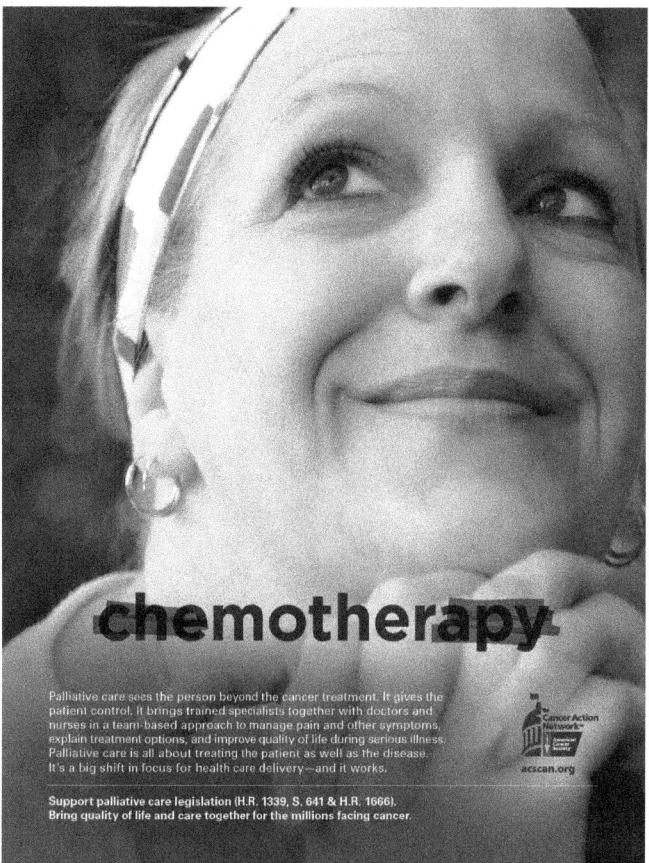

Figure 4.1 American Cancer Society Action Network palliative care campaign ad

To initiate this national campaign in 2013, two federal bills were introduced in the US Congress:

- The Palliative Care and Hospice Education and Training Act (HR1339/S641) to address the deficit in palliative care training offered in US medical schools by creating new incentives for the training and development of interdisciplinary health professionals and faculty in palliative care.

- The Patient Centered Quality Care for Life Act puts in place the building blocks of a national effort to improve the fragmented care that people with serious illnesses often experience by drawing more national attention to palliative care.

Complementing these federal bills, model state legislation has also been introduced and/or enacted in a growing number of states to increase the availability of palliative care information and services for all adults and children. Coupled with the federal bills, these state proposals will help build consistent messaging and a clear call for stakeholder action to integrate palliative care and quality of life in the fabric of care delivery across the nation. Information about the Patient Quality of Life Coalition can be found at www.patientqualityoflife.org and legislative campaign information at www.acscan.org/qualityoflife.

Conclusion

Now is the time to join forces across diseases and disciplines to spread the word about palliative care and its essential role

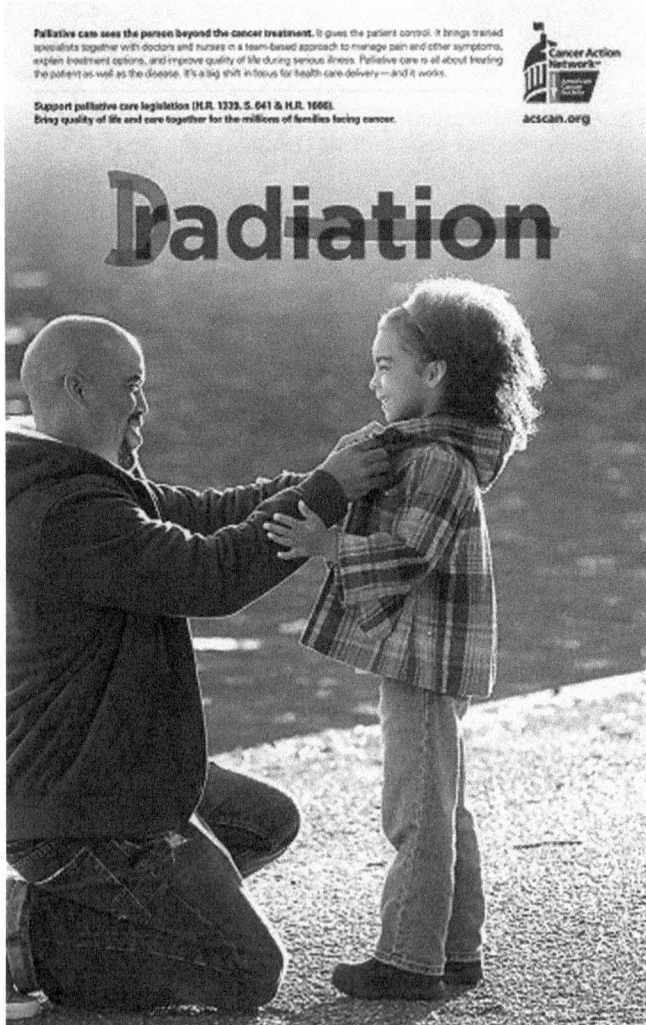

Figure 4.2 American Cancer Society Action Network palliative care campaign ad

in promoting quality of life for all seriously ill adults and children and their families. Other disease organizations are also beginning to promote earlier palliative care. For example, the American Heart Association/American Stroke Association, a member of the Patient Quality of Life Coalition, published its palliative care scientific statement in March 2014[9] and at the same time issued a press release endorsing the two federal palliative care bills.[18] The nation's most vulnerable patients are counting on us to give them the words to use while also delivering the quality care they need.

References

1. American Cancer Society Cancer Action Network. A national poll: Facing cancer in the health care system. 2010. http://www.acscan.org/healthcare/cancerpoll Accessed July 7, 2014.
2. Institute of Medicine. *Delivering High-Quality Cancer Care: Charting a New Course for a System in Crisis*. Washington, DC: National Academies Press; 2013.
3. Parikh RB, Kirch RA, Smith TJ, Temel JS. Early specialty palliative care—Translating data in oncology into practice. *N Engl J Med*. 2013;369:2347–2351.
4. Public Opinion Research on Palliative Care. 2011. https://www.capc.org/media/filer_public/18/ab/18ab708c-f835-4380-921d-fbf729702e36/2011-public-opinion-research-on-palliative-care.pdf. Accessed July 7, 2014.
5. Dalal S, Palla D, Hui L, et al., Association between a name change from palliative to supportive care and the timing of patient referrals at a comprehensive cancer center. *Oncologist*. 2011;16(1):105–111.
6. Hui DM, De La Cruz M, Mori HA, et al. Concepts and definitions for "supportive care," "best supportive care," "palliative care," and "hospice care" in the published literature, dictionaries, and textbooks. *Support Care Cancer*. 2013;21(3):659–685.
7. Institute of Medicine. *Dying in America: Improving Quality and Honoring Individual Preferences Near the End of Life*. Washington, DC: National Academies Press; 2014.
8. Smith TJ, Temin S, Alesi ER, et al. American Society of Clinical Oncology provisional clinical opinion: The integration of palliative care into standard oncology care. *J Clin Oncol*. 2012;30(8):880–887.
9. Holloway RG, Arnold RM, Creutzfeldt CJ, et al. AHA/ASA scientific statement: Palliative and end of life care in stroke: A statement for healthcare professionals from the American Heart Association/American Stroke Association. *Stroke*. 2014;45:1887–1916.
10. Vitaltalk Website. www.vitaltalk.org. Accessed July 9, 2014.
11. Palliative Care Communication Institute Website. http://www.pccinstitute.com/. Accessed October 29, 2014.
12. PREPARE Website. www.prepareforyourcare.org. Accessed July 7, 2014.
13. National Palliative Care Registry™ Annual Survey Summary. Center to Advance Palliative Care and National Palliative Care Research Center. www.registry.capc.org. Accessed September 29, 2014.
14. Feudtner C, Womer J, Augustin R, et al. Pediatric palliative care programs in children's hospitals: A cross-sectional national survey. *Pediatrics*. 2013; 132(6): 1063–1070.
15. Patient Quality of Life Coalition Website. www.patientqualityoflife.org. Accessed July 7, 2014.
16. American Cancer Society Action Network Website. www.acscan.org/qualityoflife. Accessed July 9, 2014.
17. American Cancer Society Cancer Action Network. How do you measure up? http://www.acscan.org/content/wp-content/uploads/2014/08/HDYMU-2014-Report.pdf Accessed September 29, 2014.
18. Palliative Care Bills are the right step for patients, says American Heart/Stroke Association. American Heart Association press release March 27, 2014.http://newsroom.heart.org/news/palliative-care-bills-are-the-right-step-for-patients-says-american-heart-stroke-association. Accessed September 29, 2014.

CHAPTER 5

Communication Ethics

Timothy W. Kirk, Nessa Coyle, and Matthew Doolittle

Introduction

Communication is a key mediating variable in achieving the primary goal of palliative care: optimizing quality of life by reducing suffering in patients and families experiencing serious and life-limiting illness. Through analysis of its conceptual foundation and internal values, this chapter demonstrates that palliative care is an inherently moral practice, seeking to ameliorate suffering by restoring and supporting the moral agency of patients and families. Because therapeutic communication is a necessary condition for achieving this goal, it constitutes a core ethical obligation of palliative care providers and organizations. Ethical communication among healthcare providers, and between providers, patients, and family members, can be considered a form of care, subject to the same ethical norms that pertain to all clinical care: respect personhood, minimize harm, and maximize benefit. Using the concepts of sensitivity, truthfulness, confidentiality, and deliberation, a framework for ethical communication is presented. Because an excessive focus on communication outcomes often diverts attention away from the communication process itself, raising the risk for confrontation and stalemate, the ethical framework presented here emphasizes the importance of process, suggesting that communication processes are ethically significant apart from the outcomes they may produce.

An Ethical Framework for Palliative Care Communication

This part of the chapter (a) highlights ways in which effective therapeutic communication is a necessary condition to achieve the stated ends of palliative care; (b) explains how palliative care can be considered a "moral practice"; and (c) argues that thoughtful, deliberate communication with patients, with family members, and among healthcare providers is a core ethical obligation in palliative care.

Communication as a Necessary Condition of Quality Palliative Care

The National Consensus Project for Quality Palliative Care's (NCP) definition of palliative care emphasizes that the primary aim of palliative care is to "optimize quality of life by anticipating, preventing, and treating suffering."[1(p9)] In operationalizing the definition, the NCP notes four essential features of care delivery:

- Care is provided and services are coordinated by an interdisciplinary team;
- Patients, families, palliative and nonpalliative healthcare providers collaborate and communicate about care needs;
- Services are available concurrently with or independent of curative or life-prolonging care;
- Patient and family hopes for peace and dignity are supported throughout the course of illness, during the dying process, and after death.[1(p9)]

These essential features constitute the guideposts used by the NCP to then identify the eight core domains of palliative care quality and, in so doing, provide the functional landscape in which the ethical obligation of communication takes shape.

Because palliative care is patient- and family-centered care, and because the sources and meaning of suffering, peace, dignity, and wholeness are highly variable across patients and families, successful design and delivery of palliative care depend upon careful and effective communication between the parties involved. Interdisciplinary care provision and coordination requires communication among all members of the care team, as well as between individual members of the care team, patients, and family members. Good palliative care cannot happen without such communication (see Figure 5.1).

Therapeutic communication processes by individuals and organizations are not only a functional requirement for quality palliative care but also an ethical one. To explain why this is so, it is helpful to consider palliative care as not only a clinical practice but also as a moral practice.

Palliative Care as a Moral Practice

In ethics, "moral practice" is a technical term. MacIntyre defines a moral practice as an activity in which people work together using specific skills and methods toward a shared goal.[2] The activity (practice) has three defining characteristics. First, the goal of the practice is considered good not just for the intended participants and recipients of the activity but for society at large. Second, the practice itself has internal values to which participants subscribe. Third, the capacities, skills, and patterns of behavior that facilitate that goal are valuable not only for participation in the practice but for development as a person in general. In short, becoming an expert in a moral practice is good for the practice and good for society generally. Palliative care constitutes precisely such a

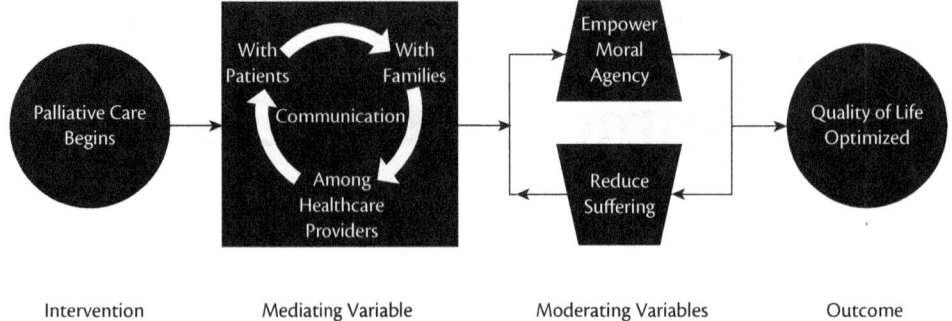

Figure 5.1 Communication as a mediating variable in achieving the goal of palliative care

practice, and therapeutic communication, necessary to achieve the goals of that practice, constitutes a core obligation within the practice.

For palliative care to count as a moral practice in the manner described earlier, two conditions need to be present. First, the goals of the practice need to be well-defined and resonant with larger social values. Second, shared internal values must be present that promote the goals of the practice, and those values need to carry normative weight. Both of these conditions are satisfied in the structure and processes of palliative care. One of the ways they are satisfied is in the commitment to preventing and relieving suffering by restoring and engaging the moral agency of patients and their family members.

Reducing Suffering By/As Restoring Moral Agency

In the public health and social psychology literatures, "agency" is a concept that describes a person's ability to develop and exercise a sense of self by engaging with the world in a manner that sets and achieves goals by doing things for oneself. *Moral* agency is a similar concept in moral philosophy and psychology. It incorporates the elements of agency noted earlier but adds a layer of value. A person's moral agency is his or her ability to identify and embrace guiding values in life and to execute decisions, participate in actions, and develop character traits that reflect and express those values.[3] One's moral agency is the condition on which one can be praised or blamed for actions, held morally responsible for good and bad decisions, and even be considered a good or bad person. For example, in palliative care a surrogate decision-maker may be labeled negatively because the direction of care he or she chooses is perceived by clinicians to be harmful for the patient. Similarly, a surrogate may be held in high regard for making a difficult decision that is considered to be in a patient's best interest. In both cases, the inclination to hold the surrogate responsible for the decision made implies that the surrogate has moral agency.

A growing body of literature in health research supports a strong connection between communication and agency. Epstein and Street[4] offer an especially clear summary of research demonstrating that healthcare provider communication with cancer patients and families can strongly affect patient agency, which in turn can significantly impact health outcomes and ability to cope. Health and ability to cope, in turn, are strong predictors of quality of life. For example, O'Hair et al.[5] have developed the Cancer Survivorship and Agency Model (CSAM), which creates a paradigm for communication processes in oncology based on evidence-based relationships between clinical communication and patient agency. This model focuses not only on maximizing health outcomes as measured by morbidity and mortality but also on empowering patients' exercise of their moral agency throughout the care continuum. In so doing, it suggests that care processes consistent with the CSAM paradigm that restore and support moral agency produce an important outcome distinct from improved survivorship: the exercise of agency itself.

Since a core goal of palliative care is the restoration and support of moral agency, a strong reason that communication in palliative care is ethically significant is precisely because of the ways in which that communication can strengthen (or weaken) patients' moral agency. As written in the NCP definition, palliative care seeks to minimize suffering to "facilitate patient autonomy, access to information, and choice."[1p9] The presumptions in this definition are (a) that patient autonomy, access to information, and choice are important predictors of an optimal quality of life; (b) that suffering is an important barrier that hinders autonomy, access to information, and choice; and (c) when suffering is minimized, patient autonomy, access to information, and choice are enhanced, thereby increasing the likelihood of optimizing quality of life. It is striking that the links in the causal chain to optimizing quality of life contained in the NCP definition resonate so strongly with promoting moral agency. That is, in identifying these three variables, this definition of palliative care strongly implies that optimizing quality of life requires optimizing moral agency.

Therapeutic Communication as a Core Ethical Obligation in Palliative Care

Insofar as communication can significantly impact care outcomes—affecting the exercise of moral agency in decisions related to treatment choices, treatment adherence, engagement of informal caregivers, and care satisfaction of patients and family members[4]—communication can be considered a form of care. As a form of care, it is subject to similar kinds of ethical evaluation and guidance as other treatment. In particular, communication in palliative care should seek to (a) discern and incorporate the values and preferences of patients and family members, thereby respecting their *autonomy* through supporting and engaging moral agency; (b) minimize the risk of avoidable harm, thereby respecting *nonmaleficence*; and (c) maximize benefit to patients and families by engaging processes and producing outcomes that are consistent with how they would define "good," thereby honoring *beneficence*.

Autonomy is rooted in personhood and moral agency.[6] Healthcare providers seek the consent of autonomous beings because such beings are recognized as persons. Persons have the right to participate in healthcare decisions because (a) such decisions impact them most directly and (b) they are best positioned to deliberate about available options and execute decisions that reflect their values and preferences. Hence, we say such persons are "autonomous" meaning, literally, that they have the ability and right to self-govern.

In this way, palliative care's commitment to restore and engage the moral agency of patients is essentially an operationalization of the ethical duty to respect patient autonomy. This requires more than seeking a patient's permission for certain care interventions in what may appear to be simple one-way communication. Rather, it requires partnering with patients and family members to help them explore their values and determine which care choices honor those values. Some patients may have a clear understanding of their values through reflection and deliberation activities in other areas of their lives. However, unless they have a long history of making complex healthcare decisions, most patients do not have much experience translating their values and beliefs into choices about clinical care. Assisting patients in exploring and translating their values into clinical decisions, through communication practices like those outlined later in this chapter, supports and engages their moral agency.

Beneficence is a core principle in contemporary healthcare ethics. A simple way to think about beneficence is that it structures ethical duties to align with the maxim, "do good."[7] What it means to do good, however, is not as straightforward as it might seem. It is only through a shared understanding of a patient's values and goals that providers and patients together have some of the information necessary to understand which outcomes count as "beneficial" or "harmful"—and therefore "good" or "bad"—for each patient. Absent such careful exploration, and subsequent documentation of what patient preferences are and why, healthcare providers risk assuming that patients' care preferences mirror what providers believe is in their best medical interest. There is little evidence, however, that such an assumption is accurate. In fact, there is some evidence for the opposite.[8]

Explanation of the likely outcomes of various care options provides important information required to help patients and families balance hoped-for benefits with possible harms. It is here that careful, consistent, and timely communication within the care team, as explained later, is requisite. The strongest prediction of likely outcomes requires collaboration between care disciplines and clinical specialties to ensure patients and providers alike are using the most complete and up-to-date information possible in decision-making. A delayed or missing MRI report, an incomplete or unread nursing note, or a complicated and unreviewed medication profile can all lead to decisions made by patients, families, and healthcare providers that may not maximize benefit.

To the extent that communication among professionals can significantly impact care and treatment decisions, which can significantly impact the risk of harm or benefit to patients, attention to such communication is an ethical obligation. Without it, providers risk violating nonmaleficience-the duty to avoid preventable harm. While beneficent intent is an important component to honoring both principles, Yeo et al. explain that intentions are not enough.[7] What makes intentions valuable is that they raise the likelihood of outcomes that are intended. Absent that link, intentions are little more than well wishes.

Well-coordinated care that engages and supports patients' moral agency, maximizes benefit, and minimizes harm requires an optimally functioning care team. Frequent and deliberate communication among healthcare providers is a defining element in such a team.

Communication Within the Team

This part of the chapter addresses communication among members of the healthcare team as a precursor for communication with patients and families, as well as challenges to such communication. It emphasizes the importance of being attentive, self-aware, and reflective regarding the emotional responses of oneself and other healthcare providers during the clinical encounter. It concludes that a conscious and deliberative team-oriented approach is one necessary for ethical communication in palliative care. A case study is used to illustrate how communication among members of a care team can break down, resulting in increased suffering of the patient and family and a team left feeling frustrated and ineffectual. The risk for such breakdown is especially high when multiple care services are involved, as was the situation in this case.

The Case of Ms. R

Ms. R is a 59-year-old married woman with an existing history of major depressive disorder and anxiety. She had been diagnosed three years previously with non-small cell lung carcinoma. Two months ago, she developed worsening disease in her lung and underwent radiofrequency ablation complicated by pneumothorax and then empyema. Approximately one month ago, Ms. R. developed mild right-sided weakness and disorientation and underwent craniotomy for a parietal lobe lesion.

Ms. R's husband was her healthcare agent, but he was largely absent. Her sister, who was constantly at the bedside or outside the room, appointed herself gatekeeper to the patient. The sister challenged and questioned every nurse and doctor going into the room, often declining care and access to the patient.

During Ms. R's long and complicated course, meetings had been held among members of the team, and with family members, but these had not clarified questions related to her care or satisfied her sister's concerns. Because of this, and because the primary team felt that a number of consulting services had been involved primarily at the request of the patient's sister, the team was reluctant to try to arrange further meetings. The number of services involved in Ms. R's care made such meetings difficult to organize and frustrating.

After a change in attending physicians, a meeting of the primary and consulting teams was held. Recommendations emerging from the meeting were then discussed at a family meeting, which included only the primary team attending, the bedside nurse, Ms. R's husband, and her sister. Consistent with the patient and sister's wishes, she was discharged home to be followed by the hospital palliative care team.

Challenges to Communication Between Healthcare Providers

Even as the Institute of Medicine[9] and the National Cancer Institute[4] call for more patient-centered communication in palliative care, economic and social factors have led to an increasing complexity in healthcare that is often difficult to reconcile with such goals. Such increased complexity has given rise to communication challenges among healthcare providers, some of which are illustrated by the case of Ms. R. Five of these challenges are addressed next.

Distrust Based on Prior Events

In the case of Ms. R, the surgical team had acknowledged and apologized for the patient's pneumothorax but not in a way that was acceptable to her sister. This negative outcome, which the sister repeatedly referred to as "an error," became a focus for her fear and rage about Ms. R's suffering and a lens through which she interpreted all of the patient's subsequent suffering. It is possible that this lens enabled her to avoid directly confronting the grave nature of her sister's cancer, but it certainly prevented her from being able to see herself as anything other than a solitary warrior and never a member of a team dedicated to treatment or to the relief of her sister's suffering.

Indeed, prior events—some known to the current provider team, some unknown—often constitute "ghosts" in relationships between palliative care providers, patients, and families. In the case of Ms. R, the negative effects of prior events were exacerbated by inconsistent communication patterns between her primary care team and the various consultants contributing to her care. The result was that physicians and nurses treating the patient were uncertain about the treatment approach. This eroded the sister's confidence in Ms. R's healthcare providers.

Challenges to Provider Self-Image

Uncertainty and confusion among Ms. R's care providers left them more vulnerable to the "attacks" of her sister and more vulnerable to a lack of confidence about the treatment plan itself. Members of staff, like the patient's sister, felt anxiety, anger, frustration, and confusion, which made caring for the patient even more difficult. Indeed, one of the major challenges of this case was that of retaining focus on the patient herself in the face of the angry, dysfunctional dynamics taking place around her.

In general, healthcare providers wish to think of themselves as benevolent and competent, especially when caring for a patient with far-advanced disease. In this case, Ms. R's sister habitually stood in the hallway outside the patient's room. As each nurse or physician attempted to enter the room to see the patient, she repeatedly reviewed details of the patient's long, fearful, and painful course. She used the second-personal pronoun in describing all of these events, so that every provider—regardless of involvement in the case—repeatedly heard such statements as, "You did this to her." The sister ended virtually every conversation with the statement, "So you're just going to do nothing then." As one of the nurses reported to the psychiatric consultant, "It's so hard to go in there. You just have to get through that before she'll let you in. Even just to change the IV. You just have to stand there and take it. And you feel like nothing." In this case, the sister perceived any delays in care as a sign of bad faith on the part of the team. Her persistent and intense focus on the idea of "error," and her perception of the universal insensitivity of the patient's healthcare team, challenged the providers' sense of competence and even their benevolence during every single clinical interaction. The nursing staff, which necessarily had the greatest number of clinical interactions with the patient, was challenged to an even greater degree than the rest of the team. Consequently, nurses were assigned to the patient for short periods of time.

In such situations, frequent rotation of nursing staff, although protective of the nurses' emotional health, increases the importance of regular communication between nurses. Face-to-face communication, as might occur during shift reports, provides an opportunity not only to share information but to process the difficult emotions associated with giving care in such a challenging climate. Shared deliberation in such conversations can inspire personal reflection on how best to refocus care efforts onto supporting the moral agency of the patient.

Family-Centered Care—Family Alliance

The paradigm of patient- *and* family-centered care highlighted in the NCP definition of palliative care rests on a sometimes difficult-to-navigate tension between the two. At varying points along the care continuum, care for the family may appear to overshadow that of the patient. However, care for the family is often integral to care of the patient. Indeed, in the psychosocial domains of palliative care, it can be helpful to consider the family as a second-order patient.[10] Such consideration recognizes that family members are usually the primary caregivers in the home and need their agency to be supported.

In the case of Ms. R, the anger and frustration expressed by her sister made it more difficult for members of the team to recognize the sister's grief. Increasingly the patient's family was viewed as an obstacle or even as an opponent, rather than a potential ally in a shared effort to reduce the suffering of the patient. The intensity of the sister's negative communication rarely diminished, but she did clearly benefit from the ability to vent her frustrations. Generally, after approximately 20 to 30 minutes of this venting, she would invite her listener to enter the room to care for the patient.

Eventually the sister became comfortable enough to report that she, herself, had lost weight and was not sleeping, saying that she felt "exhausted." She alluded to her own treatment for anxiety and the toll that her own fear about Ms. R's grave illness had taken on her. Communicating this information to nursing staff and the rest of the team was helpful in making care in this challenging case more tolerable, primarily by restoring in the healthcare providers a sense of genuine concern and benevolence that had been partially replaced by anger. Patient- and family-centered communication among the team was restored, and the foundation for a strong alliance with the family was laid.

Tension Between Stability and Change in Provider Staffing Patterns

Rotating staff schedules can significantly impact communication. It may seem intuitively true that rotation of team members constitutes a barrier to effective, consistent communication. Indeed, rotation can interfere with the development of stable clinical relationships conducive to the establishment of trust and subsequent open and honest communication. In the case of Ms. R, the attending physicians rotated on a weekly basis so that medical leadership was not consistent and the approach to care varied. This contributed to her sister's lack of trust. Continuity was provided by nursing (although working three or four 12-hour shifts a week also contributed to lack of continuity) and social work staff as well as other involved disciplines.

However, team rotation can also open opportunities for a new approach to care. In this case a new attending was able to establish a more effective communication pattern among the multiple consulting teams. By bringing healthcare team members into alignment with one another through interprofessional communication, they were better able to engage constructively with the patient and family. As such, this case illustrates how the dynamic tension between stability and change can produce both benefit and harm and thus requires ongoing attention.

Professional Hierarchy in Healthcare

Even among members of the team who may seem to share the same training and elements of the same background, the complex structure of healthcare itself creates important cultural challenges within teams. The hierarchical nature of healthcare training, and the different roles of nurses, nurse practitioners, attending physicians, social workers, chaplains, and fellows shape and complicate healthcare communication. In the case of Ms. R, fellows and nurses, who had more frequent contact with the patient and the patient's family, experienced greater distress over the lack of communication among members of the healthcare team than did supervisors and attending physicians, who had less frequent contact. The distress was magnified by a sense that the attendings did not fully understand the untenable nature of the ongoing situation.

Deliberative Decision-Making

The involvement of multiple services with numerous providers who were responsible for some portion of Ms. R's care complicated the ability not only to engage in shared decision-making with the patient and sister but even the ability of the team to devise a clear medical recommendation. Despite the challenges of moving beyond a simple patient–nurse–physician–social work model of care, teamwork is both the hallmark and the strength of the palliative care model. Deliberative processes are therefore central to palliative decision-making.[11]

Clinical deliberation has been described as a "dialectic" or a "dialogue" designed to identify "flash points" that have disrupted the care of the patient or the work of the team.[11] Healthcare providers should have regular opportunities to reflect on their own personal, cultural, or religious values, or even "prejudices."[12] Such reflection enables providers to have greater insight into what role such personal values and preferences are playing in the care they are giving patients and families. Deliberation among team members allows providers to explore and acknowledge resonance and dissonance between such values and preferences and what role—individually and collectively—they are playing in assisting or hindering understanding of the patient's narrative experience. Identifying the narrative of the family and the patient may be the most effective way of coming to understand the values of the patient and the impact of the illness. Undertaking the moral and intellectual work necessary to understand the most accessible way to present and interpret information in an individual case inherently reinforces the ethical practice of communication. It is a necessary process that requires time, space, and attention to the membership of the team included in the deliberation.

Communication With the Patient

As noted earlier, therapeutic communication is a necessary condition to achieve the goals of palliative care. This part of the chapter addresses communication with the patient within this framework. Clinical sensitivity and communication practice as well as trust and confidentiality in palliative care are emphasized. Because engaging persons at the level of their lived experience is fundamental to palliative care and demonstrates respect and caring, patient quotations are used liberally throughout this discussion.

Palliative care discussions are often about meaning, goals, and values. The following palliative care patient, a woman in her mid-40s with advanced breast cancer, describes her reaction to the way her physician discussed her prognosis—a reaction to which healthcare providers without training may not know how to respond. Feeling unprepared when receiving such a response can lead to avoidance by providers, thereby missing an important window of insight into the patient's suffering:

> My doctors succeeded in taking away all hope from me that I was going to live … they basically gave me a death sentence … it was as though the village Shaman cursed you—basically they give you no way of living past a year … no one can survive that … what happens is that you internalize it and then you die.

Next she describes a communication approach that could have left open a window of hope:

> Most people die within a year but statistics can't be applied to the individual, we all know that. There are always people who fall out of the statistics and let's hope that you are one of them.

This interaction illustrates the importance of hope in engaging this patient's agency. Through her communication and the openness of the healthcare provider to hear her suffering, an opportunity was presented to address her needs. The communication provided a direction—a road map—to reduce her suffering and support her autonomy.

Clinical Sensitivity and Communication Practice

Sensitivity in the clinical encounter relies on empathetic awareness.[13] Clinical sensitivity can be seen as sensitivity to the impact of the patient's illness on his or her overall well-being and quality of life.[14,15] It includes the meaning to individuals of what is being experienced as well as their vulnerabilities, symptoms, and suffering as illustrated here:

> There was a time when I could build you a house. But now, to put a nail in the wall—I can't do that. It's really hard. For everything, I have to ask a favor. I have to depend on people for everything. Oh, it never was like that. I don't want it to be like that.

The ability to be affected by the suffering of another, to enable such suffering to evoke an empathetic response, and to relieve pain are traditional themes in nursing and medicine.[13,14]

Receptivity and openness to another person, recognizing suffering through both verbal and nonverbal communication, and responding to it empathetically suggest an ethical responsibility to alleviate the suffering.[13,14] Attentive listening is the first step to reducing suffering. Kirk uses the term "clinical intimacy" to reflect shared meaning-making between healthcare providers and patients.[16] The need for this is reflected in this patient's plea: "I just wish the doctors would consider the whole person, you know, and not just the cancer. I mean the cancer is part of me but not the whole me. That's why Dr. X is so wonderful; because she speaks to me like another human being, not like a patient. I don't want to be 'a patient.' I want to be me."

Clinical Sensitivity and Truthfulness

Clinical sensitivity provides a backdrop for obtaining informed consent. "The main characteristic of informed consent is communication, and the quality of the communication will be determined by the quality or 'trueness' of the consent."[17(p52)] If patients are not given information, they tend to create "facts" for themselves, sometimes leading to a false set of assumptions on which they then base their healthcare decisions: "It was adenocarcinoma small cell. I extrapolated from that bit of information that it was terminal. In my case six months." Informed consent empowers patients to become participants in healthcare decisions. It protects autonomy and supports agency. It is an ethical obligation to provide as much information as patients desire about their illness and treatment.

It can be hard for healthcare providers to talk about the end of life with a patient they have cared for many years—death may be seen as a failure. That telling a patient the truth is harmful, however, has not been borne out by research primarily done with cancer patients. The opposite has been found to be true.[18,19] Telling the truth fosters trust and demonstrates respect when it is done in a compassionate and sensitive manner and is titrated to the patients' ability to absorb the information.[17] One palliative care patient put it this way: "Being able to talk about this is a really wonderful thing. It makes me able to say how I feel. It makes me say things out loud and bring them into a better clarity and makes me know myself." This patient is in essence saying that the ability to communicate with his healthcare provider facilitates his "autonomy, access to information, and informed choice"—key elements in the NCP definition of palliative care.[1(p9)]

We may know what is best for ourselves, but we cannot provide guidance for a patient unless we hear his or her voice. In the setting of palliative care and end-of-life care, it is dangerous to assume that we know what is best for the patient and how the end of that patient's life should unfold. This can lead to coercion in a setting where patients can be very dependent on their primary physician and other healthcare providers, especially when strong ideologies are held among the providers regarding what constitutes a "good death."[20] There can be a fine line between (a) supportive care that empowers the expression of self and values and (b) guidance that so strongly emphasizes one course of action that it masks patient preferences, encouraging the patient to defer choice to the healthcare provider.

Cecily Saunders summarizes an approach to sensitive communication when she says, "the real question is not 'what do you tell your patients?' but rather "what do you let your patients tell you."[21] Learning about significant areas in patients' lives—such as family, work or school, goals, and dreams—is a way for them to become known; it shows respect for what they have done and who they are. By allowing the uniqueness of each person to reveal itself, communication barriers can be broken down.

Even the most seasoned healthcare provider, however, is vulnerable to becoming overwhelmed, as revealed in a recent conversation between a surgeon and oncologist. Each spoke of his regrets about "thinking out loud" in front of a patient to whom they both had grown very close, presenting options that had almost zero possibility of prolonging or improving the patient's quality of life. On hearing the options, the patient begged for one with predictable results. The desire to "be complete" in presenting information was meeting the provider's rather than the patient's needs, and the result was communication that lacked sensitivity to those patient needs—despite genuine intent to do what was in his best interest.

Clinical Sensitivity and Nonverbal Communication

Being aware of nonverbal communication, both one's own and others', is part of clinical sensitivity. Patients are very attuned to this form of communication (posture, gaze, gestures, tone of voice, speech modulation, and duration) especially when it is at odds with their perception of the words being spoken.[17]

Nonverbal communication can convey messages of caring or the opposite. For example, responding to a patient's phone call or call light in a timely manner can convey concern and caring, while a delay without explanation can convey the opposite. Waiting several days to tell the patient of a test result suggests a lack of sensitivity to his or her apprehension and anxiety. Telling patients, without explanation, that it is fine for them to miss chemotherapy and go on holiday, when in the past they have been told that it is essential that chemotherapy be administered according to a strict protocol and they must not miss a dose, gives them a certain message.

One patient interpreted a delay in getting an appointment with his oncologist after discharge from the hospital in the following way:

> Well, if he is putting off the first appointment that long he is putting off chemo even longer. And we both know the longer we go between chemo the more chance there is for the cancer to grow. So to be out of chemo for that long is like a vote of nonconfidence.

On the other hand, giving a patient who is near death and transitioning to home hospice an outpatient appointment for two months hence is also giving a message: a window of hope, a nonverbal statement of caring and nonabandonment, an act of kindness. Nonverbal communication can be misinterpreted, however, as meaning may be interpreted differently depending on culture, gender, age, and severity of disease.[17,22]

Confidentiality in Palliative Care

Patients and families expect that information shared with healthcare providers in the clinical situation will not be shared with others unless doing so is necessary for their care. A breach of confidentiality is generally perceived as the disclosure of information to a third party not directly involved in the patient's care. This duty of confidentiality provides the basis for trust in the therapeutic relationship.[23] In other words, confidentiality in palliative care has a relationship aspect and can "serve to strengthen the trust and confidence between patients and their healthcare providers."[23(p280)] Respecting confidentiality supports patient agency and personhood. It also demonstrates integrity and generates trust. With trust comes increased confidence in a patient's care provider and the likelihood that information relevant to his or her care will be shared. Confidentiality is not and cannot be absolute between the patient and the healthcare provider, and sometimes it is necessary and legally required to break confidentiality. The patient needs to be informed, however, of the limits of confidentiality.

Professional organizations and regulatory bodies place great importance on confidentiality. Kirk outlines three basic elements that help ensure confidentiality between providers and their patients: (a) establish and follow organizational practices that effectively respect confidentiality (e.g., policies addressing disclosure, record-keeping, EHRs, e-mail/fax phone communication, use of interpreters); (b) be clear and explicit with patients and families about the principles and practices related to confidentiality in your practice environment; and (c) immediately inform patients when breaches of confidentiality occur and take action to mitigate the damages caused by such breaches.[23]

Respecting confidentiality can be complicated when care is interdisciplinary, multidisciplinary, and patient- and family-centered. Tensions can arise when there is a disparity between what the patient wants the family to know and what the family needs to know in order to take care of the patient. This becomes particularly relevant in palliative care, which by its nature involves an interdisciplinary team approach, often collaborating with outside consultants, wherein information is shared freely. This raises questions about what information and how much information should be shared within the team.

Palliative care providers are particularly vulnerable to experiencing the tension between confidentiality and necessary disclosure, as intense relationships can quickly develop between patients and providers in life-threatening circumstances. Very personal and intimate information may, for example, be shared with the nurse, with the assumption by the patient that this discussion is just between the two of them. There is an implied promise that confidences will be respected, and breaking such a promise is a betrayal of trust. Some of the information shared by the patient may be irrelevant to the patient's care and should not be shared with other team members, while some may directly impact the patient's care and must be shared with the team. For example, if a patient tells a nurse that he wants his death to be hastened because life is so untenable, the nurse, after exploring the nature of his suffering, is obliged to share that information with other members of the team, letting the patient know at the same time that this is being done and why; for example: "I can hear how great your suffering is and that we have not been able to alleviate it so far—this information is so important that I would like to share it with other members of the team so that we can come up with better ways to relieve your distress."

The following case illustrates both a lack of clinical sensitivity and observant communication practice, contrasted by an acute clinical sensitivity from another team member resulting in supportive communication. It is a reminder to each of us that we communicate all the time but sometimes are blind to the communication cues that surround us.

> Mrs. B is an 86-year-old woman with advanced dementia. She was admitted to a long-term care facility with a hospice consultation team because she could no longer be cared for at home. One afternoon she was visited by her son who lived some distance away. The nurse was glad of the opportunity to meet with the son so that she could learn more about the patient and explore the patient's values with him. They met in the patient's room sitting on either side of her bed.
>
> At one point the nursing aide entered the room, saying it was time for the patient to be changed. When she entered the room, the patient's face lit up, meeting the aide's eyes, smiling, and reaching out for her. As the son and nurse stepped into the hallway to give the patient some privacy, the aide began to sing with the patient in Spanish as she carefully turned and cleansed the patient, applied soothing lotion to her sacral area, and replaced her undergarment. The patient hummed along with the tune.
>
> At this point the nurse realized that she had been talking "over" Mrs. B, and that because she had been so intent on communicating with the son, she had not intentionally tried to communicate with the patient in any way. She had not made eye contact and had not touched her. Indeed she did not know if Mrs. B, in turn, had attempted to connect or communicate with her—the nurse—while in the room. And yet the conversation had been about the patient's preferences and values. The lack of intentional communication was indeed communication.

The ease with which the aide communicated with the patient—using loving gestures, gentle care, and song—was a vivid reminder to the nurse of the importance of connecting and communicating with all patients and not allowing labeling of "advanced dementia" to lead to the neglect of intentional communication as a basic component of palliative care.

Conclusion

This chapter has addressed how communication is a key mediating variable in achieving the primary goal of palliative care: optimizing quality of life by reducing suffering in patients and families. Because thoughtful, deliberate communication using the right principles and processes as explained here is a necessary condition for achieving this goal, it constitutes a core ethical obligation of palliative care providers and organizations. Ethical communication among healthcare providers, and between providers, patients, and family members, can be considered a form of care, subject to the same ethical norms that pertain to all clinical care: respect personhood, minimize harm, and maximize benefit. Using the concepts of sensitivity, truthfulness, confidentiality, and deliberation, a framework for ethical communication has been presented to assist care providers in identifying and engaging processes of verbal and nonverbal communication resonant with the goals and values of palliative care.

References

1. Dahlin C, ed. *The Clinical Practice Guidelines for Quality Palliative Care*. 3rd ed. Pittsburgh, PA: National Consensus Project for Quality Palliative Care; 2013.
2. MacIntyre A. The nature of the virtues. *Hastings Cent Rep*. 1981;11(2):27–34.
3. Manning RC. Toward a thick theory of moral agency. *Soc Theory Pract*. 1994;20(2):203–220.
4. Epstein RM, Street RL, Jr. *Patient-Centered Communication in Cancer Care*. Bethesda, MD: National Cancer Institute; 2007.
5. O'Hair D, Villagran MM, Wittenberg-Lyles E, et al. Cancer survivorship and agency model: Implications for patient choice, decision making, and influence. *Health Commun*. 2003;15:193–202.
6. Moorhouse A, Yeo M, Rodney P. Autonomy. In: Yeo M, Moorhouse A, Khan P, Rodney P, eds. *Concepts and Cases in Nursing Ethics*. 3rd ed. Peterborough, ON: Broadview Press; 2010:143–205.
7. Yeo M, Moorhouse A. Beneficence. In: Yeo M, Moorhouse A, Khan P, Rodney P, eds. *Concepts and Cases in Nursing Ethics*. 3rd ed. Peterborough, ON: Broadview Press; 2010:103–142.
8. Steinhauser KE, Christakis NA, Clipp EC et al. Preparing for the end of life: Preferences of patients, families, physicians and other care providers. *J Pain Symptom Manage*. 2001;22(3):727–737.

9. Institute of Medicine. *Dying in America: Improving Quality and Honoring Individual Preferences Near the End of Life*. Washington, DC: National Academies Press; 2014.
10. Lederberg MS. The family of the cancer patient. In: Holland JC, ed. *Psycho-Oncology*. Oxford: Oxford University Press; 1998:981–993.
11. Altilio T, Coyle N: The interdisciplinary team—integrating moral reflection and deliberation. In: Kirk TW, Jennings B, eds. *Hospice Ethics: Policy and Practice in Palliative Care*. New York, NY: Oxford University Press; 2014:103–117.
12. Hermsen MA, Ten Have HA. Palliative care teams: Effective through moral reflection. *J Interdiscipl Care*. 2005;19(6):561–568.
13. Blum L. *Moral Perception and Particularity*. Cambridge, MA: Cambridge University Press; 1994.
14. Nortvedt P. Clinical sensitivity: The inseparability of ethical perceptiveness and clinical knowledge. *Sch Inq Nurs Pract*. 200;15(1):25–32.
15. Nortvedt P. Sensibility and clinical understanding. *Med Health Care Philos*. 2008;11(2):209–219.
16. Kirk TW. Beyond empathy: Clinical intimacy in nursing practice. *Nurs Philos*. 2007;8(4):233–243.
17. Siminoff LA. The ethics of communication in cancer and palliative care. In: Kissane DW, Bultz BD, Butow PM, Finlay IG, eds. *Handbook of Communication in Oncology and Palliative Care*. Oxford: Oxford University Press; 2010:51–61.
18. Zhang B, Nilsson ME, Prigerson HG. Factors important to patients' quality of life at end of life. *Arch Intern Med*. 2012;172(15):1133–1142.
19. Trice ED, Prigerson HG. Communication in end-stage cancer: A review of the literature and future research. *J Health Commun*. 2009;14(S1):95–108.
20. Koesel N, Link M. Conflicts in goals of care: Are aggressive life-prolonging interventions and a "good death" compatible? *J Hosp Pall Nurs*. 2014;16(6):330–335.
21. Saunders C. The moment of truth: Care of the dying person. In: Pearson L, ed. *Death and Dying*. Cleveland, OH: Case Western Reserve University Press; 1969:49–78.
22. Schmid Mast M, Klöckner C, Hall JA. Gender, power, and non-verbal communication. In: Kissane DW, Bultz BD, Butow PM Finlay IG, eds. *Handbook of Communication in Oncology and Palliative Care*. Oxford: Oxford University Press; 2010:63–73.
23. Kirk TW. Confidentiality. In: Cherny N, Fallon M, Kaasa S, Portenoy R, Curran D, eds. *Oxford Textbook of Palliative Medicine*. 5th ed. Oxford: Oxford University Press; 2015;279–284.

CHAPTER 6

Communication in Palliative Social Work

Myra Glajchen and Susan B. Gerbino

Introduction

Social workers play a vital role in palliative and end-of-life care communication. More often than other members of the interdisciplinary team, social workers counsel patients and families at every stage of the disease trajectory, providing continuity of care across settings. Social workers bring a unique set of skills to the team, including empathic listening, assessment of the person-in-situation, and skills in conflict resolution, which are invaluable for advance care planning.[1] Although social workers play this key role, evidence-based studies related to best practices and outcomes are scant. Studies have examined social work communication with hospitalized elderly patients, patients in nursing homes, patients in Veterans' Affairs clinics, patients considering hospice, and bereaved caregivers.[2-6] In a recent survey of 1,169 practicing hospice and palliative care social workers in which they rank-ordered the frequency of their professional activities, communication-related activities were ranked highest; these included conveying psychosocial needs of patient and family, facilitating effective team communication, patient and family education, advance care planning, and participating in family meetings.[5] Unfortunately, new healthcare financing trends have reduced the sustainability and role of social workers in end-of-life care in many settings, and some of their unique practice skills have been absorbed by other disciplines. This chapter explores the critical role of communication in palliative social work, building upon previous seminal work related to the domains of palliative care and skills necessary to practice specialist-level social work, with guidance for practice, research, and education.[7]

Domain One: Structure and Processes of Care

Communication between the healthcare team, patients, and family caregivers is the hallmark of high-quality palliative and end-of-life care, and the beginning phase of illness sets the tenor for the entire process. Social workers play a key role in communication during diagnosis, care planning, and treatment.

Diagnosis

The diagnostic phase is characterized by high anxiety as patients and caregivers try to integrate new medical information in unfamiliar language, choose from a range of treatment options, and manage their reaction to the illness. The emphasis on patient-centered care and informed consent can be both empowering and demanding as patients are flooded with information, choices, and expectations for autonomous decision-making in countries where Western medicine is practiced.[8] It is unclear whether all patients can fully participate in patient-centered care and shared decision-making.[9] What we know is that the expectation for autonomous decision-making is not always culturally appropriate. Communicating with patients and families from other cultures frequently falls to the social worker.

Cancer patients report unmet needs for information about the extent of disease, prognosis, treatment options, and side effects.[10] Information about diagnosis is generally delivered by the physician with mixed results. High rates of physician interruption coupled with low rates of patient recall can leave patients feeling uncertain.[11] In one Canadian study, patient-centeredness and psychosocial focus were associated with higher satisfaction for prostate cancer patients, while shorter consultations and higher biomedical focus were related to higher anxiety.[8] Even in specialist-level palliative care, healthcare providers may give overly long, complex explanations that are too technical.[12] Social workers have a vital role in tailoring the information, helping to translate the barrage of medical information and terminology into understandable, everyday language.

Plan of Care

Social workers are taught critical thinking as a core skill. Social work practice involves the dynamic and interactive process of engagement, assessment, intervention, and evaluation at multiple levels. "Starting where the client is," social workers are trained to conduct comprehensive assessment through which they collect, organize, and interpret patient and family data; assess the patient and family's strengths and needs; and develop mutually agreed-upon intervention goals.[13] Inherent in this assessment is the skill of empathic listening. The social worker is also an expert in community resources that inform and support patients and caregivers living with advanced illness. The social worker has a dual role in communicating directly with patients and families while relaying their needs and care preferences to the team.

Information and Education

Many patients facing advanced illness make it a priority to find information so they can weigh treatment options and make informed choices. In several studies, information-seeking has been shown to benefit patients through reduced distress and increased satisfaction. Education is a frequently used, albeit undervalued, social work intervention. Providing patients with reliable, accessible information is a fundamental social work intervention that empowers patients and families, gives patients a sense of control, reduces anxiety, and helps patients to plan ahead. Information about resources, advance care planning, caregiving, and normative grief responses are common to social work practice in end-of-life care.[14]

Advance Care Planning

Effective communication is viewed as critical to patients' and families' understanding of the illness and timely advance care planning. Passage of the Patient Self-Determination Act in 1990 was designed to improve the rate of completion for advance directives, but these rates have remained low. In 2000, 15% to 20% of Americans had some form of advance directive; by 2013, the rate had risen to 26.3%.[15] Acting as core healthcare professionals in advance care planning is an important role for social workers, as seen in such programs as the Medical Orders for Life Sustaining Treatment (MOLST) program.[1]

A benchmark of good palliative and end-of-life care is the extent to which patients make informed decisions based on their preferences. In the past, physicians assumed that open communication about advanced illness would cause undue psychological distress by "denying hope," but the recent trend toward patient autonomy points to a preference for disclosure among patients. These developments highlight a clear role for social workers in the comprehensive assessment of the psychological, social, and cultural factors necessary to support patients' self-determination. Barriers to communication may include contradictory information from multiple specialists, different professional communication styles, variations in education level, culture and ethnicity, and anxiety, which affects comprehension and recall. The social worker is well positioned to provide continuity of care across different settings and providers.

Domain Two: Physical Aspects of Care

Pain and Symptom Management

Patients with advanced and life-threatening illnesses bear a heavy burden in managing physical and psychological symptoms.[16] As part of their comprehensive assessment, social workers evaluate the amount of patient and caregiver distress caused by each physical symptom, as well as the interrelationship between physical and psychosocial symptoms. A recent study involving lung cancer patients and caregivers found that psychosocial-spiritual concerns were the most distressing while physical and psychosocial concerns were interrelated.[17] These findings highlight the pivotal need for early integration of social work into the care plan.

The advent of shorter hospital stays, along with trends for outpatient treatment and preferences for home death, have shifted the burden of symptom management to the home setting. Caregivers' roles in palliative and end-of-life care can include reporting of pain and other physical symptoms, management of symptoms using medication and nonpharmacological therapies, and management of side effects.[18] Because caregivers play so vital a role in helping keep the patient comfortable, the social worker has an important task in educating caregivers about symptoms, side effects, and strategies for their amelioration.

With the widespread availability of high-tech home care and pain management, family caregivers may be expected to help manage patient-controlled analgesia pumps, epidural catheters, and home infusions.[19] The technical aspects of these interventions can be daunting. A recent survey of 1,677 family caregivers in the United States reported that 46% of caregivers performed medical and nursing tasks at home; 78% managed medications, IVs, and injections; and 35% helped with wound care.[20] In addition, because of gaps and uneven quality in insurance coverage and home care services, effective education by the palliative care social worker in these areas is crucial. The social worker has an important role to play in encompassing the patients and caregivers as the unit of care. Social workers can help patients and caregivers formulate questions for the medical staff and process instructions. Practical tasks include logistics such as coordinating medical appointments, scheduling prescription pickups, checking that medications are covered by insurance, and interacting with home care staff.[20] Communication of physical symptoms can be complicated by education, culture, and language. For example, Lin found significant correlations between caregiver concerns and hesitancy to administer analgesics in Chinese cancer patients.[21] Medical decision-making usually falls to the family unit in immigrant populations, but cultural concerns and misconceptions can represent barriers. The palliative care social worker has the training to explore the cultural context in which caregiving takes place, making a successful outcome more likely. Caregivers may play a role in providing nondrug management of physical symptoms, using massage, lotions, heat and cold compresses, guided imagery, relaxation, breathing, and meditation.[18] As such, techniques have been shown to be helpful as an adjunct to medication; the social worker can help by training patients and caregivers in these techniques or making appropriate referrals for services.

Practical Support

Most patients and family caregivers need practical help at home as the illness progresses and symptom burden peaks during the end-of-life phase. Managing practical issues is a core social work skill. For patients with large extended families, relatives may be available to help with personal care tasks such as feeding, washing, toileting, and grooming. Patients eligible for home care or those who can afford services may hire outside help to alleviate physical strain. Assistance with the practical activities of making meals, managing household tasks, and transporting the patient to and from medical appointments can be arranged. Although patients and caregivers may be reluctant to accept outside help, the presence of paid or informal aides can also provide families with social and emotional support.[19]

Care Coordination and Home Care

Comprehensive palliative care assessment should focus on attaining the best possible quality of life for patients while avoiding unwanted treatment. This level of care coordination requires excellent discharge and advance care planning. In an attempt to help patients prepare for the post-hospital experience, researchers in Oregon identified three concerns that should be addressed: understanding the disease and prognosis; assessment and management of symptom burden; and a clear follow-up plan, which specifies which member of the team to call with what kind of concern.[22] The social worker on the palliative care team has an important role in providing follow-up care, coordinating with community agencies, and serving as the point person post-discharge. Social workers have expertise in practical issues related to treatment and care at home. Screening for socioeconomic distress should be completed during initial intake and reassessed over time. Patients and caregivers should be asked what kind of help they need at home, including help with activities of daily living (including instrumental), equipment, and transportation. A home visit by a nurse or social worker can provide the team with an environmental scan.

Domain Three: Psychosocial and Psychiatric Aspects of Care

Psychosocial Distress in Patients

Anxiety, distress, depression, and mood disorders are prevalent in palliative and end-of-life care, with prevalence rates of 25% for depression and 38% for mood disorders.[23] Physicians and nurses are charged with imparting medical information, but this focus, together with patients' reluctance to express distress, can result in overlooking psychosocial concerns. Physicians report discomfort and a lack of training in the strong emotions evoked by end-of-life discussions, which can shortchange the family's emotional concerns.[24] Addressing the psychosocial aspects of illness is often a role for social work. The palliative social worker should perform a comprehensive assessment of the patient and caregiver, provide supportive counseling to alleviate mild distress, and refer patients for psychotherapy or psychiatric evaluation as needed. Other goals include reinforcing the patient's existing psychological strengths and enhancing self-efficacy.[24] The social worker should communicate back to the team to ensure that the psychosocial needs of patients are addressed. Clinical trials have shown psychological treatment is effective for patients with advanced cancer.[25] Fortunately, social workers are already trained in assessment and management of psychological distress. Ideally, psychosocial care should be integrated into medical care to promote a higher likelihood of acceptance by patients.

Psychosocial Distress in Caregivers

In highly evolved teams, a strong interdisciplinary focus encompasses the patient and caregiver as the unit of care. However, due to workforce shortages and the limited availability of specialist-level palliative care programs, no discipline is specifically accountable for caregivers' needs. Social workers should be proactive in claiming responsibility for caregivers, assessing their strengths, and communicating their needs back to the team. As the patient deteriorates, the caregiver's quality of life can worsen, with an increase in physical demands and psychological preparation for death.

The palliative social worker is trained to identify caregivers at high risk of psychosocial problems, future distress, family problems, and the need for psychosocial services. Because the psychosocial status of caregivers can fluctuate over time, frequent reassessment is essential. A well-designed, multisite, prospective longitudinal cohort study of 332 dyads comprised of advanced cancer patients and their caregivers found that end-of-life discussions were associated with less aggressive medical care in the final weeks of life, earlier hospice referrals, better patient quality of life, better caregiver quality of life, less caregiver regret, and lower likelihood of a major depressive disorder for caregivers after six months. The study's conclusions, which have been replicated, suggest that timely end-of-life discussions are associated with better outcomes for both patients and caregivers.[26]

Domain Four: Social Aspects of Care

Social and Economic Needs of Patients and Caregivers

Patients and caregivers facing advanced illness frequently experience profound financial and social strain. Financial costs include unreimbursed medical expenses such as copays, deductibles, transportation, special equipment and food, as well as home care services not covered by insurance. For these reasons, almost one-third of the families of seriously-ill adults report a loss of savings due to advanced illness.[27] Economic burden can impact healthcare decisions, so the social worker should include this domain as part of treatment planning. Given the vast numbers of patients who are uninsured, social workers must advocate on a macro level for access to healthcare. On a micro level, there are programs designed to help patients and caregivers receive care and medications. The social worker must take the lead in connecting patients to these programs.

Family Meeting

The family meeting is seen as a valuable clinical tool for communicating medical information, delineating the goals of care, and facilitating decision-making. The palliative social worker can take a leading role in organizing and structuring the meeting, ensuring that the caregivers' needs are met, and encouraging a safe setting to ask questions, process emotions, and receive support.[28] If well structured, the family meeting is an ideal forum for eliciting concerns, providing clear information about the medical condition and treatment, and granting reassurance that patient preferences will be respected.[29] Whenever possible, the patient should be included in the family meeting.

Outcome studies confirming the effectiveness of the family meeting are beginning to emerge. Positive outcomes include reducing family burden, facilitating end-of-life care decisions, and avoiding inappropriate life-sustaining therapies. A prospective study of 31 family members reported that family caregivers felt more confident dealing with their concerns after the family meeting, and a self-report instrument was effective in helping caregivers set the agenda. This suggests the important role for social workers in planning the agenda with patient and caregiver input.[30] Box 6.1 outlines important questions in family meeting research.

> **Box 6.1** Family Meeting Research Questions
>
> ♦ Is the family meeting associated with higher satisfaction?
> ♦ How can we measure outcomes from the family meeting?
> ♦ Does the family meeting cost or save money?
> ♦ Is the discussion subject to interpretation by the note-taker?
> ♦ Are outcomes affected by meeting length, space, number of participants?
> ♦ Should the family meeting be a quality indicator in palliative care?
> ♦ Are family meetings more effective if they are led by the palliative social worker?

Domain Five: Spiritual, Religious, and Existential Aspects of Care

Religious, Spiritual, and Existential Issues

Whole-person care is enhanced if spiritual and existential distress are integrated into treatment. Ideally, a trained chaplain is available to help address spiritual concerns in palliative care, but all healthcare professionals should be trained in conducting a spiritual screening so they can identify and treat spiritual distress, address the component of suffering, and refer to trained chaplains as needed.[31]

In recent years, religion and spirituality have been embraced by social work education and practice. Social workers have been encouraged to ground practice in psychosocial theory, which includes a climate of open dialogue and understanding of religious and spiritual longing and experience.[32,33] Specific social work communication skills can be used to demonstrate spiritual sensitivity, including assessment of factors such as the patient's hopes and fears, the sense of meaning attached to the person's life and death, the sense of purpose, beliefs about the afterlife, guilt, forgiveness, and life review.[34] Issues such as existential suffering, conflict in religious beliefs, or a deep-seated need for forgiveness may warrant more in-depth attention by the social worker and/or referral to a chaplain.[35] Existential despair can exacerbate depression, and elements of despair can lead to depression.

Social Work Skills

Basic social work skills such as recognizing personhood, being present, listening, affirming, and normalizing the patient experience communicate spiritual sensitivity.[35] Practically speaking, social work skills are helpful in assessing those religious beliefs that impact medical care, including those related to transfusions, mechanical ventilation, hydration and nutrition, the role of miracles, or physician-assisted death. A life review encourages terminally ill patients to complete their life affairs, reflect on the contributions they have made, and consider their legacy.[36] End-of-life patients may prefer to raise existential questions with the social worker or the chaplain as opposed to healthcare workers. Social workers should encourage patients and families to share their beliefs or spiritual concerns with the whole team, including the physician, to ensure that these issues are part of any goals of care discussion. Table 6.1 outlines communication tasks and social work communication goals in palliative care.

Domain Six: Cultural Aspects of Care

Cross-Cultural Care and Communication

Culture plays a complex role in palliative and end-of-life care and can influence decision-making. Culture and the lack of diverse language skills on the team, necessitating the use of translators, can limit the ability of patients and families to fully grasp the details of the diagnosis and prognosis, compromising informed consent and advance care planning. Yet cultural aspects that influence palliative care practice are not well understood.[37] Studies suggest that some cultures uphold filial loyalty and intergenerational assistance above formal services, resulting in reluctance to elect hospice and overreliance on family caregivers.[38] These findings highlight the important contribution social workers can make by raising issues of culture with their interdisciplinary colleagues.

Social workers are trained to work effectively with individuals and families from different age groups, ethnicities, cultures, religions, and socioeconomic and educational backgrounds. Social workers integrate knowledge about the influence of values and religion on health-related beliefs and understand how these systems affect utilization of palliative care. Many cultures maintain their own values and traditions. Cultural humility is needed so that patients and families can educate teams about what they hold most dear.

Speaking the same language as the patient and family is optimal, but understanding cultural norms goes beyond the spoken word and should include insight into beliefs related to truth-telling, emotionally laden terminology such as "cancer" and "hospice," and individual- versus family-centered decision-making. Using a person-centered care approach considers patients and caregivers as the experts. Best practices dictate that healthcare professionals show respect, develop reflective listening, be present during patient encounters, learn about the patient's healing practices, provide culturally appropriate education, and acknowledge the values of the patient and family.[39] It is noteworthy that these activities fall within the scope of social work practice.

Culturally Specific Needs of Patient and Family

Negotiating the goals of care can be complicated by language and culture. Evidence suggests that cultural differences between patients and physicians can lead to symptom underestimation.[40] Ethnic background may play a role in end-of-life decision-making: Previous studies have concluded that blacks are less likely to elect DNR and more likely to choose aggressive care at the end of life.[41] Hispanic, black, and Chinese patients are more likely to die in inpatient, rather than home-based, settings, and hospice utilization is lower for black patients. The literature about Chinese patients reports taboos against death discussion and a stated preference for patients to die in the hospital rather than at home.[42]

Immigrants have lower rates of service use after hospitalization, because linguistic barriers and mistrust of formal services can lead to confusion after hospital discharge.[43] Although medical interpreters are widely available, it may be more convenient to use family members, which can result in inaccuracies and compromise of informed consent and confidentiality. Studies abound on cultural competence for physicians in end-of-life care, with most showing

Table 6.1 Communication Tasks and Social Work Goals

Communication Task	Social Work Communication Goal
Diagnosis	Tailor information to individual and family needs
	Explain information in clear language
	Start where the patient is
	Address psychosocial concerns
Plan of care	Conduct comprehensive assessment
	Organize and interpret patient and family data
	Assess strengths and limitations
	Listen empathically
Advance care planning	Initiate discussion of advance directives
	Facilitate selection of surrogate decision-maker
	Elicit patient's and family's values
	Support patient autonomy, self-determination
	Include caregivers
	Discuss treatment options
	Communicate back to team
Information and education	Link patients and caregivers with resources
	Educate patients about illness and symptoms
	Relay preferences back to team
Pain and symptom management	Assess physical and symptom burden
	Educate about medication, side-effect management
	Teach complementary and alternative medicine techniques
Practical support	Assess home care needs
	Assess need for help with activities of daily living and instrumental activities of daily living
	Assess insurance and financial needs
	Discuss logistics
Care coordination, home care	Screen for economic distress
	Involve patients and families in discharge planning
	Discuss follow-up plan, including transportation
	Coordinate home care, community agency referral
Assessing patient distress	Assess psychosocial reaction and distress
	Provide supportive counseling
	Reinforce strengths and coping
	Alleviate mild distress
Assessing caregiver distress	Include patient and caregiver as unit of care
	Assess caregiver burden
	Identify caregivers at high risk
	Communicate caregivers' needs to team
Social and economic needs	Assess financial needs and strain
	Evaluate concerns about treatment costs
	Evaluate social support and isolation
	Evaluate work-related concerns
Religious and spiritual issues	Complete spiritual screening
	Assess degree of religiosity
	Assess use of spirituality as coping mechanism

(continued)

Table 6.1 Continued

Communication Task	Social Work Communication Goal
Existential issues	Assess suffering
	Encourage life review
	Assess guilt, regret, need for forgiveness
Culturally specific needs	Evaluate role of culture in understanding of illness
	Assess socioeconomic and social context
	Evaluate role of language
	Assess decision-making style
Cross-cultural communication	Assess acculturation
	Integrate cultural values into decision-making
	Communicate cultural values to team
	Use professional medical interpreters
End-of-life communication	Discuss practical aspects of patient's death
	Discuss hopes and fears of patient and family
	Educate about expected course
Hospice	Participate in intake assessment
	Identify psychosocial issues and concerns
	Identify high-risk family dynamics
	Evaluate home environment
Life review	Promote life review as therapeutic tool
	Promote closure and emotional resolution
	Discuss memories, regrets, accomplishments
	Help patient resolve suffering, convey final words
Bereavement	Target caregivers with high distress
	Assess previous coping
	Assess social support
	Start work during active treatment phase
	Assess meaning of the loss and of the lost person
Truth-telling and informed consent	Reinforce medical information
	Assess emotional and cognitive readiness
	Serve as role model for interdisciplinary team collaboration
	Encourage doctors to present options, risks
	Ensure open exchange between patient and team
	Support patient autonomy
Withholding and withdrawing treatment	Help patients make treatment decisions
	Support patient self-determination

lack of preparedness and discomfort when dealing with mistrust, health beliefs at odds with Western medicine, and identification of relevant customs.[43] Cultural competency, a phrase that implies that all professionals should become competent by studying various cultures rather than approaching differences with cultural humility, has become a recent target identified by the Institute of Medicine.[44] Because membership in a cultural group does not predict cultural practices, it is essential that the social worker evaluate this domain, using input from family members and communication skills with professional interpreters as needed.

Domain Seven: Care of the Imminently Dying Patient

Communicating With Patients About the End of Life

Conversations about the expected course of illness are essential in palliative care. End-of-life discussions are associated with less aggressive medical care near death, earlier hospice referrals, improved patient quality of life, and better bereavement adjustment for caregivers.[45] The team social worker has a unique combination of practical and counseling skills that can be helpful in caring for the imminently dying patient. As death approaches, the social worker can help the family consider how and where they would like the death to occur, anticipate their needs, ensure they understand treatment options, and communicate the family's concerns back to the team.

Hospice

A cross-sectional survey was completed to characterize social work outcomes in 66 member hospices. Results showed that increased social work involvement was significantly associated with lower hospice costs, better team functioning, reduced medical services; fewer visits by other team members, and increased patient satisfaction. The authors concluded that hospice outcomes would be enhanced with more full-time hospice social workers, joint interdisciplinary visits, and increased participation of social work during intake sessions.[46]

Life Review

Many terminally ill patients feel the impetus to complete their life affairs, reflect on the contribution they have made to others, and review their legacy.[47] "Life review" refers to a structured process that promotes self-reflection while recognizing the unique value of the patient's life. Patients may not wish to speak to their physicians about these matters, preferring to raise existential questions with the social worker or the chaplain. Life review is considered a critical, albeit understudied, therapeutic tool in palliative care. Through life review, the social worker can foster a sense of connectedness between patient and family, promote a measure of emotional resolution, and help identify areas of suffering.[48] Ideally, life review should take place over time, but in reality, the work may be compressed into short or single encounters. Social workers can use open-ended questions related to important memories, regrets, and accomplishments. In addition, dignity therapy, a form of individualized, short-term psychotherapy, has shown promising results for improving quality of life. In a randomized controlled trial of 441 terminally ill patients in Canada, the United States, and Australia, dignity therapy was significantly more helpful than client-centered or standard palliative care in improving quality of life, changing how their family appreciated them, improving spiritual well-being, and lessening sadness. Many social workers have been trained in dignity therapy.[49]

Bereavement

Social workers in palliative care will frequently encounter grief and bereavement before or after the death of the patient. Social workers' involvement with family caregivers across the illness trajectory positions them to deal with the meaning of the loss and of the lost person.[50] Ideally, bereavement work should begin during the active phases of palliative care and hospice treatment. Bereavement is a multifaceted experience, and every caregiver is likely to react differently.[51] Current thinking recommends preventive interventions that target high-risk caregivers based on family functioning, coping with previous loss, and social support. Social workers bring value to palliative care through comprehensive assessment skills targeting family members likely to benefit from clinical intervention. Some caregivers may have high distress or other factors that could lead to complicated grief. Specific social work skills include psychoeducation, emotional expression, cognitive-behavioral interventions, and assistance with the establishment of new life goals.[52]

Domain Eight: Ethical and Legal Aspects of Care

Advance Care Planning

Social workers play a key role in advance care planning,[53] and the practice is highly regarded by the social work discipline.[54] The National Association of Social Workers (NASW) highlights the importance of patient self-determination and decision-making. In palliative care, discussions about advance directives promote autonomy and give a semblance of control during a time of great uncertainty and strain. Because "patient autonomy" is not a culturally appropriate term for all patients, discussions must be embedded within a thorough exploration of what the patient defines as helpful.

Although research on social workers' involvement in end-of-life planning is limited, scholars have recognized the critical role of social workers on the healthcare team care team through their work in advocacy, active involvement of family caregivers, and identification and communication between patients and their healthcare agents.[55] Moreover, research suggests that social workers conduct advance directive communication with patients in multiple settings, including acute care, hospital, home care, Veteran's Administration, intensive care unit (ICU), hospice, and long-term care settings. In a qualitative study that compared differences in advance directive communication practices by nurses and social workers with hospitalized elderly patients, certain social work communication skills were identified, including initiating the topic of advance directives, providing information about advance directives, facilitating selection of a surrogate decision-maker, eliciting the patient's values, discussing treatment options, and communicating the information back to the team.[56] A cross-sectional study examined 390 social workers using a random sample of NASW members. Over 70% were involved in healthcare proxy discussions and counseling related to end-of-life planning. The social workers drew upon their training in communication and listening to understand the patients' needs, values, and wishes, along with advocacy skills to convey those to other members of the healthcare team.[57] A study exploring the services provided to the families of patients who died in the ICU found the most frequently used activities were talking about caregivers' feelings (74%), supporting the family's decisions related to the patient's care (61%), talking about what the patient valued in life (54%), reminiscing about the patient (52%), talking about spiritual and religious needs (50%), and discussing what the patient would have wanted (50%).[58]

Truth-Telling and Informed Consent

Informed consent is an essential part of patient self-determination. To ensure that the patient and family participate fully in decision-making and advance care planning, the social worker empowers patients by reinforcing the medical information, encouraging physicians to present available therapeutic options with risks and benefits, and ensuring an open exchange between patients and the healthcare team. "Truth-telling" and "breaking bad news" are used interchangeably in the literature. While these activities are viewed as clinical imperatives, they must be balanced with patients' emotional and cognitive readiness to accept and manage the information. Social workers can serve as role models for interdisciplinary collaboration by helping team members clarify their roles while advocating on behalf of patients and ensuring that the needs of patients and families take precedence.

Artificial Nutrition and Hydration, Instituting DNR Orders, and Sedation

Advance care planning in palliative care is designed to support patient autonomy and to prevent unwanted treatment. With help from the palliative care team, including the social worker, patients are given the opportunity to make their own decisions regarding treatment, resuscitation, CPR, nutrition, and hydration.[59] Several surveys have documented social workers' preparedness to involve patients and family members in decision-making at the end of life and social workers' strong belief that they should be professionally responsible for end-of-life discussions.[60] In a study comparing the attitudes of nurses and social workers in Israel, professional differences were noted, with social workers placing more emphasis than nurses on their involvement in end-of-life decision-making.[54] These findings, which reflect the differences in the professional values and experiences of both groups, encourage the use of interdisciplinary teams to improve end-of-life decision-making.

Conclusion

Social workers are uniquely qualified to improve communication in palliative and end-of-life care. Box 6.2 summarizes Elena's story and the integral role of social work during serious illness. While barriers to the delivery of social work services have not been well studied, heavy caseloads and lack of interview space have been noted as barriers to social work practice and have direct impact on social work communication.[61] In addition, although legislative gains and patient self-determination have led to a greater emphasis on the rights of patients to express their goals and preferences, patients and caregivers do not fully grasp their medical and legal options at the end of life. In many settings, the social worker must help patients understand their options regarding treatment refusal, treatment withdrawal, assisted suicide, euthanasia, and other choices and advocate with the team to ensure that the patient's choices are respected.[62] Advocacy from professional groups, buy-in from social work educators, and widespread curriculum change is needed to ensure that palliative and end-of-life care are taught at the undergraduate and graduate level of social work programs. We must train a social work workforce that is poised to meet the needs of an aging population likely to live longer with advanced illness. Last, social workers must design evidence-based studies that demonstrate the effectiveness and pivotal role of social work communication in palliative and end-of-life care across settings and throughout the continuum of illness (Box 6.2).

Box 6.2 Case Study of Elena

Elena was 50 years old when she was diagnosed with liposarcoma. Born in Cuba, Elena described herself as "mostly American with a dash of Cuba." She had come to the United States as a child, along with her older sister and parents. Her parents always longed to go back to Cuba and never felt at home in the United States. Although Elena and her sister were bilingual, her parents spoke only Spanish. Elena was a successful Wall-Street executive in a loving relationship with Karen, a teacher. After her diagnosis, Elena and Karen were married—a poignant event as they already knew Elena was very ill. Although Elena's sister embraced her when she came out, their parents had a more difficult time accepting that their daughter was gay and married to a non-Cuban. There were other areas of tension: Elena and Karen considered themselves agnostic, while Elena's parents were devout Catholics. Karen had been raised Irish Catholic but was turned off by the Church's rejection of gay marriage; Elena had never found meaning in organized religion.

During her first inpatient stay, Elena worked with an oncology social worker who was very helpful to her. Because Elena took care of herself, staying fit and eating well, her sudden diagnosis was a shock. The focus of the clinical work was on her adjustment to illness, understanding her diagnosis, supporting her family, and helping her talk to her teenage daughter, Alexis. Elena knew from the medical team that the cancer was likely to recur but rarely metastasized and the prognosis was therefore good. Being of a different generation and culture, Elena's parents were distressed by the frank exchange of information and disagreed with the decision to discuss the diagnosis and illness course with their teenager. Elena recognized this was not the "Cuban way." The oncology social worker arranged a meeting with Elena's parents and the oncologist. The social worker was instrumental in helping the physician understand the parents' cultural beliefs about "truth-telling." As Elena healed from the surgery and no further treatment was needed, they all "returned to normal."

Elena did not think about a recurrence and had two years of "blissful and purposeful denial." Things changed radically when the tumor recurred. Elena had more extensive surgery, but this time, there was no inpatient social worker and no one to attend to her psychosocial distress. The oncology social worker no longer worked at the medical center, and no further counseling was offered. Elena was in great distress, never quite believing the tumor would recur. A friend referred Elena to a social worker in private practice and the initial work began to help her process the trauma of the recurrence, the assault to her body image in the wake of large surgical scars, her belief that she was no longer sexually attractive, and the physical effects of the surgery—primarily fatigue.

Over time, Elena healed, returned to work, resumed her intimate life with Karen and her family life with Alexis. Once the therapeutic alliance was strong, she felt safe enough to invite Karen, Alexis, and her parents to meet with the social worker.

(continued)

Box 6.2 (Continued)

The fallout of caregiver burden—they had not been offered any home care—was a major theme. During the sessions, Elena's parents noticed and appreciated the loving way Karen cared for their daughter. Over the next five years, Elena underwent several more surgeries, had to stop working, and went on experimental chemotherapy on which she remained almost to the end of her life.

At that time, the social worker joined forces with the palliative care team at the hospital, particularly the social worker and the chaplain, as Elena's parents felt most comfortable speaking to "a person of God." Together, they discussed goals of care, honoring Elena's wish for the most aggressive treatment possible, along with symptom management for pain and nausea. The team worked to help Elena stay as alert as possible, in keeping with her wishes. Alexis worked with both the hospital-based and the private social worker to ensure she had support wherever her mother was—at home or in the hospital. Two weeks before she died, Elena consented to hospice care. Although the team had tried to bring hospice care into the picture much sooner, they respected Elena's preference for the very costly chemotherapy she was receiving. When Elena died, it was at home, in some pain, but on her own terms. Afterward, her wife and daughter met with the social worker for bereavement counseling before joining Gilda's Club for separate bereavement groups. At this writing, they are doing well. Elena's parents remained close to Karen and found solace in their religious practice.

References

1. Bomba PA, Morrissey MB, Leven DC. Key role of social work in effective communication and conflict resolution process: Medical Orders for Life-Sustaining Treatment (MOLST) program in New York and shared medical decision making at the end of life. *J Soc Work End Life Palliat Care*. 2011;7(1):56–82.
2. Black K. Advance directive communication practices: Social workers' contributions to the interdisciplinary health care team. *Socl Work Health Care*. 2005;40 (3):39–55.
3. Gutheil IA, Heyman, JC. Communication between older people and their health care agents: Results of an intervention. *Health Soc Work*. 2005 May;30(2):107–116.
4. Csikai EL, Martin SS. Bereaved hospice caregivers' views of the transition to hospice. *Soc Work Health Care*. 2010;49(5):387–400.
5. Weisenfluh SM, Csikai EL. Professional and educational needs of hospice and palliative care social workers. *J Soc Work End Life Palliat Care*. 2013;9(1):58–73.
6. Bhattacharya SB, Rossi MI, Mentz JM. Optimizing strategies to improve interprofessional practice for veterans, part 1. *J Multidiscip Healthc*. 2014;7:179–188.
7. Altilio T, Gardia G, Otis-Green S. Social work practice in palliative and end-of-life care: A report from the summit. *J Soc Work End Life Palliat Care*. 2007;3(4):68–86.
8. Hack TF, Ruether JD, Pickles T, Bultz BD, Chateau D, Degner LF. Behind closed doors II: Systematic analysis of prostate cancer patients' primary treatment consultations with radiation oncologists and predictors of satisfaction with communication. *Psycho-Oncology*. 2012;21(8):809–817.
9. Légaré F, Ratté S, Stacey D, Kryworuchko J, Gravel K, Graham ID, Turcotte S. Interventions for improving the adoption of shared decision making by healthcare professionals. *Cochrane Database Syst Rev*. 2010;5:CD006732.
10. Hack TF, Degner LF, Parker PA, et al: The communication goals and needs of cancer patients: A review. *Psycho-Oncology*. 2005;14:831–845.
11. Hagerty RG, Butow PN, Ellis PM, Dimitry S, Tattersall MH. Communicating prognosis in cancer care: A systematic review of the literature. *Ann Oncol*. 2005;16(7):1005–1053.
12. Billings JA, Quill TE. The initial interview in palliative care consultation. *UpToDate*. July 19, 2013.
13. University of Southern Indiana, Ten core competencies of social work practice. https://www.usi.edu/liberal-arts/social-work/cswe-accreditation. Accessed July 1, 2014.
14. Kovacs PJ. Cagle JG. Education: A complex and empowering social work intervention at the end of life. Education. *Health Soc Work*. 2009;34(1):17–27.
15. Jaya K, Rao MD, Anderson LA, Lin F-C, Laux JP. Completion of advance directives among U.S. consumers. *Am J Prev Med*. 2014;46(1):65–70.
16. Altilio T. Pain and symptom management: Clinical, policy, and political perspectives. *J Psychosoc Oncol*. 2006;24(1):65–79.
17. Otis-Green S, Sidhu RK, Del Ferraro C, Ferrell B. Integrating social work into palliative care for lung cancer patients and families: A multi-dimensional approach. *J Psychosoc Oncol*. 2014;32(4):431–446.
18. Coyle N, Glajchen M. Pain management in the home: Using cancer patients as a model. In: Benzon H, Rathmell J, ed. *Practical Management of Pain*. 5th ed. Philadelphia, PA: Elsevier, 2013:1040–1048.
19. Glajchen, M. Role of family caregivers in cancer pain. In: Bruera E, Portenoy RK, eds. *Cancer Pain: Assessment and Management*. 2nd ed. Cambridge, UK: Cambridge University Press; 2009:597–607.
20. AARP. *Home Alone: Family Caregivers Providing Complex Chronic Care*. Washington, DC: AARP Public Policy Institute; 2012.
21. Lin JG, Chen YH. The role of acupuncture in cancer supportive care. *Am J Chin Med*. 2012;40(2):219–229.
22. Benzar E, Hansen L, Kneitel AW, Fromme EK. Discharge planning for palliative care patients: A qualitative analysis. *J Palliat Med*. 2011;14(1):65–69.
23. Mitchell AJ, Chan M, Bhatti H, Halton M, Grassi L, Johansen C, Meader N. Prevalence of depression, anxiety, and adjustment disorder in oncological, haematological, and palliative-care settings: A meta-analysis of 94 interview-based studies. *Lancet Oncol*. 2011; 12(2):160–174.
24. Kissane DW, Bylund CL, Banerjee SC, et al. Patient-centered communication stands out as a crucial clinical skill to optimize outcomes: Communication skills training for oncology professionals. *J Clin Oncol*. 2012;30(11):1242–1247.
25. Deshields TL1, Nanna SK.J. Providing care for the "whole patient" in the cancer setting: the psycho-oncology consultation model of patient care. *Clin Psychol Med Settings*. 2010; 17(3):249–257.
26. Wright AA, Zhang B, Ray A, et al. Associations between end of life discussions, patient mental health, medical care near death, and caregiver bereavement adjustment. *JAMA*. 2008; 300(14):1665–1673.
27. Covinsky KE, Goldman L, Cook EF, Oye R, Desbiens N, Reding D, Fulkerson W, Connors AF Jr, Lynn J, Phillips RS. The impact of serious illness on patients' families: SUPPORT Investigators. Study to understand prognoses and preferences for outcomes and risks of treatment. *JAMA*. 1994;272(23):1839.
28. Radwany S, Albanese T, Clough L, Sims L, Mason H, Jahangiri S. End of life decision making and emotional burden: Placing family meetings in context. *Am J Hosp Palliat Care*. 2009; 26(5):376–383.
29. Gueguen JA, Bylund CL, Brown RF, Levin TT, Kissane DW. Conducting family meetings in palliative care: Themes, techniques,

and preliminary evaluation of a communication skills module. *Palliat Support Care.* 2009;7(2):171–179.
30. Hannon B, O'Reilly V, Bennett K, Breen K, Lawlor PG. Meeting the family: Measuring effectiveness of family meetings in a specialist inpatient palliative care unit. *Palliat Support Care.* 2012;10 (1):43–49.
31. Canda ER, Furman LD. *Spiritual Diversity in Social Work Practice: The Heart of Helping.* 2nd ed. New York, NY: Free Press; 2010.
32. Streets F. Overcoming a fear of religion in social work education. *J Relig Spiritual Soc Work.* 2009;28:185–208.
33. Liechty D. Sacred content, secular context: A generative theory of religion and spirituality for social work. *J Soc Work End Life Palliat Care.* 2013;9(2–3):123–143.
34. Hess, D. Faith healing and the palliative care team. *J Soc Work End Life Palliat Care.* 2013;9(2–3):180–190.
35. Puchalski C, Ferrell B, Virani R, et al. Improving the quality of spiritual care as a dimension of palliative care: The report of the Consensus Conference. *J Palliat Med.* 2009;12:885.
36. Steinhauser KE, Alexander SC, Byock IR, et al. Do preparation and life completion discussions improve functioning and quality of life in seriously ill patients? Pilot randomized control trial. *J Palliat Med.* 2008;11:1234.
37. Kao HF, An K. Effect of acculturation and mutuality on family loyalty among Mexican American caregivers of elders. *J Nurs Scholarsh.* 2012;44(2):111–119.
38. National Association of Social Workers. *NASW Standards for Social Work Practice in Palliative and End of Life Care.* Washington, DC: National Association of Social Workers; 2004.
39. Long, CO. Ten best practices to enhance culturally competent communication in palliative care. *J Pediatr Hematol Oncol.* 2011; 33(Suppl 2):S136–S139.
40. Palos GR, Mendoza TR, Liao KP, et al. Caregiver symptom burden: The risk of caring for an underserved patient with advanced cancer. *Cancer.* 2011;117(5):1070–1079.
41. Mebane EW, Oman RF, Kroonen LT, et al. The influence of physician race, age, and gender on physician attitudes toward advance care directives and preferences for end of life decision-making. *J Am Geriatr Soc.* 1999;47:579–591.
42. Nielsen LS, Angus JE, Howell D, Husain A, Gastaldo D. Patient-centered care or cultural competence: negotiating palliative care at home chinese canadian immigrants. *Am J Hosp Palliat Care.* 2015 Jun;32(4):372–329.
43. Mitchell BL, Mitchell LC. Review of the literature on cultural competence and end of life treatment decisions: The role of the hospitalist. *J Natl Med Assoc.* 2009;101(9):920–926.
44. Institute of Medicine. *Unequal Treatment: Confronting Racial and Ethnic Disparities in Health Care.* Washington, DC: National Academy Press; 2002.
45. Mack JW, Cronin A, Keating NL, Taback N, Huskamp HA, Malin JL, Earle CC, Weeks JC. Associations between end of life discussion characteristics and care received near death: a prospective cohort study. *J Clin Oncol.* 2012;30(35):4387.
46. Reese D, Raymer, M. Relationships between social work services and hospice outcomes: Results of the National Hospice Social Work Survey. *Social Work.* 2004;49(3):415–422.
47. Steinhauser KE, Christakis NA, Clipp EC, et al. Factors considered important at the end of life by patients, family, physicians, and other care providers. *JAMA.* 2000;284:2476–2482.
48. Volker DL, Limerick M. What constitutes a dignified death? The voice of oncology advanced practice nurses. *Clin Nurse Spec.* 2007;21:241–247.
49. Chochinov HM, Kristjanson LJ, Breitbart W, McClement S, Hack TF, Hassard T, Harlos M. Effect of dignity therapy on distress and end-of-life experience in terminally ill patients: A randomized controlled trial. *Lancet Oncol.* 2011;12(8):753–762.
50. Malkinson, R. Cognitive-behavioral therapy of grief: A review and application. *Res Soc Work Pract.* 2001;11(6):671–698.
51. Kris AE, Cherlin EJ, Prigerson H, et al. Length of hospice enrollment and subsequent depression in family caregivers: 13-month follow-up study. *Am J Geriatr Psychiatry.* 2006;14:264–269.
52. *NASW Standards for Social Work Practice in Palliative and End of Life Care.* Washington, DC: National Association of Social Workers; 2015.
53. Christ GH, Sormanti M. Advancing social work practice in end of life care. *Soc Work Health Care.* 1999;30(2):81–99.
54. Werner P, Carmel S, Ziedenberg H. 2004. Nurses' and social workers' attitudes and beliefs about and involvement in life-sustaining treatment decisions. *Health Soc Work.* 2004;29(1):27–35.
55. Gutheil IA, Heyman JC. Communication between older people and their health care agents: Results of an intervention. *Health Soc Work.* 2005;30(2):107–116.
56. Black K. Advance directive communication: Nurses' and social workers' perceptions of roles. *Am J Hosp Palliat Care.* 2006;23:175–184.
57. Heyman JC, Gutheil IA. Social work involvement in end-of-life planning. *J Gerontol Soc Work.* 2006;47:47–61.
58. McCormick AJ, Engelberg R, Curtis JR. Social workers in palliative care: Assessing activities and barriers in the intensive care unit. *J Palliat Med.* 2007;10:929–937.
59. Silveira MJ, DiPiero A, Gerrity MS, Feudtner C. Patients' knowledge of options at the end of life: Ignorance in the face of death. *JAMA.* 2000;284(19):2483–2488.
60. de Haes H, Koedoot N. Patient centered decision making in palliative cancer treatment: A world of paradoxes. *Patient Educ Couns.* 2003;50(1):43–49.
61. Subramanian K. The nature of social work services in a large public medical center serving an impoverished multicultural population. *Soc Work Health Care.* 2000;31:47–63.
62. Yuen JK, Reid MC, Fetters MD. Hospital do-not-resuscitate orders: Why they have failed and how to fix them. *J Gen Intern Med.* 2011;26(7):791–797.

CHAPTER 7

Communication in Palliative Medicine

Jennifer Gabbard and Thomas Smith

Introduction

Mrs. N is a 61-year-old nurse with rapidly progressive pulmonary fibrosis. She is hospitalized with profound hypoxia, an oxygen saturation of 70% on room air, and diffuse progressive fibrosis in both lungs. She has heard from the lung transplant team that she is not a current candidate for lung transplantation, but might be "if she could walk 300 or 400 feet unaided." No one directly communicated that the likelihood of her recovering to be able to walk 300 feet is extremely unlikely. Mrs. N and her family are upset because even though she has been told she is not a candidate, she cannot believe this news as she is otherwise healthy. She asks, "What am I supposed to do, go home and die?" No one on the lung transplant team has laid out a plan for her that would include double-checking again about her transplant candidacy, explaining to her that indeed she was dying and that her prognosis was weeks to months, and that she should consider hospice, spending her remaining time with family, caring for her own spirit and attending to legacy issues.

Communication is arguably one of the most important palliative care skills. Pain and symptom management are important, but being able to communicate "sad, bad, and difficult news" with empathy and complete truthfulness is also critically important.[1-6] In our experience at several institutions, and with multiple different specialties, being able to communicate information in a way that is truthful, frank, and maintains hope is one of the least-developed competencies, as shown by the case with Mrs. N.[7,8] This is not just in patients with cancer but universally across medicine; physicians must be able to convey poor or serious prognoses.

Knowledge of prognosis aids patients in their preferences regarding aggressive therapy versus supportive care.[9,10] Sadly, however, many physicians still do not have prognostic discussions with their patients. Even as increasing evidence has shown this type of practice does not deliver high-quality care, many physicians prefer nondisclosure over frank disclosure. This is likely secondary to their own discomfort with communicating difficult news along with their own inability to formulate a reliable prognosis.[5,11] One of the problems is there is no clear consensus on the definitions of the words "terminal" and "end of life," which could be used as an excuse for clinicians and patients to avoid the topic.[5] As advances in treatment options occur, making it easier to offer hope to patients at the time of diagnosis, the need for improving clinician skills in communication is crucial.[3] Patient-centered communication allows patients and families to make well-informed healthcare decisions that are consistent with their values, goals, and preferences.[12]

One of the core features of palliative medicine is communication. At least half of our consultations at Johns Hopkins involve communication about goals of care, advance directives, planning for the future, and decisions about code status. Palliative care teams are consulted for symptom assessment and management, communication of estimated prognosis, discussions about treatment options, and goals of care along with psychological support.[13-15] The majority of communication involves decisions related to advance care planning, a critical communication task that should take place during the early stages of a disease trajectory (see Figure 7.1), rather than as initial communication during an acute hosptalization.[14,16]

Communication about advance care planning involves considering decision options ahead of time, discussing the pros and cons of those options, and relaying those preferences to family members or a designated proxy. Physicians often feel unequipped to have these discussions with their patients. Research shows that the rate of advance directives discussions and documentation in outpatient primary care clinics ranges only between 3% to 30%.[17,18] The SUPPORT trial that occurred in the mid-1990s showed limited advance directive discussions and documentation of with many DNRs placed days before death.[19] More recent studies showed some improvements, with 47% of patients completing advance directives and 73% having a surrogate decision-maker, although only 30% were documented in medical records.[20] Heyland also showed that only one-fourth of patients were asked about their preferences during an acute hospitalization. Yung et al. recently found that 90% of community-dwelling elderly patients would not want aggressive care, but only 22% of patients' preference information appeared in their medical records. Allision et al. state that disregard of patients' preferences is a medical error and that our current system has not overcome the reluctance of physicians to discuss treatment wishes when confronted with patients who are seriously ill.[21] This was illustrated among admitted cancer patients; oncologists raised the subject of advance care planning with only 2 of 75 consecutive patients.[22] A study of patients with cancer with metastatic spinal cord compression showed that, because of inadequate physician–patient communication, often patients were not aware of the urgency of having an advance directive, which in turn led to delay in end-of-life palliative care.[23]

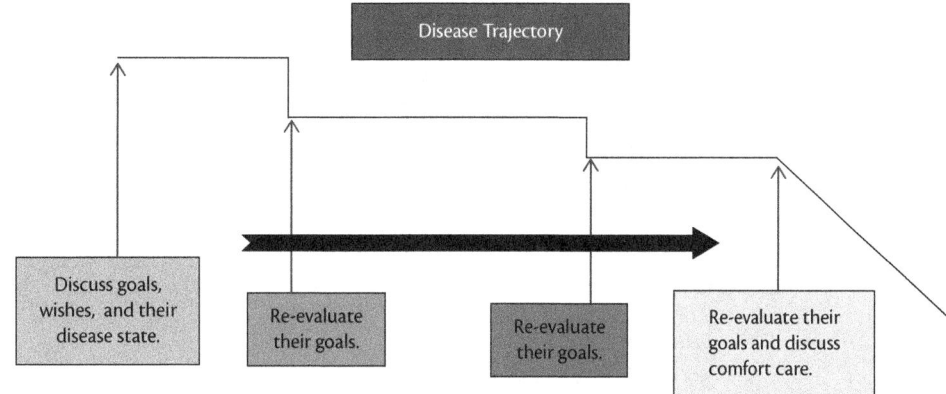

Figure 7.1 Multiple stages of a disease trajectory and life of the patient

The sad truth is that communication is lacking in the medical field in general, and palliative care physicians are stepping in and becoming responsible for a wide range of clinical communication tasks.

Why Is Improving Communication Important?

Communication is important to ensure that patients and families make well-informed decisions. Braddock showed that when reviewing 1,057 patient encounters, only 9% resulted in what was defined as an informed medical decision.[24] More recent studies by Lee and Zikmund-Fisher found that when discussing medical decisions, patient preferences were assessed only 50% of the time.[25,26] Enhancing communication between physicians and patients can ultimately lead to better symptom control, more hospice referrals, less futile chemotherapy at the end of life, better patient understanding of their disease trajectory and treatment options, better understanding of their prognosis, an increase in the number of patients dying at home and spending time with loved ones, and increased quality of end-of-life care. Figure 7.2 depicts the importance of communication, and Table 7.1 illustrates the research on why communication matters in palliative medicine.

Communication is also important to ensure patient and family understanding of disease and prognosis. In the Temel study, a randomized clinical trial comparing usual oncology care and usual oncology care plus palliative care for lung cancer patients, patients who received concurrent palliative care survived longer. This was linked to having a better understanding of the incurable nature of the disease, and those with better "prognostic awareness" of their disease received less intravenous chemotherapy in the last 60 days of life.[27] In the oncology-only group (patients who did not receive palliative care), the oncologists recorded *no* time (zero minutes on average) in communicating explicitly with patients and family members about helping them cope with their disease or in engaging family members.[28] Patients without palliative care experience more depression, more anxiety, less prognostic awareness, worse mood and quality of life, and more IV chemotherapy with little chance of success, as well as living a shorter length of time.[29–31]

Finally, physician communication has been found to be important to patient and family satisfaction with care. Patient and family satisfaction with physician communication has been correlated to decreased anxiety, improved patient satisfaction, improved perception about medical staff, better adherence to treatment, decreased length of stay in the hospital, fewer intensive care unit

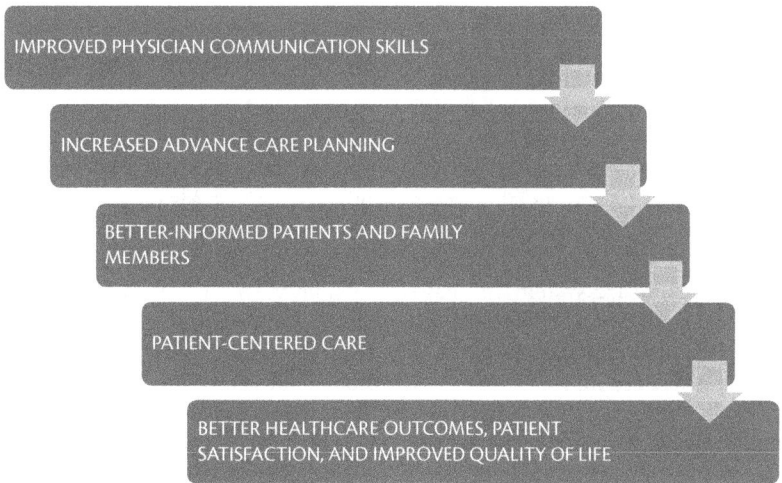

Figure 7.2 Why is communication important?

Table 7.1 Why Communication in Palliative Medicine Matters

Palliative Communication	Research Findings	Authors' Comments	Reference
Communication about symptoms	51% of patients reported at least one moderate/severe symptom	More thorough communication about symptoms is needed	Walling et al.[85]
Number of patients who had discussed hospice with *any* doctor, two months before death	Only 53% had discussed hospice with any provider two months before death	Having this discussion two months before death decreases the in-hospital death rate from 51% to 19%	Huskamp et al.[86, 87]
Number of patients who thought chemotherapy could cure their metastatic disease	69% of patients with lung cancer and 81% of those with colorectal cancer thought their chemotherapy was curative	No chance of cure	Weeks et al.[88]
Number of patients who understood that palliative radiation was not going to cure them	Only 36% of 384 lung cancer patients understood that radiation would not cure them	No chance of cure	Chen et al.[89]
Number of patients with an accurate awareness of their prognosis	16.5%; 18.5% *if* the most important doctor discussed prognosis	This was directly related to the propensity of the doctor to actually discuss prognosis	Liu et al.[9]
Number of lung and colorectal cancer patients with EOL discussion	73% overall; 55% occurred in the hospital; 27% of the time with oncologists. Most common time was 33 days before death	Most terminally ill cancer patients never discuss their death with their oncologist, even though we know such discussions do not increase anxiety or depression or take away hope	Mack et al.[47]
Prognostic awareness or knowing that one has a terminal cancer	Patients with cancer are more likely to receive EOL care that is consistent with their preferences (68%) when they have had the opportunity to discuss their wishes for EOL care with a physician	Patients who die in the hospital have more emotional and physical distress, especially ICU decedents, compared with home hospice	Mack et al.[90,91]
Regret about EOL care	At least 50% experience regret about the EOL care their loved one receives	Completion of advance care planning strongly associated with reduced caregiver distress	Garrido and Prigerson[92]

Note. EOL = end of life; ICU = intensive care unit.

(ICU) admissions, and decreased litigation.[32–35] Family satisfaction is in direct proportion to the amount of time the patient and family speak.[36,37] Also, collaboration with the primary care healthcare provider results in better patient understanding of their disease trajectory, less distress, and better quality of life at all phases of lung cancer.[38]

What Are the Barriers to Communication?

Barriers to communication include physician, patient, and healthcare factors as summarized in Table 7.2. When someone is diagnosed with a serious or life-threatening disease, it greatly impacts his or her emotional state and also has health and financial repercussions. The cost of care; a lack of understandable information about prognosis, treatment options, and likelihood of response; and lack of psychosocial support contribute to communication problems that are exacerbated in patients with advanced cancer.[12,39] Patients and families often lack experience within the healthcare system and have limited healthcare literacy, which along with the complexity of treatment options can lead to limited engagement in their healthcare decisions. In addition, there are no reimbursement incentives for physicians to engage in patient-centered communication. Physicians also lack proper training in communication.[12] In one survey of oncologists, less than 10% reported having formal training in how to convey poor prognosis, and only 32% had the chance to directly observe another provider deliver a poor prognosis to a patient during their training.[3] Advances have reduced these communication gaps by targeting deficiencies during training and have led to improvements in patient–oncologist communication but not to the point of being sufficient for optimal care.[40] Buss et al. surveyed oncology fellows and found that they felt better trained in non-palliative care communication skills (i.e., procedures) than end-of-life discussions.[41]

Importance of Prognostication

Patients and their families want to know what they have, what can be done about it, and what is going to happen to them.[42] Studies have shown at least 80% of patients want to know their prognosis.[5,43,44] Alston and colleagues surveyed 1,068 adults in the United States, and the majority wanted to be involved in the decision-making about their care (see Box 7.1), but only 47% felt their provider took into account their goals and concerns, and less than 37% were presented nontreatment options.[12,45] El-Jawahri et al. showed that only 22% of patients reported having a discussion about end-of-life preferences with their oncologist.[46] Chang et al. also showed a discord between physicians' and patients' perceptions: 62% of physicians stated they had prognostic discussions but, when surveyed, only 23% of patients reported that a prognosis discussion had taken place.[15]

Table 7.2 Key Barriers in Communication

Patient factors	♦ Patients and their families frequently tend to steer conversations away from difficult or emotionally laden topics. ♦ Patients often feel emotionally overwhelmed. ♦ Patients and their families have a tendency to overestimate the probability of a cure in difficult situations. ♦ Language barriers can create miscommunication and ambiguity about care, treatment options, and death and dying. ♦ Cultural barriers may create mistrust of physicians. ♦ Health literacy may be limited.
Physician factors	♦ Lack of proper communication skills. ♦ Fear of causing pain by conveying poor or serious prognosis. ♦ Fear they will take away a patient's hope. ♦ Trained to save lives, not trained well to manage death. ♦ Not trained to assess and manage emotions. ♦ Inability to formulate a reliable prognosis.
Healthcare factors	♦ Current reimbursement system does not incentivize clinicians to engage in patient-centered communication. ♦ Multiple transitions of care. ♦ Multiple subspecialists.

Furthermore, patients who inappropriately believe in the curability of their disease choose more aggressive treatments. In one study, two-thirds of lung and colorectal cancer patients thought they could be cured by palliative chemotherapy or radiation.[47] When 126 patients with incurable cancer were surveyed, 98% reported they would like their oncologist to be realistic about their future.[48] So, since patients want to know their prognosis, why are physicians not relaying this information to their patients? Some of the reasons are summarized in Table 7.3. Often, physicians do not communicate a poor prognosis for fear that a patient will become depressed and hopeless. However, Hagerty has shown that relaying a realistic prognosis to patients does not take away their hope as long as they feel well informed and the physician shows empathy and confirms that he or she will control their pain and symptoms.[49] Studies have shown that surrogate decision-makers feel withholding prognostic information does not help in maintaining hope but actually limits their ability to prepare and causes more stress.[50, 51] A good way to convey hope may be to say, "Though we cannot cure your disease, there are many things that we can still do to help you—let's focus on those."

Box 7.1 Key Things Patients Want Their Healthcare Provider To Do[45]
Listen to them
Tell them the truth about their diagnosis
Tell them about each treatment option and the risks and benefits of each
Explain how each treatment option will impact their quality and quantity of life
Understand their goals
Help them understand the financial impact of each treatment option
Explain nontreatment options

Another barrier to communication is a physician's own unwillingness or inability to formulate a reliable prognosis.[52] This was illustrated by a study by Christakis that showed physicians overestimate prognosis by a factor of 5.[53,54] In Phase I drug treatments, where physicians should discuss prognosis routinely as a justification for taking a new and potentially toxic drug, this occurred in only 11 of 52 encounters.[55] Ahluwalia et al. showed that when patients questioned their physicians about prognosis and future care, 84% of physicians missed the opportunity and instead responded by "terminating the conversation, hedging their responses, denying the patient's expressed emotion, or inadequately acknowledging the sentiment underlying the patient's statement."[56] (p. 445)

One study showed that 60% percent of medical oncologists prefer not to discuss "code status," advance medical directives, or even hospice until there are no more treatments to give.[57,58] This is likely one of the reasons that up to 20% of cancer patients receive chemotherapy in the last two weeks of life.[59] Jackson et al. interviewed 18 physicians who treated dying patients at five academic centers: 86% felt certain a patient's death was imminent but only 11% ever had a conversation about imminent death, and fewer than half of all patients had any physician tell them they were terminal.[60] As a result, patients lose quality time with their families and for reflection and instead spend more time in the hospital and ICU.[58] Although patients report that they want to die at home, less than 40% do, and more than 11% of patients have three or more hospitalizations in the last 90 days of their life.[61]

Patients and families want prognostic information, poor or otherwise, that supports their ability to make decisions. Surveys of patients show that higher patient satisfaction is linked to more shared decision-making. Physicians who explained the latest medical evidence, included an option for not doing disease-directed therapy, explained the benefits and risks of each option, took the time to understand the patients' goals and concerns, listened to them, used language they understood, and clearly explained their condition had higher satisfaction scores.[45]

Table 7.3 Reasons Healthcare Providers Do Not Have Truthful Discussions About Prognoses

Reason/Excuse	Assessment of Reason/Excuse	Rationale
1. People do not want this sort of information.	Incorrect	Study after study shows that most people want to know their diagnosis, what will happen to them, and what can be done to help them. Physicians who ask, "What do you know about your illness? What do you want to know?" allow patients to express their own wishes about the information they want.
2. It will make people depressed.	Incorrect	In fact, giving patients honest information may allow them and their caregivers to cope with illness better; patients who reported having end-of-life discussions had no higher rates of depression or worry, lower rates of ventilation and resuscitation, and more and earlier hospice enrollment.[58]
3. It will take away hope.	Incorrect	Hope is maintained with truthful discussions in cancer,[64,93,94] dialysis,[95] and mechanical ventilation.[50] Hope is derived not from prognostic disclosure but from the caring patient–physician relationship.[96]
4. Involvement of hospice or palliative care will reduce survival.	Incorrect	Multiple studies suggest that survival is equal or better with hospice or palliative care.[31,97–101]
5. We do not really know the patient's prognosis.	False	Most of the time, physicians provide no estimate[46] or a conscious overestimate[53] and give the least information to those with the worst prognosis.[53,102]
6. Talking about prognosis is not culturally appropriate.	Incorrect	Patients of different ethnic and cultural backgrounds often have different preferences for information, but nothing is universal,[103] so it is always appropriate to ask.
7. We do not like to have these discussions, and they are hard on us.	True	Most physicians and oncologists find breaking bad news to be stressful and unsatisfying.[104–106] Physicians who have long-term relationships with patients are most likely to overestimate survival.[53] In one study, lying to a simulated 26-year-old brain tumor patient about her dismal prognosis was less troubling than telling her the truth.[107] The reasons patients prefer to discuss advance directives with a physician they have not met was that "It would be too difficult on my usual doctor."[22]

This approach also saves money, or, as we explain, "it provides better care at a cost we can afford." A 2008 study showed that the addition of palliative care to standard hospital care led to better established goals of care early in the hospital course, decreased ICU cost, and thus helped the patient avoid unnecessary tests and treatments that were not in accordance with his or her goals. Thus improving physician–patient communication ultimately led to decreased overall hospital cost.[58,62–64]

The Importance of an Interdisciplinary Team Approach

Palliative care has been a leader in introducing the importance of the interdisciplinary team approach, and studies have shown that interdisciplinary teams are linked to improved patient satisfaction.[65] No single healthcare provider can meet all of the complex needs of patients and family members who may require a range of treatments, care services, social support, physical needs, and spiritual care. Spiritual care is an integral part of each interdisciplinary team. Patients at the end of life want to communicate about their fears, hope, and spirituality and look to their physician to approach the subject of spirituality.[66,67] In 2006, a study by Mako and colleagues showed that in patients with advanced-stage cancer, 96% reported experiencing spiritual pain that was not adequately addressed.[68] Delgado-Guay et al. showed that spiritual pain impacted physical symptoms (58%) and emotional symptoms (76%) of patients, greatly impacting quality of life.[69] Thus having a chaplain as a part of the interdisciplinary team can ensure that spiritual care is provided to patients. An interdisciplinary team approach allows for patient-centered care that enhances communication and allows for shared decision-making.

Communication Can Be Learned, Unlearned, and Relearned

Based on the emerging literature on the importance of communication, medical education is now implementing requirements for teaching communication skills to medical students and residents; this skill is now considered a core competency.[70–72] Physicians with communication expertise spend twice as much time on advance directive discussions, engage in more partnership-building with patients and families, allow time for the patient and family to talk, and discuss more lifestyle and psychological issues.[73,74]

One model often used to teach communication is the SPIKES protocol, as seen in Figure 7.3.[3] There are several excellent protocol approaches to cultivating prognostic awareness.[38] For example, the Japanese SHARE (**S**upportive environment, **H**ow to deliver bad news, **A**dditional information, and **R**eassurance and **E**motional support) model appears to be more effective than SPIKES and takes just one day.[75] An online curriculum, COMFORT™ SM (**C**ommunication, **O**rientation and Opportunity, **M**indful presence, **F**amily, **O**penings, **R**elating, and **T**eam) is freely available on the web and shows improved communication scores in four of seven available modules from pre- and posttest.[76] Figure 7.4 depicts trigger points for communication: as a disease progresses, when the prognosis changes, and when performance status declines.[77,78]

A Cochrane review of 43 randomized trials showed positive effects of communication training on consultations, including

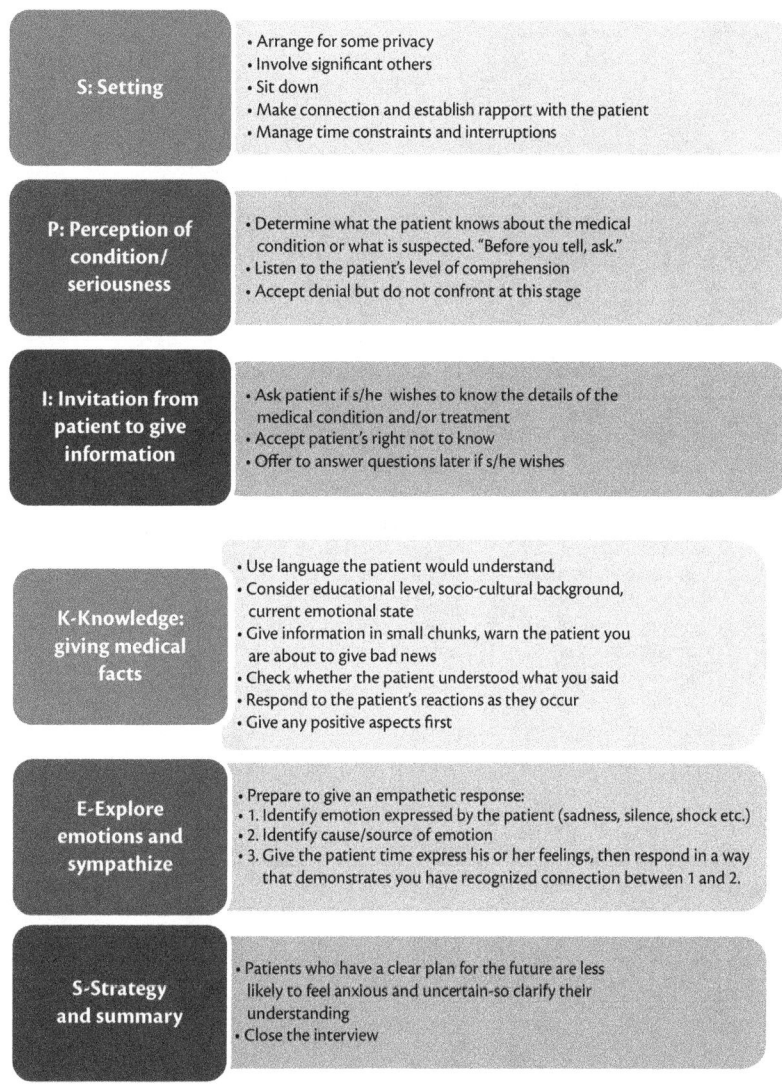

Figure 7.3 Six steps of SPIKES
Baile WF, Buckman R, Lenzi R, Glober G, Beale EA, Kudelka AP. SPIKES: A six-step protocol for delivering bad news: Application to the patient with cancer. *The Oncologist*. 2000;5(4):302–311.

"clarifying patients' concerns and beliefs; communicating treatment options; increasing providers' empathy; and patients' perception of providers' attentiveness to them and their concerns as well as their diseases progresses." (p. 2) In addition, short-term training of less than 10 hours was as effective as more prolonged training.[79] A recent study that examined a two-day communication skills training workshop program based on patient preferences showed improvement in oncologists' communication performances, especially skills of emotional support and consideration for how to deliver information.[80] Thus the training does not have to be extensive but still can have a profound effect. Table 7.4 lists some programs that are available to help improve communication skills.

There is also evidence that communication skills training is associated with better communication but could also lead to emotional exhaustion at three months' time.[81] Similarly, a highly effective communication skills training program for oncologists improved skills but expressions of empathy declined substantially, suggesting that oncologists were learning to protect themselves from too much emotional involvement.[2] Other studies have shown that communication skills training can improve communication skills but lack enhancement in empathy.[82] Whether these disadvantages can be overcome is not known. Recent randomized trials of interventions among ICU physicians that slightly reduced depersonalization, emotional exhaustion, and burnout have not been tested in those who do palliative care or oncology but are at least somewhat promising.[83]

Conclusion

As emphasized in this chapter, improving physician–patient communication and delivering goal-directed care is essential to delivering high-quality healthcare. Patient-centered communication allows patients and families to make well-informed healthcare decisions that are consistent with their values, goals, and preferences. There is no evidence that realistic prognostic discussion causes depression, shortens life, or takes away hope, thus it

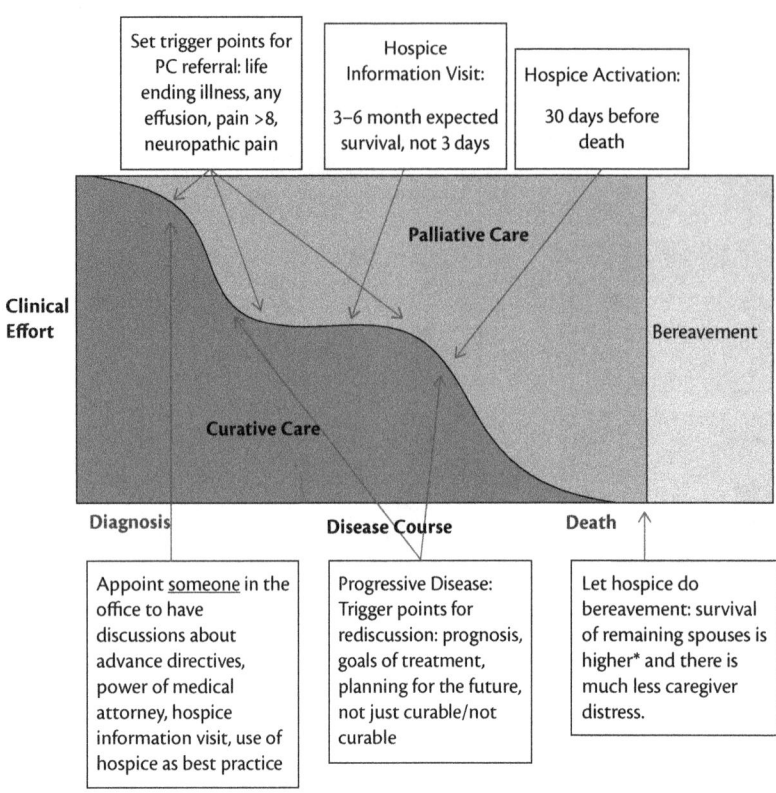

Figure 7.4 Modifying practice patterns to improve patient outcomes. PC = palliative care

Table 7.4 Readily Available Communication Programs

Program	Website	Cost	Evidence
End-of-Life Nursing Education Consortium	www.aacn.nche.edu/elnec	Many modules available for free; nominal charge for courses	Studies show improved communication skills and comfort.[108]
Oncotalk	http://depts.washington.edu/oncotalk/	Most modules available online free of charge	Substantial improvements in learner skills; e.g., after Oncotalk 56% of participants used the word "cancer" compared with 16% before.[109]
Comskil training program	https://www.mskcc.org/events/cme/clone-communication-skills-program-oncology/form-7	$1,200—Attending faculty $480—Trainees	Participants have shown significant gains in self-efficacy regarding communicating with patients in various contexts.[110]
Education in Palliative and End-of-life Care Communicating Bad News	http://epec.net/stpage2.php	Free downloads	
COMFORT Curriculum	www.pccinstitute.com	Free downloads	Improved communication scores in four of seven available modules from pre- and posttest.[76]
Tough Talk: Helping Doctors Approach Difficult Conversations	http://depts.washington.edu/toolbox/toc.html	Free downloads and toolkit	
Palliative medicine communication course	www.dom.pitt.edu/dgim/spc/communication_course.html	$1,200 for three days	
I*CARE program	http://www.mdanderson.org/education-and-research/resources-for-professionals/professional-educational-resources/i-care/index.html	Free online CME credit through video courses that focus on patient–doctor communication	
CareSearch	www.caresearch.com.au	Free online interactive learning modules	

Note. CME = continuing medical education.

is hard to argue against honest communication about prognosis.[49,64,84] Communication is a learned skill, with multiple ways to learn and teach. Shorter, simple residential and online courses can improve the way we communicate successfully.

References

1. Fallowfield L, Jenkins V. Communicating sad, bad, and difficult news in medicine. *Lancet*. 2004;363(9405):312–319.
2. Fallowfield L, Jenkins V, Farewell V, Solis-Trapala I. Enduring impact of communication skills training: Results of a 12-month follow-up. *Br J Cancer*. 2003;89(8):1445–1449.
3. Baile WF, Buckman R, Lenzi R, Glober G, Beale EA, Kudelka AP. SPIKES: A six-step protocol for delivering bad news: Application to the patient with cancer. *Oncologist*. 2000;5(4):302–311.
4. McCarthy M. US health system is not meeting patients' needs at end of life, says expert committee. *BMJ*. 2014;348:g5739.
5. Rich BA. Prognosis terminal: Truth-telling in the context of end-of-life care. *Camb Q Healthc Ethics*. 2014;23(2):209–219.
6. Bostick NA, Sade R, McMahon JW, Benjamin R. Report of the American Medical Association Council on Ethical and Judicial Affairs: Withholding information from patients: Rethinking the propriety of "therapeutic privilege." *J Clin Ethics*. 2006;17(4):302–306.
7. Campbell TC, Carey EC, Jackson VA, et al. Discussing prognosis: Balancing hope and realism. *Cancer Journal* (Sudbury, Mass.). 2010;16(5):461–466.
8. Von Roenn JH, von Gunten CF. Setting goals to maintain hope. *J Clin Oncol*. 2003;21(3):570–574.
9. Liu PH, Landrum MB, Weeks JC, et al. Physicians' propensity to discuss prognosis is associated with patients' awareness of prognosis for metastatic cancers. *J Palliat Med*. 2014;17(6):673–682.
10. Glare PA, Sinclair CT. Palliative medicine review: Prognostication. *J Palliat Med*. 2008;11(1):84–103.
11. Lamont EB, Christakis NA. Prognostic disclosure to patients with cancer near the end of life. *Ann Intern Med*. 2001;134(12):1096–1105.
12. Patient-centered communication and shared decision making. In: Committee on Improving the Quality of Cancer Care: Addressing the Challenges of an Aging Population, Board on Health Care Services, Institute of Medicine, Levit L, Balogh E, Nass S, et al., eds. *Delivering High-Quality Cancer Care: Charting a New Course for a System in Crisis*. Washington, DC: National Academies Press; 2013. http://www.ncbi.nlm.nih.gov/books/NBK202146/
13. Weissman DE. Consultation in palliative medicine. *Arch Intern Med*. 1997;157(7):733–737.
14. National Consensus Project for Quality Palliative Care. clinical practice guidelines for quality palliative care. www.nationalconsensusproject.org. Accessed August 30, 2014.
15. Chang A, Datta-Barua I, McLaughlin B, Daly B. A survey of prognosis discussions held by health-care providers who request palliative care consultation. *Palliat Med*. 2014;28(4):312–317.
16. National Comprehensive Cancer Network. Practice guidelines in oncology: Palliative care. http://www.nccn.org/professionals/physician_gls/f_guidelines.asp Accessed August 30, 2011.
17. Wheatley E, Huntington MK. Advanced directives and code status documentation in an academic practice. *Fam Med*. 2012;44(8):574–578.
18. Hayek S, Nieva R, Corrigan F, et al. End-of-life care planning: Improving documentation of advance directives in the outpatient clinic using electronic medical records. *J Palliat Med*. 17(12): 1348–1352.
19. SUPPORT Principal Investigators. A controlled trial to improve care for seriously ill hospitalized patients. *JAMA*. 1995;274(20):1591–1598.
20. Heyland DK, Barwich D, Pichora D, et al. Failure to engage hospitalized elderly patients and their families in advance care planning. *JAMA Intern Med*. 2013;173(9):778–787.
21. Allison TA, Sudore RL. Disregard of patients' preferences is a medical error: Comment on "Failure to engage hospitalized elderly patients and their families in advance care planning." *JAMA Intern Med*. 2013;173(9):787.
22. Dow LA, Matsuyama RK, Ramakrishnan V, et al. Paradoxes in advance care planning: The complex relationship of oncology patients, their physicians, and advance medical directives. *J Clin Oncol*. 2010;28(2):299–304.
23. Guo Y, Palmer JL, Bianty J, Konzen B, Shin K, Bruera E. Advance directives and do-not-resuscitate orders in patients with cancer with metastatic spinal cord compression: Advanced care planning implications. *J Palliat Med*. 2010;13(5):513–517.
24. Braddock CH, 3rd, Edwards KA, Hasenberg NM, Laidley TL, Levinson W. Informed decision making in outpatient practice: Time to get back to basics. *JAMA*. 1999;282(24):2313–2320.
25. Lee CN, Chang Y, Adimorah N, et al. Decision making about surgery for early-stage breast cancer. *J Am Coll Surg*. 2012;214(1):1–10.
26. Zikmund-Fisher BJ, Couper MP, Singer E, et al. Deficits and variations in patients' experience with making 9 common medical decisions: The DECISIONS survey. *Med Decis Making*. 2010;30(5 Suppl):85s–95s.
27. Temel JS, Greer JA, Admane S, et al. Longitudinal perceptions of prognosis and goals of therapy in patients with metastatic non-small-cell lung cancer: Results of a randomized study of early palliative care. *J Clin Oncol*. 2011;29(17):2319–2326.
28. Smith AK. Palliative care: An approach for all internists: Comment on "Early palliative care in advanced lung cancer: A qualitative study." *JAMA Intern Med*. 2013;173(4):291–292.
29. Greer JA, Pirl WF, Jackson VA, et al. Effect of early palliative care on chemotherapy use and end-of-life care in patients with metastatic non-small-cell lung cancer. *J Clin Oncol*. 2012;30(4):394–400.
30. Irwin KE, Greer JA, Khatib J, Temel JS, Pirl WF. Early palliative care and metastatic non-small cell lung cancer: Potential mechanisms of prolonged survival. *Chron Respir Dis*. 2013;10(1):35–47.
31. Temel JS, Greer JA, Muzikansky A, et al. Early palliative care for patients with metastatic non-small-cell lung cancer. *N Engl J Med*. 2010;363(8):733–742.
32. Lautrette A, Ciroldi M, Ksibi H, Azoulay E. End-of-life family conferences: Rooted in the evidence. *Criti Care Med*. 2006;34(11 Suppl):S364–S372.
33. Tulsky JA. Interventions to enhance communication among patients, providers, and families. *J Palliat Med*. 2005(8 Suppl 1):S95–S102.
34. Huffines M, Johnson KL, Smitz Naranjo LL, et al. Improving family satisfaction and participation in decision making in an intensive care unit. *Crit Care Nurse*. 2013;33(5):56–69.
35. Aslakson R, Cheng J, Vollenweider D, Galusca D, Smith TJ, Pronovost PJ. Evidence-based palliative care in the intensive care unit: A systematic review of interventions. *J Palliat Med*. 2014;17(2):219–235.
36. McDonagh JR, Elliott TB, Engelberg RA, et al. Family satisfaction with family conferences about end-of-life care in the intensive care unit: Increased proportion of family speech is associated with increased satisfaction. *Crit Care Med*. 2004;32(7):1484–1488.
37. Stapleton RD, Engelberg RA, Wenrich MD, Goss CH, Curtis JR. Clinician statements and family satisfaction with family conferences in the intensive care unit. *Crit Care Med*. 2006;34(6):1679–1685.
38. Aubin M, Vezina L, Verreault R, et al. Family physician involvement in cancer care and lung cancer patient emotional distress and quality of life. *Support Care Cancer*. 2011;19(11):1719–1727.
39. National Cancer Institute. Cancer health disparities. http://www.cancer.gov/cancertopics/factsheet/disparities/cancer-health-disparities Accessed January 5, 2015.
40. Pham AK, Bauer MT, Balan S. Closing the patient-oncologist communication gap: A review of historic and current efforts. *J Cancer Educ*. 2014;29(1):106–113.
41. Buss MK, Lessen DS, Sullivan AM, Von Roenn J, Arnold RM, Block SD. Hematology/oncology fellows' training in palliative care: Results of a national survey. *Cancer*. 2011;117(18):4304–4311.

42. Bernacki RE, Block SD. Communication about serious illness care goals: A review and synthesis of best practices. *JAMA Intern Med.* 2014;174(12):1994–2003.
43. Butow PN, Dowsett S, Hagerty R, Tattersall MH. Communicating prognosis to patients with metastatic disease: What do they really want to know? *Support Care Cancer.* 2002;10(2):161–168.
44. Hagerty RG, Butow PN, Ellis PA, et al. Cancer patient preferences for communication of prognosis in the metastatic setting. *J Clin Oncol.* 2004;22(9):1721–1730.
45. Alston C, Paget L, Halvorson GC, et al. Communicating with patients on health care evidence: Discussion paper. Washington, DC: Institute of Medicine; 2012. http://www.iom.edu/~/media/Files/Perspectives-Files/2012/Discussion-Papers/VSRT-Evidence.pdf. Accessed March 1, 2014.
46. El-Jawahri A, Traeger L, Park ER, et al. Associations among prognostic understanding, quality of life, and mood in patients with advanced cancer. *Cancer.* 2014;120(2):278–285.
47. Mack JW, Cronin A, Taback N, et al. End-of-life care discussions among patients with advanced cancer: A cohort study. *Ann Intern Med.* 2012;156(3):204–210.
48. Peppercorn JM, Smith TJ, Helft PR, et al. American society of clinical oncology statement: Toward individualized care for patients with advanced cancer. *J Clin Oncol.* 2011;29(6):755–760.
49. Hagerty RG, Butow PN, Ellis PM, et al. Communicating with realism and hope: Incurable cancer patients' views on the disclosure of prognosis. *J Clin Oncol.* 2005;23(6):1278–1288.
50. Apatira L, Boyd EA, Malvar G, et al. Hope, truth, and preparing for death: Perspectives of surrogate decision makers. *Ann Intern Med.* 2008;149(12):861–868.
51. Iverson E, Celious A, Kennedy CR, et al. Factors affecting stress experienced by surrogate decision makers for critically ill patients: Implications for nursing practice. *Intensive Crit Care Nurs.* 2014;30(2):77–85.
52. Luckett T, Phillips J, Agar M, Virdun C, Green A, Davidson PM. Elements of effective palliative care models: A rapid review. *BMC Health Serv Res.* 2014;14:136.
53. Christakis NA, Lamont EB. Extent and determinants of error in doctors' prognoses in terminally ill patients: Prospective cohort study. *BMJ.* 2000;320(7233):469–472.
54. Christakis N. *Death Foretold: Prophecy and Prognosis in Medical Care.* Chicago, IL: University of Chicago Press; 2001.
55. Jenkins V, Solis-Trapala I, Langridge C, Catt S, Talbot DC, Fallowfield LJ. What oncologists believe they said and what patients believe they heard: An analysis of phase I trial discussions. *J Clin Oncol.* 2011;29(1):61–68.
56. Ahluwalia SC, Levin JR, Lorenz KA, Gordon HS. Missed opportunities for advance care planning communication during outpatient clinic visits. *J Gen Intern Med.* 2012;27(4):445–451.
57. Mack JW, Smith TJ. Reasons why physicians do not have discussions about poor prognosis, why it matters, and what can be improved. *J Clin Oncol.* 2012, 30(22):2715–2717.
58. Harrington SE, Smith TJ. The role of chemotherapy at the end of life: "When is enough, enough?" *JAMA.* 2008; 299(22):2667–2678.
59. Meier DE. Increased access to palliative care and hospice services: Opportunities to improve value in health care. *Milbank Q.* 2011;89(3):343–380.
60. Sullivan AM, Lakoma MD, Matsuyama RK, Rosenblatt L, Arnold RM, Block SD. Diagnosing and discussing imminent death in the hospital: A secondary analysis of physician interviews. *J Palliat Med.* 2007;10(4):882–893.
61. Teno JM, Gozalo PL, Bynum JP, et al. Change in end-of-life care for Medicare beneficiaries: Site of death, place of care, and health care transitions in 2000, 2005, and 2009. *JAMA.* 2013;309(5):470–477.
62. Morrison RS, Penrod JD, Cassel JB, et al. Cost savings associated with US hospital palliative care consultation programs. *Arch Intern Med.* 2008;168(16):1783–1790.
63. Morrison RS, Dietrich J, Ladwig S, et al. Palliative care consultation teams cut hospital costs for Medicaid beneficiaries. *Health Aff (Millwood).* 2011;30(3):454–463.
64. Smith TJ, Dow LA, Virago E, Khatcheressian J, Lyckholm LJ, Matsuyama R. Giving honest information to patients with advanced cancer maintains hope. *Oncology.* 2010;24(6):521–525.
65. Leclerc BS, Blanchard L, Cantinotti M, et al. The effectiveness of interdisciplinary teams in end-of-life palliative care: A systematic review of comparative studies. *J Palliat Care.* 2014;30(1):44–54.
66. Puchalski C, Ferrell B, Virani R, et al. Improving the quality of spiritual care as a dimension of palliative care: The report of the Consensus Conference. *J Palliat Med.* 2009;12(10):885–904.
67. Pearce MJ, Coan AD, Herndon JE, 2nd, Koenig HG, Abernethy AP. Unmet spiritual care needs impact emotional and spiritual well-being in advanced cancer patients. *Suppor Care Cancer.* 2012;20(10):2269–2276.
68. Mako C, Galek K, Poppito SR. Spiritual pain among patients with advanced cancer in palliative care. *J Palliat Med.* 2006;9(5):1106–1113.
69. Delgado-Guay M, Parsons H, Hui D, et al. The impact of spirituality, religiosity, and spiritual pain in coping strategies and quality of life (QOL) of caregivers of advanced cancer patients (CACP) in the palliative care (PC) setting (717). *J Pain Symptom Manage.* 2011;41(1):282.
70. Kalet A, Pugnaire MP, Cole-Kelly K, et al. Teaching communication in clinical clerkships: Models from the Macy Initiative in Health Communications. *Acad Med.* 2004;79(6):511–520.
71. Duffy FD, Gordon GH, Whelan G, et al. Assessing competence in communication and interpersonal skills: The Kalamazoo II report. *Acad Med.* 2004;79(6):495–507.
72. Henry SG, Holmboe ES, Frankel RM. Evidence-based competencies for improving communication skills in graduate medical education: A review with suggestions for implementation. *Med Teach.* 2013;35(5):395–403.
73. Roter DL, Larson S, Fischer GS, Arnold RM, Tulsky JA. Experts practice what they preach: A descriptive study of best and normative practices in end-of-life discussions. *Arch Intern Med.* 2000;160(22):3477–3485.
74. Detering KM, Hancock AD, Reade MC, Silvester W. The impact of advance care planning on end of life care in elderly patients: Randomised controlled trial. *BMJ.* 2010;340:c1345.
75. Tang WR, Chen KY, Hsu SH, et al. Effectiveness of Japanese SHARE model in improving Taiwanese healthcare personnel's preference for cancer truth telling. *Psycho-Oncology.* 2014;23(3):259–265.
76. Wittenberg-Lyles E, Goldsmith J, Ferrell B, Burchett M. Assessment of an interprofessional online curriculum for palliative care communication training. *J Palliat Med.* 2014;17(4):400–406.
77. Keating NL, Beth Landrum M, Arora NK, et al. Cancer patients' roles in treatment decisions: Do characteristics of the decision influence roles? *J Clin Oncol.* 2010;28(28):4364–4370.
78. Smith TJ, Longo DL. Talking with patients about dying. *N Engl J Med.* 2012;367(17):1651–1652.
79. Dwamena F, Holmes-Rovner M, Gaulden CM, et al. Interventions for providers to promote a patient-centred approach in clinical consultations. *Cochrane Database Syst Rev.* 2012;12:Cd003267.
80. Fujimori M, Shirai Y, Asai M, et al. Development and preliminary evaluation of communication skills training program for oncologists based on patient preferences for communicating bad news. *Palliat Support Care.* 2014;12(5):379–386.
81. Fujimori M, Oba A, Koike M, et al. Communication skills training for Japanese oncologists on how to break bad news. *J Cancer Educ.* 2003;18(4):194–201.
82. Liu X, Rohrer W, Luo A, Fang Z, He T, Xie W. Doctor-patient communication skills training in mainland China: A systematic review of the literature. *Patient Educ Couns.* 2014;98(1):3–14.
83. West CP, Dyrbye LN, Rabatin JT, et al. Intervention to promote physician well-being, job satisfaction, and professionalism: A randomized clinical trial. *JAMA Intern Med.* 2014;174(4):527–533.

84. Innes S, Payne S. Advanced cancer patients' prognostic information preferences: A review. *Palliat Med.* 2009;23(1):29–39.
85. Walling AM, Weeks JC, Kahn KL, et al. Symptom prevalence in lung and colorectal cancer patients. *J Pain Symptom Manage.* 2015;49(2):192–202.
86. Huskamp HA, Keating NL, Malin JL, et al. Discussions with physicians about hospice among patients with metastatic lung cancer. *Arch Intern Med.* 2009;169(10):954–962.
87. Kumar P, Temel JS. End-of-life care discussions in patients with advanced cancer. *J Clin Oncol.* 2013;31(27):3315–3319.
88. Weeks JC, Catalano PJ, Cronin A, et al. Patients' expectations about effects of chemotherapy for advanced cancer. *N Engl J Med.* 2012;367(17):1616–1625.
89. Chen AB, Cronin A, Weeks JC, et al. Expectations about the effectiveness of radiation therapy among patients with incurable lung cancer. *J Clin Oncol.* 2013;31(21):2730–2735.
90. Mack JW, Weeks JC, Wright AA, Block SD, Prigerson HG. End-of-life discussions, goal attainment, and distress at the end of life: Predictors and outcomes of receipt of care consistent with preferences. *J Clin Oncol.* 2010;28(7):1203–1208.
91. Wright AA, Keating NL, Balboni TA, Matulonis UA, Block SD, Prigerson HG. Place of death: Correlations with quality of life of patients with cancer and predictors of bereaved caregivers' mental health. *J Clin Oncol.* 2010;28(29):4457–4464.
92. Garrido MM, Prigerson HG. The end-of-life experience: Modifiable predictors of caregivers' bereavement adjustment. *Cancer.* 2014;120(6):918–925.
93. Smith TJ, Dow LA, Virago EA, Khatcheressian J, Matsuyama R, Lyckholm LJ. A pilot trial of decision aids to give truthful prognostic and treatment information to chemotherapy patients with advanced cancer. *J Support Oncol.* 2011;9(2):79–86.
94. Mack JW, Wolfe J, Cook EF, Grier HE, Cleary PD, Weeks JC. Hope and prognostic disclosure. *J Clin Oncol.* 2007;25(35):5636–5642.
95. Davison SN, Simpson C. Hope and advance care planning in patients with end stage renal disease: Qualitative interview study. *BMJ.* 2006;333(7574):886.
96. Harris JC, DeAngelis CD. The power of hope. *JAMA.* 2008;300(24):2919–2920.
97. Connor SR, Pyenson B, Fitch K, Spence C, Iwasaki K. Comparing hospice and nonhospice patient survival among patients who die within a three-year window. *J Pain Symptom Manage.* 2007;33(3):238–246.
98. Saito AM, Landrum MB, Neville BA, Ayanian JZ, Weeks JC, Earle CC. Hospice care and survival among elderly patients with lung cancer. *J Palliat Med.* 2011;14(8):929–939.
99. Saito AM, Landrum MB, Neville BA, Ayanian JZ, Earle CC. The effect on survival of continuing chemotherapy to near death. *BMC Palliat Care.* 2011;10:14.
100. Christakis NA, Iwashyna TJ. The health impact of health care on families: A matched cohort study of hospice use by decedents and mortality outcomes in surviving, widowed spouses. *Soc Sci Med.* 2003;57(3):465–475.
101. Smith TJ, Temin S, Alesi ER, et al. American Society of Clinical Oncology provisional clinical opinion: The integration of palliative care into standard oncology care. *J Clin Oncol.* 2012;30(8):880–887.
102. Lee SJ, Loberiza FR, Rizzo JD, Soiffer RJ, Antin JH, Weeks JC. Optimistic expectations and survival after hematopoietic stem cell transplantation. *Biol Blood Marrow Transplant.* 2003;9(6):389–396.
103. Blackhall LJ, Murphy ST, Frank G, Michel V, Azen S. Ethnicity and attitudes toward patient autonomy. *JAMA.* 1995;274(10):820–825.
104. Foley K, Gelband H, eds. *Improving Palliative Care for Cancer.* Washington, DC: National Academy Press; 2001.
105. Gordon EJ, Daugherty CK. "Hitting you over the head": Oncologists' disclosure of prognosis to advanced cancer patients. *Bioethics.* 2003;17(2):142–168.
106. Rogg L, Aasland OG, Graugaard PK, Loge JH. Direct communication, the unquestionable ideal? Oncologists' accounts of communication of bleak prognoses. *Psycho-Oncology.* 2010;19(11):1221–1228.
107. Panagopoulou E, Mintziori G, Montgomery A, Kapoukranidou D, Benos A. Concealment of information in clinical practice: Is lying less stressful than telling the truth? *J Clin Oncol.* 2008;26(7):1175–1177.
108. Barrere C, Durkin A. Finding the right words: The experience of new nurses after ELNEC education integration into a BSN curriculum. *Medsurg Nurs.* 2014;23(1):35–43, 53.
109. Back AL, Arnold RM, Baile WF, et al. Efficacy of communication skills training for giving bad news and discussing transitions to palliative care. *Arch Intern Med.* 2007;167(5):453–460.
110. Bylund CL, Brown RF, Bialer PA, Levin TT, Lubrano di Ciccone B, Kissane DW. Developing and implementing an advanced communication training program in oncology at a comprehensive cancer center. *J Cancer Educ.* 2011;26(4):604–611.

CHAPTER 8

Communication in Palliative Nursing

Constance M. Dahlin

Introduction

Mike is a registered nurse in the neurological outpatient clinic. Sarah Smith is a 46-year-old woman with progressive weakness and difficulty swallowing. Mike is meeting her for the first time when she comes in for a complete work-up for diagnostic purposes.

MIKE: Good morning, Ms. Smith. My name is Mike, and I am a registered nurse. I work with the neurological team. I will be your primary nurse.
SARAH: Good morning. What is a primary nurse?
MIKE: It means I will be the main nurse you deal with. But I work with a team, so when I am not here, the rest of the team will be there for you. How are you doing today?
SARAH: I am a little nervous. There is so much going on, and I have seen so many people. I keep getting asked questions and doing tests.
MIKE: I can imagine that has been hard. In order for me to get to know you, can you tell me the history of your weakness?
SARAH: Well, over the last three or four months, I started to have more difficulty walking with weakness and tiredness. I thought I was working too hard, was just stressed, and needed a vacation. But time off did not help. I also began to start coughing, when I drank certain liquids. That was scary.
MIKE: So when did you contact your healthcare team about these symptoms?
SARAH: After two months, when nothing helped.
MIKE: Do you have any friends or family who are part of your care?
SARAH: My family is there for me.
MIKE: Are they here with you today?
SARAH: No, I am here alone today.
MIKE: Okay. Do you want to include them in today's visit with the team by phone?
SARAH: I had not thought of that; that would be helpful, so they can hear everything.
MIKE: What else do you need right now, before we start to review everything?
SARAH: Nothing, right now.
MIKE: Okay, feel free to interrupt me, or ask any questions at any point.

The American Nurses Association (ANA) defines nursing as "the protection, promotion, and optimization of health and abilities, prevention of illness and injury, alleviation of suffering through the diagnosis and treatment of human response, and advocacy in the care of individuals, families, communities, and populations."[1–3] While the science of nursing is grounded in nursing process, the art of nursing lies in caring, compassion, and communication.[4] A palliative care patient has many areas to which the nurse must attend: the patient's and family's response to a serious illness, management of the effects of a serious and often life-limiting illness, administration of treatments related to the condition as well as side effects, and the patient's and family's psychosocial issues of coping with serious illness and the inherent losses.[5] The nurse accompanies the patient and family through the illness journey providing support, caring, compassion, continuous presence, and hope.[4]

Nurse communication is the basis of quality palliative care, and a nurse's ability to collaborate within the circle of care that includes the patient, family, and healthcare team is essential. In palliative care, relief of suffering is achieved through person-centered and family-focused assessment and attention to all the aspects of quality of life—the spiritual, emotional, and social aspects of care as well as the physical and psychological. Indeed, through compassionate care and communication, the nurse is able to create a protective environment in which the patient and family can deal with the crisis and stress resulting from an advanced illness diagnosis.[6] In the report, *Dying in America: Improving Quality and Honoring Individual Preferences Near the End of Life,* communication is emphasized as an essential component to providing respectful care, delivering pain and symptom management, and alleviating suffering while honoring a patient's values, goals, and preferences.[7]

The ANA's Nursing: Scope and Standards of Practice directly addresses a nurse's responsibility to (a) assess communication format preferences of patients, families, and colleagues; (b) assess his or her own communication skills; (c) convey information to patients, families, and the interdisciplinary team; (d) maintain communication to promote safe and effective transfers of care; and (e) provide professional perspective in healthcare discussions.[1] The ANA also addresses the nurse's responsibility for the care of patients with serious advanced illness in two documents. In the *Nursing Care and Do Not Resuscitate (DNR) and Allow Natural Death (AND) Decisions* Position Statement, the organization clearly states, "Nurses must advocate for and play an active role in initiating discussions about DNR with patients, families, and members of the health care team."[8] The *Registered Nurses' Roles and Responsibilities in Providing Expert Care and Counseling at the End of Life* Position Statement further describes the goal of

> **Box 8.1** Hospice and Palliative Nurses Association Communication Competencies for Palliative Nursing[11]
>
> The hospice and palliative registered nurse communicates effectively in a variety of formats in all areas of practice.
>
> The hospice and palliative registered nurse uses effective verbal, nonverbal, and written communication with patients and families, interdisciplinary team members, and the community in order to therapeutically address and accurately convey the palliative needs of patients and families.
>
> The hospice and palliative registered nurse communicates with the patient, family, the interdisciplinary team, and healthcare providers regarding patient care and the provision of that care. The nurse facilitates an interdisciplinary process.
>
> Extracted from ANA and HPNA (2014).[11]

nursing involvement as "The counseling a nurse provides regarding end-of-life choices and preferences for individuals facing life-limiting illness, as well as throughout the patient's life span, honors patient autonomy, and helps to prepare individuals and families for difficult decisions that may lie ahead."[9]

Within the specialty of palliative nursing, the Hospice and Palliative Nurses Association (HPNA) in collaboration with the ANA delineates communication throughout palliative nursing. In *Palliative Nursing: Scope and Standards of Practice*, communication is an essential competency and is expected in all aspects of care.[10] Box 8.1 provides an overview of HPNA's Palliative Nursing Communication Competencies. The HPNA position statement *The Nurse's Role in Advanced Care Planning* also acknowledges the critical role of the hospice and palliative nurse to advocate, educate, and support a patient's right to self-determination, autonomy, and dignity. In particular, the nurse's recognition of the patient as

Table 8.1 Nurse Communication Tasks Delineated by the National Consensus Project for Quality Palliative Care *Clinical Practice Guidelines*[12]

Domain	Communication Focus	Nurse Actions
Domain 1—Structure and Processes	◆ Emphasis on interdisciplinary team engagement, collaboration with patients and families, and coordinated assessment and continuity of care across healthcare settings	◆ Participates in assessment of the patient to determine evolving needs and preferences of the patient and family, with recognition of the complex, competing, and shifting priorities in goals of care ◆ Collaborates to contribute to the evolving care plan ◆ Participates in team discussions and reviews care plan ◆ Seeks skill development in communication
Domain 2—Physical Aspects of Care	◆ Collaborative assessment and treatment of physical symptoms, treatment options for common conditions, in context of respect for goals of care of the patient and family	◆ Uses symptom assessment instruments for consistent evaluation ◆ Identifies and utilizes tools for adults with cognitive impairment and of neonates, children, or adolescents when necessary
Domain 3—Psychological and Psychiatric Aspects of Care	◆ Collaborative assessment process of psychological concerns and psychiatric diagnoses, treatment options for common conditions, in context of respect for goals of care of the patient and family	◆ Uses verbal, nonverbal, and/or symbolic means appropriate to the patient, with particular attention to patients with cognitive impairment and the developmental stage and cognitive capacity of neonates, children, and adolescents
Domain 4—Social Aspects of Care	◆ Interdisciplinary and collaboration engagement with patients and families to identify and support patient and family strengths	◆ Communicates within the circle of care—patient, family, and healthcare team
Domain 5—Spiritual, Existential, and Religious Aspects of Care	◆ Interdisciplinary exploration, assessment, and attention to spiritual issues of the patient and family	◆ Communicates with the patient and family in respectful manner with attention to religious and spiritual beliefs, rituals, and practices
Domain 6—Cultural Aspects of Care	◆ Assessment of culture as a source of resilience and strength for the patient and family	◆ Elicits cultural identifications, strengths, concerns, and needs of the patient and family with sensitivity. ◆ Communicates in a language and manner that the patient and family understand
Domain 7—Care of the Patient at End of Life	◆ Communicates signs and symptoms of the dying process to patient, family, and all other involved health providers, as well as family guidance as to what to expect in the dying process and the post-death period	◆ Identifies and communicates the signs and symptoms of patients at the end of life ◆ Meets the physical, psychosocial, spiritual, social, and cultural needs of patients and families
Domain 8—Ethical and Legal Aspects of Care	◆ Ongoing discussion about goals of care along with completion and documentation of advance care planning ◆ Identification and resolution of commonly encountered ethical issues as well as complex legal and regulatory issues that arise in palliative care	◆ Promotes understanding of the patient's preferences for care across the care continuum ◆ Articulates complex situations and problem-solves with interdisciplinary team

Note. Created from National Consensus Project 2013.[12]

an individual with diverse personal, religious, and cultural value systems is emphasized in the development of respectful relationships with patients, families, and colleagues.[11] Implied within this statement is the recognition that the nurse must differentiate his or her own individual values from those of the patient and family. In appreciation and support of the patient's and family's values, preferences, and wishes, the nurse is the ultimate advocate.

Finally, the National Consensus Project for Quality Palliative Care's *Clinical Practice Guidelines* emphasizes the importance of communication across the eight domains of palliative care. From person-focused and family-centered care planning, to physical and psychological symptom assessment, to social, spiritual, and cultural aspects of care throughout the stage of advanced illness, communication serves as the basis of palliative nursing.[12] Indeed, communication is the cornerstone of palliative care and acts as a healthcare intervention in and of itself.[13] Table 8.1[12] summarizes nurse communication tasks delineated by the *Clinical Practice Guidelines*.

Nurse Communication

The nurse plays a pivotal role in accompanying the patient through an illness journey, providing care that creates a healing environment. Often, the nurse is the initial direct professional caregiver and the first to identify issues for patients with life-threatening illness. Undoubtedly, early nurse–patient communication is critical to alleviate physical and psychosocial distress in a sustained fashion.[14] Through patient care and constant clinical presence, either at the bedside or office, the nurse often has the best opportunity to listen and attend to the patient's hopes, fears, dreams, and regrets. This patient rapport affords hospice and palliative nurses the unique role of facilitating care throughout the illness trajectory. Indeed, the nurse's presence may be a healing intervention all of its own. Nonetheless, important features of communication include providing information about treatment options and advance care planning while considering the patient's values, preferences, and beliefs. The nurse may encounter other issues related to goals of care, conflict between the wishes of the patient and those of the family, and opinions about the use of life-sustaining measures.

On both sides of the nurse–patient relationship, the importance of communication cannot be underestimated. Patients and families state that communication is one of the most important clinical skills.[15] Nurses acknowledge that it is their most important competency.[16] Within the nurse–patient relationship, the nurse employs a variety of communication modalities—verbal interaction, nonverbal modalities, and therapeutic presence. Verbal skills include keen conversational proficiency in areas such as conversational style, facilitative communication, active listening, voice tone, word choice, and even humor.[17] Nonverbal communication takes place through two modalities: (a) the physical—eye contact, smile, the use of touch, and (b) the interactive engagement styles—encouragement, presence, empathy, and respect.[17] These communication elements form the core of therapeutic presence or deliberate-focused attention. It has been suggested that the most beneficial nursing communication includes facilitative communication that incorporates the therapeutic use of both self- and patient-centered care.[18]

Communication is essential to establish a trusting relationship and improve the patient's experience.[19,20] The therapeutic use of self involves the creation of a trusting relationship in which a patient can discuss any topic without judgment; establishing mutual respect between the patient, the family, and the nurse; and promoting continuity of care, as well as allowing time for full exploration of values, concerns, and understanding of perspectives. Therapeutic presence includes attending to suffering, affirming the patient's self-worth and dignity, decreasing isolation, facilitating identification and clarification of treatment goals, promoting advance care planning and enhancing holistic care,[21] along with other behaviors such as active and passive listening and supportive counseling.[22] This presence results in empathy and understanding of suffering—specifically creating a psychologically safe space to discuss difficult issues.[14] This therapeutic relationship provides the nurse with the context to assess the patient's and family's response to the diagnosis or the particular events within a patient encounter.

Similar to Maslow's hierarchy of needs, there is a hierarchy of communication between nurses and patients. The most fundamental communication level begins with the nurse's assessment of the patient's daily living activities or the explanation of health-related tasks. On a simple level, this may involve small talk or discussion of basic treatment issues, such as pain medication schedules, daily living activities, or personal care. Examples include:

Introductions: My name is Sam, and I am your nurse today.

Directions: I will be taking your vital signs; please tell me which arm to use.

Closed-ended questions: Do you take any medications? How often?

On a higher level, nurses may assess pain, symptoms, and treatments through either open or closed questions. Open-ended questions are best, in which the nurse approaches the patient in a manner that allows the patient to honestly evaluate his or her response to treatments. In this way, the nurse may gain more specific information concerning treatment effectiveness, distress, or pain. Examples of opening questions include:

What concerns do you have about the disease/treatment/medication?

How do you think the treatment is working?

How is your pain/symptom affecting you/your family?

How is your pain/function affecting your quality of life?

What is your average day/night like?

The highest and most complex level of communication is the existential level. Communication at this level is sensitive, and the patient reveals a sense of self, often nuanced around existential aspects of end of life, including disclosure, the search for meaning, and suffering.[20] Exploration at this level can help a patient live with a life-threatening illness, achieving both quality of life and psychological healing.[23] Examples include:

What sustains you in difficult times?

Where do you find support?

What brings you joy/comfort?

What gives you meaning in life?

What are you most proud of?

Goldsmith and colleagues describe nurse interactions consisting of both task and relational communication.[24] Tasks include offering information and providing physical care, whereas relational includes providing support, comfort, and caring. Although rarely emphasized but implied, emotional intelligence is essential for communication and relationship-building. The process of emotional intelligence includes the ability to (a) correctly identify one's own emotions, (b) use emotions to facilitate reasoning, (c) understand emotions, and (d) manage emotions.[25] Within nursing, emotional intelligence pertains to self-awareness of emotional responses and the ability to cope with suffering as well as comfort level in addressing suffering in all its manifestations.[14] This may affect the ability to offer therapeutic presence in difficult situations such as: the patient with intractable pain, symptoms, and complex family issues; the patient who is dying with necrotic wounds; the patient who is dying from copious bleeding; or the young patient with horrible fungal lesions.

The Nurse–Patient Relationship

Palliative care communication begins with the patient and family at diagnosis and continues with the family through the death of the patient and into bereavement. Research has examined communication in the nurse–patient encounter. One study on the focus of nursing communication grouped nurse–patient encounters into the following themes: exploration of patient concerns, provision of support, enhancement of disclosure, educational preparation, and referral for further counseling, as appropriate.[26] Another study examined patient perceptions of nursing communication to determine elements that would be perceived as positive or negative. Satisfactory encounters included a nurse's use of compassion, responsiveness, and dedication, whereas unsatisfactory communication included sparseness, conflict, contradiction, increasing only when things were close to the end.[27]

The nurse–patient relationship is comprised of three stages: introductory, middle, and termination.[28] The introductory phase is the formation of the nurse–patient relationship during which the nurse and patient shape their relationship. The middle phase is the working relationship, in which the essence of care occurs; it centers on treatment planning, then moves to pain and symptom management, and last to the meaning of life, legacy work, and family work. The termination phase is the third and final phase, in which the patient and nurse separate due to death or change of care location. Tasks for each phase are summarized in Table 8.2.[28]

The initial communication or introductory phase starts at diagnosis with the introduction of the nurse as a member of the care team. Over the first several encounters, the patient and nurse establish a working relationship. Mutual assessment occurs as the nurse and the patient learn about each other's styles. The patient determines the nurse's communication style and begins to work within that context.[28] Specifically, the nurse assesses the patient's communication requirements in terms of learning styles and information needs. Nursing tasks include exploring the patient's understanding of his or her illness, his or her personality and coping styles, identifying the patient's values and care preferences, and determining whether any advance care planning documents exist.

Patient education is based on learning style. Types of learning styles include visual, auditory, or kinesthetic (a mixture of both). The nurse's learning style often differs from the patient's learning style. Nursing assessment of learning style includes fundamental communication issues such as literacy, numeracy (capacity for numerical thought and expression), and native language. In addition, the nurse factors in the patient's age and cognitive development, which affects the patient's ability to learn and to understand the seriousness of the illness. Children and patients with cognitive impairment may need concurrent support from family or other support persons.

The secondary stage of the nurse–patient relationship is the working phase and often extends over long periods of time, from months to years. During this time, the nurse focuses on the disease trajectory of the life-limiting illness, offering supportive care. This care centers on the impact of and the patient's adaptation to the diagnosis of the serious, life-threatening illness. Communication between the patient and the nurse covers a range of topics, including information on the condition, treatment, and disease management.[29] Through assessment and therapeutic presence, the nurse

Table 8.2 Stages of the Nurse–Patient Relationship[28]

Stage	Nurse Tasks	Patient Tasks
Initial or Introductory Phase	1. Exploring patient/family understanding of illness 2. Determining personality, coping, and learning styles 3. Eliciting presence of advanced care planning	1. Establishing trust and understanding with the nurse
Working Phase	1. Monitoring patient response to illness 2. Providing clinical care 3. Delivering treatment 4. Offering illness/treatment education	1. Establishing care plan in collaboration with team 2. Participating in care 3. Providing information on response to therapy
Termination	1. Saying goodbye 2. Telling the patient what he or she meant to them or taught them 3. Assisting with transition	1. Saying goodbye 2. Showing appreciation to nurse and other staff 3. Assisting with transition

Note. Adapted from Perrin (2010).[28]

gains insight into patient and family coping and provides a supportive environment in which patients are able to articulate their needs, concerns, and perceptions of care.

During the working phase, the nurse focuses on three critical communication tasks in palliative and end-of-life care: (a) creating an environment conducive to communication, (b) promoting physician and patient interaction, and (c) facilitating family and patient interaction.[30] This is best achieved through a primary nursing model that allows the nurse to have a consistent and constant relationship with the patient. The nurse's steady presence in team meetings regarding changes in the patient's condition, disease progression, treatment modifications, and end-stage disease is paramount. The nurse participates in team discussions, provides consistent information to the healthcare team, and facilitates follow-up using similar language and shared information used in the team discussion.

As the patient enters the dying process, the termination phase commences and the nurse and the patient begin to separate. The nurse supports patient and family decision-making, provides information about the dying process, and offers consolation in anticipatory grieving. The nurse is continually present for the patient and family in the difficult times.[27] In addition, he or she ensures the patient's comfort, dignity, and avoidance of suffering. The nurse acknowledges his or her relationship with the patient and its changing nature. The nurse and the patient often engage in appreciation of each other. For the patient, this may take the form of expressing gratitude for the nurse's care; for the nurse, he or she may express what the patient has meant to the nurse and lessons learned in the course of the patient's care. In this way, the nurse and patient achieve closure for their relationship, as the patient dies.

The Nurse–Family Relationship

During the illness, nurse–family communication centers on alleviation of the patient's physical and psychological pain and symptoms. During and immediately following the patient's death, the nurse engages in a parallel process with the family and the patient, assisting the family with closure, while also assisting the patient's transition from life to death. Finally, the nurse provides grief and bereavement resources for the family.

Since palliative care is family-centered, the nurse must also consider the needs of the patient's family system. Evidence suggests that families desire consistent and routine communication with a compassionate presence.[31] Family members value helpful explanations and consistency with detailed explanations. One study found that families preferred and valued the following behaviors: (a) being kept informed, (b) receiving assurance, (c) having a compassionate presence from nurses, (d) receiving assistance from nurses in the facilitation of final acts, and (e) having acts that honor the patient's dignity.[15] On the other end of the spectrum, families feel frustrated by sparse or infrequent communication, contradictory communication, conflicting communication between providers, or communication that occurs only when a situation is very serious.[27]

Nurses must balance between patient and family care needs, offering comfort or promoting control. This may be a challenge as families may cause conflict, induce anxiety, or promote excessive or unfounded optimism.[32] In particular, families may interfere with patient autonomy, particularly if families disagree with patient choices. Another challenge is communication norms within a family system. Patients and families may protect each other from painful information. Usually, it is best to focus on the patient's needs and wishes and to continually bring those to the forefront of conversations. Informing and reminding the family of the patient's wishes helps ensure that these wishes form the basis of care. If a nurse is told not to discuss certain topics, he or she should explore and examine the reason for the request with the person making the request.[33] Overall, the nurse acts as a patient advocate within the family, while simultaneously acting as a patient and family advocate within the healthcare system.

Common Conversations for Nurses

For nurses, common conversations include initiating and participating in advance care planning and family meetings and sharing poor or serious prognoses/diagnoses. Note that there may be differences in how conversations occur at the registered nurse level and the advanced practice nurse level, which is predicated on scope of practice. Advance care planning conversations entail three components. The first is the delegation of a surrogate decision-maker, also known as a healthcare durable power of attorney or a healthcare proxy. Here the nurse elicits from the patient whom the patient would like to act in his or her best interest, if he or she is unable to do so. A question the nurse may ask is, "Have you ever thought about whom you would want to make decisions, if you were unable to do so?" As part of the process, the nurse encourages the patient to talk with the surrogate decision-maker about his or her wishes. It is important for nurses to convey the message that the advance care planning process allows patients more autonomy over their healthcare.[34] This is one way nurses can empower patients.

The second element of advance care planning conversations includes advance directives or living wills. These documents state or explain the patient's wishes for medical care, if he or she is unable to offer direction. The nurse asks, "Have you completed any forms about your treatment preferences in various health situations?" There is not one universally recognized form in every state, because each state differs in its recognition of advance directives and surrogate decision-makers. Common documents include *Making Choices*[35] and a companion guide for the role of the nurse in advance care planning from Gunderson Health System,[36] *Five Wishes* from Aging with Dignity,[37] and *Advance Directives* from Project Grace.[38] Many are available in languages other than English. Each form has its own advantages and disadvantages in terms of specificity and complexity. It is best for nurses to get to know one form and use it consistently.

The third element of advance care planning is the completion of a document that records the patient's wishes regarding life-sustaining treatments, both in the acute setting or outside the hospital. Inpatient orders are recorded as code status. Out-of-hospital orders include documents known as comfort care orders, allow natural death orders, or provider/physician/medical orders for life-sustaining treatment forms. These documents vary by state, specificity, and which life-sustaining measures are included. They are not stand-alone documents and should accompany advance directives and surrogate decision-making forms.

When providing information and assisting completion of out-of-hospital orders, the nurse faces the challenge of providing realistic information and statistics about the success of cardiac/pulmonary resuscitation in persons with advanced, serious, life-limiting illness. In addition, due to cultural and generational differences, the nurse must determine whether to discuss the overall treatment in the context of the patient's definition of quality of life or by specific life-sustaining intervention. As a result, these conversations are often nuanced and best done with the patient and his or her family. Everyone present then hears the patient's goals, wishes, and preferences, which promote consistent understanding.

Family meetings are a vehicle for comprehensive, respectful, thorough, and timely communication between patients, families, and healthcare providers. The registered nurse and the advanced practice nurse can facilitate family dialogue on a range of topics.[23] Subject matters range from disease-specific information, disease trajectory, treatment options, caregiving issues, psychosocial support, discharge planning, and death planning.[39] There are several steps for effective meetings. First, the nurse considers the patient's and family's environment, specifically ensuring patient and family physical and emotional comfort when initiating discussions. Second, the nurse is deliberate in setting the right atmosphere in which patient–family discussions occur. Third, the nurse asks for permission to talk. Fourth, the nurse begins a meeting with open-ended questions, listening, and validating through verbal and nonverbal communication. Fifth, the nurse elicits both patient and family concerns and fosters hope.[6]

Giving prognosis or sharing a serious illness diagnosis often includes discussions about disease progression, recurrence, or advanced illness. The nurse first needs to offer a warning comment such as, "I thought I would have better news," "I have difficult news to share," or "Unfortunately, I have bad news." The nurse then gives the medical information. At that point, the nurse is silent and waits for the patient and family to respond. Thereafter, the nurse responds to any emotional affect and offers support. Depending on the situation, the nurse may offer more information. Usually, however, the patient and family are in a state of shock or surprise and unable to absorb anything beyond the new information. The nurse should offer follow-up support and a plan for future conversations. It is then incumbent for the nurse to share the patient response with the team.

Role of the Nurse on the Interdisciplinary Team

In order to promote comprehensive palliative care and continuity of care, collaboration with other healthcare providers is essential. The nurse must work within an interprofessional team. Since palliative care members work together on patient and family issues, communication is vital to create a consistent plan of care. There may be team members who do not understand the value of communication for the team and for effective healthcare.[40] The Institute of Medicine describes how effective communication is part of team-based healthcare.[40] Moreover, effective communication ultimately improves both the quality of healthcare and patient care as well as team collaboration.[41]

Nurses are consistently rated by the public as one of the most trusted members of the healthcare team.[42] From home, to outpatient clinics, to the hospital, along with homeless shelters, long-term care facilities, and correctional facilities, nurses have the most consistent and continual presence for patients and families throughout the healthcare continuum. They are afforded many opportunities to initiate and stimulate conversations about goals of care, treatment, and prognosis. By virtue of their position, nurses make important observations about patient and family concerns. In this way, nurses act as translators between care providers and between team members and patients and families.[43,44]

Communication must be a shared value within a care team with a mutual commitment to team-based care. The team must have consistent channels for candid and complete communication.[40] Specifically, all team members are accountable for promoting the values of honesty, creativity, humility, and curiosity, both within the team and in patient care.[32] In this way, the team prioritizes and continually refines its own communication skills. In practice, this is achieved by sustained and deliberate strategies such as creating regular meeting times and scheduled interactions, having private space to interact, and providing support for face-to-face meetings. Such meetings include communication training, clinical care discussions, and team process, although there are separate meetings for each area.[45] Communication within the team is achieved through attention to team processes related to clinical care, team process in performing the work, and interpersonal interactions. With clear communication practices, a team can more effectively examine the collaboration of the team in all aspects of care: clinical, educational, and administrative realms. It should be noted that team communication is always a work in progress and needs the team members' focused attention.

Barriers to Nurse Communication

Communication barriers for nurses range from personal to educational and professional factors. Personal challenges include an individual's personality, cultural norms, and fears.[46] Shy or introverted nurses may be uncomfortable asking too many questions as they feel they are being too inquisitive or intrusive. Another nurse may have been raised in a culture in which it is inappropriate to ask personal questions or probe certain topics such as advanced illness, death, and dying. Or perhaps asking patients and families any questions on uncomfortable topics may cause the nurse personal distress.

The issue of confident and competent nursing practice as well as comfort in being true to one's own emotions brings its own challenge. In palliative nursing, the nature of the topics are inherently difficult, since they deal with diagnosis, advanced disease, dying, and death. A nurse may fear failure as a provider with any display of emotions in front of a patient, family, or other healthcare provider. In order to keep the facade of strength, the nurse may avoid any emotionally laden conversations. Finally, the nurse may have experienced a significant unresolved loss. This may make it impossible to attend for him or her to emotional laden issues or conversations such as loss, grief, death, or dying[45] for fear they will evoke too much emotion.

Educational challenges in palliative nursing are significant. Little is known about communication in nursing or the unique elements of nursing communication, since the majority of research in healthcare communication has focused on physicians.[46] This results in a lack of information that could promote excellence in nursing specific communication. Moreover, few schools of nursing offer discrete skills in the care of seriously ill patients, let alone palliative care. Ironically, the result is that although nurses are essential care providers, they have had little exposure to death, dying, and communication.[16,47] Finally, in the younger generation of nurses, communication occurs through social media, that is, through the written word via texting, e-mailing, tweeting, and chat forums. Given that there is no place even in the larger global community to practice verbal communication skills, many younger nurses have had little exposure to or practice with verbal communication, resulting in discomfort. Moreover, many of these nurses have difficulty translating the rules of social media and technology into the professional realm of healthcare.

Professional issues result from inadequate nursing education and role ambiguity. With little to no preparation, nurses often learn palliative communication skills through trial and error with patient care, rather than by mentored leaning. Because of lack of experience, some nurses worry that they do not have the skill or correct verbiage to engage the patient and family in palliative care topics. Specifically, they may fear that bringing up issues related to death and dying will cause too much emotional distress to the patient and family.[45] Some nurses are concerned that talking about palliative issues will result in patient and family conflict.[32] The consequence is either that they learn on their own or they do "just-in-time" learning for a particular situation but do not have an overall concept of clinical communication.

Within the professional role of nursing and healthcare, nurses may feel a lack of autonomy or authority within an organization or a professional culture to talk about difficult issues.[43] Even when nurses are comfortable communicating about palliative topics, they often feel marginalized or disempowered to have difficult conversations because only physicians are allowed to initiate these conversations in their setting.[43] Being constrained by their colleagues or their institution means that nurses perceive that initiating palliative care conversations with patients and/or families will cause discord with their colleagues.[34] This leads to poor healthcare delivery since communication is vital to quality care.

Last, many nurses lack perspective about the importance of palliative care communication.[34] Nurses may underestimate the importance of their role or decide that avoiding palliative communication is less labor intensive. Though communication is clearly embedded in nursing practice under the roles of clinical care, advocacy, and education, many nurses deliberately abdicate their important communication role. The result is a loss of the nurse's potential engagement with patients on meaningful and necessary topics. But, more important, the patient receives inadequate care and support at the time he or she may need it most.

Nurses as Change Agents

Palliative nurse communication promotes better outcomes and higher patient family satisfaction.[48] Moreover, it can promote quality of life through less aggressive care and improve bereavement care for families. Many opportunities exist for skilled nursing communication to improve individual patient care as well as clinical care. Current efforts to improve nursing communication include education, role preparation, and cultural changes. End of Life Nursing Education Consortium (ELNEC) courses within an organization, either as a part of orientation or as ongoing education, may be an effective method to improve nursing communication.

The first place to promote quality nursing communication is within nursing education. Many baccalaureate programs are filled with the essentials of biology, physiology, pathophysiology, and nursing skills. Few programs focus on communication or even use a communication skills lab. In addition, case studies focusing on necessary elements of communication in palliative care scenarios are uncommon for undergraduates. Nurses therefore have little opportunity to practice their communication skills until they start seeing patients. When they are assigned palliative patients in clinical rotations, the emphasis is on evaluating the nurse's success/performance with regard to clinical skills rather than their communication skills. Again, there is little experience in palliative communication. When nurses graduate, they may be in preceptorships or orientation partnerships. This may be the first time they have to deal with palliative patients and issues. Therefore, the value of nursing communication as a skill must be demonstrated through mentoring during entry of the novice or advanced beginner into palliative nursing.[49]

Communication within the workplace sets an important tone. A culture of respect for all disciplines within the care team is paramount. Providing communication education empowers nurses to actively participate in teams. Communication as part of orientation and ongoing education is important too. It allows the nurse to utilize communication as a therapeutic and essential aspect of palliative nursing. It promotes an open environment, thereby improving care. The result is more effective nursing communication as a whole, which positively affects nurse retention.[25]

An environment with skilled nurse communicators benefits patients as well. An organization that believes in advance care planning can promote early conversations to guide care. Nurses are empowered by education in advance care planning conversations as this is part of the nursing process. Nurses who encourage palliative conversations early in the disease trajectory ultimately promote patient autonomy, facilitating patients as full partners in their care by understanding their choices. Additionally, these conversations allow the formation of supportive relationships before advanced disease develops and enables proactive patient/family education.[22]

Conclusion

The basis of nursing is to protect, promote, and optimize health; prevent illness and injury; and alleviate suffering.[1,2] Communication is the foundation of palliative care and forms the basis of palliative nursing. Through therapeutic presence and skilled communication strategies, nurses establish strong nurse–patient relationships. Facilitative communication allows nurses to promote informed patient and family decision-making around their healthcare treatment options. The result is empowered patient and families as active participants in their care. Additionally, palliative care is by nature interdisciplinary, and nurses have a prominent role in the collaborative care of patients. Team collaboration, along with skilled communication, enhances the quality of patient care. The nurse is essential in achieving this outcome through the art of caring, compassion, and communication.

References

1. American Nurses Association. *Nursing: Scope and Standards of Practice*. 2nd ed. Silver Spring, MD: American Nurses Association; 2010.
2. American Nurses Association. *Social Policy Statement*. Silver Spring, MD: American Nurses Association; 2010.
3. American Nurses Association. What is nursing? http://www.nursingworld.org/especiallyforyou/what-is-nursing. Published 2013. Accessed September 26, 2014.
4. Palos G. Care, compassion, and communication in professional nursing: Art, science, or both. *Clin J Oncol Nurs*. 2014;18(2):247–248.
5. Chochinov H, Hassard T, McClement S, et al. The landscape of distress in the terminally ill. *J Pain Symptom Manage*. 2009;38(5):641–649.
6. Dahlin C, Wittenberg E. Communication in palliative care: An essential competency for nurses. In: Ferrell BR, Coyle N, Paice N, eds. *Oxford Textbook of Palliative Nursing*. 4th ed. New York, NY: Oxford University Press; 2015;81–109.
7. Institute of Medicine. *Dying in America: Improving Quality and Honoring Individual Preferences Near End of Life*. Washington, DC: National Academies Press; 2014.
8. American Nurses Association. Position statement: Nursing care and do not resuscitate (DNR) and allow natural death (AND) decisions. http://www.nursingworld.org/MainMenuCategories/EthicsStandards/Ethics-Position-Statements.aspx. Published 2012. Accessed September 26, 2014.
9. American Nurses Association. Position statement—Registered nurses' roles and responsibilities in providing expert care and counseling at the end of life. http://www.nursingworld.org/MainMenuCategories/EthicsStandards/Ethics-Position-Statements/etpain14426.pdf. Published 2010. Accessed September 26, 2014.
10. American Nurses Association and Hospice and Palliative Nurses Association. *Palliative Nursing: Scope and Standards of Practice: An Essential Resource for Hospice and Palliative Nurses*. 5th ed. Silver Spring, MD: American Nurses Association and Hospice and Palliative Nurses Association; 2014.
11. Hospice and Palliative Nurses Association. Position statement: The nurse's role in advanced care planning. www.hpna.org/DisplayPage.aspx?Title=Position. Published 2011. Accessed September 26, 2014.
12. National Consensus Project for Quality Palliative Care. *Clinical Practice Guidelines for Quality Palliative Care*. 3rd ed. Pittsburgh, PA: National Consensus Project; 2013.
13. Gramling R, Norton S, Ladwig S, et al. Direct observation of prognosis communication in palliative care: A descriptive study. *J Pain Symptom Manage*. 2013;45(2):202–212.
14. Lynch M, Dahlin C, Hultman T, Coakley E. Palliative care nursing: Defining the discipline? *J Hosp Palliat Nurs*. 2011;13(2):106–111.
15. Williams B, Lewis D, Burgio KL, Goode P. "Wrapped in their arms": Next-of-kin's perceptions of how hospital nursing staff support family presence before, during, and after the death of a loved one. *J Hosp Palliat Nurs*. 2012;14(8):541–550.
16. White K, Coyne P. Nurses' perceptions of educational gaps in delivering end-of-life care. *Oncol Nurs Forum*. 2011;38(6):711–717.
17. Martins C, Basto M. Relieving the Suffering of end of life patients: A grounded theory study. *J Hosp Palliat Nurs*. 2011;13(3):161–171.
18. Cloyes K, Berry P, Reblin M, Clayton M, Ellington L. Exploring communication patterns among hospice nurses and family caregivers. *J Hosp Palliat Nurs*. 2012;14(6):426–437.
19. Buckman R. *Practical Plans for Difficult Conversations in Medicine*. Baltimore, MD: Johns Hopkins University Press; 2010.
20. Ferrell BR, Coyle N. *The Nature of Suffering and the Goals of Nursing*. New York, NY: Oxford University Press; 2008.
21. Krammer L, Hanks-Bell M J, Cappleman J. Therapeutic Presence. In: Panke J, Coyne P, eds. *Conversations in Palliative Care*. 3rd ed. Pittsburgh, PA: Hospice and Palliative Nurses Association; 2011:45–52.
22. Boyd D, Merkh K, Rutledge D, Randall V. Nurses' perceptions and experiences with end-of-life communication and care. *Oncol Nurs Forum*. 2011;38(3):229–239.
23. Dahlin C, Kelley J, Jackson V, Temel J. Early palliative care for lung cancer: Improving quality of life and increasing survival. *Int J Palliat Nurs*. 2010;16(9):420–423.
24. Goldsmith J, Ferrell B, Wittenberg-Lyles E, Ragan S. Palliative care communication in oncology nursing. *Clin J Oncol Nurs*. 2012;17(2):163–167.
25. Codier E, Munero L, Frietas E. Emotional intelligence abilities in oncology and palliative care. *J Hosp Palliat Nurs*. 2011;13(3):183–188.
26. Sheldon L, Hilaire D, Berry D. Provider verbal response to patient distress cure during ambulatory oncology visits. *Oncol Nurs Forum*. 2011;38(3):369–375.
27. Waldrop D, Meeker MA, Kerr C, Skretny J, Tangeman J, Milch R. The nature and timing of family-provider communication in late-stage cancer: A qualitative study of caregivers' experiences. *J Pain Symptom Manage*. 2012;43(2):182–194.
28. Perrin K. Communicating with seriously ill and dying patients, their families and their health care providers. In: Matzo M, Sherman DW, eds. *Palliative Care Nursing: Quality Care to the End-of-Life*. 3rd ed. New York, NY: Springer; 2010:169–185.
29. Carter N, Bryant-Lukosius D, Dicenso A, Blythe J, Neville A. The supportive care needs of men with advanced prostate cancer. *Oncol Nurs Forum*. 2011;38(2):189–198.
30. Pierce S. Improving end-of-life care: Gathering questions from family members. *Oncol Nurs Forum*. 1999;34(2):5–14.
31. Hebert R, Schulz R, Copeland V, Arnold R. Preparing family caregivers for death and bereavement: Insights from caregivers of terminally ill patients. *J Pain Symptom Manage*. 2009;37(1):3–12.
32. Beckstrand R, Collette J, Callister L, Luthy K. Oncology nurses' obstacles and supportive behaviors in end-of-life care: Providing vital family Care. *Oncol Nurs Forum*. 2012;39(5):E398–E406.
33. Wittenberg-Lyles E, Goldsmith J, Ferrell B, Ragan S. *Communication in Palliative Nursing*. New York, NY: Oxford University Press; 2012.
34. Cohen A, Nirenberg A. Current practices in advance care planning: Implications for oncology nurses. *Clin J Oncol Nurs*. October 2011;15(5):547–553.
35. Gundersen Health System. Making choices information booklet. https://glrespectingchoices.dcopy.net/product/mc530-e-making-choices-information-booklet. Accessed September 19, 2014.
36. Gundersen Health System. Respecting choices: Role of the nurse. https://glrespectingchoices.dcopy.net/product/rc-006-role-of-the-nurse. Accessed June 17, 2015.
37. Aging with Dignity. Five wishes. http://www.agingwithdignity.org/five-wishes.php. Accessed September 19, 2014.
38. ProjectGRACE. Advance directives. https://www.empathchoicesforcare.org/Advance-Directives. Accessed June 17, 2015.
39. Coyle N, Kissane DW. Conducting a family meeting. In: Kissane DW, Bultz BD, Butow PM, Finaly IG, eds. *Handbook of Communication in Oncology and Palliative Care*. New York, NY: Oxford University Press; 2010:165–175.
40. Mitchell P, Wynia R, Golden B, et al. *Core Principles & Values of Effective Team-Based Health Care*. Washington, DC: Institute of Medicine; 2012.
41. Freise C, Manojlovich M. Nurse-physician relationships in ambulatory oncology settings. *J Nurs Scholarsh*. 2012;44(3):258–365.
42. Gallup. Honesty and ethics rating of clergy slides to new low. http://www.gallup.com/poll/166298/honesty-ethics-rating-clergy-slides-new-low.aspx. Published December 13, 2013. Accessed September 26, 2014.
43. Slatore CG, Hansen L, Ganzini L, et al. Communication by nurses in the intensive care unit: Qualitative analysis of domains of patient-centered care. *Am J Crit Care*. 2012;21(6):410–418.
44. Heft P, Chamness A, Terry C, Uhrich M. Oncology nurses's attitudes towards prognosis-related communication: A pilot mailed

survey of Oncology Nursing Society Members. *Oncol Nurs Forum.* 2011;38(5):468–474.
45. Andershed B, Ternestedt BM. Being a close relative of a dying person: Development of concepts, "involvement in the light and the dark." *Cancer Nurs.* 2000;23(2):151–159.
46. Clayton M, Reblin M, Carlisle M, Ellington L. Communication behaviors and patient and caregiver emotional concerns: A description of home hospice communication. *Oncol Nurs Forum.* 2014;41(3):311–321.
47. Ferrell BR, Virani R, Grant M. Analysis of end-of-life content in nursing textbooks. *Oncol Nurs Forum.* 1999;26(5): 869–876.
48. Baer L, Weinstein E. Improving oncology nurses' communication skills for difficult conversations. *Clin J Oncol Nurs.* 2013;17(3):E45–E51.
49. Peereboom K, Coyle N. Facilitating goals-of-care discussions for patients with life-limiting disease: Communication strategies for nurses. *J Hosp Palliat Nurs.* 2012;14(4):251–258.

CHAPTER 9

Communication in Palliative Care Chaplaincy

George F. Handzo

Introduction

Now when Job's three friends heard of all this evil that had come upon him, they came each from his own place ... They made an appointment together to come to show him sympathy and comfort him. And when they saw him from a distance, they did not recognize him. And they raised their voices and wept, and they tore their robes, and sprinkled dust on their heads toward heaven. And they sat with him on the ground seven days and seven nights, and no one spoke a word to him, for they saw that his suffering was great. Job 2:11–13[1]

A Note on Terminology

While more formal definitions are proposed later in this chapter, for the purposes of parsimony the term "spirituality" is used here to include the domains called "religion" and "existential."

Basics of Chaplaincy Communication in Palliative Care

Wittenberg-Lyles and colleagues have defined communication as "the mutual creation of meaning."[2] This definition fits palliative chaplaincy very well, as arguably the aim of professional healthcare chaplaincy is to help those the chaplain communicates with find and affirm meaning in their particular situation. Indeed, one of the best-known chaplaincy education and research organizations in the United States at one time had as its byline "Finding Meaning, Bringing Comfort."

Finding meaning is particularly important in the context of suffering of any kind. John Bowker wrote in his seminal book *The Place of Suffering in the Religions of the World* that suffering is the central challenge of all religions of the world, and the central challenge of any religion may be to help people find meaning in suffering.[3] Rabbi Kushner is among many who have written books on the struggle to find meaning in suffering.[4]

Park and Folkman in their seminal theoretical paper on meaning-making posit several components with direct implications for communication in chaplaincy.[5] They propose two levels of meaning—global and situational. Global meanings include a person's most basic values and beliefs about the way the world works. The authors particularly name religion as a global meaning system that helps deal with suffering and loss. Situational meaning is given to some particular event such as a major illness or a death. When a person's global and situational meaning are in conflict, dissonance occurs, which causes suffering. The major task of communication in healthcare chaplaincy is to help reduce a patient's or family caregiver's suffering by helping them reduce or eliminate the dissonance between the religious, spiritual, or existential aspects of their global meaning systems and the situational meaning they attribute to their current situation. Rabbi Kushner's book was so popular largely because even the title expresses a basic dissonance between common global and situational meanings. Kushner's God was omnipotent, all-knowing and totally beneficent, and yet Kushner's young son died from a terrible degenerative disease that caused tremendous suffering.

Mrs. S. was a young mother with strong conservative Christian beliefs including, like Kushner, that God would protect those who believed in him and keep them from harm. She dealt with the fact that her 4-year-old son had cancer by continuing to believe that God would cure him eventually and that the suffering she and her son were enduring was a test from God of their faith. Eventually the healthcare team told Mrs. S. that her son was going to die and had only days or weeks to live. Despite this communication, Mrs. S. was still adamant that a miracle cure would happen. Alarmed by what they feared would be Mrs. S's reaction when her son died, the chaplain was called. Consistent with good chaplaincy practice, the chaplain listened to her, affirmed the strength of her faith, and did not try to convince her that she was wrong. He continued to visit and build a relationship of trust and respect.

One morning, the healthcare team again called the chaplain with the news that Mrs. S had suddenly gone from being very anxious to seemingly at peace. When the chaplain visited her, she explained her changed mood.

"I realized that I have really been very selfish in trying to hang on to my son. I now realize God clearly has other plans for my son that are beyond my ability to know. I just need to trust that God plans are the best plans."

Indeed, Mrs. S, absent the necessity of defending her faith or feeling that her beliefs were not respected, was able to, in that space, find a way to reconcile the situational meaning of her son's impending death with her global meaning system, which included a foundational belief in the goodness of her God.

Wittenberg-Lyles and colleagues also make the point that every communication has two levels—the content or task level and the relationship level. They roughly equate the verbal part of the communication to the content and the nonverbal to the relationship.[2] In that dyad, one might describe chaplaincy and spiritual care in general as primarily about relationship-building and very little about content.[6] Healthcare chaplains often talk about their central or foundational "task" being active listening or presence and responding in ways that clearly put the patient in control of the conversation.[7] In one study in which chaplains self-reported their interventions with hospitalized patients, 70% of the interventions were characterized as either "emotional enabling" or "empathetic listening."[8] Massey and colleagues developed the first evidence-informed taxonomy for what chaplains do and found that most of the interventions they identified had to do with asking, assisting, and facilitating.[9] Those that related to "providing" were mostly religious in nature, such as providing religious items. The goal of chaplaincy communication is to create a relationship within which patients or family members feel free to find their own meaning, discover their own interior and exterior resources, and feel safe to explore topics and feelings that they have heretofore avoided. This strategy is consistent with the need to reconcile levels of meaning as described by Park and Folkman. It is also consistent with the patient- and family-centered approach of palliative care, which emphases listening to the patients' and family members' values and beliefs and then helping them to incorporate those values and beliefs into the patient's care plan.

Complementary to this approach is the prohibition in the professional chaplains' Code of Ethics in North America against proselytizing or otherwise imposing one's beliefs on those with whom the chaplain communicates.[10] Again, this is in line with the chaplain helping patients or family members find their own beliefs rather than telling them what they should believe or even what they might consider believing. This prohibition emerges both from this patient-centered stance and from the realization of the power differential between patient and healthcare provider. This power disparity is often emphasized if the chaplain is a clergyperson of the patient's faith tradition.

It should be noted here that the term "chaplain" itself actually encompasses at least two distinct groups of practitioners within healthcare. The primary group normally participating on palliative care teams is the chaplain who serves all patients on a given team or nursing unit regardless of their faith affiliation or lack of it. This person's job generally might be described as helping patients and family members discover and use their own spiritual and religious resources in the service of their healing or coping. They are sometimes also called "multifaith" chaplains or "interfaith" chaplains to underline that they do not serve patients of only one denomination. The second group is generally clergy appointed by local faith communities to serve patients of that denomination. Their focus is largely or completely centered on helping their coreligionists use the values, beliefs, and rituals of the particular tradition. Their communication tends to include language and meanings unique to that tradition. Since the practice of communication in palliative chaplaincy is largely built on the multifaith chaplain model, that is the role that is discussed in the rest of this chapter.

A somewhat stylized example of these two dynamics in chaplaincy care often plays out as follows:

PATIENT: Chaplain, I've been wondering why I got cancer. I'm a good person and I take care of myself.
CHAPLAIN: Are you thinking this doesn't seem right?
PATIENT: Yeah, something like that.
CHAPLAIN: Uh, huh. (Silence)
PATIENT: Well, maybe there are some things in the world that God doesn't control for some reason we don't understand.
CHAPLAIN: Maybe so.
PATIENT: Well, I guess I need to think about this further.
CHAPLAIN: Sounds good. I'll look forward to hearing your thoughts.

Communicating About Spirituality/Religion

While chaplains talk to patients and their caregivers about a variety of topics, their unique contribution is to talk to them about spiritual/religious/existential concerns.[11] This is a singular challenge from a communication point of view. Religion and spirituality are often talked about in a language other than the language of science, which is the native tongue of all of the other disciplines in palliative care.[12]

For example, members of a healthcare team were becoming frustrated with a patient's family because they did not seem to be hearing or accepting the communication that their mother was going to die. They responded that they trusted that God was going to "heal" her. A conversation and assessment by the chaplain determined that the family did understand the team's communication very well and understood that the team might be correct. However, whereas the healthcare team assumed the family was using "healing" purely in a physical sense, the family, while not giving up on that possibility, were also hoping for "healing" in a spiritual or existential sense as their mother passed from this life to what they believed would be the next life.

Spirituality is often spoken of in the language of story or poetry or expressed in a nonverbal art form. Thus it is not unusual for chaplains to sing with patients or to sit with them in silence. Compassion has been seen as a spiritual intervention with both verbal and nonverbal components.[13] Spirituality is experienced as much as it is talked about. Yet spirituality is important to patients, and they want to talk about it with their caregivers.[14,15]

Research indicates patients' demand for spiritual care is high and increasing. One study found that 88% of patients in a palliative care unit with end-stage cancer expressed the desire to work with a chaplain.[16] The study also found that roughly 50% of patients indicated that they would like the chaplain to provide a sense of "presence," listen to them, visit with them, or accompany them on their spiritual journey in the context of illness.

Increasing research in the field of spiritual struggle indicates its importance and prevalence during times of stress such as illness.[17] Ai and colleagues found strong evidence for a link between spiritual struggle and poor health outcomes.[18,19] Conversely, Balboni and colleagues found that when patient's spiritual needs are met in the context of advanced cancer, the patients are less likely to die in an intensive care unit (ICU) and likely to spend more time in hospice.[20] Another study reported that 41% of inpatients desired a discussion of religion/spirituality concerns while hospitalized, but only half of those reported having such a discussion.[21] Having the discussion was positively correlated with patient satisfaction.

Healthcare team members are called upon to assess spiritual need but do not know how to begin the conversation.[22] They are accustomed to providing answers or at least reassurance, rather than allowing for the issues to unfold in the relationship.[23,24] The difference between the language of science and the language of spirituality—often coupled with the lack of realization on either the staff's or the patient's part that they are speaking, at least in part, different languages—makes communication around spiritual issues difficult.

Integration of spiritual and medical language is a communication problem on multiple levels. Much of the terminology, including the word "spiritual," does not have widely accepted definitions even among chaplains. Communicating can also entail having multiple goals.[25] Communication involving faith can include the purpose of communicating with a God or Higher Power, the purpose of communicating with a faith community, and the purpose of reinforcing for oneself one's own faith and belief, and reflection on these purposes can occur at the same time. As already illustrated with the case above, communication can be informed by a worldview grounded in foundational meanings and can be based on the "truths" of scientific research or the "truths" of faith. These worldviews then influence situational meanings and thus the ways people communicate about those situations. As an example, the scientific worldview might be concerned about whether it is acceptable to pray for healing in the context of a fatal illness.[26] The faith-based worldview would never be concerned with that question, because faith holds that healing is always possible. A final difficulty for the healthcare team can be the reality that faith can be negative and punitive of self or others and an impediment to participation in the treatment process.[27]

The Emergence of Chaplaincy as a Profession

In most of the English-speaking world and elsewhere, chaplaincy is emerging as the profession best fit to take the lead in providing for the spiritual dimension, of care.[28,29,30] One conceptualization of modern healthcare chaplaincy is that the chaplains are able and willing to be the spiritual care lead on the palliative care team. They are trained to help patients and families of any faith or no faith deal with issues within the spiritual domain of care. As discussed, the professional chaplain achieves this goal by focusing on helping the patient or family member discover his or her own spiritual resources and assist with utilizing those resources. While Job's friends eventually gave in and tried to "help" by providing an answer, their initial instinct was to just be with Job in silence and let him express his suffering; this is what a professional chaplain today would try to do.

In the process of professionalization, healthcare chaplaincy in North America has acquired more of the hallmarks of a profession, including credentials for certification, a code of ethics, and standards of practice.[31] There has recently been much debate in the field about the advisability or even the possibility of building an evidence base for chaplaincy communication, with some arguing that building evidence and systematically improving the quality of chaplaincy communication is necessary for its status as a profession and will help patients[32,33,34] and others raising the danger that this process will rob spiritual care of an essence that enables it to provide the benefit it does.[35]

Chaplaincy has developed its own training model focused around communication issues, including reflective listening and creating space for patients to express themselves safely and find their own meaning and comfort. This method, called "clinical pastoral education," is described in depth in Chapter 37. Although many of these issues are not characterized this way in chaplaincy circles, they involve such issues as the chaplain being primarily a receiver rather than a sender of communication as Wittenberg-Lyles has described. Self-disclosure is generally minimized in favor of having patients or family members talk about themselves. Likewise, advice-giving or teaching is minimized unless specifically requested. The discipline of when to keep silent is also important.[36] Students also concentrate on understanding and minimizing the ways their styles of communicating actually impede communication between themselves and the patient.

Although Afifi's precise categories are not generally named in chaplaincy training, most of the same concepts apply.[37] For instance, touch is a very important and often difficult to negotiate nonverbal communication technique. On the one hand, chaplains recognize the power of touch. In some traditions it is believed that "laying on of hands" has the power to heal or to literally transmit healing energy. On the other hand, in some cultures touching, especially between sexes, is highly restricted and could be offensive. Likewise, space, especially between people, is highly culture sensitive, and chaplains are taught to approach people with caution and remain aware of their apparent comfort level regarding the distance between them. Normal chaplaincy practice is to be at eye level with the patient, which, if the patient is lying down in bed, means sitting or kneeling if necessary. Chaplains are taught to be aware of the power differential between themselves and the patient so not to add to what is unavoidable in that regard. Clothing or uniform is also important. Wearing clothing associated with one's faith group, such as the collar of a Christian clergyperson, on the one hand helps communicate to the patient who the visitor is. On the other hand, the collar can be a barrier to communication between the chaplain and non-Christians. Some Jewish female chaplains wear a yarmulke at all times. While this is a non-issue for almost all patients, it can be highly offensive to observant Jews, as only men are supposed to wear a yarmulke in that tradition. Finally, while chaplains need to obey all infectious disease restrictions, they must be very aware of the barriers to communication imposed by artifacts like masks, gowns, and gloves.

The Problem of Definition

DeVries and colleagues have described some of the problems with definition in chaplaincy that make communication difficult.[38] They point out that since chaplaincy is not yet fully regarded as a profession, others are free to define who can use the title and also what those people can do. It is then very difficult for those to whom chaplains relate, whether they be patients, family members, or members of other disciplines, to know precisely what a chaplain is. VandeCreek also points out the problems related to a lack of a definition of spiritual care and how definitions shared with hospital administrators, clinicians (especially nurses), and patients can affect the contributions that chaplains can make.[39] The Association of Professional Chaplains in the United States has taken several steps to improve this situation, including defining a set of qualifications for being called a "Board-Certified Chaplain" and defining several sets of Standards of Practice, each tailored to a different care setting.[40]

Most of the definitions are aimed at clearly differentiating terms that are often confused or used interchangeably such as "religion" and "spirituality" or "spiritual care," "chaplaincy care," and "pastoral care." Definitions that now have gained some acceptance in the field are summarized in Table 9.1. Figure 9.1 is a graphic representation of the relationships between a number of these concepts.

Table 9.1 Definitions

Religion	An organized system of beliefs, practices, rituals, and symbols designated (a) to facilitate closeness to the sacred or transcendent (God, higher power, or ultimate truth/reality) and (b) to foster understanding of one's relationship and responsibility to others living in a community[65]
International defintion of spirituality	A dynamic and intrinsic aspect of humanity through which persons seek ultimate meaning, purpose, and transcendence and experience relationship to self, family, others, community, society, nature, and the significant or sacred[66]
Spiritual Care	That care which recognizes and responds to the needs of the human spirit when faced with trauma, ill health, or sadness and can include the need for meaning, for self-worth, to express oneself, for faith support, perhaps for rites, prayer, or sacrament, or simply for a sensitive listener[67]
Chaplaincy Care	Care provided by a board-certified chaplain or by a student in an accredited clinical pastoral education program[68]
Pastoral Care	Now understood as a term that comes out of the Christian tradition and generally describes the care given by a faith leader to members of his or her community[69].
Spiritual Assessment	A more extensive (in-depth, ongoing) process of active listening to a patient's story as it unfolds in a relationship with a professional chaplain and summarizing the needs and resources that emerge in that process[70]

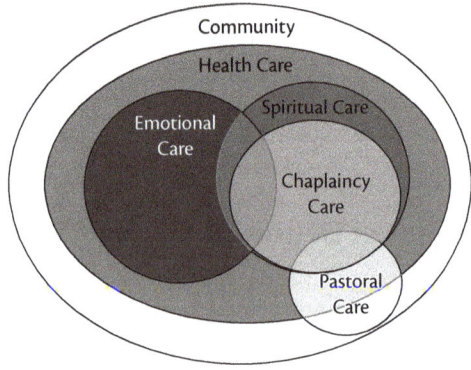

Figure 9.1 Relationship of spiritual care concepts
Developed by David Fleenor, BCC, and George Handzo, BCC.

The Problem of Scope

Since a clear description of what chaplains do is lacking and the term poorly defined, even by chaplains, there is much room for miscommunication about the scope of chaplains.[41] Patients and families often perceive chaplains as presiding over end-of-life situations and thus may be very concerned if a chaplain visits unannounced. When chaplains do try to communicate about what they do, they often use jargon such as "being present" and "being with the patient where they are," which sometimes confuses patients, families, or other staff. Especially in the environment in which productivity and adding value are so important, chaplains often do not communicate well what they produce. Many chaplains are trying to reduce the perception that they deal only with religious issues by using the term "spiritual care" more often. However, again, without defining "spiritual care," this shift is not clear and actually may communicate to people who want "religious services" that this is not what chaplains do.[42] The matter is made worse by the fact that very rarely do any two chaplains, even within the same institution, define what they do in the same words. This variation in communication means that staff may get used to one chaplain and understand what he or she does, but the next one may do things differently, possibly in a way not to their liking.

Finally, even if chaplains as a profession come to a common understanding of what they do, they must translate that into the medical language of the team and use medical processes. For instance, most members of the medical team use diagnostic terminology to describe what is going on with the patient and communicate about the treatment plan. Chaplains have resisted this "medicalizing" of what they do, but one list has been developed by the National Comprehensive Cancer Network (NCCN) in the United States. "Diagnoses" include guilt, hopelessness, grief, concerns about death and afterlife, conflicted or challenged belief system, loss of faith/doubts, concerns about meaning/purpose in life, concerns about relationship to deity, conflict between religious beliefs and recommended treatment, and conflict with/loss of religious community.[43]

The lack of specificity of role has opened the door for conflicts with other disciplines such as social work.[44] However, all palliative care models include spiritual care and have begun to work toward a better definition of chaplains' scope of practice and how that relates to the roles of other disciplines.[12,43] Leveraging the generalist-specialist model generally used in healthcare, the professional chaplain's role is to be the spiritual care specialist on the team, with all other members of the team being spiritual care generalists. Thus all members of the team would be expected to communicate with patients and family members about spiritual issues at some level, but they would refer to the chaplain for more complex issues.

There is no accepted taxonomy of chaplaincy interventions with patients and families especially as tied to assessments and outcomes. In the United States, Peery has proposed an extensive list that covers the scope of what chaplains do focusing on interventions that rely on relationships such as "facilitating" and "enabling."[45] A large sample gathered in New York City of chaplain's self-reported interventions generally confirmed this list.[9] Massey and colleagues in the Chicago area involved almost 60 chaplains in developing and testing for validity a list of what chaplains do focusing on the ICU.[10] The list was divided into effects, methods, and interventions. Again, most of the effects could be characterized as the products of relationships such as "helping someone feel comforted" and "lessening the feelings of isolation." Many of the interventions chaplains do to achieve these effects fall under the general rubric of reflective listening and emotional support. However, Piderman and colleagues at Mayo Clinic studied a highly religious population and found that the two major reasons patients there wanted chaplains to visit were to "remind me of God's care and presence" and "provide support for family and friends." This is quite a different finding than the other studies.[46]

Internationally, a list produced in England is much more task-oriented in that it includes many more activities focused on the delivery of religious services.[35] This finding may reflect the chaplaincy system in the United Kingdom, which is still much more denominational than it is multifaith focused. Showing the variation by country, surveys of cancer patients in Israel reveal that those who use chaplaincy services focus on spiritual interventions such as meditation and request religious services much less often than in the United States or United Kingdom.[47] Kelly and colleagues in Scotland have leveraged the power of listening by placing chaplains in community clinics to do "Community Chaplaincy Listening."[48] Research on this intervention is ongoing, but results to date seem to indicate that patient and physician satisfaction is high, which is notable given the very secular nature of the country; some tangible results may be fewer physician visits and a reduction in need for anxiety medication. The project also demonstrates the usefulness of this kind of intervention in the outpatient setting, as has been shown elsewhere in a palliative care setting.[49]

Professional chaplains do not generally engage in teaching patients about belief unless the patient specifically asks for it. Any intervention a chaplain would make under the broad category of counseling is, likewise, focused on helping the patients and family members come to their own understandings and conclusions, rather than giving them answers.

The chaplain's skill in communication and emphasis on listening and nonjudgmental presence comes into play when helping patients and caregivers deal with spiritual distress. The chaplain's primary goal in these situations is to help patients find their own meaning and discover their own resources through listening to and reflecting on their individual life story. The chaplain might use appropriate readings or music to assist in this process. For patients who would like ongoing counseling, the chaplain might refer to community resources such as community clergy, pastoral counselors, or spiritual directors.

All chaplains are also trained in religious interventions. These fall into two categories. The first type of intervention is those that the chaplain performs as a clergyperson with a person of his or her own faith group. In this case, the chaplain operates as a clergyperson of that faith group. The second type of intervention does not necessarily require the chaplain and the patient to be of the same faith group. For instance, professional chaplains are trained to pray with people of any faith. They can often read from the patient's sacred texts or help the patient find music or other spiritual resources. Chaplains occasionally officiate at weddings and funerals—sometimes for patients of their own faith and sometimes not. The relationship issue is also apparent here in that families often choose a chaplain of another faith to do a funeral for a loved one. This is often the result of a close relationship they perceive the chaplain to have had with the patient or the fact that it was the chaplain who was present with them when their loved one died and immediately after.[50]

Emerging Best Practice

One of the major changes in professional healthcare chaplaincy is the issue of outcomes and accountability. Since chaplaincy has been about relationships as opposed to tasks, it has been difficult to talk about what outcomes might be important. However, without specific outcomes, chaplains cannot communicate what they produce to the healthcare team. In response, Lucas posited a model now called Outcome-Oriented Chaplaincy in which the patient is actively engaged in deciding outcomes and determining to what extent those outcomes are met.[51,53] Thus communication between the chaplain and the patient on the issue of outcomes is essential. In this emerging system, relationships are means to generate outcomes that align with the rest of the care plan.

Another change has been the focus on spiritual distress and spiritual needs rather than simply on the desire of a patient to talk to a chaplain. This change also is related to outcomes and accountability focused on meeting spiritual need and reducing spiritual distress. This shift is facilitated by the documentation of the self-reported spiritual distress, which has exceeded 90% in at least one sample,[17] and of the interconnectedness of spirituality as a part of the lives of many patients, especially near the end of life.[52] Gaudette has documented a relationship of anxiety to spiritual distress in palliative care patients.[53] Part of the problem remaining for documentation of outcomes is that while "spiritual/religious practices" are high on the list of spiritual needs, the two most mentioned needs were "love and belonging" and "meaning and purpose," which are very hard to measure as outcomes.[54] They do, however, reinforce the basic relational nature of chaplaincy.

This focus on spiritual needs and spiritual distress has also placed an emphasis on screening for spiritual distress and including spiritual issues in a patient's complete history. Both spiritual screening and history tools have focused on discovering the importance of spirituality for the patient and to what extent spiritual coping is helping the patient at that moment.[15,55] The goal is to help those who need assistance receive it as soon as possible.

The issue of documentation raises the issue of confidentiality. Some chaplains do not chart their conversations with the patient because they say these are "protected" by clergyperson confidentiality, and therefore they cannot document anything they learn from the patient. Historically, "clergy confidentiality" refers to the information that someone seeking forgiveness shares with a clergyperson within the context of ritual confession. It has also often been understood as part of a pastoral relationship in which someone seeks religious counsel from his or her community's leader in the areas of marriage or child-rearing. While every US state has different understandings of what "clergy–communicant" confidentiality is and how it is to be determined and protected, it is typically applicable to religious community relationships when a clergy/religious leader is employed by the congregation/synagogue/temple and serving in the role as pastor, rabbi, priest, and so on. Thus it is much different than most conversations between a patient and a healthcare chaplain.

Nevertheless, many patients and chaplains do not understand the difference between confidential clergy communication and normal communication with a chaplain and expect a higher level of confidentiality from the chaplain than they expect from other members of the healthcare team. Further, many chaplains are not trained in how to document conversations and do not understand what information is included or, more important, what information should be left out. For example, the chaplain may not understand that, while it might be helpful to document that the patient had a conversation with the chaplain about past events that the patient considered sinful, it would generally be not only improper but useless to document the nature of that sinfulness.

One way to negotiate what really is a potential problem for patients is to bring the patient into the decision-making process of what information should be documented and what should be left out. A chaplain might seek the patient's permission to document in the following way.

CHAPLAIN (TO PATIENT): Mrs. S, we have talked about a lot issues in this visit that seem very important to you, including issues that are important to you as you make decisions about your care. I think that the other people caring for you on this healthcare team would very much like to know about these issues so they can also take them into account and respect them as they discuss your care with you. It would help if I could write about these issues in your medical record so the other members of the team could read about them. I assure you that only those actually taking care of you will read this material. Would it be okay if I did that?

Chaplain as Member of the Healthcare Team

Healthcare, especially in palliative care, is becoming transdisciplinary, which means that all members of the team will be trained to participate in the patient's care across all domains. In particular, all caregivers will have a role in spiritual care. As previously stated, the chaplain is the spiritual care specialist on the team, and all others are spiritual care generalists.

The importance of the generalist role in making referrals to chaplains has been highlighted by Fitchett and colleagues, who found that those who have the greatest spiritual need are the least likely to request a chaplain.[56] Grossoehme describes nurses and chaplains as collaborators in the delivery of spiritual care, with chaplains helping nurses to more fully succeed in their role.[57]

The chaplain as spiritual care specialist has several distinct roles on the team; perhaps the most important is the chaplain's role as subject matter expert. Other disciplines, especially nursing, have communication with patients around spiritual issues such as forgiveness but often have no particular training in how to deal with this material.[58] Chaplains can help other disciplines build skill and confidence in spiritual communication.

Another component of communication with patients and families involves understanding the family's culture that guide spiritual beliefs and practices. In the United States, the chaplain is often regarded as the "culture broker" on the team.[59] As the culture broker, the chaplain assists the patient, family, and healthcare team navigate any cultural, ethnic, or religious issues that may hinder communication between and among them. They can also assist the institution and staff in becoming more friendly and accommodating to patients, family members, and staff from various cultures in the community. Because chaplains are experts in helping people identify and articulate their beliefs, they can also aid healthcare team members in accommodating those beliefs and various cultural practices. It is also part of the chaplain's role to be aware of and in relationship with the religious resources in the community, which can be called on as needed.

One specific area of care that often involves both teaching staff and dealing with cultural issues falls in the broad category of ethical issues. These also could be considered to fall within the NCCN diagnosis of "conflict between religious beliefs and recommended treatment." Sometimes this conflict between the healthcare team and the patient/family is caused by miscommunication or incomplete communication—especially when bad news is involved. In some of these situations, the chaplain can be the translator between medical language and lay language. The chaplain can help the patient process bad news both cognitively and emotionally so that conflicts are not based on misunderstandings or lack of understanding of the information being communicated.

Because chaplains are seen as religious people, patients may feel they are more neutral or trustworthy than others on the healthcare team. One particular opportunity for this chaplain role can be in helping facilitate family meetings. The chaplain may be, especially for the family in which religion is important, the most appropriate facilitator for the meeting. Another opportunity arises when there is a conflict between what the healthcare team perceives as the best interests of the patient or even the expressed interests of the patient and the expressed wishes of the family.[60] An underutilized role of the chaplain is as communication facilitator between faith communities/institutions and his or her healthcare colleagues. This can lead to improved relationships between religious institutions and healthcare institutions. A particular service that would benefit both congregations and hospitals would involve the chaplain conducting events that help members understand and start to think about advance directives and other treatment decision issues.[61]

A particular instance of conflict between the team and the family occurs when the family wants to continue treatment in hopes of a miracle in the face of the healthcare team's clearly communicated recommendation that all aggressive treatment be discontinued. This situation often requires extreme sensitivity to keep the family's trust while helping them come to terms with the certainty of their loved one's death. As part of this strategy, Hess has posited a collaborative model of divine intervention that can be useful, as God is seen working both through faith and through medicine.[62] Cooper has posited the AMEN model (**A**ffirm, **M**eet, **E**ducate, **N**o matter what), which also partners with the patient toward a solution rather than risking creating an adversarial relationship.[63] In both cases, the chaplain's skill in relationship-building and helping families work through their values and beliefs may be critical.

It is also important to recognize barriers to this kind of chaplain role. One study found that the major barrier identified by staff is training.[23] Thus the role of the chaplain as trainer is critical. There also can be issues with power dynamics and trust stemming from the perception that chaplains are not clinically trained as are those in other disciplines. While this differentiation is less true than previously, the chaplains often are not proficient in speaking or understanding medical language. Chaplains need to speak both "medical" and "spiritual."

Finally, chaplains are unique on the team in that it is not only permitted but encouraged for them to provide professional care within their scope of practice to other members of their team. This puts chaplains in something of a dual role in relationship to the rest of their team that has to be carefully negotiated but also recognizes that spirituality is a major support for many staff as well as for many patients and family members.[64]

Conclusion

Communication is foundational to professional healthcare chaplaincy and essential for building a trusting relationship between the chaplain and the patient or family caregiver. Unlike other disciplines or even community clergy, the healthcare chaplain is primarily a listener rather than an information provider. The goal is for patients to discover their own spiritual and religious resources and utilize them in the service of their healing. In the process, the chaplain can facilitate communication between the patient/family and the team on care planning and other issues.

References

1. *The Holy Bible*, English Standard Version. Wheaton, IL: Crossways; 2001.
2. Wittenberg-Lyles E, Goldsmith J, Ferrell B, Ragan S. *Communication in Palliative Nursing*. New York, NY: Oxford University Press; 2012.
3. Bowker J. *Problems of Suffering in the Religions of the World*. New York, NY: Cambridge University Press; 1970.
4. Kushner, H. *When Bad Things Happen to Good People*. New York, NY: Anchor Books; 2004.
5. Park C, Folkman S. Meaning in the context of stress and coping. *Rev Gen Psychol*. 1997;1(2):115–144.
6. Edwards A, Pang N, Shiu V, Chan C. The understanding of spirituality and the potential role of spiritual care in end-of-life and palliative care: A meta-study of qualitative research. *Palliat Med*. 2010;24(8):753–770.
7. Kidd R. Foundational listening and responding skills. In: Roberts S, ed. *Professional Spiritual & Pastoral Care: A Practical Clergy and Chaplain's Handbook*. Woodstock, VT: Skylight Paths Publishing; 2012:92–105.
8. Handzo GF, Flannelly KJ, Kudler T, et al. What do chaplains really do? II. Interventions in the New York Chaplaincy Study. *J Health Care Chaplain*. 2008;14(1):39–56.
9. Massey K, Barnes M, Summerfelt WT. What do I do? Developing a taxonomy of chaplaincy activities and interventions in spiritual care in ICU palliative care. Paper presented at Caring for the Human Spirit: Driving the Research Agenda for Spiritual Care in Health Care; March 2014; New York, NY.
10. Association of Professional Chaplains. Common code of ethics for professional chaplains. http://www.professionalchaplains.org/Files/professional_standards/professional_ethics/apc_code_of_ethics.pdf. Accessed June 11, 2014.
11. Handzo GF, Koenig HG. Spiritual care: Whose job is it anyway?. *South Med J*. 2004;97(12):1242–1244.
12. Sexton C. Words and the chemistry of the soul at the end-of-life. *J Pastoral Care Counsel*. 2009;63(1–2):18.1–3.
13. Halifax J. A Heuristic model of enactive compassion. *Curr Opin Support Palliat Care*. 2012;6(2):228–235.
14. Borneman T, Ferrell B, Puchalski C. Evaluation of the FICA Tool for Spiritual Assessment. *J Pain Symptom Manage*. 2010;20(2):163–173.
15. Balboni T, Vanderwerker L, Block S, et al. Religiousness and spiritual support among advanced cancer patients and associations with end-of-life treatment preferences and quality of life. *J Clin Oncol*. 2007;25(5):555–560.
16. Galek K, Mako C, Poppito SR. Spiritual pain among patients with advanced cancer in palliative care. *J Palliat Med*. 2006;9(3):1106–1113.
17. Pargament KI, Murray-Swank NA, Magyar GM, Ano GG. Spiritual struggle: A phenomenon of interest to psychology and religion. In: Miller ER., Delaney HD. eds. *Judeo-Christian Perspectives on Psychology*. Washington, DC: American Psychological Association; 2005:245–268.
18. Ai AL, Pargament KI, Appel HB, Kronfol Z. Depression following open-heart surgery: Path model involving interleukin-6, spiritual struggle, and hope under preoperative distress. *J Clin Psychol*. 2010;66(10):1058–1075.
19. Ai AL, Pargament K I, Kronfol Z. Tice TN. Appel H. Pathways to post-operative hostility in cardiac patients: Mediation of coping, spiritual struggle and interleukin-6. *J Health Psychol*. 2010;15:186–195.
20. Balboni T, Balboni M, Paulk M, et al. Support of cancer patients' spiritual needs and associations with medical care costs at the end of life. *Cancer*. 2011;117(23):5383–5391.
21. Williams J, Meltzer D, Arora V, Chung G, Curlin F. Attention to inpatients' religious and spiritual concerns: Predictors and association with patient satisfaction. *J Gen Intern Med*. 2011;26(11):1265–1271.
22. Balboni M, Sullivan A, Amobi A, et al. Why is spiritual care infrequent at the end of life? Spiritual Care perceptions among patients, nurses, physicians and the role of training. *J Clin Oncol*. 2013;31:4461–4467.
23. Ferrell B, Otis-Green S, Baird P, Garcia A. Nurses' responses to requests for forgiveness at the end-of-life. *J Pain Symptom Manage*. 2014;47(3):631–641.
24. Ellington L, Reblin M, Ferrell B, et al. The religion of "I don't know": Naturalistic observation of spiritual conversations occurring during cancer home hospice nurse visits. *Omega*. March 9, 2015. Advance online publication.
25. Tracy K, Coupland N. Multiple goals in discourse: An overview of issues. *J Lang Soc Psychol*. 1990;9:1–13.
26. Taylor EJ, Outlaw FH, Bernardo TR, Roy A. Spiritual conflicts associated with praying about cancer. *Psycho-Oncology*. 1999;8:386–394.
27. Pargament K. *The Psychology of Religion and Coping*. New York, NY: Guilford Press; 1997.
28. Puchalski C, Ferrell B. *Making Health Care Whole: Integrating Spirituality into Patient Care*. West Conshohocken, PA: Templeton Press; 2010.
29. National Consensus Project for Quality Palliative Care. Clinical practice guidelines for quality palliative care. 3rd ed. www.nationalconsensusproject.org/Guidelines_Download2.aspx. Published 2013. Accessed May 30, 2014.
30. Swift C, Handzo G, Cohen J. Healthcare chaplaincy. In: Cobb M, Puchalski C, Rumbold B, eds. *Oxford Textbook of Spirituality in HealthCare*. New York, NY: Oxford University Press; 2012:185–190.
31. Association of Professional Chaplains. Standards of practice for professional chaplains. http://www.professionalchaplains.org/content.asp?pl=198&sl=200&contentid=200. Accessed June 17, 2015.
32. Berlinger N. The nature of chaplaincy and the goals of QI: Patient-centered care as professional responsibility. *Hastings Cent Rep*. 2008;38(6):30–33.
33. O'Connor T. The search for truth: The case for evidence based chaplaincy. *J Health Care Chaplain*. 2002;13(1):185–194.
34. Carey L, Cobb M, Equeall D. From "pastoral contacts" to "pastoral interventions." *Scot J Hlthcare Chaplaincy*. 2005;8(2):14–20.
35. Nolen S. Re-evaluating chaplaincy: To be, or not . . . *Health and Social Care Chaplaincy*. 2013;1(1):49–60.
36. Moriichi S. Re-discovery of silence in pastoral care. *J Pastoral Care Counsel*. 2009;63(1–2):3.1–6.
37. Afifi WA. Nonverbal communication. In: Whaley BB, Samter W, eds. *Explaining Communication: Contemporary Theories and Exemplars*. Mahwah, NJ: Lawrence Erlbaum; 2007:39–60.
38. de Vries R, Berlinger N, Cadge W. Lost in translation: The chaplain's role in health care. *Hastings Cent Rep*. 2008;38(6):23–27.
39. VandeCreek L. Defining and advocating for spiritual care in the hospital. *J Pastoral Care Counsel*. 2010;64(2):5.1–10.
40. Association of Professional Chaplains. BCCI certification. http://bcci.professionalchaplains.org/content.asp?pl=25&contentid=25. Accessed June 24, 2014.
41. Cramer E, Tenzek KE, Allen M. Translating Spiritual care in the chaplain profession. *J Pastoral Care Counsel*. 2013;67(1):1–15.
42. Cadge W. *Paging God: Religion in the Halls of Medicine*. Chicago, IL: University of Chicago Press; 2012.
43. National Comprehensive Cancer Network. Distress management guidelines. http://www.nccn.org/professionals/physician_gls/f_guidelines.asp Accessed June 14, 2014.
44. Wittenberg-Lyles E, Oliver DP, Demiris G, Baldwin P, Regehr K. Communication dynamics in hospice teams: Understanding the role of the chaplain in interdisciplinary team collaboration *J Palliat Med*. 2008;11(10):1330–1335.
45. Peery B. Outcome oriented chaplaincy: Intentional caring. In: Roberts S, ed. *Professional Spiritual and Pastoral Care: A Practical Clergy and Chaplain's Handbook*. Wooodstock, VT: Skylight Paths; 2012:342–361.

46. Piderman K, Marek D, Jenkins S. Johnson M, Buryska J, Mueller P. Patient's expectations of hospital chaplains. *Mayo Clin Proc.* 2008;83(1):58–65.
47. Schultz M, Lulav-Grinwald D, Bar-Sela G. Cultural differences in spiritual care: Findings of an Israeli oncologic questionnaire examining patient interest in spiritual care. *BMC Palliat Care.* 2014:13(1):19.
48. Bunniss S, Mowat H, Snowden A. Community chaplaincy listening: Practical theology in action. *Scot J Hlthcare Chaplaincy.* 2013;16:42–51.
49. Glombicki JS, Jeuland J. Exploring the importance of chaplain visits in a palliative care clinic for patients and companions. *J Palliat Med.* 2013;17(2):131–132.
50. Handzo G, Puchalski C. The role of the chaplain in palliative care. In: Cherney N, Fallon M, Kaasa S, Portenoy R, Currow D, eds. *Oxford Textbook of Palliative Medicine.* 5th ed. New York., NY: Oxford University Press; in press.
51. VandeCreek L, Lucas A. *The Discipline for Pastoral Care Giving: Foundations for Pastoral Care Giving.* Binghamton, NY: Haworth Press; 2012.
52. Asgeirsdottir GH., Sigurbjörnsson E, Traustadottir R, Sigurdardottir V, Gunnarsdottir S, Kelly E. In the shadow of death: Existential and spiritual concerns among persons receiving palliative care. *J Pastoral Care Counsel.* 2014;68(1):1–11.
53. Gaudette H, Jankowski K. Spiritual Coping and anxiety in palliative care patients: A pilot study. *J Health Care Chaplain.* 2013;19(4):131–139.
54. Flannelly K.J, Galek K, Bucchino J, Vane A. The relative prevalence of various spiritual needs. *Scot J Hlthcare Chaplaincy.* 2006;9(2):25–31.
55. Fitchett G, Risk JL. Screening for spiritual struggle. *J Pastoral Care Counsel.* 2009;62(1,2):1–12.
56. Fitchett G, Meyer PM, Burton LA. Spiritual care in the hospital: Who requests it? Who needs it? *J Pastoral Care.* 2000;54(2):173–186.
57. Clung E, Grossoeheme D, Jacobson A. Collaborating with chaplains to meet spiritual needs. *Medsurg Nursing.* 2006;15(3):147–156.
58. Ferrell B, Otis-Green S, Baird P, Garcia A. nurses' responses to requests for forgiveness at the end-of-life. *J Pain Symptom Manage.* 2014;47(3):631–641.
59. Tinoco L, ed. *Providing Cultural and Linguistically Competent Care.* Oak Brook, IL: Joint Commission; 2006.
60. Smith AK, Lo B, Sudore R. When previously expressed wishes conflict with best interests. *JAMA Intern Med.* 2013;173(13):1241–1245.
61. Burns G. A life-context approach to developing end-of-life decisions. *Chaplaincy Today.* 2000;24(1):-23–25.
62. Hess D. Faith healing and the palliative care team. *J Soc Work End Life Palliat Care.* 2013;9:2–3:180–190.
63. Cooper RS, Ferguson A, Bodurtha J, Smith T. AMEN in challenging conversations: Bridging the gaps between faith, hope, and medicine. *J Oncol Pract.* June 2014. Advance online publication.
64. Overvold J. Weaver AJ. Flannelly KJ. Koenig HG. A study of religion, ministry and meaning in caregiving among health professionals in an institutional setting in New York City. *J Pastoral Care Counsel.* 2005;59(3):225–235.
65. Koenig HG. King DE. Carson VB. *Handbook of Religion and Health.* 2nd ed. New York, NY: Oxford University Press; 2012.
66. Puchalski C, Vitillo R, Hull S, Reller N. Improving the spiritual dimension of whole person care: Reaching national and international consensus. *J Palliat Med.* 2014;17(6):642–656.
67. *Spiritual Care Matters: An Introductory Resource for All NHS Scotland Staff.* Edinburgh: National Health Service Education for Scotland; 2009.
68. Peery B. What's in a name? *PlainViews.* 2009;6(2). http://plainviews.healthcarechaplaincy.org/articles/Whats-in-a-Name. Accessed June 24, 2014.
69. LaRocca-Pitts M. Agape Care: A. *PlainViews.* 2006;3(2). http://plainviews.healthcarechaplaincy.org/articles/Agape-Care-A-Pastoral-and-Spiritual-Care-Continuum. Accessed June 24, 2014.
70. Fitchett G, Canada AL. The role of religion/spirituality in coping with cancer: Evidence, assessment, and intervention. In: Holland JC, ed. *Psycho-Oncology.* 2nd ed. New York, NY: Oxford University Press; 2010:440–446.

CHAPTER 10

Communication in Clinical Psychology

Sunita K. Patel, Stephanie Davidson, and Jeanelle Folbrecht

Introduction

The practice of palliative care is emerging as a critical component in contemporary healthcare, which increasingly seeks to address patients' quality of life issues concurrently with management of medical or physical symptoms.[1] Originally viewed as relevant primarily in treating suffering at the end of life, palliative care is now increasingly viewed as encompassing a broader continuum in the treatment of chronic and progressive illnesses. This expansion beyond the end-of-life phase appears to be partially fueled by changing demographic trends, including a rising older population with chronic health conditions that necessitate increased palliative care services. Further, advances in modern medicine have increased the timeframe from onset of a progressive health condition to death with a course that is often punctuated by episodes of acute illness and partial recovery, requiring palliative care interventions.[2]

Within this evolving context, the World Health Organization (WHO) revised its original definition of palliative care to: "the active total care of patients whose disease is not responsive to curative treatment. Control of pain, of other symptoms, and of psychological, social, and spiritual problems is paramount. The goal of palliative care is achievement of the best quality of life for patients and their families."[3] Such a definition, with its focus on symptom reduction and optimal quality of life, invites contributions from a range of healthcare disciplines, including psychologists. Traditionally, physicians, nurses, social workers, and the clergy have been members of the interdisciplinary palliative care team in a typical hospice setting, while psychologists often provided concurrent care to the same patient population from different settings.

Psychologists are trained and involved in the provision of interventions to individuals with chronic medical illnesses such as heart disease, AIDS, cancer, dementia, and chronic pain.[4] The recent expansion of palliative care presents exciting opportunities for contributions from psychologists who are already skilled in addressing many of the psychological challenges encountered by patients with progressive, debilitating disease. In 2008, the National Consensus Project for Quality Palliative Care updated quality care guidelines to include psychological and psychiatric aspects of care for optimal quality of life outcomes. The guidelines recommend assessment and treatment of psychological reactions such as stress, anticipatory grieving, and poor coping, as well as psychiatric diagnoses such as depression, anxiety, and delirium, based on the goals and needs of the patient.[5] Psychologists, by training, are poised to work within the interdisciplinary team to meet these essential aspects of quality palliative care.

Psychologists in the palliative setting work with the patient, the family, and the interdisciplinary team to mitigate psychological factors that elicit suffering or interfere with medical therapies and aim to facilitate coping and improve symptom management. This approach is distinct from psychologists in a primary care setting where the focus is behavioral prevention or management of disease, or the mental health setting in which the focus is long-term treatment for psychiatric disorders.[6] In the palliative care setting a psychologist does not typically provide treatment with the intent of "curing" or resolving the psychiatric condition; instead treatment is undertaken for other purposes, such as improving treatment adherence, facilitating sound decision-making around treatment choices, assisting the interdisciplinary team with behavioral management, and reducing psychosocial complications that could prolong hospitalization.

A key component of the psychologist's role in a palliative care program is that of a contributing member to the larger interdisciplinary team focused on shared palliative care goals for the patient and family.[7] As a member of the interdisciplinary team, psychologists have both unique and overlapping functions with other members who may also provide psychosocial support and interventions, although perhaps under different circumstances and with a different focus.[8,9]

Although psychologists may have some roles and skill sets that overlap with other team members, they also bring specialized knowledge and expertise in psychological constructs and theoretical frameworks that view the patient as an interactive member of larger systems (e.g., family, community, and the healthcare systems, etc.).[10,11] The patient is understood as having the capacity to both influence and be influenced by the various dynamics in his or her internal or external environment but also as in need of assistance to realize the various options. With this background, the psychologist's role extends beyond assessment and treatment of the patient to include educating team members on how best to understand and manage the patient's manifestation of psychological and behavioral difficulties.[10,11]

The key roles a palliative care psychologist contributes to the interdisciplinary team are

1. To conduct comprehensive assessments of the patient and family.
2. To provide targeted short-term treatment to address specific concerns of relevance in a palliative care setting.
3. To provide education and support to the patient's family or caregivers congruent with the palliative care goals.
4. To contribute to the optimal functioning of the interdisciplinary care team, which may involve communication, education, support, and facilitation of self-care.

Key Role #1: Provision of Assessment Services

Assessment Aims

Psychologists typically conduct assessments after another member of the interdisciplinary team (e.g., physician, social worker, etc.) has identified concerns about the patient's psychosocial health. The initial assessment focuses on identifying the patient's primary biological, psychological, and social concerns and detailing the associated symptoms, duration, and situational factors that contribute to the difficulties that have been identified by the palliative care team. Such descriptive information leads to diagnostic clarifications, including differentiation between normal responses to stressors that may improve with limited intervention versus meeting criteria for psychiatric conditions that warrant more intense treatment approaches.[10–12]

Patients with complex presenting problems require the psychologist's assessment to be comprehensive enough to pinpoint the underlying beliefs, conflicts, and dynamics driving the distress and other symptoms that the patient outwardly expresses to the world. The assessment must also remain sufficiently focused on specific problems in order to formulate interventions that are targeted and relevant to the patient's current health status.

Among the myriad of troubling biopsychosocial factors that may be revealed via the comprehensive assessment, the psychologist needs to identify and prioritize which specific problems may be a target for intervention while the patient is under the care of the palliative team. In the course of this determination, the psychologist will consider programmatic and interdisciplinary team objectives so that treatment goals are aligned and synergistic with interventions from other team members. Further, in assessing patients referred by other members of the palliative care team, the psychologist may need to periodically assess team expectations of his or her role with the patient, as it may be necessary to address any unrealistic expectations such as desiring a previously antagonistic patient to become the "model" participant after short-term psychological intervention.

Assessment Approaches

Assessment may involve a combination of interview and self-report questionnaires. Psychological assessment that is intended as systematic or routine screening of a large number of patients generally employs validated questionnaires with previously established "cut-off" scores or key items that serve as "red flags" to signal further assessment.[13,14] In contrast, the comprehensive assessment of a patient conducted by a psychologist is conducted as part of an interpersonal interview process that is also intended to establish a therapeutic relationship with the patient.

The comprehensive assessment may require more than one provider–patient visit and may also involve communication with the patient's family or primary caregiver. In the case of young children, the very sick, disabled, or elderly, the psychologist's primary source of information is often someone other than the patient. In addition, while the patient's well-being is always of central importance, psychologists may also assess the needs and coping abilities of primary caregivers in order to understand how their functioning may impact the patient's adjustment. Depending on the reasons for referring the patient for psychological assessment, the psychologist may also consider bedside nurses or other healthcare providers as sources of information to understand the specific triggers that might be exacerbating the patient's difficulties.

Psychologists may incorporate a more extensive psychometric approach in situations requiring integration of objective data that can be compared against population norms, such as in evaluating neurocognitive dysfunction, comparing a patient's symptoms or functional status to specific patient populations, or deciphering personality and behavioral traits to estimate the patient's risk for psychosocial complications such as noncompliance with complex medical regimens, and so on. In the cancer setting, in which screening for psychosocial distress is now considered the sixth vital sign in patient assessment, preliminary data suggests it is feasible to detect interval changes in distress among end-of-life patients with standardized screenings.[15] Measuring interval changes using psychometric tools was thought to be more informative than relying on a distress level obtained from a single assessment.[16] Psychologists are versed in the tradition of behavioral measurement and consider issues such as the measure's validity, reliability, sensitivity, specificity, and applicability as they integrate the patient's data for clinical purposes.[13]

Assessment Domains

In addition to identifying the patient's symptoms (fear, worry, guilt, loneliness, anger, pain, sleeplessness, etc.) and specific concerns ("I might die," "I am a burden on my husband," "I have no control," "the nurses don't like me," etc.), psychologists assess a broad range of areas deemed helpful in understanding the individual patient's psychosocial risk and protective factors that may contribute to health outcomes. The following are key domains of assessment to gain a comprehensive picture of the patient's functioning within the context of self, family, community, and the palliative care setting:

- The patient and family's premorbid functioning including prior medical and psychiatric illness, substance use history, and identification of psychological vulnerabilities such as tendency to cope by aggressive acting out or self-blaming depressive thoughts and the like, as well as lifestyle activities, degree of self-sufficiency, and developmental status for disabled or pediatric patients
- The patient or family's health literacy and ability to understand medical language and make informed decisions related to the patient's health

- The patient's perceptions of his or her illness trajectory, including level of optimism versus pessimism regarding his or her ability to adapt, as well as level of motivation and engagement for self-care and adherence to medical therapies
- The patient and family's perception of the patient–healthcare team communication, responsiveness, and relationship, including comfort in making requests
- Information about family constellation and history including cultural and spiritual background; relationships with partners, siblings, and/or parents; and information about past trauma or stressful life events
- Information about patient and family resources, including socioeconomic and occupational status; English-language proficiency of relevant caregivers; acculturation level of immigrant families; access to resources such as insurance, housing, assistance with daily living activities if needed, and so on.
- The extent of social support available to the patient and family from the spouse, children, extended family, or the community in which the patient resides
- The patient and family's responsiveness and ability to benefit from standard treatment approaches

Case Example of Assessment Focused on Psychiatric Diagnosis

Bob, a 32-year-old patient with refractory leukemia, was transferred from an outside hospital for a clinical trial in preparation for bone marrow transplant. Bob was initially pleasant but quickly became agitated and accused nurses of laziness, complained about inadequate care by personal care assistants, and frequently demanded to see the floor supervisor to complain. After he had "fired" several nurses and demanded one-to-one nursing care, psychology was consulted to assist with Bob's difficult behavior. When the psychologist assessed Bob, she observed very rapid and pressured speech. He perseverated on what he felt was the incompetence of staff and feelings of injustice related to his care both at his previous hospital and during his current hospitalization. He had difficulty answering the psychologist's questions and his thoughts would go on tangents, but he would resist redirection. Bob moved his legs and arms constantly and spoke in a very loud voice, contributing to the perception that he might be or become aggressive. He believed that he was given cancer by God so that he might be able to save his family and spoke of the influence he hoped to have on his family's errant behavior. His caretaking team interpreted Bob's behavior as rude, entitled, and purposeful and therefore responded to his outbursts and demands in an argumentative fashion, further escalating his behavior. The results of the psychological assessment, however, suggested that Bob was suffering from a coexisting psychiatric illness. The psychologist worked to educate nursing on the nature of what appeared to be a manic episode of bipolar disorder, which included helping the team to differentiate his agitated and demanding behavior from mere entitlement and disrespect. Working with the nursing team, a plan was put into place that included education on ways to interact with Bob to reduce his agitation and prevent escalation of behavior. The psychologist also discussed Bob's symptoms with the larger healthcare treatment team and recommended delay of the planned treatment of a bone marrow transplant until his symptoms were under better control. This recommendation considered the patient's safety by highlighting psychological factors that could negatively impact his ability to undergo a complex medical procedure while also considering the well-being of other patients and staff. Following communication of the assessment-derived recommendations, the psychologist remained available to the medical and nursing teams and worked with Bob in person and by phone to manage his agitated state. Unfortunately, Bob refused to engage in ongoing management of his manic symptoms and was therefore not eligible for transplant.

Key Role #2: Provision of Treatment Services

Psychologists provide evidence-based psychotherapy to reduce suffering and manage symptoms. They treat emotional difficulties such as depression, anxiety, and posttraumatic stress disorder. Within the palliative care setting, they manage the impact of these emotional factors on physical symptoms such as pain, nausea, poor sleep, and fatigue. Best-practice techniques such as motivational interviewing, mindfulness techniques, and cognitive-behavioral skills, including cognitive restructuring, relaxation, and guided imagery exercises, are among the tools that are part of a psychologist's training used in the palliative care of patients.[4,6]

Psychologists, by training, are focused on creating a strong therapeutic relationship with patients that encourage them to disclose and articulate their innermost thoughts and needs without shame or fear of censure. The therapeutic relationship is the basis for trust in treatment and fosters an environment that demonstrates the desire of the psychologist and, by extension, the team, to support the patient as he or she strives to grieve, adjust, and come to terms with the confines of illness. Psychologists "walk with" the patient as he or she processes and transitions through the evolving illness trajectory and help ground the patient by focusing on the established treatment goals.

Typically, patients work with the psychologist to address problems with adjustment to illness. Challenges with adjustment are often characterized by anxiety about treatment or existential concerns and depressive symptoms, including decreased motivation, tearfulness, and sadness. Some patients also exhibit problematic behaviors that interfere with treatment such as problems with compliance or acting out.[10–12] Treatment by the psychologist in the palliative care program is typically short term with a duration ranging from a single session to multiple visits across several weeks delivered by the bedside and focused on goals that are relevant/feasible for the patient to achieve.

Goal-Setting and Problem-Solving

Psychological interventions in palliative care are targeted to address specific problems and have well-defined goals. Goal-setting is a collaborative process with the patient and family that allows the palliative care team to ensure that the patient's preferences and values are at the center of care and creates a shared mission for all involved. Goals are best achieved when they are specific, realistic, and time-limited. Once set, these goals can be modified based on the changing needs of the patient. It is also useful to break down larger goals into component parts, which helps give the patient a sense of accomplishment and empowerment with each meaningful success. Smaller goals also allow patients to pace themselves appropriately, making it more likely that he or she will be successful.[12]

Once goals are defined, the team can then focus on helping the patient in solving problems and addressing barriers that impede progress toward a particular goal. Some patients may have adequate premorbid problem-solving skills but difficulty drawing on that knowledge due to stress or cognitive changes related to their illness. Others may lack strategies for solving problems even prior to illness and therefore require explicit assistance. Through modeling, support, and directive instruction, psychologists can help patients learn and apply problem-solving skills.[17] Once learned, these strategies empower patients with a greater sense of control and confidence and reduce the feeling of being overwhelmed.[12]

Psychotherapy

The psychologist draws from a number of evidence-based theoretical frameworks of human behavior to shape and deliver the interventions to the patient, as well as to help patients understand how the treatments will benefit them. The following are common approaches used in the palliative care setting.

Cognitive Behavioral Therapy

The goal of cognitive behavioral therapy in the course of advancing illness is to utilize tools that can modify dysfunctional thinking and behavior that have been known to increase emotional distress.[12,17] These interventions have been found to be useful in treating anxiety and depression and in symptom management in palliative care settings.[18,19] Although these types of interventions have been found to be successful, it is important to note that as a patient's illness progresses, he or she may be unable to engage in behavioral interventions or in this type of cognitive exploration due to increasing fatigue and frailty, changes in mental status, and rapidly increasing physical symptoms.[12]

Existential Psychotherapy

Existential therapy is focused on helping patients confront the basic struggles of being human. According to existential therapists, the challenges of human existence are the inevitability of death, the ultimate freedom that comes from the need for structure and a sense of being grounded, our inherent isolation, which means that humans come into the world alone and will ultimately leave alone, and the desire to find meaning for how and why one should live the life that one is given.[20] In a palliative care setting the psychologist will help the patient confront these struggles by defining the meaning of his or her life in order to find an acceptance of death. Patients who are able to reach a state of peaceful awareness of their impending death have been found to experience lower rates of psychological distress, higher rates of advance care planning, better quality of death as reported by their caretakers, and better physical and psychological outcomes for their caregivers.[21] Several therapeutic approaches have been developed to help patients develop insight related to the meaning of their lives, including dignity therapy and meaning-centered psychotherapy.[22,23]

Psychotherapy at the End of Life

As patients begin to prepare for the end of their lives, psychologists can work with them to help them achieve what Farber and Farber describe as a respectful death.[24] The Respectful Death Model of Care seeks to develop a relationship between providers, patients, and families that is based on the agreement that professionals will care for the patient and family up until death and into bereavement, that the patient and family will be invited to bring up all topics of importance to them whether medically related or not, and that all parties will remain conscious of the patient and family experience and the meaning of the care to the providers as it changes within in the context of a progressing illness.[25] Psychologists are also able to help identify important issues for the patient, including what aspects of treatment the patient feels can protect his or her dignity, how the patient wants to spend the time that remains, and what important aspects of the dying process the patient wants to control. In addition, a psychologist can assist patients in communicating effectively with the family to address unresolved problems, including those that center on challenges with forgiveness, separation, and loss.[25,26]

Case Example of Short-Term, Goal-Oriented, Cognitive Behavioral Therapy, and Existential Therapy Interventions

Amy, a 39-year-old with lymphoma, was initially seen for psychotherapy on an outpatient basis to prepare for a stem cell transplant. The patient shared that she was experiencing a great deal of anxiety about her treatment choices. The psychologist worked with Amy to help her make a list of pros and cons, which helped her to decide to move forward with the process. Amy was also taught to record her worries about transplant and to challenge unrealistic concerns with the facts that she had learned about the transplant process. Unfortunately, prior to the initiation of her transplant, Amy was admitted to the hospital with dysphasia, vision problems, and increasing difficulty hearing on the left side due to progressive disease involving multiple cranial nerves. Due to these physical limitations, she had to be taken off her antidepressant medications, which caused an increase in anxiety related to withdrawal. The patient was also placed on steroids, which further increased her symptoms of anxiety. While the psychiatrist worked on providing psychotropic interventions to assist with anxiety control, the psychologist worked with her by teaching relaxation and meditation techniques to address anxiety and decrease physical discomfort. A focus on problem-solving helped Amy identify activities that would assist her in gaining a greater sense of control, including helping her set a visitation schedule for family that would offer her the greatest level of support during the most difficult periods of the day. She also benefited from the ability to set daily goals that were attainable and helped her to feel that she was working toward getting out of the hospital in order to continue to receive hospice services at home. During this time, Amy expressed many existential concerns as she prepared to transition to hospice. The psychologist coordinated care with the chaplain to begin to address these worries by focusing on meaningful relationships for the patient and on important conversations and interactions that she wanted to have with family and friends. One particularly helpful set of conversations focused on helping the patient to share her funeral wishes with her closest family member.

Case Example of Assessment/Intervention by a Palliative Psychologist as Part of an Interdisciplinary Pediatric Team

Alex, a 25 year-old male who had received a bone marrow transplant to treat acute lymphocytic leukemia, was admitted to the hospital several months posttransplant for "failure to thrive." He complained of nausea, was not eating, and was losing a great deal of weight. The medical team presumed the cause was graft versus host disease, a possible risk of transplant in which the engrafted bone marrow cells attach to the recipient. The clinical social worker noted additional symptoms of anhedonia and social withdrawal and asked the medical team to consult psychology to rule out the possibility that depression might be contributing to the patient's presentation. During a clinical interview, the psychologist discovered grief related to the loss of a romantic relationship and additional symptoms of depression. Alex initially tried to hide these symptoms partially due to anger but eventually revealed that he felt he had no control over his life and was worried that he would not be able to make it to his sister's wedding one week later. He additionally had a conditioned response of gagging when in the presence of food, contributing to the perception of nausea and actual weight loss. Describing the nature of Alex's depression to his physician, working with the patient and physicians to establish a team approach to medical decision-making, and using behavioral methods to reduce negative responses to food resulted in avoiding unnecessary tests, early discharge, and, most important, Alex's attendance at his sister's wedding.

Key Role #3: Involvement With Patients' Family Systems

Family is an important resource for the patient's psychosocial adjustment to the illness trajectory. As such, it is valuable to assess and understand the family's dynamics, belief systems, and cultural factors. Culturally defined health beliefs and practices may explain behaviors such as nonadherence to prescribed therapies, the extent and quality of involvement with the patient's care or treatment decisions, and relationships with healthcare staff.[27] In addition, while the patient's well-being is always of central importance, psychologists may need to assess the needs and coping skills of primary caregivers in order to understand how their functioning may impact the patient's adjustment. The patient's illness can, over time, strain family relationships, and partners or siblings of pediatric patients may experience feelings of neglect or loss of companionship, with subsequent impact on the patient's adjustment.[28] By the same token, family members have also expressed that the illness experience resulted in an increased closeness.[29]

Supporting Patient–Family Communication

Communication in families with a member suffering from a life-impacting or life-limiting illness often take on a unique pattern influenced by many factors but particularly by the age of the patient and the culture of the family. Often family members and patients are aware of the likelihood of death but do not discuss their fears or concerns with one another. This has been described at the "law of double protection."[30] This pattern of mutual isolation and protection may be present in varied patient groups, including pediatric cases and the elderly. Loving and well-meaning families avoid discussion of the reality of the illness and death for fear they will upset their loved one and discourage them in a way that will cause loss of hope and the will to live. Some cultures believe that discussing death invites death itself through discouragement and loss of will. Often it is felt that avoiding such painful topics also helps avoid emotional pain, but too often such avoidance invites a sense of isolation. Another cultural phenomenon in the discussion of life-threatening illness is the "third person" phenomenon in which families cannot bring themselves to address anxieties regarding probable death with the patient directly but instead invite others such as friends or healthcare providers to do so to assure their loved one's peace and to ease discomfort without violating cultural norms or risking conflict.

The palliative psychologist has a powerful opportunity to assess the patient's anxiety, explore taboos regarding open discussion of death and dying, and work with the patient and family toward communication aimed at reducing anxiety, increasing awareness of the patient's wishes, and facilitating meaningful interactions between family members. To do so requires rapport with the patient and family and skill in eliciting the patient and family's understanding of the seriousness and probable outcome of the illness and assessing differences in evaluation between the family and the medical care team. Often families are acutely aware of the medical team's beliefs about the seriousness of the patient's illness or the possibility of futility of care but prefer to "remain positive" or wait for a positive change in the patient's situation due to faith. The psychologist can facilitate communication between the medical team and family toward increased understanding of both perspectives and active consideration of the patient's goals and wishes. The psychologist in such emotionally charged situations is called upon to tolerate strong emotions while assisting others to do the same, while guiding the patient and family toward meaningful discussions in a culturally sensitive way.

These discussions can become challenging to navigate within the end-of-life context; psychologists work to help patients process and communicate their preferences and needs to the family and medical team. As such, they assess the patient's awareness, beliefs, and fears with regard to his or her illness. Although patients may not talk about the gravity of their illness, they are often aware and sometimes fearful of illness and death. Psychologists can help patients by encouraging the expression of emotion rather than stifling it. Often, caring family members and even some professionals see a patient's sadness or anger and try to calm them without first understanding the concerns or frustration that brings out the emotion. Providing means of emotional expression through therapeutic interactions can result in a decrease in distress as well as very meaningful and comforting conversations. For children, these interactions would include play, art, storytelling, and other means of working with them at their level of expression.

Psychologists can also look for opportunities for patients to exert control and gain a sense of mastery in their environment. Opportunities for making decisions, voicing wishes, and exercising appropriate control can reduce feelings of hopelessness, bolster a sense of self-efficacy, and improve mood and adjustment. Helping family members learn how to support patients as they work to maintain a level of independence can also be extremely important for both adults and children.

Case Example of Treatment of Family Dynamics With Adult Patients

Carolyn was a 64-year-old female diagnosed with metastatic lung cancer. She was referred for psychotherapy to address symptoms of depression. When the psychologist met with both she and her husband, it was revealed that Carolyn was very angry about her recent diagnosis as she had just retired and was looking forward to a new beginning after a difficult time in her marriage. She described herself as a private person and shared the resentment she felt that others were so distressed by her diagnosis that they were not able to consider that she might want to keep aspects of her treatment private and might want to spend time with others focused on topics other than cancer. She was particularly angry with her husband whom she felt was encouraging ongoing prayer and conversation about her illness despite her resentment. Couples counseling techniques focused on improving communication were utilized to help the patient and her husband understand how this diagnosis had impacted them as a unit and as individuals. Each of them explored ways to better support one another and themselves. Carolyn's husband was able to acknowledge his fears about losing his wife and how those fears had influenced his desire to push her to act as if she were well despite how she might have been feeling. Both Carolyn and her husband were able to recognize how her prognosis had impacted their daily interactions and were able to change some problematic patterns of interacting that had begun to develop since her initial diagnosis. As a couple they were able to focus on short-term goals that would allow them to enjoy their time together within the bounds of the patient's physical limitations. The two were able to begin discussions about Carolyn's desires for her care at the end of life so that she could feel comfortable that her wishes would be respected while her husband gained a clearer understanding of her needs. During the course of treatment, it became clear that Carolyn's husband was not taking care of his own emotional and physical needs. Through counseling he was able to understand the importance of self-care in his role as caregiver and obtained appropriate medical care. He was also able to recognize unhealthy patterns of coping and was able to engage in new strategies.*

Case Example of Navigating Family Dynamics With Pediatric Patients

The psychologist was called to see an 11-year-old child diagnosed with advanced cancer because she was having frequent, recurring nightmares resulting in refusal to sleep, daytime sleepiness, and increased distress and anxiety. Further, the palliative physician needed information to help differentiate her daytime sleepiness from avoidance of sleep at night versus overmedication for pain. The psychologist's assessment revealed that the child internalized and avoided expressing both physical and emotional symptoms of discomfort, possibly resulting in the disturbing dreams. Education regarding the normal pattern of communication within families of seriously ill children and recommendations for eliciting and exploring the patient's current awareness of her illness, beliefs about their cause, general fears and concerns, as well as fears and concerns about death was provided to the family and the medical team. A plan was developed for both individual therapy with the psychologist to explore concerns and wishes and training of the family to increase their ability to tolerate difficult emotions and begin to explore the child's concerns as a means of providing comfort.

Key Role #4: Psychologist as an Integrated Member of the Interdisciplinary Palliative Care Team

Communication Around Patient Care Issues

Communication between members of the interdisciplinary team that is characterized by mutual trust and respect is essential for quality patient-based care and coordinating end-of-life related care. Psychologists contribute to this process by communicating with other members about their patient-related interactions and also by making themselves readily available to other providers for discussion. Psychologists are involved in regular meetings with palliative team members and psychosocial rounds that are useful for sharing medical and psychosocial information in order to develop a unified treatment approach and care plan for patients and families. Based on these interactions with the interdisciplinary team and their interactions with the patient, psychologists can become aware of the need for enhanced or changed communication and can work with the relevant parties toward such changes. Ongoing communication about patient-related issues with other members also serves to facilitate "synergy" in the delivery of intervention services and minimize inadvertently working at cross-purposes. Communication within the interdisciplinary team may also result in more efficient use of psychosocial services as increased awareness of interventions being offered by other providers allows the psychologist (or other providers) to provide more targeted treatments or sometimes be more able to attend to the needs of family members.

Provision of Education as a Team Member

A psychologist's role as a member of the interdisciplinary team may involve providing education to other members in various forms. He or she can help the team to recognize how psychological and behavioral factors are impacting a patient who is being cared for by the team. Often, understanding the reasons underlying problematic behavior from challenging patients can help team members retain compassion and better tolerate "problematic" patients. A psychologist's education includes helping team members learn to assess psychological and psychiatric issues and to recognize behaviors and family dynamics that could impact the treatment being provided. Most important, the psychologist can help the team recognize how these challenges are interfering with reaching goals set by the patient and family and can propose strategies for the team to better meet the needs of the family unit. Psychologists also participate in more explicit forms of education activities ranging from training other providers in specific skills, such as relaxation training, to offering seminars on behavioral methods to assist with sleep, fatigue, pain, treatment adherence, provider stress management, patient–provider communication, and so on.[4,10-12]

Provision of Staff Support and Facilitation of Self-Care as a Team Member

Compassionate individuals who value meaningful interactions are typically attracted to working in the palliative health setting; however, these are also the palliative care providers who are at risk for high occupational stress and burnout precisely due to the nature of the work to which they are drawn. Constant exposure to death, inadequate time with dying patients, growing workload, increasing number of deaths, communication difficulties with the patient and family, and inadequate coping with elicited emotions such as grief, depression, and guilt in caring for patients can lead to compassion fatigue and vicarious trauma.[31-34] Psychologists are able to assist providers in recognizing their personal needs for support and help normalize the emotional responses elicited in caring for very sick or terminal patients and their families.

The factors involved in mitigating the impact of stress are generally twofold. The first category is comprised largely of personal protective characteristics or choices that support emotional well-being such as self-awareness, cognitive mindset, and behavioral choices to engage in practices to promote well-being. The second category is comprised of factors influenced by the environment, including training and education, atmosphere or culture of the workplace and team, and psychological interventions aimed at promoting mindfulness and attention to grief. The psychologist can play a valuable role in developing strategies to impact the functioning of the interdisciplinary palliative care team and the well-being of its members. Using their training in the impact of cognitive beliefs on emotions and behavior, psychologists may engage providers in cognitively reframing stressful events to a more empowering perspective. For example, helping the provider refocus on the personal values being served by caring for patients can enhance a sense of purpose and improve job satisfaction.[35] The psychologist may further facilitate stress management among members of the palliative care team by fostering an environment where the team acknowledges and supports each other to reduce provider burnout issues. Toward this end, the psychologist may initiate meetings for the team to pause and acknowledge stress or conflict among members and assist the team toward problem-solving and conflict resolution.

Case Example of Facilitation of Communication Among Team Members

A disagreement among team members over the management of a particular patient's pain was discovered during sign-out. The two physicians had had similar disagreements regarding the philosophy of pain management previously, and this discussion was quickly moving toward polarizing the two parties. Discussion of specific cases was leading to personalization on part of the physicians and impacting both their frustration and the cohesiveness of the team. Recognizing the conflict and the impact on the team, the physicians invited the palliative psychologist to assist them in resolving the conflict. To minimize depersonalization, the discussion focused on managing differences in pain management practices during transfers of patient in general rather than the specific case. The physicians and psychologist identified ways the entire team could support the physicians in working with patients with challenging pain, personalities, or family dynamics. Communication regarding values in patient pain management resulted in greater understanding and healthy debate rather than personalization. Tension between the physicians was reduced, understanding of the challenges in working with difficult situations increased, and team interdependence led to greater engagement among team members.

Palliative Psychology Training and Competencies

Psychologists working in palliative care begin their training by obtaining a doctoral degree (PhD or PsyD) in psychology. The focus of the programs is on the diagnosis of mental health conditions, assessment of neurobehavioral and personality factors, and the provision of mental health services to a range of patient populations. It is typically at the postdoctoral level that psychologists begin to specialize in a specific area of practice beyond the basic emphasis on either clinical or counseling psychology. While the first set of skills is typically clear, with approved training programs and licensure requirements for psychologists, there is little guidance on the range of specific skills needed to work in palliative care programs and little or no widely available certification process. A number of psychology doctoral programs have specialized tracks that focus on health psychology or related competencies in preparation for working in medical settings. More recently, postdoctoral training programs focused on training opportunities for psychologists in palliative care have been developed, such as those offered through the Veterans Administration, The Ohio State University Medical Center, and James Cancer Hospital.[36] Psychologists can also obtain preparation to work in palliative care programs through a number of web-based training programs, such as those offered by Education in Palliative and End-of-Life Care,[37] the California State University Institute for Palliative Care (San Marcos),[38] the University of Washington Center for Palliative Care Education (HIV/AIDS specific),[39] and the National Hospice and Palliative Care Organization (pediatric specific).[40]

Challenges and Future Directions

Psychologists' ability to substantially contribute toward quality care of patients and families in palliative medicine is increasingly recognized, with practice guidelines from the National Consensus Project recommending that interdisciplinary teams be able to meet the psychological and psychiatric symptoms of patients in the palliative care setting. Challenges for the discipline of psychology in palliative care include organizational and financial resources and insurance reimbursement issues that limit the availability of psychologists designated to palliative care programs. Further, high volume in medical centers may reduce the availability of psychologists to even those patients who are referred for such services.

Over the next decade we anticipate continued evolution of the psychologist's role in palliative care. Palliative psychologists will continue to clarify and define their contributions separate from other members of the palliative team, as well as from other psychologists who provide assessment and treatment services to patients with chronic health issues in medical settings.

Future directions for psychologists should include integration of clinical research to empirically determine the models of care and intervention that are optimally efficacious so as to replace the models that are only marginally successful in meeting patient, provider, and institutional objectives. Further, given the changing healthcare systems where resource allocation requires increased justification, it will be important to demonstrate clear medical or financial benefits of psychosocial involvement.

References

1. National Institutes of Health. NIH State-of-the-Science Conference Statement on improving end-of-life care. *NIH Consensus and State-of-the-Science Statements* 2004;21(3):1–26.
2. Clark D, Hockley J, Admedzai, S, eds. *New Themes in Palliative Care*. Buckingham, UK: Open University Press; 1997.
3. World Health Organization. WHO definition of palliative care. http://www.who.int/cancer/palliative/definition/en. Accessed June 30, 2014.
4. Brown R, Freeman W, Brown R, et al. The role of psychology in health care delivery. *Prof Psychol Res Pr*. 2002;33(6):536–545.
5. Hultman T, Reder ER, Dahlin C. Improving psychological and psychiatric aspects of palliative care: The National Consensus Project and the National Quality Forum Preferred Practices for Palliative and Hospice Care. *Omega*. 2008;57(4):323–339.
6. Haley W, Larson D, Kasl-Godley J, Neimeyer R, Kwilosz D. Roles for psychologists in end-of-life Care: Emerging models of practice. *Prof Psychol Res Pr*. 2003;34(6):626–633.
7. Block SD. Psychological issues in end-of-life care. *J Palliat Med*. 2006;9(3):751–772.
8. Breitbart W. Psycho-oncology and palliative care: Opportunity for integration. *Palliat Support Care*. 2004;2(2):113–114.
9. O'Connor M, Fisher C. Exploring the dynamics of interdisciplinary palliative care teams in providing psychosocial care: "Everybody thinks that everybody can do it and they can't." *J Palliat Med*. 2011;14(2):191–196.
10. Payne S, Haines R. Doing our bit to ease the pain. *Psychologist* 2002;15:564–567.
11. Payne S, Haines R. The contribution of psychologists to specialist palliative care. *Int J Palliat Nurs*. 2002;8(8):401–406.
12. Cathcart F. The contribution of clinical psychology to palliative care. In: Hanks G, Cherny NI, Chistakis NA, Fallon M, Kaasa S, Portenoy RK, eds. *Oxford Textbook of Palliative Medicine*. 4th ed. New York, NY: Oxford University Press; 2009:258–264.
13. Kelly B, McClement S. Measurement of psychological distress in palliative care. *Palliat Med*. 2006; 20: 779–789.
14. Jacobsen PB, Wagner LI. A new quality standard: The integration of psychosocial care into routine cancer care. *J Clin Oncol*. 2012;30(11):1154–1159.
15. Bultz BD, Carlson LE. Emotional distress: The sixth vital sign—future directions in cancer care. *Psycho-Oncology*. 2006;15(2):93–95.
16. Patel SK, Fernandez N, Wong A, et al. Changes in self-reported distress in end-of-life pediatric cancer patients and their parents using the pediatric distress thermometer. *Psycho-Oncology*. 2014;23(5):592–596.
17. Beck JS. *Cognitive Therapy: Basics and Beyond*. New York, NY: Guilford Press; 1995.
18. Anderson T, Watson M, Davidson R. The use of cognitive behavioural therapy techniques for anxiety and depression in hospice patients: A feasibility study. *Palliat Med*. 2008;22(7):814–821.
19. Turk DC, Feldman, CS. A cognitive-behavioural approach to symptom management in palliative care: Augmenting somatic interventions. In: Chochinov HC, Breitbart W, eds. *Handbook of Psychiatry in Palliative Medicine*. New York, NY: Oxford University Press; 2000:223–240.
20. Yalom ID. *Existential Psychotherapy*. New York, NY: Basic Books; 1980.
21. Ray AB, Block SD, Friedlander RJ, Zhang B, Maciejewski PK, Prigerson HG. Peaceful awareness in patients with advanced cancer. *J Palliat Med*. 2006;9(6):1359–368.
22. Breitbart W, Poppito S, Rosenfeld B, et al. Pilot randomized control trial of individual meaning-centered psychotherapy for patients with advanced cancer. *J Clin Oncol*. 2012;30(12):1304–1309.
23. Chochinov HM, Kristjanson LJ, Breitbart W, et al. Effect of dignity therapy on distress and end-of-life experience in terminally ill patients: A randomised control trial. *Lancet Oncol*. 2011;12:753–762.
24. Farber A, Farber S. The respectful death model: Difficult conversations at the end of life. In: Katz RS, Johnson TA, eds. *When Professionals Weep*. New York, NY: Routledge; 2006:221–236.
25. Vachon MLS. The emotional problems of the patient in palliative medicine. In: Hanks G, Cherny NI, Chistakis NA, Fallon M, Kaasa S, Portenoy RK, eds. *Oxford Textbook of Palliative Medicine*. 4th ed. Oxford: Oxford University Press; 2009:1410–1436.
26. Greenstein M, Breitbart W. Cancer and the experience of meaning: A group psychotherapy program for people with cancer. *Am J Psychother*. 2000;54(4):486–500.
27. De Trill M, Kovalcik R. The child with cancer: Influence of culture on truth-telling and patient care. *NY Acad Sci*. 1997;809:197–210.
28. Alderfer MA, Long KA, Lown EA, et al. Psychosocial adjustment of siblings of children with cancer: A systematic review. *Psycho-Oncology*. 2010;19(8):789–805.
29. Ostroff J, Ross S, Steinglass P. Psychosocial adaptation following treatment: A family systems perspective on childhood cancer survivorship. In: Baider L, Cooper C, Kaplan De-Nour A, eds. *Cancer and the Family*. 2nd ed. Chichester, UK: John Wiley & Sons; 2000:155–173.
30. Grootenhuis MA, Last BF. Children with cancer. *Recent Results Cancer Res*. 2006;168:73–79.
31. Kearney MK, Weininger RB, Vachon ML, Harrison RL, Mount BM. Self-care of physicians caring for patients at the end of life: Being connected . . . a key to my survival. *JAMA* 2009;301(11):1155–1164, E1151.
32. Stamm BH. Measuring compassion satisfaction as well as fatigue: Developmental history of the Compassion Satisfaction and Fatigue Test. In Figley CR, ed. *Treating Compassion Fatigue*. New York, NY: Brunner-Routledge; 2002:107–119.
33. Figley CR. *Compassion Fatigue: Coping with Secondary Traumatic Stress Disorder in Those Who Treat the Traumatized*. New York, NY: Brunner/Mazel; 1995.
34. Wittenberg-Lyles E, Goldsmith J, Ferrell B, Ragan S. *Communication in Palliative Nursing*. New York, NY: Oxford University Press; 2012.
35. Chittenden EH, Ritchie CS. Work-life balancing: Challenges and strategies. *J Palliat Med*. 2011;14(7):870–874.
36. Center to Advance Palliative Care Website. http://www.capc.org. Accessed June 30, 2014.
37. Education in Palliative and End-of-Life Care Website http://www.epec.net. Accessed June 30, 2014.
38. California State University Institute for Palliative Care Website. http://www.csupalliativecare.org. Accessed June 30, 2014.
39. University of Washington Center for Palliative Care Education Website. http://depts.washington.edu/pallcare/about/index.shtml. Accessed June 30, 2014.
40. National Hospice and Palliative Care Organization Website. http://www.nhpco.org/childrenspediatricschipps/professional-education. Accessed June 30, 2014.

CHAPTER 11

Cultural Humility

Kathryn Neubauer, William Dixon, Rosalie Corona, and Joann Bodurtha

Introduction

In the next 50 years, nearly half of the US population will no longer be white, non-Hispanic.[1] In 2013, 19 of the 25 largest US counties were majority-minority.[2] The need to provide health services to patients of diverse cultures and languages will continue to increase. For example, by 2060 Latinos are estimated to make up 31% of the US population.[1] The Asian American population also continues to experience significant growth. Given these demographic changes, enhanced appreciation of the values, social practices, rituals, and forms of expression that persons of varied race/ethnicities, geographies, religions, socioeconomic status, and other group identities bring to the table also needs to grow.[3] If culture and behaviors are recognized as essential elements of health and disease, a workforce that is open to understanding and working with the unique, shared, and differing attributes of patients and families is essential.

While exploring cultural generalizations may provide an opportunity to learn more about others, stereotyping can inhibit that knowledge. Diversity within a group is often greater than it is between groups. As such, empathy and individual consideration must always provide the underpinnings to relationships within the delivery of healthcare. Technological developments in communication and transportation may facilitate connections around the world for many, but cultural codes, family traditions, and experiences continue to powerfully influence daily life, systems of care, available options, and individual choices.[4-6] Cross-cultural encounters benefit from a patient focus that is not prescribed by an ethnic group focused pedagogy or jumping to conclusions.[7] As Brody and Hunt stated, "Every physician-patient encounter is a cross-cultural exercise—even if the physician grew up on the same street in the same town."[8]

Some have suggested that the assimilation of the "melting pot" in the United States has transitioned to a "salad bowl" of diversity impacted by ongoing migration, pre- and post-migration stressors, and varied degrees of assimilation and acculturation.[9] Healthcare providers need to better understand others' values and behaviors, as they affect many of the expectations providers have about patient and family communication. For example, initiating questions and making eye contact can vary remarkably and shape interactions especially in stressful times.

The potentially vulnerable stages of life in which palliative care takes place require self-awareness across all modalities of communication used to engage the uniqueness of cultures to deliver quality care.[10] Cultural humility does not provide a recipe for handling all situations, but it does provide an umbrella framework for the varied terms and communication behaviors that demonstrate respect for the role of culture in all of our lives. For cultural awareness and sensitivity antecedents to cultural humility, see definitions in Box 11.1).[9,11-15]

The co-existing framework of competencies, potentially implying a mastery of what is a lifelong learning process, has also evolved to incorporate the ongoing process of developing self-awareness, knowledge, and skills in order to be able to apply them in culturally diverse individual and organizational situations.[16] Curricula and resources have been developed that include specialty-focused materials, courses, models, immersion experiences, distance learning, simulations, and other approaches.[17-19] This chapter describes the historical background of cultural humility, provides insights into cultural perspectives and related challenges in palliative care, and presents a perspective on the agenda for moving forward. Also included are a skills guide showcasing exemplary practices, exercises, and educator tools.

Historical Background

Cultural humility provides a framework encouraging enhanced patient/family–provider communication that is known to support improved care.[20] The multiple impacts of culturally aware communication and connectedness in improving health outcomes and reducing health disparities are receiving increasing emphasis.[21-23] Healthcare disparities, "differences in access to or availability of facilities and services, and the variation in rates of disease occurrence and disabilities between socioeconomic and/or geographically defined population groups," can arise from differences in race, ethnicity, culture, socioeconomic status, sexual orientation, insurance coverage, and much more.[24] When race/ethnic discordance between provider and patient/family is present, it has been shown that provider–patient communication is less open, and the provider is less likely to give patients choices and control over their medical care and/or responsibility for their health decisions.[25] This is true even when controlling for education level of the patient. Differences in expectations and preferences, influenced by religion, race, culture, and geography, may impact providers' and patients' approaches to end-of-life discussions.[26]

> **Box 11.1** Terms Central to Culture and Healthcare[9,11-15]
>
> **Cultural awareness**—An essential skill in the provision of culturally appropriate services, cultural awareness entails an understanding of how a person's culture may inform his or her values, behavior, beliefs, and basic assumptions.[11]
>
> **Cultural brokering**—Cultural brokering has been defined as "bridging, linking or mediating between groups or persons of different cultural backgrounds to effect change."[12]
>
> **Cultural competence**—On the individual level, cultural competence has been defined as "the act whereby a healthcare professional develops an awareness of one's existence, sensations, thoughts, and environment without letting these factors have an undue influence on this for whom care is provided."[13] Cultural competency is the acceptance and respect for difference, a continuous self-assessment regarding culture, an attention to the dynamics of difference, the ongoing development of cultural knowledge, and the resources and flexibility within service models to meet the needs of minority population.[14]
>
> At the organization level, cultural competence requires that organizations
>
> - have a defined set of values and principles and demonstrate behaviors, attitudes, policies, and structures that enable them to work effectively cross-culturally.
> - have the capacity to (a) value diversity, (b) conduct self-assessment, (c) manage the dynamics of difference, (d) acquire and institutionalize cultural knowledge and (e) adapt to diversity and the cultural contexts of the communities they serve.
> - incorporate the above in all aspects of policymaking, administration, practice, and service delivery and involve systematically consumers, key stakeholders, and communities.
>
> **Cultural safety**—"an environment that is spiritually, socially and emotionally safe, as well as physically safe for people; where there is no assault challenge or denial of their identity, of who they are and what they need. It is about shared respect, shared meaning, shared knowledge and experience of learning together."[15 (p213)]
>
> **Cultural sensitivity**—Cultural sensitivity is a set of skills that enables a person to learn about and get to know people who are different from him or her, thereby coming to understand how to serve them better within their own communities.[9]

Healthcare providers may have unintentional personal biases and beliefs that influence their practices.[27] Biases are found across a range of healthcare providers. In a survey completed by nurses about challenges to culturally appropriate care, three common challenges emerged: the extent of diversity, the lack of resources to provide the most appropriate care, and caregiver's personal beliefs and biases.[28] This study and others demonstrate the many factors contributing to healthcare providers' unintentional biases. The patient/family's ethnic, cultural, and personal background influences the interpretation of symptoms, understanding of the disease, and expectations of treatment. Healthcare providers may lack an understanding of cultural, ethnic, and personal backgrounds and how they affect disease and treatment.[29] Healthcare providers are tasked with navigating the complex interplay of their patients' conceptions of health and disease with their own beliefs and values.[30] As local and national concerns about health disparities increase, different models and frameworks have been proposed to help educate healthcare providers in this area.

Cultural Competency

In the early 1990s, initial efforts to address cultural and ethnic healthcare disparities focused on training healthcare providers to demonstrate enhanced cultural competency. The *Merck Manual of Diagnosis and Therapy* presented its first "Cross-Cultural Issues in Medicine" chapter in 1992.[31] In an important 1996 editorial, Lavizzo-Mourey and Mackenzie conceptualized cultural competence as the inclusion and integration of health-related beliefs and cultural values, disease incidence and prevalence, and treatment efficacy in the healthcare for all patients.[32] The authors emphasized the importance of knowing distinct cultural beliefs and values and the incidence and prevalence of certain medical conditions in various populations. Similar definitions and descriptions of cultural competence were soon developed by others.[29,32-34]

Curriculum guides were developed, including the Society of Teachers of Family Medicine's endorsement of "Recommended Care Core Curriculum Guidelines on Culturally Sensitive and Competent Health Care."[35] In 2000, the Office of Minority Affairs in the US Department of Health and Human Services issued National Standards for Culturally and Linguistically Appropriate Services (CLAS) for healthcare organizations that received federal funds (https://www.thinkculturalhealth.hhs.gov/content/clas.asp).[36] Although private providers were not required to adhere to these standards, they were strongly encouraged to adopt them.[37] In 2001 the National Association of Social Workers published the *NASW Standards for Cultural Competence in Social Work Practice,* which is based on the 2000 policy statement "Cultural Competence in the Social Work Profession" from the NASW policy. This was the first publication to define the standards of cultural competence in social work. Sue and Sue's first edition of *Counseling the Culturally Diverse: Theory and Practice* became a widely used resource in psychology and the social sciences with emphasis on the therapists' own awareness of their assumptions, values, and biases; understanding of the worldview of culturally diverse clients; and the development of appropriate intervention strategies and techniques.[38] The American Psychological Association also set standards for cultural competence and diversity in guiding the professional activities of psychologists.[39]

Attention to the underlying causes of health disparities increased over this time period. A 1999 article in the *Journal of the American Medical Association* found that African American patients participated less in visits with white doctors than white patients did.[25] In 2000, undergraduate and graduate medical education programs began to address this issue more formally as medical education accreditation committees began requiring that all students be exposed to and learn to treat patients from cultures different than their own.[33] The federal government issued its first "National Healthcare Disparities Report" in 2003 providing a broad overview of the disparities spanning different racial, ethnic, and socioeconomic groups. The government continued to

Table 11.1 Examples of Targeted Communication Patterns in Cultural Competency Training

Communication Patterns	Examples
Communication style: Direct or indirect	Some cultural groups ascribe to a more direct communication style while others may employ a more indirect style of communication where the words chosen require interpretive understanding.
Nonverbal communication (e.g., eye contact, smiling, laughing)	In some Asian cultures, for example, smiling or laughing are viewed as signs of weakness or may convey embarrassment or shyness.
Physical distance in social interactions	In some cultural groups (e.g., Latinos, African Americans), maintaining a closer distance when communicating is important whereas other cultural groups (e.g., European Americans) may prefer and expect larger distances.
Silence	Silence can mean different things for different people. For some silence may be an invitation for the listener to take a turn, whereas for others silence may signify an agreement, privacy, or respect.
Turn-taking	In groups that adhere to a hierarchical family orientation, encouragement of speaking among children or individuals with a lower hierarchical status is not encouraged. In contrast, many American families encourage children to speak up and share their thoughts, feelings, and opinions.

produce these reports and began tracking progress on resolving these disparities.[40]

The cultural competency perspective emphasizes the importance of all providers having the knowledge, awareness, and skills to address the concerns of persons of varied cultural backgrounds. Medical schools have increased the number of lectures and courses dedicated to teaching students about cultural norms, beliefs, and illnesses specific or common in certain cultures.[34,41] Immersion programs, where health professional students do a clinical rotation either internationally or in a locally native population, have become more common. In 1982, only 6% of medical students did an international immersion program compared to 38% in 2002.[34] Likewise, nursing schools started programs to help diversify both faculty and student populations.[42,43] In 1999, the textbook *Transcultural Concepts in Nursing Care* focused on theories, models, and recent research into transcultural nursing care.[44] Training often focused on helping healthcare providers understand differences among racial/ethnic groups and developing skills and awareness for addressing those differences in healthcare settings (see Table 11.1 for examples of differences targeted in cultural competency training).

Cultural Humility: Background and Training Tools

Cultural competency training was designed to increase knowledge and alter behaviors, but in many care settings providers paid variable attention to attitudes involved in patient–provider and family–provider relationships.[45] Education directed at competencies in more hierarchical settings and traditions often accentuated factual data for each racial/ethnic/and cultural group with discrete end points, such as the context of an examination. Knowing which medical conditions are more prevalent in certain cultures or the beliefs of the majority of that culture does not translate into understanding how patients' personal backgrounds and cultures influence what they value in their medical care.[45] Additionally, healthcare providers knowledgeable about different cultures and races/ethnicities may assume they know what is important to a patient of a specific racial/ethnic group or culture and not take into account his or her individual background and history. Perhaps most important of all is that communication training is devoid of accommodating the individual in cultural competence.

For this reason, education, though still variable across disciplines, institutions, and instructional units, has increasingly integrated the concept of cultural humility in cultural competence training.[46] Tervalon and Murray-Garcia's seminal paper was ultimately pivotal in the emergence of this broader umbrella framework identified as cultural humility, especially in physician training. Cultural humility places self-awareness at the forefront and suggests that even if providers know some facts about health and disease within a group, they must dialogue with the patient and family to know if those hypotheses are correct. Providers are encouraged to practice in a way that is open to learn from the patient about what their cultural background means to them. As an example, a social worker cannot define a Mexican American patient only by general facts learned about Mexican Americans. Rather, an individual patient's culture is personal and will incorporate being Mexican American, a father, a husband, a night student, and many other aspects of his life. Cultural humility teaches that healthcare providers optimally allow each patient to inform the provider as to the important aspects of the patient's personal culture, so that the healthcare provider and patient form a mutually respectful and humble partnership, working towards the patient's better health. Tervalon and Murray-Garcia point to three important parts of cultural humility. The first describes lifelong learning and critical self-reflection, the second recognizes and mitigates power imbalances in the patient–provider relationship, and the third discusses institutional consistency (see Table 11.2 for a list of skills to help achieve these goals).

Cultural humility involves teaching healthcare providers to be humble enough to admit they do not know about every cultural group or how the different identity areas may intersect (e.g., how race/ethnicity may intersect with gender and socioeconomic status) and how these aspects affect their individual patients. Providers make a commitment to learn these aspects as they are encountered, with ongoing self-reflection. This includes being aware that their own personal beliefs and biases affect how they provide healthcare. This concept of unconscious bias is illustrated in a study that evaluated pain treatment in extremity fractures in Latino patients versus white patients with the same fractures. In this study, Latino patients were twice as likely as white patients to

Table 11.2 Cultural Humility Concepts With Exemplary Tool/Skill

Cultural Humility Concept	Cultural Humility Tool/Skill Example
Self-awareness	Use *open-ended questions* to learn more about a family's perceptions about illness, treatment decisions, death/dying to allow for more in depth response.
	Observe *family interactions* (e.g., Who attends the meetings with the healthcare provider and what is their relationship to one another? Who does the talking "for" the family and does that person encourage opinions from others?)
	Learn to *rephrase* to show you are listening to what someone has shared with you.
	Engage in *reflective journaling* to develop self-awareness and recognition of changing world views.
Power imbalances	*Observe family interactions* to gain some insight into whether family dynamics are hierarchical, which may suggest some power imbalances within the family.
	Ask open-ended *questions* to better understand the patients' and their families decision-making preferences

receive no pain treatment.[47,48] In a follow-up study to determine whether the ethnic difference in adequacy of pain treatment was due to differences in healthcare provider pain evaluation, the study found no difference in healthcare provider pain rating between Latino and white patients. Despite no differences in how physician's rated patients' pain, for the same pain rating Latino patients received less pain medicine. Thus the study results suggest there must be another reason for pain treatment differences, including potential implicit and explicit biases.[48] Two strengths of cultural humility include the provider avoiding assumptions about the patient/family and also avoiding culturally biased treatment.

Cultural humility requires healthcare providers to recognize the power imbalances inherent in every patient–provider relationship, as well as within families. Culture, race/ethnicity, language, sexual orientation, ability/disability, socioeconomic status, and position inextricably impact this relationship. Awareness of power differentials, community participation, and collective decision-making may receive more emphasis in cultural humility training. Providers need to be both teachers and students in this relationship and recognize that they are still learning about their patients' beliefs and attitudes and how these influences affect patients' views on their medical treatments. Tervalon and Murray-Garcia also call on healthcare institutions to recognize imbalances and reflect on their practices and demographics to better serve their communities. Family medicine education has particularly championed the adoption of the cultural humility framework.[8,49] Others have been strong advocates for humility as a critical element in the training of global healthcare professionals.[42,50]

Cultural Humility and Palliative Care: A Self-Awareness Perspective

Cultural humility is central to palliative and end-of-life care. Quality palliative care must attend to provider–patient/family cultural, ethnic, and personal differences. In "Strategies for Culturally Effective End-of-Life Care," Crawley et al. posit that in end-of-life care there may be "values and social expectations that are so ingrained in physicians as to be unquestioned but may be alien to patients from different cultural backgrounds."[51(p673)] The palliative care team needs to ensure its members' practices are rooted in sensitivity to individual and family cultural and personal beliefs when engaging end-of-life decisions. Palliative care requires that the patient–provider relationship is a dynamic human-to-human relationship.[52] Mitigating power imbalances is especially important, necessitating that the patient become the teacher and the provider become the learner to optimize end-of-life care.

Within the context of palliative care, healthcare providers may want to explore their own attitudes and beliefs about illness and dying. Considering this from the perspective of one's family can be a good starting point. For example, questions providers can ask themselves may be: What does my family believe happens to an individual after death? How are those who have passed remembered or considered in the family? What are my family's rituals or preparations for dying? They should also consider generational differences in these attitudes and beliefs. For example: Do children and adults in my family have different expectations and beliefs? How did my beliefs change or remain the same as I got older? In addition to considering generational differences, providers should consider whether beliefs and attitudes may differ between men and women. Are certain behaviors done differently in the different contexts? Other contextual factors are also important, and may prompt question such as: How does my cultural upbringing intersect with my gender and religiosity in influencing my beliefs and behaviors? Again, there is great intersectionality here, and continuing to add layers will help providers recognize their own attitudes and beliefs. Practicing cultural humility also requires providers to be open to an ongoing process. Attitudes may shift based on each family and each patient/family encounter.

Cultural humility and the commitment to address power imbalances in the patient–provider dynamic requires lifelong dedication to self-evaluation and critique.[45] Every person receiving care represents a fragment of the culture that has informed and shaped who they are. When facing serious or life-threatening illness such as cancer, the individual and family will face a staggering amount of medical information, numerous clinical encounters, and many decisions. Effective cross-cultural communication among these seriously ill adults, their families, and healthcare providers is critical for effective pain management, discussions of death and dying, improved symptom management, emotional adjustment, greater patient and family satisfaction with care, as well as provider perceptions influencing dignity at end of life.[53,54] Becoming a student of the patient and not separating from his or her suffering is the goal.[55] For example

When a Cambodian hospice patient was asked if he had pain, he pointed to his heart. The clinician assumed that the patient was having cardiac pain and further assessment and treatment focused on eliminating the cardiac pain, without effective results. Upon further discussions with the family, the healthcare providers learned that the patient's "heart pain" referred to his health and how painful it was to both he and his family to see him so ill, as well as his worries about his family and the burden his illness placed on them. For Cambodians, the heart symbolizes love, kindness, willingness to help others, and health.[56]

The assumed meaning of the hand over the heart represents an example of underdeveloped cultural humility in narrowly defining heart pain in biologic terms.

Sharma et al. discusses the importance of the following in cross-cultural family meetings in which the patient, family, and healthcare team members may all come from different cultural backgrounds:

♦ Explicitly assessing patient and family preferences related to the communication of "difficult news," including the right of informed refusal

♦ Exploring the family's preferred role in decision-making (individual autonomy vs. family-centered decision making)

♦ Exploring patient and family values and preference, including religious and spiritual beliefs that may impact end-of-life preferences, filial roles, respect for authority, and attitudes toward advance directives

♦ Understanding and supporting the family's treatment decisions (including accommodating desires for more aggressive care and use of respectful negotiation when this is contraindicated)

♦ Using of compassion, kindness, and respect to help build trust[57]

Cultural humility also takes into consideration the importance of health literacy. Health literacy is

> the degree to which individuals have the capacity to obtain, process, and understand the basic health information and services needed to make appropriate health decisions. It is influenced by multiple factors, including patient-provider communication skills, patient knowledge of health topics, culture, requirements of the health care system, situation and context, disabilities.[58(p3)]

Brain death may look different from the perspectives of a neurology textbook and the Internet, yet cultural humility in assessing the use of different information sources may impact shared decision-making.

Time, openness, and a nonjudgmental presence are required in order for providers to more fully listen to what is central and sacred to patients. Assessing the patient and family's physiological, emotional, and spiritual needs allows the palliative care team to know the person and not just the disease. Hearing the patient's story is not equivalent to taking a medical history.[59] The story of a patient and family can quickly be diminished once the healthcare conversation turns to symptoms, disease, and tests and focuses less on the person as a whole.

The language a healthcare team uses with patients and families is central to considerations of cultural humility. The meanings of "hospice" and "palliative care" may be confusing to patients and families or may include erroneous information. All members of the palliative care team can assist in making sure that words are understood with clarifying questions and repeat visitation. Language differences can span the continuum of a different lexicon to the different uses of the same lexicon. The utilization of trained interpreters or cultural brokers can increase patient satisfaction by interpreting and assessing patient and family needs.[58] Using family members as interpreters can confuse their role in the family unit and raise issues of confidentiality and legality in federally funded healthcare. Additionally, family members may not know how to interpret medical information the healthcare provider is trying to convey, and/or they may modify such information to protect the patient. Instead, when family members are present who speak both languages, they may be asked to supplement the primary translation and support the patient and other members of the family.[58] Providers need to be discerning about how family involvement can shape any patient interaction.

Barriers to Cultural Humility Training and Awareness

Any concept such as cultural humility that includes empathy, communication, teamwork, and lifelong learning has built-in challenges that need to be considered by those who work in palliative care. First, learners may have had limited experiences with other cultures in what is intrinsically already a difficult and stressful task.[60] Second, many providers lack training in end-of-life care, even if healthcare workers deal with death in their practice. Third, there are time and practical constraints for conversations with patients and families. And finally, racism, religious hegemony, and multiple cultural prejudices continue to exist.[61]

Training is appropriately offered as one strategy to address some of these challenges to the practice of cultural humility, but it has its own issues. For example some students may deny, minimize, or resist cultural influences in healthcare. Raising awareness and changing attitudes may be more difficult for students resistant to a discussion of diversity, bias, and social problems that exist.[62] In addition, healthcare profession students' resistance may be influenced by the timing and the context in which they are taught cross-cultural communication skills. For medical students, these skills are usually presented in first- or second-year medical school courses at a time when students may not have had sufficient patient contact, may not recognize the value of these skills in optimizing healthcare for all patients, or may have had little opportunity to practice these skills.[62,63]

Healthcare providers may not have thought much about their own deaths and/or done much death-inventory work. Treating and palliating patients and families may be difficult for oncologists who lack experience and observation of end-of-life communication strategies across cultures.[64] The American Medical Association and the National Medical Association have consistently called for improvements in the cultural competency of healthcare providers with CLAS standards providing a framework for the development of continuing medical education and medical school curricula.[36] Additionally, in 2010 the Joint Commission released standards to encourage effective communication, cultural competence, and patient- and family-centered care.[65] Accreditation standards govern the majority of health profession programs and include at least one cultural competency goal in the curricular expectations. While these requirements vary by discipline, more clinical programs generally incorporate cultural competency into multiple program aspects. Cultural humility must also be added to the curriculum to enhance communication among healthcare providers, patients, and families.

Table 11.3 Exercises and Instructions for Instructors, Examples, and Potential Tools

Information	Goals	Website
Organizations and programs	Value diversity; cultural self-assessment; manage dynamics of difference; institute cultural knowledge; adapt to diversity	http://nccc.georgetown.edu/information/organizations.html
Providers and practitioners	Acknowledge cultural differences; understand own culture; engage in self-assessment; acquire cultural knowledge and skills; view behavior within a cultural context	http://nccc.georgetown.edu/information/providers.html
Faculty and trainers	Understand and articulate the rationale for cultural and linguistic competence; elicit "buy-in" from faculty, staff, community; incorporate into curricula and training programs; contribute to body of knowledge for competence	http://nccc.georgetown.edu/information/faculty.html
Families, youth, and communities	Advocate for themselves, families, and communities; build and sustain consumer demand for culturally and linguistically competent service systems; serve as a source of knowledge and support; continue to learn; partner with providers, policymakers, and other families; participate in governing boards; participate in research	http://nccc.georgetown.edu/information/families.html
Projects and Initiatives	Children and Youth with Special Health Care Needs, The National SUID/SIDS Project, Division of MCH Workforce Development, Child and Adolescent Mental Health	http://nccc.georgetown.edu/projects/index.html
Distance Learning	Assist in incorporating cultural and linguistic competence into users' work; provide areas of defined areas of knowledge, skills, and awareness; offer articles, publications, other multimedia resources, self-discovery strategies	http://nccc.georgetown.edu/distance.html
Self-Assessments	Lead to development of short- and long-term goals, measurable objectives; identify fiscal and personnel resources and enhanced community partnerships; provide a vehicle to measure outcomes	http://nccc.georgetown.edu/resources/assessments.html
Date Vignettes	Help increase understanding of racial and ethnic disparities in achieving the Maternal and Child Health Bureau's Six Core Outcomes for Children and Youth and Special Health Care Needs	http://nccc.georgetown.edu/data_vignettes/index.html

Note. National Center for Cultural Competence materials (http://nccc.georgetown.edu/).[69]

In order for healthcare providers to receive cultural humility communication training as well as have time for self-reflection, they may have to take time away from patients. The cost of time away from seeing patients and lack of incentive to participate pose a major barrier to healthcare providers' availing themselves of such training. In addition, healthcare providers may have the misconception that patient-centered communication results in longer patient visits when, in fact, effective communication may result in shorter, more efficient visits.[66,67] Medical interns spend just 12% of their time examining and talking with patients and more than 40% of their time behind a computer. Indeed, the study found interns spent nearly as much time walking (7%), as they did caring for patients at the bedside.[68] See Table 11.3,[69] Box 11.2,[70–72] 11.3,[73,74] 11.4,[19,37,49,52,75–79] and 11.5[80] for resources for teaching cultural humility.

Box 11.2 Guides to Teaching Cultural Humility Online[70–72]

- Teaching Cultural Humility and Competence: A Multidisciplinary Course for Public Health and Health Services Students[70]
  - http://jdc.jefferson.edu/cgi/viewcontent.cgi?article=1027&context=hplectures
- Teaching Cultural Humility and Competence. Lessons Learned from Developing and Teaching a Multi-Disciplinary Online Course[71]
  - Interdisciplinary course to teach cultural humility. Describes the goals of the course, how they went about creating the course, and the pilot study.
  - The website describes the course in detail and includes a thorough summary PowerPoint presentation.
  - http://dx.confex.com/dx/10/webprogram/Paper2888.html
- Teaching Cultural Humility[72]
  - PowerPoint presentation on how to apply different technologies to teaching cultural humility online.
  - Objective is to "apply the Process of Cultural Competence in the Delivery of Health Care Services to teaching clinical professional cultural humility."
  - http://coltt2011.pbworks.com/f/Teaching%20Cultural%20Humility%20On%20Line%20Notes.pdf

Box 11.3 Guides to Teaching Cultural Humility Through Writing or Self-Reflection[73,74]

- Teaching Cultural Sensitivity Through Literature and Reflexive Writing[73]
  - Physician educator at Loyola explains a course on teaching cultural sensitivity
  - http://virtualmentor.ama-assn.org/2007/08/medu1-0708.html
- Reflective Journaling and Development of Cultural Humility in Students[74]
  - Teaches students through journaling in an immersion program with a low socioeconomic and diverse cultural group
- Are You Practicing Cultural Humility? The Key to Success in Cultural Competence (California Health Advocates, Medicare: Policy, Advocacy and Education; April 2007)
  - Exercises in self-reflection
  - Defines cultures and discusses cultural humility and Tervalon and Murray-Garcia
  - www.cahealthadvocates.org/news/disparities/2007/are-you.html
- Cultural Humility Considerations in Health Outreach to Address Obesity and Overweight.
  - Self-reflection questions
  - Importance of cultural humility in counseling and patient education
  - http://outreach-partners.org/resources/outreachconnection/74

Box 11.4 Guide for Integrating Cultural Humility into Clinical Rotations for Providers[9,37,49,52,75–79]

- The American Psychological Association (APA) offers the Cultural Formulation Interview (including the Informant version) and the Supplementary Modules to the Core Cultural Formulation Interview for further research and clinical evaluation. They should be used in research and clinical settings as potentially useful tools to enhance clinical understanding and decision-making and not as the sole basis for making a clinical diagnosis. Additional information can be found in *DSM-5* in the Section III chapter "Cultural Formulation." The APA requests that providers and researchers provide further data on the usefulness of these cultural formulation interviews at http://www.dsm5.org/Pages/Feedback-Form.aspx.[19]
  - Measures: Cultural Formulation Interview
  - Rights granted: This material can be reproduced without permission by researchers and by providers for use with their patients. Rights holder: American Psychiatric Association

  To request permission for any other use beyond what is stipulated above, contact: http://www.appi.org/CustomerService/Pages/Permissions.aspx
- Bridging the Gap: A Curriculum to Teach Residents Cultural Humility.[49]
  - Second-year family medicine resident yearlong diversity curriculum
  - Includes multiple elements (e.g., diversity bingo, book discussion, panel discussions, simulated patients, home visits, The Color of Fear™ video)
- Towards Cultural Competency in End-of-Life Communication Training.[75]
  - Geriatric fourth-year medical student clerkship
  - Palliative care based and "fosters cultural sensitivity and humility"
  - Communication workshop for culturally responsive palliative care and end-of-life care
  - Includes role-playing and feedback on breaking bad news and withdrawal/withholding treatment
- Transcultural Nursing: Assessment & Intervention[76]
  - Gives models for assessment and intervention for caring for diverse patients
- Clinical Practice Guidelines for Quality Palliative Care.[77]
  - National Consensus Project for Quality Palliative Care
  - Applicable to all medical providers
  - http://www.nationalconsensusproject.org/NCP_Clinical_Practice_Guidelines_3rd_Edition.pdf

(continued)

Box 11.4 Continued

- NASW Standards for Cultural Competence in Social Work Practice.[37]
  - http://www.socialworkers.org/practice/standards/NASWCulturalStandards.pdf
- Initiative for Pediatric Palliative Care: An Interdisciplinary Educational Approach for Healthcare Professionals[52]
- Integrating Cultural Competency and Humility Training into Clinical Clerkships: Surgery as a Model.[78]
  - Cultural humility training in third- and fourth-year medical students directed to clerkship directors and curriculum committees
  - Proposed first- and fourth-year medical student cultural competency and cultural humility survey evaluations to assess cultural competency and cultural humility training provided by the medical institution.
- Cultural Humility Task Force at San Francisco General Hospital Department of Psychiatry
  - Gives example of institution teaching cultural humility
  - "Provides leadership to the department in maintaining a focus on the importance of future in clinical work; and to advance the importance of cultural humility through organizing trainings, workshops and culturally focused seminars."
  - http://psych.ucsf.edu/sfgh/chtf/

  Other resources
- Twelve Tips for Teaching Diversity and Embedding it in the Medical Curriculum.[79]

Box 11.5 National Standards for Culturally and Linguistically Appropriate Services in Healthcare[80]

Standard 1: Healthcare organizations should ensure that patients/consumers receive from all staff members effective, understandable, and respectful care that is provided in a manner compatible with their cultural health beliefs and practices and preferred language.

Standard 2: Healthcare organizations should implement strategies to recruit, retain, and promote at all levels of the organization a diverse staff and leadership that are representative of the demographic characteristics of the service area.

Standard 3: Healthcare organizations should ensure that staff at all levels and across all disciplines receive ongoing education and training in culturally and linguistically appropriate service delivery.

Standard 4: Healthcare organizations must offer and provide language assistance services, including bilingual staff and interpreter services, at no cost to each patient/consumer with limited English proficiency at all points of contact, in a timely manner during all hours of operation.

Standard 5: Healthcare organizations must provide to patients/consumers in their preferred language both verbal offers and written notices informing them of their right to receive language assistance services.

Standard 6: Healthcare organizations must assure the competence of language assistance provided to limited English proficient patients/consumers by interpreters and bilingual staff. Family and friends should not be used to provide interpretation services (except on request by the patient/consumer).

Standard 7: Healthcare organizations must make available easily understood patient-related materials and post signage in the languages of the commonly encountered groups and/or groups represented in the service area.

Standard 8: Healthcare organizations should develop, implement, and promote a written strategic plan that outlines clear goals, policies, operational plans, and management accountability/oversight mechanisms to provide culturally and linguistically appropriate services.

Standard 9: Healthcare organizations should conduct initial and ongoing organizational self-assessments of CLAS-related activities and are encouraged to integrate cultural and linguistic competence-related measures into their internal audits, performance improvement programs, patient satisfaction assessments, and outcomes-based valuations.

Standard 10: Healthcare organizations should ensure that data on the individual patient's/consumer's race, ethnicity, and spoken and written language are collected in health records, integrated into the organization's management information systems, and periodically updated.

Standard 11: Healthcare organizations should maintain a current demographic, cultural, and epidemiological profile of the community as well as a needs assessment to accurately plan for and implement services that respond to the cultural and linguistic characteristics of the service area.

Standard 12: Healthcare organizations should develop participatory, collaborative partnerships with communities, and utilize a variety of formal and informal mechanisms to facilitate community and patient/consumer involvement in designing and implementing CLAS-related activities.

Standard 13: Healthcare organizations should ensure that conflict and grievance resolution processes are culturally and linguistically sensitive and capable of identifying, preventing, and resolving cross-cultural conflicts or complaints by patients/consumers.

Standard 14: Healthcare organizations are encouraged to regularly make available to the public information about their progress and successful innovations in implementing the CLAS standards and to provide public notice in their communities about the availability of this information.

From: National Standards for Culturally and Linguistically Appropriate Services in Health Care; US Department of Health and Human Services Office of Minority Health, March 2001.

Conclusion

The larger exigencies of healthcare are at the nexus of both cultural humility and palliative care. These include establishing trust relationships in evolving administrative structures and stressful times, listening and legislating effectively in polarized media and political environments, addressing the needs of changing families and migration with constrained resources in underresourced communities, and growing diversity in the workforce.[81-89] The gap between diversity in the palliative care workforce, its involved disciplines, and the increasingly diverse mix in the US population has been well-recognized, particularly by nursing.[16] The American Academy of Hospice and Palliative Medicine is seeking to address diversity and cultural issues through committee, programmatic, and communication work.[90] The relatively slow pace of change in organizational structures, especially at the leadership level, may require an additional level of commitment and cultural brokering to effect change. Additionally, individual provider knowledge and familiarity with cultural humility varies just as widely as provider understandings of palliative care communication. The framework of cultural humility essentially provides a path forward toward resilience in times of difficulty, rapid change, compounding economic costs, and conflicts.

References

1. US Census Bureau. Interim projections by age, sex, race, and Hispanic origin: 2000-2050. http://www.census.gov/population/projections/files/methodology/idbsummeth.pdf Accessed September 16, 2014.
2. Fact finder. US Census Bureau. http://factfinder2.census.gov/faces/nav/jsf/pages/searchresults.xhtml?refresh=t. Accessed August 6, 2014.
3. Giger J, Davidhizar RE, Purnell J, Harden JT, Phillips J, Strickland O. American Academy of Nursing expert panel report: Developing cultural competence to eliminate health disparities in ethnic minorities and other vulnerable populations. *J Transcult Nurs.* 2007;18(2):95-102.
4. Idler EL, Benyamini Y. Self-rated health and mortality: A review of twenty-seven community studies. *J Health Soc Behav.* 1997;38(1):21-37.
5. Kreuter MW, McClure SM. 2004 The role of culture in health communication. *Annu Rev Public Health.* 2004; 25:439-455.
6. Kagawa-Singer M1, Kassim-Lakha S. A strategy to reduce cross-cultural miscommunication and increase the likelihood of improving health outcomes. *Acad Med.* 2003;78(6):577-587.
7. Chang E, Simon M, Dong X. Integrating cultural humility into health care professional education and training. *Adv Health Sci Educ Theory Pract.* 2010;17:269-278.
8. Brody H, Hunt L. Moving beyond cultural stereotypes in end-of-life decision making. *Am Fam Physician.* 2005;71:429.
9. National Association of Community Health Centers, Community Healthcorps. Prescription 4: Cultural sensitivity. http://www.communityhealthcorps.org/client/documents/Prescription-4-Cultural-Sensitivity-Member.pdf. Published August 2008. Accessed September 19, 2014.
10. Roter D. Three blind men and an elephant: Reflections on meeting the challenges of patient diversity in primary care practice. *Fam Med.* 2002;34(5):390-393.
11. Centre for Cultural Diversity and Ageing. http://www.culturaldiversity.com.au/. Updated 2010. Accessed September 15, 2014.
12. Jezewski MA. Culture brokering in migrant farmworker health care. *West J Nurs Res.* 1990 Aug;12(4):497-513.
13. Purnell L, Palunka B, eds. *Transcultural Health Care; A Culturally Competent Approach.* 3rd ed. Philadelphia, PA: F.A. Davis; 2003.
14. Cross TL, Bazron B, Dennis K, Isaacs M. *Towards A Culturally Competent System of Care: A Monograph on Effective Services for Minority Children Who Are Severely Emotionally Disturbed.* Washington, DC. CASSP Technical Assistance Center, Georgetown University Child Development Center; 1989.
15. Williams SW, Hanson LC, Boyd C, et al. Communication, decision making and cancer: What African Americans want physicians to know. *J Palliat Med.* 2008;11(8):1221-1226.
16. McGee P, Johnson M. Developing cultural competence in palliative care. *Br J Community Nurs.* 2013;18(6):296-298.
17. Lipson JG1, DeSantis LA. Current approaches to integrating elements of cultural competence in nursing education. *J Transcult Nurs.* 2007;18(1 Suppl):10S-20S; discussion 21S-27S.
18. Roberts SG1, Warda M2, Garbutt S3, Curry K. The use of high-fidelity simulation to teach cultural competence in the nursing curriculum. *J Prof Nurs.* 2014;30(3):259-265.
19. American Psychological Association. DSM-5 Cultural Formulation Interview. http://www.mhima.org.au/mhima-latest-news/dsm-5-cultural-formulation-interview-cfi-is-available-online Accessed September 26, 2014.
20. Fuentes JN, Boylan LS, Fontanella JA. Behavioral indices in medical care outcome: The working alliance, adherence and related factors. *J Gen Intern Med.* 2009;24:80-85.
21. Ursua RA, Auilar DE, Wyatt LC, et al. A community health worker intervention to improve management of hypertension among Filipino Americans in New York and New Jersey: A pilot study. *Ethn Dis.* 2014;24:67-76.
22. Cooper LA, Roter DL, Carson KA, et al. A randomized trial to improve patient-centered care and hypertension control in underserved primary care patients. *J Gen Intern Med.* 2011;26:1297-1304.
23. Saha S, Korthuis PT, Cohn JA, Sharp VL, Moore RD, Beach MC. Primary care provider cultural competence and racial disparities in HIV care and outcomes. *J Gen Intern Med.* 2013;28:622-629.
24. Medical Subject Headings (MeSH). US National Library of Medicine Website. http://www.nlm.nih.gov/mesh/. Accessed July 27, 2014.
25. Cooper-Patrick L, Gallo JJ, Gonzales JJ, et al. Race, gender, and partnership in the patient-physician relationship. *JAMA.* 1999;282(6):583-589.
26. Frost DW1, Cook DJ, Heyland DK, Fowler RA. Patient and healthcare professional factors influencing end-of-life decision-making during critical illness: A systematic review. *Crit Care Med.* 2011 May;39(5):1174-1189.
27. Hagiwara N, Penner LA, Gonzalez R, Eggly S, Dovidio JF, Gaertner SL, West T, Albrecht TL. Racial attitudes, physician-patient talk time ratio, and adherence in racially discordant medical interactions. *Soc Sci Med.* 2013 Jun;87:123-131.
28. Hart P, Marena N. Cultural challenges and barriers through the voices of nurses. *J Clin Nurs.* 2013; Aug(15-16):2223-2232.
29. Betancourt JR, Green AR, Carillo JE, Ananeh-Firempong O. Defining cultural competence: A practical framework for addressing racial/ethnic disparities in health and health care. *Public Health Rep.* 2003;18:293-302.
30. Wear D. Insurgent multiculturalism: Rethinking how and why we teach culture in medical education. *Acad Med.* 2003;78:549-554.
31. Beers MH, Berkow R, Merck Research Laboratories. *The Merck Manual of Diagnosis and Therapy.* 16th ed. Whitehouse Station, NJ: Merck Research Laboratories; 1992.
32. Lavizzo-Mourey R, Mackenzie ER. Cultural competence: Essential measurements of quality for managed care organizations. *Ann Intern Med.* 1996;124:919-921.
33. Horowitz S. Cultural competency training in U.S. medical education: Treating patients from different cultures. *Alternat Ther Health Med.* 2005; 11(6): 290-294.
34. Champaneria MC, Axtell S. Cultural competence training in U.S. medical schools. *JAMA.* 2004;291:2142.

35. Like RC, Steiner RP, Rubel AJ. STFM core curriculum guidelines: Recommended core curriculum guidelines on culturally sensitive and competent health care. *Fam Med*. 1996;28:291–297.
36. US Department of Health & Human Services. The National Standards for Culturally and Linguistically Appropriate Services in Health and Health Care. https://www.thinkculturalhealth.hhs.gov/content/clas.asp. Published 2010. Accessed June 6, 2014.
37. National Association of Social Workers. *NASW Standards for Cultural Competence in Social Work Practice*. Washington, DC: National Association of Social Workers. 2001. http://www.naswdc.org/practice/standards/NASWculturalstandards.pdf. Accessed August 27, 2014.
38. Sue DW, Sue D. *Counseling the Culturally Diverse: Theory and Practice*. 6th ed. Hoboken, NJ: John Wiley; 2013.
39. American Psychological Association Website. http://www.apa.org/search.aspx?query=cultural%20competence%20standard&fq=DocumentTypeFilt:%22Guidelines%22. Accessed September 26, 2014.
40. US Department of Health & Human Services. *2012 National Healthcare Disparities Report*. Rockville, MD. Agency for Healthcare Research and Quality. http://www.ahrq.gov/research/findings/nhqrdr/nhdr12/2012nhdr.pdf. Published 2013. Accessed May 6, 2014.
41. Dogra N, Reitmanova S, Carter-Pokras O. Teaching cultural diversity: Current status in U.K., U.S., and Canadian medical schools. *J Gen Intern Med*. 2009;25(Suppl 2):164–168.
42. Levi A. The ethics of nursing student international clinical experiences. *Obstet Gynecol Neonatal Nurs*. 2009;38:94–99.
43. Pacquiao, D. The relationship between cultural competence education and increasing diversity in nursing schools and practice settings. *J Transcult Nurs*. 2007;18:28S–37S.
44. Andrews M, Boyle J. Transcultural concepts in nursing care. *J Transcult Nurs*. 2002;13(3):178–180.
45. Tervalon M, Murray-García J. Cultural humility versus cultural competence: A critical distinction in defining physician training outcomes in multicultural education. *J Health Care Poor Underserved*. 1998 May; 9(2):117–125.
46. Isaacson M. Clarifying concepts: Cultural humility or competency. *J Prof Nurs*. 2014;30:251–258.
47. Todd KH, Samaroo N, Hoffman JR. Ethnicity as a risk factor for inadequate emergency department analgesia. *JAMA*. 1993;269(12):1537–1539.
48. Todd KH, Lee T, Hoffman JR. The effect of ethnicity on physician estimates of pain severity in patients with isolated extremity trauma. *JAMA*. 1994;271(12):925–928.
49. Juarez JA, Marvel K, Brezinski KL et al. Bridging the gap: A curriculum to teach residents cultural humility. *Fam Med*. 2006;38(2):97–102.
50. Cruess SR, Cruess RL, Steinhart Y. Linking the teaching of professionalism to the social contract: A call for cultural humility. *Med Teach*. 2010;32:357–359.
51. Crawley LM, Marshall PA, Lo B, Koening BA. Strategies for culturally effective end-of-life care. *Ann Intern Med*. 2002;136:673–679.
52. Browning DM, Solomon MZ. Initiative for Pediatric Palliative Care (IPPC) Investigator Team. The initiative for pediatric palliative care: An interdisciplinary educational approach for healthcare professionals. *J Pediatr Nursing*. 2005;20(5):326–334.
53. Periyakoil VS, Stevens M, Kraener H. Multicultural long-term care nurses' perceptions of factors influencing patient dignity at the end of life. *J Am Geriatr Soc*. 2013;61:440–446.
54. Williams R. Cultural safety: What does it mean for our work practice? *Aust NZ J Public Health*. 1999;23:213–214.
55. Austerlic S. Cultural humility and compassionate presence at the end of life. Santa Clara, CA: Markkula Center for Applied Ethics. http://www.scu.edu/ethics/practicing/focusareas/medical/culturally-competent-care/chronic-to-critical-austerlic.html. Published February 2009. Accessed June 21, 2014.
56. Coolen PR. Cultural relevance in end-of-life care. Ethno Med Website. https://ethnomed.org/clinical/end-of-life/cultural-relevance-in-end-of-life-care. Published May 1, 2012. Accessed September 2, 2014.
57. Sharma RK, Dy SM. Cross-cultural communication and use of the family meeting in palliative care. *Am J Hosp Palliat Care*. 2011 Sep;28(6):437–444.
58. EPEC^{TM}_O: National Cancer Institute at the National Institutes of Health. Education in palliative and end-of-life care for oncology: Cultural considerations when caring for African Americans. Bethesda, MD: National Cancer Institute.
59. Frank AW. *The Wounded Storyteller: Body, Illness, and Ethics*. Chicago, IL: University of Chicago Press; 1995.
60. Surbone A. Cultural aspects of communication in cancer care. *Support Care Cancer*. 2008;16(3):235–240.
61. Drisdom S. Barriers to using palliative care: Insight into African American Culture. *Clin J Oncol Nurs*. 2013;17:376–380.
62. Boutin-Foster C, Foster JC, Konopasek L. Physician, know thyself: The professional culture of medicine as framework for teaching cultural competence. *Acad Med*. 2008;83(1):106–111.
63. Crosson JC et al. Evaluating the effects of cultural competency training on medical student attitudes. *Fam Med*. 2004;36:199–203.
64. Granek L, Krzyzanowska MK, Mazzotta P, Tozer R. Oncologists' strategies and barriers to effective communication about the end of life. *J Oncol Pract*. 2013;9(4):129–135.
65. Quinn GP, Jimenez J, Meade CD, et al. Enhancing oncology health care providers sensitivity to cultural communication to reduce cancer disparities: A pilot study. *J Cancer Educ*. 2011;26:322–325.
66. Levinson W, Lesser CS, Epstein RM. Developing physician communications skills for patient centered care. *Health Aff (Millwood)*. 2010;29(7):1310–1318.
67. Epstein RM, Street RL. *Patient-Centered Communication in Cancer Care: Promoting Healing and Reducing Suffering*. NIH Publication No. 07-6225. Bethesda, MD: National Cancer Institute; 2007.
68. Block L, Habicht R, Wu AW, Desai SV, Wang K, Silva KN, Niessen T, Oliver N, Feldman L. In the wake of the 2003 and 2011 duty hours regulations, how do internal medicine interns spend their time? *J Gen Intern Med*. 2013;28(8):1042–1047.
69. National Center for Cultural Competence, Georgetown University Website. nccc.georgetown.edu/. Accessed May 23, 2014.
70. Simmons C, Chernett NL, Yuen E, Toth-Cohen S. Teaching cultural humility and competence: A multi-disciplinary course for public health and health services students. Philadelphia PA: Thomas Jefferson University. http://jdc.jefferson.edu/cgi/viewcontent.cgi?article=1027&context=hplectures. Accessed June 16, 2015.
71. Yuen C, Toth-Cohen S, Simmons C. Teaching cultural humility and competence. Lessons Learned from developing and teaching a multi-disciplinary online course. Philadelphia, PA: Thomas Jefferson University; 2010. http://dx.confex.com/dx/10/webprogram/Paper2888.html
72. Baker V. Teaching cultural humility. Paper presented at Colorado Teaching and Learning with Technology Conference, August 4, 2011. http://coltt2011.pbworks.com/f/Teaching%20Cultural%20Humility%20On%20Line%20Notes.pdf
73. Roy R. Teaching cultural sensitivity through literature and reflexive writing. *AMA J Ethics*. 2007;9(8):543–546.
74. Schuessler JB, Wilder B, Byrd LW. Reflective journaling and development of cultural humility in students. *Nursing Educ Persp*. 2012;33 96–99.
75. Lubimer KT, Wen AB. Towards cultural competency in end-of-life communication training. *Hawaii Med J*. 2011;70(11):239–241.
76. Giger JN. *Transcultural nursing: Assessment & intervention*. 6th ed. St. Louis: MO: Elsevier/Mosby; 2013.
77. *Clinical practice guidelines for quality palliative care*. 3rd ed. Pittsburgh, PA: National Consensus Project for Quality Palliative

Care; 2013. http://www.nationalconsensusproject.org/NCP_Clinical_Practice_Guidelines_3rd_Edition.pdf
78. Butler PD, Swift M, Kothari S, et al. Integrating cultural competency and humility training into clinical clerkships: Surgery as a model. *J Surg Educ*. 2011;68(3):222–230.
79. Dogra N, Reitmanova S, Carter-Pokras O. Twelve tips for teaching diversity and embedding it in the medical curriculum. *Med Teach*. 2009;31:990–993.
80. US Department of Health and Human Services, Office of Minority Health. What is cultural competency? http://minorityhealth.hhs.gov/omh/browse.aspx?lvl=1&lvlid=6. Published 2005. Accessed August 3, 2014.
81. Broom A, Good P, Kirby E, Lewin Z. Negotiating palliative care in the content of culturally and linguistically diverse patients. *Int Med J*. 2013;43:1043–1046.
82. Cruz-Oliver DM, Talamantes M, Sanchez-Reilly S. What evidence is available on end-of-life (EOL) care and Latino elders? A literature review. *J Hosp Palliat Med*. 2014;31:87–97.
83. Frey R, Gott M, Raphael D, Black S, Teleo-Hope, Lee H, Wang Z. "Where do I go from here"? A cultural perspective on challenges to the use of hospice services. *Health Soc Care Community*. 2013;21:519–529.
84. Gorospe E. Establishing palliative care for American Indians as a public health agenda. *The Internet Journal of Pain, Symptom Control and Palliative Care*. 2005; 4(2). http://ispub.com/IJPSP/4/2/8930. Accessed June 21, 2014.
85. Johnston ME, Herzig RM. The interpretation of "culture": Diverging perspectives on medical provision in rural Montana. *Soc Sci Med*. 2006;63:2500–2511.
86. Lyckholm LJ1, Coyne PJ, Kreutzer KO, Ramakrishnan V, Smith TJ. Barriers to effective palliative care for low-income patients in late stages of cancer: Report of a study and strategies for defining and conquering the barriers. *Nurs Clin North Am*. 2010;45(3):399–409.
87. Maddalena V, Bernard W, Davis-Murdoch S, Smith D. Awareness of palliative care and end-of life options among African Canadians in Nova Scotia. *J Transcult Nurs*. 2013;24:144–152.
88. Quinones-Gonzalez. Bridging the communication gap in hospice and palliative care for Hispanics and Latinos. *Omega*. 2013;67:193–200.
89. Shahid S, Bessarab D, vanSchalk K, Aoun S, Thompson S. Improving palliative care outcomes for Aboriginal Australians: Service providers' perspectives. *BMC Palliat Care*. 2013;12:26–36.
90. Beresford, L. Disparities, diversity, and palliative care. American Academy of Hospice and Palliative Medicine Website. http://aahpm.org/quarterly/su14-feature. Accessed September 26, 2014.

CHAPTER 12

Health Literacy and Communication in Palliative Care

Wen-ying Sylvia Chou, Anna Gaysynsky, and Alexander Persoskie

Introduction

Palliative care—patient and family-centered care that optimizes quality of life by anticipating, preventing, and treating suffering—needs to be integrated into the care of all serious illnesses in order to reduce pain and distress and ensure that the physical and psychosocial needs of patients and caregivers are addressed. However, there are significant obstacles to the delivery of patient-centered palliative care, with many of these challenges arising from communication problems and the fact that the healthcare system assumes too much concerning the health literacy of individuals. Palliative care communication requires not only that patients and caregivers have an adequate understanding of the condition and their medical options but also that the healthcare system is ready and equipped to optimally accommodate various health literacy levels and elicit and respond to the values of patients and caregivers.

To date, health literacy definitions abound and vary greatly in scope. This chapter follows the US Department of Health and Human Services definition of health literacy as the "degree to which individuals have the capacity to obtain, process and understand basic health information and services needed to make appropriate health decisions."[1] Assessing health literacy calls for a consideration of an individual's ability in relation to the complexity of the tasks at hand, as well as the context-specific demands placed on their "functional literacy."[2] In other words, throughout this chapter, health literacy is discussed not only as a patient- or caregiver-level characteristic but also as an attribute of the healthcare system as a whole.

Limited health literacy is a major issue in the United States. It is estimated that nearly half of all American adults have limited health literacy.[3] In the United States, prevalence of low health literacy is highest among racial/ethnic minorities, those with limited education, the elderly, and people with certain disabilities.[4,5] However, limited health literacy affects people from all walks of life and across socioeconomic levels.[5] Having limited health literacy hinders individuals' ability to access and navigate the healthcare system, make appropriate health decisions, and act on health information. The deleterious impact of limited health literacy has been documented across a variety of health domains, and palliative care is no exception. For instance, patients with limited health literacy may lack knowledge about medications and other modes of treating chronic pain,[6] which may lead to suboptimal pain management.

Using a multilevel ecological framework, this chapter first highlights connections between health literacy and palliative care across a wide variety of health areas, including (a) palliative care utilization; (b) communication between providers, patients, families and other caregivers; and (c) self-care and caregiving outside the clinical setting. Examples of health literacy intervention efforts, including tools and approaches at multiple levels of influence, are then highlighted. The chapter concludes with a discussion of research and practice priorities around palliative care communication, including the role of technology and new media, patient navigation, and expanding the focus of palliative care services and research beyond advanced cancer.

The Role of Health Literacy in Palliative Care Communication

In what ways does health literacy affect palliative care? To what extent is health literacy accountable for disparities that exist in patients' palliative care preferences and decisions? How can it help explain and address disparities in palliative care outcomes? We have adapted and modified Paasche-Orlow and Wolf's health literacy conceptual framework,[2,7] which considers limited health literacy not merely as an individual-level problem affecting the patient or caregiver but as a challenge facing healthcare providers and health systems in effectively communicating with patients. Specifically, this view of health literacy incorporates more than the individual's cognitive and functional skills in healthcare decision-making; it also takes into account the contextual demands placed on the individual by a specific clinical condition, the communication characteristics of medical culture, and the way clinical services are structured.[8]

Such an approach recognizes that limited health literacy is not just a product of individual deficits. It also reflects healthcare trends toward greater patient engagement in care (which requires that patients and caregivers have the ability to obtain, analyze, and act on complex health information), the increasing specialization and fragmentation of care, and the increasing complexity of medical treatments. In light of this, health literacy interventions must move beyond efforts intended to address individuals' abilities to consider the complexity of tasks required of patients and families, the ability of providers to engage with patients, and other features of the community and healthcare system that support patient-centered care.

Paasche-Orlow and Wolf's original framework suggested three points in the healthcare process that were affected by health literacy. Considering palliative care, we have modified the framework to include the following topics: (a) access to and utilization of palliative care, (b) clinical interactions in palliative care, and (c) self-care and caregiver support. In this section, we discuss salient factors and exemplary research to date in each of these domains.

Access to and Utilization of Palliative Care

Limited health literacy may impede individuals' access to and utilization of palliative care services, resulting in unnecessary suffering. At the most basic level, lack of knowledge about available hospice and palliative care services means patients do not request or access these services.[9] Educating individuals about the role and function of palliative care, and addressing common misconceptions regarding these services, may be one of the simplest ways to facilitate access to palliative care and reduce disparities in the utilization of these services.[9,10]

Limited health literacy can also hinder palliative care use in less direct ways. For instance, research indicates that financial considerations (as opposed to true patient preferences) keep many low-income individuals from utilizing palliative care services.[10] Many individuals lack the health literacy necessary to understand available healthcare coverage options, which may prevent them from taking advantage of Medicaid or other programs for which they are eligible.[2] In effect, the inability to navigate the complicated insurance and healthcare systems may make palliative care inaccessible.

Even when palliative care is accessible and affordable, limited health literacy can still prevent individuals from obtaining services. Poor information exchange and impaired decision-making have been shown to be a direct result of limited health literacy.[11,12] In order to make palliative care decisions that are in line with their values, patients need to process a wealth of information, including accurate prognostic information, the meaning and value of palliative care, the types of services that are available, as well as the costs and benefits of their other options.[13] Many critically ill patients have inadequate knowledge and unrealistic expectations regarding care, may be unclear about their personal values and how these relate to different treatment options, and may have inadequate support resources to facilitate decision-making.[14]

In addition to individual-level characteristics, factors within healthcare systems can also impact palliative care access and utilization for patients with limited health literacy. To begin with, healthcare systems are complex, and navigation requires a level of literacy that most patients do not have. Healthcare settings are uncomfortable and potentially threatening environments in which help-seeking could expose patients' reading and communication difficulties, leading to stigmatization and even shame.[15] Complicated forms, unclear verbal directions, signage and placards, as well as written materials containing advanced vocabulary and medical jargon all create barriers to care.[7] For example, studies suggest that the legal language of standard advance directives may pose a barrier to the completion and understanding of these forms,[16] potentially preventing individuals from receiving the type of care they desire at the end of life.

Clinical Interactions in Palliative Care

Limited health literacy is linked to poor patient–provider communication, in part due to insufficient or inaccurate understanding of the illness.[1] Limited health literacy is also associated with lower patient participation and less engagement in decision-making.[2,17] Specifically, individuals with limited health literacy have been observed to ask fewer questions and receive less information during clinical interactions, due to fear, embarrassment, or low self-efficacy.[17]

Shame can also induce individuals to attempt to hide their limited literacy from providers (e.g., by claiming to have forgotten their reading glasses)[18] and to feign understanding of important information. As one teenage patient commented, "[health professionals] never explain anything properly. It's always their own big words and I just say, 'Yeah, okay' and I go home and I'm like, 'I don't know what that meant.'"[15] It can therefore be extremely difficult for providers to both identify patients who have poor health literacy and recognize when these patients have failed to comprehend a critical piece of information.

Many approaches to assessing health literacy have been proposed, including the Rapid Estimate of Adult Literacy in Medicine, the Test of Functional Health Literacy in Adults, and the Newest Vital Sign (NVS).[19] One study also suggested that a simple question such as "How confident are you filling out medical forms by yourself?" can be used to identify patients with limited or marginal health literacy skills.[19] However, formal assessments of health literacy are usually reserved for research purposes and not conducted as part of routine clinical interactions.[20] Additionally, although one study found no evidence that assessing patient literacy with the NVS caused patients to feel ashamed,[21] it is important that these tools be deployed in a sensitive manner in order to avoid inadvertently causing harm to patients. Alternatively, providers and health systems can put measures in place that can help all individuals—not just those with low literacy—to better understand health information, thereby eliminating the need to assess the capabilities of individual patients.

These efforts are important because characteristics of healthcare providers and the healthcare system as a whole contribute to suboptimal patient–provider communication. For example, implicit and explicit biases can prevent providers from engaging in patient-centered communication even when they are aware of a patient's level of health literacy. Studies have shown that providers may perceive patients who have limited health literacy as incompetent or uninterested and therefore provide them with less information and attention.[17] Providers' use of complex medical jargon and unclear presentation of numerical information can further impede communication.[7,22] The findings of one study perfectly encapsulate the extent of the communication chasm that exists between providers and patients: even when physicians in this study believed they were using "everyday language" to communicate, patients did not perceive this to be the case.[1]

Communication problems can result in a misalignment of goals and knowledge between providers and patients/caregivers. In palliative care, common areas of misalignment stemming from poor communication include discrepant understandings of diagnosis or prognosis, differential understanding of treatment options, and misunderstanding of patient preferences. These differences have been well documented in the literature. For example, Quirt et al. found that only 64% of patients with advanced cancer agreed with their physician about the extent of their disease, and in those cases where there was disagreement, most patients underestimated the extent of their disease.[23]

Even more alarming is the observation that providers may be communicating prognostic information in such a way that patients fail to realize a discussion is even occurring. For instance, Curtis et al. reported poor concordance in end-of-life discussions between patients with AIDS and their physicians, with physicians believing they had delivered prognostic information more frequently than patients perceived they had received it.[24] Similarly, another study of patients with terminal illness found that in 46% of patient/clinician pairs the clinician reported having communicated the fatal nature of the disease, while the patient reported that no such discussion occurred.[25] Poor understanding of disease status can be especially detrimental to decision-making at the end of life, whereby election to receive aggressive life-prolonging measures (vasopressor support, additional chemotherapy, cardiopulmonary resuscitation, etc.) can further diminish quality of life and dignity.[13]

This lack of concordance between patients and providers is not limited to prognosis: misunderstandings regarding treatment goals frequently occur as well. For example, in an Australian study of cancer patients, only 60% of patients were able to correctly state the goal of their treatment, with 17% of patients receiving palliative therapy incorrectly believing their treatment would either cure or prevent the recurrence of their cancer and 32% of patients receiving curative care believing their treatment was palliative in nature. This was in stark contrast to the perceptions of the physicians in this study, who believed that nearly all of their patients understood both their diagnosis and the type of treatment they were receiving.[26]

Health providers also frequently have misperceptions regarding their patients' wishes and have difficulty in judging patient preferences.[27] For example, in Haidet et al.'s study of metastatic cancer patients, physicians incorrectly identified patients' cardiopulmonary resuscitation preferences in 30% of cases, and there was surprisingly little difference in ability to correctly identify patient preferences between physicians who reported having had discussions about prognosis with their patients and those who did not.[28]

Self-Care and Caregiver Support in Palliative Care

A great deal of palliative care occurs outside the walls of the clinic, where patients, families, and other caregivers take on important tasks such as symptom management and medication administration.[29] Individuals with limited health literacy tend to have less practical and instrumental knowledge and may not possess the skills needed for the day-to-day management of serious illness. They may have limited knowledge and understanding of symptoms, biometric data, and medication dosage and may be unable to carry out a healthcare plan, make appropriate decisions, and seek medical attention when needed. Compounding these self-care challenges is the fact that limited health literacy patients are also more likely to rely on care and support from family and friends who themselves have inadequate health literacy and do not have the resources or knowledge to properly assist in palliative care tasks.[2]

Providers and the overall healthcare system may further contribute to difficulties with patient self-care and caregiving at the end of life. Once patients leave the clinical care setting, many hospital-based palliative care teams cease to play active roles in patient care, such that any gaps in discharge planning or transitioning to home care create problems for families that they must face without adequate support.[30] Caregivers of terminally ill patients frequently report the need for more support and information as they take on an increasing number of complex tasks. However, this information is often not provided, leaving caregivers inadequately prepared for their roles.[31]

Another system-level barrier to self-care and caregiving for individuals with low health literacy is the growing use of technology-mediated communication, such as the use of online prescription refills and mobile symptom-monitoring tools, in clinical settings. Healthcare systems adopting these communication platforms may not be mindful of the additional challenges these tools may generate for patients with limited health literacy, particularly in accessing and successfully using these technologies.[32]

Addressing Health Literacy in Palliative Care: Strategies and Tools

As health literacy barriers have come to the forefront of the US public health agenda, researchers, healthcare providers, and actors in both the public and the private sectors are amassing a toolkit of approaches to address health literacy across care settings. The following is a summary of the key tools and strategies for enhancing health literacy being implemented at multiple levels of the social-ecological model that have the potential to enhance the utilization, quality, and equity of palliative care services.

Tools Aimed at Patients and Caregivers

At the most basic level, minimizing the negative impact of limited health literacy requires tailoring the format and modality of information presentation. General principles have been proposed for health-literate communication, most of which apply to palliative care. According to these guidelines, information should be clear, brief, free of medical jargon, and focused on actionable information relevant to patients' concerns.[1] Materials should also be linguistically and culturally sensitive and developed with the help of members of the target population. In terms of written information specifically, health literacy scholars have focused on increasing readability, for example through the use of short sentences and paragraphs,[33] ample white space, large font sizes, and text-enhancing graphics and illustrations.[1]

Studies suggest that patient education materials designed according to these principles are more acceptable to patients across the continuum of health literacy. For example, one study compared a standard advance directive—written at a 12th-grade reading level—with one redesigned to enhance readability. The redesigned version was written at a 5th-grade reading level, used a larger font, contained graphics, and incorporated input from patients and providers. The document was judged by all participants—particularly those with low health literacy—to be easier to understand and more useful for end-of-life decision-making. These alterations also increased utilization: individuals who were presented with the redesigned form were more likely than those presented with a standard form to complete an advance directive 6 months poststudy.[16]

However, improving readability does not necessarily eliminate knowledge gaps associated with limited health literacy. For example, in the advance directive study discussed previously, both the standard and the redesigned document led to similar knowledge gains about advance directive topics.[16] As Davis and colleagues observe, "simplifying materials makes them more appealing, less frightening, and easier to read; however, when used alone, a simply written pamphlet or consent document does not significantly improve patient comprehension nor does it adequately inform."[1] Addressing limited health literacy requires moving beyond the layout of written materials.

Nonprint presentation formats such as audio and video recordings have been found to be effective in palliative care communication, particularly with complex issues such as prognosis and treatment preferences.[34,35] For example, one study demonstrated the utility of a video format in eliciting patient preferences for advance care related to dementia: when the individuals in the study were presented with a verbal description of advanced dementia and three available care options (life-prolonging, limited, or comfort care), only 50% of participants expressed a preference for comfort care.[34] However, after the same participants viewed a video depicting a patient with advanced dementia and the different treatments associated with the three care options, 89.2% stated a preference for comfort care.[34] Viewing this video also eliminated the tendency for African Americans, Latinos, and those at lower educational levels to opt for life-prolonging care at greater rates.[35] These results suggest that video formats may enhance understanding of end-of-life care options, including palliative care.

Strategies have also been proposed to facilitate patient understanding of medical information received during clinical encounters, including recording medical consultations for later review, providing visual aids, and encouraging patients to have a preferred support person present for important discussions.[36] Depending on the context, specific communication tools may also be available, such as question prompt lists, which are structured lists of questions patients can use during consultations with providers. Question prompt lists have been found to facilitate patient–provider communication and empower patients when having difficult conversations around prognosis and end-of-life issues.[37]

Another critical tool that may aid critically ill individuals in making treatment decisions is the patient decision aid (PtDA). PtDAs contain structured and personalized information about treatment options, with the aim of facilitating communication and reducing decision burden.[14,38] Despite the potential of PtDAs to help people with low health literacy, however, a recent review concluded that PtDAs are typically designed without special attention to the needs of these individuals (e.g., very few PtDAs are explicitly tested with limited health literacy populations or designed to conform to literacy criteria).[39] The review offered recommendations for making PtDAs more accessible and comprehensible for low health literacy individuals: for example, ensuring that they are written at or below the 8th-grade level, using a "higher is better" frame, and displaying numerical information in tables or pictographs rather than as part of the text.[39]

Patient navigators—trained, culturally competent personnel who help patients and families address barriers to healthcare—offer another approach to address limited health literacy at the level of patients and their family. The unique skills and functions of navigators allow them to address the needs of limited health literacy individuals, for example by providing patient education in a manner that is culturally sensitive, supportive, and empowering.[40] Furthermore, navigators are poised to address health literacy across the entire care continuum, from educating the community about palliative care before a health crisis occurs to helping individuals overcome barriers to access and utilization of palliative care services by acting as advocates once patients are in a health system.[40] In doing so, navigators can help ensure that palliative care is "appropriately integrated from diagnosis on and not considered a secondary form of care."[41]

While most of the strategies discussed here are framed in terms of improving care for patients, it should be noted that many of these strategies can also help caregivers with limited health literacy. Caregiver support in palliative care is especially vital because caregivers are often required to take on complex medical tasks with inadequate information or training.[42] Group-based education programs on caregiving and coping with loss have been shown to be effective in fulfilling caregivers' unmet needs and improving their care competence and preparedness.[29] Ultimately, these types of interventions may improve not only the palliative care received by patients but also the physical, mental, and psychosocial health of caregivers.

Tools at the Care Setting Level

Increasing recognition of the fact that health literacy arises as much from the demands of the healthcare system as from individuals' limitations has prompted providers, researchers, and health systems to begin evaluating and implementing system-level changes needed to achieve organizational health literacy.[43] Several best-practice recommendations have been suggested for providers in communicating with limited health literacy patients. One resource encourages providers to plan sufficient time for consultations, slow down their rate of speech, use short sentences and familiar words, limit the information they provide to a maximum of three main points when possible, and allow patients to record the exchange so they can review what was said at a later time.[5]

Communication of prognostic information and treatment options remains a significant challenge in palliative care. A part of this challenge stems from numeracy demands in clinical interactions. Since verbal descriptions of probability (e.g., *unlikely, possible, almost certain*) are subject to different interpretations, communicating probabilistic information generally requires the use of numbers.[44] However, many limited health literacy patients and caregivers have difficulty understanding and using numeric information, making it imperative for providers to follow evidence-based practices for enhancing patient comprehension of this information.[45]

The literature on risk communication emphasizes the fact that the numeric format in which information is presented can either facilitate or hinder patient comprehension.[46] For example, probabilistic information presented as a frequency (e.g., "3 out of 10 patients experience side effects") is generally easier to comprehend than that presented as a percentage (e.g., "30% of patients experience side effects").[47] Additionally, when comparing treatment options, risks described in terms of their absolute levels (e.g., "the number of patients who experience the side effect would increase from 1 in 1,000 to 2 in 1,000") are preferable to those described in terms of relative levels (e.g., "the risk would double"), as the latter may lead patients to overestimate the magnitude of the risk difference.[47] Healthcare providers should also use a consistent denominator when comparing risks (e.g., "1 in 100" vs. "10 in 100") to avoid confusing patients.[48]

Supplementing numeric data with graphs or other visual displays has been found to facilitate comprehension of this information.[47] The type of visual display used depends on the nature of the information to be presented. For example, bar graphs are useful for making comparisons between different risk levels, line graphs are well suited for showing temporal trends in risk, and pictographs (also called icon arrays or image matrices) displaying, for example, the ratio of affected to unaffected individuals are best for conveying the probability of a single risk or benefit.[44,46] However, because pictographs display the number of people affected (i.e., the numerator) in addition to the number unaffected and use a frequency rather than probability format, they are usually the favored visual format for presenting risk information.[46]

Providers should also be mindful of the fact that the way they describe, or "frame," treatment options can have a profound effect on the choices made by patients and caregivers. For example, patients tend to perceive treatments more positively when outcomes are described in terms of survival rates as opposed to death rates,[45] and such effects are more common in patients who are less numerate.[49] Therefore, when opposite but equivalent frames exist for quantifying an outcome, providers are encouraged to present risk information using both frames to avoid biasing patients' decisions.[48]

While it is important that providers follow best practices for presenting information, it is equally important that they assess whether the information was indeed communicated effectively. One approach to evaluating whether information was imparted successfully is to ask patients, "What is your understanding of your illness?" Research suggests that patients who respond without naming their diagnosis or describing prognosis tend to have a poor understanding of their condition.[50] Another related, well-used method for evaluating patient understanding is the "teach-back" method, where a patient is asked to explain discussed information to the clinician. Note that this method is meant only to help providers gauge how well they are communicating and should *not* be used as a test of patient knowledge.

Even when best practices in risk communication are employed and/or patients have adequate health literacy and understand the information provided, patients and caregivers can still feel overwhelmed and have difficulty making appropriate decisions, given the inherently uncertain nature of disease trajectories and treatment paths. Particularly in end-of-life contexts, information about prognosis and treatment options may be hard for patients and caregivers to accept and process. In attempting to be informative, providers may end up presenting patients with too much information (e.g., too many numbers, too many choices); instead, they should consider focusing only on information most critical to patients' decision-making.[45] In order for us to move toward true patient-centered palliative care, it is important that providers avoid overwhelming patients and caregivers with a barrage of information and instead seek to understand the priorities and values of patients and their families (e.g., quality vs. quantity of life) and explain how they might best achieve their goals, given the options available.[13]

Incorporating health literacy into medical training is another important method for improving patient–provider communication in the palliative care context. Some have suggested including health literacy training in accreditation standards for medical education and testing for health literacy awareness in board examinations.[51] One promising training program carried out in Canada in 2008 aimed to provide physicians with the skills and confidence they needed to support patients in making decisions regarding place of care at the end of life.[52] The intervention consisted of an online tutorial describing decision-support principles and case studies, a skill-building workshop involving role-play and expert feedback, and a follow-up call to reinforce workshop principles.[52] Compared to a control group, clinicians in the training program were able to provide higher quality decision support and address a greater number of patient needs postintervention.[14] However, more research is needed to test the effectiveness and feasibility of particular training regimens, including Internet-based programs.

As a complement to provider training, healthcare organizations can employ specialized counselors to improve communication with patients (especially those with low health literacy) regarding palliative care services. One large hospital in Georgia has pioneered a new approach to palliative care provision by giving counselors a central role on palliative care teams.[53] In this model, counselors initiate contact with patients and families, discuss care options using health literacy principles, attend to the psychosocial needs of patients/caregivers, and coordinate clinical visits to ensure continuity of care. Trained counselors can adequately address end-of-life needs because they do not face the same time constraints and competing priorities that prevent healthcare providers from focusing on communication and patient education. Early evidence indicates that this approach is effective, particularly in terms of reducing conflict, communication deficits, and knowledge gaps.[53]

More broadly, assessing an organization's response to health literacy needs is an important step toward improving care quality.[43] The Office of Disease Prevention and Health Promotion offers several tools to help health organizations meet the needs of low literacy populations. For example, a self-assessment tool for hospitals and health centers includes an action plan for reducing literacy barriers that can help organizations decrease the health literacy demands experienced by patients in these settings.[54] In conducting these types of audits, organizations should also evaluate the existence of system-level supports that can make services more health literate, such as the provision of sufficient time for consultations and the presence of incentives for excellent communication with patients.[8] Finally, rather than viewing limited health literacy as the "exception to the rule," health organizations should adopt universal precautions (e.g., eliminating meaningless choices, simplifying forms) that reduce the cognitive burden placed on all patients and ensure the comprehension of key information. Such strategies would benefit patients at all levels of education and literacy.[8]

Tools at the Community Level

As people interact with medical topics more frequently outside of healthcare settings, unique opportunities exist at the community level for improving health literacy related to palliative care. For example, many Americans, particularly those from a lower socioeconomic background, get their health information from television.[1] The media play an important role in educating the public about various health topics, including end-of-life issues,[55] and therefore have the potential to impact knowledge and attitudes about palliative care. The public health community can leverage the reach and influence of the news and entertainment media to better inform the public about palliative care services.

Leveraging existing social networks (e.g., faith-based organizations, work places, community centers, etc.) may be another effective way to communicate information about palliative care to the public.[56] One way to do this involves working with community-based organizations to host educational meetings and providing materials on palliative care for the organizations to distribute to their members. This approach has the benefit of reaching individuals (who may later become caregivers or patients) that are unaware of palliative care and who would not seek out this information on their own. Moreover, this strategy allows the materials to be tailored for the health literacy level and culture of the population served by each organization.[57] Faith-based organizations, in particular, offer a promising venue for community-based palliative care education. Religious leaders are often called upon in end-of-life situations, but many of these leaders are not sufficiently knowledgeable about palliative care services.[58] Partnering with clergy and providing them with education and training in the area of palliative care is a promising approach for reaching individuals in the community.[55]

Tools at the National and State Policy Level

Because of the enormous public health and economic costs associated with low health literacy, policymakers have been asked to address health literacy through a range of interventions.[43,59] One approach open to policymakers is realigning payment systems so they incentivize organizations and providers to address health literacy issues.[8] This might be done by providing reimbursement for time devoted to culturally competent patient education or by providing liability insurance discounts to providers who receive training on patient-centered communication techniques.[60] According to Paasche-Orlow and Wolf, incentives that encourage entire organizations to address health literacy issues (e.g. rewards for investing in education and patient self-management technologies) are also needed.[8] In the United States, it has also been suggested that moving away from the fee-for-service model altogether would go a long way toward fostering patient-centered communication in all aspects of health (including palliative care).[60]

One of the other tools available at this level is the legislation and implementation of training and care standards in health settings. For example, several US states have mandated the training of health professionals in cultural competence; making health literacy training a requirement for all health professionals in the same way could have significant implications for patient–provider communication and quality of care.[7] However, the evidence base on the effectiveness of such initiatives is currently lacking, and a more rigorous assessment of these policies is called for.[7]

Policymakers can also affect change through their funding decisions. Increased funding for multidisciplinary research on communication and health literacy is needed in order to stimulate the development of effective interventions and to generate an evidence base for eliminating health disparities.[51,59] The government could also advance research in this field by appropriating funds to establish centers of excellence as test-beds and early adopters of innovations to improve health literacy.[59] Further research in this area is especially vital in the context of palliative care, where relatively little work on health literacy has been done to date.

More generally, increased support for safety-net hospitals and clinics that serve low health literate individuals is important to ensure that services and training are adequate to address this population's needs.[8] Clinics and agencies that care for vulnerable populations, such as the Ryan White Care Act Programs and the Indian Health Service, would benefit from specialized funding to implement proven interventions and best practices for improving health literacy.[59]

Taking a long-term perspective, state policies related to education can help ensure that future generations are better equipped with the foundational skills required to successfully navigate the healthcare system and make appropriate medical decisions. To this end, health literacy standards should be incorporated into learning goals and assessments across all levels of the education system.[51] Given that educational attainment has long been linked with health outcomes, improving the quality of education should be recognized as integral to public health.[7]

Outside the formal education system, adult education classes and public libraries also have untapped potential for increasing the health literacy of the public and educating those most in need about important health issues.[3,61] Introducing palliative care topics in these settings, and long before important decisions need to be made, can help make future discussions less uncomfortable and prepare individuals to identify preferred and appropriate care for themselves and their loved ones when the need arises.

Priorities in Research and Practice

The last section of this chapter is devoted to a discussion of current gaps and emerging areas that deserve further attention in palliative care communication research and practice. They include considerations for using technologically mediated communication, increasing access to and acceptability of palliative care, and moving research and practice beyond cancer care settings. However, it is important to remember that underlying all of these efforts should be a focus on ascertaining patient values throughout the care process, so that we can alleviate unnecessary suffering through patient-centered palliative care.

Considering Emerging Technologies and Media

The growth of the Internet, mobile technology, wearable censors, and social media has created new opportunities for communicating about health, improving health literacy, as well as interacting with the healthcare system, and these opportunities also extend to palliative care communication and service delivery. The overall US Internet access rate is estimated to be at 87%, and the Internet serves as a common source of health information.[62] While the Internet provides rapid access to a large amount of information, effectively engaging with online health information requires adequate health literacy.[1] Simply supplying palliative care information or enabling online access to such information would not necessarily help those with limited health literacy; in fact, it may exacerbate disparities if individuals with limited literacy find online information confusing or overwhelming. Furthermore, user-centered design is crucial for ensuring that technology-mediated tools are accessible, beneficial, and equitable. Czaja et al. found that even well-educated seniors with prior computer experience had difficulty navigating and accessing information on the Medicare website and concluded that less computer literate individuals could be expected to experience even greater difficulty using the site.[63]

Despite these challenges, new technologies do offer opportunities for delivering health literate interventions. Technologies such as automated telephone calls/reminders, integrated electronic health record systems, and computerized agents can facilitate patient education and improve care in a cost-effective way.[7] For instance, in a pilot study on the use of a computerized conversational agent during the informed consent process, Bickmore et al. found that limited health literacy patients preferred using technology for this purpose and gained an equivalent amount of knowledge regardless of whether they used the technology or spoke to a real person.[64] However, much more work remains to be done in this area to identify the specific features of technology-mediated innovations that patients and their families find useful and engaging.[2]

Emerging social media platforms—characterized by the multidirectional flow of user generated content—enable individuals to exchange health information, including information related to palliative care such as methods for pain management, end-of-life options, and bereavement. More generally, research indicates that patients use social media sites to exchange medical information and discuss their illnesses and treatments.[65] It is important for researchers to explore the content and communication processes in these peer-to-peer exchanges and to leverage the spaces "where people are," as these methods can generate insight about the lived palliative care experiences of patients and their loved ones. For example, a review on the use of blogs in the palliative care context found that critically ill patients used blogs to exchange both emotional support and information with other people who were in similar situations and that, for at least some patients, the process of blogging was empowering.[66]

Increasing Access to and Utilization of Palliative Care

Increasing appropriate use of palliative care is vital, as it has been shown to enhance patient quality of life, improve symptom management, reduce the number of tests and procedures endured, and increase the satisfaction of patients, providers, and family caregivers.[67] One possible way to achieve this is by increasing the use of patient navigators, as described earlier. Hauser et al. recommend that navigators receive specific training in palliative care in order to enable them to assist patients and their families at more advanced stages of disease.[41] Examples of the types of services patient navigators might provide include screening patients and caregivers for symptoms like pain or depression, initiating discussions around advanced care planning, and providing timely referrals to needed palliative care services.

Employing navigators who can effectively communicate with patients is especially important because of the way palliative care is currently discussed, which may itself pose a barrier to the use of these services. Even the very term "palliative care" is ambiguous, as few individuals are aware of the broad range of services it covers,[68] and many associate it with death and dying. Indeed, the in-depth interviews conducted by Kendall et al. suggest that patients find palliative care unacceptable because, in their minds, the concept is inextricably linked to imminent death.[69] Some research suggests that patient narratives, or "role-model stories" that describe the positive experiences real individuals have had with palliative care can improve knowledge and attitudes toward this type of care and may also aid low health literacy individuals with the recall of important health information.[38,70]

There have also been calls to "rebrand" palliative care and avoid complicated, official medical terminology in discussions of this topic with lay audiences.[71] One suggestion has been to replace the term "palliative care" with the term "supportive care" because this phrase may have fewer undesirable connotations. In fact, one survey showed that many US providers perceive the term "palliative care" to be a barrier to referral (because they believe that it leads to patient distress) and would be more inclined to refer a patient with early-stage cancer to a service named "supportive care."[72] Indeed, after the Cleveland Clinic changed the name of its outpatient palliative care center to the Supportive Care Center, patient referrals to the center grew by 41% and the average timing of referrals increased from 4.7 to 6.2 months before death.[73]

Moving Beyond Cancer Care Settings

Most palliative care studies to date, including those on health literacy, focus on patients with cancer.[74] This may be a result of the relative abundance of research funding for cancer compared to other diseases, or it may simply reflect the reality of palliative care utilization: approximately half of patients receiving hospice and palliative care services have cancer diagnoses.[9] Research is needed to develop appropriate palliative care services for non-cancer patients and to better communicate the benefits of palliative care to these patients and their families.[75] These efforts are especially important because different diseases follow different trajectories and require different services and communication approaches.[76]

Additionally, compared to cancer, the public may be less informed about other diseases and may have a different set of expectations around living and dying from these conditions, necessitating targeted educational efforts to increase utilization of palliative care services in patients with these diseases. These realities also mean that providers and the healthcare system as a whole need to focus on individual patients and families, rather than on diseases—eliciting goals, values, and preferences and empowering patients to make informed decisions.[76] In this way, all patients, regardless of literacy level or diagnosis, will be able to choose the type of care that reflects what they truly want and obtain services that will reduce their suffering and distress.

Lessons from Recent Caregiving Experiences

We wrote the final version of this chapter while accompanying a dear friend on her end-of-life journey. Her experience of living with advanced cancer and desperately seeking treatment options underscored the complexity of palliative care decisions and the enormous health literacy demands placed on patients and caregivers by the healthcare system. This young and brilliant scientist, barely in her 30s and at the height of her career, was thrown at the mercy of a fragmented healthcare system upon diagnosis and, subsequently, recurrence. Being armed with advanced degrees, self-efficacy, insurance coverage, and a highly health-literate support network did not shield her from the serious problems patients encounter when the traditional disease treatment model no longer serves their needs. In fact, communication breakdowns at multiple levels and at various points of care, as well as challenges encountered during transitions between different treatment settings, left us wondering about the additional burdens limited health literacy imposes on individuals and their loved ones in similar situations.

Aspects of this real-world cancer journey are highly relevant to our discussion of health literacy and palliative care, and we hope that by citing this experience we can begin to elucidate some of the tremendous challenges in reconciling a theoretical definition of "patient-centered palliative care" with the practical delivery of care that truly reflects and respects patient values. First, for a young, previously healthy individual whose expressed goal is to continue any and all possible treatment paths in order to buy more time, discussing the possibility of palliative care or hospice is enormously challenging. There is no clear "right time" to have a conversation about palliative care options in this kind of situation, and there can be resistance on multiple levels (from the patient, caregivers, and even the clinical care team) to initiating a patient-centered conversation about palliative care.

Exacerbating this problem is the fact that, in advanced diseases, a large number of providers from different disciplines (e.g., oncology, radiology, nutrition) and even different institutions are typically involved in care. Patients commonly do not have a single point of contact, and no single provider is responsible for communicating with the patient or initiating difficult palliative care conversations. Delivering prognostic news and discussing disease outlook is admittedly difficult, even for experienced providers, but the fact that this aspect of the job is rarely well defined or clearly delegated inhibits important discussions from taking place and prevents critically ill individuals from utilizing palliative care services that may improve their quality of life.

As stated earlier, we believe that in order to deliver true patient-centered care that is in line with patient preferences, communication efforts that aim to elicit and optimally respond to patient and caregiver values and priorities are crucial. However, it is important to point out that the reality of an advanced disease entails many uncertainties, and there are important differences across patients in terms of their values and goals. These realities can lead to a significant amount of tension between respecting patient preferences and attempting to provide palliative care when curative options are no longer available.

Conclusion

In conclusion, as Dr. Atul Gawande articulated in a *New York Times* article in 2014, "in medicine and society, we have failed to recognize that people have priorities that they need us to serve besides just living longer.... And the best way to learn those priorities is to ask about them."[77] His reflections point to the importance of communication about palliative care and the role health literacy plays in this process. To deliver care that reflects the values and preferences of patients and their loved ones, the healthcare system must support and enable providers (whether they are physicians, nurses, or patient navigators) to ascertain their patients' understanding of health and disease, as well as their goals, fears, and priorities. Engaging in this process with vulnerable, low health literacy patients is even more challenging—and even more necessary—if we hope to achieve the goal of effective, patient-centered, and equitable palliative care.

References

1. Davis TC, Williams MV, Marin E, Parker RM, Glass J. Health literacy and cancer communication. *CA Cancer J Clin*. 2002;52(3):134–149.
2. Paasche-Orlow MK, Wolf MS. The causal pathways linking health literacy to health outcomes. *Am J Health Behav*. 2007;31 Suppl 1:S19–S26.
3. Kindig DA, Panzer AM, Nielsen-Bohlman L. *Health Literacy: A Prescription to End Confusion*. Washington, DC: National Academies Press; 2004.
4. *The Current State of Health Care for People with Disabilities*. Washington, DC: National Council on Disability; 2009.
5. Reisfield GM, Wilson GR. Health literacy in palliative medicine #153. *J Palliat Med*. 2008;11(1):105–106.
6. Devraj R, Herndon CM, Griffin J. Pain awareness and medication knowledge: A health literacy evaluation. *J Pain Palliat Care Pharmacother*. 2013;27(1):19–27.
7. Paasche-Orlow MK, Wolf MS. Promoting health literacy research to reduce health disparities. *J Health Commun*. 2010;15 Suppl 2:34–41.
8. Paasche-Orlow MK, Schillinger D, Greene SM, Wagner EH. How health care systems can begin to address the challenge of limited literacy. *J Gen Intern Med*. 2006;21(8):884–887.
9. Matsuyama RK, Balliet W, Ingram K, Lyckholm LJ, Wilson-Genderson M, Smith TJ. Will patients want hospice or palliative care if they do not know what it is? *J Hosp Palliat Nurs*. 2011;13(1):41–46.
10. Lewis JM, DiGiacomo M, Currow DC, Davidson PM. Dying in the margins: understanding palliative care and socioeconomic deprivation in the developed world. *J Pain Symptom Manage*. 2011;42(1):105–118.
11. James BD, Boyle PA, Bennett JS, Bennett DA. The impact of health and financial literacy on decision making in community-based older adults. *Gerontology*. 2012;58(6):531–539.
12. Ishikawa H, Yano E, Fujimori S, et al. Patient health literacy and patient–physician information exchange during a visit. *Fam Pract*. 2009.
13. Gillick MR. Decision making near life's end: a prescription for change. *J Palliat Med*. 2009;12(2):121–125.
14. Murray MA, Stacey D, Wilson KG, O'Connor AM. Skills training to support patients considering place of end-of-life care: a randomized control trial. *J Palliat Care*. 2010;26(2):112–121.
15. Easton P, Entwistle VA, Williams B. How the stigma of low literacy can impair patient-professional spoken interactions and affect health: Insights from a qualitative investigation. *BMC Health Serv Res*. 2013;13(1):319.
16. Sudore RL, Landefeld CS, Barnes DE, et al. An advance directive redesigned to meet the literacy level of most adults: A randomized trial. *Patient Educ Couns*. 2007;69(1–3):165–195.

17. Douma KF, Koning CC, Zandbelt LC, de Haes HC, Smets EM. Do patients' information needs decrease over the course of radiotherapy? *Support Care Cancer.* 2012;20(9):2167-2176.
18. Parker R. Health literacy: A challenge for American patients and their health care providers. *Health Promot Int.* 2000;15(4):277-283.
19. Wallace LS, Rogers ES, Roskos SE, Holiday DB, Weiss BD. Brief report: Screening items to identify patients with limited health literacy skills. *J Gen Intern Med.* 2006;21(8):874-877.
20. Schlichting JA, Quinn MT, Heuer LJ, Schaefer CT, Drum ML, Chin MH. Provider perceptions of limited health literacy in community health centers. *Patient Educ Couns.* 2007;69(1):114-120.
21. VanGeest JB, Welch VL, Weiner SJ. Patients' perceptions of screening for health literacy: Reactions to the newest vital sign. *J Health Commun.* 2010;15(4):402-412.
22. Thorne S, Hislop TG, Kuo M, Armstrong EA. Hope and probability: Patient perspectives of the meaning of numerical information in cancer communication. *Qual Health Res.* 2006;16(3):318-336.
23. Quirt CF, Mackillop WJ, Ginsburg AD, et al. Do doctors know when their patients don't? A survey of doctor-patient communication in lung cancer. *Lung Cancer.* 1997;18(1):1-20.
24. Curtis JR, Patrick DL, Caldwell E, Greenlee H, Collier AC. The quality of patient-doctor communication about end-of-life care: A study of patients with advanced AIDS and their primary care clinicians. *AIDS.* 1999;13(9):1123-1131.
25. Fried TR, Bradley EH, O'Leary J. Prognosis communication in serious illness: Perceptions of older patients, caregivers, and clinicians. *J Am Geriatr Soc.* 2003;51(10):1398-1403.
26. Gattellari M, Butow PN, Tattersall MH, Dunn SM, MacLeod CA. Misunderstanding in cancer patients: Why shoot the messenger? *Ann Oncol.* 1999;10(1):39-46.
27. Hancock K, Clayton JM, Parker SM, et al. Discrepant perceptions about end-of-life communication: A systematic review. *J Pain Symptom Manage.* 2007;34(2):190-200.
28. Haidet P, Hamel MB, Davis RB, et al. Outcomes, preferences for resuscitation, and physician-patient communication among patients with metastatic colorectal cancer. *Am J Med.* 1998;105(3):222-229.
29. Hudson P, Quinn K, Kristjanson L, et al. Evaluation of a psycho-educational group programme for family caregivers in home-based palliative care. *Palliat Med.* 2008;22(3):270-280.
30. Benzar E, Hansen L, Kneitel AW, Fromme EK. Discharge planning for palliative care patients: A qualitative analysis. *J Palliat Med.* 2011;14(1):65-69.
31. McCorkle R, Pasacreta JV. Enhancing caregiver outcomes in palliative care. *Cancer Control.* 2001;8(1):36-45.
32. Kim E-H, Stolyar A, Lober WB, et al. Challenges to using an electronic personal health record by a low-income elderly population. *J Med Internet Res.* 2009;11(4):e44.
33. Payne S, Large S, Jarrett N, Turner P. Written information given to patients and families by palliative care units: A national survey. *Lancet.* 2000;355(9217):1792.
34. Volandes AE, Paasche-Orlow M, Gillick MR, et al. Health literacy not race predicts end-of-life care preferences. *J Palliat Med.* 2008;11(5):754-762.
35. Volandes AE, Ferguson LA, Davis AD, et al. Assessing end-of-life preferences for advanced dementia in rural patients using an educational video: A randomized controlled trial. *J Palliat Med.* 2011;14(2):169-177.
36. Lee SJ, Back AL, Block SD, Stewart SK. Enhancing physician-patient communication. *ASH Education Program Book.* 2002(1):464-483.
37. Dimoska A, Tattersall MH, Butow PN, Shepherd H, Kinnersley P. Can a "prompt list" empower cancer patients to ask relevant questions? *Cancer.* 2008;113(2):225-237.
38. Bekker H, Winterbottom A, Butow P, et al. Do personal stories make patient decision aids more effective? A critical review of theory and evidence. *BMC Med Inform Decis Mak.* 2013;13(2):1-9.
39. McCaffery K, Holmes-Rovner M, Smith S, et al. Addressing health literacy in patient decision aids. *BMC Med Inform Decis Mak.* 2013;13(2):1-14.
40. Fischer SM, Sauaia A, Kutner JS. Patient navigation: A culturally competent strategy to address disparities in palliative care. *J Palliat Med.* 2007;10(5):1023-1028.
41. Hauser J, Sileo M, Araneta N, et al. Navigation and palliative care. *Cancer.* 2011;117(15 Suppl):3585-3591.
42. Harrop E, Byrne A, Nelson A. "It's alright to ask for help": Findings from a qualitative study exploring the information and support needs of family carers at the end of life. *BMC Palliat Care.* 2014;13:22.
43. Koh HK, Berwick DM, Clancy CM, et al. New federal policy initiatives to boost health literacy can help the nation move beyond the cycle of costly "crisis care." *Health Aff.* 2012;31(2):434-443.
44. Lipkus IM. Numeric, verbal, and visual formats of conveying health risks: Suggested best practices and future recommendations. *Med Decis Making.* 2007;27(5):696-713.
45. Nelson W, Reyna VF, Fagerlin A, Lipkus I, Peters E. Clinical implications of numeracy: Theory and practice. *Ann Behav Med.* 2008;35(3):261-274.
46. Fagerlin A, Zikmund-Fisher BJ, Ubel PA. Helping patients decide: Ten steps to better risk communication. *J Natl Cancer Inst.* 2011;103(19):1436-1443.
47. Gigerenzer G, Edwards A. Simple tools for understanding risks: From innumeracy to insight. *BMJ.* 2003;327(7417):741.
48. Fagerlin A, Ubel PA, Smith DM, Zikmund-Fisher BJ. Making numbers matter: Present and future research in risk communication. *Am J Health Behav.* 2007;31 Suppl 1:S47-S56.
49. Peters E, Västfjäll D, Slovic P, Mertz CK, Mazzocco K, Dickert S. Numeracy and decision making. *Psychol Sci.* 2006;17(5):407-413.
50. Morris DA, Johnson KS, Ammarell N, Arnold RM, Tulsky JA, Steinhauser KE. What is your understanding of your illness? A communication tool to explore patients' perspectives of living with advanced illness. *J Gen Intern Med.* 2012;27(11):1460-1466.
51. Parker RM, Ratzan SC, Lurie N. Health literacy: A policy challenge for advancing high-quality health care. *Health Aff.* 2003;22(4):147-153.
52. Murray M, O'Connor A, Stacey D, Wilson K. Efficacy of a training intervention on the quality of practitioners' decision support for patients deciding about place of care at the end of life: A randomized control trial study protocol. *BMC Palliat Care.* 2008;7(1):1-9.
53. Babcock CW, Robinson LE. A novel approach to hospital palliative care: An expanded role for counselors. *J Palliat Med.* 2011;14(4):491-500.
54. Office of Disease Prevention and Health Promotion. *National Action Plan to Improve Health Literacy.* Washington, DC: US Department of Health and Human Services; 2010.
55. Crawley L, Payne R, Bolden J, et al. Palliative and end-of-life care in the African American community. *JAMA.* 2000;284(19):2518-2521.
56. Selsky C, Kreling B, Luta G, et al. Hospice knowledge and intentions among Latinos using safety-net clinics. *J Palliat Med.* 2012;15(9):984-990.
57. Maltby BS, Fins JJ. Informing the patient-proxy covenant: An educational approach for advance care planning. *J Palliat Med.* 2004;7(2):351-355.
58. Reese DJ, Ahern RE, Nair S, O'Faire JD, Warren C. Hospice access and use by African Americans: Addressing cultural and institutional barriers through participatory action research. *Soc Work.* 1999;44(6):549-559.
59. Vernon JA, Trujillo, A., Rosenbaum, S., & DeBuono, B. *Low Health Literacy: Implications for National Health Policy.* Washington, DC: Department of Health Policy, School of Public Health and Health Services, George Washington University; 2007.
60. *"What Did the Doctor Say?:" Improving Health Literacy to Protect Patient Safety Health Care at the Crossroads.* Oakbrook Terrace, IL: Joint Commission; 2007.

61. Office of Disease Prevention and Health Promotion. *National Action Plan to Improve Health Literacy*.Washington, DC: US Department of Health and Human Services; 2010.
62. Health fact sheet. Pew Research Center Website. http://www.pewinternet.org/fact-sheets/health-fact-sheet/. Accessed September 15, 2014.
63. Czaja SJ, Sharit J, Nair SN. Usability of the Medicare health web site. *JAMA*. 2008;300(7):790–792.
64. Bickmore TW, Pfeifer LM, Paasche-Orlow MK. Using computer agents to explain medical documents to patients with low health literacy. *Patient Educ Couns*. 2009;75(3):315–320.
65. Sugawara Y, Narimatsu H, Hozawa A, Shao L, Otani K, Fukao A. Cancer patients on Twitter: A novel patient community on social media. *BMC Res Notes*. 2012;5(1):699.
66. Ngwenya NB, Mills S. The use of weblogs within palliative care: A systematic literature review. *Health Informatics J*. 2014;20(1):13–21.
67. Hyer L, Babcock CW, Robinson LE, Ackermann R. Transitions model: Melding of psychotherapy and palliative care using teams. *Clin Gerontologist*. 2011;34(5):379–398.
68. McIlfatrick S, Hasson F, Noble H, et al. How well do the general public understand palliative care? A mixed methods study. *BMJ Support Palliat Care*. 2014;4(Suppl 1):A2.
69. Kendall M, Carduff E, Lloyd A, et al. Different dyings: Living and dying with cancer, organ failure and physical frailty. *BMJ Support Palliat Care*. 2014;4(Suppl 1): A12-A3.
70. Enguidanos S, Kogan AC, Lorenz K, Taylor G. Use of role model stories to overcome barriers to hospice among African Americans. *J Palliat Med*. 2011;14(2):161–168.
71. Wells J. Is it time to rebrand palliative care? http://www.ehospice.com/ArticleView/tabid/10686/ArticleId/10006/language/en-GB/View.aspx. Accessed September 3, 2014.
72. Fadul N, Elsayem A, Palmer JL, et al. Supportive versus palliative care: What's in a name? A survey of medical oncologists and midlevel providers at a comprehensive cancer center. *Cancer*. 2009;115(9):2013–2021.
73. Davis MP, Bruera E, Morganstern D. Early integration of palliative and supportive care in the cancer continuum: Challenges and opportunities. *Am Soc Clin Oncol Educ Book*. 2013:144–150.
74. Gibbs LM, Addington-Hall J, Gibbs JSR. Dying from heart failure: Lessons from palliative care: Many patients would benefit from palliative care at the end of their lives. *BMJ*. 1998;317(7164):961.
75. Addington-Hall J, Fakhoury W, McCarthy M. Specialist palliative care in nonmalignant disease. *Palliative Med*. 1998;12(6):417–427.
76. Murtagh F, Preston M, Higginson I. Patterns of dying: Palliative care for non-malignant disease. *Clinical Med*. 2004;4(1):39–44.
77. Gawande A. The best possible day. *The New York Times*. October 5, 2014.

Appendix A
Health Literacy Considerations for Special Populations

Individuals With Limited English Proficiency

In the United States, people with limited English proficiency (LEP) are also more likely to have lower health literacy, and individuals with both LEP and low health literacy are a particularly vulnerable group.[1] However, few patient-education materials in the United States have been translated into languages other than Spanish, despite the large population of immigrants from Asia and other places, effectively making crucial health information inaccessible to these populations. Conversely, merely translating materials is not sufficient either, as many LEP individuals have limited literacy in their native language as well.[2] LEP patients also report having more difficulties communicating with medical providers.[2] Usually, this problem is addressed through the use of interpreters who translate the provider's instructions. However, health literacy is rarely taken into account during this process, with the result that the verbatim translations are still often too complex and full of jargon.[2] For effective communication to take place, literacy and language barriers need to be addressed concurrently.

As the LEP population in the United States continues to grow, efforts to address language and literacy barriers in the healthcare setting will only become more vital.[1] In the palliative care context specifically, where word choice is crucial, if translations (of written or oral information) are not executed thoughtfully, they may actually increase communication barriers. For instance, the word *hospicio* in Spanish is commonly understood as "orphanage" or "place for poor people"[3] and does not convey a positive, or even neutral, message about hospice as a setting for end-of-life care.

Incarcerated Individuals

There is a high level of morbidity and mortality among the US prison population, as well as an increasing number of older inmates, which makes the need to address palliative care in the correctional setting especially pressing.[4] Providing quality palliative care is challenging even under the best circumstances but is even more so in the prison setting. Among the challenges in this environment is the fact that many inmates have cognitive deficits, learning disabilities, and very low levels of literacy: it has been estimated that close to two-thirds of inmates lack basic literacy skills.[5] Beyond low levels of general literacy, inmates have also been shown to have little knowledge of basic medical terminology, anatomy, or therapeutic procedures, which inhibits their ability to communicate effectively with their providers, make appropriate healthcare decisions, and advocate for care that is aligned with their values.[5]

The very limited understanding of disease held by many incarcerated individuals combined with the lack of trust prison inmates have in the correctional system as a whole (including providers who work in these settings) presents a serious barrier to providing palliative care in the prison context. In the words of one prison doctor, inmates expect to be cured when they are sick and when they are told that a cure is not possible, "their first thought is that the department just doesn't want to spend the money."[4] This attitude and lack of trust also pushes the prisons themselves to provide aggressive care (even when it is futile and possibly even unwanted) in their attempt to protect themselves from accusations that they are denying treatment to ill inmates.[4] Initiatives to educate inmates about health and palliative care will be crucial for members of this population to be able to make informed choices about their care. Intervention planners also need to be aware that the circumstances of the inmate population differ significantly from those of the free-living population, and solutions need to be specifically designed to suit their unique needs. For instance, an issue unique to the prison context is the fact that inmates have very restricted Internet access, which limits their ability to obtain their own information on medical topics, including palliative care.[4]

Individuals With Disabilities

Individuals with communication disorders—such as impaired hearing or eyesight and aphasia—face special health literacy challenges. Communication barriers for persons with disabilities have been well documented.[6] For instance, one study identified limited literacy and language skills, as well as limited access to health practitioners fluent in sign language, as barriers to receiving appropriate palliative and end-of-life care for members of the deaf community in Canada.[7] Another issue for this population is that frequently used idioms and many advanced medical terms do not have equivalent counterparts in sign language, which makes explaining concepts related to palliative care especially challenging.[7]

Having a visual impairment can also hinder individuals from obtaining and processing health information and navigating the healthcare system (e.g., due to the inability to read signage in a medical office). In the United States, the Americans with Disabilities Act was designed to ensure that individuals with disabilities (as well as low English proficiency) have access to health information and assistance in healthcare settings; nevertheless, barriers for these populations continue to exist.[6] Clearly, healthcare systems need to make additional efforts to better accommodate the needs of individuals with disabilities—for instance by providing health materials and forms in different formats (such as Braille, large-print, and auditory).[8]

Individuals With Cognitive Impairments

Cognitive issues can complicate communication and decision-making around palliative care. For example, people with severe dementia lack the capacity required to make decisions about their care and treatment near the end of life.[9] Therefore, discussions and decisions around palliative and end-of-life care need to occur as early as possible in the disease trajectory—while these individuals are still able to communicate their preferences.[9] Additionally, cognitive impairment is not an issue limited to patients suffering from Alzheimer's and similar diseases; many palliative care patients (including those with cancer) exhibit evidence of cognitive impairment, and this has important implications for the delivery of quality care, for example in regard to the recognition and management of symptoms.[10] Therefore, it is crucial to initiate conversations about palliative care as early as possible, regardless of the patient's diagnosis.

Appendix A References

1. Sentell T, Braun KL. Low health literacy, limited English proficiency, and health status in Asians, Latinos, and other racial/ethnic groups in California. *J Health Commun.* 2012;17 Suppl 3:82–99.
2. Andrulis DP, Brach C. Integrating literacy, culture, and language to improve health care quality for diverse populations. *Am J Health Behav.* 2007;31 Suppl 1:S122–S133.
3. Selsky C, Kreling B, Luta G, et al. Hospice knowledge and intentions among Latinos using safety-net clinics. *J Palliat Med.* 2012;15(9):984–990.
4. Linder JF, Meyers FJ. Palliative care for prison inmates: "Don't let me die in prison." *JAMA.* 2007;298(8):894–901.
5. Enders SR, Paterniti DA, Meyers FJ. An approach to develop effective health care decision making for women in prison. *J Palliat Med.* 2005;8(2):432–439.
6. Office of Disease Prevention and Health Promotion. *National Action Plan to Improve Health Literacy.* Washington, DC: US Department of Health and Human Services; 2010.
7. Maddalena V, O'Shea F, Murphy M. Palliative and end-of-life care in Newfoundland's deaf community. *J Palliat Care.* 2012;28(2):105–112.
8. Harrison TC, Mackert M, Watkins C. Health literacy issues among women with visual impairments. *Res Gerontol Nurs.* 2010;3(1):49–60.
9. Sampson EL. Palliative care for people with dementia. *Brit Med Bull.* 2010;96(1):159–174.
10. Pereira J, Hanson J, Bruera E. The frequency and clinical course of cognitive impairment in patients with terminal cancer. *Cancer.* 1997;79(4):835–842.

Appendix B
List of Key Health Literacy Resources
General

Health.gov Website

http://www.health.gov/communication/literacy/
This section of the health.gov website features a variety of content related to health literacy, including tools, research, and resources.

Centers for Disease Control and Prevention Website

http://www.cdc.gov/healthliteracy/index.html
The Centers for Disease Control and Prevention hosts a site devoted to health literacy, which provides information about health literacy and tools for improving public health practice through the application of health literacy principles.

National Action Plan to Improve Health Literacy

http://www.health.gov/communication/HLActionPlan/pdf/Health_Literacy_Action_Plan.pdf
This report, from the US Department of Health and Human Services, provides a blueprint for improving the way health information is communicated to the public and ensuring that Americans obtain the literacy skills they need to help them live healthier lives. The action plan outlines seven goals designed to improve health literacy in the United States, along with suggestions for strategies to achieve these goals.

Health Literacy: A Prescription to End Confusion

www.iom.edu/report.asp?id=19723
This report by the Institute of Medicine reviews the scientific knowledge base related to health literacy and provides recommendations for creating a more health-literate society.

Health Literacy Interventions and Outcomes: An Updated Systematic Review

http://www.ahrq.gov/research/findings/evidence-based-reports/er199-abstract.html#Report
This systematic review by the Agency for Healthcare Research and Quality summarizes evidence regarding the impact of health literacy on healthcare service use and health outcomes and evaluates the effectiveness of interventions designed to improve outcomes among individuals with low health literacy.

Simply Put

http://www.cdc.gov/healthmarketing/pdf/Simply_Put_082010.pdf

This guide from the Centers for Disease Control and Prevention provides practical strategies for creating materials that are easy to understand and accessible.

Toolkit for Making Written Material Clear and Effective

https://www.cms.gov/WrittenMaterialsToolkit/
This resource from the Centers for Medicare and Medicaid Services provides information on making written materials easier for people to read, understand, and use.

For Health Providers/Organizations

American Medical Association Website

http://www.ama-assn.org/ama/pub/about-ama/ama-foundation/our-programs/public-health/health-literacy-program.page
The website of the American Medical Association contains information on the way health literacy affects diagnosis, treatment, and patient safety and also provides resources for providers and organizations seeking to learn more about the topic.

AHRQ Health Literacy Universal Precautions Toolkit

http://www.ahrq.gov/professionals/quality-patient-safety/quality-resources/tools/literacy-toolkit/index.html
This toolkit, prepared for the Agency for Healthcare Research and Quality, allows providers to assess and improve the health literacy of their services.

Health Literacy Online

http://www.health.gov/healthliteracyonline/Web_Guide_Health_Lit_Online.pdf
This guide, produced by the Office of Disease Prevention and Health Promotion, provides tips for creating user-friendly websites and delivering online health information in an effective way.

Health Resources and Services Administration Website

http://www.hrsa.gov/publichealth/healthliteracy/
This website offers information about health literacy as well as a free, online training course titled "Effective Communication Tools for Healthcare Professionals," which addresses cultural sensitivity, health literacy, and limited English proficiency.

Advancing Effective Communication, Cultural Competence, and Patient- and Family-Centered Care—A Roadmap for Hospitals

http://www.jointcommission.org/assets/1/6/ARoadmapforHospitalsfinalversion727.pdf
This guide from The Joint Commission provides recommendations to assist hospitals improve the way they communicate with patients, including addressing their health literacy needs.

For the Public

Mayo Clinic Website

http://www.mayoclinic.org/patient-care-and-health-information
The Mayo Clinic hosts a website that provides a wealth of easy-to-understand information on a wide array of health and medical topics, including palliative care (http://www.mayoclinic.org/tests-procedures/palliative-care/basics/definition/prc-20013733)

The Ohio State University Medical Center Website

https://patienteducation.osumc.edu/Pages/Home.aspx
This website features materials on thousands of health-related topics (including end-of-life issues), all written below the 8th-grade reading level.

Literacy Assessment Tools

Newest Vital Sign

http://www.pfizerhealthliteracy.com/physicians-providers/newest-vital-sign.html
This screening tool identifies patients at risk for low health literacy. The NSV takes only a few minutes to administer and is therefore suitable for use in clinical settings (a Spanish-language version of the tool is also available).

Rapid Estimate of Adult Literacy in Medicine–Short Form

http://www.ahrq.gov/populations/sahlsatool.htm
The REALM–SF is a seven-item word-recognition test that can provide clinicians with an assessment of patients' health literacy level. The REALM–SF has been validated and field tested in diverse research settings.

Test of Functional Health Literacy in Adults

http://www.peppercornbooks.com/catalog/information.php?info_id=5
The TOFHLA measures the functional health literacy level of patients (including their numeracy and reading comprehension abilities) using real healthcare materials (e.g., instructions for diagnostic tests). However, although the TOFHLA is comprehensive, it may be too lengthy for use in routine clinical encounters.

CHAPTER 13

Patient- and Family-Centered Written Communication in the Palliative Care Setting

Antoinette Mary Fage-Butler and
Matilde Nisbeth Jensen

Introduction

The purpose of this chapter is to provide an overview of how written communication can support the needs of palliative care patients. There is growing awareness that a patient-centered perspective is valuable for all patients, but it is all the more important in the palliative care setting, where fundamental existential choices about how to live, maintain quality of life, and die are often compromised. Palliative care has evolved as a discipline that primarily emphasizes or assumes live interactions.[1] However, as we illustrate in this chapter, written printed materials and online communication are also very important aspects of patient-centered palliative care. We illustrate how written communication can support the needs of palliative care patients via three text types: professional–patient emails, end-of-life leaflets, and online patient–patient forums. Throughout the chapter we also focus, where relevant, on the provision of patient-centered written materials for caregivers. By "caregivers" we mean the "family, informal caregivers, and friends" of palliative care patients.[2] Following a discussion of how the three text types can support patient-centered palliative care, we address the question of health literacy in relation to the three text types, considering how they may support patient empowerment. The chapter concludes with recommendations intended to support healthcare professionals in optimizing palliative care communicative practice and suggestions for future research.

The Importance of Patient-Centered Texts for Patients

Palliative care has been defined by the National Consensus Project (NCP) for Quality Palliative Care[3] as follows:

> Palliative care means patient and family-centered care that optimizes quality of life by anticipating, preventing, and treating suffering. Palliative care throughout the continuum of illness involves addressing *physical, intellectual, emotional, social, and spiritual needs and to facilitate patient autonomy, access to information and choice.* [our italics]

In this characterization of palliative care, which we draw on throughout this chapter, the focus on meeting the heterogeneous needs of patients and on facilitating autonomy, access to information, and choice clearly reflects the health communication paradigm of patient centeredness. In the palliative care setting, where patients' needs are often particularly complex and profound, autonomy is at stake through medicalization, pain, and weakness, and treatment options may be few or nonexistent, the value of patient centeredness as a supportive and empathetic approach to health communication[4] is clear. Indeed, patient centeredness has been described as an ethical approach to health communication[5] that can address the humanistic lacunae of biomedicine.[6] As a health communication paradigm, patient centeredness underlines the centrality of individual patients' needs and perspectives,[7] where the patient is theorized as a person whose human needs should be met in the clinical situation.[8,9] Just as palliative care aims to "facilitate patient autonomy, access to information and choice," patient centeredness underlines the importance of providing patients with clear information about their illness and its treatment,[10] as well as healthcare professionals sharing power and responsibility to enhance patients' autonomy and choice.[7,11] As pointed out by the NCP, palliative care is relevant throughout the continuum of an illness, but patients' needs and their possibilities for autonomy do change in line with the trajectory of a progressive illness.

Although patient centeredness has mainly been associated with the clinical situation,[12] there is increasing awareness that patient centeredness is a health communication paradigm that is also relevant for written communication.[13] Research shows that patients who receive one-way written communication want to be addressed in ways that respect their perspectives and acknowledge their needs.[14] In the palliative care context, this would mean that attempts should be made to meet patients' psychosocial needs in written communication,[6] characterized by the NCP[3] as *intellectual, emotional, social, and spiritual.* Moreover, we argue that patient-centered texts may even support patients' *physical* needs, particularly for pain relief or symptom control. This is because through improved knowledge, patients may be able to identify other possibilities for care that would ease symptoms such as pain. Also, greater choice and autonomy, which are associated with patient-centered communication, can result in the experience of fewer symptoms and better quality of life.[15] Before we examine written texts for palliative care patients and their caregivers, considering how they may meet their complex needs, we first address the concept of health literacy.

Health Literacy and Written Palliative Care Communication

Health literacy is very relevant for written health communication generally, particularly given the established causal relationship between low health literacy levels and poor health[16] and because it is a necessary prerequisite for patient engagement and empowerment.[17]

Health literacy is often viewed as a quantifiable construct that can be measured through tests such as the Test of Functional Health Literacy in Adults (TOFHLA) or Rapid Estimate of Adult Literacy in Medicine (REALM).[18] However, we argue that taking a patient-centered approach, which entails seeing health literacy as a dynamic, situated construct, is preferable. First, an individual patient's health literacy level is likely to alter depending on subject matter, as individuals who are motivated to know as much as possible about their own or their loved one's condition equip themselves with specialized medical terminology.[19] Second, psychological factors may affect the measurement of health literacy levels, as emotional involvement when one's own health is at stake can negatively affect one's ability to understand written texts.[20]

Although we argue that a patient's health literacy level may fluctuate relative to contextual and personal circumstances, we acknowledge that there are lower and higher health literacy levels that are reflective of patients' linguistic abilities, engagement, and even the state of their health. Given that lower health literacy can bar patients from accessing important information and support, patients with lower health literacy levels need particular focus in palliative care communication. Thus, later in this chapter, we include a discussion of how the various written text types discussed in this chapter might operationalize a patient-centered approach to health literacy.

Text Types for Written Palliative Care Communication

Compared to oral health communication, written health communication has received limited research attention.[21] However, in recent years, research into written health communication has gained momentum in line with greater societal focus on patient empowerment, patients' desire for more information and their increased access to it on the Internet, as well as the growing prevalence of the idea that care is discursively coproduced between patients and healthcare professionals.[22] Clerehan[21] has argued for a tripartite division of written health communication:

1. One-to-one: for example, a healthcare provider responds to the needs of an individual patient (known or unknown to them)
2. One-to-many: for example, a healthcare provider communicates to a group (who may, for instance, have a disease in common)
3. Many-to-many: for example, a bank of providers share advice or responses to a group (usually online)

In this chapter, we discuss in turn three text types that reflect these three categories. The first is email communication between a healthcare professional and a patient (or caregiver); the second exemplifies one-to-many communication via end-of-life leaflets; and the third illustrates an example of many-to-many communication, exemplified through online patient–patient forums for palliative care patients. Specifically, we examine which of the needs of palliative care patients outlined in the NCP definition[3] can be met by these text types. This means that for each text type, we discuss only the patient needs that can be addressed by the text type in question. We structure the discussion to illustrate the positive qualities of each text type in relation to meeting patients' needs before illuminating potential pitfalls. After the discussion of the three text types, we then explore patient empowerment and health literacy relative to these text types.

One-to-One Communication in Palliative Care: Email

Email is increasingly being integrated into provider–patient communication, including in the palliative care setting.[23] It can provide a supportive communication channel for terminally ill patients,[24] and both patients and healthcare professionals agree that it can be especially valuable for patients with chronic diseases[25-27] as it facilitates two-way updates and monitoring that can improve the quality of care.[27-29]

In our integrative literature review on the advantages and disadvantages of email communication for patients generally,[30] we found that patients identify numerous advantages with email, including improved convenience and access, more frequent and better informational exchanges, freedom from the medical gaze, and the potential to level out power imbalances. We also identified a number of primarily medium-related disadvantages for patients. In the following, we discuss how email may specifically address palliative care patients' needs.

Addressing Physical Needs

As argued in the introduction to this chapter, written communication may support palliative care patients' *physical* needs indirectly. For example, access to expert biomedical knowledge and advice between scheduled clinical encounters is vital for patients with cancer.[31] Patients are often concerned about physical symptoms and treatment side effects, particularly as side effects may worsen after patients are discharged from the hospital.[32] Email can thus indirectly support patients' physical needs as it makes prompt communication with healthcare professionals possible.[33]

Addressing Intellectual Needs and Access to Information

Studies of cancer patients' use of email have found that informational needs that are unmet in the offline encounter can be addressed by email.[32,34] As email increases accessibility,[23-25] it can lead to greater two-way information flow between healthcare professional and patient. This is especially relevant for palliative care patients, who have a "continuous need to have their symptom experience confirmed, explained, and understood as something 'normal' and especially as a 'side effect' of medication and not a sign of relapse or sensations unrelated to the disease."[34(p111)] Email offers the possibility of not only more frequent communication between patient and healthcare professional but also more patient-centered communication. First, email offers patients the opportunity to express thoughts, articulate concerns, and ask questions without the tight time constraints of the face-to-face encounter.[23,31] This might be especially relevant in relation to sensitive or embarrassing issues as patients may feel more comfortable expressing themselves in writing than in the face-to-face consultation.[24,25,34] Second, email can be very valuable when speech is problematized as in Kagan et al.'s study[35] of cancer patients' use of email after neck or head surgery. Third, having a written record aids recall, both for the patient and the healthcare professional,[33,35] and can improve communication with caregivers.[25,29,31] A written record supports patients who may find it hard to understand or write down accurately what healthcare professionals say in clinics or over the phone,[31,36] and patients appreciate being able to print out a hard copy to which they can refer.[36] In this way, email can have a positive effect on the clinical follow-up, as it frees time for other matters.[24]

Studies have also found that email can be valuable to palliative care patients in relation to concerns they may have about the impact of their illness on their lives,[34,37] reflected in questions such as "May I take a bath in the sea?' or "May I play golf?"[34] It is important to point out that the information requested here is very patient-specific and can hardly be anticipated in written mass-communicated materials.

Addressing Emotional Needs

There is increasing evidence that email can address palliative care patients' emotional needs[25,32,38] by "providing a medium through which patients can express worries and concerns, and physicians can be patient-centered in response."[39(p36)] The written medium of email communication can also help caregivers express their concerns with a healthcare professional without the patient being present.[29]

David et al. in their study on the possibilities of meeting breast cancer patients' psychosocial needs by using email for counseling showed that "email can establish communication with psychosocially disadvantaged breast cancer patients who are not being reached by conventional avenues of therapy."[38(p11)] In another study, email helped a patient communicate about the suffering induced by her terminal illness after other communication modes had failed.[24] Moreover, as email communication facilitates more frequent patient–provider communication, it can function as reassurance as some patients have reported that, having sent an email, they considered the responsibility to lie with their healthcare professional to a higher degree.[37] Another advantage of email is that, because the patient can communicate away from an institutional setting, it may hinder further medicalization and pathologization of the patient, which can be important for patients' sense of identity. Furthermore, Grimsbø et al.[39] found email communication might make healthcare professionals better at picking up on emotional cues and concerns as these may be more explicitly expressed by patients when they have to write their messages instead of speaking, and both parties have more time to express themselves and to respond.

Potential Pitfalls

As illustrated, email can contribute positively to patient-centered communication, but it has its limits. Not all patients have email access or sufficient computer literacy, and not all are physically able to use this form of communication, particularly in the terminal stages of palliative care. Some patients do not find email advantageous because of worries about confidentiality,[36] and others have expressed concerns about the lack of human contact as email can seem impersonal.[25,36] Email communication can also lead to misunderstandings,[25,35] which may not be corrected because the asynchronous nature of the medium makes it impossible to give instant feedback.[31,36] Because of its asynchrony, email is also unsuitable for urgent issues[23] in palliative care, and delayed or missing email responses can have negative consequences for existing provider–patient relations.[24] In Dilts et al.'s[33] study, for example, cancer patients indicated that they would be unwilling to wait longer than 24 hours for a response to emails. Special consideration also needs to be paid to healthcare providers' concerns about overburdening and reimbursement. Safeguards in relation to patients' expectations and providers' conditions of the communication need to be put in place at policy level to protect both patient and provider.

One-to-Many in Palliative Care: End-of-Life Leaflets

Numerous types of one-to-many text types exist, including texts related to medicines, diseases, procedures, and, unique to the palliative care setting, end-of-life leaflets. We focus only on this latter type. Such texts are one of the most common ways in which family caregivers of palliative patients are provided with information.[40] The texts are produced by a variety of senders—for example, palliative care organizations, psychological institutions, and hospices. They exist as online resources and printed leaflets, and they inform patients and caregivers about what to expect and what issues to be aware of when death is imminent. More specifically, they provide important information about the process of dying as well as directing patients' and caregivers' attention to important decisions that need to be made, which is valuable given modern society's lack of understanding and tabooization of death.[41]

As Clerehan et al.[42] assert, leaflets in general are an "important adjunct" to oral communication with healthcare professionals, and they need to be *useful* and *understandable* for patients. However, in the case of end-of-life leaflets, ensuring their usefulness for all patients and caregivers may be difficult as their informational needs and abilities are unique and fluctuating. As Payne et al.[43] point out, caregivers frequently need to obtain information about how to manage care or access services in circumstances that are personally challenging. The understandability of end-of-life leaflets is also paramount. End-of-life issues are both complex and emotive, so materials should be written in a way that promotes understanding.[41] The stakes are high with this kind of communication: if caregivers do not understand the materials, they may not be able to provide adequate end-of-life care for their loved ones.[40]

Addressing Physical Needs

Although leaflets cannot meet palliative care patients' physical needs directly, they do so indirectly. End-of-life leaflets for caregivers play a very important role in providing information that relates to pain relief and other symptom management in the final stages of life.[40]

Addressing Intellectual Needs and Access to Information

Kehl and McCarty[40] underline caregivers' need for information and appropriate communication. In a study of 150 end-of-life leaflets from US hospices, 100 documents were found to contain information about preparing for approaching death, 33 contained information about signs and symptoms of approaching death, and 9 described what to do at the time of death.[40] Kehl et al.[44] in their description of the written materials used by hospices to prepare families for dying in the home setting found that more than 90% of the hospices studied had materials that addressed the signs of impending death. At the same time, however, they identified information that was missing in these materials—information about symptoms that are distressing to both patient and caregivers or that "may not be critical to the patient's comfort, but can be especially distressing to family members,"[44(p970)] suggesting that some informational needs were not addressed in this text type.

Addressing Emotional and Spiritual Needs

Quality information can benefit caregivers emotionally, as families that are better prepared for the passing of their loved ones have more confidence in their caregiving abilities and obtain better closure, whereas lack of preparedness has been associated with complicated grief, anxiety, and depression.[44] Of the 150 texts in their study, Kehl and McCarty[40] found that only a few related to emotional and spiritual responses to dying (five documents) and approaching death awareness (three documents). Again, for such texts to be useful, they need to meet the emotional and spiritual needs of their intended audiences, such as addressing the emotional impact of the responsibilities involved in 24-hour caregiving. Not only should these lacunae in information provision be addressed, but end-of-life leaflets should also employ a more patient- and family-centered approach to the information provided, in line with a more patient-centered approach to palliative communication.[44,45]

Potential Pitfalls

The quality of end-of-life leaflets is not merely related to the usefulness of the content they convey; it is also closely related to their comprehensibility. Therefore such texts need to be "easily understood by families under high levels of stress to improve the experiences of both patients and families."[40(p248)] Research using readability formulas demonstrates a discrepancy between the readability of written patient information and actual literacy skills in general.[41] This is all the more worrying as many caregivers are over 65 years old, and there is a correlation between older age and lower health literacy levels. This is further exacerbated by the physical and emotional stress of caregiving, as the impending death of a family member can negatively affect health literacy.[40] Although hospice personnel may be available to answer questions, caregivers with poor reading comprehension may be embarrassed to ask for help with understanding end-of-life leaflets.[40]

Many-to-Many Communication in Palliative Care: Online Patient–Patient Forums

Other than giving rise to email communication between healthcare professionals and patients, the Internet has also made it possible for palliative care patients and their caregivers to communicate with their peers via online forums. The patient forum is interesting to explore as it is a health communication medium that supports health communication without a professional necessarily being present. In these forums, patients and caregivers can seek and receive condition-related information, advice, and support from others who have similar experiences, as well as share their own. Such forums have been welcomed by many patients but criticized by some healthcare professionals. In the following, we present how these forums might positively address patients' and their caregivers' needs before discussing potential pitfalls.

Addressing Physical Needs

Although Barak et al.[46] point out that online forums primarily offer "relief and improved feelings" as opposed to clearly therapeutic effects, online may provide patients with specific advantages in relation to their physical needs. Online forums make it possible for patients to access a repertoire of patient-tested techniques with which to manage treatment.[47,48] This links to the idea that patients have experiential knowledge[49] that complements healthcare professionals' biomedical knowledge. Moreover, in a similar way to email, online forums can be accessed by patients in their own homes, thus mitigating the effects of debilitating conditions or deteriorating health.

Addressing Intellectual Needs and Access to Information

According to cancer e-patient Dave de Bronkert, "Patients know what patients need to know."[50] This underlines the immense potential of online forums to address patients' intellectual and informational needs on sites where health information is shared and "decentralized" or detached from an expert source.[51] Online forums are extremely valuable because of the ongoing, pressing need for high-quality information provision in the palliative care setting.[46] They have also been found to help patients manage the extensive health-related information available online as patients provide other patients with advice on how to navigate and interpret the vast array of sources,[52] guiding participants toward key resources.[53] In the early stages of palliative care, patients may benefit from information from other forum participants on how best to navigate healthcare systems such as which clinic to attend, which professionals to consult, or which treatments to request or avoid. Indeed, the efficiency and patient centeredness of offline health consultations may increase as patients are better informed about what questions to ask, medical terms to use, and symptoms or side effects to mention to their healthcare provider.[54] With regard to the quality of these forums, as Barak et al.[46] observe, much of the information is "not erroneous or harmful," contrary to some healthcare professionals' concerns.[55–57] Significantly, Esquivel et al.[58] found that only 10 of 4,600 postings on an unmoderated Internet cancer forum were false or misleading, and 7 of these false or misleading statements were corrected within an average of 4 hours and 33 minutes, suggesting that patients are capable of moderating sites.

Caregivers of patients can also benefit greatly from online forums, as their ongoing need for relevant information may otherwise not be met.[51] As Kinnane and Milne point out, online forums are extremely beneficial to caregivers as "there is sharing of 'helpful' information, for example, web sites, reading materials and experiences."[2(p1132)] Knapp[47] also points out that in the pediatric palliative care setting, online parent–parent communication might also improve parents' understanding so that their offline communication with their children's healthcare professional is improved. Thus online forums can provide caregivers with practical and specific information and experiences, which is supportive of patient- or caregiver-centered communication.

Addressing Emotional, Social, and Spiritual Needs

Online forums provide patients with many advantages regarding the expression of their feelings about their illness and disease trajectory. A study of palliative care patients' discourse in an online forum by Schwartz and Lutfiyya[59] found that online forums give patients the opportunity to verbalize the significance of their suffering in a confidential manner, thus avoiding boring, annoying, or worrying people in their offline surroundings.[60] It has also been found that patients' engagement in online patient–patient communication is motivated by their need to communicate with others experiencing similar problems—a need that is sometimes met with difficulty in offline settings. In this regard, it is relevant that online patient forums have been described as spaces where solidarity and positive regard are shown.[61] In their study of participation in online forums, van Uden-Kraan et al.[60] describe "emotional empowerment" as the process through which information is exchanged, emotional support is encountered, and recognition is gained by sharing experiences.

Forums can also address patients' social needs as their illnesses may increasingly restrict participation in offline social activities. Alemi et al. argue that "often, chronically ill patients intentionally disrupt these relationships, because they cannot meet the expectations of the group and because they seek new friends who have access to information about their illness."[62(p41)] Ziebland and Wyke[54] similarly argue that illness very often brings a sense of isolation and dislocation from the past and the future. In health-related social networks, online community members can indeed develop close relationships, sometimes referring to each other as "family."[63] They can derive emotional and social support and empowerment from sharing their health experiences with other community participants.[63] Caregivers also receive many social benefits from online forums where they are able to "provide and receive peer support."[2] Parents of pediatric palliative care patients who participate in online forums "may reduce feelings of isolation and increase emotional support and empowerment."[47(p70)]

Spirituality has been defined as the ways humans satisfy the need to transcend or rise above the everyday materials or sensory experience[64] and patients' and their caregivers' spiritual needs, which are recognized as being similar,[65] can also be met in online forums. Specifically, caregivers receive "spiritual support" through prayers for the group or received from the group; both patients and their caregivers also receive messages of encouragement during difficult times (such as health deterioration or death).[2]

Potential Pitfalls

Despite their many advantages, there are a number of limitations associated with online patient forums in the palliative care setting. In the terminal stages of an illness, a patient may no longer be physically able to engage in online forums. This was a reason proposed for the observed low level of participation of pancreatic cancer patients in an online forum.[66] Others have observed that there might be symptom restrictions to computer use for conditions such as in the case of Parkinson's disease.[67] Similar to email communication, participation in online patient–patient written communication requires Internet access and computer literacy, so not all patients or caregivers can avail of online forums. Moreover, many of the existing forums are in English, which can be another exclusionary parameter. As for any written communication, the absence of nonverbal cues might lead to misunderstandings.[67] It has also been argued that online relationships are less valuable than offline ones, that they detract from offline social involvement with friends,[54] and that vulnerable patients might be affected by other members' departure.[67] These criticisms are, however, countered by Heidelberger et al.,[63] who argue that online social health networks are an extension, not a replacement, of patients' existing social networks.

Another concern with online forums relates to fears that patient forums propagate cyberchondria, hypochondria brought on by an imbalanced, unqualified reading of online biomedical information,[68,69] leaving patients anxious and possibly distorting their offline decisions.[54] The negative impact of information in online forums has been documented: Sandaunet,[70] for example, found that one of the reasons that breast cancer patients withdrew from an online self-help group was that they wanted to avoid exposure to worrying information about breast cancer.

Conclusion

As defined by the NCP,[3] patient-centered palliative care should facilitate patient autonomy, access to information, and choice. These aims reflect the goals of *patient empowerment*,[12] and empowerment is a very valuable outcome for palliative care patients who feel increasingly disempowered by their illness. Each of the three categories of written health communication described by Clerehan[21] and exemplified in the three text types that we presented in this chapter have the potential to support the empowerment of patients and their caregivers. Patients find that emailing their healthcare professionals facilitates greater knowledge and understanding of their condition. Moreover, greater access and convenience mean that email communication is on patients' terms to a far greater degree; patients gain in autonomy as email can help them express their individual concerns; and because of increased timely communication, patients may be better equipped to deal with their health situation. End-of-life leaflets can support both patient and caregiver as they have educational value, providing important information about the very difficult decisions, circumstances, and existential challenges around imminent death. Finally, with regard to patient forums, Bos et al.[71] have argued that Web 2.0 supports the empowerment of patients by patients (as opposed to empowerment of patients by healthcare professionals, which is how patient empowerment is normally defined), reflected in the concept Patient 2.0 Empowerment. Active participation in online forums can equip patients with greater competence to "tell their story," which can help improve communication with healthcare professionals.[54] Not only has receiving help from online forums been found to be empowering, but so too is sharing information that can help others.[46]

We have also taken up the question of health literacy needs in relation to written materials for palliative care patients in this chapter. Our main argument is that it is important to make a distinction between communication for a mass audience and communication between individuals. The target audience of texts such as end-of-life leaflets is large and heterogeneous. It is therefore not possible to tailor to patients' and caregivers' individual health literacy levels. While some argue that documents should be understood by 90% of the population,[72] we argue that they should be clear and understandable for all. We therefore recommend that written materials be produced using the skills of language, communication, or document-design experts, as medical professionals may lack the skills required to produce optimally comprehensible texts.[73–75] We suggest applying what Askehave and Zethsen have termed a lowest common denominator approach for texts intended for a mass audience, where the author must constantly question whether something can be simplified or explained.[76] Like others who have problematized an overreliance on readability formulas because of issues of validity,[21,77] we suggest that leaflets intended for a mass audience be user-tested and amendments made on the basis of patients' feedback. In relation to end-of-life leaflets, it has been suggested that removing medical terms may improve the readability of these texts.[40] However, this could mean that caregivers would not encounter the medical terms they need for effective communication with hospice staff, so a better suggestion may be to include medical terms in end-of-life leaflets and explain them within the text.[40] In relation to individualized communication, such as email with patients, we suggest a more dynamic approach to health literacy. Although it is often recommended that medical terms be avoided when communicating with patients,[78,79] some patients (such as some e-patients) have very high health literacy levels in relation to their specific condition.[80,81] It would therefore be very valuable for a healthcare professional to tailor his or her communication to match the individual patient's health literacy level; evidence suggests that healthcare professionals are able to align their terminology in email communication.[82] A similar suggestion is made by Wittenberg-Lyles et al.,[83] who advocate an adaptive use of medical terminology in oral communication in the palliative care setting.

The findings presented in this chapter have a number of implications for professional practice (see also Table 13.1). As email communication with healthcare professionals can help to meet patients' informational and emotional needs, we encourage healthcare professionals to engage in email communication with patients who express a wish for this while bearing in mind the potential pitfalls associated with this medium. Moreover, although healthcare professionals by definition are not involved

Table 13.1 Summary of Key Learning Points for Palliative Care Health Providers

Patient- and family-centeredness	A patient- and family-centered approach to written communication is invaluable in the palliative care setting for many communicative and ethical reasons. Is the text in question meeting patients' and carers' intellectual, emotional, social, and spiritual needs, as defined by the National Consensus Project?
Health literacy	Although health literacy is generally regarded as a quantitative measure of a demographically defined group or a population's health literacy skills, healthcare providers should ♦ be aware of the changing, situation-related, and highly individual nature of patients' health literacy. ♦ try to ascertain the patient's or family caregiver's health literacy needs and preferences to maximize the quality of communication. ♦ communicate in accordance with the patient's or carer's health literacy needs and preferences, using the relevant text type.
One-to-one communication: Email	In an age when email is increasingly used to correspond with patients, we encourage healthcare providers to ♦ engage in email communication with palliative care patients who express a wish for this, while bearing in mind the potential pitfalls associated with this medium. ♦ tailor their communication to match the individual patient's health literacy level; an adaptive use of medical terminology is suggested.
One-to-many communication: End-of-life leaflets	End-of-life materials should reflect patients' and family caregivers' needs, and thus we recommend ♦ that written materials be produced drawing on the skills of language, communication, and document-design experts. ♦ the application of a "lowest common denominator" approach to texts intended for a mass audience to ensure that as many patients and family caregivers as possible can access the text. ♦ relevant medical terms be included but explained in the text.
Many-to-many communication: Online patient–patient forums	Research indicates that palliative care patients derive many benefits from online forums, particularly in relation to empowerment and engagement, and that the knowledge on online forums is generally accurate. We encourage healthcare providers to ♦ visit relevant patient forums to gain insight into patients' needs. ♦ inform palliative care patients about condition-related forums that may support their informational and relational needs. ♦ engage in open dialogue with patients about patients' use of forums given the rise of e-medicine and the emergence of the palliative care e-patient.

in patient–patient communication in online forums, we think it could be valuable for them to visit relevant patient forums to gain insights into palliative care patients' needs. Encouraging patients to use these forums would also benefit patients, given the emotional and social support and information that they can provide. By encouraging patients' participation in online networks, healthcare professionals may learn sooner from their better-informed patients about relevant symptoms and worries, which could lead to more accurate diagnoses, treatment, and support, with significant human and economic benefits. We also suggest that healthcare professionals engage in open dialogue with patients about their use of the Internet. As pointed out earlier, worries about cyberchondria and the biomedical accuracy of online health information have been voiced, but if patients communicate with their healthcare professionals about what they find online, many of these potentially negative aspects can be avoided.

The findings of this chapter also point toward future research avenues in written palliative care communication. Further research is required to ensure that leaflets meet patients' and their caregivers' needs in relation to the aims of patient centeredness, patient empowerment, and health literacy, and in this regard, it would be particularly valuable to ask patients and their caregivers for their perspectives. Moreover, researchers have been slow to adopt the online patient forum as a locus of empirical investigation, probably because there is "little commercial or professional interest in evaluating 'pure' virtual communities and 'unsophisticated' peer to peer interventions such as mailing lists, as opposed to more complex interventions."[57(p3)] However, patient forums provide a rich and authentic source of patients' perspectives.

In this chapter, we presented three written text types, discussed their advantages and disadvantages in meeting patients' and their caregivers' needs, and considered them from the angles of patient centeredness, patient empowerment, and health literacy. Maintaining and consolidating the ongoing focus on patients' and their caregivers' needs and integrating patients to a greater extent into health communication is valuable not only because of ethical imperatives but also because palliative care patients, like chronic patients more generally, are an essential, but underused, resource in healthcare.[80]

References

1. Reis A, Pedrosa A, Dourado M, Reis C. Information and communication technologies in long-term and palliative care. *Procedia Technology*. 2013;9:1303–1312.
2. Kinnane NA, Milne DJ. The role of the Internet in supporting and informing carers of people with cancer: A literature review. *Support Care Cancer*. 2010;18(9):1123–1136.
3. National Consensus Project for Quality Palliative Care. *Clinical Practice Guidelines for Quality Palliative Care*. 3rd ed. Pittsburgh, PA: National Consensus Project; 2009.
4. de Haes H, Koedoot N. Patient centered decision making in palliative cancer treatment: A world of paradoxes. *Patient Educ Couns*. 2003;50(1):43–49.
5. Duggan PS, Geller G, Cooper LA, Beach MC. The moral nature of patient-centeredness: Is it "just the right thing to do"? *Patient Educ Couns*. 2006;62(2):271–276.
6. Engel GL. The need for a new medical model: A challenge for biomedicine. *Science*. 1977;196(4286):129–136.
7. Laine C, Davidoff F. Patient-centred medicine: A professional evolution. *JAMA*. 1996;275(2):152–156.
8. Mead N, Bower P. Patient-centredness: A conceptual framework and review of the empirical literature. *Soc Sci Med*. 2000;51:1087–1110.
9. Balint E. The possibilities of patient-centered medicine. *J R Coll Gen Pract*. 1969;17(82):269.
10. Little P, Everitt H, Williamson I, et al. Observational study of effect of patient centredness and positive approach on outcomes of general practice consultations. *BMJ*. 2001;323:908–911.
11. Mead N, Bower P. Patient-centred consultations and outcomes in primary care: A review of the literature. *Patient Educ Couns*. 2002;48(1):51–61.
12. Holmström I, Röing M. The relation between patient-centeredness and patient empowerment: A discussion on concepts. *Patient Educ Couns*. 2010;79(2):167–172.
13. Fage-Butler AM. Including patients' perspectives in patient information leaflets: A polyocular approach. *Fachsprache*. 2013;35(3–4):140–154.
14. Raynor DT, Blenkinsopp A, Knapp P, et al. A systematic review of quantitative and qualitative research on the role and effectiveness of written information available to patients about individual medicines. *Health Technol Assess*. 2007;11(5):iii, 1–160.
15. Stewart M, Brown JB, Donner A, et al. The impact of patient-centered care on outcomes. *Fam Pract*. 2000;49(9):796–804.
16. Bostock S, Steptoe A. Association between low functional health literacy and mortality in older adults: Longitudinal cohort study. *BMJ*. 2012;344:1–10.
17. Ishikawa H, Yano E. Patient health literacy and participation in the health-care process. *Health Expect*. 2008;11(2):113–122.
18. Ownby RL, Acevedo A, Waldrop-Valverde D, Jacobs RJ, Caballero J. Abilities, skills and knowledge in measures of health literacy. *Patient Educ Couns*. 2014;95(2):211–217.
19. Dahm MR. Does experience change understanding? The effects of personal experiences on patients' knowledge of medical terminology. Paper presented at: Conference of the Australian Linguistic Society. La Trobe University, Melbourne, Australia, 2009.
20. Wright P. Designing healthcare advice for the public. In: Durso F, ed. *Handbook of Applied Cognition*. Chichester, UK: John Wiley & Sons; 1999:695–724.
21. Clerehan R. Quality and usefulness of written communication for patients. In: Chou W-Y, Hamilton H, eds. *Routledge Handbook of Language and Health Communication*. London: Routledge; 2014:212–227.
22. Godbold N. Developing relationships to counter patient isolation and support "empowerment" in health care. In: Godbold N, Vaccarella M, eds. *Autonomous, Responsible, Alone: The Complexities of Patient Empowerment*. London: Interdisciplinary Press; 2012.
23. Katzen C, Solan M, Dicker A. E-mail and oncology: A survey of radiation oncology patients and their attitudes to a new generation of health communication. *Prostate Cancer Prostatic Dis*. 2005;8(2):189–193.
24. Strasser F, Fisch M, Bodurka DC, Sivesind D, Bruera E. E-motions: Email for written emotional expression. *J Clin Oncol*. 2003;20(15):3352–3355.
25. Atherton H, Sawmynaden P, Sheikh A, Majeed A, Car J. Email for clinical communication between patients/caregivers and healthcare professionals. *Cochrane Database Syst Rev*. 2012;11:CD007978.
26. Wong RK, Tan JS, Drossman DA. Here's my phone number, don't call me: Physician accessibility in the cell phone and e-mail era. *Dig Dis Sci*. 2010;55(3):662–667.
27. Patt MR, Houston TK, Jenckes MW, Sands DZ, Ford DE. Doctors who are using e-mail with their patients: A qualitative exploration. *J Med Internet Res*. 2003;5(2).
28. McGeady D, Kujala J, Ilvonen K. The impact of patient–physician web messaging on healthcare service provision. *Int J Med Inform*. 2008;77(1):17–23.
29. Cornwall A, Moore S, Plant H. Embracing technology: patients', family members' and nurse specialists' experience of communicating using e-mail. *Eur J Oncol Nurs*. 2008;12(3):198–208.

30. Fage-Butler AM, Nisbeth Jensen M. The relevance of existing health communication models in the email age: An integrative literature review. *Commun Med* 2014;11(3).
31. Moore S, Sherwin A. Improving patient access to healthcare professionals: A prospective audit evaluating the role of e-mail communication for patients with lung cancer. *Eur J Oncol Nurs*. 2004;8:350–354.
32. Andersen T, Ruland CM. Cancer patients' questions and concerns expressed in an online nurse-delivered mail service: Preliminary results. In: Saranto K, Flatley Brennan P, Park H-A, Tallberg M, Ensio A, eds. *Connecting Health and Humans*. Amsterdam: IOS Press; 2009:149–153.
33. Dilts D, Ridner SH, Franco A, Murphy B. Patients with cancer and e-mail: Implications for clinical communication. *Support Care Cancer*. 2009;17(8):1049–1056.
34. Grimsbø GH, Finset A, Ruland CM. Left hanging in the air: Experiences of living with cancer as expressed through e-mail communications with oncology nurses. *Cancer Nurs*. 2011;34(2):107–116.
35. Kagan SH, Clarke SP, Happ MB. Head and neck cancer patient and family member interest in and use of e-mail to communicate with clinicians. *Head Neck*. 2005;27(11):976–981.
36. Hsiao AL, Bazzy-Asaad A, Tolomeo C, Edmonds D, Belton B, Benin AL. Secure web messaging in a pediatric chronic care clinic: A slow takeoff of "kids' airmail." *Pediatrics*. 2011;127(2):e406-e413.
37. Andreassen HK. What does an e-mail address add? Doing health and technology at home. *Soc Sci Med*. 2011;72(4):521–528.
38. David N, Schlenker P, Prudlo U, Larbig W. Online counseling via e-mail for breast cancer patients on the German Internet: Preliminary results of a psychoeducational intervention. *Psychosoc Med*. 2011:8.
39. Grimsbø GH, Ruland CM, Finset A. Cancer patients' expressions of emotional cues and concerns and oncology nurses' responses, in an online patient–nurse communication service. *Patient Educ Couns*. 2012;88(1):36–43.
40. Kehl KA, McCarty KN. Readability of hospice materials to prepare families for caregiving at the time of death. *Res Nurs Health*. 2012;35(3):242–249.
41. Ache K, Wallace L. Are end-of-life patient education materials readable? *Palliat Med*. 2009;23(6):545–548.
42. Clerehan R, Buchbinder R, Moodie J. A linguistic framework for assessing the quality of written patient information: Its use in assessing methotrexate informtion for rheumatoid arthritis. *Health Educ Res*. 2005;20(3):334–344.
43. Payne S, Large S, Jarrett N, Turner P. Written information given to patients and families by palliative care unites: A national survey. *The Lancet*. 2000;355(9217):1792.
44. Kehl KA, Kirchhoff KT, Finster MP, Cleary JF. Materials to prepare hospice families for dying in the home. *J Palliat Med*. 2008 11(7) 969–972.
45. King DA, Quill T. Working with families in palliative care: One size does not fit all. *J Palliat Med*. 2006 9(3):704–715.
46. Barak A, Boniel-Nissim M, Suler J. Fostering empowerment in online support groups. *Comput Human Behav*. 2008 24(5):1867–1883.
47. Knapp C. e-Health in pediatric palliative care. *Am J Hosp Palliat Care*. 2010;27(1) 66–73.
48. Graffigna G, Libreri C, Bosio C. Online exchanges among cancer patients and caregivers: Constructing and sharing health knowledge about time. *Qualitative Research in Organizations and Management: An International Journal*. 2012 7(3):323–337.
49. Caron-Flinterman JF, Broerse JEW, Bunders JFG. The experiential knowledge of patients: A new resource for biomedical research? *Soc Sci Med*. 2005;60(11):2575–2584.
50. de Bronkert D. Meet e-patient Dave. http://www.ted.com/talks/dave_debronkart_meet_e_patient_dave. Filmed 2011. Accessed Sepetmber 8, 2014.
51. Ginossar T. Online participation: A content analysis of differences in utilization of two online cancer communities by men and women, patients and family members. *Health Commun*. 2008;23(1):1–12.
52. Swan M. Emerging patient-driven health care models: An examination of health social networks, consumer personalized medicine and quantified self-tracking. *Int J Environ Res Public Health*. 2009;6(2):492–525.
53. Lindsay S, Smith S, Bellaby P, Baker R. The health impact of an online heart disease support group: A comparison of moderated versus unmoderated support. *Health Educ Res*. 2009;24(4):646–654.
54. Ziebland S, Wyke S. Health and illness in a connected world: How might sharing experiences on the Internet affect people's health? *Milbank Q*. 2012;90(2):219–249.
55. Deshpande A, Jadad AR. Trying to measure the quality of health information on the Internet: Is it time to move on? *J Rheumatol*. 2009;36(1):1–3.
56. Lewis T. Seeking health information on the Internet: Lifestyle choice or bad attack of cyberchondria? *Media, Culture & Society*. 2006;28(4):521–539.
57. Eysenbach G, Powell J, Englesakis M, Rizo C, Stern A. Health related virtual communities and electronic support groups: Systematic review of the effects of online peer to peer interactions. *BMJ*. 2004;328(7449):1166.
58. Esquivel A, Meric-Bernstam F, Bernstam EV. Accuracy and self correction of information received from an Internet breast cancer list: Content analysis. *BMJ*. 2006; 32(7547):939–942.
59. Schwartz KD, Lutfiyya ZM. "In pain waiting to die": Everyday understandings of suffering. *Palliat Support Care*. 2012;10(01):27–36.
60. van Uden-Kraan CF, Drossaert CH, Taal E, Shaw BR, Seydel ER, van de Laar MA. Empowering processes and outcomes of participation in online support groups for patients with breast cancer, arthritis, or fibromyalgia. *Qual Health Res*. 2008;18(3):405–417.
61. Morrow PR. Telling about problems and giving advice in an Internet discussion forum: Some discourse features. *Discourse Studies*. 2006;8(4):531–548.
62. Alemi F, Mosavel M, Stephens RC, Ghadiri A, Krishnaswamy J, Thakkar H. Electronic self-help and support groups. *Med Care*. 1996;34(10):32–44.
63. Heidelberger CA, El-Gayar O, Sarnikar S. Online health social networks and patient health decision behavior: A research agenda. Paper presented at: System Sciences, 44th Hawaii International Conference, 2011.
64. Mitchell G, Murray J, Hynson J. Understanding the whole person: Life-limiting illness across the life cycle. In: Mitchell G, ed. *Palliative Care: A Patient-centered Approach*. Oxon, UK: Radcliffe; 2008:79–107.
65. Taylor EJ. Spiritual needs of patients with cancer and family caregivers. *Cancer Nurs*. 2003;26(4):260–266.
66. Grant MS, Wiegand DL. Palliative care online: A pilot study on a pancreatic cancer website. *J Palliat Med*. 2011;14(7):846–851.
67. Attard A, Coulson NS. A thematic analysis of patient communication in Parkinson's disease online support group discussion forums. *Comput Human Behav*. 2012;28:500–506.
68. Starcevic V, Berle D. Cyberchondria: towards a better understanding of excessive health-related Internet use. *Expert Rev Neurother*. 2013;13(2):205–213.
69. White RW, Horvitz E. Cyberchondria: Studies of the escalation of medical concerns in web search. *ACM Transactions on Information Systems (TOIS)*. 2009;27(4):1–37.
70. Sandaunet AG. The challenge of fitting in: Non-participation and withdrawal from an online self-help group for breast cancer patients. *Sociol Health Illn*. 2008;30(1):131–144.
71. Bos L, Marsh A, Carroll D, Gupta S, Rees M. Patient 2.0 empowerment. Paper presented at: Proceedings of the International Conference on Semantic Web and Web Services. Las Vegas, NV, 2008.

72. Raynor DT. Testing, testing. The benefits of user-testing package leaflets. *Regul Focus.* 2008:16–19. file:///C:/Users/ewittenberg/Downloads/focus_Apr08_16-19.pdf. Last accessed June 16, 2015.
73. Askehave I, Zethsen KK. Translating for laymen. *Perspectives: Studies in Translatology.* 2002;10(1):15–29.
74. García-Izquierdo I, Montalt V. Equigeneric and intergeneric translation in patient-centred care. *Hermes [Special Issue: Health Communication.* Ed. M Pilegaard]. 2013;51:39–51.
75. Nisbeth Jensen M, Zethsen KK. Translation of patient information leaflets: Trained translators and pharmacists-cum-translators—a comparison. *Linguistica Antverpiensia New Series. Themes in Translation Studies [Special issue: Translation and Knowledge Mediation in Medical and Health Settings.* Ed. V Montalt, M Shuttleworth] 2012;11:31–49.
76. Askehave I, Zethsen KK. Communication barriers in public discourse. *Document Design.* 2003;4(1):23–42.
77. Schriver K. The mechanism used by readability formulas makes them unreliable: Readability formulas in the new millennium: What's the use? *ACM J Computer Documentation.* 2000;24(3):138–140.
78. Koch-Weser S, DeJong W, Rudd RE. Medical word use in clinical encounters. *Health Expect.* 2009;12(4):371–382.
79. Dahm MR. Coming to terms with medical terms—exploring insights from native and non-native English speakers in patient-physician communication. *Hermes.* 2012;49 79–98.
80. Ferguson T. *E-patients:* How they can help us heal healthcare. http://e-patients.net/e-Patients_White_Paper.pdf. Published 2007. Accessed September 8, 2014.
81. Fage-Butler AM, Nisbeth Jensen M. Medical terminology in online patient-patient communication: Evidence of high quality?. *Health Expect.* 2015. [Epub ahead of print]. doi: 10.1111/hex.12395.
82. Jucks R, Bromme R. Choice of words in doctor-patient communication: An analysis of health-related internet sites. *Health Commun.* 2007 21(3) 267–277.
83. Wittenberg-Lyles E, Goldsmith J, Oliver DP, Demiris G, Kruse RL, Van Stee S. Using medical words with family caregivers. *J Palliat Med.* 2013 16(9):1135–1139.

CHAPTER 14

Health Disparities

Susan Eggly, Lauren M. Hamel,
Louis A. Penner, and Terrance L. Albrecht

Introduction

Accumulating evidence demonstrates that palliative care is a critical component of high quality, patient-centered care.[1-3] The early introduction of palliative care for patients with life-limiting disease leads to significant improvements in patients' quality of life and less aggressive care at the end of life.[4] The use of treatments, services, and communication practices related to palliative and hospice care varies by patient population. Systematic variation in health status and/or healthcare by patient population represents differences and/or disparities between populations. Differences are genetic or biological factors associated with a specific population or populations that affect the health risk or health status of that population's members. Disparities, on the other hand, are systematic differences in the mental or physical health or health risks in which members of social groups, such as racial/ethnic minorities, systematically experience worse health or greater health risk than other groups. Such disparities may result from inequitable economic, political, social, communication, and/or psychological processes.[5-8]

Health disparities are well documented in many populations and medical contexts and have been the subject of research and policy for the past two decades.[6,8-10] This chapter discusses palliative care disparities that disproportionately burden adult members of racial/ethnic minorities in the United States. The focus is on racial/ethnic minorities rather than other populations because the vast majority of existing research compares palliative care in non-Hispanic white populations with African American and, to a lesser extent, Hispanic and Asian populations.[11] There are some exceptions, such as studies that examine patient race/ethnicity as well as other variables such as patient socioeconomic status and geographic location. For example, Nayar and colleagues studied days in an intensive care unit (ICU), emergency room visits, and inpatient admissions as indicators of the quality of end-of-life (EOL) care among Medicare beneficiaries with lung cancer. Findings showed variation in the quality of care by patient race/ethnicity, socioeconomic status, and whether the patient lived in a rural or urban area.[12] However, research on populations other than adult racial/ethnic minorities and on other specific aspects of palliative care is quite limited.

This chapter uses the term "palliative care" to refer broadly to all aspects of EOL care, including hospice. The majority of research on palliative care disparities is in hospice—a type of palliative care that emphasizes relief or symptom control rather than curative treatment, recommended for patients with a life-threatening illness who are anticipated to live for less than 6 months.[13] Thus this chapter focuses largely on disparities found in hospice care.

The discussion begins with disparity patterns in various palliative care domains among racial/ethnic groups, including the use of services; geographic or medical setting; pain management; disenrollment from hospice; populations other than African Americans, Hispanics, and Asians, including children; and advance directives. Next, the factors that contribute to these disparities are explored through the use of a conceptual model of societal, interpersonal communication, and individual factors. Finally, we review communication approaches and strategies that may mitigate disparities. The chapter concludes with a discussion of current research limitations, making recommendations for policy, practice, and future research.

Disparities in Palliative Care Use

Studies consistently show that minorities experience poorer access to healthcare than their white counterparts. Reasons for this include low socioeconomic status, distance from providers, insurance type or lack of insurance, and health literacy.[8,10] Not surprisingly, this finding persists in the context of palliative care. Studies among Medicare beneficiaries have consistently demonstrated lower rates of hospice use among members of racial/ethnic minority groups than for whites across diagnoses, geographic areas, and settings of care, including nursing homes.[11-18] Johnson et al.[11] report that among Medicare beneficiaries who died in 2010, 45.8% of whites used hospice compared to 34% of African Americans, 37% of Hispanics, 28.1% of Asian Americans, and 30.6% of Native North Americans. Most studies largely focus on cancer, given that cancer is the most common diagnosis for patients in hospice,[19] but several studies of hospice use by patients with cardiovascular disease show similar disparities.[14,18] For example, a study of 98,258 Medicare beneficiaries with heart failure showed that African Americans and Hispanics were much less likely to use hospice than white patients, even after adjusting for income, urban dwelling, severity of illness, and medical comorbidities.[18]

Consistent with research clearly showing that white patients are more likely to use palliative care, racial/ethnic minorities are more likely to receive aggressive, high-intensity care, as indicated by number of hospitalizations, use of an ICU and visits to an emergency room at the end of life, and dying in a hospital. Smith et al.[17] examined racial/ethnic differences in the use of hospice and high-intensity care at the end of life in 40,960 non-Hispanic white, non-Hispanic black, Hispanic, and Asian Pacific Islander Medicare beneficiaries with advanced cancer who died between 1992 and 1999. High-intensity care was indicated by receipt of chemotherapy in the last 14 days of life and/or fewer than two hospitalizations, more than 14 days in the hospital, and admission to an ICU in the last month of life. Findings showed that 42.0% of white patients enrolled in hospice compared to 36.9% of African Americans, 32.2% of Asians, and 37.7% of Hispanics. Also, although disparities between white and Hispanic patients disappeared after adjustment for clinical and socio-demographic factors, higher proportions of African American and Asian patients received high-intensity care, as compared to white patients, even when these factors were controlled.

Researchers have also examined specific aspects of palliative care use, such as medical setting, geographic location, and socio-demographic status. For example, after controlling for demographics, diagnoses, function, patient preferences, and facility resources, nursing-home residents in facilities having higher proportions of African American residents had greater odds of hospitalization.[20] In a study of geographic and race/ethnic disparities in access to EOL care, Nayar et al.[12] examined 91,039 Medicare beneficiaries with lung cancer who died in 2008. Findings were mixed regarding high-intensity care for patients who resided in rural versus urban geographic areas, but racial minorities had more days in an ICU, had more visits to an emergency room, had more inpatient days, and were less likely than white patients to use hospice. Similarly, Hardy et al.[13] found that in urban and rural areas, African Americans, Hispanics, and Asian/Pacific Islanders were much less likely than whites to receive hospice services and that patients with lower socioeconomic status were also much less likely to receive hospice services. Johnson et al.[16] also studied hospice use by patient race and geographic area by examining intercounty variation among Medicare beneficiaries who died in 2008 in North and South Carolina. Findings differed somewhat from those of other studies—the use of hospice by African American and white patients was similar in most counties, but in counties where a disparity was found, more resources to deliver high-intensity care were available, and African Americans were more likely to use these services.

Other specific aspects of disparities in palliative care that have been studied include pain management; disenrollment from hospice; populations other than African Americans, Hispanics, and Asians, including children; and advance directives. A critical component of palliative care is pain management, but little disparity research has been conducted specifically on the assessment and treatment of pain at the end of life.[21] Abundant evidence exists outside of this context, however, demonstrating disparities in the assessment and treatment of cancer and non-cancer pain for African Americans and Hispanics, as compared to whites, as well as access to pharmacies that stock adequate supplies of pain medications.[21-24] In a systematic review of the influence of patient race/ethnicity on pain assessment and treatment, Cintron et al.[23] found racial/ethnic disparities in the access to and use of effective treatment of pain—African Americans and Hispanics are more likely to have their pain underestimated by providers, less likely to receive opioid analgesics, and more likely to have their pain undertreated or untreated, compared to whites. In a critical review of the literature on racial/ethnic disparities in pain, Anderson et al.[21] specifically discussed the small body of research on palliative care. These authors suggest that, although the literature is sparse and findings somewhat mixed, racial/ethnic disparities exist in the assessment and treatment of pain at the end of life, possibly due in part to minority patients' underuse of palliative and hospice services.

With regard to disenrollment from hospice, Unroe et al.[14] found that African Americans with heart failure enrolled in hospice are more likely to disenroll as compared to whites. African Americans who left hospice during their first admission were less likely at the end of life to have access to comprehensive services that hospice programs provide and were more likely to receive high-intensity services. Others have found that African Americans are more likely than whites to leave hospice to pursue life-prolonging therapies.[25] Kapo et al.[26] conducted a retrospective review of a cohort of patients enrolled in university-affiliated hospice in southeastern Pennsylvania. Findings showed that African Americans who left hospice during their first admission, either voluntarily or because they were no longer eligible, were significantly less likely to return than other patients. They were therefore less likely to have access to the comprehensive services provided by hospice, including nursing care, pain and symptom management, education, and family support.

Few studies have been conducted on race/ethnic minorities other than African Americans, Hispanics, and Asians. In a notable exception, Kitzes and colleagues[27] studied EOL care among American Indians and Alaska Natives. In one study, authors examined medical records of 2,521 adult American Indians who died in New Mexico between 1994 and 1998. They also conducted interviews with hospital administrative staff and cultural advisers at selected Indian Health Service facilities regarding EOL care at their facilities. Findings showed little attention to palliative care services in medical records (e.g., referrals to hospice) or in hospital policies and procedures. Although the study was conducted on patients who died over a decade ago, authors note the paucity of palliative care studies in this population and suggest these findings be used to accelerate efforts to study and improve palliative care in this patient population. In a later study,[28] these authors investigated potential benefits of palliative care consultations with staff trained in effective techniques and preferred patterns of communication among members of Southwestern native communities. Findings demonstrated that, contrary to common beliefs about Native Americans, patients and families were willing to participate in these discussions, but disparities in rates of "do not resuscitate" and hospice use among Native Americans, as compared to non-Native Americans, were not affected by the discussions.

Similarly, few studies have examined racial/ethnic disparities in palliative care among pediatric populations.[29] A relatively small, retrospective, single-center study of children who died of cancer or stem cell transplant suggested that race/ethnicity was significantly associated with hospice enrollment. The association persisted even after controlling for payer status, patient diagnosis, and religion, although in a slightly different manner than with adult patients.[30] Specifically, Latinos enrolled in hospice significantly more often than other patients; however, 34% of Latinos and 50% of non-Latinos had withdrawn from hospice at the time of death.

Although few researchers have specifically examined racial/ethnic disparities in the use of advance directives, several describe variability in this practice.[31–35] To address this ethnic/racial variation, Zaide et al.[32] examined whether a palliative care consultation would influence rates of completion of advance directives (defined for this study as advance directives, "do not resuscitate," and "do not intubate" orders) in a diverse population of patients seen by a palliative care service at a tertiary care hospital in New York. Although the consultation was associated with increased completion of advance directives in all groups, findings showed that white patients were more likely to complete advance directives than African American patients both before (25.7% vs. 12.7%) and after (59.4% vs. 40.8%) the consultation. However, black–white differences in the completion of advance directives decreased following the consultation, prompting the authors to suggest that a palliative care consultation "levels the playing field" in this context. This study and many others highlight the difficulties in disentangling specific practices, such as the use of advance directives, from other palliative care practices or, more important, from individual preferences, beliefs, and attitudes about EOL care. For example, in one study examining the use of advance directives in African American and white patients, whites were almost four times more likely to have an advance directive than African Americans, but they were also found to have more positive attitudes and beliefs about hospice care.[31] In another study of a faith-based intervention to promote advance care planning among African Americans,[33] most study participants believed the intervention was effective in promoting awareness of advance care planning, but only 25% were willing to complete an advance directive after the intervention. In focus groups and interviews with study participants, the authors found that beliefs and attitudes, such as a value on prolonging life and mistrust in doctors and hospitals, presented a critical barrier to advance directives.

Factors Contributing to Disparities in Palliative Care

Clearly, there are significant and widespread racial/ethnic disparities in the use of palliative care in the United States. This chapter focuses next on investigating the numerous, complex, and overlapping factors that contribute to these disparities. To do this, we provide a conceptual model of the multilevel factors that contribute to these disparities (see Figure 14.1).

The model begins by examining societal-, hospital-, and provider-level factors, such as the availability of services, costs related to care, and hospital staff diversity and sensitivity to the needs of minorities. Second, the model turns to patient and family individual-level factors. These include: socio-demographic characteristics, preferences for care, knowledge of care, religious/spiritual beliefs about death and the end of life, and expectations of family members' role in EOL care. Finally, we discuss patient and provider interpersonal communication factors, including attitudes and perceptions of each other, care, and clinical communication.

Societal-, Hospital-, and Provider-Level Factors

First, the use of palliative care for any individual depends on available services and an individual's ability to pay for those

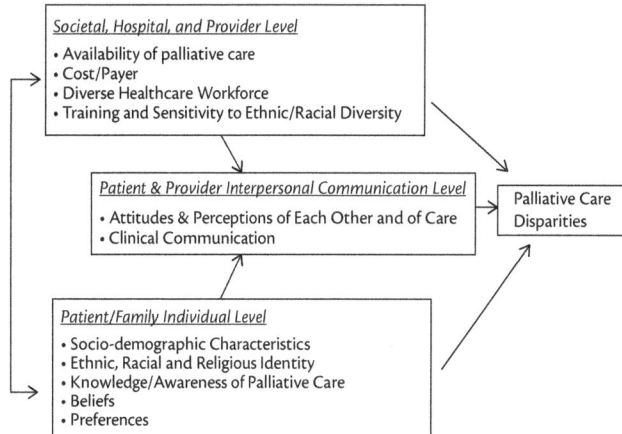

Figure 14.1 A multilevel model of factors contributing to palliative care disparities

services. Availability of services varies by geographic area, a fact that disproportionately affects minorities, residents of rural areas, and people with low income.[15,16,24,36] Second, with regard to cost, most insurance plans cover most or all of the costs of palliative care. However, many people in the United States, and particularly members of minority groups and those with lower economic status, lack comprehensive insurance.[19,35] Further, insurance coverage is only part of the financial cost of healthcare. In a study of 1,447 family members of deceased persons from 22 states, Welch et al.[35] found that although rates of being insured did not differ between African American and white decedents, there were differences in whether a person was covered by a single government-sponsored source of health insurance (e.g., Medicare or Medicaid alone), a combination of plans (e.g., Medicare plus a supplement), or private insurance. African Americans were more likely to have a single plan (39.4% vs. 16.5%) compared to whites. Moreover, African American family members were more than twice as likely to report the decedent had used all or most of his or her savings to pay for care, and it was very or somewhat difficult for the decedent and the family to cover the cost of care during the last year of life.

Third, an important factor in a patient's ability to use palliative care is the availability of an ethnically/racially diverse staff.[11] A diverse staff may be more appealing to minorities and more likely to provide referrals to minorities, have interpreters, and have outreach efforts into diverse communities, which may increase minority enrollment into palliative care.[37,38]

Patient/Family Individual-Level Factors

The vast majority of research on racial/ethnic disparities in palliative care is devoted to factors related to individual patients and their families. Socio-demographic characteristics, such as age, race, ethnicity, gender, income, and education, play a critical role in disparities in palliative and other forms of healthcare. This chapter summarizes the evidence on racial/ethnic differences regarding the influence of communication in patient and family preferences, knowledge, and spiritual/religious beliefs and decisions in general and the use of palliative care, specifically.

Preferences for EOL care vary by patient race/ethnicity. African Americans are more likely than members of other racial/ethnic groups to prefer life-sustaining treatments.[31,34,39] Barnato et al.[40]

conducted a survey of more than 2,000 Medicare beneficiaries nationally to better understand racial/ethnic differences in EOL care preferences. The majority of respondents across groups said that if they knew they had a terminal illness and had less than a year to live, they would want to die at home, without life-prolonging drugs with uncomfortable side effects or mechanical ventilation to extend life by a week or a month. However, preferences differed for EOL treatment by racial/ethnic group—minorities were more likely to prefer high-intensity options than whites. Specifically, 17.7% of African Americans and 15.2% of Hispanics reported wanting to die in a hospital, as compared to 8% of non-Hispanic whites. Similarly, more African Americans (28.1%) and Hispanics (21.2%) than whites (15%) reported they would want life-extending drug treatment with uncomfortable side effects. On the other hand, fewer African Americans (49.3%) and Hispanics (56.6%) than whites (74.2%) reported they would want palliative medications that might be life shortening. Finally, African Americans were much more likely than whites to want to receive ventilator support to extend life for a week or a month.

Several scholars have sought to determine the reasons for these disparities. Knowledge is clearly a critical factor,[41] and, compared to whites, non-whites generally lack knowledge of palliative care and advance directives.[34,42] Confusing terminology, where to find services, and payment options have prevented minority group members from using palliative care services.[43–45] Johnson and colleagues[41] surveyed 200 older primary care patients about their exposure to hospice information and found that African Americans reported significantly less exposure to information than whites. These authors also found that greater exposure to information about hospice was associated with more positive beliefs about hospice care, suggesting that interventions to increase knowledge may reduce palliative care disparities. However, there are limitations to simply providing information—additional factors also have to be considered, including patient ability to speak, read, and understand English; level of health literacy; and beliefs about death.[33,46] Health literacy has been found to present a barrier independent of other factors.[46,47] Volande et al.[46] conducted an intervention designed to increase knowledge about dementia in the hopes of influencing preferences for EOL care in a population of primary care patients at six outpatient clinics in the Boston area. The intervention included a verbal explanation of dementia and related treatments and was followed by a two-minute video of a white patient with advanced dementia. Although unadjusted analyses showed that African Americans were more likely to prefer aggressive care following the verbal explanation, adjusted analyses showed that level of health literacy, and not race, was an independent predictor of EOL care preferences. Interestingly, following the video portion of the intervention, differences in preferences by race and literacy level disappeared.[46]

A conflict between patients' and their families' religious/spiritual beliefs, the expectations for the role of family members, and the goals of palliative care may influence decisions about palliative care use among minorities.[31,33,48–50] Garrido and colleagues[50] conducted a study of more than 300 adults aged 55 years and older from diverse racial and socioeconomic groups to determine how religious affiliation and religious importance affected advance care planning. They found that the more an individual believed God holds ultimate control over life, the less likely he or she was to engage in advance care planning. Similarly, Crawley et al.[51] suggested that a predominant belief among some African Americans that suffering and death are meant to be endured as a part of spiritual commitment may conflict with palliative care goals. Accepting hospice care may be perceived as accepting death, equated with giving up, and may not be consistent with some spiritual/religious beliefs.[44,45]

Some groups hold expectations that family members should be cared for by other family members, and the use of hospice care may violate that expectation.[44,45] Kwak and colleagues[34] found that Asians and Hispanics were more likely to prefer family-centered decision-making, which was perceived to be at odds with palliative care. It is important to note here that there is variation within racial groups related to cultural values, demographics, the level of acculturation, and knowledge of palliative care options.[34]

Patient and Provider Attitudes, Perceptions, and the Quality of Clinical Communication

A related but distinct level of influence on the use of palliative care is the attitudes and perceptions of patients and providers and the communication that occurs between them throughout screening, diagnosis, and treatment phases of care. In this section, we summarize the influence of these factors on palliative care use in minority groups.

Patient Attitudes: Mistrust and Concerns About Discrimination

A major patient factor associated with the reduced use of palliative care among African Americans is mistrust in medical institutions and providers.[49,52] These attitudes, derived in great part from the legacy of racism and poorer healthcare for minorities in the United States,[8,53] have been associated with patient preferences and decisions about EOL care.[36,49,54,55] Specifically, there are concerns about receiving inferior care if an advance directive is signed,[44,45] that limiting intensive and aggressive treatment may be a form of injustice,[36,51] and about the economic motives of healthcare providers.[56] Possibly, mistrust increases the likelihood of African American patients' undergoing aggressive treatment at the end of life, including ICU admission, using feeding tubes, undergoing CPR, and not enrolling in hospice.[40,57]

Patient Perceptions of Care and Communication

Studies have described variation in the perception of hospice care and communication quality experienced by patients of differing racial/ethnic groups. Welch et al.[35] interviewed 1,578 family members of African American and white decedents to investigate differences in perceptions of EOL care and found significant differences by patient race. Family members of African American decedents, compared to those of white decedents, were substantially less likely to rate the overall quality of the care they received at the last place of care as excellent or very good. Also, family members of African American decedents reported more problems with communication with healthcare providers, with being kept informed, and with receiving support for their family members. Problems with communication at the last place of care included not having spoken with any physician despite having wanted to do so and concerns about the communication quality when communication occurred. These findings are not surprising in light of research suggesting that communication differs in clinical interactions with African American versus white patients. Compared to patient–physician clinical interactions with white patients, interactions with African

American patients are shorter, patients have less positive affect and ask fewer questions, and physicians are more contentious and provide less information. Also, following the visits, African American patients have less trust in physicians and understanding of the diagnosis and treatment.[58-65] However, in a recent study of physicians-in-training, Long et al.[66] report results that conflict with prior research on the association of race/ethnicity and quality of EOL communication. Findings related to patient/family member perceptions of EOL communication provided by physicians-in-training showed that racial minority status, lower income, and lower education level were associated with significantly higher ratings of communication about EOL care. The authors speculate that a reason for this unexpected finding may be that patients with higher education and income levels have greater expectations for the quality of communication and that physicians-in-training may not have the experience or skills to engage in the in-depth discussions desired by these patients and family members.

Provider-Level Factors: Biases and Poor Quality Interpersonal Communication

An important contributor to disparities in palliative care is at the level of providers, who are the primary source of palliative care information and referrals. Palliative care involves disciplines such as nursing, social work, and chaplaincy, but most research on disparities in this context is focused on physicians.

Physician attitudes toward minorities and toward discussing death and EOL have been shown to influence clinical communication and, in turn, contribute to disparities in palliative care. Physicians, like other professionals, have unconscious biases that affect their treatment decisions, their communication with patients, and patients' perceptions of them.[67,68] Few studies are available investigating the relationship between physician attitude, patient race/ethnicity, and clinical discussions about palliative or hospice care. Ache and colleagues[69] found that African American physicians, compared to white physicians, more often feel their patients are reluctant to discuss hospice care. They also found that the physician attitudes and recommendations may interact with patient race, influencing EOL conversations and potentially contributing to disparities in these conversations.[69] Physicians and other providers report discomfort with EOL conversations and fear they may be reducing their patients' hope.[70] However well-intended, physicians' attitudes and behaviors likely put some patients at a disadvantage in terms of their ability to make adequate preparations for EOL care consistent with their needs and preferences.

Racial/ethnic communication disparities in the broader healthcare literature have been established,[7,59,62] but studies examining disparities in patient–provider palliative care communication are limited.[66] The work that has been conducted suggests that African Americans are more likely to experience poorer quality and quantity of clinical communication at the end of life when compared to whites.[35]

Recommendations for Future Research and Communication Interventions to Address Palliative Care Disparities

This section summarizes research limitations and makes suggestions for future research to address ethnic/racial disparities in palliative care and inform interventions to reduce or eliminate disparities. Then we summarize communication approaches that may be useful in addressing this critical aspect of patient care.

Recommendations for Future Research

Perhaps the most apparent research limitation is the focus on hospice and on cancer to the exclusion of other aspects of palliative care and other potentially life-limiting diagnoses. More research is needed on, for example, pain management, variation in services by geographic and medical setting, and advance care planning.

Second, as we have noted, the majority of research on disparities in palliative care compares non-Hispanic white populations with African Americans and, to a lesser extent, Hispanics and Asians. There is a great need to investigate the palliative care needs of additional populations, such as members of religious and ethnic minorities other than African Americans, Hispanics, and Asians; immigrants; children; patients with mental or physical disabilities; veterans; and patients who identify as lesbian, gay, bisexual, and/or transgender. Further, with very few exceptions, most research compares populations as a whole and ignores heterogeneity within populations.

Third, research on the effect of clinical communication on palliative care is quite limited and largely consists of opinion pieces and literature reviews. The evidence that does exist indicates that disparities may be present in palliative care discussions with providers and patients from varying racial/ethnic backgrounds. Clinical communication has been shown to influence treatment decisions and health outcomes in other care settings,[71-73] thus it is reasonable to think it influences care and outcomes in this context. For example, studies using video and audio recordings of oncology and primary clinic visits with African American and white patients document differences in patient–provider communication by patient race and suggest ways in which communication may influence outcomes.[59,63,74,75]

Fourth, there is a great need for larger, more diverse samples and for longitudinal designs. Of critical importance, descriptive studies need to be used to inform randomized controlled trials of interventions to improve care. Similarly, the research largely lacks theoretical focus or conceptual frameworks. The application of theories from the fields of communication, social psychology, and similar fields may improve our understanding of the causes palliative care disparities and suggest interventions.[3,7,74,76] This chapter suggests a model (see Figure 14.1) of the multilevel factors that contribute to palliative care disparities, including the influence of patient–provider interpersonal communication, that could potentially be useful for better understanding relationships between and among factors and ultimately lead to a comprehensive approach to providing high-quality palliative care across patient populations.

Fifth, most research in this area focuses on patient and family factors, implying that they are to blame for disparities in palliative care. However, minority members' attitudes such as mistrust in medical care are derived from a history of poor care, and thus it is the responsibility of medical institutions to implement policies and practices to earn the trust of minority communities. Research on the effect of hospital practices, such as diversity in the workforce, availability of interpreters, palliative care consults, educational programs, community outreach, and culturally sensitive care, is needed to better understand ways to earn the trust

Table 14.1 Suggestions for Communication Sensitive to the Needs of Patients' Cultural/Individual Preferences[81]

Cultural/Individual Preference	Examples of Language to Use
Direct or indirectness in communication	How much do you want to know about your medical condition?
Whether to involve family members	Would you prefer that I discuss your medical condition with you directly or with a family member?
Decision-making preference	Do you want to make decisions yourself, after I have given you all the options, or would you prefer that I suggest what I think is the best option?
Advance care planning	If you became unable to make healthcare decisions, who would you want to make them for you?
Social, educational, and family factors	Tell me a little about your family.
Religious and spiritual factors	Is there anything I should know about your religious or spiritual views, as we discuss your medical condition?

of ethnic/racial minority communities to improve their access to high quality palliative care.

Communication Interventions to Address Palliative Care Disparities

The responsibility for improving practices to reduce or eliminate disparities in palliative care lies largely with medical institutions, hospitals, researchers, and providers, rather than with the patients and families who bear the burden of the disparities. Our suggestions for communication approaches to reduce or eliminate palliative care disparities are consistent with Ferrell's[3] summary of recommendations for improving the quality of palliative care in cancer, which is adapted from the Institute of Medicine report on the quality of cancer care in the United States.[2] We focus on three kinds of approaches: hospital and provider interventions to improve the quality of clinical communication, patient and family interventions to improve access to information, and outreach efforts to improve knowledge in minority communities.

Provider communication can affect patient perceptions and use of palliative care.[28,77] Several publications are available suggesting specific communication strategies for approaching EOL communication with patients and families.[78–80] For example, Ngo-Metzger and colleagues[81] provide guidelines for patient-centered communication at the end of life and suggests ways to avoid stereotyping and be sensitive to patients' cultural and individual preferences. Also, promising models for provider training are available[82–87] (see Table 14.1).

Close family members often act as caretakers; thus family members should also be the focus of interventions and included in the palliative care referral process and decision-making.[19,88] Interventions for patients and their families might include decision aids and question prompt lists focused on EOL decisions. These interventions have been shown to facilitate family conversations about EOL decisions and to improve the quality of communication in patient/family–provider interactions. For example, Clayton et al.[89] developed and tested a question prompt list to improve Australian patients' and families' ability to gain access to information about palliative care during clinical visits and to facilitate their ability to express to providers their preferences and concerns about palliative care. These kinds of interventions have generally not been developed in collaboration with or specific to the needs of minority populations, but given the research on disparities in communication in racially discordant interactions, interventions focused on specific populations are emerging in other contexts.[90]

Conclusion

This chapter summarized patterns of disparities in palliative care in the United States and proposed a conceptual model for better understanding the numerous and complex factors that contribute to these disparities. Recommendations are made on how hospitals, providers, and researchers can address and overcome these disparities. The Institute of Medicine, professional organizations, and researchers have clearly stated that these and other health and healthcare disparities are preventable.[6,8] Effective and compassionate communication regarding palliative care can enable all patients to make informed choices about their care.

References

1. Ferrell B, Connor SR, Cordes A, et al. The national agenda for quality palliative care: The National Consensus Project and the National Quality Forum. *J Pain Symptom Manag.* 2007;33(6):737–744.
2. Levit L, Balogh E, Nass S, Ganz PA, eds. *Delivering High-Quality Cancer Care: Charting a New Course for a System in Crisis.* Washington, DC: National Acadamies Press; 2013.
3. Ferrell BR, Smith TJ, Levit L, Balogh E. Improving the quality of cancer care: Implications for palliative care. *J Palliat Med.* 2014;17(4):393–399.
4. Temel JS, Greer JA, Muzikansky A, et al. Early palliative care for patients with metastatic non-small-cell lung cancer. *N Engl J Med.* 2010;363(8):733–742.
5. Braveman P. Health disparities and health equity: Concepts and measurement. *Annu Rev Public Health.* 2006;27:167–194.
6. Siegel R, Ward E, Brawley O, Jemal A. Cancer statistics, 2011: The impact of eliminating socioeconomic and racial disparities on premature cancer deaths. *CA Cancer J Clin.* 2011;61(4):212–236.
7. Penner LA, Hagiwara N, Eggly S, Gaertner SL, Albrecht TL, Dovidio JF. Racial healthcare disparities: A social psychological analysis. *Eur Rev Soc Psychol.* 2013;24(1):70–122.
8. Smedley BD, Stith AY, Nelson AR. *Unequal Treatment: Confronting Racial and Ethnic Disparities in Health Care.* Washington DC: National Academies Press; 2003.
9. *Crossing the Quality Chasm: A New Health System for the 21st Century.* Washington, DC: Institute of Medicine Committee on Quality Health Care in America; 2001.
10. Agency for Healthcare Research and Quality. 2013 National Healthcare Disparities Report. 2014. http://www.ahrq.gov/

research/findings/nhqrdr/nhdr13/2013nhdr.pdf. Accessed June 18, 2015.
11. Johnson KS. Racial and ethnic disparities in palliative care. *J Palliat Med.* 2013;16(11):1329-1334.
12. Nayar P, Qiu F, Watanabe-Galloway S, et al. Disparities in end of life care for elderly lung cancer patients. *J Comm Health.* 2014;39(5):1012-1019.
13. Hardy D, Chan W, Liu CC, et al. Racial disparities in the use of hospice services according to geographic residence and socioeconomic status in an elderly cohort with nonsmall cell lung cancer. *Cancer.* 2011;117(7):1506-1515.
14. Unroe KT, Greiner MA, Johnson KS, Curtis LH, Setoguchi S. Racial differences in hospice use and patterns of care after enrollment in hospice among Medicare beneficiaries with heart failure. *Am Heart J.* 2012;163(6):987-993 e983.
15. Cohen LL. Racial/ethnic disparities in hospice care: A systematic review. *J Palliat Med.* 2008;11(5):763-768.
16. Johnson KS, Kuchibhatla M, Payne R, Tulsky JA. Race and residence: Intercounty variation in black-white differences in hospice use. *J Pain Symptom Manage.* 2013;46(5):681-690.
17. Smith AK, Earle CC, McCarthy EP. Racial and ethnic differences in end-of-life care in fee-for-service Medicare beneficiaries with advanced cancer. *J Am Geriatr Soc.* 2009;57(1):153-158.
18. Givens JL, Tjia J, Zhou C, Emanuel E, Ash AS. Racial and ethnic differences in hospice use among patients with heart failure. *Arch Intern Med.* 2010;170(5):427-432.
19. Carrion IV, Park NS, Lee BS. Hospice use among African Americans, Asians, Hispanics, and whites: Implications for practice. *Am J Hosp Palliat Care.* 2012;29(2):116-121.
20. Mor V, Papandonatos G, Miller SC. End-of-life hospitalization for African American and non-Latino white nursing home residents: Variation by race and a facility's racial composition. *J Palliat Med.* 2005;8(1):58-68.
21. Anderson KO, Green CR, Payne R. Racial and ethnic disparities in pain: Causes and consequences of unequal care. *J Pain* 2009;10(12):1187-1204.
22. Shavers VL, Bakos A, Sheppard VB. Race, ethnicity, and pain among the U.S. adult population. *J Health Care Poor Underserved.* 2010;21(1):177-220.
23. Cintron A, Morrison RS. Pain and ethnicity in the United States: A systematic review. *J Palliat Med.* 2006;9(6):1454-1473.
24. Morrison RS, Wallenstein S, Natale DK, Senzel RS, Huang LL. "We don't carry that"—failure of pharmacies in predominantly nonwhite neighborhoods to stock opioid analgesics. *N Engl J Med.* 2000;342(14):1023-1026.
25. Johnson KS, Kuchibhatla M, Tanis D, Tulsky JA. Racial differences in hospice revocation to pursue aggressive care. *Arch Intern Med.* 2008;168(2):218-224.
26. Kapo J, MacMoran H, Casarett D. "Lost to follow-up": Ethnic disparities in continuity of hospice care at the end of life. *J Palliat Med.* 2005;8(3):603-608.
27. Kitzes J, Berger L. End-of-life issues for American Indians/Alaska Natives: insights from one Indian Health Service area. *J Palliat Med.* 2004;7(6):830-838.
28. Marr L, Neale D, Wolfe V, Kitzes J. Confronting myths: The Native American experience in an academic inpatient palliative care consultation program. *J Palliat Med.* 2012;15(1):71-76.
29. Linton JM, Feudtner C. What accounts for differences or disparities in pediatric palliative and end-of-life care? A systematic review focusing on possible multilevel mechanisms. *Pediatrics.* 2008;122(3):574-582.
30. Thienprayoon R, Lee SC, Leonard D, Winick N. Racial and ethnic differences in hospice enrollment among children with cancer. *Pediatr Blood Cancer.* 2013;60(10):1662-1666.
31. Johnson KS, Kuchibhatla M, Tulsky JA. What explains racial differences in the use of advance directives and attitudes toward hospice care? *J Am Geriatr Soc.* 2008;56(10):1953-1958.
32. Zaide GB, Pekmezaris R, Nouryan CN, et al. Ethnicity, race, and advance directives in an inpatient palliative care consultation service. *Palliat Support Care.* 2013;11(1):5-11.
33. Bullock K. Promoting advance directives among African Americans: A faith-based model. *J Palliat Med.* 2006;9(1):183-195.
34. Kwak J, Haley WE. Current research findings on end-of-life decision making among racially or ethnically diverse groups. *Gerontologist.* 2005;45(5):634-641.
35. Welch LC, Teno JM, Mor V. End-of-life care in black and white: Race matters for medical care of dying patients and their families. *J Amer Geriatr Soc.* 2005;53(7):1145-1153.
36. Born W, Greiner KA, Sylvia E, Butler J, Ahluwalia JS. Knowledge, attitudes, and beliefs about end-of-life care among inner-city African Americans and Latinos. *J Palliat Med.* 2004;7(2):247-256.
37. Reese DJ, Melton E, Ciaravino K. Programmatic barriers to providing culturally competent end-of-life care. *Am J Hosp Palliat Care.* 2004;21(5):357-364.
38. Lorenz KA, Ettner SL, Rosenfeld KE, Carlisle D, Liu H, Asch SM. Accommodating ethnic diversity: A study of California hospice programs. *Med Care.* 2004;42(9):871-874.
39. Anthony DL, Herndon MB, Gallagher PM, et al. How much do patients' preferences contribute to resource use? *Health Affairs.* 2009;28(3):864-873.
40. Barnato AE, Anthony DL, Skinner J, Gallagher PM, Fisher ES. Racial and ethnic differences in preferences for end-of-life treatment. *J Gen Intern Med.* 2009;24(6):695-701.
41. Johnson KS, Kuchibhatla M, Tulsky JA. Racial differences in self-reported exposure to information about hospice care. *J Palliat Med.* 2009;12(10):921-927.
42. Matsuyama RK, Balliet W, Ingram K, Lyckholm LJ, Wilson-Genderson M, Smith TJ. Will patients want hospice or palliative care if they do not know what it is? *J Hosp Palliat Nurs.* 2011;13(1):41-46.
43. Rhodes RL, Teno JM, Connor SR. African American bereaved family members' perceptions of the quality of hospice care: Lessened disparities, but opportunities to improve remain. *J Pain Symptom Manage.* Nov 2007;34(5):472-479.
44. Spruill AD, Mayer DK, Hamilton JB. Barriers in hospice use among African Americans with cancer. *J Hosp Palliat Nurs.* May 2013;15(3):136-144.
45. Drisdom S. Barriers to Using Palliative Care: Insight Into African American culture. *Clin J Oncol Nurs.* Aug 2013;17(4):376-380.
46. Volandes AE, Paasche-Orlow M, Gillick MR, et al. Health literacy not race predicts end-of-life care preferences. *J Palliat Med.* 2008;11(5):754-762.
47. Melhado L, Bushy A. Exploring uncertainty in advance care planning in African Americans: Does low health literacy influence decision making preference at end of life? *Am J Hosp Palliat Care.* 2011;28(7):495-500.
48. Balboni TA, Balboni M, Enzinger AC, et al. Provision of spiritual support to patients with advanced cancer by religious communities and associations with medical care at the end of life. *JAMA Intern Med.* 2013;173(12):1109-1117.
49. Crawley LM. Racial, cultural, and ethnic factors influencing end-of-life care. *J Palliat Med.* 2005;8(Suppl 1):S58-S69.
50. Garrido MM, Idler EL, Leventhal H, Carr D. Pathways from religion to advance care planning: Beliefs about control over length of life and end-of-life values. *Gerontologist.* 2013;53(5):801-816.
51. Crawley L, Payne R, Bolden J, et al. Palliative and end-of-life care in the African American community. *JAMA.* 2000;284(19):2518-2521.
52. Gross CP, Smith BD, Wolf E, Andersen M. Racial disparities in cancer therapy: Did the gap narrow between 1992 and 2002? *Cancer.* 2008;112(4):900-908.
53. Skloot R. *The immortal life of Henrietta Lacks.* New York: Crown; 2010.
54. Krakauer EL, Crenner C, Fox K. Barriers to optimum end-of-life care for minority patients. *J Am Geriatr Soc.* 2002;50(1):182-190.

55. Watkins YJ, Bonner GJ, Wang E, Wilkie DJ, Ferrans CE, Dancy B. Relationship among trust in physicians, demographics, and end-of-life treatment decisions made by African American dementia caregivers. *J Hosp Palliat Nurs.* 2012;14(3):238–243.
56. McAteer R, Wellbery C. Palliative care: Benefits, barriers, and best practices. *Am Fam Physician.* 2013;88(12):807–813.
57. Perry WR, Kwok AC, Kozycki C, Celi LA. Disparities in end-of-life care: A perspective and review of quality. *Popul Health Manag.* 2013;16(2):71–73.
58. Jean-Pierre P, Fiscella K, Griggs J, et al. Race/ethnicity-based concerns over understanding cancer diagnosis and treatment plan. *J Natl Med Assoc.* 2010;102(3):184–189.
59. Eggly S, Harper FW, Penner LA, Gleason MJ, Foster T, Albrecht TL. Variation in question asking during cancer clinical interactions: A potential source of disparities in access to information. *Patient Educ Couns.* 2011;82(1):63–68.
60. Cooper LA, Roter DL, Johnson RL, Ford DE, Steinwachs DM, Powe NR. Patient-centered communication, ratings of care, and concordance of patient and physician race. *Ann Intern Med.* 2003;139(11):907–915.
61. Johnson RL, Roter D, Powe NR, Cooper LA. Patient race/ethnicity and quality of patient-physician communication during medical visits. *Am J Public Health.* 2004;94(12):2084–2090.
62. Gordon HS, Street RL, Jr., Sharf BF, Souchek J. Racial differences in doctors' information-giving and patients' participation. *Cancer.* 2006;107(6):1313–1320.
63. Siminoff LA, Graham GC, Gordon NH. Cancer communication patterns and the influence of patient characteristics: Disparities in information-giving and affective behaviors. *Patient Educ Couns.* 2006;62(3):355–360.
64. Song L, Hamilton JB, Moore AD. Patient-healthcare provider communication: Perspectives of African American cancer patients. *Health Psychol.* 2011;31(5):539–547.
65. Eggly S, Barton E, Winckles A, Penner LA, Albrecht TL. A disparity of words: Racial differences in oncologist-patient communication about clinical trials. *Health Expect.* 2013. Advance online publication.
66. Long AC, Engelberg RA, Downey L, et al. Race, income, and education: Associations with patient and family ratings of end-of-life care and communication provided by physicians-in-training. *J Palliat Med.* 2014;17(4):435–447.
67. Penner LA, Dovidio JF, West T, et al. Aversive racism and medical interactions with black patients: A field study. *Ann Behav Med.* 2010;39:24–24.
68. van Ryn M, Saha S. Exploring unconscious bias in disparities research and medical education. *JAMA.* 2011;306(9):995–996.
69. Ache KA, Shannon RP, Heckman MG, Diehl NN, Willis FB. A preliminary study comparing attitudes toward hospice referral between African American and white American primary care physicians. *J Palliat Med.* 2011;14(5):542–547.
70. Casarett DJ, Quill TE. "I'm not ready for hospice": Strategies for timely and effective hospice discussions. *Ann Intern Med.* 2007;146(6):443–449.
71. Epstein RM, Street R.L J. *Patient-Centered Communication in Cancer Care: Promoting Healing and Reducing Suffering.* Bethesda, MD: National Cancer Institute; 2007.
72. Kelley JM, Kraft-Todd G, Schapira L, Kossowsky J, Riess H. The influence of the patient-clinician relationship on healthcare outcomes: A systematic review and meta-analysis of randomized controlled trials. *PLoS One.* 2014;9(4):e94207.
73. Albrecht TL, Eggly SS, Gleason ME, et al. Influence of clinical communication on patients' decision making on participation in clinical trials. *J Clin Oncol.* 2008;26(16):2666–2673.
74. Street RL, Jr., Gordon H, Haidet P. Physicians' communication and perceptions of patients: Is it how they look, how they talk, or is it just the doctor? *Soc Sci Med.* 2007;65(3):586–598.
75. Hagiwara N, Penner LA, Gonzalez R, et al. Racial attitudes, physician-patient talk time ratio, and adherence in racially discordant medical interactions. *Soc Sci Med.* 2013;87:123–131.
76. Penner LA, Gaertner S, Dovidio JF, et al. A social psychological approach to improving the outcomes of racially discordant medical interactions. *J Gen Intern Med.* 2013;28(9):1143–1149.
77. Loggers ET, Maciejewski PK, Jimenez R, et al. Predictors of intensive end-of-life and hospice care in Latino and white advanced cancer patients. *J Palliat Med.* 2013;16(10):1249–1254.
78. Back AL, Arnold RM, Baile WF, Tulsky JA, Fryer-Edwards K. Approaching difficult communication tasks in oncology. *CA Cancer J Clin.* 2005;55(3):164–177.
79. Levetown M. Communicating with children and families: Fom everyday interactions to skill in conveying distressing information. *Pediatrics.* May 2008;121(5):e1441–1460.
80. Clayton JM, Hancock KM, Butow PN, et al. Clinical practice guidelines for communicating prognosis and end-of-life issues with adults in advanced stages of a life-limiting illness, and their caregivers. *Med J Aust.* 2007;186(12 Suppl):S77, S79, S83–S108.
81. Ngo-Metzger Q, August KJ, Srinivasan M, Liao S, Meyskens FL, Jr. End-of-life care: Guidelines for patient-centered communication. *Am Fam Physician.* 2008;77(2):167–174.
82. Kissane DW, Bylund CL, Banerjee SC, et al. Communication skills training for oncology professionals. *J Clin Oncol.* 2012;30(11):1242–1247.
83. Back AL, Arnold RM, Baile WF, et al. Efficacy of communication skills training for giving bad news and discussing transitions to palliative care. *Arch Intern Med.* 2007;167(5):453–460.
84. Bylund CL, Brown RF, Bialer PA, Levin TT, Lubrano di Ciccone B, Kissane DW. Developing and Implementing an advanced communication training program in oncology at a comprehensive cancer center. *J Cancer Educ.* 2011;26(4):604–611.
85. Brown RF, Bylund CL. Communication skills training: Describing a new conceptual model. *Acad Med.* 2008;83(1):37–44.
86. Goldsmith J, Wittenberg-Lyles E. COMFORT: Evaluating a new communication curriculum with nurse leaders. *J Prof Nurs* 2013;29(6):388–394.
87. Wittenberg-Lyles E, Goldsmith J, Richardson B, Hallett JS, Clark R. The practical nurse: A case for COMFORT communication training. *Am J Hosp Palliat Care.* 2013;30(2):162–166.
88. Carr D. Racial differences in end-of-life planning: Why don't blacks and Latinos prepare for the inevitable? *Omega.* 2011;63(1):1–20.
89. Clayton JM, Butow PN, Tattersall MH, et al. Randomized controlled trial of a prompt list to help advanced cancer patients and their caregivers to ask questions about prognosis and end-of-life care. *J Clin Oncol.* 2007;25(6):715–723.
90. Eggly S, Tkatch R, Penner LA, et al. Development of a question prompt list as a communication intervention to reduce racial disparities in cancer treatment. *J Cancer Educ.* 2013;28:282–289.

CHAPTER 15

The Role of Communication and Information in Symptom Management

Gary L. Kreps and Mollie Rose Canzona

Introduction

Symptom management is a primary function of palliative care. However, delivering multidimensional, coordinated care that addresses the concerns of patients and families is challenging.[2,3] Patients often experience a wide variety of interrelated physical, psychological, and relational problems as a result of disease processes or treatments. Symptoms and side effects, which are referred to in this chapter as negative effects, can cause suffering, reduce quality of life, and interfere with healing processes. The progression of major diseases typically leads to uncomfortable symptoms, such as pain, nausea, fatigue, insomnia, fever, skin irritations, incontinence, digestive problems, dizziness, hair loss, and a number of additional physical and sexual dysfunctions. Often, these negative effects become even more troublesome for patients and families than the primary healthcare problems they are coping with.[3] Invasive and high-risk treatments, including surgery, radiotherapy, and chemotherapy, can lead to debilitating negative effects for individuals confronting serious illness such as cancers, heart disease, strokes, and other neurological and chronic diseases. These physical problems/conditions are often accompanied by or provoke psychological difficulties for patients, such as depression, irritability, fear, paranoia, and even dementia.[4]

Helping patients and family members effectively manage negative effects is essential to preserving their personal comfort and their physical and psychological well-being.[5] Without attention to careful and effective symptom management, negative effects can make the lives of patients and families tremendously stressful, painful, and frustrating, as well as minimize their abilities to cope effectively with their major health problems.[5] Creative and adaptive intervention strategies are required to meet the unique needs of different patients.

Understanding the Nature of Negative Effects

Negative effects contain both physical and psychosocial dimensions.[6] The physical dimension refers to the physiological presence of pain, discomfort, or dysfunction. Patients also experience negative effects on a psychosocial level as they attach symbolic meaning to those physiological processes. Physical causes of discomfort from negative effects is interpreted symbolically by individuals (often in very idiosyncratic ways) as psychological discomfort.[7,8] For example, the experience of pain, a common negative effect, is an important biological process in which the body sends neural messages about abnormal processes, intrusions, and threats. However, pain also promotes symbolic awareness of these problems and encourages attempts to identify the root causes of pain and the development of strategies for relieving these root causes. Individuals who experience chronic pain (physical dimension) may also develop depression or anxiety (symbolic dimension) as they work (often unsuccessfully) to understand and address these changes.

In addition, psychological interpretations of discomfort derive from biological reactions to physical threats as well as from our reactions to unpleasant feelings and emotions. Humans have developed the ability to mirror physical discomfort phenomena symbolically to make sense of psychological distress. Yet physical and psychological causes of discomfort actually feel like identical phenomena to most people. It is often difficult to distinguish between physical and psychological causes of discomfort; they both feel bad. For example, common healthcare situations, such as sounds (the dentist's drill), sights (blood), or messages ("the lab tests show your tumor is malignant") can trigger feelings of pain, nausea, or anxiety. In essence, there are many different physical and symbolic sources for discomfort in the modern world, especially within the healthcare system, and symptom management must be designed to address both physical and symbolic dimensions of negative effects.[6] Symptom management is a high-priority issue for those confronting serious chronic diseases, debilitating illnesses, and intrusive mental health problems such as depression, anxiety, and posttraumatic stress disorder.

The Family and Negative Effects

Negative effects pose challenges for the well-being of patients and families. Patients experiencing debilitating and poorly controlled negative effects may feel like they are losing control over their lives, and the burden associated with increased dependence can tax family caregivers and relationships.[9] Often, even when patients and families are utilizing palliative care services, a family caregiver is relied on to provide significant practical and emotional support to patients.[10] Burke et al.'s examination of family caregivers of heart failure patients discovered that caregivers perceive themselves as healthcare managers, healthcare plan enforcers, advocates for their loved one's quality of life, and experts on the realities of living with heart failure. Notably, they experienced distress when the expectations of that role exceeded their ability to perform.[11]

Patients' serious or complex health issues are a source of physical, psychological, social, functional, and spiritual burden for family caregivers.[12] Family members may experience a range of physical and symbolic problems ranging from sleeplessness, weight loss, fatigue, social isolation, depression, anxiety, burnout, and general deterioration of health.[13] It is important for palliative care providers to appreciate the effects illness and health conditions have on families in order to deliver care that improves quality of life for patients and family members.[14]

Individual Difference and Negative Effects

Each patient and family member represents a unique case for palliative care providers. These cases may vary significantly based on the nature of negative effects, individual differences, and the social worlds in which those individuals are embedded. For example, the experience of certain negative effects has additional deleterious symbolic dimensions due to cultural norms that suggest these problems are particularly socially unacceptable (stigmatized). The negative effects of incontinence, impotence, or even nausea are not only troubling; they are also embarrassing problems for those who suffer from them. The fear of loss of bladder or bowel control in public places can cause tremendous stress and additional discomfort for patients.[14,15,16] Even more innocuous negative effects, such as fatigue or skin irritations, can be embarrassing and stressful. These negative effects cause additional symbolic trauma for sufferers that compound the problems and lead to fear, alienation, and stress. Palliative care programs need to be designed to help those who suffer from these socially stigmatized negative effects cope with the symbolic stress these problems can cause.

The interpretation of negative effects is subjective and different for each person and each situation. When we are fully occupied with an engrossing and stimulating activity, we may not be as aware of physical discomfort as we might be when there is low stimulation. The perceptions of discomfort that we were able to habituate while busy often come to the forefront when there are not competing foci, particularly at night when there is often a high level of suffering from negative effects such as pain, nausea, and anxiety. Further, the same negative effects may be perceived dissimilarly by different individuals in different situations. Some people have a greater tolerance for negative effects than others. Effective symptom management must take these subjective interpretations of negative effects into account and develop individually and situationally appropriate strategies for addressing the ways each patient/family understands and navigates negative effects.

Symptom Management and Negative Effects

Managing the interactions between physiological and psychosocial dimensions (or symbolic dimensions) of these problems is complex. Surgical procedures are invasive and can lead to additional sources of discomfort for patients, particularly during the often long and uncomfortable process of rehabilitation from surgery.[17,18] Surgical procedures can also have unpleasant side effects (including risks of infection and long-term physical limitations) that can lead to new sources of anxiety and distress.[19]

Many negative effects, such as insomnia, nausea, and pain management, are regularly treated pharmacologically with prescribed, over-the-counter, and even self-prescribed illicit drugs and alcohol.[20,21] While many prescribed drugs are initially effective at reducing pain and suffering from negative effects, their continued use can also lead to additional problems (such as fatigue, anxiousness, digestive problems, and serious addictions), exacerbate other negative effects, or lead to interaction effects and polypharmacy with other drugs or treatments being used.[22] The interaction effects between many medications can be particularly problematic, and new healthcare problems establish a spiral of interventions and thus a spiral of negative effects. While strategic and informed pharmacology is definitely an important part of symptom management, medications can rarely be used alone, because drugs that address physiological issues are not particularly good at treating the symbolic dimensions of negative effects (e.g., depression, anxiety).

The best care strategies are designed to address both the physical and the psychological dimensions of healthcare problems.[23] Improving quality of life for patients is not an easy task. Understanding how communication functions in patient/family sense-making and response to negative effects in the delivery of palliative care/training and in the use of strategic and innovative healthcare interventions can help providers deliver multidimensional care to patients and their families.

Communication and Patient Response to Negative Effects

While the physiological response to negative effects is typically uncomfortable, a patient's interpretation of that discomfort is modified by a variety of internal and external factors that can either intensify or de-intensify suffering. For example, some internal (psychological) factors that can exacerbate the experience of discomfort may include feelings of depression, fatigue, uncertainty, loss of control, anxiety, fear, hopelessness, and loneliness. External (environmental) factors that can exacerbate perceptions of discomfort may include harsh lighting, unsettling noises, strong and unappealing scents, crowding, and jostling.

All of these internal and external factors that can exacerbate the perception of discomfort can be moderated (to a greater or lesser extent) through communication. Communication is a primary social mechanism for forming and influencing the creation of meaning.[24] Whether negative effects are caused by intrusive physical phenomena or emotional reactions to difficult situations (symbolic dimensions), communication provides a channel for influencing symbolic dimensions of health and illness.[1,25] There are direct links between communication and psychology in which the messages we perceive influence the meanings we create.[26] For example, messages that demonstrate encouragement, acceptance, compassion, respect, friendship, love, and support can promote feelings of being supported, being in control, a sense of self-efficacy, and personal resilience that can help people cope with negative effects.[27–29] Messages should minimize discomfort and maximize meaning in order to help patients and families improve quality of life.[8] Communication is a central mechanism through which palliative care providers can help shape patient outcomes.

Communication and the Delivery of Palliative Care

Effective symptom management is designed to treat both the physiological and the symbolic aspects of pain.[30] A large body of research has shown that communication between patients and families and providers is a critical factor in the delivery of high-quality care.[31] Often patients and families are not prepared to handle the challenges of illness and palliative care and look to providers to shepherd them through the process.[32] Patients and families have tremendous needs for relevant, accurate, and timely information to make the best health decisions and to coordinate the delivery of care.

Communication has been shown to help patients continually adapt to negative effects by increasing understanding about the causes of these problems, their unique patterns of incidence, and the best strategies for symptom management.[6,33] Providing relevant health information to patients and families can help them take charge of their healthcare problems. For many patients and families who prefer an active partnership with their healthcare providers, this can promote coping.[34] However, it should be noted that while delivering relevant and appropriate health information is usually helpful, providers should avoid the assumption that patients and families all desire a large share of decision-making power. Many cultural, ethnic, and minority groups differ in their preferences for autonomy and control.[35]

Research has shown that there are numerous barriers to communication in the delivery of care, including intercultural communication challenges, limited communication skills by both patients and families and providers, differential levels of health literacy, time constraints, poor access to relevant health information, political struggles and power differentials between healthcare providers and patients and families, low levels of interprofessional cooperation between members of healthcare teams, and lack of interpersonal sensitivity in healthcare interactions.[36–39] The communication barriers limiting the delivery of effective healthcare reduce the effectiveness of symptom management. In many cases, the ways that care is delivered can actually initiate and exacerbate other negative effects.[4,6]

However, patient–provider communication can promote coordinated care, informed health decision-making, and reduction of medical errors.[40] Arora's comprehensive review of the literature showed that physicians' communicative behavior (specifically, establishing effective interpersonal relationships, facilitating active exchange of relevant health information, and encouraging patient involvement in decision-making) had a positive impact on patient attitudes, self-efficacy, resilience, and ultimately health outcomes.[41] Healthcare providers can use strategic health communication to help patients and their families who are experiencing significant pain and discomfort by providing timely, accurate, and sensitive information to promote palliative care.[42] Active communication can also help patients, families, and providers work together to reduce pain and suffering.[6] Communication in healthcare enables (a) the development of relational interdependence between healthcare patients, families, and providers; (b) all stakeholders to gain access to relevant and timely health information; (c) channels for feedback to promote adaptation in palliative care; (d) coordinated verbal and nonverbal communication; (e) the use of communication technologies to support palliative care; and (f) consumer empowerment in pain and symptom management.[43]

Kreps proposed a model of communication and symptom management (see Figure 15.1) that illustrates the interdependence between the patient, the patient's providers, and the patient's friends and family. This model suggests that for effective

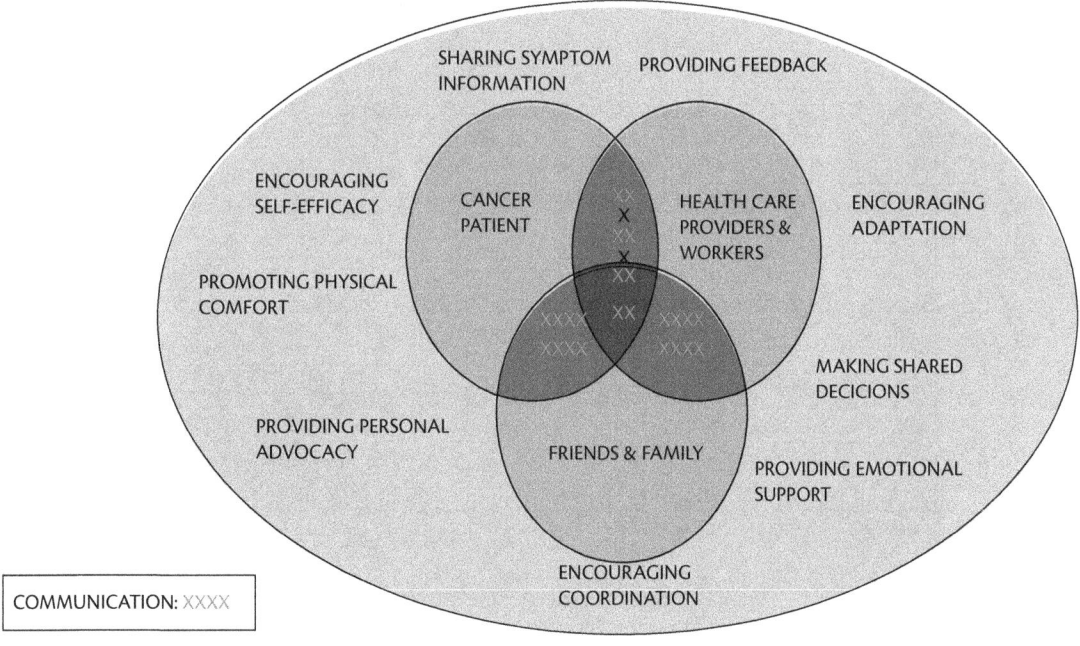

Figure 15.1 Communication and symptom management model

symptom management there must be active lines of communication between these people. Communication enables these partners in the healthcare enterprise to share relevant symptom information about the experience of negative effects so that cause, intensity, and intervention strategies may be understood in order to provide the greatest relief.[43] Communication is also needed to provide critical feedback about the utility of current symptom management strategies. Communication can encourage active adaptation to a patient's changing symptom management needs as well as making decisions about symptom management. The provision of emotional support and coordination of care is essential to managing negative effects.[44,45] Partners can also use their strategic communication skills to provide personal advocacy for the patient, promote physical and psychological comfort, and encourage patient self-efficacy. Further, partners can assist in the process of training patients with recurrent negative effects to develop strategies for tuning out (habituating) the discomfort or focusing their minds on other thoughts. While interventions on interpersonal and group levels are effective in improving communication about negative effects, there is also a need for evidence-based intervention strategies to implement at the system level.

Supportive and informative interaction has been found to be a powerful therapeutic process for promoting active symptom management and reducing symbolic feelings of suffering.[46] However, access to therapeutic and informative health communication, particularly at the specific points in time when symptom management support is most needed, is often limited for many sufferers. There is a tremendous need to increase access to relevant, supportive, and strategic health communication to promote symptom management.

Strategic Communication and Symptom Management

The symbolic dimensions of health problems, such as negative effects, are best addressed through strategic health communication processes.[23,47] Several promising health communication interventions have been developed for promoting effective symptom management.[48] Some of these interventions, which have been shown to promote positive coping with negative effects, are designed to train healthcare providers to communicate more effectively with patients to identify and mediate discomfort as part of larger palliative care programs.[42,49] Work has also been done to inform the creation and training of multidisciplinary and interdisciplinary palliative care teams.[2,50] Palliative care education programs coordinate care among healthcare providers to communicate with patients in ways that promote effective symptom management.[48]

Other interventions are designed to provide negative effect sufferers with more information about their healthcare problems and strategies for coping with negative effects. For example, a broad range of websites is dedicated to providing patients, families, and healthcare providers with education and support about symptom management. Some of these websites are summarized in Table 15.1.

The amount of external oversight concerning the accuracy, timeliness, completeness, and accessibility of the information provided on these websites varies considerably. Without the involvement of care providers, patients and families must make their own decisions about whether the symptom management information they find on these websites is appropriate for them

Table 15.1 Websites Offering Symptom Management Education and Support

Website	Description
http://www.pallcarevic.asn.au/families-patients/information/pain-symptom-relief/	Palliative Care Victoria offers information about pain and symptom relief, relationships, care planning, talking to doctors, and loss, in addition to personal stories, web resources, and financial assistance.
http://www.msfocus.org/symptom-mgmt.aspx	The Multiple Sclerosis Foundation offers information about a variety of symptom management techniques, including acupressure, the Alexander Technique applied kinesiology, and sound and music therapy.
http://www.ucsfhealth.org/programs/cancer_symptom_management/	UCSF Medical Center offers a special program in symptom management that addresses physical and emotional symptoms of cancer. This site also provides information on Art for Recovery, Healing through Dance, and restorative movement classes.
http://university.asco.org/symptom-management	The American Society of Clinical Oncology offers an online curriculum of five learning modules in symptom management for patients with serious or life-threatening disease.
http://www.cancer.gov/cancertopics/coping	The National Cancer Institute offers resources for coping with cancer, including information related to managing physical effects, managing emotions, finding healthcare services, financial information, preparing for end of life, as well as information for caregivers, family, and friends.
http://www.dbsalliance.org/site/PageServer?pagename=wellness_symptom_management	The Depression and Bipolar Support Alliance offers a symptom management worksheet patients and families can complete and discuss with healthcare providers.
http://www.stoppain.org/palliative_care/content/symptom/pain.asp	The Department of Pain Medicine and Palliative Care provides information regarding methods to alleviate pain and sources of pain for cancer patients and AIDS patients.
http://hepc.liverfoundation.org/treatment/while-on-treatment/managing-side-effects/	The American Liver Foundation offers information about potential negative effects for patients undergoing Hepatitis C therapy.
http://www.webmd.com/pain-management	WebMD offers a Pain Management Center where patients and families can access information about symptoms, diagnoses, and treatment of negative effects.

and what the best strategies are for implementing these symptom management recommendations. Physicians, nurses, social workers, pharmacists, and other healthcare professionals can help patients and families make sense of and apply symptom management information gathered on the Web.[51] Some healthcare providers and healthcare systems enable patients to consult with providers online, making it relatively quick and easy to find help interpreting web-based information about symptom management.

Although some providers may find this challenging,[52] the best strategy to ensure patients and families understand and properly use the symptom management information they gather online is to discuss the information with their healthcare providers.[53] A trusted healthcare professional can help them make sense of the symptom management information and advise them about the best strategies for utilizing the information for managing pain.[54]

A number of promising health communication interventions have been designed to promote awareness and coordination in facilitating prompt response to negative effect incidents. For example, Berry et al. introduced a computerized format for self-reporting pain assessment, *PAIN Report It*, that has been shown to help patients gain personal control over symptom management and share real-time information about pain incidence and treatment with their providers.[55] Computerized self-report systems like this can promote coordination of efforts in responding quickly to severe pain incidents.[56]

In addition, online diaries for tracking negative effects incidence and management can help patients and providers identify unique patterns, as well as report incidents in real time.[57] This diary data can predict when negative effect incidents are likely to occur and plan advance strategies for quick and decisive symptom management interventions. Evidence suggests that when providers make time to factor summary diary information into patient care, they can be particularly useful for empowering patients to better understand unique patterns of pain and its severity, as well as develop prevention plans.[58,59]

Other work has focused on the development of computerized assessment programs for measuring pain and discomfort.[58] Electronic questionnaires and web-based applications have been used to track, store, and share negative effects information with healthcare providers.[60] The use of handheld devices has made the collection of negative effects information portable for patients and families who experience these events at different times and different places.[61] Applications and texting capabilities enable efficient storage and processing of negative effects incident information, as well as the ability to share this information immediately with others.[62]

Patients and families have long been engaging peer support groups to cope with serious health problems.[63] The advent of online social support groups has made it easier for people to connect with others over long distances, especially when support group members may find it difficult to travel, as is the case for many people with serious health problems and hard-to-manage negative effects.[64] Research has shown that online support groups can help patients and family manage negative effects.[65] Table 15.2 lists several active and available support groups.

Online support groups allow negative effect sufferers (and their caregivers) to connect with others who are experiencing similar health issues and to share relevant information and develop strategies for managing difficult symptoms.[66] The social networking site Facebook is the dominant social networking platform, with 71% of online adults as account holders.[67] Many disease- or condition-specific open access and private/membership groups have appeared on Facebook in recent years. These groups offer information and support for patients and families with life-threatening and life-limiting health issues.[68] The asynchronous nature of these online support groups means that group members can post messages whenever they need support or information; they do not need to wait for specific group meeting times. Evidence has suggested that the information provided on these online support groups is of very high quality, and group participation provides many benefits to users.[69]

Telehealth information systems also have a long history of providing health professional advice and care to patients and families in remote areas where limited health services are available.[64] These telehealth systems have been used effectively to deliver symptom management interventions.[70] Research has shown that telehealth management interventions have resulted in significant improvements in anxiety levels and appetite for palliative care patients who may not have had access to in-person care.[71]

Table 15.2 Online Support Groups for Pain Management Information

Website	Description
http://www.drugs.com/answers/support-group/side-effect/	Drugs.com offers an online forum where users can discuss their experience with negative effects and medications.
http://www.cancer.org/treatment/treatmentsandsideeffects/complementaryandalternativemedicine/mindbodyandspirit/support-groups-cam	The American Cancer Society provides information related to the structure and topics of support groups (including online) for patients and families considering participation.
http://forums.webmd.com/3/breast-cancer-exchange/forum/4085/6	WebMD offers specialized support communities by cancer type. This forum for breast cancer offers patients an opportunity to discuss negative effects as a result of cancer and radiation, chemotherapy, surgery, and adjuvant therapies.
https://www.inspire.com/groups/cancer-treatment/topics/side-effects-of-treatment/	The Inspire Cancer Treatment online support group offers users the opportunity to discuss the impact of cancer and its treatments on their health and quality of life.

New Directions for Communication and Symptom Management

While current communication programs for the management of negative effects have been promising, we are just beginning to design and implement powerful strategic communication intervention programs for palliative care.[48] For example, the future is promising for the development of smart, interactive, and comprehensive health information systems that will travel with patients wherever they go (mobile health), automatically monitoring consumer health status (real-time data capture), sharing relevant health information with all members of the symptom management team (interprofessional coordination), and delivering symptom management support to patients and families when and where they need it.[64] The integration of artificial intelligence into the design of health information systems will allow health communication programs to interact sensitively, meaningfully, and persuasively with patients and families about symptom management needs and concerns. For instance, human-computer interfaces can be used to customize health-related reminders for patients and families and offer avatars (graphical representation of a person) that can act as relational agents by generating customized information that can be communicated to patients and families.[71] E-health information systems can be tailored to provide personalized information to patients and families based on their unique experiences and information needs.[72]

New embedded information technologies that are either worn on patient clothing or implanted within their bodies have the potential for continuously collecting physiological information that will enable proactive prediction of negative effects events and allow early response interventions to prevent suffering.[64] These imbedded information systems could be designed to deliver relevant health information to patients and stimulate their neural pathways to minimize symptoms, and perhaps even administer needed medications to sufferers. The growth of nanotechnology is making smaller and less invasive embedded information technologies increasingly feasible for use as integrated health information systems to support symptom management. For example, Abraham and colleagues tested the use of wireless pulmonary artery pressure monitoring system in patients with heart failure. They found all devices were successfully implanted and provided accurate information without serious device-related complications.[73]

The development and implementation of online palliative care training systems can help healthcare providers and patients/families develop communication competencies to support effective symptom management. Similar health communication education programs have already been designed and implemented to train healthcare providers to communicate effectively with culturally diverse, low health literacy, and low English proficiency patients (see http://ftp://ftp.hrsa.gov/healthliteracy/training.pdf). E-health systems that use sensitive and strategic health communication practices to support patients can increase both the quality of care for negative effects and enhance patient—and family caregiver—symptom management practices. Although access to technology use (particularly mobile phones) is increasing in traditionally underserved groups such as racial and ethnic minorities,[75] particular attention must be taken to ensure that symptom management support technologies are made available and accessible to vulnerable and hard-to-reach populations.[75] Moore and colleagues found that using a bidirectional text messaging system for underserved patients with chronic disease was not only feasible but improved patients' reported self-management and information awareness.[75]

Conclusion

The future for the development of health communication interventions for promoting symptom management is bright. Creative technology developers are designing new tools and programs for supporting effective health communication that will help meet the information needs of patients who confront serious negative effects and the caregivers who help them. Health technology will become a central part of effective, far-reaching, and proactive palliative care communication.

References

1. McCusker M, Ceronsky L, Crone C, et al. *Palliative Care for Adults*. 5th ed. Bloomington, MN: Institute for Clinical Systems Improvement; 2013.
2. Ledford CJW, Canzona M, Cafferty L, Virgina K. Negotiating the equivocality of palliative care: A grounded theory of team communicative processes in inpatient medicine. *Health Commun*. in press.
3. Pachman DR, Barton DL, Swetz KM, Loprinzi CL. Troublesome symptoms in cancer survivors: Fatigue, insomnia, neuropathy, and pain. *J Clin Oncol*. October 20, 2012;30(30):3687–3696.
4. Given CW, Given BA. Symptom management and psychosocial outcomes following cancer. *Semin Oncol*. 2013:40(6):774–783.
5. Meier DE, Brawley OW. Palliative care and the quality of life. *J Clin Oncol*. 2011;29:2750–2752.
6. Kreps GL. Communication and palliative care: E-health interventions and pain management. In: Moore RJ, ed. *Handbook of Pain and Palliative Care: Biobehavioral Approaches for the Life Course*. New York: Springer; 2012:43–51.
7. Simard S, Savard J, Ivers H. Fear of cancer recurrence: Specific profiles and nature of intrusive thoughts. *J Cancer Surviv*. 2010;4(4):361–371.
8. Lengacher C, Shelton M, Reich R, et al. Mindfulness based stress reduction (MBSR(BC)) in breast cancer: Evaluating fear of recurrence (FOR) as a mediator of psychological and physical symptoms in a randomized control trial (RCT). *J Behav Med*. 2014;37(2):185–195.
9. Bajwah S, Higginson IJ, Ross JR, et al. The palliative care needs for fibrotic interstitial lung disease: A qualitative study of patients, informal caregivers and health professionals. *Palliat Med*. 2013;27(9):869–876.
10. Manzanec P, Buras D, Hudson J, Montana B. Transdisciplinary pain management. *J Hosp Palliat Nurs*. 2002;4(4):228–234.
11. Burke RE, Jones J, Ho PM, Bekelman DB. Caregivers' perceived roles in caring for patients with heart failure: What do clinicians need to know? *J Cardiac Fail*. 2014(10):731–738.
12. Grant M, Sun V, Ferrell B, et al. Family caregiver burden, skills preparedness, and quality of life in non-small cell lung cancer. *Oncol Nurs. Forum*. July 2013;40(4):337–346.
13. Hudson PL, Thomas K, Trauer T, Remedios C, Clarke D. Psychological and social profile of family caregivers on commencement of palliative care. *J Pain Symptom Manage*. 2011;41(3):522–534.
14. Wittenberg-Lyles E, Goldsmith J, Parker Oliver D, Demiris G, Rankin A. Targeting communication interventions to decrease oncology family caregiver burden. *Semin Oncol Nurs*. 2003(28):262–270.
15. Donovan KA, Boyington AR, Judson PL, Wyman JF. Bladder and bowel symptoms in cervical and endometrial cancer survivors. *Psycho-Oncology*. 2014;23(6):672–678.

16. Knarr J, Musil C, Warner C, Kless J, Long J. Female stress urinary incontinence: An evidence-based, case study approach. *Urol Nurs*. 2014;May;34(3):143–151.
17. Short R, Vetter TR. Acute to chronic pain: Transitions in the post-surgical patient. In: Moore RJ, ed. *Handbook of Pain and Palliative Care: Biobehavioral Approaches for the Life Course*. New York, NY: Springer; 2011:295–330.
18. Sehgal N, Falco F, Benjamin A, Henry J, Josephson Y, Manchikanti L. Rehabilitation treatments for chronic musculoskeletal pain. In: Moore RJ, ed. *Handbook of Pain and Palliative Care: Biobehavioral Approaches for the Life Course*. New York, NY: Springer; 2011:583–614.
19. Adler B, Yarchoan M, Adler JR. Neurosurgical interventions for the control of chronic pain conditions. In: Moore RJ, ed. *Handbook of Pain and Palliative Care: Biobehavioral Approaches for the Life Course*. New York, NY: Springer; 2011:565–582.
20. Kuehn B. SAMHSA: Pain medication abuse a common path to heroin. *JAMA*. October 9, 2013;310(14):1433–1434.
21. Moos R, Brennan P, Schutte K, Moos B. Older adults' health and late-life drinking patterns: A 20-year perspective. *Aging Mental Health*. January 2010;14(1):33–43.
22. Molton IR, Terrill AL. Overview of persistent pain in older adults. *Am Psychol*. 2014;69(2):197–207.
23. Hallford DJ, McCabe MP, Mellor D, Davison TE, Goldhammer DL. Depression in palliative care settings: The need for training for nurses and other health professionals to improve patients' pathways to care. *Nurse Educ Today*. 2012;32(5):556–560.
24. Öhlén J, Wallengren Gustafsson C, Friberg F. Making sense of receiving palliative treatment: Its significance to palliative cancer care communication and information provision. *Cancer Nurs*. 2013;36(4):265–273.
25. Karademas EC, Paschali A, Hadjulis M, Papadimitriou A. Maladaptive health beliefs, illness-related self-regulation and the role of the information provided by physicians. *J Health Psychol*. August 7, 2014. Advance online publication.
26. Pollo A, Benedetti F. Pain and the placebo/nocebo effect. In: Moore RJ, ed. *Handbook of Pain and Palliative Care: Biobehavioral Approaches for the Life Course*. New York: Springer; 2011:331–346.
27. Barber F. Effects of social support on physical activity, self-efficacy, and quality of life in adult cancer survivors and their caregivers. *Oncol Nurs Forum*. September 2013;40(5):481–489.
28. Greeff A, Thiel C. Resilience in families of husbands with prostate cancer. *Educ Gerontol*. March 2012;38(3):179–189.
29. Molina Y, Yi J, Martinez-Gutierrez J, Reding K, Yi-Frazier J, Rosenberg A. Resilience among patients across the cancer continuum. *Clin J Oncol Nurs*. February 2014;18(1):93–101.
30. Disler RT, Currow DC, Phillips JL, Smith T, Johnson MJ, Davidson PM. Interventions to support a palliative care approach in patients with chronic obstructive pulmonary disease: An integrative review. *Int J Nurs Stud*. 2012;49(11):1443–1458.
31. Epstein RM, Street RL. The values and value of patient-centered care. *Ann Fam Med*. 2011;9(2):100–103.
32. Considine J, Miller K. The dialectics of care: Communicative choices at the end of life. *Health Commun*. 2010;25:165–174.
33. Schapira M, Steensma DP. Truth telling and palliative care. In: Moore RL, ed. *Handbook of Pain and Palliative Care: Biobehavioral Approaches for the Life Course*. New York, NY: Springer. 2012:35–42.
34. McCormack LA, Treiman K, Rupert D, et al. Measuring patient-centered communication in cancer care: A literature review and the development of a systematic approach. *Soci Sci Med*. 2011;72(7):1085–1095.
35. Evans BC, Ume E. Psychosocial, cultural, and spiritual health disparities in end-of-life and palliative care: Where we are and where we need to go. *Nurs Outlook*. 2012;60(6):370–375.
36. Kwon JH. Overcoming barriers in cancer pain management. *J Clin Oncol*. 2014;32(16):1727–1733.
37. Baldwin P, Wittenberg-Lyles E, Parker Oliver D, Demiris G. An evaluation of interdisciplinary team training in hospice care. *J Hosp Palliat Nurs*. 2011;13(3):172–182.
38. Campbell V. The challenges of cancer pain assessment and management. *Ulster Med J*. 2011;80(2):104–106.
39. Oishi A, Murtagh FE. The challenges of uncertainty and interprofessional collaboration in palliative care for non-cancer patients in the community: A systematic review of views from patients, carers and health-care professionals. *Palliat Med*. October 2014;28(9):1081–1098.
40. Duggan A Thompson T. Provider-patient interaction and related outcomes. In: Thompson TL, Parrott R, Nussbaum JR, eds. *Routledge Handbook of Health Communication*. 2nd ed. New York, NY: Routledge; 2011:414–428.
41. Arora NK. Interacting with cancer patients: The significance of physicians' communication behavior. *Soc Sci Med*. 2003;57:791–806.
42. Goldsmith J, Ferrell B, Wittenberg-Lyles E, Ragan S. Effective communication in palliative care. *Clin J Oncol Nurs*. 2013;17:163–164.
43. Kreps GL. The role of communication in cancer pain and symptom management. *Psycho-Oncology*. 2004;13(1):35.
44. Mazor KM, Beard RL, Alexander GL, et al. Patients' and family members' views on patient-centered communication during cancer care. *Psycho-Oncology*. 2013;22:2487–2495.
45. Wittenberg-Lyles E, Goldsmith J, Ragan SL The COMFORT initiative: Palliative nursing and the centrality of communication. *J Hosp Palliat Nurs*. 2010;12(5):282–292.
46. Meier DE, Isaacs SL, Highs E. *Palliative Care: Transforming the Care of Serious Illness*. San Francisco, CA: Jossey-Bass; 2010.
47. Green K, Tuan T, Hoang TV, Thi Trang NN, Thanh Ha NT, Hung ND. Integrating palliative care into HIV outpatient clinical settings: Preliminary findings from an intervention study in Vietnam. *J Pain Symptom Manage*. 2010;40(1):31–34.
48. Epstein AS, Morrison RS. Palliative oncology: Identity, progress, and the path ahead. *Ann Oncol*. 2012;23(Suppl 3):43–38.
49. Wittenberg-Lyles E, Goldsmith J, Parker Oliver D, Demiris G, Rankin A. Targeting communication interventions to decrease oncology family caregiver burden. *Semin Oncol Nurs*. 2003(28):262–270.
50. Sivell S, Lidstone V, Taubert M, Thompson C, Nelson A. Identifying the key elements of an education package to up-skill multidisciplinary adult specialist palliative care teams caring for young adults with life-limiting conditions: An online Delphi study. *BMJ Support Palliat Care*. March 26, 2014. Advance online publication.
51. Russ H, Giveon SM, Catarivas MG, Yaphe J. The effect of the Internet on the patient-doctor relationship from the patient's perspective: A survey from primary care. *Israel Med Assoc J*. April 2011;13(4):220–224.
52. D'Agostino TA, Ostroff JS, Heerdt A, Dickler M, Li Y, Bylund CL. Toward a greater understanding of breast cancer patients' decisions to discuss cancer-related Internet information with their doctors: An exploratory study. *Patient Educ Couns*. October 2012;89(1):109–115.
53. Simon C, Schramm S, Hillis S. Patient Internet use surrounding cancer clinical trials: Clinician perceptions and responses. *Contemp Clin Trials*. May 2010;31(3):229–234.
54. Cooley DL, Mancuso AM, Weiss LB, Coren JS. Health-related Internet use among patients of osteopathic physicians. *Am Osteopath Assoc*. August 2011;111(8):473–482.
55. Berry DL, Wilkie DJ, Thomas CR Jr., Fortner P. Clinicians communicating with patients experiencing cancer pain. *Cancer Invest*. 2003;21(3):374–381.
56. Page DB, Weaver F, Wilkie DJ, Simuni T. A computerized survey of pain in Parkinson's disease patients: A pilot feasibility study. *Parkinsonism Relat Disord*. February 2010;16(2):139–141.
57. Connelly M, Bromberg MH, Anthony KK, Gil KM, Franks L, Schanberg LE. Emotion regulation predicts pain and functioning in children with juvenile idiopathic arthritis: An electronic diary study. *J Pediat Psych*. January–February 2012;37(1):43–52.

58. Marceau LD, Smith LD, Jamison RN. Electronic pain assessment in clinical practice. *Pain Manage*. 2011;1(4):325–336.
59. Stinson JN, Stevens BJ, Feldman BM, et al. Using an electronic pain diary to better understand pain in children and adolescents with arthritis. *Pain Manage*. 2011;1(2):127–137.
60. Lalloo C, Kumbhare D, Stinson JN, Henry JL. Pain-QuILT: Clinical feasibility of a web-based visual pain assessment tool in adults with chronic pain. *J Med Internet Res*. 2014;16(5):e127.
61. Jibb LA, Stevens BJ, Nathan PC, Seto E, Cafazzo JA, Stinson JN. A smartphone-based pain management app for adolescents with cancer: Establishing system requirements and a pain care algorithm based on literature review, interviews, and consensus. *JMIR Res Protoc*. 2014;3(1):e15.
62. Johansen MA, Henriksen E, Horsch A, Schuster T, Berntsen GK. Electronic symptom reporting between patient and provider for improved health care service quality: A systematic review of randomized controlled trials. Part 1: State of the art. *J Med Internet Res*. 2012;14(5):e118.
63. Cowan P. Support groups for chronic pain. In: Moore RJ, ed. *Handbook of Pain and Palliative Care: Biobehavioral Approaches for the Life Course*. New York, NY: Springer; 2011:639–648.
64. Kreps GL, Neuhauser L. New directions in e-health communication: Opportunities and challenges. *Patient Educ Couns*. 2010;78:329–336.
65. Ruland CM, Andersen T, Jeneson A, Moore S, Grimsbø GH, Børøsund E, Ellison MC. Effects of an Internet support system to assist cancer patients in reducing symptom distress: A randomized controlled trial. *Cancer Nurs*. 2013;36(1):6–17.
66. Wright KB, Rains S, Banas J. Weak tie support network preference and perceived life stress among participants in health-related, computer-mediated support groups. *J Comp Med Commun*. 2010:15: 606–624.
67. Duggan M, Smith A. Social media update 2013. Pew Research Center. http://www.pewinternet.org/2013/12/30/social-media-update-2013/. Published December 30, 2013.
68. Greene J, Choudhry N, Kilabuk E, Shrank W. Online social networking by patients with diabetes: A qualitative evaluation of communication with Facebook. *J Gen Intern Med*. 2011;26(3):287–292.
69. Chung JE. Social interaction in online support groups: Preference for online social interaction over offline social interaction. *Comput Human Behav*. 2013;29(4):1408–1414.
70. Edirippulige S, Martin-Khan M, Beattie E, Smith AC, Gray LC. A systematic review of telemedicine services for residents in long term care facilities. *J Telemed Telecare*. April 23, 2013. Advance online publication.
71. Kreps GL, Neuhauser L. Artificial intelligence and immediacy: Designing health communication to personally engage patients and families and providers. *Patient Educ Couns*. 2013;92:205–210.
72. Klasnja P, Pratt W. Healthcare in the pocket: Mapping the space of mobile-phone health interventions. *J Biomed Inform*. 2012;45(1):184–198.
73. Abraham WT, Adamson PB, Hasan A, et al. Safety and accuracy of a wireless pulmonary artery pressure monitoring system in patients with heart failure. *Am Heart J*. 2011;161(3):558–566.
74. Kreps GL, Gustafson D, Salovey P, Perocchia RS, Wilbright W, Bright MA, Muha C. The NCI Digital Divide Pilot Projects: Implications for cancer education. *J Cancer Educ*. 2007; 22(1):S56-S60.
75. Moore SL, Fischer HH, Steele AW, et al. A mobile health infrastructure to support underserved patients with chronic disease. *Healthcare*. 2014;2(1):63–68.

CHAPTER 16

Patient Experience of Illness

Terry Altilio and Meagan Lyon Leimena

Introduction

To enter the world of illness, we invite you to immerse yourself in the landscape where sick persons and healthcare providers meet. The experience through which you understand your illness is inherently connected to your circumstances and surroundings, and, like many others, the hospital becomes the complex setting where you are ushered into the land of a specific disease state. The immersion into medical culture might include a prolonged hospital stay or a shockingly short one, a posthospital plan such as a subacute rehabilitation facility or the introduction of community-based services such as hospice. Depending on the resources of your country and community, you may not enter a hospital and be cared for in a clinic with support of healers, family, and friends, and there may be no expectation of health services at home or medications to relieve your symptoms. If you live in a country where starvation is rampant, your anorexia and fear of weight loss may not disturb others; rather, these symptoms may be met with a peculiar calm and absence of outrage that surrounds children and adults dying from starvation in your community. In cultures where shared food and meals have great meaning, your inability to eat may create turmoil much beyond the symptom itself.

Return to the image of entering a hospital with unrelenting symptoms and catastrophic thoughts about their meaning. In exchange for having a provider interpret and fix your symptoms, you surrender your clothes, privacy, personal space, and bodily autonomy to an eager or exhausted provider whose complex mission is to move from symptom to diagnosis to treatment plan in the shortest time possible. Your emotional reaction to sharing your body may vary depending on whether you think of your body as a closed, private system or an open system that links you to environment and relationship.[1] Nonetheless, the focus is on the body and may never lead to a "bridge that links, body to self and society."[1(pxiii)] You sleep in a foreign bed, share a room with a stranger, see unusual sights, hear a cacophony of sounds, and meet a flood of healthcare providers repeating questions in their well-intended efforts to establish a diagnosis. Sharing a room may be particularly comforting, or you may experience the lack of privacy as stressful and intrusive. Perhaps the gender, race, ethnicity, or age of the professionals who care for and touch you are unfamiliar or uncomfortable. Perhaps you are embarrassed, ashamed, or confused by your symptoms and disease and the anxiety, distress, or tears that you cannot control. Your time is not your own; nights and days become confused as sleep is interrupted by unfamiliar sounds or by staff, always for important purposes. Autonomous activities such as using the bathroom and taking medications must now involve forethought as you are dependent on others for assistance. If your primary language is other than that of your providers, you struggle to understand and respond as interpreters are not always available, and engaging your family to assist in translation may further assault your sense of autonomous self. No matter what language, the words providers use to describe what is happening to your body might be incomprehensible or meaningless. You may or may not feel able to ask questions consequent to your values and relationships with authority figures. Or you delay asking questions because you are truly afraid to know the answers. The familiar sights, sounds, textures, and cadence to your life are changed, replaced by the hum of an intricate institution where you are, by virtue of your presence there, defined by your illness. Your identity as a whole, composite person might feel shattered as the bits and pieces that make up the kaleidoscope of your life are suddenly out of control.

This chapter provides context and considerations for the practice of palliative care in current healthcare systems. Opportunities and challenges for palliative care providers, patients and families are examined to better understand different roles and influences on the patient's experience of illness. Theoretical frameworks are also reviewed, including explanatory models, mini-ethnographies, and the roles of language and metaphors for their utility in making sense of the experience of illness. Case narratives throughout the chapter provide illustrations of theories and their application, intervention techniques, and scenarios for careful consideration in the palliative care environment.

The Patient Experience of Illness

Patients and families enter the lives of healthcare professionals and the structures of healthcare institutions most often out of necessity. They bring their worries, symptoms, and diseases as well as their unique histories, fears, hopes, and beliefs to the systems where providers diagnose, diseases are managed, and care is provided. Just as patients hear through a distinctive filter, specialist healthcare providers listen through unique training and professional filters, which focus on diagnosis, prognostication, and treatment plans. At times the professional and institutional filters are myopic, influenced by a disproportionate emphasis on outcome or philosophies of care that cloud efforts to grasp the person's singular, lived experience of illness.

In a specialty such as palliative care, the work is both enriched and complicated by the expectation that care will be delivered through a team process where specialists have shared knowledge informed by disciplinary expertise. The roles, responsibilities, and expectations of various disciplines may enhance or deter their ability to "unpack" personal bias and judgment while eliciting and holding the illness experience. Additionally, palliative care is practiced in a variety of settings subject to influences—political, financial, and professional—that, with attention, can become less compelling and controlling to allow the purest version of patient's experience of illness. Kleinman and others encourage us to consider macro and micro, social, institutional, and political forces that influence those who provide care for patients and families. The insight gained through this kind of analysis can enhance our participation as empathic witness and enrich communication—not only in the words used but, perhaps more important, in the way we listen. Taken together, these efforts can lead to care that is patient-centered in its truest form.

Palliative care and the domains that support this specialty provide a framework for healthcare professionals that integrate disease processes and outcomes, as well as the psychological, social, cultural, environmental, and political processes informing the dynamic illness experience of patients and their families. One cannot talk about a person's experience of illness without considering the context in which it occurs. On the macro level, context may relate to access, social justice, regulation, politics, privilege, and power. At the same time, culture, language, values, and beliefs affect personhood and, on a micro level, affect institutions, healthcare professionals, patients, and families. The focus of this chapter is to bring a sampling of these variables to light so their impact might be identified and become a focus of reflection and deliberation.[2]

The narrative of Mrs. R illustrates subtle and meaningful variations in the illness experience represented through exploration of advance directives. Unique illness experiences can be a compilation of much more than disease and treatment, as they reflect an individual life in process in the setting of family, friends, and community. Acknowledgment and appreciation of the opportunities for shared understanding can create a partnership between patient and healthcare teams leading to a clearer sense of how to align patient values with the delivery of palliative care services.

The Reciprocity of Illness Experience

Mrs. R, age 65, is diagnosed with progressing amyotrophic lateral sclerosis. She is working with her team to explore advance directives and the role her adult children might play in decision-making. She chooses her sister as her healthcare agent and is reluctant to engage her children further in discussion or planning. She summarizes her decision and distress by the simple words, "I can see my own suffering reflected in their eyes," an awareness that concentrates complex feelings and opens a path to further understand and attend to both individual and shared grief and worry. Mrs. R's selection of her sister does not reflect her children's unwillingness or inability to act as her agent but rather her desire as a mother to contain the distress her illness has caused and affirm the authority and presence of her sister as a source of support to them in the future. In Mrs. R's experience of illness, the assigning of a healthcare agent has meaning much beyond the signature—it invites discussion of family structure, legacy, grief, fear, and hope in the setting of a mother with a progressive disease.

Exploring literature related to the patient experience reveals an eclectic array of authors who enrich our thoughtfulness and stimulate our curiosity as we approach the person at the core of palliative practice. Complementing the writings of these authors are the narratives of patients and families, such as Mrs. R, who live through the experience of illness. This chapter integrates ideas and perspectives from Arthur Kleinman, Susan Sontag, Anatole Broyard, and others who invite us to focus on the unique person and their world of illness. These ideas and perspectives gain further authenticity through the narratives of patients, families, and healthcare providers.

To aid in the integration of ideas, Table 16.1 defines concepts reflected and personalized through the narratives of patients, families, and healthcare professionals. A recurrent theme in this chapter is the importance of words and language, their explicit and implicit meaning, in the social exchanges occurring between providers and patients. Key concepts woven into this chapter are isolated in Table 16.1 with the goal of enhancing consideration of their meaning and implications in the practice of high-quality palliative care. Words have great power and are a currency of healthcare interactions in particular. Mindfulness about the words and concepts used in practice, education, and discussion of theory are essential to palliative care as a specialty of intention with respect for all persons.

Kaleidoscope as Metaphor

When looking through a kaleidoscope, one finds a complex, shifting pattern that seems to be an apt representation of the landscape where patients and providers move as they travel beyond diagnosis of disease to an understanding of illness. Simply put, the allure and attraction of a kaleidoscope emanates from ever-changing reflections created from mirrors, glass, and beads—patterns that are made possible within a cylindrical structure that holds and encloses the reflecting materials.[3] In the setting of a person's experience of illness, these colorful and varied patterns might represent the ecological and psycho-social-spiritual influences within which a disease process is integrated and managed over time. These engaging patterns are enriched by considerations such as language used by patients and healthcare professionals to shape the narratives, metaphors, and meanings attributed to specific diseases, including implicit and explicit judgments and assumptions about behavioral influences in such diseases as HIV and lung cancer. The external structure is formed by macro considerations, including media, politics, and culture, both personal and institutional, that undergird all social interactions. In addition to well-recognized structural influences such as time, technology, and access to care, there are more subtle social constructs such as ethnocentrism and hegemony, privileged values, and philosophies of care that may quietly impact how healthcare exchanges occur between patients and professionals. The changing images of the kaleidoscope is where the challenges, complexity, beauty, and invitation to patients themselves, their caregivers, and healthcare professionals lie. It is in the deconstructing of these images that we give form to the shadows that often infuse the patient experience of illness and the relationships with healthcare professionals.

The World of Illness and Challenge of Metaphor

In 1989 Anatole Broyard published an essay about the discovery of his prostate cancer leading to a finer appreciation of both his body and existence. Through the experience of his illness, including physical challenges and interventions leading to the relief of suffering, he developed a heightened sense of self.

> I realize of course this elation is just a phase, just a rush of consciousness, a splash of perspective, a hot flash of ontological alertness. But I'll take it, I'll use it. I will use everything I can while

Table 16.1 Key Concepts

Delegitimzation	The experience of having one's perceptions of illness systematically disconfirmed[9(p347–348)]
Disease	Alteration in biological structure or functioning; what providers create in the recasting of illness in terms of theories of disorder; the problem from the practitioner's perspective[1(p5)]
Emotional resilience	Being able to function in a steady or objective fashion while also experiencing the emotional core of provider–patient interactions
Empathic witness	Existential commitment to be with the sick person and to facilitate his or her building of an illness narrative that will make sense of and give value to the experience[1(p54)]
Ethnography	Description by an anthropologist of the lives and world of the members of a society with consideration of social and psychological themes; story that includes myths, rituals, daily activities and problems[1(p230)]
Explanatory model	Notions patients, families, and providers have about a specific illness episode[1(p121)]. Explanatory models are in response to questions about patients' perceptions, feelings, and understanding of their illness; see Kleinman's eight questions in Table 16.2.
Illness	Human experience of symptoms and suffering; how the sick person and the members of his or her family or wider social network perceive, live with, and respond to symptoms and disability[1]
Medical gaze (also clinical or observing gaze)	Process by which healthcare providers and medical institutions disaggregate the body and the personhood or sense of self[5]
Narrative humility	An approach to witnessing patient stories that acknowledges that the story belongs entirely to the patient, is subjective, and can never be fully known or understood by the healthcare professional; invites self-awareness and critique for the professional, acknowledging the inherent imbalance in the healthcare professional–patient relationship.
Patient-centered care	Care that is respectful of and responsive to individual patient preferences, needs, and values, and ensures that patient values guide all clinical decisions
Sense of coherence	Factors influencing a patient's experience of illness, including comprehensibility (events are logical and make sense), manageability (feeling that one can cope or manage illness-related events), and meaningfulness (life makes sense, challenges have purpose and it is worth meeting them)[8(p15)]
Remoralization	Clinical actions focused on gaining control over fear, coming to terms with anger at functional limitation and restoring confidence in body and self; educating sick persons; helping patients prepare for death[1(p39)]

I wait for the next phase. Illness is primarily a drama and it should be possible to enjoy it as well as to suffer it. I see now why the romantics were so fond of illness- the sick man sees everything as metaphor. In this phase I am infatuated with my cancer. It stinks of revelation.[4]

Broyard's perspective reinforces the notion that a patient's individual experience of illness is one to be honored and explored with curiosity to fully appreciate its meaning.[4] Similarly, the idea of narrative humility calls on the healthcare professional to humbly witness the patient's story as entirely his or her own and worthy of time and attention. However, at the same time, there are a myriad of challenges facing today's providers as they engage the patient's story and support the patient's experience in modern healthcare systems. In *The Birth of the Clinic*, Michel Foucault describes the concept of "clinical or observing gaze" where the patient's body and sense of self become separated by professionals working within the demands of the healthcare system. The process can be one of painful dehumanization for both healthcare professionals and patients.[5] Emotional resilience—achieving balance and perspective in the face of the physical, emotional, and practical strains of the work—might feel like a challenge for providers where pressures are often surreptitious in their effects.[6]

In her classic work, *Illness as Metaphor*, Susan Sontag explores metaphors and presents a detailed history of cancer and tuberculosis examining themes such as strength, weakness, energy, and effort and inviting readers to consider the function of disease-related metaphors on society and the illness experience of the person.[7] Sontag shows that metaphors contribute to mystery, fantasy, and fables around diseases, further isolating or objectifying those who are sick. For some, metaphoric descriptions are self-generated and represent the struggle to bring order to chaos. For others, metaphors are introduced by another—usually healthcare professionals or family members—in an effort to be helpful and to meet a shared or individual need to gain mastery in a situation of uncertainty. The challenge for palliative care providers lies in discovering the effectiveness of metaphor in a unique person's narrative: Are they comfortable or empowering? Are they incongruous with the nature of a specific person, leaving them blamed, defeated, or demoralized? For example, the war and sports metaphors often integrated into cancer language may leave many energized and inspired while leaving others isolated or compromised as they attempt to assume a posture that is incompatible with their personhood. "Losing the battle" with cancer and being "a warrior" while being offered a treatment the success of which is described as a "Hail Mary pass" may speak clearly and coherently to those for whom football and war are comfortable metaphors, but others may be left feeling isolated and confused.

A Mini-Ethnography

In exploring the choice of metaphors and the efforts of people to regain authority as they live with disease, the work of Arthur Kleinman is informative. Kleinman introduces the concept of mini-ethnography, the purpose of which is to encourage healthcare professionals to place themselves in the lived experience of patient and family, cognitively, emotionally, and with imagination.[1(p180)] He speaks of the ritual of documentation as "an act of transformation" through which symptoms and illness become disease and persons become patients. Kleinman invites providers to move beyond checklists, lab reports, and templates to recover the ability to listen with awe to the patient's words. This can lead to and beyond diagnosis to aspects of illness that form a kaleidoscopic pattern that may lead to a more appropriate plan of care.

This invitation has setting- and discipline-specific challenges. In a hospital setting, the care of patients is often shared across disciplines and specialties. The focus for primary physicians may be diagnostic, moving from symptoms to disease to treatment plan and discharge. Nurses and aides often have ongoing and intimate contact in the normal course of their work, which can provide a platform for listening to and joining with the aspects of patient experience that move beyond disease to person. Chaplains and social workers share the benefit and burden of conversation—listening and responding—as their primary tool. In some settings this role and responsibility is undervalued, especially if we allow the external structure of the kaleidoscope to control the internal patterns of practice until we no longer recognize the language, values, and focus of our work. In countries where regulations have proliferated, patients are customers, and hospice is an industry, spending time in conversation has been devalued. Yet in the palliative care world, where a priority focus has become advance directives, goals, code status, and decision-making, respecting the process and pace of patients and families is essential, given that these aspects of practice are intimately woven with culture, family dynamics, community, access to care, social justice, and spiritual and religious values. This interesting and dynamic domain of palliative care invites healthcare professionals to engage in a process that moves beyond the essential health information to explore the cognitive, emotional, social, and spiritual aspects of person and social network and to imagine the impact of this work not only in the present but also in the future family legacy.

Aaron Antonovsky developed a concept called "sense of coherence" during a study of menopausal women of different ethnic groups, which included concentration camp survivors.[8] Antonovsky focused his attention on the overall good health of some survivors, shifting from pathogenesis to salutogenesis—a focus on sickness to a focus on health and well-being. Sense of coherence has been described as:

> a global orientation that expresses the extent to which one has a pervasive, enduring though dynamic, feeling of confidence that the stimuli deriving from one's internal and external environments in the course of living are structured, predictable and explicable (comprehensibility); the resources are available to one to meet the demands posed by these stimuli (manageability) and that these demands are challenges worthy of investment and engagement (meaningful).[8(p15)]

While Antonovsky's coherence scales and concepts have not been integrated into palliative literature and the idea of predictability may seem antithetical, the additional lens of "coherence" may be a useful construct within which to frame the process and experience of illness. The ability to comprehend, manage, and find meaning interfaces with Kleinman's invitation to act as empathic witnesses and make an "existential commitment to be with the sick person and to facilitate his or her building of an illness narrative that will make sense of and give value to the experience."[1(p54)] For some, regaining a sense of coherence may come through cognitive mastery of information, while for others, placing their experience within the context of their culture, family, or spiritual belief system may be the platform from which they find mastery and meaning. The following narratives describe patient family experiences where clues to coherence range from shaving cream to tattoos.

Magic Cream

Mr. Carl is a 61-year-old Africa American admitted for pain management and "failure to thrive." He has lung cancer, for which he received many years of disease-modifying therapies. In his initial visit with the palliative consult team, there is an introductory discussion about a healthcare agent and goals of care, building upon the work begun by his oncologist. Mr. Carl chooses his brother, James, as his agent, and a family meeting is arranged. Both James and Mr. Carl are distressed. James is frustrated by his brother's lack of appetite, noting that his eating and drinking improve when he is with family. This observation is troubling as James hears a complex message—one that not only validates the importance of family but also implies that Mr. Carl's nutrition and perhaps his survival is dependent on his family's presence. James protects himself from this disarming responsibility by saying that Mr. Carl just needs to "try harder." Mr. Carl avoids eye contact and moves uncomfortably. Efforts to understand his nonverbal communication finally reveals his main priority—"I need to shave."

The palliative physician offers a razor, but Mr. Carl states that he needs his magic cream. James, in an immediate effort to please his older brother, leaves to find the shaving cream in Mr. Carl's apartment where he lives in a supportive housing complex. Goals and code status will have to wait until Mr. Carl's most important need is met. While there are many ways to interpret Mr. Carl's response, the symbolic significance of magic cream—its relationship to history, culture, generations, and dignity—becomes clear when he explains that black men with tightly wound hair shave in a particular way. Moreover, he learned this as a child "looking up" at older men—he learned by looking. James understands the symbolic significance and responds to his older brother out of love and the desire to make a difference in his life. In a rather poignant twist, James also finds hidden cigarettes in his search for the cream, which only reinforces the idea that Mr. Carl just needs to try harder. The consequent distress creates another avenue upon which to explore the cognitive appraisal and emotional responses of each man, as well as their relationship and respective grief processes. In describing James's distress, Mr. Carl calmly notes that "some habits that you learn are good ones, and others are not." Magic cream and cigarettes are symbols of coherence anchored in childhood memory. This narrative reflects the interconnection of disease, symptoms, meaning, social relationships, culture, and history and represents how the healthcare professional's response to a patient request can lead to a beginning restoration not only of a thread of coherence but also the authority of personhood.

An Illustrated Man

This patient invites exploration of illness and personal narrative through observation and curiosity about tattoos. Mr. G is 38 years old, single, and the father of two children ages 5 and 7 years. His mother and brothers are active advocates and caregivers, vigilant in their effort to protect and support. Mr. G has tattoos on his arms and legs representing religious icons, his children, and his prison experiences. As dialogue about the tattoos unfolds, the mythology surrounding Mr. G's image emerges. His identity and sense of self is informed by the images reflected—he is strong, a fighter, a father, and a devoted son with a commitment to religious ritual. The suffering of symptoms and imagining of his death and separation from his children and family is fully informed by a shared expectation that he will "fight." As his disease progresses, he is cared for at his mother's home by a hospice program. On the last night of his life and with a conscious awareness that he is dying, he reverses his do not resuscitate decision, requests that his mother call the emergency medical team, and dies in an emergency room with every effort being made to restart his heart.

A Theoretical Frame for Patients' Experience of Illness

Kleinman offers an explanatory model of illness as a foundation for understanding how the patient experiences illness episodes.[1(p121)] An explanatory model is inherently personal, shaped by an individual lens that interprets everything from the meanings of physical sensations and symptoms to chosen words and gestures. An essential aspect of this model is the patient's narrative—the opportunity to "tell their story," which might include perceptions about the attributed meaning of illness, ideas about treatment, and the disparate emotions associated with being ill. Equally important is the healthcare professional's reception of the patient's story, reinforcing the reciprocal nature of the provider–patient relationship. How a story is received, validated or invalidated, plays an important part in the patient's overall illness experience and has the potential to shape decision-making around treatment options and advance directives. Consider the power of the provider's response when a patient is sharing a story that involves socially taboo behaviors that are now associated with the physical symptoms of illness. Perhaps these symptoms are understood as punishment for behaviors such as smoking, alcohol use, or sexual activity. Imagine the significant influence a palliative care professional might have as he or she contributes to a patient's story about whether or not shortness of breath and emphysema are punishment for smoking cigarettes. Further, consider the power of consciously or unconsciously transmitted messages from healthcare professionals and family around diseases affected by lifestyle, such as diet, exercise, or habits and the potential for patients to feel judged or diminished.

Kleinman highlights the particular challenge for chronic pain patients in having their stories heard and their credibility validated by friends, family, and healthcare professionals.[1(p127–129)] The challenge of delegitimization of pain exists, especially for patients who suffer from pain of unknown etiology as they make desperate efforts to convince others of their illness experience.[9] These patients might be denied the empathy afforded to others with more obvious sources of pain and suffering, creating additional distress. The experience of not being believed can threaten one's very personhood, especially when one values integrity and finds oneself in significant pain in the setting of judgment or accusations by professionals. Patients bring their whole selves to their clinical encounters, including their experiences with power, oppression, privilege, and authority, and there is risk of generating further isolation and replicating negative experiences when suffering is not validated. At times, the "whole self" extends beyond the body and psyche to place and possessions. When this is not recognized, interventions intended to be helpful may inadvertently delegitimize the experience of others. Invitations to explore individual narratives anchored in place and possession may be discovered through questions or less traditional paths, as the two following patients demonstrate.

A Hospital Bed: Challenge to Personhood

Mrs. M is a 75-year-old married mother of four and grandmother of eight, referred for home hospice care. A social worker and nurse visit her at home and, in describing benefits offered to complement her care, they are taken aback by her distress at the idea of a hospital bed and suggestion of a home health aide. A bed in the living room will ease the challenge of walking the steps, and an aide will complement the care of family. The message of helpfulness is "heard" as a desire to change the structure of space and relationships. Placing a bed in her living room on the first floor disrupts a space that is imbued with a meaning and purpose and is incongruous with the home she has created. She will not allow a bed in the living area and intends to continue to share a bed with her husband. Offering an aide is "heard" as a message that her children are not doing a good job and a challenge to the family value that children, not strangers, care for their parents.

The Poster on the Wall

Mrs. H is an 82-year-old mother and grandmother who is Spanish speaking. Struggling with nausea, vomiting, and pain, she lies in bed, with flat affect, facing a lovely colorful poster hung by her children. Her son is eager for her symptoms to improve so she can resume dialysis. Upon request, the interpreter is asked to translate the words on the poster. The message is one of "fighting to overcome" with the expectation that hopefulness and strength will prevail—a message that seems discordant given Mrs. H's condition. A private conversation with Mrs. H reveals that she is feeling isolated and defeated by the expectations of her children as she is quite settled with the awareness she is dying. This is the beginning of necessary therapeutic work to attempt to align expectations and hopes.

In contrast to delegitimization, Kleinman calls upon each healthcare professional to serve as "empathic witness" in response to the patient's unique narrative, an important but complex task in modern medical systems with frequent challenges to time, continuity, and emotional investment in patient care. This is a call to be present and open, reserve judgment, and solicit the individual experience without immediately objectifying "the typical pain patient" or "classic case of addiction." This objectification and distancing can be seen clearly when providers refer to patients by their disease process as in "sicklers" or "addicts" and label patients by their treatments choices as "Bed 13 is a DNR." Kleinman has developed a series of questions to help healthcare professionals better elicit and understand the experiences of their patients.[10] His questions, illustrated in Box 16.1 are provided as a diagnostic invitation rather than a checklist, to explore the illness experience of the patient as a whole person in the context of his or her belief system and values. This approach provides potential to reduce confusion and look into the kaleidoscope together, rather than allowing competing interests to create distance between patient and professional.

> **Box 16.1** Kleinman's Explanatory Model Questions[10(p255–256)]
>
> 1. What do you think caused your problem?
> 2. Why do you think it started when it did?
> 3. What do you think your sickness does to you?
> 4. How severe is your sickness? Do you think it will last a long time, or will it be better soon in your opinion?
> 5. What are the chief problems your sickness has caused for you?
> 6. What do you fear most about your sickness?
> 7. What kind of treatment do you think you should receive?
> 8. What are the most important results you hope to get from treatment?

When Explanatory Models Collide—An Opportunity

Mr. Z, a low-income, divorced man with metastatic laryngeal cancer, returns to live with his mother after years of homelessness and substance use. His progressive disease has led to dependence, loss of autonomy, and a perceived reduced quality of life, and he expresses a desire to limit life-extending treatments. He chooses not to be resuscitated while hospitalized with symptoms including pain and nausea, symbolic of progressing disease. His mother, guided by strong faith and a commitment to her son's survival, disagrees and expresses the desire for escalation of all care options and full resuscitative measures. As he transitions to inpatient hospice and becomes unable to communicate, his mother remains steadfast in her commitment to keep him alive at all costs. There are significant challenges in communication and decision-making as Mr. Z declines and the hospice staff advocates for his autonomy while attempting to support a mother losing her only son. Table 16.2 explores some of the individual and system-level issues around end-of-life care from the perspectives of the patient, his mother, and the hospice staff with an explanatory model of care that invites intervention and negotiation with the goal of ameliorating suffering. Often the key to appropriate interventions and negotiation may be found in conflicting explanatory models that are unrecognized and cause enormous distress.

Empathic Witness and Beyond

Palliative care serves patients and their families along the continuum of illness embracing a wide range of serious diseases. At times, palliative teams enter at a point of crises and the work is intense and immediate. In other instances, relationships between providers and patients and families extend over a long period of time, and providers work within the grey areas of disease and implicit uncertainty. Balancing roles of participant and observer, healthcare work requires we respond to the unique experience of suffering, and contain our biases in order to discover the path most coherent with the unique values, beliefs, and history of patients and families. Just as movement of the bits and pieces in the kaleidoscope impact living with illness, so are healthcare professionals asked to respond to the changing patterns and pressures, micro and macro, with expertise, steadiness, and compassion.

As patients seek meaning in the evolving experience of illness, therapeutic modalities have been developed to enhance the expertise of healthcare professionals who join with patients and families as empathic witness and guide. For example, meaning-based therapy, dignity therapy, and schema-based interventions have all been integrated into the skill sets of palliative care providers. Meaning-based therapy begins with a person's narrative and integrates cognitive and existential strategies. Schema therapy emanates from the work of Jeffrey Young and is an outgrowth of cognitive therapy, emphasizing the adaptive or maladaptive schemas as organizing principles for understanding experience.[11] Dignity therapy is designed to assist patients in discussion of meaningful aspects of life and to

Table 16.2 Explanatory Model of End-of-Life Care for Mr. Z

Constructs	Patient	Mother	Hospice Staff
Sources of distress	Loss of quality of life and pleasure; conflict and ambiguity about honoring mother and personal wishes; desire to redeem himself in mother's eyes	Religious beliefs about sanctity of life; desire to keep son alive, make up for lost time; experience of marginalization due to poverty led to wish for all available intervention options	Concern about mother's "denial" of son's condition and commitment to honor patient's wishes; perceived selfishness in extending son's suffering
Pain experience	Trach and PEG result in physical pain; emotional distress associated with disappointing mother; anticipatory fear and anxiety related to potential pain associated with further intervention	Pain and suffering are an acceptable part of faith based life; pain is a reasonable trade-off for life and provides potential for redemption in the afterlife	Staff desire to ameliorate patient physical pain and increase medication
Communication and language issues	Disease progression limits communication; expressive facial features remain a mode of communication until they are no longer interpretable, creating additional loss for mother and leaving interpretation of pain and suffering to mother and staff	Significant distress around hospice staff's use of the word "terminal"; faith and hope language essential to her process; ambiguity fosters hope and certainty interpreted as usurping the will of God	Strong commitment to counterperceived denial and protect patient from further suffering; help prepare her for loss by using language such as "terminal" and inviting mother to "let go," which was totally incongruous with her beliefs and emotional responses

document legacy.[12] Aspects of these therapeutic systems can be woven into the everyday practice of palliative care professionals who with active listening and observational skills can identify opportunities to explore and enhance meaning and personhood. Remoralization, a concept and intervention, invites opportunities to enhance personhood and deputize existing skills and strengths to assist the patient in processing his or her illness experience.[1(p39)] Mr. F's story highlights the role of understanding and harnessing the skills and values of an individual as he or she processes illness-related changes. This can be especially useful with reframing and goal-setting in the face of changing functional and role status.

Work as a Metaphor
Mr. F is shocked by a recent diagnosis of lung cancer metastatic to his brain. Only 60 years old, he managed recurrent headaches for months until he could see a doctor and undergo a cascade of tests. Mr. F has worked as a plumber with the same company for 25 years; the sense of balance his work brings to his life and coworker relationships is essential. While he describes no family or close friends, he agrees to appoint a friend as healthcare agent, a process that challenges his preference for privacy and invites him to explore a schema of mistrust evolving from familial betrayals experienced early in life. Mr. F describes himself as independent, stubborn, and self-sufficient. He takes pride in applying the lessons of his work, namely fixing problems and understanding systems, to his life and illness. Over the course of a prolonged hospitalization, Mr. F's condition declines precipitously and he becomes angry and frustrated by his need to receive care and depend on others—a dependence that represents loss of autonomy and a shattered sense of self. The palliative social worker works with Mr. F to reframe his feelings of dependency by reviewing the relationship with his healthcare agent as one of deep loyalty and caring and offers the idea that allowing his friend to participate is not a burden but rather an opportunity and expression of their friendship. As his disease progresses, he describes feeling less of himself, unrecognizable lying in a hospital bed needing help to eat, and, on one occasion, crying in an uncharacteristic show of emotion about his inability to "solve the problems" of his disease and the loss of his work. In an effort to preserve coherence of self, he maintains a singular focus on returning home, choosing all resuscitative measures and exhausting any treatment options. Attempts to mediate goals include unitizing his valued problem-solving skills to focus on possible alternatives such as subacute rehabilitation as a path to gradual enhanced self-care. Mr. F's condition changes precipitously, and he dies alone in the intensive care unit in the presence of technology and healthcare professionals making every effort to "solve the problem" of his dying.

The Value of Story

Often the discovery of meaning and the recovery of personal authority emanates from shared stories. For many, storytelling has been an essential part of our lives since childhood. Patients, families, and healthcare professionals often use stories to master losses, recover or discover meaning, and affirm and reaffirm aspects of personhood and history in the setting of illness that forces a detour from an assumed path of one's life. In palliative care, storytelling is often the vehicle through which patients and families help healthcare professionals grasp the history, values, and experiences that inform their decision-making. Storytelling and story teaching are two interventions with formal structures and a literature to describe their use with persons who are ill.[13] Arthur W. Frank, a Canadian sociologist, writes of the significance and value of illness narratives as a path to rediscovering voice. While storytelling is often through voice or the written word, there are other interesting avenues for exploring, introducing, or sharing of a story that have meaning and provide insight to a person's choices and responses to illness.

Heaven and Hell
Mr. J is 27 years old and dying of AIDS. He has isolation precautions in the hospital and is too weak to get out of bed. When asked about resuscitation, he consistently indicates that he wants physicians to attempt resuscitation. His weakness reflects in his voice as well as his body, which makes it difficult to "hear" his fears and turmoil related to his anticipated death. He accepts an invitation to phone his sister and cousin, and, while he listens more than he speaks, he is clearly heard to say "heaven and hell" during the conversation. In a clinical leap of faith the palliative social worker respectfully and tentatively proposes that perhaps the suffering Mr. J has experienced in his life will enable him a space in heaven. Palliative care professionals preoccupied with aspects of care such as advance care planning and resuscitation sometimes mask and divert from the true and deep terrors that need to be engaged in order to join in the patient's experience of illness and perhaps influence their course.

Conclusion

The patient's experiences of illness are as unique as the images one sees when looking into a kaleidoscope: colorful, complex, rich, and evolving. Palliative care professionals are afforded great privilege by the possibility of accompanying patients, over time, through their illness journeys across settings and the continuum of illness. A central aspect of the patient's experience is their ability to tell their story and be heard, whether through a formal narrative intervention with a social worker; in a quiet moment in a hospital hallway with a nurse, physician, or chaplain; or in shared expression with a music therapist. There is power in the opportunity for healthcare professionals and patients to join together to process and make meaning out of an illness experience. By remaining open and humble, providers can create or contribute to the space patients and families inhabit within their illnesses. Sometimes this is achieved by paying attention to the environment patients create with their belongings or the words they use. Narrative can be crafted in many different ways and all are meaningful. Theoretical frameworks and therapeutic modalities exist to inform thinking, but there is also space within the specialty of palliative care for less tangible but equally valuable guidance. The ability to listen with humble openness, to offer reflection without judgment, and to be an empathic witness to the range of emotions between suffering and joy in the whole experience of illness, by the whole person who lives it, is a privilege of palliative care.

Further Reading

Campion-Smith C, Austin H, Criswich S, Dowling B, Francis G. Can sharing stories change practice? A qualitative study of inter-professional narrative-based palliative care course. *J Interprof Pract.* March 2011;25(2):105–111.

Frank, AW. *The Wounded Storyteller: Body, Illness and Ethics.* Chicago: University of Chicago Press; 2013.

Kleinman, A. Caregiving: The odyssey of becoming more human. *Lancet.* 2009;373(9660):292–293.

References

1. Kleinman A. *The Illness Narratives: Suffering, Health and the Human Condition.* New York, NY: Basic Books; 1988.
2. Hermsen MA, Ten Have HA. Palliative care teams: Effective through moral reflection. *J Interpr of Care.* 2005;19(6):561–568.
3. Kaleidoscope. In: *How Products Are Made*, Vol. 6 http://www.madehow.com/Volume-6/Kaleidoscope.html#ixzz35hirhyNN. Accessed June 20, 2014.
4. Broyard A. About men; Intoxicated by my illness. *The New York Times.* November 12, 1989. http://www.nytimes.com/1989/11/12/magazine/about-men-intoxicated-by-my-illness.html#. Accessed June 25, 2014.
5. Foucault M. *The Birth of the Clinic: An Archaeology of Medical Perception.* Sheridan Smith, AM, trans. New York, NY: Vintage Books; 1975.
6. Coulehan JL. Tenderness and steadiness: Emotions in medical practice. *Lit Med.* 1995;14(2):222–236.
7. Sontag S. *Illness as Metaphor and AIDS And its Metaphors.* New York, NY: Picador USA; 1978.
8. Antonovsky A. *Unraveling the Mystery of Health: How People Manage Stress and Stay Well.* San Francisco, CA: Jossey-Bass; 1987.
9. Ware NC. Suffering and the social construction of illness: The delegitimation of illness experience in chronic fatigue syndrome. *Med Anthropol Q.* 1992;6(4):347–361.
10. Kleinman A. Culture, illness and cure: Clinical lesions from anthropologic and cross-cultural research. *Annals Int Med.* 1978;88:251–258.
11. Parsonnet L, Lethborg C. Addressing suffering in palliative care: Two psychotherapeutic models. In: Altilio T, Otis-Green S, eds. *Oxford Textbook of Palliative Social Work.* New York, NY: Oxford University Press; 2011:191–200.
12. Chochinov HM, Kristjanson LJ, Breitbart W, McClement S, Hack TF, Hassard T, Harlos M. Effect of dignity therapy on distress and end-of-life experience in terminally ill patients: A randomised controlled trial. *Lancet Oncol.* 2011;12(8):753–762.
13. Davidson MR. A phenomenological evaluation: Using story telling as a primary teaching method. *Nurse Educ Pract.* 2004;4(3):184–189.

CHAPTER 17

Family Member Experience of Caregiving

Maryjo Prince-Paul and Karen S. Vrtunski

Introduction

Meet Sally. She is 52 years old, has been married 27 years, and works as a middle manager for a nonprofit organization in a metropolitan area in the Midwest. She is the middle child of three with an older sister living in California and a younger brother living nearby. Sally has two adult children who both live on their own, one in Texas and the other in Colorado. Sally's father and mother are 86 and 82 years, respectively. They have been married for 59 years and live in the family home in a small town about two hours away. Her father is independent while her mother has struggled for a number of years with several chronic conditions, including heart failure, hypertension, and diabetes and a most recent diagnosis of advanced lung cancer. Her mother has had two minor strokes, and her health has been slowly and steadily deteriorating, most notably in the past three years. Her father has gradually assumed more and more responsibility for meeting the couple's daily needs, like shopping and cooking, running errands, and getting to physician appointments. For everything beyond these basic functions, her parents look to Sally for help. They depend on her to arrange for housekeeping needs, to assist with managing finances, to interpret and advocate for their multiple care providers, and to advise them on how to best maintain their ability to live in their home. She has always been their "go-to girl." Sally loves her parents deeply, she adores her husband, and she enjoys her work. At the same time, she often feels that she has to choose among the three since she does not have enough time or energy to tend to her parents, to give her work her focused attention, and to spend time investing in her marriage. Plus, she finds herself feeling uncomfortable and awkward with the reversal of roles, particularly with her mother. It never even occurs to Sally that she has absolutely no time to spend with her friends, to exercise, or to read a book. She moves from one responsibility to the next and is constantly exhausted.

The National Alliance for Caregiving[3] and the American Association of Retired Persons[1] report an estimated 65.7 million caregivers like Sally make up 29% of the US adult population. These informal caregivers, who are unpaid family and friends, provide care to loved ones who are ill, disabled, or aged. The pressures of family caregiving are part of their daily life. Family caregivers monitor chronic and sometimes acute medical conditions and may provide long-term care in the home. Unfortunately, family caregivers of those with chronic and life-limiting illnesses often receive little preparation, information or support to perform their caregiving duties[4,5] and are unarmed to navigate a dynamic, complex, and challenging healthcare system. Although they often provide the most intense, around-the-clock care, the significance of their role and their own care-related needs are often overlooked. Therefore, family caregiver needs, including communication, deserve a closer look in order to improve outcomes and sustain quality of life of both caregiver and care recipient.

What Is a Family Caregiver?

To define family caregiving, we turned to several well-known national advocacy groups as well as esteemed caregiver researchers. The Administration on Aging defines a caregiver as "anyone who provides assistance to another in need."[1,6] The National Alliance for Caregiving and the American Association for Retired Persons (AARP)[1] define caregiving as caring for an adult family member or friend. Horowitz's[7] description of informal or family caregiving has been widely accepted in the research community and provides clarity about role function within the family caregiving domain. The dimensions of a family caregiver proposed by Horowitz include direct care, emotional care, medication care, and financial care. Choi and colleagues[8] identified family caregivers as eligible in their study of caregiver/patient dyads in a medical intensive care unit if they were nonprofessional and unpaid while no legal relation or cohabitation with the patient was required. Although there is not a universally accepted definition for "family caregiver," most definitions adopt a lifespan perspective that includes children and youth as both caregivers and care recipients.[9] For the purpose of this writing, we follow the consensus guidelines and operational definition of the landmark report of the National Consensus Development Conference for Caregiver Assessment, part of the National Family Caregivers Association.[2] A *family caregiver* is

> broadly defined and refers to any relative, partner, friend or neighbor who has a significant personal relationship with, and provides a broad range of assistance for, an older person or an adult with a chronic or disabling condition. These individuals may be primary or secondary caregivers and live with, or separately from, the person receiving care.[2]

The Pre-Illness Relationship

The paths to becoming a caregiver are many and varied. For some, there is a definitive moment in time—a significant event—marking the need for family to assume the caregiver role.

For example, a loved one may suddenly become incapacitated due to illness or may experience an acute, severe exacerbation of a more chronic condition that substantially increases dependence on others for support. Alternatively, the transformation to caregiving may be a more gradual process, as when a longstanding, chronic condition slowly and incrementally makes daily tasks difficult or impossible to accomplish without assistance from others. No matter the path, each individual's response to the call to care for another is unique and, to a great degree, impacted by a range of personal characteristics such as age, gender, physical health, living arrangement, cost of care, employment status, role and family relationships, and family functioning.[10] For example, if a potential caregiver is at an age and stage of life requiring care and support of children, taking on the role of caring for a seriously ill loved one may result in significant and unexpected challenges as attempts are made to balance multiple and competing demands and responsibilities.

In terms of living arrangements, while moving a care recipient into the caregiver's home may enhance safety and allow for more convenient care provision, it also carries the potential for unintended consequences for all involved due to disruptions in physical environment and household routines. Additionally, history, quality, and nature of pre-existing family roles and relationships are likely to have a significant impact on an individual's response to the demands of care, making care easier and more natural for some and more challenging for others.[10] Such personal characteristics known to influence a caregiver's capacity and willingness to take on caregiving have been described by some as *contextual*. In their updated and expanded conceptual model for the cancer family caregiving experience, Fletcher et al.[11] outlined contextual factors as one of three elements in their stress process model. In their view, "context" refers to characteristics that are well established and grounded in history, noting that some are fixed (i.e., gender, race and ethnicity, type of relationship), some are stable yet changeable (i.e., personality, living arrangements, socioeconomic status), and some are changeable depending on circumstances (i.e., physical health, work, financial well-being, social support, family functioning, relationship quality). Their model proposes a relationship among these various factors that shapes the caregiver's experience of stress in his or her role.[11] It is clear that thorough assessment of caregivers is an essential component of quality palliative care, and numerous tools are available throughout the caregiving literature.

The Changing Relationship and Changing Role

Balancing many roles, including those that are new and unfamiliar, family caregivers assume a difficult task and one that becomes more complex when faced with limited or inaccessible resources. Relationships that were once defined outside of the context of a helper relationship shift to include the new role of caregiver and become interweaved with different meanings and roles. Depending on the established family role relationship, family caregiving may present itself as stressful but normative. With feelings of obligation, family caregivers may assume these roles as part of the expectation that exists within the family unit. However, as the demands of the caregiver role exceed the multiple demands of their other social and family roles, caregivers often experience burden, distress, and conflict.

More than half of family caregivers in the United Sates are employed outside the home; these caregivers are typically early to middle-age women (average age 49 years old) caring for aging parents (average age 69 years old) while they concurrently care for their children and, in some cases, their grandchildren.[12-14] Female caregivers are more likely than males to make alternate work arrangements, such as taking a less demanding job (16% females vs. 6% males), forgoing work entirely (12% vs. 3%), or losing job related benefits (7% females vs. males 3%).[1] Young working women who are also family caregivers may suffer a particularly high level of economic hardship due to their caregiving. These demands may influence their perception of burden and increase psychological and physical distress, especially in the end-of-life setting.[15]

This duality of worker–caregiver role produces a feeling of being overwhelmed, torn between roles, and worrying about loved ones while at work. As these family caregivers continue to negotiate the balance and prioritize the "trade-offs," the effects of stress may produce family conflict and impair the way the family unit functions within its environmental context.[16] Reducing work/family conflict for employed caregivers might lower caregiver distress. It is vital that healthcare professionals proactively assess early adult caregivers in the context of their life situations, not merely their caregiving role, and to equally assess their multiple role demands.

The cancer family caregiving literature has profoundly described how relationships and roles change after a cancer diagnosis ensues. These studies have also described the role-related psychosocial (social isolation), physical (negative health effects), and communication (personal and health system) concerns that coincide with the cancer experience.[16-20] In all five studies mentioned here, the caregiver/care receiver relationship was affected as a direct consequence of assuming the caregiver role.

That said, the family's historical relationship norms, in terms of communication patterns and role, prior conflicts, social networks, relationship quality, trust, power distribution, and grief reactions to previous death experiences, influence how roles and relationships may change along the illness trajectory or as death draws near.[21] Kramer and colleagues[21] examined the extent and nature of family conflict in low-income older adults with advanced chronic disease in their last 6 months of life. Family conflict was present among 55% of the sample; consequences of this conflict included a delay in timely care planning, decreased quality of care, and increased distress among the patient, family caregiver, and interdisciplinary team.

The transition to the final stage of life is inherently difficult and largely misunderstood. Communication about the end of life remains a highly charged and difficult aspect of patient care, especially for family caregivers. One of the most difficult challenges that all family caregivers face is when their loved one begins to lose an appetite and lacks the desire to eat.[22] As with most advanced illnesses, the physiological responses of weight loss and loss of appetite are common symptoms that are part of the cachexia/anorexia syndrome. Because eating is central to the human condition, as well as culturally and symbolically important, family caregivers can experience emotional tension and distress, including feelings of anger and worry, which may ultimately lead to conflicts when loss of appetite ensues.[22–25] Palliative care providers have a unique opportunity to help guide discussions about these emotionally laden issues that bear great significance to the role and relational change that occur as illnesses progress.

When facing the inevitable terminal illness of a loved one, family members often spend considerable time reviewing painful aspects of the past with feelings of guilt, regret, shame, conflicts, or failures and a possibly a desire to repair the relationship. With the unique relationship that each patient and caregiver has, incumbent upon the strain and stress that is innate with an impending loss, family caregivers may find it difficult to effectively cope with the impending life changes, including the chronicity of care. If the relationship has been one in which indirect or passive communication was the norm, roles may be deeply entrenched, and this may result in conflict with regard to the delegation of the role responsibilities formally assumed by the ill family member. The dynamics, roles, responsibilities, and communication in times of crisis or in the face of advanced illness may exacerbate a lack of tolerance for differences in opinion, place of care, goal-setting, and advance care planning.[26] In contrast, these challenges may also offer opportunities for growth, healing, and reconciliation. Results from a study conducted by Exline and colleagues[27] with family caregivers of hospice patients suggested the importance of addressing relational conflicts and forgiveness issues—but only after assessing their importance to the family members. Although communication is at the core of end-of-life care, interpersonal hurts and offenses can be challenging to address. By drawing from research on forgiveness, interdisciplinary team members, patients, and family caregivers can gain knowledge to facilitate communication and emotional healing in end-of-life contexts.[28] Psychosocial interventions for family members who are in the midst of role transformation and learning to negotiate a new relationship with their loved one have the potential to provide sustainable support and have been shown to be most efficacious for family caregivers of chronic illnesses.[16,21]

Impact of Caregiving

As in many chronic conditions, caregiving has benefits and burdens. On the one hand, it presents an opportunity to foster interconnectedness with another human being, yet it is also associated with significant burden, change in role, increased distress, and poor health outcomes for the caregiver.

Caregiver Physical Well-Being

The most commonly reported physical effects of the illness on caregivers are sleep problems and fatigue.[29,30] Family caregivers may also experience cardiovascular effects from stress and increased blood pressure and heart rate.[31] These physiological responses may be even greater in those caregivers who witness suffering in their loved ones. Family caregivers may also be at an increased risk for infections due to the effects of stress hormones on disease processes, exacerbations of their own chronic conditions, and eruptions of previously stable autoimmune disorders.[32,33] Additionally, it has been shown that as patient illness progresses, family caregivers experience significant negative physical health consequences.[33,34] Overall, all of these studies indicate that a subgroup of family caregivers is at risk for negative physical health outcomes. High levels of caregiving demands, coupled with increased psychological distress and physiological demand, provides a fertile ground to be at risk for increased mortality. A landmark study titled "The Caregiver Health Effects Study," conducted by Schulz and Beach,[35] attempted to test the relationship between caregiving and mortality. This prospective, population-based, cohort study conducted with approximately 400 spousal caregivers and 400 matched controls suggested that a caregiver experiencing mental or emotional distress is an independent risk factor for mortality among elderly spousal caregivers.

Caregiver Social Well-Being

It may seem obvious that caregiving has an impact on one's ability to sustain social connections and engage in outside social activities—there are only so many hours in the day, and there are limits to physical and emotional energy, even for those who are strong and healthy. In their most recent survey of family caregivers titled "Caregiving in the U.S.,"[1] the National Alliance for Caregiving and AARP found that half (53%) report that their responsibility for care interferes with their time with friends and other family members, with 47% of this group further expressing high levels of emotional stress. Through periodic interviews over time with a sample of caregivers of patients with cancer, Stamataki et al.[36] found that most of the caregivers in their study experience change in their friendships and social interactions, with some caregivers admitting to self-isolation and others feeling abandoned by those around them, distressed by what they perceive as avoidance and distancing from others. Another qualitative study that examined the narratives of a small number of Swedish caregivers of palliative care patients suggests that caregivers sometimes have the sense that they have left their prior life behind without being able to find a replacement for what has been lost, a state that the authors characterize as living in liminality.[37] These caregivers express that they feel as though they live within an "existential loneliness in their caregiving roles ... it means to integrate the private with the public but, sadly at the same time, deconstruction of the self into a nothingness."[37(p282)]

Caregiver Psychological Well-Being

Palliative care providers are all too aware of the impact that caregiving can have on one's emotional health—they see the effects in their everyday interactions with patients and families. What may be less obvious is how to identify individuals at risk for negative effects, as well as how to prevent, mitigate, and at the very least support caregivers as they struggle to balance the many demands of their lives. With approximately 61.6 million people in the United States providing care for an adult with limited functional ability some time during 2009, at an estimated value of $450 billion,[38] increasing our understanding of the mental health needs of caregivers is critical not only for individuals providing care but also for care recipients and the entire palliative care system.

Researchers are beginning to look more closely at the psychological side of caregiving. Since 1988, in every study that Northouse and her research team have conducted, family caregivers have reported receiving less emotional support than patients.[30,39,40] This program of research provides stark data to support that family caregivers lack the support they need to deal with their own emotional distress. Their examination of quality of life and mental health of caregivers of outpatients with advanced cancer[41] identified a relationship between better quality of life for caregivers and better caregiver mental health, well-being of care recipient, and absence of caring for other dependents. Additionally, they found that caregiver mental health was worse for female caregivers, for those caring for patients with worse emotional health, for those spending more time in caregiving, and when the caregiver experienced changes in employment.[41]

A small, qualitative study of caregiver dyads examined how each experienced and managed various tasks and changes associated with advanced illness.[26] The interviews with patients and caregivers suggest a three-part process—suffering, struggling, and settling. The authors describe suffering as having physical, emotional, and spiritual components, offering that suffering can be shared by both and/or can be reciprocal in nature. The struggling phase is characterized by movement between enduring and fighting, while settling is experienced as a shift to more acceptance and focus on comfort as opposed to cure. These three phases are not viewed as linear; rather, it is suggested that patients and caregivers seem to move back and forth between suffering and struggling, with the settling phase more likely to be achieved if certain conditions are present, such as receiving clear and consistent health status information, trust of providers, acknowledgement that illness is terminal, engagement in advance care planning, and having social and spiritual support.[26]

Others have suggested that each caregiver be approached from an individualized and unique perspective. The work of Montgomery and Koslowski[42] emphasizes the uniqueness of each caregiving situation, cautioning healthcare providers to resist the temptation to generalize even the most credible, evidence-based caregiver research results in too broad a fashion. They suggest that consideration be given to a collection of individual circumstances and experiences. For example, how one comes to be a caregiver, expectations surrounding the care situation, specific cultural and historical factors present within a particular family, and, not insignificantly, how an existing role relationship between caregiver and care recipient (i.e., daughter and mother) is transformed through the process of providing care. They propose that assuming the role of caregiver requires not only a change in one's behavior (i.e., performing care tasks) but also a shift in the definition of the relationship with the care recipient—resulting in the creation of a new role identity for the caregiver. When this new role and resulting care responsibilities conflict significantly with what the caregiver perceives her or his role should be, the result is role incongruence and distress for the caregiver. The authors also state that a caregiver experiencing this kind of role incongruence has three possible courses of action toward resolution: (a) change caregiving behavior to be more consistent with existing role definition, (b) change self-appraisal and reframe beliefs around the role and tasks of caregiving, or (c) embrace a new identify that better aligns with the caregiving role and resulting care responsibilities.[42]

Family Caregiving, Positive Responses, and Benefit Finding

The positive effects and rewards resulting from the caregiving experience are not as well identified or systematically evaluated. Being a family caregiver may be distressing and involve burden, but, at the same time, the caregiving role may offer an opportunity to experience a renewed sense of accomplishment and an overall sense of strength and purpose. In a recent study conducted by Henriksson et al.,[43] palliative family caregivers reported being helpful to their loved ones, recognizing the experience as a privilege, and perceiving the ability to bring happiness during a difficult time. Levels of caregiver self-esteem, confidence, and competence mediate the relationship between care-related stress and poor psychological well-being.[43,44] Kim and colleagues[45] identified six domains of benefit finding associated with 896 family caregivers of cancer survivors, including a greater acceptance of things, increased empathy, a greater appreciation of others, closer family relationships, improved self-awareness, and a renewed prioritization of goals.

However, most studies that have paid attention to the positive aspects of the family caregiving have been conducted with bereaved family caregivers, and thus a retrospective view has been examined.[46] Because these results may be reflective of the family caregivers reconstructed meaning of the situation, (e.g., diminishing the negative and highlighting the positive aspects), this should be recognized as a limitation to a generalized understanding of benefit finding and positive responses in a concurrent family caregiving experience.

Although these data are encouraging and aim to shed light on the positive rewards of caregiving, Stajduhar et al.[47] suggests that healthcare providers should use caution in explicitly encouraging caregivers to think positively, as this action may have a harmful effect on those caregivers who are already strained by the caregiving experience. Both the challenges and rewards of caregiving should be considered when the healthcare provider is tailoring interventions; positive responses within the context of communication should support and strengthen the caregiver–care recipient relationship.

Situational Factors Impacting the Caregiver Experience

In spite of the evidence that caregivers want and need adequate and effective support from healthcare professionals, findings from AARP[48] paint an alarming picture of the caregiver condition. In a survey of 1,677 family caregivers across the United States, nearly half (46%) of family caregivers reported performing medical and/or nursing tasks for loved ones with multiple chronic physical and cognitive conditions, tasks that may include overseeing complex medication regimes, handling mobility assistive devices, operating specialized medical equipment, providing wound care, and managing incontinence. More than half of these caregivers also reported that they provide this support because other options were not available. Caregivers also reported that they receive either very little or no training to prepare them for these complex tasks, in spite of emergency department visits and hospital stays.

Both patients and caregivers identify practical support and financial help as major unmet needs.[49] Assistance in paying for care may be available for patients meeting certain physical and financial requirements. Many disease-specific associations (e.g., Alzheimer's Association, American Cancer Society, Leukemia and Lymphoma Society, Amyotrophic Lateral Sclerosis/ALS Society) provide information and resources specifically geared toward caregivers. The Veterans Health Administration is an additional resource for financial assistance in paying for care (e.g., Aid and Attendance Pension).

While the social and emotional costs of caregiving may be difficult to quantify, the impact on financial well-being is quantifiable. Key results from a report recently published by MetLife Mature Market Institute[50] include concerning statistics: (a) one-fourth of adult children provide personal care and/or financial assistance to a parent, a figure that has tripled in the past 15 years; (b) an estimate of aggregate lost wages, pension, and Social Security benefits for these caregivers is almost $3 trillion; (c) for women, it is estimated that leaving the labor force early due to caregiving responsibilities results in $142,693 in lost wages, $131,351 in lost Social Security benefits, and $50,000 in lost pensions for a total of $324,044; men experience $89,107 in lost wages, $144,609 in lost Social Security benefits, and $50,000 in lost pensions for a total of $283,716.[50]

AARP recently recommended policy actions to encourage more financial support for caregivers; these include (a) ensure that new models of care under the Affordable Care Act speak to "person and family-centered care planning," (b) improve the Family and Medical Leave Act by requiring paid leave for caregivers, (c) increase funding for the National Family Caregiver Support Program, (d) protect family caregivers from the negative impact on Social Security benefits that results from reducing leaving employment to provide care, and (e) promote new models of care that include partnership and assistance for family caregivers.[38] Advocacy at the local, state, and national level is needed to encourage policymakers to take these and other recommendations to heart.

As previously outlined, reducing work hours or leaving the workforce results in significant and long-lasting costs for a caregiver. In addition to outlining the reality of these costs, a MetLife report encourages more awareness and action for companies around the challenges that their caregiving workers experience, suggesting that they make provisions for adequate retirement planning, offer accommodations to employees who provide care to a loved one, and promote self-care opportunities for workers.[50] It is encouraging that several companies and organizations have joined together with the common commitment of addressing employed caregiver challenges. The National Alliance for Caregiving recently joined with the Respect a Caregiver's Time (or ReACT) to identify workplaces with innovative practices and policies designed to address and support their caregiving employees.

Caregivers seem hungry for information and guidance from the healthcare system that can support them in their role. Van Ryn and colleagues[51] studied caregivers of newly diagnosed cancer patients and discovered that nearly half of the caregivers reported needing, but not receiving, training for administering medications, managing nausea and pain, changing dressings, and managing other physical symptoms. In addition to these clinically meaningful results, family caregivers also wanted more information about how to deal with their loved ones' emotional concerns, including depression, anxiety, and uncertainty. Efforts to develop and deliver family caregiver education, training, and assistance are numerous, giving rise to questions regarding the effectiveness of current efforts. In a review of the literature, Ventura et al.[49] found that palliative care patients and caregivers report a range of unmet needs, including those involving communication, spiritual and psychosocial, practical, informational, and respite needs, along with needs due to isolation and loss of autonomy. A notable finding from their synthesis across 15 studies was that patients and caregivers alike identified open communication with healthcare providers more frequently than any other need.[49] Continued advocacy is greatly needed in order to encourage the routine integration of useful, practical techniques for communication throughout education and training curricula for all healthcare professionals (i.e., physicians, nurses, social workers, home care aides, therapists, and other allied health professionals).

Family Assessment Tools

The ability of the healthcare professional to identify, involve, assess, plan, and intervene with the family caregiver is paramount to improve outcomes and quality of life. Caregiver assessment is an essential component of the comprehensive care of the patient and family unit, including the assessment of frail elders and adults with chronic or limited life expectancies, particularly dementia.[2]

With the potential for such a range of personal and contextual factors to influence a caregiver's experience, the importance of comprehensive, holistic, and ongoing assessment of a caregiver's strengths, challenges and resources cannot be overemphasized. A complete, thorough assessment of the psychosocial needs of both the patient and the family is a critical point for determining effective interventions, even (or perhaps especially) at times of crisis. It is essential to establish a fundamental understanding of the patient and family, what they see as their needs, and where the healthcare provider can be most useful in meeting those needs. Elements of a thorough caregiver assessment include caregiver physical, emotional, and cognitive capacity; family communication patterns; language preferences and degrees of literacy; family cultural values, beliefs, and practices; family experiences with illness and loss; family psychosocial and financial supports; family behavioral and mental health; risk of abuse, neglect or exploitation; and goals of care.

Table 17.1 identifies a sample of assessment tools specific to the family caregiver. However, it is important to note that none of these instruments address all of the major dimensions of family caregiver needs that have been identified in the literature: cognitive/informational, communication, daily activity, emotional, financial/legal, medical, social/relationship, and spiritual needs.[52] Moreover, quality tools are not available to provide good measures of communication for family member experiences, and current measures mostly include a singular item to assess communication, focusing primarily on information. Much more work is needed in this area.

Table 17.1 Family Caregiver Assessment Tools (Selected Examples)

	Author	Intended Measurement	Communication Context	Number of Items	Population	Internal Consistency
Needs Assessment of Family Caregivers-Cancer (NAFC-C)	Kim et al.[52]	Family caregivers' needs across stages of survivorship phases	2 items: "talking to him/her about his/her concerns"; "communicating with his/her medical staff"	27 (four dimensions, eight subfactors)	Caregivers of cancer survivors	$\alpha = .56–.86$
Caregiver Competence Scale (CCS)	Pearlin et al.[58]	Caregivers' perceived adequacy of performance	0 items	4	Caregivers of patients with dementia; caregivers of patients in palliative care	$\alpha = .86$
Rewards of Caregiving Scale (RCS)	Archbold and Stewart[60]; Hudson et al.[59]	Rewards of caregiver learning; rewards of being there; rewards of meaning for oneself	1 item: "Is just *being there* for him/her rewarding?"	10 (three subscales)	Caregivers of patients with dementia	$\alpha = .93$
Family Assessment Collaboration to Enhance End of Life Support (FACES)	Townsend, Ishler et al.[61]	Caregiver strain and resources in families	1 item: "I have someone I can confide in abut my experiences caring for my relative/friend"	23	Family caregivers of older adults receiving home hospice services	Not reported
Preparedness of Caregiving Scale (PCS)	Archbold et al.[62]	Caregivers' readiness to provide care	0 items	8	Caregivers of frail, elderly persons living at home; caregivers of patients in palliative care	$\alpha = .93$

Evidence-Based Interventions for Family Caregivers in Palliative Care

A number of evidence-based interventions for enhancing the caregiving experience are available for use in the delivery of palliative care. We have summarized four such approaches in Table 17.2. Among the interventions available, we chose to highlight these because of their unique approach, the inclusion of communication as an intervention and/or outcome, and the robust nature of their testing.

Future Directions and Conclusion

Family caregivers represent the backbone of health and social care delivery in countries throughout the world, including Western or developed countries. Family caregivers, as well as those receiving care, must be considered an integral part of the interdisciplinary healthcare team and should be involved in all components of healthcare management and care-related decisions. As we look to the future, leaders in the medical, nursing, social work, and allied health professions should examine curricula and clinical fellowships to determine how they are acknowledging, assessing, supporting, and training family caregivers. Educational, clinical, didactic, technical, and communication skills are needed. Healthcare providers are at the helm of professional care provision and will need to serve as leaders in practice settings to advocate for family caregivers and identify and provide evidence-based interventions.

Future research is also needed to tease out the complexities of specific communication needs and tailored interventions, as well as health and quality of life outcomes of family caregivers. According to the International Palliative Care Family Career Research Collaboration, part of the European Association for Palliative Care, research priorities in family caregiving must take shape in order to guide clinical practice.[53] Results from a recent survey conducted by this group suggest the following priority research areas: intervention development and testing, minority and rural caregiver groups, access to services, unmet needs, bereavement, experience and implications of the caregiver role, and development of assessment tools.[53]

From a public policy perspective, some have recommended improvements to the Family and Medical Leave Act in the United States, which has been in existence for more than two decades now as a way for workers in organizations/companies with 50 or more employees to have up to 12 weeks of unpaid leave for personal illness or to care for an ill family member without putting their jobs or benefits in jeopardy. Some suggest that the act needs to be expanded to cover relationships not currently recognized under the law, to provide paid leave for caregiving in addition to job and benefit protection, and to provide protection when an employee's care responsibilities continue beyond 12 weeks.[38] Moreover, state and federal policymakers should proactively consider requesting family caregivers to assist in the development of new models of care that focus on care coordination, quality improvement, and reimbursement. Most important, though, all providers and payers should recognize that the unit of care is the care recipient and the family caregiver. This builds on the foundational principle of the hospice and palliative care movement that has long embraced the patient/family as interdependent care.

Table 17.2 Evidence-Based Interventions for FCGs

	Purpose	Population	Duration	Protocol	Intervention Strategies	Outcomes
Bowman et al.[54] Coping and Communication Support	To affect quality of care and quality of life outcomes for FCGs from diagnosis through end of life	132 FCGs for patients with advanced cancer	6 weeks	1. Randomized controlled study 2. Initial meeting in-person and follow-up primarily by telephone with 24/7 availability	Supportive listening; education; cognitive problem-solving; validation; case management; behavioral; Web-based guidance; referral	FCGs had few physical and psychosocial difficulties; did not report high levels of burden; reported caregiving demands most frequently as problematic throughout 6 weeks of protocol
Montgomery et al.[55] Tailored Caregiver Assessment and Referral®	To enhance practitioners' skills in effectively and efficiently targeting services to benefit FCGs	266 FCGs; 52 care managers	9 months	Randomized controlled study; initial and up to 3 follow-up interviews at 3-month intervals;	Six-step process: conduct assessment; transfer key information to summary sheet and score/interpret; follow decision algorithm to identify goals, strategies, and resources targeted to their needs/preferences; consult with caregiver to review/discuss; create care plan from assessment and discussion; conduct follow-up assessment at 3-month intervals	Intervention-group FCGs experienced significant decrease in scores on all areas measured over time while control-group FCGs had an increase; Intervention-group FCGs had substantially lower levels of depressive symptoms
Northouse et al.[56] FOCUS (Family Involvement, Optimistic Attitude, Coping Effectiveness, Uncertainty Reduction, Symptom Management)	To improve appraisal variables, coping resources, symptom distress, and quality of life in men with prostate cancer and their spouses	235 patients with prostate cancer and their spouses	12 months	Randomized controlled study; baseline assessment with follow-up at 4, 8, and 12 months	Supportive-educative program; three 90-minute home visits and two 30-minute telephone sessions, spaced two weeks apart, delivered between baseline and 4 months; 5 core areas: family involvement; optimistic attitude; coping effectiveness; uncertainty reduction; symptom management	Intervention patients reported less uncertainty, better communication with spouses at 4 months only; intervention spouses reported higher quality of life, more self-efficacy, better communication, less negative appraisal of caregiving, less uncertainty, less hopelessness, less symptom distress at 4 months with some effect sustained to 8 and 12 months
Porter et al.[57] Coping Skills Training (CST)	To provide coping skills training for patients and FCGs together to (a) enhance FCG's interpersonal communication around illness and care, (b) encourage ongoing reinforcement for newly acquired coping skills; (c) enhance FCGs' confidence in their ability to help the patient cope	233 patients with lung cancer and their FCGs	8 months	Randomized controlled study with intervention group receiving CST, control group receiving education/support; telephone sessions with patient and FCG dyad; frequency of sessions tapered from weekly to biweekly to monthly	1. Progressive muscle relaxation; relaxation mini-practices 2. Pleasant imagery; activity-rest cycle; cognitive restructuring 3. Problem-solving 4. Pleasant activities 5. Communication; smoking cessation; maintenance enhancement strategies Education/support basic information on lung cancer; treatment of lung cancer; nutritional needs; physical comfort measures; medical approaches to pain/symptom management; palliative care; hospice care	Both groups saw improvements with CST; most beneficial in cancer stages II and III and education/support more beneficial in stage I

Note. FCG = family caregiver; CST = Coping Skills Training.

References

1. Caregiving in the U.S.: Executive Summary. National Alliance for Caregiving and AARP. http://assets.aarp.org/rgcenter/il/caregiving_09_es.pdf. Published November 2009. Accessed January 2, 2015.
2. National Family Caregivers Association Website. http://www.caregiveraction.org/ Accessed October 2, 2014.
3. National Alliance for Caregiving Website. http://www.caregiving.org/ Updated 2011. Accessed July 7, 2014.
4. Northouse LL, Katapodi MC, Song L, Zhang L, Mood DW. Interventions with family caregivers of cancer patients: Meta-analysis of randomized trials. *CA Cancer J Clin*. 2010;60(5):317–339.
5. Tamayo GJ, Broxson A, Munsell M, Cohen MZ. Caring for the caregiver. *Oncol Nurs Forum*. 2010;37(1):E50–E57.
6. Administration on Aging Website. http://www.aoa.gov/. Accessed June 18, 2015.
7. Horowitz A. Family caregiving to the frail elderly. *Annu Rev Gerontol Geriatr*. 1985;5:194–246.
8. Choi J, Hoffman LA, Schulz R, et al. Health risk behaviors in family caregivers during patients' stay in intensive care units: A pilot analysis. *Am J Crit Care*. 2013;22(1):41–45.
9. Talley RC, Montgomery JV, eds. *Caregiving Across the Lifespan: Research Practice Policy*. New York, NY: Springer; 2013.
10. Given GW, Given BA, Sherwood P, DeVoss D. Early adult caregivers: Characteristics, challenges, and intervention approaches. In: Talley RC, Montgomery JV, eds. *Caregiving Across the Lifespan: Research, Practice, Policy*. New York, NY: Springer; 2013:81–104.
11. Fletcher BS, Miaskowski C, Given B, Schumacher K. The cancer family caregiving experience: An updated and expanded conceptual model. *Eur J Oncol Nurs*. 2012;16(4):387–398.
12. Musil C, Warner C, Zauszniewski J, Wykle M, Standing T. Grandmother caregiving, family stress and strain, and depressive symptoms. *West J Nurs Res*. 2009;31(3):389–408.
13. Conway-Giustra F, Crowley A, Gorin SH. Crisis in caregiving: A call to action. *Health Soc Work*. 2002;27(4):307–311.
14. Jayani R, Hurria A. Caregivers of older adults with cancer. *Semin Oncol Nurs*. 2012;28(4):221–225.
15. Burns CM, LeBlanc TW, Abernethy A, Currow D. Young caregivers in the end-of-life setting: A population-based profile of an emerging group. *J Palliat Med*. 2010;13(10):1225–1235.
16. Williams A, Bakitas M. Cancer family caregivers: A new direction for interventions. *J Palliat Med*. 2012;15(7):775–783.
17. Morgan MA, Small BJ, Donovan KA, Overcash J, McMillan S. Cancer patients with pain: The spouse/partner relationship and quality of life. *Cancer Nurs*. 2011;34(1):13–23.
18. Williams A, McCorkle R. Cancer family caregivers during the palliative, hospice, and bereavement phases: A review of the descriptive psychosocial literature. *Palliat Support Care*. 2011;9(03):315–325.
19. Lowson E, Hanratty B, Holmes L, et al. From "conductor" to "second fiddle": Older adult care recipients' perspectives on transitions in family caring at hospital admission. *Int J Nurs Stud*. 2013;50(9):1197–1205.
20. Clemmer SJ, Ward-Griffin C, Forbes D. Family members providing home-based palliative care to older adults: The enactment of multiple roles. *Can J Aging*. 2008;27(3):267–283.
21. Kramer BJ, Boelk AZ, Auer C. Family conflict at the end of life: Lessons learned in a model program for vulnerable older adults. *J Palliat Med*. 2006;9(3):791–801.
22. Wallin V, Carlander I, Sandman P, Ternestedt B, Håkanson C. Maintaining ordinariness around food: Partners' experiences of everyday life with a dying person. *J Clin Nurs*. 2014;23(19–20):2748–2756.
23. Johansson AE, Johansson U. Relatives' experiences of family members' eating difficulties. *Scand J Occup Ther*. 2009;16(1):25–32.
24. Locher JL, Robinson CO, Bailey FA, et al. Disruptions in the organization of meal preparation and consumption among older cancer patients and their family caregivers. *Psycho-Oncology*. 2010;19(9):967–974.
25. Raijmakers NJ, Clark JB, van Zuylen L, Allan SG, van der Heide A. Bereaved relatives' perspectives of the patient's oral intake towards the end of life: A qualitative study. *Palliat Med*. 2013;27(7):665–672.
26. Meeker MA, Waldrop DP, Schneider J, Case AA. Contending with advanced illness: Patient and caregiver perspectives. *J Pain Symptom Manage*. 2014;47(5):887–895.
27. Exline JJ, Prince-Paul M, Root BL, Peereboom KS. The spiritual struggle of anger toward God: A study with family members of hospice patients. *J Palliat Med*. 2013;16(4):369–375.
28. Exline JJ, Prince-Paul M, Root BL, Peereboom KS, Worthington EL, Jr. Forgiveness, depressive symptoms, and communication at the end of life: A study with family members of hospice patients. *J Palliat Med*. 2012;15(10):1113–1119.
29. Miaskowski C, Dodd M, Lee K, et al. Preliminary evidence of an association between a functional interleukin-6 polymorphism and fatigue and sleep disturbance in oncology patients and their family caregivers. *J Pain Symptom Manage*. 2010;40(4):531–544.
30. Northouse L, Williams AL, Given B, McCorkle R. Psychosocial care for family caregivers of patients with cancer. *J Clin Oncol*. 2012;30(11):1227–1234.
31. Monin JK, Schultz R, Martire LM, Jennings JR, Lingler JH, Greenberg MS. Spouses' cardiovascular reactivity to their partners' suffering. *J Gerontol B Psychol Sci Soc Sci*. 2010;65B(2):195–201.
32. Rohleder N, Marin TJ, Ma R, Miller GE. Biologic cost of caring for a cancer patient: Dysregulation of pro- and anti-inflammatory signaling pathways. *J Clin Oncol*. 2009;27(18):2909–2915.
33. Bevans M, Sternberg EM. Caregiving burden, stress, and health effects among family caregivers of adult cancer patients. *JAMA*. 2012;307(4):398–403.
34. Vitaliano PP, Zhang J, Scanlan JM. Is caregiving hazardous to one's physical health? A meta-analysis. *Psychol Bull*. 2003;129(6):946–972.
35. Schulz R, Beach SR. Caregiving as a risk factor for mortality: The Caregiver Health Effects Study. *JAMA*. 1999;282(23):2215–2219.
36. Stamataki Z, Ellis JE, Costello J, Fielding J, Burns M, Molassiotis A. Chronicles of informal caregiving in cancer: Using "the cancer family caregiving experience" model as an explanatory framework. *Support Care Cancer*. 2014;22(2):435–444.
37. Dahlborg Lyckhage E, Lindahl B. Living in liminality—being simultaneously visible and invisible: Caregivers' narratives of palliative care. *J Soc Work End Life Palliat Care*. 2013;9(4):272–288.
38. Feinberg L, Reinhard SC, Houser A, Choula R. Valuing the invaluable: 2011 update: The growing contributions and costs of family caregiving. AARP Public Policy Institute; 2011. http://assets.aarp.org/rgcenter/ppi/ltc/i51-caregiving.pdf. Accessed June 18, 2015.
39. Northouse LL. Social support in patients' and husbands' adjustment to breast cancer. *Nurs Res*. 1988;37(2):91–95.
40. Northouse LL, Mood DW, Montie JE, et al. Living with prostate cancer: Patients' and spouses' psychosocial status and quality of life. *J Clin Oncol*. 2007;25(27):4171–4177.
41. Wadhwa D, Burman D, Swami N, Rodin G, Lo C, Zimmermann C. Quality of life and mental health in caregivers of outpatients with advanced cancer. *Psycho-Oncology*. 2013;22(2):403–410.
42. Montgomery R, Kosloski K. Caregiving as a process of changing identity: Implications for caregiver support. *Generations*. 2009;33(1):47–52.
43. Henriksson A, Carlander I, Arestedt K. Feelings of rewards among family caregivers during ongoing palliative care. *Palliat Support Care*. 2013:1–9.
44. Hudson P, Thomas T, Quinn K, Cockayne M, Braithwaite M. Teaching family carers about home-based palliative care: Final results from a group education program. *J Pain Symptom Manage*. 2009;38(2):299–308.

45. Kim Y, Schulz R, Carver CS. Benefit-finding in the cancer caregiving experience. *Psychosom Med.* 2007;69(3):283–291.
46. Wong WK, Ussher J, Perz J. Strength through adversity: Bereaved cancer carers' accounts of rewards and personal growth from caring. *Palliat Support Care.* 2009;7(2):187–196.
47. Stajduhar K, Funk L, Toye C, Grande G, Aoun S, Todd C. Part 1: Home-based family caregiving at the end of life: A comprehensive review of published quantitative research (1998–2008). *Palliat Med.* 2010;24(6):573–593.
48. Reinhard SC, Levine C, Samis S. Home alone: Family caregivers providing complex chronic care. AARP Public Policy Institute; 2012. http://www.aarp.org/content/dam/aarp/research/public_policy_institute/health/home-alone-family-caregivers-providing-complex-chronic-care-rev-AARP-ppi-health.pdf. Accessed June 18, 2015.
49. Ventura AD, Burney S, Brooker J, Fletcher J, Ricciardelli L. Home-based palliative care: A systematic literature review of the self-reported unmet needs of patients and carers. *Palliat Med.* 2014;28(5):391–402.
50. The MetLife study of caregiving costs to working caregivers. MetLife Mature Market Institute; 2011. https://www.metlife.com/mmi/research/caregiving-cost-working-caregivers.html#key findings. Accessed June 18, 2015.
51. van Ryn M, Sanders S, Kahn K, et al. Objective burden, resources, and other stressors among informal cancer caregivers: A hidden quality issue? *Psycho-Oncology.* 2011;20(1):44–52.
52. Kim Y, Kashy DA, Spillers RL, Evans TV. Needs assessment of family caregivers of cancer survivors: Three cohorts comparison. *Psycho-Oncology.* 2010;19(6):573–582.
53. Hudson PL, Thomas K, Trauer T, Remedios C, Clarke D. Psychological and social profile of family caregivers on commencement of palliative care. *J Pain Symptom Manage.* 2011;41(3):522–534.
54. Bowman KF, Rose JH, Radziewicz RM, O'Toole EE, Berila RA. Family caregiver engagement in a coping and communication support intervention tailored to advanced cancer patients and families. *Cancer Nurs.* 2009;32(1):73–81.
55. Montgomery RJ, Kwak J, Kosloski K, O'Connell Valuch K. Effects of the TCARE(R) intervention on caregiver burden and depressive symptoms: Preliminary findings from a randomized controlled study. *J Gerontol B Psychol Sci Soc Sci.* 2011;66(5):640–647.
56. Northouse LL, Mood DW, Schafenacker A, et al. Randomized clinical trial of a family intervention for prostate cancer patients and their spouses. *Cancer.* 2007;110(12):2809–2818.
57. Porter LS, Keefe FJ, Garst J, et al. Caregiver-assisted coping skills training for lung cancer: Results of a randomized clinical trial. *J Pain Symptom Manage.* 2011;41(1):1–13.
58. Pearlin LI, Mullan JT, Semple SJ, Skaff MM. Caregiving and the stress process: An overview of concepts and their measures. *Gerontologist.* 1990;30(5):583–594.
59. Hudson PL, Aranda S, Hayman-White K. A psycho-educational intervention for family caregivers of patients receiving palliative care: A randomized controlled trial. *J Pain Symptom Manage.* 2005;30(4):329–341.
60. Archbold P, Stewart B. *Family Caregiving Inventory.* Portland: Oregon Health Sciences University; 1996.
61. Townsend AL, Ishler KJ, Vargo EH, Shapiro BM, Pitorak EF, Matthews CR. The FACES project: An academic-community partnership to improve end-of-life care for families. *J Gerontol Soc Work.* 2007;50(1–2):7–20.
62. Archbold PG, Stewart BJ, Greenlick MR, Harvath T. Mutuality and preparedness as predictors of caregiver role strain. *Res Nurs Health.* 1990;13(6):375–384.

CHAPTER 18

Family Caregiver Communication Goals and Messages

Joy Goldsmith

They were unusually close. And unusually happy. After 18 years of marriage, Suze could recall only one fight with Red—that occurred over a missing box of envelopes. Their days were spent trying to get to one another in the evenings for long, leisurely sessions of cooking, dinner, and planning for a less hectic and more enjoyable early retirement. They liked each other deeply and enjoyed each other with abandon. Suze held heavy responsibility for her invalid 69-year-old mother and had done so for a decade. Gale, her mom, was an alcoholic, six feet tall, and weighing under 80 pounds. She was bed-bound but happy in her house, working crosswords, and spending the days with her dog.

Introduction

The story of Suze unfolds over the course of this chapter. Her goals, communication needs, and decisions made with healthcare providers are clearly driven by her family and her relationships. Likewise, this chapter features the importance of the family but particularly the family caregivers who are placed by circumstance and family systems in the decision-making position for loved ones who are seriously, chronically, or terminally ill. Embedded throughout the chapter, the eight domains within the National Consensus Project's[1] document, titled *Clinical Practice Guidelines for Quality Palliative Care,* are highlighted. Underscored within this framework is the positioning of family care and caregiver communication that is central to the work of palliative care.

- Domain 1: Structure and Processes of Care—Emphasizes the importance of the interprofessional team in coordinating palliative care. Unique to palliative care is the clinical importance of "engagement and collaboration" among team, patient, and family.
- Domain 2: Physical Aspects of Care—Promotes proactive assessment and management of physical symptoms. Attention to these symptoms requires communication effectiveness that is inclusive of family caregiver involvement.
- Domain 3: Psychological and Psychiatric Aspects—Stresses the significance of collaborative assessment and including the patient and his or her family in these discussions so their goals of care can be articulated and honored.
- Domain 4: Social Aspects of Care—Stresses the importance of interprofessional engagement to support the existing processes and skills of a family.
- Domain 5: Spiritual, Religious, and Existential Aspects of Care—Underscores the significance of the interprofessional nature of the care team, especially those in chaplaincy service, to assess and coordinate spiritual care, honoring spiritual/religious rituals and practices of patients and families.
- Domain 6: Cultural Aspects of Care—Requires that healthcare teams understand and honor the patient/family culture, including linguistic competence, and promote services that accommodate each unique family's cultural background.
- Domain 7: Care of the Patient at the End of Life—Emphasizes interprofessional communication and documentation of the signs and symptoms of impending death. Of particular importance is guiding the family in knowing what to expect in the death and post-death processes.
- Domain 8: Ethical and Legal Aspects of Care—Features advance care planning, including ongoing discussions about goals of care with patients and especially family caregivers.

Each of these eight domains either implies or explicitly articulates the exigency of attending to the family caregiver(s) in attaining excellence in palliative care. Central ideas about family goals, family patterns, and caregiver types follow a review of the state of the science about family communication concerning goals and interaction in the context of palliative care. The story of Suze and Red highlights the central chapter themes, including transitions and goals of care, private information in families, patterns of communication within families, and finally a new typology of caregivers and supporting resources for healthcare professionals.

After an early retirement from local banking, Red was enjoying the experience of designing, managing, and caring for his now three-year-old vineyard. This would be the enterprise that would allow Suze to retire early. The last several years featured weekends full of extra work and no time for rest. But they were on the brink of experiencing the first season of a fully functioning winery.

On a cool February afternoon, Red and his business partner, Blare, were placing a final row of steel stakes into the ground for additional spring planting. Red was using a post-pounder to force the steel into the earth. In one swift move, Red clipped the top of a post with the bottom of the pounder, sending the device crashing into the left side of his head. Though no one knew at the time, skull fractures severed two arteries, causing a catastrophic and irreversible epidermal hematoma to the left parietal area of the skull. Blare knew the accident involved the post-pounder but only caught sight of the accident from the side. Red fell to the ground, unconscious for a few moments, and then came around and walked to the nearby truck under his own power.

Suze was chatting with visitors at the winery. Blare came in and told her that Red had been in an accident and that she should drive him to the ER to get checked out. Blare assured her that Red was talking and lucid. She was pleased to find this was the case when she reached Red in the truck.

On the way to the community hospital ER, she was scared and nervous. Suze playfully tested him on her birthday, their anniversary date, what he had for lunch. He was lucid, and this gave her comfort. Red seemed unsure about what had occurred in the accident. He wondered if he had hit some electrical source during his work, as his left arm was jolted on the ride with a racing paralyzing pain. He complained of pain on the left side of his head. She tried to rub it, and he pulled away. She felt a slight, hard ridge but no bump was visible—no swollen rise in the tissue.

Once in the ER, they were quickly moved to an examination room. Red complained more and more of pain and a profound sense that something was very wrong. Suze went in the hall to ask for more help. When she returned, he was drenched with sweat. His last words were, "Something is wrong. I need help." He never regained consciousness.

Centering Family Communication in Palliative Care

Patients and family caregivers enduring a terminal or chronic illness or, in Red's case, a terminal event, share a unique interdependent relationship. A serious diagnosis or sudden injury frequently leads to increased interaction between family members and the potential for shifting roles.[2-4] Each individual affects the other; therefore, healthcare teams should treat and assess the family caregiver and the patient together as one dyad. Patients and caregivers who experience communication challenges or fail to effectively communicate are at risk for poor health outcomes.[5] Insufficient communication can cause proxy decision-makers to experience disagreement in making decisions or render them unable to provide medical care that is satisfactory and consistent with the patient's preferences.[6-8]

Scholarship exploring the experience of family during illness and terminality posits five major themes central to patients and their caregivers: sensitive communication is number one.[9] Studies exploring illness as a family experience assert that communication is one of the important constructs in the function of family.[10-12] Research also indicates that communication between family caregiver and patient is lacking in satisfaction and effectiveness.[4,13]

Not only do family caregivers and patients express a desire for improved communication, but communication is a proven contributing factor in several health outcomes.[4,14] Negative biomedical outcomes based on ineffective communication include depression, feelings of abandonment, weight gain, increased alcohol intake, and reduced physical activity.[5] Positive communication outcomes include better pain management, fewer conflicts with physicians, improved decision-making, and an overall state of mental well-being.[15,16]

Family caregivers are less confident in navigating the emotional needs of patients and more comfortable with physical needs. Family conflicts and features of communication can emerge or become exaggerated in the context of illness. The growing role of the family caregiver has given rise to typology research addressing family management and coping[17] as well as family functioning[18] in the context of palliative care. Family communication difficulties are frequent, such as differing communication styles, hiding feelings from each other, avoiding particular topics, and the re-emergence of previous conflicts.[16] Few theory-based tools have been developed to allow healthcare professionals to assess communication patterns or styles of caregivers or patients.[4,15] Understanding family goals, family privacy needs, and communication patterns would lead to better understanding, problem identification, assessment of unmet needs, and overall improved support for both the family caregiver and patient.

Family members play an influential role in decisions about palliative care, impacting the selection of clinicians, hospital, and treatment options.[19-21] Families must negotiate communicative tasks such as treatment side effects, schedules, and allocating family responsibilities.[22] Family caregivers are vital collaborators during cancer care, because they often provide patient information (e.g., medical history, patient preferences), receive directions from the healthcare team (e.g., medication instructions, care tasks to be done), and facilitate communication between the patient, healthcare providers, and other family members.[23-25] Northouse and colleagues found a significant reciprocal relationship between cancer patients and their caregivers when it comes to emotional distress.[5]

Clinical communication with caregivers is also considered instrumental in establishing and promoting caregiver quality of life.[26] Caregivers endure immense demands and reduced quality of life, which is correlated with a sense of inadequacy and lowered self-efficacy, causing higher levels of distress than their ill loved one experiences.[27] Caregiver burdens include a sense of isolation, the pressure to produce hope for the patient and family, guilt over feeling angry about demand load, loss in witnessing the degradation of the patient, and resentment when they are not valued or are taken for granted.[28] As patient symptom burden increases and physical functioning decreases, caregiver burden rises.[5] Similarly, a caregiver's quality of life is a product of overall physical, psychological, social, and spiritual well-being.[29,30] By exploring the ability of the family caregiver to understand the diagnosis and provide care, the professional healthcare team can ensure that the caregiver's concerns are also recognized and addressed.[15]

As healthcare delivery shifts away from inpatient settings, patients are sent home from difficult and often toxic treatments with little or no trained healthcare; instead, they are left to rely on an informal family caregiver.[16] Family caregivers now perform the caretaking administration once performed by a healthcare professional. While some are well suited, many family caregivers lack the preparation and confidence to administer care yet find themselves central to the complex logistics and care coordination for their loved one.[15,31,32] Research has proven that assuming the role of caregiver leads to feeling distressed and overloaded, which decreases a caregiver's emotional, physical, social, and spiritual well-being.[4,5]

Multiple Goals

Goals of care and navigating the desires of patient/family are central to successful palliative care. A discussion of patient/family uncertainties can reveal multiple goals and dilemmas about goals that are tied to uncertainty. Attempting to understand what the competing goals are for caregivers and patients, and what goals have not yet been realized, is a powerful tool in supporting care decisions. Once uncertainty is acknowledged and conflicting goals are identified, healthcare professionals can better assist the patient and family in making goals of care decisions.

Multiple goals theory is based on the idea that everyone is navigating more than one objective within any communication event. At the minimum, any individual is simultaneously attempting to achieve tasks as well as engage/manage relational goals. For example, if a family caregiver is navigating a loved one's shift from a critical care ward to a rehabilitation facility, his or her interaction with a nurse will include communication that addresses the nuts and bolts of time and cost but also the connection shared with that very nurse. In short, within the course of an interaction, people have more than one purpose; this is the basic premise of goal multiplicity.

Embracing goal multiplicity accepts that goals and conversation are tightly intertwined and that people almost always want more than one thing when they engage in interaction together.[33] Every person accomplishes, or attempts to accomplish, multiple goals in interactions. Sometimes these goals are emergent, and sometimes people enter an interaction knowing very clearly what they need/want to achieve. The strategies that people use to manage and accomplish these goals remain ambiguous and of special interest to communication researchers, especially in the context of health.

These identity/relationship concerns become their own cluster of goal multiplicity in an interaction. New goals also emerge as each speaker/partner makes certain conversational moves throughout the course of interaction. Because communicators pursue multiple and often competing goals, problems and dilemmas can be common in interaction. Add to this the context of palliative care, and unexamined, unrealized, and conflicting goals quickly become confounding for family caregivers charged with decision-making responsibilities.

Decisions about goals are based on relationships, level of uncertainty, and/or a need to reduce uncertainty.[33] Multiple goals need to be recognized. Listening to what the patient/family have to say and the questions they ask presents rich narrative information concerning goal pursuits and uncertainty. Goal multiplicity is common to everyone; however, family patterns are specific to individual family structures. Attending to the specifics of a family's use of information, as well as their communication patterns, can inform the way goals are understood and pursued by the palliative care team.

Communication Privacy Management

A CT scan was performed within minutes of Red losing consciousness at the ED, and he was directly airlifted to the nearest trauma center for brain surgery. Following soon after by car, Suze arrived to find a young woman from their hometown awaiting her in the neurosurgical trauma center. Now addressed as Dr. Schmidt, this young woman from Suze's hometown had become a neurologist and indicated she had seen Red's scan. She assured Suze that he would do well in surgery. Suze, relieved, caught her breath and felt hopeful in her wait. The surgery was not long—a few hours. A surgeon came to meet with her. A man in a green suit jacket—someone she immediately identified as the chaplain, accompanied him. And then her life changed.

The surgeon advised Suze that Red had suffered a severe traumatic injury to the brain and that he would likely never recover and was showing all the indications of brain death. He recommended that she withdraw life support. Suze asked if there was even a chance that he could recover—even a 1% chance. The surgeon stared back and said, "Yes, there is a 1% chance I suppose." And then he left. He never inquired about Suze or took additional time to be present in the delivery of this bombshell news. As far as Suze knew during her wait, Red would recover. The chaplain then approached her. She was devastated, in complete shock, and furious that the chaplain was sent to communicate compassion on behalf of the surgeon. She couldn't get away from him fast enough. Over the next 36 hours, the chaplain approached her two more times, and finally she directly told him not to engage her further.

The intimacy of palliative care creates an environment for frequent and even unsolicited patient and family disclosure of very personal and private information. Every healthcare professional makes decisions about how to navigate private family information and also how to use it. Communication privacy management outlines how individuals become owners of private information and how this ownership impacts private disclosures.[34]

Family members can stand in shock as physicians or other clinicians share the chronic or terminal status of a loved one. When the physician leaves, it can be the nurse, social worker, or chaplain who is left to explain the unfolding information, answer questions, and help families process the meaning of a change in health status. As such, team members impact the actual *process* of telling and revealing the *content* of private information, as well as facilitate an understanding of meaning for people connected to that private information.[35]

It is not uncommon for family or patient to ask healthcare team members to share or withhold private health information, such as a diagnosis or a recurrence, or a change in status or care plan.[36] Families have a relational history of avoiding or engaging difficult topics or speaking indirectly or directly about serious topics. The decision to reveal private information about the disease, disease trajectory, and/or prognosis can create a privacy dilemma.[37] When a privacy dilemma occurs, team members are placed in a challenging situation with potential communication difficulties.

Consider the following circumstance. When private information is given to a social worker, such as a diagnosis the patient is not capable of comprehending, the social worker is given the tasks of interpreting the information, carrying the burden or responsibility of knowing the information, and delivering the message to others.[37] In essence, team members take on a unique role within each family, as they steward private health information in the delivery of palliative care.

Communication conflicts can emerge as family members try to protect a patient or other family member from private information. It is not unusual for families to request that the use of palliative care and hospice services be withheld from the patient.[36] Families sometimes instruct healthcare providers not to mention diagnosis/recurrence, not to tell the patient he or she will not recover, and not to talk about transitions to different care locations including hospice in front of the patient.[38] There are instances in which honoring these requests can create less effective palliative care for patients and their families. The need to recognize culturally driven goals is imperative in understanding some privacy requests[39] and navigating those cultural needs while delivering the best care possible.

Often, the coordination of what is acceptable and what is not between individuals is unclear, and privacy expectations clash. In the case of Suze and Red, Suze clashed with the chaplain in his attempts to provide support. Including him in the prognostic conversation and his following overtures to discuss life-support withdrawal violated what Suze thought was acceptable. The culture of cure can reconfigure previously established privacy rules within a family. Differing communication expectations about private information creates turbulence, especially in the context of terminal news disclosures.

Once an individual tells someone private information, that individual assumes responsibility for that information (i.e., they must decide if they will keep it secret or share it with others). The presence of the chaplain in the terminal diagnosis disclosure meeting between Suze and the surgeon made it clear that he was now a sharer of this private information. Healthcare teams manage one-on-one and group boundaries of private information. When a patient is chronically or terminally ill/diagnosed, each family member itemizes different elements that become private in the midst of knowing a loved one is changing/dying. These communication dynamics merge with a family member's goals for the patient, for the life of the family, for the caregiver him or herself—profoundly affecting the care that is ultimately delivered to the patient. Goals, private health information, and the communication climate of the family itself shape the way difficult news is processed and the ways in which it is translated into decision-making for the caregiver(s).

Family Communication Patterns

Because of the variation in communication valued and established within a family, the ways in which family members talk to each other about illness and loss exemplifies a family's particular and established communication climate.[40] Family communication patterns theory details how family conversation (what is shared and how frequently it is shared) and family conformity (sharing family values, attitudes, and beliefs) range from high to low to form four specific family communication patterns.[41-45]

First, families have rules that govern appropriate topics for family conversation. Family conversation can vary from free, spontaneous interaction between family members (high) to limitations on family topics and time spent communicating with each other (low).[12] Families with high family conversation patterns tend to talk openly about death, dying, cancer, and illness. Families with high communication prior to the disease maintain the pattern throughout the illness, as the situation underscores preexisting interaction patterns.[46] On the other hand, families with low family conversation patterns engage less frequently, or not at all, in discussions about illness/trauma and have a more difficult time making care decisions and executing transitions in care. By avoiding talk about illness/loss, some family caregivers feel they are protecting the patient or other family from sad conversations, as noted in the previous section.[40] Notably, families who have a history of family communication constraints, such as topics that have been prohibited and/or roles in the family that are intractable, are more likely to experience family conflict during serious illness.[47]

Second, the dimension of conformity establishes and protects the hierarchy or structure in a family. Family members with high conformity feature uniform beliefs and family values emphasizing family harmony. Harmony and roles/positions in the family are prioritized above all else. Specifically, hierarchical roles within the family are often emphasized over conversation and disclosure. Conversely, families with low conformity have less emphasis on obedience to parents/elders and more emphasis on specific situational needs or changes.[48]

> In a state of shock, Suze only knew that she had to give Red a chance to prove he would not recover. She asked for two more CT scans over the course of the next two weeks and told herself that if these tests were not demonstrating progress of any kind, she would withdraw support.

> Blare, Red's partner and Suze's brother, wanted to be supportive and present for Suze. But Suze preferred to navigate these decisions alone, as she had always done with her mom's care. In doing so, she relied on her own relationship with Red to guide the twists and turns of three weeks of decision-making and waiting. Red would not want to live in a compromised state. Over and over she remembered the surgeon saying that 1% was always a possibility. With the compassionate care and skill of several trauma nurses, Suze decided to withdraw life support. She did not consult with family. Despite the presence of Red's siblings, Suze acted alone in making her decision about his care.

Suze and her family can be placed into the family communication pattern that features minimal conversation and high defenses around roles and attitudes. High conversation and high defenses produces family communication that is frequent but protects immovable attitudes and beliefs within a family. In a family that instead possesses high conversation and low conformity, many things are discussed with frequency, as family members work less to protect the "way things are" and use communication to share multiple perspectives and differences. Finally, some families have a lack of coordination and connection. They share minimal interaction and differ vastly in their beliefs, attitudes, and role understanding.

> Red's life support was withdrawn in the brain trauma care unit. Bryan, the nurse with whom Suze had shared most of her thinking, brought blankets for Red. Finally, his feet could be warmed and covered. They were no longer a barometer that told the story of his failing organs. Bryan acquired a soft chair from the waiting

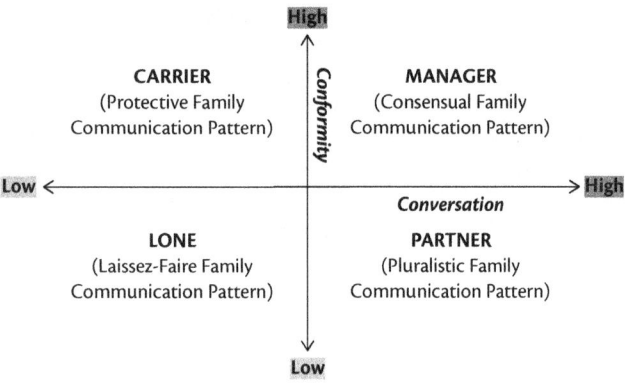

Figure 18.1 Caregiver communication typology

room and forced it into the small space around the bed. After 4 hours of standing, Suze finally sat down. Bryan had described to her what changes she might see in Red and that there was no way to estimate how long it would take him to die after withdrawal. Bryan brought her water, juice, and some food and asked every time if she thought Red was in pain. As his breathing became labored, Suze would answer "yes"—yes, she did think he was in pain. Bryan increased the morphine with each discussion. Red's respirations became erratic and his legs strained, as his breathing became increasingly shallow. After 13 hours of vigil, several minutes would pass between respirations. Suze could not watch anymore. She knew Red was gone. She had not slept in 72 hours. With Bryan's support, she chose to leave before Red was pronounced dead.

Caregiver Types

The family patterns of conversation and conformity are extended into a caregiver communication typology intended to produce practical interventions for family caregivers and their healthcare teams.[49,50] The article establishing the typology identifies four types (Carrier [low conversation high conformity]; Manager [high conversation high conformity]; Lone [low conversation low conformity]; Partner [high conversation low conformity]) that correlate with the previous section about family communication climates/patterns. See Figure 18.1 for a visual representation of how the patterns conjoin with the concept of caregiver types, as well as Table 18.1 for characteristic responses of each type.

Carrier

Carrier caregivers emerge from a family characterized by low conversation and high conformity. Relying heavily on the patient to determine caregiving decisions, the role of the Carrier is highly dependent on family obligation to provide care. The Carrier emphasizes the willingness and practice of providing total care *for* the patient as designed *by* the patient. When talking about topics that are avoided and suppressed with the patient, the Carrier consistently identifies avoidance concerning dying and death topics. Carriers also exhibit a heavy reliance on and compliance with healthcare orders. In the following, Dan is an example of a Carrier.

Dan's wife had left him and their daughter, Julianna, when she was only three. Since then, he had been the primary parent and had done everything to fill the roles of both mom and dad. At birth, Julianna was healthy, but her mother presented with the first signs of Huntington's disease. After some years of struggling with her diagnosis, she removed herself from the family. Now at age 29 and in the fifth year of her own Huntington's diagnosis, Julianna was experiencing frequent hospitalizations and struggling to manage her prescribed medication regimens. Dan wanted to make Julianna as happy as possible, having watched her suffer with a terminal illness and knowing about the difficult existence of her mother. In the latest crisis, Julianna refused a new treatment protocol, and Dan accommodated her wishes. In a conversation with her long-time physician, Dan shared that he wanted to follow Julianna's wishes and support whatever choices she made.

As a Carrier caregiver, Dan met with the healthcare team and protected Julianna's wishes, though these communication behaviors did not facilitate the best care for her. The healthcare team could have benefited this family unit by meeting with Dan, understanding his goals and communication about his daughter's illness, their lives outside of the illness, and supporting his caregiving style with interventions that focused on Dan's role as her sole parent.

Manager

Manager caregivers develop in families with high conversation and high conformity. The Manager caregiver becomes the

Table 18.1 Caregiver Types and Common Response

Caregiver Assessment[a]	Caregiver Type	Common Response
To provide the very best patient care, I also need to pay attention to my patient's caregivers. Can you tell me a bit about how you are feeling/doing?	Carrier	I'm fine. I'm worried about how best to take care of him or her.
	Manager	I feel good. I feel like we have a game plan for moving forward.
	Partner	I've been so worried and so stressed, but I have support.
	Lone	I'm a mess. I can't get any help from anyone.
Do you have your own physician? Is he or she aware of your caregiving situation?	Carrier	My family has been going to Dr. X for a long time, and she knows what's going on.
	Manager	Yes, I have a physician. But this is not about me. It's about my mom.
	Partner	I have a great family doctor but I haven't had a reason to see her.
	Lone	I don't usually see a doctor unless I have to.

[a] Based on Adelman RD, Tmanova LL, Delgado D, Dion S, Lachs MS. Caregiver burden: A clinical review. *JAMA*. 2014;311(10):1052–1060. doi: 10.1001/jama.2014.3

family medical expert. As one patient explained, she took a supplement encouraged by her caregiver because "he's pretty much my doctor." Physician credibility is important, yet manager caregivers dominate high conversation topics by focusing on their own knowledge and decisions.[51] The caregiver's research role usurps patient or other family member preferences, and high conversation is fortified by the caregiver's display of evidence as well as personal credibility. Overprotection of the patient is a common byproduct of high conformity and can truncate the ability of the patient to process his or her own health information and life changes. Though this caregiver emerges from a family pattern that is high conversation, the range of topics can be restricted by the high level of conformity; "There are no decisions to be made . . . we all just agree," a patient might say of his or her caregiver. Consequently, high conformity is sustained by the advocacy and research role of the Manager caregiver.[51] Inclusive discussion about care plans, treatment choices, and dying do not generally occur. Jules is a Manager caregiver.

> Jules had taken care of her mother from the start. A long-time smoker and overeater, Layla had suffered from multiple comorbidities since Jules was a teenager. Of the four children, Jules was the oldest and had always provided physical and social support to help her mom through the challenges of diabetes, high blood pressure, chronic bronchitis, and now end-stage COPD. Early on, Jules became highly skilled at navigating doctor's appointments, clinicians, and the day-to-day care at home. As Layla's health declined, Jules read that the use of oxygen could weaken the COPD patient if provided too early in the disease process, and the longer the delay in using this support, the longer the patient's lifespan. She let the rest of the family know this discovery and that she would let the medical team know their intent to delay this intervention at the next appointment.

By circumstance, Jules was the Manager caregiver in this family dating back to her early youth. She emerged as the decision-maker and leader. The pattern had only intensified as her mother's constellation of health issues widened. The Manager, like Jules, concludes that a certain care choice will happen, regardless of other family or patient ideas and in spite of the healthcare team. In short, the Manager can be the most formidable challenge of all caregiver types. This family and patient benefit from engagement by the team. The team can create communication circumstances in which other ideas and questions can be voiced, such as a family meeting. The Manager needs affirmation, but the concerns of other family members as well as the patient also need attention.

Lone

Lone caregivers derive from families with low conversation and low conformity. In other words, this family type has little time or shared experience together. These caregivers focus on hope found in biomedical treatments and typically, have lower health literacy and sole responsibility in all aspects of patient care.[49] The Lone caregiver sees his or her role as a biomedical task. Patients describe Lone caregivers as preoccupied with eating schedules and medicine administration. The patient and caregiver rarely share conversation about pain, quality of life, or advance directives. Rather, they rely on instructions provided by the healthcare team. Low conversation is compounded by overreliance on a physician-based plan of care decisions. There is less need to discuss disease process, plans/place of care, or quality of life concerns, as the physician's recommendation is considered best for the patient. Other family members do not play a role in the day-to-day care of the patient, because this family shares almost no communication or ritual/role structures. Given the (a) reliance on physician decision-making and (b) tendency to passively receive medical decision-making from the healthcare team, as the patient's illness recurs or worsens, Lone caregivers report being unsatisfied with their healthcare experiences[51] once in bereavement. This caregiver type experiences burden well beyond the other three types, has little identity outside of his or her loved one's illness, and experiences a very low quality of life. Van is an example of this type of caregiver.

> Van had fallen in love with Jake, an Iraqi war veteran who suffered from profound posttraumatic stress disorder and all of its related costs, including alcohol and drug dependence. Unmarried, Van attempted to care for Jake without family support from either side. Jake had two previous wives and two children from his first marriage. His father lived nearby but offered little support. The stability in his care came from the local Veterans Administration, especially behavioral health. One nurse and one social worker were essential to his day-to-day progress and survival. After a routine blood draw, Jake was diagnosed with leukemia. Van immediately took up the additional weight of this new medical challenge but with no additional support or resource to aid her. She often felt defensive with the behavioral health support team and was suspicious of the treatment options presented by the oncology team.

Van had no support from family to distribute and share caregiver burden. Like most Lone caregivers, this left her with little time and energy to attend to anything but Jake's myriad health challenges. She functioned with lower health literacy due to burden and lack of time. Because of her disconnected family experience and solitary efforts of care, Van was not skilled at partnering or trusting the healthcare team. Attending to the caregiver with a force of interventions including counseling, respite, and end-of-life planning is essential for caregivers such as Van.

Partner

Partner caregivers come from families with high conversation and low conformity. In these families, the patient is highly involved in the direction of the care but is not an individual actor in the decision-making process. The subject of dying and death are part of the conversations within this family. As a patient described a five-year prognosis, she noted "I have my cremation taken care of . . . put me in there whenever you're done looking at me in the box." Caregivers of this type describe pliability in the pursuit of care tasks and responsibilities.[51] Unique to the Partner is the inclusion of personal burden in his or her talk with the patient and other family members. Including a topic this sensitive underscores the range of conversation topics embraced by this family pattern, as well as an ability to navigate conflict and difference. Partners have the distinction of partnering well with healthcare teams. Ozzie's daughters are an example.

> Ozzie, a survivor of D-Day, was suffering late-stage dementia, in addition to end-stage lung cancer. His three daughters phoned or met daily to plan meal rotations and, more and more frequently,

the rotation for nighttime care. The oldest daughter took the lead but relied on the others for schedule support, financial support of their father, and feedback about ideas concerning home health and hospice. Ozzie was not coherent and had not been for several months. The family had navigated two house fires, one catastrophic, as a result of Ozzie's smoking. He could no longer stay at home alone. His food and liquid intake was waning dramatically. The daughters were open about their dad's slowing functions and how they wanted better care for him than the care their mother had experienced 10 years earlier. Ideas and resources shared by the team's social worker gave the daughters tremendous support, as they entered the final phase of Ozzie's life and considered end-of-life challenges. They frequently sought out feedback from their dad's healthcare team and were eager to take on new ways of working together.

All family patterns and caregiver types experience high conflict and anxiety during chronic, serious, and terminal illness/trauma. The Partner caregiver typically demonstrates resilience due to the frequency of interaction and the sharing of roles and tasks within the family unit. In this family, the caregiver finds a place for difference, discussion, negotiation, and, most important, change. Ozzie's oldest daughter had a variety of support from her siblings, as they shared tasks and skills. But most notably, this family sought out ideas and team strategies from the professionals caring for their loved one. Like Ozzie, the patients of this type of caregiver are given attention in terms of their spiritual and social well-being not at the expense of their physical needs but in a manner that richly recognizes aspects of quality of life not present for other caregiver types.

The Family Caregiver Communication Tool

Family care can be improved with attention to family communication and caregiver types. For a family with a Manager caregiver, healthcare team communication with family members beyond that of the lead caregiver is important in discovering other perspectives and needs in the family system. For example, during family meetings, team members can be assigned to various family members with the aim of representing multiple needs at the meeting. Carriers benefit from mediation of patient–caregiver communication. Team members should assist with discussions as well as encourage the Carrier to seek support inside and outside of the family to process the work of caregiving. Partners benefit from healthcare teams that have clearly established care procedures and decision-making. This kind of caregiver does partner with the team itself. Lone caregivers require intervention by all team members. Information and resources should be prioritized and spiritual and social support emphasized.

As an outgrowth of the caregiver research detailed in this chapter, the Family Caregiver Communication Tool (FCCT) can help healthcare teams identify types and employ targeted family caregiver interventions for families that have a palliative-appropriate patient. The FCCT is a cognitive measure of communication patterns dependent upon the frequency, range, and congruence of communication within the family. The two dimensions of family conversation and family conformity are operationalized in a brief series of questions that can be easily scored. Family caregiver conversation includes (a) the frequency of interaction and (b) the range of topics discussed in interactions about caregiving and care decisions. Family congruence includes conformity in attitudes, values, beliefs, and roles exhibited by family members in the context of caregiving. The goal of FCCT is to ascertain a caregiver's communication pattern and specific caregiver type.

Conclusion

Clinical imperatives of a typology of caregiver communication include giving providers an awareness of caregiver type and most appropriate caregiver support, as this may improve caregiver/patient quality of life and outcomes. Access to caregiver-specific training and support in order to mitigate caregiver burden and provide the most appropriate communication intervention is currently an area of necessity.[52] Scholars assert that intervention by healthcare professionals is required to help family caregivers recognize their own needs for outside help.[53] Thus it is essential that efforts be focused on socializing caregivers into their roles in a manner that normalizes intervention and aid from appropriate and targeted sources (see Table 18.2 for digital communication interventions to support caregivers).

Palliative care communication is in its infancy. Controlled trials and communication-centered outcomes are still required to accurately understand and create the most useful communication interventions for caregivers. The FCCT and caregiver typology is positioned to capture reliable data and move systematized work of caregiver communication interventions forward.

Caregiver education represents a current and future opportunity for creating and enacting communication interventions to advance the work of palliative care. Northouse et al.[5] finds that interventions to enhance caregiver knowledge and coping increases caregiver self-efficacy and quality of life. Empowering family caregivers with the knowledge about this typology and other resources will increase opportunity, coping, and health literacy, as the family increasingly assumes the weight of patient care responsibilities.

Based on this and the indexing research on caregiver types, the creation of a caregiver communication tool for use by clinicians and eventually caregivers can move this research to team-based palliative care contexts. Similarly, if patient and caregiver are treated as one unit as the Consensus Guidelines suggest, a system change initiative that includes a plan of care for the family caregiver could be initiated as normative practice in palliative care.

. . .

Coda

Days, weeks, and months after Red's death, Suze revisits over and over her feeling of being abandoned by the surgeon. Her lingering angst centers on the communication shared with him. She feels strongly that the surgeon avoided her and increased the trauma of making the choice to withdraw life support sooner by providing the "1%" escape hatch. It was all on her—to allow Red to die. This thought is her unsettled anxiety in bereavement: that she had to remove support and end his life alone.

Table 18.2 Family Caregiver Digital Resources

Resource	Description	Website	Google Play Link
Cancer Terms Pro: A Comprehensive Oncology Glossary	Database of thousands of oncology terms and definitions	https://itunes.apple.com/us/app/cancer-terms-pro-a-comprehensive/id353869108?mt=8	N/A
CareZone	A comprehensive information manager for caregivers—securely stores medical records of multiple people, in addition to photos, a personal journal, and a calendar to coordinate tasks	https://itunes.apple.com/us/app/carezone-family-organizer/id552197945?mt=8	https://play.google.com/store/apps/details?id=com.carezone.caredroid.careapp
CaringBridge	Allows users to make a private website to share health updates with friends and family	https://itunes.apple.com/app/caringbridge/id365726944?rnt=8	https://play.google.com/store/apps/details?id=com.caringbridge.app
Chemo Brain Doc Notes	Offers memos and voice recording to organize health questions before an appointment and record provider responses	https://itunes.apple.com/app/chemo-brain-doc-notes-free/id766256080?mt=8	https://play.google.com/store/apps/details?id=com.crowdcare.docnotesfree
Clinical Trial Seek	Provides information on clinical trials and permits patients and caregivers to search for potential trials based on location, disease type, trail phase, and eligibility requirements	https://itunes.apple.com/us/app/clinical-trial-seek/id550482779?mt=8	https://play.google.com/store/apps/details?id=com.novartis.clinicaltrials
CURE Magazine for iPad	Access to CURE, a free publication with the latest cancer information for patients, survivors, and caregivers	https://itunes.apple.com/us/app/cure-magazine-for-ipad/id396123859?mt=8	N/A
iPharmacy: Drug Guide & Pill Identifier	Allows users to identify a pill by shape, color, and bar code and lists available prices and discounts for medications	https://itunes.apple.com/us/app/ipharmacy-drug-guide-pill/id368679506?mt=8	https://play.google.com/store/apps/details?id=com.sigmaphone.topmedfree
Microsoft HealthVault	Stores medical information and records for multiple people, which can be shared with others	https://itunes.apple.com/us/app/microsoft-healthvault/id546835834?mt=8	N/A
My Cancer Manager	Tracks common emotional health concerns of cancer patients and caregivers—insomnia, depression, pain, and anxiety—as well as other stressors such as finances, nutrition, and family	https://itunes.apple.com/us/app/cancerhelp/id402342273?mt=8#	N/A
My Pillbox	Reminds when and how to take medication, as well as when to refill their prescription	N/A	https://play.google.com/store/apps/details?id=com.tobeamaster.mypillbox
Pain Care	A pain journal that records painful episodes, medications, and possible triggers, which can be shared with the physician to tailor chronic pain management	https://itunes.apple.com/app/id347787779	https://play.google.com/store/apps/details?id=com.stanislav.android

Note. N/A = Not Available.

References

1. Dahlin C, ed. *Clinical Practical Guidelines for Quality Palliative Care.* 3rd ed. Pittsburgh, PA: National Consensus Project; 2013.
2. Kissane D, Block S, Burns W, Patrick JD, Wallace CS, McKenzie DP. Perceptions of family functioning and cancer. *Psycho-Oncology* 1994;3:259–269.
3. Kissane D, McKenzie M, McKenzie D, Forbes A, O'Neill L, Bloch S. Psychosocial morbidity associated with patterns of family functioning in palliative care: Baseline data from the family focused grief therapy controlled trial. *Palliat Med.* 2003;17:527–537.
4. Siminoff LA, Zyzanski SJ, Rose JH, Zhang AY. The Cancer Communication Assessment Tool for Patients and Families (CCAT-PF): A new measure. *Psycho-Oncology* 2008;17:1216–1224.
5. Northouse L, Katapodi MC, Schafenacker A, Weiss D. The impact of caregiving on the psychological well-being of famiy caregivers and cancer patients. *Semin Oncol Nurs.* 2012;28:236–245.
6. Emanuel E, Emanuel L. Proxy decision making for incompetent patients: An ethical and empirical analysis. *JAMA.* 1992;267:2067–2071.
7. Winzelberg G, Hanson L, Tulsky J. Beyond autonomy: Diversifying end-of-life decision-making approaches to serve patients and families. *J Am Geriatr Soc.* 2005;53:1046–1050.
8. Nolan M, Kub J, Hughes M, et al. Family health care decision making and self-efficacy with patients with ALS at the end of life. *Palliat Support Care.* 2008;8:273–280.
9. Tallman K, Greenwald R, Reidenouer A, Pantel L. Living with advanced illness: A longitudinal study of patient family, and caregiver needs. *Perm J.* 2012;16:28–35.
10. Skinner H, Steinhauer P, Sitarenious G. Family Assessent Measure (FAM) and process model of family functioning. *J Fam Theory Rev.* 2000;22:190–210.
11. Beavers H, Hampson R. The Beavers System Model of Family Functioning. *J Fam Theory Rev.* 2000:22(2):128–143.

12. Fitzpatrick MA. Family communication patterns theory: Observations on its development and application. *J Fam Commun.* 2004;4:167–179.
13. Boehmer U, Clark J. Communication about prostate cancer between men and their wives. *J Fam Pract.* 2001;50:226–231.
14. Mallinger J, Griggs J, Sheilds C. Family communication and mental health after breast cancer. *Eur J Cancer.* 2006;15:355–361.
15. Given B, Given C, Sherwood P. Family and caregiver needs over the course of the cancer trajectory. *J Support Oncol.* 2012;10:57–64.
16. Northouse L. Helping patients and their family caregivers cope with cancer. *Oncol Nurs Forum* 2012;39:500–506.
17. Lindsey-Davis L, Chestnutt D, Molloy M, Deshefy-Longhi T, Shim B, Gillis C. Adapters, strugglers, and case managers: A typology of spouse caregivers. *Qual Health Res.* 2014;24:1492–1500.
18. Schuler T, Zaider T, Li Y, Hichenberg S, Masterson M, Kissane D. Typology of perceived family functioning in an American sample of patients with advanced cancer. *J Pain Symptom Manage.* 2014;48:281–288.
19. Teno J, Carridge B, Casey V, et al. Family perspectives on end-of-life care at the last place of care. *JAMA.* 2007;291:88–93.
20. Hubbard G, Illingworth N, Rowa-Dewar N, Forbat L, Kearney N. Treatment decision-making in cancer care: The role of the carer. *J Clin Nurs.* 2010;19:2023–2031.
21. Zhang AY, Siminoff LA. Silence and cancer: Why do families and patients fail to communicate? *Health Commun.* 2003;15:415–429.
22. Friesen P, Pepler C, Hunter P. Interactive family learning following a cancer diagnosis. *Oncol Nurs Forum.* 2002;29:981–987.
23. Ellington L, Reblin M, Clayton M, Berry P, Mooney K. Hospice nurse communication with patients with cancer and their family caregivers. *J Palliat. Med.* 2012;15:262–268.
24. Li H, Stewart BJ, Imle MA, Archbold PG, Felver L. Families and hospitalized elders: A typology of family care actions. *Res Nurs Health.* 2000;23:3–16.
25. Eggly S, Penner L, Greene M, Harper F. Information seeking during "bad news" oncology interactions: Question asking by patients and their companions. *Soc Sci Med.* 2006;63:2974–2985.
26. Tamayo GJ, Broxson A, Munsell M, Cohen MZ. Caring for the caregiver. *Oncol Nurs Forum.* 2010;37:E50–E57.
27. Collinge W, Kahn J, Walton T, et al. Touch, caring, and cancer: Randomized controlled tiral of a multimedia caregiver education program. *Suppor Care Cancer.* 2013;21:1405–1414.
28. Williams A, Bakitas M. Cancer family caregivers: A new direction for interventions. *J Palliat Med.* 2012;15:775–783.
29. Ferrell B. From research to practice: Quality of life assessment in medical oncology. *J Support Oncol.* 2008;6:230–231.
30. Kitrungroter L, Cohen MZ. Quality of life of family caregivers of patients with cancer: A literature review. *Oncol Nurs Forum.* 2006;33:625–632.
31. Cameron J, Franche R, Cheung A, Stewart D. Lifestyle interference and emotional distress in family caregivers of advanced cancer patients. *Cancer.* 2002;15:521–527.
32. Rabow M, Hauser J, Adams J. Supporting family caregivers at the end of life: "They don't know what they don't know." *JAMA.* 2004;291:483–491.
33. Tracy K, Coupland N. Multiple goals in discourse: An overview of issues. *J Lang Soc Psychol.* 1990;9:1–13.
34. Helf P, Petronio S. Communication pitfalls with cancer patients: "Hit and run": Deliveries of bad news. *J Am Coll Surg.* 2007;205:807–8111.
35. Petronio S. *Boundaries of Privacy: Dialectics of Disclosure.* Albany: State University of New York Press; 2002.
36. Gentry J. "Don't tell her she's on hospice": Ethics and pastoral care for famlies who withhold medical information. *J Pastoral Care Counsel.* 2008;62:421–426.
37. Petronio S, Lewis S. Medical disclosures in oncology: Families, patients, and providers. *J Fam Theory Rev.* 2010;2:175–196.
38. Planalp S, Trost MR. Communication issues at the end of life: Reports from hospice volunteers. *Health Commun.* 2008;23:222–233.
39. Wittenberg-Lyles E, Goldsmith J, Ferrell B, Ragan S. *Communication in Palliative Nursing.* New York, NY: Oxford University Press; 2012.
40. Caughlin JP, Mikucki-Enyart S, Middelton A, Stone A, Brown L. Being open without talking about it: A rhetorical/normative approach to understanding topic avoidance in families after a lung cancer diagnosis. *Commun Monogr.* 2011;78:409–436.
41. Fitzpatrick MA, Ritchie L. Communication schemata within the family: Multiple perspectives on family interaction. *Human Commun Res.* 1994;20:275–301.
42. Harris J, Bowen DJ, Badr H, Hannon P, Hay J, Regan Sterba K. Family communication during the cancer experience. *J Health Commun.* 2009;14(Suppl 1):76–84.
43. Koerner AF, Fitzpatrick MA. Family communication patterns theory: A social cognitive approach. In: Braithwaite D, Baxter L, eds. *Engaging Theories in Family Communication: Multiple Perspectives.* Thousand Oaks, CA: SAGE; 2006:50–65.
44. McLeod J, Chaffee S. Interpersonal approaches to communication research. *Am Behav Sci.* 1973;16:469–99.
45. Ritchie L, Fitzpatrick MA. Family communication patterns: Measuring interpersonal perceptions of interpersonal relationships. *Commun Res.* 1990;17:523–544.
46. Syren SM, Saveman BI, Benzein EG. Being a family in the midst of living and dying. *J Palliat Care.* 2006;22:26–32.
47. Kramer BJ, Kavanaugh M, Trentham-Dietz A, Walsh M, Yonker JA. Predictors of family conflict at the end of life: The experience of spouses and adult children of persons with lung cancer. *Gerontologist.* 2009;50:215–225.
48. Koerner AF, Fitzpatrick MA. Toward a theory of family communication. *Commun Theory.* 2002;12:70.
49. Wittenberg-Lyles E, Goldsmith J, Parker Oliver D, Demiris G, Rankin A. Targetting communicaiton interventions to decrease caregiver burden. *Semin Nurs Oncol.* 2012;28:262–270.
50. Wittenberg-Lyles E, Goldsmith J, Demiris G, Oliver DP, Stone J. The impact of family communication patterns on hospice family caregivers: A new typology. *J Hosp Palliat Nurs.* 2012;14:25–33.
51. Goldsmith J, Wittenberg E, Small Platt C, Iannarino N, Reno J. Family caregiver communication patterns in oncology: Advancing a typology. *Psycho-Oncology:* In press.
52. Oliver DP, Wittenberg-Lyles E, Demiris G, Washington K, Porock D, Day M. Barriers to pain management: Caregiver perceptions and pain talk by hospice interdisciplinary teams. *J Pain Symptom Manage.* 2008;36:374–382.
53. Murphy M, Escamilla M, Blackwell P, et al. Assessment of caregivers' willingness to participate in an interntion research study. *Res Nurs Health.* 2007;30:347–355.

CHAPTER 19

Cultural Considerations in Palliative Care and Serious Illness

Guadalupe R. Palos

Introduction

Culture drives communication across an individual's lifespan. It is widely recognized that palliative care is a cultural event. Thus an attempt to understand how cultural systems shape a person's expectations for patient–provider–family communication about palliative care seems logical. Recent trends in American society support the critical need for intercultural communication in order to deliver safe and high-quality palliative care. A review of the literature indicates four key trends that support the need to understand cultural systems and engage in culturally competent communication about palliative care. First, the United States is undergoing tremendous demographic shifts that will have a profound impact on palliative care and services. These shifts include a progressive increase in the number of older Americans[1] and a rise in the ethnic and racial heterogeneity of the nation.[2] Second, patients and families often report illness and symptoms that do not fit "biomedical textbook explanations."[3,4] Suffering is an example of a concept that can be a source of confusion in a provider–patient discussion. Third, provider–patient communication significantly impacts medical care and treatment outcomes.[5–7] When barriers to communication exist, it increases the likelihood that a patient will not complete or return for his or her treatment.[5,6] Finally, it is well documented that certain subgroups carry a disproportionate burden of disparities in the use, access, and delivery of healthcare, which include palliative care and services.[8–10]

The primary justification supporting the need to address culture in palliative care arises from America's changing demographics. This country is a mosaic of ethnic groups, racial groups, cultures, and religions. Based on US Census data, by 2050 over 42% of older Americans will belong to a racial or ethnic group.[1] Another demographic shift that will affect palliative care is the increasing ethnic and racial diversity of the US population. The US Census projects that by 2060 57% of America's population will be minorities.[2] Much of this growth stems from the migration of people from other countries to the United States. Newly arriving immigrants and refugees bring their own cultural meaning of illness, disease, suffering, and death. However, individuals born and raised in the United States possess their own cultural attitudes, behaviors, and values toward these concepts. Regardless of origin, these cultural systems shape the subjective experience of patients and their families. Culture influences the views, behaviors, decisions, and communication about palliative care of patients, families, and healthcare providers. In the United States, the healthcare system is based on a Eurocentric or Western biomedical model, which values individualism, self-determination, and open disclosure.[11] These values are often incongruent with the family-centered cultures that value collectivism, shared decision-making, and respectful communication.[12] To achieve optimal intercultural communication about palliative care, providers must focus on individuals' cultural values and less so on their ethnic or racial background.

It is well documented there are often differences between a patient's and a provider's interpretation and explanation of illnesses or symptoms.[4,13] An example of a potential source of cultural miscommunication is the phenomena of suffering. The concept of suffering, whether physical or emotional, is a basic tenet of life. Every culture explains suffering in its own manner and ties the experience to its religious, spiritual, or indigenous beliefs. The attitude of a cultural group toward suffering is also closely tied to its cultural system or worldview.[4] In a healthcare encounter, the provider, patient, and family each have a different understanding of suffering and its treatment. The subjective nature of suffering will affect patient–provider communication about palliative care since the patient's self-report is critical in managing physical and psychological symptoms. The confluence of these diverse cultural worldviews can impact patient/family trust and acceptance of the information related to palliative care, treatment goals, and outcomes. Thus, to promote communication about palliative care, healthcare providers must consider how a patient's culture influences his or her perceptions about illness and suffering. These factors, in part, support the need for culturally competent provider practice and communication.

Despite the growing evidence of the benefits of palliative care, the support of legislative policies and regulatory mandates and the recent efforts to provide equitable access to healthcare, there is empirical evidence suggesting disparities in palliative care across several areas, including communication, symptom management, and satisfaction.[9,10,14–16] As healthcare providers, we must understand that palliative care based on a Western biomedical model will not meet the needs of our nation's mosaic of cultures. All cultures form their own cultural roles, expectations, and views toward their social networks, support systems, and communities. These culturally based systems help shape decisions about their healthcare and more specifically about their palliative care experience. However, many ethnic and minority populations do not define or view palliative care in the same manner as the American mainstream does. The preference of many cultural groups is to use their own long-standing cultural values, beliefs, practices, and attitudes to guide their communication, decision-making, and interactions with healthcare providers trained in a Western biomedical model.

This chapter addresses how cultural value systems of patients and their families impact communication and decisions related to the access and delivery of palliative care. First, an overview of palliative care definitions is provided followed by key cultural terms and concepts. The chapter then provides emergent evidence suggesting cultural groups encounter disparities in palliative care communication and symptom management. The next section describes trends that influence access to palliative care and cultural determinants that shape the subjective meaning of this type of care among multicultural populations. Finally, using a case study to illustrate cultural characteristics of communication, the chapter concludes with a description of intercultural communication practices in palliative care.

Advances in Palliative Care

In 2002 the National Consensus Project for Quality Palliative Care was created, and it established three major goals: (a) to build a national consensus on the principles and philosophy of palliative care; (b) to create and distribute national clinical guidelines to ensure standard and high quality palliative care; and (c) to promote recognition, reimbursement, and accreditation for palliative care. The consensus group further posited that palliative care was essential across setting, chronicity, or acuity of different chronic diseases and stage of treatment.[17] Palliative care was further established with the National Quality Forum's (NQF) release of national clinical guidelines for quality palliative care, recognizing the critical role of patient–family–provider communication across eight domains of care.[18] Culture was identified as a core domain, and the NQF-endorsed practice for quality palliative care includes cultural assessment.

Significant advances have been made in the care and delivery of evidence-based palliative care. Interestingly, there are multiple definitions of palliative care, which vary by organization. The National Consensus Quality definition of palliative care is consistent with the one used by the NQF and the Centers for Medicare and Medicaid Services, which states:

> Palliative care means patient and family-centered care that optimizes quality of life by anticipating, preventing, and treating suffering. Palliative care throughout the continuum of illness involves addressing physical, intellectual, emotional, social, and spiritual needs to facilitate patient autonomy, access to information, and choice.[19]

The World Health Organization defines palliative care as an approach to relieve suffering and to improve quality of life.[20] The Center to Advance Palliative Care views palliative care as a medical specialty targeting the needs of people with serious illnesses who require symptom management, whatever the diagnosis.[21] The National Consensus for Quality Palliative Care believes that "palliative care is both a philosophy of care and an organized structured system for delivering care."[18] The NQF states that palliative care encompasses patient- and family-centered care that enhances quality of life by managing suffering across the trajectory of a patient's illness.[17] The importance of palliative care was further established in 2012, when the American College of Surgeons Commission on Cancer released accreditation standards that endorsed palliative care services. These standards support the interpretation of comprehensive palliative care that ranges from screening to end of life.[22]

Culture and Palliative Care

As the field of palliative care continues to grow, and attention to cultural aspects of care are prioritized and emphasized, intercultural communication becomes an even more important part of patient–family–provider interactions. One way to develop competence in intercultural communication is to be aware of key terms and concepts relevant to this topic. A list of key terms and concepts about culture can be found in Table 19.1.

Concepts of worldviews and explanatory models of illness provide a framework for understanding more about the intersection between culture and palliative care. A worldview is how people see the world, and thus it shapes the reality of one's life, particularly during times of crisis, such as when one develops a serious illness. This concept allows people to determine their behavior, make decisions, and form their cultural systems. Whenever a patient and provider interact in a clinical encounter, their communication is based on the worldviews formed through their own life experiences, professional training and experience, and cultural values and beliefs. For example, a person's worldview will frame his or her attitudes toward health, suffering, and decisions about palliative, hospice, and end-of-life care. Many studies have shown that culture or worldview also impacts the preferences of seriously ill patients for life-sustaining techniques, aggressive treatments, and advance directives.[23,24] Furthermore, providers' worldviews, race, or biases can influence their decisions to explain palliative care to patients and their families. Providers' views can also affect the treatment they render to minority patients and whether such treatment is based on minority patients' wishes.[25,26] In sum, worldviews are influenced by a person's personal biases toward ethnic or racial groups; preferences for end-of-life care; satisfaction with care; and spiritual, religious, or indigenous beliefs and practices.

America's increasing globalization and aging population will impact the worldview or cultural meaning assigned to a palliative care experience.[27] Kluckhohn and Strodtbeck expand on this concept by suggesting that worldviews are based on five determinants: (a) human nature—how people view being human; (b) man and nature—how people view themselves in relation to nature; (c) time—how individuals view the past, present, and future; (d) activity—how people view being and doing; and (e) relational—how people view their interpersonal social relationships with family and other social support networks.[28] A person's worldview provides the lens from which to define health, illness, death, and dying. It also shapes how people understand

Table 19.1 Definitions of Key Terms and Concepts Relevant to Culture and Palliative Care

Term	Definition
Ancestry[49]	Refers to a person's ethnic roots, heritage, or the place of birth of the person's parents or ancestors before coming to the United States
Culture	Serves as the blueprint that provides an individual's meaning for being and for living one's life
Cultural meaning systems	Cognitive structures that influence how people view or perceive clinical reality
	Shapes clinical reality through culture-based idioms and culture-based subjective experience related to illness and symptoms
Ethnicity	Shared culture and way of life especially reflected in language, folkways, religious, and institutional forms; material culture such as clothing and food; and cultural products such as music, literature, and art
	Often viewed as a social class and/or associated with political and social persecution
Explanatory models of illness[50,51]	Culturally based concepts that individuals use to define and explain the causes, treatment, and effects of illness to themselves
Intercultural Communication[52]	Discusses the knowledge, motivation, skills to interact effectively and appropriately with members of different cultures
	Also referred to cross-cultural competence
Origin[49,53]	Viewed as the heritage, nationality, country of birth of the person, or the person's ancestors before arriving in the United States
Race[54]	Refers a social definition of race recognized in this country. It is not meant to define race biologically, anthropologically, or genetically.
Illness or symptoms[13,27,55]	Represents the human experience and lived reality of the symptoms, suffering, and process of adaptation for patients and family members
	Describes a network of meanings for the sufferer: fears and expectations about illness, social reactions of friends, life stresses, and therapeutic experiences

and respond to health messages. Explanatory models can interact, overlap, or at times contradict or compete with one another. For example, including healing or dying rituals delivered by indigenous healers may clash with healthcare providers who base their palliative care on a biomedical model of medicine. Explanatory models can influence how patients, families, and providers feel about communication, expectations, preferences, decision-making, advance care planning, and grief/mourning. Figure 19.1 illustrates the multiple levels and interactions of worldviews and how they impact palliative care.

Disparities in Palliative Care

Disparities in healthcare may pertain to the differences in the morbidity, mortality, and burden of diseases and other unfavorable outcomes among specific groups. It is well documented that certain groups, including the aging, medically underserved, physically disabled, and ethnic and racial minorities, suffer a disproportionate burden of ill health, reduced survival rates, and poor quality of life.[14,29] There is also increasing evidence that these same groups experience disparities in access to palliative care and variance in outcomes such as provider communication, symptom management, and even death. Several studies show ethnic minorities such as African Americans and Latinos/Hispanics receive poorer assessment and treatment of pain and other symptoms for chronic, acute, or cancer-related pain.[15,30,31]

Additionally, there is limited research focusing on the underlying causes contributing to disparities in palliative care by subgroups of culture, race, ethnicity, or socioeconomic status.[10,14,32] This limitation suggests these groups are more likely to receive inadequate assessment, management, and delivery of palliative and end-of-life care. For instance, groups such as African Americans and Latinos, which are collectivistic, have certain preferences toward caring for a loved one with a serious illness, such as avoiding the use of an advance directive or how and to whom bad news is disclosed.[33,34] Although there is limited research on Asians' preferences for palliative and end-of-life care, a few studies have found that Asians are less likely to enroll in hospice care and are more likely to die in a hospital when compared to white, non-Hispanic patients.[35,36] The lack of evidence-based studies can undermine clinical practice, since best practices do not exist for culturally appropriate assessment, management, and delivery of palliative care.

There is mounting evidence that palliative care disparities exist in communication of medical information. For example, the Institute of Medicine report, *Unequal Treatment*, identified that language barriers contributed to disparate care in non-English speaking groups.[29] For instance, many providers are unfamiliar with how to communicate with diverse ethnic or cultural groups about end-of-life decisions, advance directives, or code status guidelines. Another challenge in communication is avoiding stereotyping or generalizing about the preferences or expectations of specific cultural groups. For example, in several Asian cultures, disclosure of a diagnosis of a serious illness or other types of bad news to a patient is considered cruel, disrespectful, or even inhumane.[37] One systematic review concluded that language barriers were associated with less understanding of a provider's explanation of services, fewer frequent clinic visits, and less satisfaction with care.[38] This knowledge gap reflects the urgent need to better understand how cultural factors impact patient–provider communication.

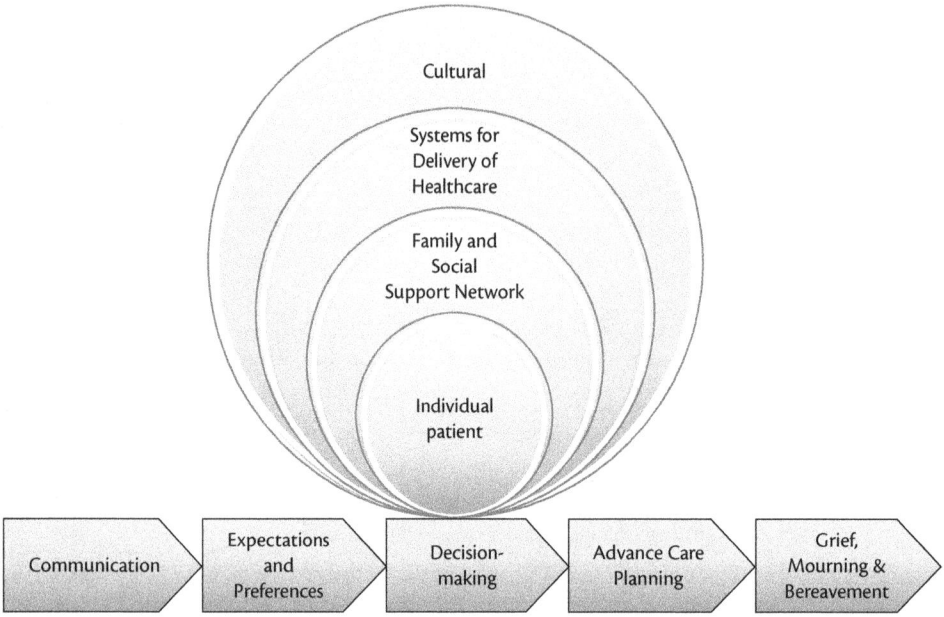

Figure 19.1 Schema of cultural worldviews multiple levels and interactions influencing palliative care and intercultural communication.

Social Determinants of Palliative Care

Health Access and Care Utilization

Several studies document lower usage rates of palliative care and hospice services among African Americans, Latinos, Asians, and even older adults regardless of diagnoses, care settings, or geographic location.[35,39,40] It is true that we will all die, yet the goal of a "good death," its timing, and the experience of grief and bereavement is influenced by utilization of services and care that help facilitate these events. Healthcare utilization by many cultural groups is influenced by such factors as insurance status, income level, lack of a usual source of care, and cultural factors.[14,41] In fact, some research suggests that people living in poverty, having a lower socioeconomic status, or living with similar inequalities die younger than wealthy people in higher classes.[42] Additional evidence indicates ethnic and racial minorities are the least likely to receive specialized palliative care.[43] Other factors that influence healthcare utilization include limited English proficiency, perceived provider bias, and location of care.[44,45] Factors that impede healthcare utilization patterns have an impact on the quality and safety of palliative care received by diverse ethnic and racial groups.

Acculturation

Acculturation is another major determinant affecting the lives and health of many ethnic subgroups, including immigrants and refugees. Acculturation has been defined as maintaining one's original culture and establishing bonds with the new culture.[46] The level of acculturation achieved by a person with strong cultural heritage will affect palliative care across the spectrum of care. For example, immigrant Latinos may often prefer to use indigenous remedies and cures to manage a serious illness and symptoms, while more acculturated Latinos prefer to have their illness managed using the Western biomedical model of care. Yet, with the increased acceptance of hospice care within the United States, more acculturated members of the same cultural group believe a death at home with hospice care can be a better experience than a hospital death.

Cultural Determinants

Culture is a fundamental tenet of palliative care. Hence an optimal model of palliative care must consider the important influence of culture when an individual is faced with a serious illness or limited time to live. The World Health Organization's definition of palliative care includes goals such as (a) regard basic dying as a normal process of life, (b) neither hasten nor postpone death, and (c) offer a support system to help the family cope during the patient's illness and their own bereavement.[20] However, patients and their families differ in how they interpret, react to, and accept these goals. Differences occur in their acceptance of uncertainty or loss of control, desire to talk about unfavorable outcomes, and readiness to face the reality of a pending death. Healthcare professionals face tremendous challenges in providing culturally appropriate and personalized care to patients and families with their own unique worldviews.

Although there is great heterogeneity among cultural groups, there are a core group of cultural determinants. These determinants include ethnic or cultural identity, communication, social organization, space and time orientation, spirituality and religion, and death and dying.[47,48] Understanding the role and importance of these determinants will help healthcare providers when advocating for patients and their families, encouraging adherence to symptom management and treatment plans, and accessing timely and quality palliative care. There are six cultural characteristics that can significantly impact care, decisions, and communication in the palliative care experience. Table 19.2 lists and provides a description of each cultural characteristic.

These cultural characteristics are critical aspects of providing high-quality and comprehensive palliative care. Two key points are also important: first, these characteristics must be taken into

Table 19.2 Cultural Characteristics of Multicultural Palliative Care

Cultural Characteristic	Description
Ethnic identity	Cultural or ethnic group an individual self identifies with. Factors influencing the self-categorization include country of origin, degree of acculturation, reasons for migration, and current geographic residence
Communication	Verbal and nonverbal preferences for sending and receiving information. Includes preferences for communication style, language, tone, and eye contact
Social organization	Networks, groups, and family structure that a person identifies with and uses as sources of social support. Focus on roles and status of elders, spouse, children, respected extended family, and other sources of support networks (i.e., church, tribes, enclaves)
Time and space	Individual's and cultural groups' views toward past, present, and future time. Also pertains to the amount of physical or socially accepted space when communicating between individuals
Religion, spirituality, and taboos	Source of religious or spirituality used as a source of strength, reference for meaning of life, interpretation of indigenous practices and rituals
Death and dying practices	Beliefs and practices toward dying, death, and the afterlife as well as norms for expressing grief, mourning, and bereavement

account by all members of the palliative care team, and second, providers often overlook how their own personal and professional cultural worldviews affect their clinical care and decisions. Healthcare providers need to develop their skills and knowledge through ongoing training. Acquiring multicultural palliative skills is an ongoing and lifelong process.

The following narrative seeks to illustrate how cultural considerations impact palliative care communication.

Case Study

Mr. G, a 57-year-old Hispanic man, born and raised in the United States, is married with two children and owns his own business. He has a history of hypertension and diabetes, which has been well-managed with medication, diet, and exercise. Mr. G. understands the importance of managing his health problems and watching for unusual signs or symptoms, particularly of diabetes. His insurance is adequate but limits access to specialists. Mr. G. would like to get a second opinion about his increasing episodes of shortness of breath and fatigue. With the new Health Care Reform Act, he changes insurance carriers and makes an appointment with a cardiologist. The new physician informs Mr. G. that he has severe blockage in his arteries requiring immediate bypass surgery. Mr. G tells the physician he must discuss the plans with his family, make arrangements with his brother to cover his business, and process the information regarding his illness and its treatment.

He decides to have the surgery. The day after the operation, Mr. G is recovering well and enjoying a family visit with his wife and children when he suddenly suffers a stroke. Several medical complications during the stroke leave him in a coma. Mr. G. is transferred to intensive care where hospital policies restrict the number and type of visitors as well as visiting hours. Eventually Mr. G.'s condition worsens because of his other chronic conditions. His diabetes affects the circulation in his legs necessitating full amputation of both legs.

Mr. G. has eight siblings who monitor his care and treatment decisions. Over the course of his illness, the number and type of providers involved in Mr. G's care continues to grow. There are at least three referring physician specialists, various shifts of nurses, and other support staff, who pose a growing number of choices regarding Mr. G.'s treatment. Mr. G.'s wife asks one brother to serve as the family spokesperson when communicating with the team. Since the day of the unexpected stroke, discussions between Mr. G.'s family and the large healthcare team have been uncomfortable and unproductive. The family was unprepared for this unfortunate turn of events and believes the information given by the various physicians has been conflicting and confusing. Despite Mr. G.'s declining health status, the family is adamant that all physicians do whatever they can to save his life. The healthcare team is concerned about the worsening status of their patient. Mr. G.'s brother convinces his wife to ask for a social worker to facilitate communication among the physicians, nursing staff, and Mr. G.'s brother's wife, children, and brother.

The social worker convenes a family meeting. During the meeting, Mrs. G and the family tell the healthcare team that no matter what type of physical limitations Mr. G. will experience, they expect the team to keep him alive. One physician asks the family to consider Mr. G.'s quality of life since he has been in a coma for a month, has had amputation of both lower extremities, and suffered severe brain damage due to the stroke. The social worker asks the family if Mr. G. had advance directives. They inform her there are no directives on record, and, even if there were, they still want to do whatever is necessary to keep him alive. They share stories with the team about friends who were in comas, woke up, and are now alive. They believe Mr. G will have the same outcome. The wife tells the team, "Even with my husband's problems, he will still be alive. That's all that matters." The meeting ends without resolution on what to do next other than continue providing medical care to Mr. G.

This narrative illustrates that families' and providers' worldviews differ in how they approach (a) health/illness, (b) advance directives, (c) decision-making, (d) expectations and preferences, (e) communication, and (f) mourning and grief. This family's experience and response to this situational crisis is also reflected in the following quote from Meyerstein's discussing the impact of illness on families:

> Patient and family members wander in unfamiliar territory, facing strange hospital environments, foreign "medicalese" and confusing procedures. Family members are thrown off their familiar path and have difficulty finding their way back. While the detour has different

meanings for individual family members, sustaining one's spirits and preserving identity in the face of illness is a challenge.[34]

Understanding the general nuances of these cultural phenomena can be helpful to providers when communicating and making decisions with culturally diverse patients and families about palliative care needs. Table 19.3 provides a summary of the issues the family faced, the cultural characteristics from which the issues originated, and assessment strategies to help enhance intercultural communication between the family and providers.

Practice Implications

America is becoming increasingly heterogeneous, thus increasing the likelihood that healthcare providers will be called upon to care for a patient and family with unique worldviews toward palliative care. The combination of these nuances coupled with the complexity of palliative care require healthcare providers to integrate explanatory models of illness, death, and dying with biomedical models of care in their consultations with culturally diverse populations.

Methods to reduce disparities in palliative care must be multilevel and culturally appropriate. Six recommendations may help develop cultural competency in the delivery of palliative care: these include (a) providing culturally competent training programs for providers, staff, and administrators to increase their knowledge and skills in this area; (b) providing an interpreter or translation services for different languages, including American Sign Language; (c) coordinating care with traditional healers (when preferred by patients and their families); (d) integrating

Table 19.3 Intercultural Communication in the Case of Mr. G

Issue	Cultural Characteristic	Intercultural Communication
Patient and family are of Latino heritage whose worldviews of health and illness may be a combination of traditional cultural values and biomedical model of care	Ethnic identity NCP guideline states: "the cultural background, concerns, and needs of the patient and family are elicited and documented"[18(p57)]	Patient–family–provider clarification of the patient's and his or her family's self-reported ethnic identify would help guide planning and management during this hospitalization. Although intake forms may state: Latino/Hispanic male, discussion on how this label is operationalized by the family would be helpful.
Verbal and nonverbal communication impacted the family's perceptions of the patient's condition and prognosis. The need to have so many different providers made it difficult to establish trust and an open relationship, which was needed in this family crisis.	Communication NCP guideline: "Communication should occur in a language and manner that the patient and family understand"[18(p57)]	Family conferences with each referring physician as well as an interdisciplinary meeting between all providers and family members would be helpful from the moment the crisis began. Providers could schedule regular meetings at times when the family could find time in their daily routine. Entire team could communicate across disciplines/shifts regarding who the family's spokesperson is, language preference, and initiation of preferences for scheduling family conferences
Mr. G. had a nuclear and extended family, which formed a collective group to help shape decision-making and communication.	Social organization NCP guidelines state: "Communication in all forms, with the patient and family is respectfully towards their cultural preferences regarding disclosure, truth-telling, and decision-making"[18(p57)]	Acknowledgement and inclusion of the collective as a whole in this crisis would aid in establishing trust and rapport with the family Even with HIPAA regulations, just asking about the family and acknowledging their roles would be meaningful to cultural groups who value collectivism.
After Mr. G. transfers to the ICU, the family's time with him is extremely limited due to his poor condition and strict policies regarding number of visitors and visiting hours.	Time and space NCP guidelines state: "Cultural needs identified by the team and family are addressed in the interdisciplinary team care as outlined in Domain 1"[18(p57)].	Social worker or case manager could advocate for staff to relax the policies given the worsening condition of the patient. In addition, a designated staff member could serve as the "go-to person" for the family regarding changes in the patient's status.
Family had strong beliefs and faith but did not have a regular faith-based facility.	Religion, spirituality, and taboos NCP Domain 5: Spiritual, religious, and existential aspects of care[18(p48)]	Once religious preferences are confirmed with the family, providers could ask the family if they wished to have a member of clergy speak with the family or pray for the patient. Clergy could also be invited to family conferences to help families deal with bad news about the patient's conditions.
Family's preferences and expectations for the staff are to keep Mr. G alive no matter how bad his condition becomes. Family is using their worldview and narratives from social support networks to build hope that Mr. G. will come out of his coma.	Death and dying practices NCP guidelines state "program aims to respect and accommodate the range of language, dietary, and rituals practices of the patient and their family"[18(p57)]	Communication among the patient, the family, and providers about living wills and advance directives with the patient before his surgery would help family and staff in managing and treating the patients during the various episodes of crisis. Palliative care communication initiated at admission would also help the family understand the purpose of advance directives and goals of palliative care, and assess the family's worldviews toward end-of-life care.

Note. NCP = National Consensus Project.

community health workers or patient navigators to provide cultural linkages, build trust, and help with provider–patient communication; (e) including family, friends, and other members of the extended kinship network to help make decisions and encourage adherence with appointments or treatment regimens; and (f) recruiting and retaining minority personnel.

Conclusion

Culture impacts every patient–family–provider meeting, and each group brings its own unique background to the encounter. Thus the potential for cultural clash and ineffective communication during these encounters is a reality. In fact, conflicting worldviews have been cited as barriers in establishing effective provider–patient relationships. Poor provider–patient communication can also contribute to disparities in palliative care. Thus these factors support the need for healthcare providers to communicate, assess, and provide care that is culturally and linguistically appropriate. Nonetheless, it is challenging to translate these goals into standard models of palliative care. One way to achieve these goals is to regard patient/family cultural worldviews toward palliative care as a positive strength that, as a collective partnership with healthcare providers, can be used to help the patient achieve an optimal quality of life across the palliative care trajectory.

References

1. Vincent GVV. *The Next Four Decades: The Older Population in the United States: 2010–1050.* Washington, DC: US Department of Commerce; 2010.
2. US Census Bureau. US Census Bureau projections show a slower growing, older, more diverse nation by 2060. http://www.census.gov/newsroom/releases/archives/population/cb12-243.html. Published December 12, 2012. Accessed July 20, 2014.
3. Groce NE, Zola IK. Multiculturalism, chronic illness, and disability. *Pediatrics.* May 1993;91(5):1048–1055.
4. Dimou N. Illness and culture: Learning-differences. *Patient Educ Couns.* September 1995;26(1–3):153–157.
5. Arora NK. Interacting with cancer patients: The significance of physicians' communication behavior. *Soc Sci Med.* September 2003;57(5):791–806.
6. Schouten BCM, L. Cultural differences in medical communication: A review of the literature. *Patient Educ Couns.* 2006;64:21–34.
7. Bullock K. Promoting advance directives among African Americans: A faith-based model. *J Palliat Med.* February 2006;9(1):183–195.
8. Johnson KS. Racial and ethnic disparities in palliative care. *J Palliat Med.* November 2013;16(11):1329–1334.
9. Laguna J, Enguidanos S, Siciliano M, Coulourides-Kogan A. Racial/ethnic minority access to end-of-life care: A conceptual framework. *Home Health Care Serv Q.* 2012;31(1):60–83.
10. Evans BC, Ume E. Psychosocial, cultural, and spiritual health disparities in end-of-life and palliative care: Where we are and where we need to go. *Nurs Outlook.* November–December 2012;60(6):370–375.
11. Barclay JS, Blackhall LJ, Tulsky JA. Communication strategies and cultural issues in the delivery of bad news. *J Palliat Med.* August 2007;10(4):958–977.
12. Palos G. Cultural heritage: cancer screening and early detection. *Semin Oncol Nurs.* May 1994;10(2):104–113.
13. Larsen PD. Chronicity of illness. In: Lubkin IM, Larson PD, eds. *Chronic Illness: Impact and Interventions.* Sudbury, MA: Jones & Bartlett; 2009:3–25.
14. Johnson KS. Racial and ethnic disparities in palliative care. *J Palliat Med.* November 1, 2013;16(11):1329–1334.
15. Anderson KO, Green CR, Payne R. Racial and ethnic disparities in pain: Causes and consequences of unequal care. *J Pain.* December 2009;10(12):1187–1204.
16. Mack JW, Weeks JC, Wright AA, Block SD, Prigerson HG. End-of-life discussions, goal attainment, and distress at the end of life: Predictors and outcomes of receipt of care consistent with preferences. *J Clin Oncol.* March 1 2010;28(7):1203–1208.
17. National Quality Forum. *A National Framework and Preferred Practices for Palliative and Hospice Care Quality.* Washington, DC: National Quality Forum; 2006.
18. National Consensus Project. *Clinical Practice Guidelines for Quality Palliative Care.* 2nd ed. Pittsburg, PA: National Consensus Project for Quality Palliative Care; 2009.
19. Federal Register. Medicare and Medicaid Programs: Hospice conditions of participation; final rule. Vol. 732008:109–322.
20. World Health Organization. Cancer control: Knowledge into action. http://www.who.int/cancer/modules/en/. Accessed July 20, 2014.
21. Center to Advance Palliative Care. Defining palliative care. http://www.capc.org. Accessed July 20, 2014.
22. Commission on Cancer. Cancer Program Standards 2012. Version 1.2.1: Ensuring patient-centered care. http://www.facs.org/cancer/coc/programstandards2012.html. Published January 21, 2014. Accessed July 20, 2014.
23. Mack JW, Paulk ME, Viswanath K, Prigerson HG. Racial disparities in the outcomes of communication on medical care received near death. *Arch Intern Med.* September 27, 2010;170(17):1533–1540.
24. Braun UK, McCullough LB, Beyth RJ, Wray NP, Kunik ME, Morgan RO. Racial and ethnic differences in the treatment of seriously ill patients: A comparison of African-American, Caucasian and Hispanic veterans. *J Natl Med Assoc.* September 2008;100(9):1041–1051.
25. Burgess DJ, van Ryn M, Crowley-Matoka M, Malat J. Understanding the provider contribution to race/ethnicity disparities in pain treatment: Insights from dual process models of stereotyping. *Pain Med.* March–April 2006;7(2):119–134.
26. Cintron A, Morrison RS. Pain and ethnicity in the United States: A systematic review. *J Palliat Med.* December 2006;9(6):1454–1473.
27. Flanagan AY. *Families of Chronically Ill Patients.* Sacramento, CA: CME Resource/NetCE; 2011.
28. Kluckhohn FS, F. *Variations in value orientations.* Evanston, IL: Row, Peterson; 1961.
29. Smedley BD, Stith A, Nelson AR. *Unequal treatment: Confronting racial and ethnic disparities in health care.* Washington, DC: National Academies Press; 2003.
30. Green CR, Anderson KO, Baker TA, et al. The unequal burden of pain: Confronting racial and ethnic disparities in pain. *Pain Med.* September 2003;4(3):277–294.
31. Higginson IJ, Gomes B, Calanzani N, et al. Priorities for treatment, care and information if faced with serious illness: A comparative population-based survey in seven European countries. *Palliat Med.* February 2014;28(2):101–110.
32. Bullock K. The influence of culture on end-of-life decision making. *J Soc Work End Life Palliat Care.* 2011;7(1):83–98.
33. Carr D. Racial differences in end-of-life planning: Why don't blacks and Latinos prepare for the inevitable? *Omega.* 2011;63(1):1–20.
34. Mazanec PM, Daly BJ, Townsend A. Hospice utilization and end-of-life care decision making of African Americans. *Am J Hosp Palliat Care.* December 2010;27(8):560–566.

35. Ngo-Metzger Q, Phillips RS, McCarthy EP. Ethnic disparities in hospice use among Asian-American and Pacific Islander patients dying with cancer. *J Am Geriatr Soc*. January 2008;56(1):139–144.
36. Lackan NA, Eschbach K, Stimpson JP, Freeman JL, Goodwin JS. Ethnic differences in in-hospital place of death among older adults in California: Effects of individual and contextual characteristics and medical resource supply. *Med Care*. February 2009;47(2):138–145.
37. Matsumura S, Bito S, Liu H, et al. Acculturation of attitudes toward end-of-life care: A cross-cultural survey of Japanese Americans and Japanese. *J Gen Inter Med*. July 2002;17(7):531–539.
38. Yeo S. Language barriers and access to care. *Ann Rev Nurs Res*. 2004;22:59–73.
39. Greiner KA, Perera S, Ahluwalia JS. Hospice usage by minorities in the last year of life: Results from the National Mortality Followback Survey. *J Am Geriatr Soc*. July 2003;51(7):970–978.
40. Connor SR, Elwert F, Spence C, Christakis NA. Racial disparity in hospice use in the United States in 2002. *Palliat Med*. April 2008;22(3):205–213.
41. Connolly A, Sampson EL, Purandare N. End-of-life care for people with dementia from ethnic minority groups: A systematic review. *J Am Geriatr Soc*. February 2012;60(2):351–360.
42. Viswanath K. & Ackerson LK. Race, ethnicity, language, social class, and health communication inequalities: A nationally representative cross-sectional study. *PLoS One*. 2011;6(1):e14450.
43. Lau R, O'Connor M. Behind the rhetoric: Is palliative care equitably available for all? *Contemp Nurse*. December 2012;43(1):56–63.
44. Ramirez AG, Wildes K, Talavera G, Napoles-Springer A, Gallion K, Perez-Stable EJ. Clinical trials attitudes and practices of Latino physicians. *Contemp Clin Trials*. July 2008;29(4):482–492.
45. Saha S, Fernandez A, Perez-Stable E. Reducing language barriers and racial/ethnic disparities in health care: An investment in our future. *J Gen Intern Med*. November 2007;22(Suppl 2):371–372.
46. Berry JW. Acculturation: Living successfully in two cultures. *Int J Intercult Rel*. 2005;Nov;29(6):697–712.
47. Caballero AE. Understanding the Hispanic/Latino patient. *Am J Med*. October 2011;124(10 Suppl):S10–S15.
48. Palos GR. Culture and pain assessment in Hispanic patients. In: Payne R, Patt RB, Hill CS, eds. *Assessment and treatment of cancer pain*. Seattle, WA: IASP Press; 1998:35–51.
49. People and Households: Ancestry. US Department of Commerce. http://www.census.gov/population/ancestry/. Accessed January 20, 2013.
50. Kleinman A. *Patients and healers in the context of culture*. Berkeley: University of California Press; 1980.
51. Shaw SJ, Armin J, Torres CH, Orzech KM, Vivian J. Chronic disease self-management and health literacy in four ethnic groups. *J Health Commun*. 2012;17(Suppl 3):67–81.
52. Wiseman RL. Intercultural communication competenence. In: Gaudykunst WB, Mody B, eds. *Handbook of International and Cultural Communication*. 2nd ed. Thousand Oaks, CA: SAGE; 2002:207–224.
53. Humes KR, Jones NA, Ramirez RR. *Overview of Race and Hispanic Origin. 2010*. C2010BR-02. Washington, DC: US Census Bureau; 2011.
54. People and Households: Race. US Department of Commerce. http://www.census.gov/population/race/. Accessed January 20, 2013.
55. Good BJ, Delvecchio-Good MJ. The meaning of symptoms: A cultural hermeneutic model for clinical practice. In: Eisenberg L, Kleinman A, eds. *The Relevance of Social Science for Medicine*. Boston, MA: Reidel; 1981:165–196.

CHAPTER 20

Family Conversations About In-Home and Hospice Care

Wayne A. Beach, Kyle Gutzmer, and David M. Dozier

Introduction

In *A Natural History of Family Cancer*,[1] the story is told of how family members talk about and through terminal illness on the telephone. Over 13 months and across 61 phone calls, from diagnosis through treatment to the eventual death of a wife/mother/sister (two hours following the last recorded call), these materials provide rare insight into communication throughout a family cancer journey. The recordings are unique and critically important because they represent the only known corpus, in the history of the social and medical sciences, of an actual family who somehow coped with, but understandably could not fully control, "the trials, tribulations, hopes and triumphs of cancer."[1(p10)]

As with most if not all medical diagnoses, the course and trajectory of cancer is replete with uncertainties and fears about unknown futures.[2] Few guarantees can be provided that complete remission and healing will occur. For this family, death ensued as a loved one's life was lost to a spreading disease that lengthy and concerted medical interventions could not overcome. While this families' recorded experiences offer remarkable and even extraordinary glimpses of the human social condition, these conversations are at the same time altogether routine and "strikingly familiar to all who have encountered them."[1(p9)] With nearly 600,000 annual cancer deaths (> 1,500 each day) in the United States,[3] communication about cancer is exceedingly normal. And like many patients and family members facing terminal illness, hospice care was involved in the later stages of life to assist with caregiving, management of pain and suffering, symptom control, and creation of a supporting environment promoting comfort and compassion for others in need. In 2012, approximately 1.1 million deaths were managed under the auspices of hospice.[4] This is not intended to diminish the many challenges faced by this particular family or the interactional orientations and practices used to manage recurring problems. Rather these conversations offer a rich resource for understanding social life in the very midst of an ongoing family crisis and provide important case studies about ordinary family experiences for palliative care researchers and clinical professionals. When actual patient and family communication is closely examined, key insights and intervention strategies become available in new and profound ways. From close examination of interactional materials, enhanced knowledge and understandings can be utilized to improve communication skills and thus provide unique opportunities to deliver palliative care more compassionately and effectively.

By examining naturally occurring interactions, and making these materials available to diverse health and palliative care communities, we extend previous work that examines critical topics such as patient–provider interactions,[5] pressures on family relationships,[6] stressors inherent to caring for dying patients,[7] how emotional moments can facilitate connections between patients and physicians,[8] and routine problems associated with delivering and receiving bad news.[9-11] It is also clear that end-of-life discussions are essential for improving quality of care,[12] including communicating a hope to patients that is not located in physical outcomes alone.[13]

However, there are considerable methodological limitations that constrain direct access to naturally occurring interactions. For example, morbidity and mortality are often main outcome measures of palliative care. Jocham et al. write, "traditional indicators of the health intervention outcomes, namely mortality and morbidity, are insufficient or inadequate: hence, there is a need to extend the scope of research in palliative care by addressing different objectives."[14(p7)] They recommend including evaluation measures of patient quality of life, including psychological and social dimensions such as communication.

Limitations also exist with survey-based methodologies for assessing communication throughout palliative care. Previous communication research focused on palliative and cancer care has mostly utilized patients' self-reports.[1,15] As de Haes and Teunissen observe, "few studies focus on what happens in communication in palliative care … the practice of palliative communication thus remains unseen."[15(pp348-349)] Similarly, Back and colleagues[11] suggest that surveys assessing miscommunication about prognosis are limited. Because "the actual conversation was not analyzed, it is unclear what the physician said or whether the physician allowed a misconception to persist. Thus, although these studies suggest that communication could be improved, the reasons it failed are unclear."[11(p1902)] The authors indicate that examination of real-time, grounded communication is necessary in order to more accurately assess communication in these settings.

Recent efforts to examine audio recordings of patient–caregiver dyads and hospice nurses in home settings have begun to remedy these methodological limitations. Attention has been given to how patients and caregivers express concerns and display distress and, in response, how nurses manage these emotions.[16,17]

In this chapter we address three primary resources for promoting research and education across palliative care networks. First, we examine what has not been available in palliative care research and practice: a series of recorded and transcribed conversations between family members, which represent scenes involving the trials and growth opportunities of transitions to in-home and hospice care. Interactions about daily circumstances include sharing perspectives on the mother's dire health condition, challenges associated with caring for a dying loved one at home, and the significant contributions of a hospice nurse, who has recently entered their lives to deliver support and medical expertise. Second, we describe how these family phone conversations have been adapted into a professional theatrical production titled *When Cancer Calls. . . .*[18] Funded by the National Institutes of Health/National Cancer Institute (CA144235), thousands of audience members (patients, family members, and healthcare professionals) have reported being significantly impacted by experiencing this production in which all dialogue is drawn from real-time, naturally occurring phone conversations comprising a family cancer journey. Third, readers are provided with a glimpse of audience members' reactions, drawn from a sampling of post-viewing talkback and focus group sessions. These comments highlight the power of integrating the social sciences with the arts and offer testimony to why all persons dealing with health and illness (personally and professionally) can benefit from viewing and talking about *When Cancer Calls . . . .* The chapter concludes with implications for integrating these conversational and theatrical resources into palliative care research, education, and training.

Scenes From Family Conversations About In-Home and Hospice Care

The following analyses of four transcribed excerpts are drawn from a single phone call involving a father, son, and mother (dying cancer patient). Mom is in her early 50s and was diagnosed with what she described to Son (call #2) as a "large cell cancer." Other conversations between Dad and Son suggest that the primary site for Mom's cancer was her lungs. Despite radiation, chemotherapy, and various medications, the cancer quickly spread to her adrenal glands, kidneys, and spine. It is not known exactly when a terminal diagnosis was rendered by physicians, but throughout this journey her husband of 30 years was her primary caregiver. In his late 20s, and within two months of Mom's diagnosis, Son moved from San Diego to Texas to continue his graduate education. He regularly calls for updates about Mom's condition.

Prior to Excerpt 1 Mom had, for some time, been in and out of the hospital to receive extensive radiation treatments in hopes of minimizing tumor growth. These treatments were progressively ineffective. Frequent infections also required intravenous antibiotics. More recently, attempts to manage Mom's pain involved various combinations of pills, liquids, injections, and increased dosages of morphine to reduce her discomfort. As worsening conditions reduced her strength and mobility, and the continual use of a wheelchair became necessary, decisions were made to keep her in the hospital for an extended period to more closely monitor and accommodate her failing health. The clinical interactions comprising these events were not recorded, as a part of the family phone call corpus. However, discussions must have occurred between healthcare staff, Mom, and Dad that eventually advised releasing Mom from the hospital, preparing for in-home care, and overviewing (perhaps encouraging) the probability of hospice involvement.

"Normally, as hospice care is provided only during the last six weeks of a patient's life, the doctor's recommendation marks a significant development in the family cancer journey. A shift from *curative* to *palliative* occurs, and in the case of this family, a critical juncture is arrived at: it is realized, and acted upon, that because her disease is not curable, ensuring her comfort must be given increasing and focused attention. Yet, even though the expectation of death looms, and she is beyond medical recovery, considerable and ongoing interactional work (e.g., regarding hope, acceptance, grief, and very practical matters of day-to-day care) occurs and is designed to organize the environment needed to progressively move toward, and beyond, death."[1(pp183–184)]

We employ conversation analysis, a rigorous research method for closely examining how speakers make available their moment-by-moment understandings of unfolding interactions.[19–21] Emphasis is given to how participants work together to produce and manage social actions that, by definition, cannot be produced alone.[22–23] A priority for conversation analysis is to provide warrantable claims about how primary practices and patterns of everyday communication are "grounded in the conduct of the parties, not in the beliefs of the writer."[24(p476)] As in the following, naturally occurring transcriptions of audio and video recordings are made available for inspection and specialized transcription notation symbols are used for analyses (see appendix).

"They Will Not Just *Ware*house Her."

In Excerpt 1, Dad and Son focus on the hospital to home transition. These moments vividly portray the kinds of normal misunderstandings and caregiving problems that arise when family members experience in-home care. This phone call occurred soon after Mom was released from the hospital and at the onset of hospice care. While the family members by now fully recognized that tumor control was unsuccessful and that Mom was dying, they were, of course, not aware (as Excerpt 3 reveals) that her death would occur in only three to four weeks. The difficult realities of in-home care are previewed in lines 1 through 7.

1) SDCL: Malignancy #41: 4–5

```
1   SON:   I understand mother is home?
2   DAD:   Yes she is.
3   SON:   A:nd how is that going.
4   DAD:   A:::hhh (.) tough.
5   SON:   pt On everybody on her on you, o:n who?
6   DAD:   All of the above.
7   SON:   Oka:y.
8   DAD:   Uhm. =
9   SON:   = Is it w—i—this sounds terrible t'say (0.2) is it *worth* it?
10         (0.3)
11  DAD:   It's not a choice.
12  SON:   Okay.
13  DAD:   They *dis*charged her.
14  SON:   O:h.
15  DAD:   They will not just *ware*house her.
16  SON:   O::h okay.
17  DAD:   Doctor said you know, take her home (.) handle her with hospice
18         and she can be the:re. And know she'll probably like the
19         surroundings better etcetra. And she wasn't overly thrilled but,
20         .hhh hhh you know.
21  SON:   Hmm.
```

When Son asks Dad how Mom's being home is "going," Dad reports "A:::hhh (.) tough" (lines 3–4). When Son next asks who it is "tough" on (line 5), Dad responds with "All of the above" (lines 5–6). In response to this news,[25] and with some dysfluency (i.e., cut-off words) indicating the delicacy of his question, Son next asks, "is it *worth* it?" (line 9). It is important to clarify, based on earlier calls, Son is well aware of the extensive efforts needed to adequately care for Mom. He also knows that for many months following Mom's diagnosis, trained healthcare professionals in a hospital setting have provided systematic and technical efforts to treat her cancer. Son is thus not questioning the critical need to provide quality care for Mom but the decision to move her home, knowing (and now realizing) that the burdens of doing so will be considerable "on everybody." But when Dad states, "It's not a choice" (line 11) and "They *dis*charged her" (line 13), it is clear that Son was *not* aware of these circumstances. Based on his change-of-state "O:h."[26] in line 14, he apparently was not informed about who had made these consequential decisions or when they were made. Son was living in Texas throughout most of these phone calls, and Mom and Dad were living in California. As Son's "is it *worth* it?" in line 9 illustrates, updating and responding to good and bad news[27] over time, and especially long distance on the telephone, requires extensive efforts by families to inform, and at times clarify possible sources of confusion, about a loved one's health condition and care status.

With Dad's "They will not just *ware*house her" (line 15), an inhumane institutional image is invoked, depicting some kind of impersonal repository, where patients are placed as dying is underway. He also displays recognition that by "not" warehousing her, healthcare team members can and do promote humane concerns that dying occur with comfort and dignity. Dad continues (lines 17–19) by reporting the doctor's advice to take Mom home, "handle her with hospice," and provide more comfortable surroundings as her dying progresses. However, Dad also reports that Mom was not particularly "thrilled" about going home. As later calls reveal, Mom was worried that home care would not provide adequate pain management, as well as about her lack of ability to adequately respond to needs that were increasingly troubling (e.g., sleeping, eating, and nausea). Dad also had a full-time job, and it was not yet clear who was to be spending time with Mom in his absence (e.g., her sister, friends, hospice nurse). These are normal ambiguities that need to be addressed as transitions to home and hospice care occur.

"I Kinda Screwed Up the Medication"

One routine problem experienced by family members involves learning how to administer medications. In the following excerpt, Dad's story about "I kinda screwed up the medication" (line 5) exemplifies one of the primary reasons Mom was not "thrilled" about being discharged from the hospital: the possibility of inadequate pain management. Here, Dad's mistake was rooted in his understanding that the doctor's instructions (lines 5–9) for giving Mom pain pills "three times a day" translated into "breakfast, lunch, and supper" (line 11).

2) SDCL: Malignancy #41: 6–7

```
1   DAD:   And then we came home, and ah (0.2) e:::h she spends a lot of
2          time sleeping, or at least dozing partially because of the medication
3          etcetra.
4   SON:   Sure.
5   DAD:   I kinda screwed up the medication on Friday because (.) doctor
6          wrote out the whole set of instructions on all the pills that she takes
7          and how often and all that stuff. .hh *I* don't know—I guess in my
8          mind, I hadn't thought it through too well. But she said y'know,
```

	9		particular pain medicine should be three times a day.
	10	SON:	Mm [hm.
	11	DAD:	[Y'know fine—breakfast, lunch, and supper.
	12	SON:	O:h so you didn't have anything to go through the night with.
	13	DAD:	Yeah [()] =
	14	SON:	[Oops.]
	15	DAD:	= Took y'know—like the best shot at it and missed.
	16	SON:	Mm hm.
	17	DAD:	Four or five o clock in the morning everything hurt like hell, and
	18		she's frantic and all that kind of business. (.) *So* I gave her a couple
	19		a pain pills and then (.) that *cal*med her down a little. But it still
	20		hurt. An' then Saturday morning there was u:h gal who does-
	21		some *kin*d of a visiting nurse. But this was an introduction and
	22		so forth for the hospice stuff.
	23	SON:	Mm hm.
	24	DAD:	So she was here some. (.) She said well, let's give her two more.
	25		We gotta get the pain to calm down. An' then *she* went through
	26		and explained to me y'know, this is got to be two pills every eight
	27		hours and now we're on a six a.m., two p.m., ten p.m. She says you
	28		gotta wake her up, give her the pills, and let her go right back to
	29		sleep.
	30	SON:	Mm hm.
	31	DAD:	(Pills) are t*i*me release morphine and it's got to be very specifically,
	32		you know.
	33	SON:	Mm hm. hhhh
	34	DAD:	Hours between-.hh *oh* okay that leveled that out and the rest of the
	35		stuff you know is *not* so critical because they're a couple of
	36		antibiotics and they're normal (medications) an' that kind of junk.

The problem with Dad's commonsense solution (i.e., a pill with every meal) was quickly surmised by Son, as he realized that Mom had no pain medications through the night (line 12). His following "*O*ops" (line 14) relies on a common practice indicating the occurrence of (typically) unintentional mistakes. As Dad describes, he took his "best shot at and missed" (line 15), well-intended actions that nevertheless caused Mom to "hurt" and be "frantic" (lines 17–20).

The remainder of this excerpt (lines 20–36) focuses on how a newly assigned hospice nurse introduces the care that will be provided, helps Dad figure out how to "get the pain to calm down" (line 25), and overviews a schedule for giving Mom her pills every eight hours—even if she has to be awakened in the middle of the night (which was news to Dad). From Dad's reporting, it is clear that the timing and expertise of the nurse's involvement was critical for providing quality care for Mom and also for minimizing stress and anxiety triggered by not knowing how best to care for her needs. The medical expertise attributed to the nurse stands in stark contrast to Dad's own lay language and orientations—for example, "all that stuff. .hh *I* don't know—I guess" (line 7), "hospice stuff" (line 22), "the rest of the stuff" (lines 34–35), and "that kind of junk" (line 36).

From Excerpt 2, it is apparent that being a lay family member, untrained in the technical details of in-home medical care, can result not only in mistakes made (and owned) but in glossed language displaying a lack of knowledge about fundamental caregiving procedures.

"What's the Doctor Saying . . . You Do This for the Ones You Love"

The following extended excerpt provides a lens revealing three contiguous, interrelated, and key dimensions of family members' experiences: (a) trying to figure out how long Mom has to live (lines 1–13); (b) attempting to diagnose her deteriorating medical condition (lines 15–39); and (c) Assessing how Dad is doing, the moral choices and obligations, and practical consequences of caring for a loved one at home (lines 40–72).

3) SDCL: Malignancy #36: 12–14

	1	SON:	So what's—what's the doctor sa:ying hh in terms of.hh you know
	2		what's going on ti:me wise and all the rest of this *business*.
	3	DAD:	We have no: time estimate. The gal ask—asked me that *y*esterday-
	4		you know, did the doctor give you any indication as tuh.hh
	5		wh*a*t kinda time frame we're looking at. An' I said *n*ope, zilch.
	6		She said you know, take her ho:me. She can do as well the:re.
	7		We'll keep her medicated an' comfortable. We got an appointment
	8		with the doctor in no::w, two weeks I guess. But um, I have no idea
	9		what the time frame is.=
	10	SON:	=Wo::w. .pt .hhh *Ph*ew, (0.2) Yuck, huh.

11	DAD:	(At the rate) it's—it's deter*i*orating a:h (.) my guess is it's still
12		y'know gonna be between now an' the end of the year. But I
13		certainly don't know that based on a damn thing other than that.
14	SON:	Well you know, you start to wonder how much more can fall
15		apart and jus—an' still be alive.
16	DAD:	Mm hm.
17	SON:	You know 'cuz Je:sus, everything seems to be sh*o*t, yiknow. .hh
18		I mean at some point you're gonna have to wonder.hhh hh if
19		there's gonna be even anything *i*n there to start *p*ushing these pills
20		around, you know.
21	DAD:	Well you know, her heart's still strong and some of the rest of the
22		things are still strong. So until some vital—vital organ really goes
23		to hell—a::h you know you—I don't know what (.) what the a:h (.)
24		what the hell you call that y'know how you would die of bo:ne
25		decay.
26	SON:	.hh Yeah, you wouldn't *d*ie necessarily of that although you jus'
27		[hurt like hell.]
28	DAD:	[()]
29	SON:	Yeah.
30	DAD:	But you know that's—that's not crucial.=
31	SON:	=No.=
32	DAD:	=And that's where a l*o*t of the tumors *a*re at this point. Y'know
33		spi:ne, hip, legs—an' that kind of business. (0.4) Y'know h*e*ll that's-
34	SON:	You would think the spine could be the sort of thing that
35		would dis*r*upt-
36	DAD:	Well ultimately it'll start pressin' on the co:rd and cause nerve
37		problems.=
38	SON:	= Yeah. =
39	DAD:	= But you know I don't know what that will do.
40	SON:	Je:ez. .hhh *hh* pt So are you—are you doin alright? (.) Under the
41		circumstances—pardon.
42	DAD:	Most of the time. A::h, you—you can't (.) can't dwell on it if you will
43		jus' because you drive yerself *c*razy. So you say okay (.) it's under
44		control for now. I will do what I have to do and that is keep her
45		comfortable, keep her fed, y'know keep her warm all that kind of
46		stuff it makes it easier—as easy as I can.
47	SON:	Mm hm. And that's really about it, huh.
48	DAD:	Yeah, like grandmother with Aunt Ester.=
49	SON:	=Yeah.
50	DAD:	I a—I y'know a::h, hell of a lot of life *isn't* a choice y'know, and you
51		do this for the ones you love. An' so it's y'know, b*i*ll payin' time.
52	SON:	Yeah.hhh hh *whew*.
53	DAD:	And yes it gets tough at times y'know, 'cuz you're tryin' to be
54		nice an' you're tryin' like *hell* because you hover:, or you get hell
55		because you're not doin' what she wants, or you know. But (.)
56		y'know, she asks for somethin' and then okay I'll go do that.
57		And by the time you get back, that's not what she wanted an' =
58	SON:	= Mm hm. =
59	DAD:	= whatever. =
60	SON:	= Yeah.
61	DAD:	A:nd (.) it's not *r*ational behavior so you—y'know you gotta stop-
62		think wai:t a minute (what's goin on,) stay pleasant overall an'
63		and don't get all bent out of shape over it.
64	SON:	Right.
65	DAD:	And I don't always do that too gracefully.
66	SON:	Heh [heh heh.]
67	DAD:	[Heh heh.]
68	SON:	That's right, this is gonna *t*each ya tolerance like nothing else in
69		the world, huh.
70	DAD:	Oh yeah, yeah I guess.
71		(0.3)
72	DAD:	A:::h well.

Because there are so many important moments in this excerpt, it is not possible here to even begin to unpack how Dad and Son navigate their way through this series of critical topics. Only selected observations are offered in the following about each of the three sets of actions already previewed.

How Long Does Mom Have to Live?

In lines 1–2, Son's question assumes that the doctor has informed Dad about how long Mom has to live. But Dad's "We have no: time estimate." (line 3) makes clear that the doctor knowingly, and/or willingly, did not speculate about Mom's remaining time. It is unclear whether the "We" references just the family or includes the doctor and hospital nurse, but Dad's next "The gal" (line 3) does refer to the hospice nurse. Both the son's and the nurse's questions, as well as Dad's overall demeanor, exemplify how those involved in caring subordinate themselves to medical authority:[28-29] Doctors are more frequently treated as experts, capable of discerning time remaining until death. For example, Dad does not render his own specific opinion in lines 3–9 but does report (lines 7–9) an upcoming appointment with the doctor. And on lines 11–13, his "guess" (see also lines 8–9)—that Mom will die between now and the end of the year—is followed with a strong caveat of not knowing a "damn thing other than that"(though, in retrospect, we can conclude that Dad's prediction was correct: Mom died in late November).

However, slightly less than one month earlier, during phone call #12, Dad and Son were speculating that Mom might die "over the Christmas holidays or something."[1(p199)] Yet the same doctor's ability to render an accurate prognosis was discounted by Dad's stating "she's only got an *ed*ucated crystal ball."[1(p199)] So it is clear that Dad and Son have a history of recognizing that predicting time of death is fraught with ambiguities and inaccuracies. These instances add another case study, but an interactionally grounded set of actual circumstances to long-standing discussions about how time until death gets managed in palliative care.[10,11,15]

Note that talk about how long another has to live is not only subject to miscalculation but can be difficult and stressful for those coming to grips with the inevitable unpredictability of dying and death. Son's triggered response, "= Wo::w. .pt .hhh *Phew.* (0.2) Yuck, huh." (line 10), offers a series of response cries[30] reflecting the power and significance of being caught up within moments assessing the duration of Mom's life.

Making Sense of Mom's Deteriorating Condition

One version of "lay diagnosis" draws attention to how patients and family members not formally trained in biomedicine attempt to describe and understand phenomena such as the nature and impact of disease on bodies, organs, and neurological systems.[31] In lines 15–39, that is essentially what Dad and Son are doing, as they "wonder" (lines 13 and 18), speculate about, and with "I don't know" (lines 23 and 39), generally claim insufficient knowledge[32] about physiological deterioration of organs, bone decay, and spinal and nerve problems. Despite the knowledge and ability to understand the delicate and often complex organization of biomedicine, attempts to do so are a preoccupation with patients and family members. Subordination to medical experts occurs, in large part, as a consequence of this fundamental lack of knowledge, which also creates windows of opportunity for doctors, nurses, and other healthcare staff to inform and educate about bodily processes.

Dad and Son know that Mom's condition is deteriorating but not how her condition is failing or the rate of deterioration. And not having the knowledge that comes from the kinds of cases healthcare staff have previously managed, which may facilitate (but not guarantee) prediction and basic understandings of the underlying mechanisms causing death, underlies the inability of Dad and Son to prognosticate Mom's death with any sense of accuracy. Importantly, however, patients and family members are often curious about these details, which may or may not be addressed openly with doctors and nurses, depending on what topics are raised and how participants pursue and/or avoid addressing biomedical concerns that arise.

Moral Choices, Obligations, and Consequences

In the final section of Excerpt 3 (previous lines 40–72), as Son shifts to "are you doin alright?," the attempts to figure out Mom's bodily systems are rather abruptly closed down in favor of how Dad is coping with these difficult challenges. Unlike biomedical systems, Dad's personal experiences provide a basis for epistemic authority: He is able to access and speak more directly about his daily caregiving incidents and choices. Though seemingly not intentional, Dad lays out a moral framework guiding his caring for Mom.

In marked contrast to Bergman's depiction of gossip as revealing a "morally contaminated character,"[33(p99)] Dad exudes a self-effacing, humble, and committed mode of social conduct characterizing what *love does*:[34]

- He tries not to dwell too much on his problems, which would "drive yourself crazy" (line 43) but strives instead to recognize that his caregiving is under control, as he "does what I have to do" in caring for Mom: provide comfort, food, and warmth (lines lines 43–46).

- He recognizes that a "hell of a lot of life *isn't* a choice," this is what people do for "the ones you love," and that it's "*bill* payin' time" (lines 50–51)—bills being inevitable but typically not-looked-forward-to obligations comprising everyday living.

- When wrongly blamed for simply trying to help Mom out (lines 53–57), he gives priority to forgiving and working to remain "pleasant overall" (lines 61–52).

- He also displays the value of being graceful, in admitting failures (line 65).

To summarize, a discourse of caregiving morality is sketched and made available to Son.[35-36] These actions display reasonable, honest, and decent concerns for Mom and family. In response, Son recognizes the power and importance of learning "tolerance" (lines 68–69).

Overall, Excerpt 3 provides deep and otherwise inaccessible insight into how Dad and Son commiserate about inherent uncertainties of dying and eventual death. Deference to, and thus reliance on, medical authority is necessary for family members. Yet it is also possible to inquire about, and portray a basic moral philosophy of, what it can mean to accept the responsibility of remaining stable in the midst of doing what one can to provide loving care.

"It's Nuts Around Here . . . It Hurts . . . and They Help Me a Lot"

During Excerpts 1–3, Mom had been sleeping. She is now awake and is able to speak with Son. Just prior to line 1, Son had informed Mom that he will be traveling home for Christmas.

4) SDCL: Malignancy #36: 28–29

```
1   MOM:   Well I don't know what to say. All I know is it's nuts around here.
2   SON:   Mm hm. (.) pt So what are ya doin' with yerself during the day,
3          mostly sleeping?
4   MOM:   Yeah. .hh hh Oh jeez it hurts uu:gh. It just hurts when I do things
5          like lay down—lay down. An' it hurts when I do this, it hurts when I
6          do that. Nothin' I can do.
7   SON:   Huh. Just everything hurts, huh.
8   MOM:   Yeah.
9   SON:   Have they gotcha on somethin that—that ke[eps that down I hope.]
10  MOM:                                           [Oh yeah. Oh yeah.]
11  SON:   Oh that's good.
12  MOM:   Yeah, fer sure.
13  SON:   Otherwise it would probably drive you nuts huh.
14  MOM:   It would certainly.
15  SON:   Heh heh heh. I understand you have someone coming by now
16         like uh a, nurse 'er something.
17  MOM:   Yep.
18  SON:   Whuttiz she do.
19  MOM:   Yesterday she kinda talked a lot.
20  SON:   Oh heh heh heh. .hh hh Well shoot you could uh—=
21  MOM:   Yeah [()
22  SON:        [=You could do—you can get a lotta people to do that.
23         Just turn on the radio hu[h.
24  MOM:                            [Right. An' we jus' sit there an' talk.
25  SON:   Mm hm. (.) Well I suppose that's nice though. An' having somebody
26         to talk to (.) y'know does she—is she going to do that regularly is
27         that-
28  MOM:   Yeah. And they help me a lot.
29  SON:   Part of the [plan.
30  Mom:               [() Yeah it's like one—one knows when she comes in
31         an' she does somethin'.
32  SON:   Mm hm.
33  MOM:   It's a regular thing. Um, she'll come in every once in a while.
34  SON:   Mm hm.
35         (2.0)
36  SON:   Well that's kinda nice though I mean at least you got.hh
37         somebody—an' you're not gonna be snotty with her like Aunt Ester
38         was with the one that came to see her, huh.
39  MOM:   Right.
40  SON:   Huh heh heh heh heh.
```

Mom's response to son's "Christmas" announcement (line 1) does not express the kind of enthusiasm mothers would normally share with their children when hearing about plans for a visit. There are three primary and legitimate reasons that explain Mom's lack of excitement.

First, she begins by stating that she does not know what to say, and that "it's nuts around here." In this way Mom indirectly informs Son that it is not normal, but chaotic, in the house now. Mom not only displays recognition that she has been released for in-home care but that such care requires coordination and visits from new people (e.g., the hospice nurse). In reality, their home is being transformed into a caring facility capable of managing Mom's failing health. It would thus be understandable, from Mom's point of view, that she does not know what to say about a changed and "nuts" home that Son is planning to visit. In this important sense, it is not likely to be the typical (and hoped-for) relaxing and peaceful Christmas visit (approximately six weeks away).

Second, Mom continues by repeatedly stating that "it hurts," and there's "Nothin' I can do" (lines 4–6). At the time of this call, Mom had just awakened and (as evident when hearing the call) was also heavily medicated for the pain she was experiencing. Considerable and ongoing pain certainly curbs Mom's ability and motivation to be able, or willing, to create a home holiday environment.

Third, a "business as usual" versus "business at hand"[37] contrast is at play in this episode. With Son's prior announcement that he is planning to come home for Christmas, he initiates a "business as usual" topic and orientation to family matters: a son plans to come home from college for Christmas vacation. We can only speculate that Son may have announced such plans so as to add normality, even hopefulness, to these trying family experiences. As discussed previously from Excerpt 3, Dad and Son had discussed the possibility of Mom dying over the Christmas holidays. But, of course, Mom was not aware of this discussion, and Son may well be making plans as usual, until events might alter regular scheduling (as indeed they did, since, as noted, Mom died in late November). In any case, and as evident in Mom's responses, an abnormal "business at hand" is in play (i.e., managing Mom's chronic and likely terminal illness) that justifiably trumps regular scheduling.

Given the "nuts" home environment, Mom's pain and medication, and a natural (even habituated) tendency by Son to make plans "as usual," it can now be seen that, and how, a mother's response to her son's (otherwise innocuous) vacation offering has little fervor. These are the kinds of impacts and interactional predicaments that emerge whenever family members are faced with significant changes in life-world experiences. Bad news events can "rupture" ordinary communication[27,38–40] and significantly alter social relationships, including (as in this case) normal routines for handling routine family affairs.

The remainder of Excerpt 4 involves discussion about a series of topics related to in-home hospice care: the nurse being able to manage the pain (lines 9–14); regular visits by the hospice nurse who talks (line 19) yet helps Mom "a lot" (line 28); and how nice it is for Mom to have a skilled medical professional who also provides good company (lines 25 and 36). As Son puts it, these activities are "Part of the plan." (line 29), an assessment Mom next (line 30) agrees with and a particularly apt way of describing primary goals of hospice and palliative care.

It should also be noted that it is exceedingly normal for these family members to be humorous throughout otherwise serious topics, such as Son's attempt to compare a nurse's "talked a lot" (line 19) with "Just turn on the radio." (line 23). Or how nice it is for Mom to have someone spend time with her and provide medical care, but only in hopes that Mom will not be "snotty with her like Aunt Ester" (line 37). In both instances, Son laughs (lines 20 and 40) and Mom does not, one of many curious set of occurrences in laughter involving attempted humor that are not closely examined herein[41,42] yet are prominent features of talk about cancer and most other illness journeys.

When Cancer Calls: Moving From Empirical Description to Creating an Effective Health Intervention and Campaign

The scenes we have briefly examined here are drawn from only portions of a single phone call. Analyzed chronologically, as a series of key moments occurring within a month of Mom's death, they reveal the considerable power and potential impact they might have on patients, family members, healthcare professionals, and community members whose lives have been touched by cancer (and other illnesses). Early on in the research process, students and colleagues exposed to a broader range of recorded and transcribed materials expressed being profoundly influenced by these natural interactions. Their observations and reactions often triggered revealing stories about their personal experiences with cancer (as patients, family members, friends, co-workers). Over time, opportunities to solicit reactions from diverse healthcare professionals and community members confirmed how personalized responses can yield important and long-term realizations about how to manage and improve cancer communication (in homes and clinics).

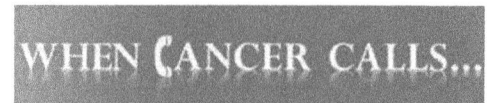

Figure 20.1 Logo for theatrical production

The close analytical examination of communication patterns during family cancer phone calls—the discovery phase of a social scientific investigation—has now been expanded by designing unique educational materials for local, national, and global health communities. A project titled Conversations About Cancer was created, initially funded by the American Cancer Society (98-172-01) and (as noted) currently supported by the National Institutes of Health/National Cancer Institute. The corpus of phone calls have been reduced in length, from approximately 7½ hours to 80 minutes, and developed into a professional theatrical production, *When Cancer Calls . . .* : (Figure 20.1).

All dialogue in this production is drawn from actual phone calls. The exceptional power of the arts is harnessed as an innovative learning tool to extend empirical research, explore ordinary family life, and expose often taken-for-granted conceptions of cancer, health, and illness. Adapting these phone conversations to a stage production reflects the National Cancer Institute's emphasis on (a) building better understanding and improving health communication to minimize cancer burdens and (b) encouraging creative communication initiatives to reduce suffering, promote healing outcomes, and enhance quality of life for patients, survivors, family members, and health professionals throughout cancer journeys. By integrating education and entertainment ("edutainment"), one primary goal is to create a resource that permits meaningful dialogue about delicate, complex, and frequently misunderstood communication challenges arising from cancer diagnosis, treatment, and prognosis.

Phase I and Phase II Trials

A Phase I feasibility study in San Diego and Denver, viewed live and as a DVD screening, revealed highly significant audience impacts:[18]

- Over 80% of all audience members agreed that this family's cancer journey was authentic, interesting, and relevant for "people like me."
- Despite the mother's death, 74% indicated that the performance was uplifting and inspiring, while only 10% considered the play "too depressing."

- From pre- to post-measures, agreement increased significantly for 14 of 15 opinions about cancer, family, and communication (one-tailed paired sample *t* test, alpha = .05). From pre- to post-, the importance of 7 of 10 key communication activities increased significantly.

A Phase II multicity, randomized control effectiveness and dissemination trial was completed very recently. Findings from this larger and even more diverse audience base are currently being analyzed. However, it is clear that our national trial confirms Phase I effectiveness through continued and highly significant findings.

National and global implications for this health intervention are considerable[43] and as patients and family members rely on communication to manage acute, chronic, and terminal conditions across an array of medical conditions. Research and educational applications are relevant for physicians, nurses, social workers, counselors, therapists, and others representing diverse medical and health professions.

Reactions from Focus Group and Talkback Sessions

Following each live performance or DVD screening, conversations are facilitated during talkback or focus group meetings. These conversations provide unique opportunities for audience members to not only give feedback but to connect their viewing experiences with everyday life events comprising cancer journeys. A host of other illnesses and medical challenges also are raised. We have discovered that while cancer is the primary health threat, understanding how communication is a resource for traveling through time, space, and illness together—regardless of the specific disease, treatment procedures, and eventual health outcomes. From these triggered conversations, discussions routinely focus on how *When Cancer Calls . . .* could be helpful for not only enhancing awareness about the importance of family communication but for improving communication skills for patients, family members, and healthcare providers.

The remainder of this chapter provides a small sampling of audience members' comments, following viewings of *When Cancer Calls . . . .* The collective voices of patients, family members, providers, and theater professionals only begin to highlight the potential of *When Cancer Calls . . . .* Research and education in hospice and palliative care, diverse medical fields, and other allied professions can benefit from innovations that focus on patient–family–provider relationships as the primary unit of analysis for investigating communication. Alone and taken as a whole, however, these individuals' narratives clearly reveal the importance of self-reported experiences and recommendations as extremely rich resources for better understanding the social dimensions of cancer (and many other illnesses).

Audience members' reactions and comments are presented next, each meaningful on its own merits yet with cumulative impacts when read as a series of collective voices. Following these narratives, various topics, themes, and implications are revisited in the conclusion and discussion for this chapter.

Patients and Survivors

I think the medical profession definitely should see this because they would be more compassionate . . . Doctors, nurses, social workers . . . medical training and residency for oncology.

I'm going to celebrate my five-year anniversary of breast cancer in May and I just have to say, I don't think about it that much, and I was just crying through the whole thing. It was a real catharsis. But it was just an unbelievable play. So well done . . . I could just go on and on. Thank you so much. It was beautiful.

I had eight surgeries and my kids, my son and my daughter, were in denial. So they never were around me. And my baby, who's 27 now, he was [but] he didn't know how to take it . . . And I think it should be shown to other families . . . I would love to have my children see this now, even though I've already done what I've done . . . You know there's still hope . . .

I'm gonna start talking with my children about my cancer. I want them to maybe take this journey with me. And before this play I didn't want them taking this journey. It was my problem, my issue, and I had to deal with it. I didn't want to burden anyone else. But this play really changed my feelings on that. So now my children are gonna have a say in how my journey goes. So thank you very, very much.

Family Members

I think the "Big C" here is really communication, not cancer.

[I was] deeply moved by the reality of [the] performance, and the modulation and the full weight. This was an enormous gift to me . . .

I just want to thank everybody first of all because this was an amazing experience . . . I think it was an excellent piece of work and I encourage those who are continuing this process to do so. It's the type of thing that I think will allow people like me to heal.

I realized how important every little piece of communication is, and how important things you didn't think were important are important . . . To watch the communication was amazing, and it was really wonderful.

My mom died in 1971 of cancer and I might as well have been 17 sitting right here today, because it was so profoundly connected to my experience. Even though it wasn't exactly my experience, it was exactly my experience.

Every oncologist should see a condensed version of this, and every trainee in whatever program. Anybody in the oncology field . . . in targeted support groups, in other targeted mechanisms . . . it's a marvelous tool.

I've worked for ABC television but this didn't feel like it was a manufactured production. I understood this to be something that was from the actual reality of what this family's experience was. I think it's beautiful as it is.

It prompts us to all think about our own experiences and how we related to it. And how we can help others relate to it, either in our family or our circle of friends.

Doctors

What can I learn about this as a provider? It's not a perspective that we get to see . . . 95% of care occurs outside of the clinic setting. That stuck with me. So we don't get to see that, what happens outside of the clinic setting.

What I liked about this is the honesty of dealing with the whole subject of cancer. I think it's very difficult to find artistic presentations where cancer is considered and even portrayed. I see that the amount of conversation that it has generated here would be done by individuals, with their families, if this kind of thing was more broadly expressed in the country—and more frequently. So you could say, did you see that cancer play? Oh yeah, I did, and you could do that with people who have cancer that you know and love. It brings it into something that you could talk to them about. And that can start a conversation, and that catalyzes a great number of things.

[I liked] just about everything: The empathy and their worries, the narration, the story line. Everything.

I think it has value from a provider's standpoint, to take into consideration what families are dealing with on the other side. So I think it definitely has value that way.

Nurses

It gives permission to communicate, which is so vital...

I worked in hospice, but there's a lot that you don't see when you're not there with the family interaction.

And I think as providers, we sometimes don't have a lot of outlets for... the emotional piece of our jobs. Because what we do is we take care of people with cancer. And I think this would be a good thing to use in groups of just healthcare providers... have a place to actually discuss it and to get conversations going. Because we all need to be able to talk about it... Everyone can talk about what that brought back for them.

I happen to be a healthcare provider, and I think often people forget the family. They don't realize maybe they don't have the disease, but yet they are going through it.

I worked in hospice for oncology, and all I could think of when I was watching it was the experience of my family, and kind of that uncertainty about what turn is this patient gonna take next in anyone who is terminally ill.

And I used to work hospice too, and I mean, people with cancer would truly relate to this. But there's so many horrible diseases: Huntington's, and end stage liver disease, and Alzheimer's. I mean there's, you know, there's just a multitude... I think it could be [useful beyond cancer]...

We could use it in every terminal disease, that it almost focus(es) more on how you deal with death, rather than the entire journey of the cancer.

... when you get outside of that family, it seems really odd to mingle and jokes, but within that family it's normal. And I think this might be a good thing for families and patients going through that to feel that, and understand we're not total sadists. There's nothing wrong with us that we're able to joke about this, that it's a normal coping mechanism.

Theater Professionals

For caregivers involved primarily in palliative care, this could be very useful... Because it presents a manner of coping, and the implication (is) that there are resources that can be used... What I'm saying is, for anybody who is not familiar enough with the interpersonal dynamics of what families experience, this could be really, really useful.

I just kept thinking: Could you imagine what this could do for an awful lot of people? Because society doesn't really give us the tools to cope with this kind of situation... This could be so helpful, the idea that we're all (part of) an experience that's collective.

Our research team is very interested in identifying these "collective" reactions to *When Cancer Calls*..., as well as more individual and even idiosyncratic depictions of how cancer journeys get managed. By closely examining transcriptions of post-production talkback sessions and focus group meetings, we are in the midst of developing a grounded-theoretic approach for identifying specific and more generalized types of descriptions offered by audience members.[44] Specific categories are being developed that will eventually be translated into guidelines for improving communication in palliative care and related health professions. Emphasis will be given to developing best practices for addressing the kinds of issues and concerns evident within family members' stories triggered by viewings of *When Cancer Calls*....

Conclusion

When actual family phone conversations are closely examined, even from a single call involving talk about transitioning to in-home and hospice care, access is provided to a social world we claim to know and understand but, in reality, is routinely overlooked and taken for granted. From the excerpts presented here, it is possible to gain a new and deeper appreciation for the real-time challenges involved when facing terminal cancer as a family. These challenges are situated in a complex fabric of potential misunderstandings, problems, burdens, fears, and uncertainties that are routinely triggered when dying and death occur. At the same time, they provide unique opportunities for patients, family members, and health professionals to rely on communication to remedy mistakes, provide comfort and support during delicate moments, help reduce uncertainties and fears, and boost hope in the midst of possible despair.

Certain problems will persist, such as inevitable asymmetries between lay versus medical expertise/knowledge, as well as frustrations arising from the inability to accurately predict how and when death will occur. Yet in the very midst of such confusion and turmoil, progress can be made: Patience and tolerance can be refined, moral compasses tested and calibrated, and love enacted that might otherwise not be available as a resource for journeying through life and death together. However, especially for interdisciplinary teams, the time and support needed to achieve compassionate communication should not be underestimated.[44] The effective management of delicate and often chronic issues, such as major depression, are directly tied to how social relationships are enacted in home and inpatient palliative care.[45]

When Cancer Calls... provides a triggering device for gaining access to actual communication defining these social relationships. By integrating the social sciences and the arts, the general public and healthcare professionals are now able to be drawn into this family's cancer journey. At the same time, many are also "transported"[46] into prior and present life-world experiences involving their own experiences as they manage daily circumstances occasioned by disease, illness, and health.

Much remains to be learned from such a rich corpus of research materials—family phone calls that are one of a kind yet appear to be universally appealing to diverse audiences nationwide. As evident from audience members' reactions provided here (i.e., from patients, family members, doctors, nurses, and theatre professionals), it is fortunate that these raw materials have been developed into *When Cancer Calls*.... Patients, family members, and providers alike value cathartic opportunities to express their feelings, to recognize that their experiences are shared by others, and to gain a newfound appreciation and ability to make sense of the importance of communication. Screenings provide "a marvelous tool" for increasing understandings and compassion throughout care and for being a "catalyst" for ongoing conversations about

Table 20.1 Educational Interventions for Palliative Care Networks: Using *WCC* as a Triggering Device for Addressing Communication Issues

Participants	Proximal Benefits	Long-Term Benefits
Patients and Family Members	In home and/or hospice settings, view *WCC* and utilize talkback sessions to identify specific communication issues that help and hinder care	Implement counseling sessions and/or workshops to address communication problems (e.g., denial or unwillingness to accept or talk about illness, caregiver stress, adult/children conflicts, fears, uncertainties, hopes)
Patients, Family Members, Providers, and Interdisciplinary Teams	Use *WCC* screenings to stimulate dialogue between lay and professional staff about communication throughout cancer (and other illness) journeys	Train providers to become more sensitive to concerns of patients/family members, so as to develop communication skills for pursuing shared treatment goals and health outcomes
Providers and Interdisciplinary Teams	Screen *WCC* for healthcare providers to provide an outlet for sharing emotional experiences and communication encounters	Use initial talkback sessions to identify and brainstorm ways to improve communication within organizational cultures, in order to enact strategies for providing higher quality care for patients and family members

Note. WCC = *When Cancer Calls* . . . [46]

illness and care. Audience members frequently and strongly recommend that others experience *When Cancer Calls* . . . , either personally and/or when used as a powerful tool for systematic education and training (see Table 20.1).

These activities function as innovative interventions for impacting and improving communication skills throughout palliative care. Numerous benefits have been described by patients, families, and providers working across allied health professions: personal healing, enhancement of skills for communicating in the family and clinic, coming to grips with often ambiguous emotions, ability to meaningfully affect change in diverse relationships (families and friendships alike), and giving priority to being compassionate as a needed set of communicative practices and activities.

These important social and health outcomes can be assessed as *When Cancer Calls* . . . continues to develop momentum. With broad dissemination beyond research protocols enacted for Phase I feasibility and Phase II effectiveness trials, collaborations with palliative centers and systems will provide exciting opportunities to focus on specific communication concerns that inhibit and enhance personalized care. By closely attending to communication as the basis of care throughout end-of-life phases, more systematic attention can be given to resolving interactional and medical problems, maintaining family relationships, enhancing patient–family–provider relationships, implementing creative decisions, and promoting the ability to remain life-affirming and hopeful in the face of terminal illness.

References

1. Beach WA. *A Natural History of Family Cancer: Interactional Resources for Managing Illness.* Cresskill, NJ: Hampton Press; 2009.
2. Beach WA, Dozier, DM. Uncertainties, fears, and hopes: Patient-initiated actions and doctors' responses during oncology interviews. *J of Health Commun.* In press.
3. American Cancer Society. Cancer facts and figures 2013. http://www.cancer.org/research/cancerfactsstatistics/cancerfactsfigures2013/ Accessed August 29, 2014.
4. National Hospice and Palliative Care Organization. *NHCPO's Facts and Figures: Hospice Care in America.* Alexandria, VA: National Hospice and Palliative Care Organization; 2013
5. Beach WA, ed. *Handbook of Patient-Provider Interactions: Raising and Responding to Concerns about Life, Illness, and Disease.* New York, NY: Hampton Press; 2013.
6. Mack W, Grier HE. The day one talk. *J Clin Oncol.* 2004;22:563–566.
7. Hudson P. Positive aspects and challenges associated with caring for a dying relative at home. *Int J Palliat Nurs.* 2004;10:58–65.
8. Back AL, Arnold RM. "Yes it's sad, but what should I do?" Moving from empathy to action in discussing goals of care. *J Palliat Med.* 2014;17:141–144.
9. Wenrich MD, Curtis JR., Shannon SE, Carline JD, Ambrozy DM, Ramsey PG. Communicating with dying patients within the spectrum of medical care from terminal diagnosis to death. *Arch Intern Med.* 2001;161:868–874.
10. Fallowfield L, Jenkins V, Beveridge H. Truth may hurt but deceit hurts more: Communication in palliative care. *Palliative Med.* 2002;16:297–303.
11. Back A L, Anderson WG, Bunch L, Marr LA, Wallace JA, Yang HB, Arnold RM. Communication about cancer near the end of life. *Cancer.* 2008;113(7 Suppl):1897–1910.
12. Mack JW, Cronin A, Taback N, et al. End-of-life care discussions among patients with advanced cancer. *Ann Intern Med.* 2012;156:204–210.
13. Steinhauser KE, Christakis NA, Clipp EC, Mcintyre L. Factors considered important at the end of life by patients, family, physicians, and other care providers. *JAMA.* 2014;284:2476–2482.
14. Jocham HR. Dassen T, Widdershoven G, Ruud H. Evaluating palliative care: A review of the literature. *Palliat Care Res Treat.* 2009;3:5–12.
15. De Haes H, Teunissen S. Communication in palliative care: A review of recent literature. *Curr Opin Oncol.* 2005;17:345–350.
16. Reblin M, Cloyes KG, Carpenter J, Berry PH, Clayton, MF, Ellington L. Social support needs: Discordance between home hospice nurses and former family caregivers. *Palliat Support Care.* in press.
17. Clayton MF, Reblin M, Carlisle M, Ellington L. Communication behaviors used to elicit and address cancer patient/caregiver emotional concerns: A description of home hospice communication. *Oncol Nurs Forum.* 2014;41(3):311–321.
18. Beach WA, Buller MK, Dozier D, Buller D, Gutzmer K. Conversations about Cancer (CAC): Assessing feasibility and audience impacts from viewing *The Cancer Play. Health Commun.* 2014;29(5):462–472.
19. Atkinson JM, Heritage J, eds. *Structures of Social Action: Studies in Conversation Analysis.* Cambridge, UK: Cambridge University Press; 1984.
20. Heritage J, Maynard DW, eds. *Communication in Medical Care: Interactions Between Primary Care Physicians and Patients.* Cambridge, UK: Cambridge University Press; 2006.

21. Sidnell, J, Stivers T, eds. *Handbook of Conversation Analysis*. Cambridge, UK: Blackwell-Wiley; 2013.
22. Beach WA, Andersen J. Communication and cancer? Part I: The noticeable absence of interactional research. *J Psychosoc Oncol*. 2003;21:1–23.
23. Beach WA, Andersen J. Communication and cancer? Part II: Conversation analysis. *J Psychosoc Oncol*. 2004;21:1–22.
24. Schegloff EA. A tutorial on membership categorization. *J Pragmatics*. 2007;39:462–482.
25. Beach, WA. Between dad and son: Initiating, delivering, and assimilating bad cancer news. *Health Commun*. 2002;14:271–299.
26. Heritage, J. A change-of-state token and aspects of its sequential placement. In: Atkinson, JM, Heritage J, eds. *Structures of Social Action*. Cambridge, UK: Cambridge University Press; 1984:299–345.
27. Maynard DW. *Good News, Bad News: Conversational Order in Everyday Talk and Clinical Settings*. Chicago, IL: University of Chicago Press; 2003.
28. Heritage J. Revisiting authority in physician-patient interaction. In: Duchan JF, Kovarsky D, eds. *Diagnosis as Cultural Practice*. New York, NY: Mouton de Gruyter; 2005:83–102.
29. Beach WA. Doctor-patient interactions. In: Tracy K, ed. *Encyclopedia of Language and Social Interaction*. Thousand Oaks, CA: SAGE; in press.
30. Goodwin C. Transparent vision. In: Ochs E, Schegloff EA, Thompson, SA, eds. *Interaction and Grammar*. Cambridge, UK: Cambridge University Press; 1996:370–404.
31. Beach WA. Introduction: Diagnosing lay diagnosis. *Text*. 2001;21: 13–18.
32. Beach WA, Metzger TR. Claiming insufficient knowledge. *Human Commun Res*. 1997;23:562–588.
33. Bergman J. *Discreet Indiscretions: The Social Organization of Gossip*. New York, NY: Aldine de Gruyter; 1993.
34. Goff B. *Love Does: Discover a Secretly Incredible Life in an Ordinary World*. Dallas, TX: Thomas Nelson, 2012.
35. Bergman J, Linnell P, eds. *Special Issue: Morality in Discourse. Res Lang Soc Interac*. 1998;31(3–4).
36. Heritage J, Lindstrom A. Motherhood, medicine, and morality: Scenes from a medical encounter. *Res Lang Soc Interact*. 1998;31:397–438.
37. Button G, Casey N. Topic initiation: Business-at-hand. *Res Lang Soc Interac*. 1988–1989;22:61–91.
38. Maynard DW. On co-implicating recipients in the delivery of diagnostic news. In: Drew P, Heritage J, eds. *Talk at Work: Interactions in Institutional Settings*. Cambridge, UK: Cambridge University Press; 1992:331–358.
39. Maynard DW. On "realization" in everyday life: The forecasting of bad news as a social relation. *Am Sociol Rev*. 1996;61:109–131.
40. Maynard DW. The news delivery sequence: Bad news and good news in conversational interaction. *Res Lang Soc Interac*. 1997;30:93–130.
41. Glenn P. *Laughter in Interaction*. Cambridge, UK: Cambridge University Press; 2003.
42. Glenn P, Holt E. *Studies of Laughter in Interaction*. New York, NY: Bloomsbury, 2013.
43. Beach WA, Gutzmer K, Dozier D, Buller MK, Buller D. Conversations about Cancer (CAC): A global strategy for accessing naturally occurring family interactions. In: Kim DK, Singhal A, Kreps G, eds. *Global Health Communication Strategies in the 21st Century: Design, Implementation, and Evaluation*. Bern, Switzerland: Peter Lange; 2014:101–117.
44. Perry R. Communication and compassion need time and support: Insights from end of life care. *Int J Ther Rehabi.l* 2013;20:478–479.
45. Irwin S, Sanjhai R, Bower K, Palica J, Sanjay SR, Maglione JE, Soskins M, Bettterton AE, Ferris FD. Psychiatric issues in palliative care: Recognition of depression in patients enrolled in hospice care. *J Palliat Med*. 2008;11:158–163.
46. Beach WA, Moran BM, Dozier DM, Buller MK, Gutzmer K, Parsloe S. *When Cancer Calls . . . :* Creating reality theatre about family cancer and implications for entertainment education (EE). 2014; unpublished manuscript.

Appendix: Transcription Notation Symbols

In data headings, "SDCL" stands for "San Diego Conversation Library," a collection of recordings and transcriptions of naturally occurring interactions; "Malignancy #" represents the title and number of call in the data corpus; page numbers from which data excerpts are drawn are also included, and line numbers represent ordering in the original transcriptions. The transcription notation system employed for data segments is an adaptation of Gail Jefferson's work described in *A Natural History of Family Cancer*.[1] The symbols may be described as follows:

:   *Colon(s)*: Extended or stretched sound, syllable, or word.

_   *Underlining*: Vocalic emphasis.

(.)   *Micropause*: Brief pause of less than (0.2).

(1.2)   *Timed Pause*: Intervals occurring within and between same or different speaker's utterance.

(( ))   *Double Parentheses*: Scenic details.

( )   *Single Parentheses*: Transcriptionist doubt.

.   *Period*: Falling vocal pitch.

?   *Question Marks*: Rising vocal pitch.

↑↓   *Arrows*: Pitch resets; marked rising and falling shifts in intonation.

° °   *Degree Signs*: A passage of talk noticeably softer than surrounding talk.

=   *Equal Signs*: Latching of contiguous utterances, with no interval or overlap.

[ ]   *Brackets*: Speech overlap.

[[*Double Brackets*: Simultaneous speech orientations to prior turn.

!   *Exclamation Points*: Animated speech tone.

-   *Hyphens*: Halting, abrupt cut off of sound or word.

> <   *Less Than/Greater Than Signs*: Portions of an utterance delivered at a pace noticeably quicker than surrounding talk.

$ *Smile Voice*: Laughing/chuckling voice while laughing and talking.

OKAY *CAPS*: Extreme loudness compared with surrounding talk.

hhh .hhh *H's*: Audible outbreaths, possibly laughter. The more h's, the longer the aspiration. Aspirations with periods indicate audible inbreaths (e.g., .hhh). H's within (e.g., ye(hh)s) parentheses mark within-speech aspirations, possible laughter.

pt   *Lip Smack*: Often preceding an inbreath.

hah *Laugh Syllable*: Relative closed or open position of laughter.

heh

hoh

CHAPTER 21

Chronic Obstructive Pulmonary Disease and Heart Disease

Niharika Ganta and Laura P. Gelfman

Introduction

Chronic obstructive pulmonary disease (COPD) and heart failure (HF) are the two most prevalent chronic, progressive life-limiting diseases affecting Americans today.[1] The American Lung Association estimates that approximately 24 million Americans are living with COPD, the third leading cause of death in the United States, with 134,676 dying from the disease in 2010.[2] Similarly, HF affects 5.1 million people in the United States.[3] The incidence of HF increases with age; nearly 10 per 1,000 people after 65 years of age are diagnosed with HF.[4] Furthermore, HF is associated with a high mortality; one in nine death certificates in 2009 mentioned HF.[3] Furthermore, patients living with COPD or HF are commonly hospitalized. COPD accounted for 715,000 hospital discharges in 2010, with 65% of these discharges in people over the age of 65.[2] HF is one of the most common causes of hospitalization among adults over age 65.[5]

Because these serious illnesses have such high prevalence, symptom burden, increased utilization, and healthcare cost, communication becomes a critical aspect of care for patients living with these illnesses. This chapter describes the specific palliative care needs of patients with advanced HF and patients with severe COPD, outlines effective communication strategies to address these needs, and discusses opportunities for improving the quality of communication among patients with these advanced illnesses, their family members, and their healthcare providers. The definitions of advanced HF and COPD are given in Table 21.1.

Palliative Care Needs of This Population

In both illnesses, patients tend to have multiple comorbidities and high symptom burden including pain, dyspnea, emotional distress, and fatigue.[6–9] Patients with HF or with COPD and their caregivers alike report stress, social isolation, depressive symptoms, and diminished quality of life.[10–15] Furthermore, caregivers who report depressive symptoms and poor health-related quality of life are at increased risk of mortality and morbidity.[16,17] The high prevalence, associated symptom burden, and healthcare utilization of these two illnesses lead to immense economic burden. The National Institutes of Health reported the total healthcare costs of COPD in the United States to be $29.5 billion in 2010 with another $20.4 billion lost in productivity.[18] Similar to COPD, the cost of caring for patients with HF is estimated to be $32 billion annually.[19]

Studies demonstrate that patients with COPD have the same, if not greater physical, social, and emotional needs as patients with inoperable non-small-cell lung cancer.[7,9] The sources of suffering for patients with severe COPD include dyspnea, depression, anxiety, social isolation, functional disability, difficulty sleeping, and nutritional deficiencies.[6,7,9,20] In spite of this burden, fewer than 50% of patients with COPD get relief from dyspnea during their last 6 months of life.[9] Similarly, patients with advanced HF have a symptom burden comparable to patients living with advanced cancer.[21,22] Patients with HF suffer from pain, dyspnea, sleeping difficulties, spiritual distress, depression, isolation, functional disability, and fatigue.[21,22] Interestingly, the Study to Understand Prognoses and Preferences for Outcomes and Risks of Treatments revealed that patients with COPD were much more likely to receive invasive mechanical ventilation, cardiopulmonary resuscitation, or tube feeding before dying than patients with lung cancer, despite both groups being equally likely to prefer care that focused on comfort rather than extending life—and having approximately equal survival.[23]

With this disparity between treatment preferences and treatment received, patients with these advanced illnesses and their family members report the need for improved communication. COPD or HF patients and their family members want more information regarding their disease, prognosis, progression of disease, and what the end of life will look like.[24,25] In an effort to alleviate this disparity, medical specialty societies, including the American Thoracic Society, the American College of Cardiology, and the American Heart Association,[26–28] have called for a more holistic approach to these serious illnesses, an increase in both patient and caregiver education, as well as communication regarding the unpredictable illness trajectory.

Communication Challenges in Patients with Severe COPD or Advanced HF

Healthcare providers caring for patients with COPD or HF face unique communication challenges. One of the challenges is the unpredictable illness trajectory of both diseases, characterized by long-standing chronic illness with progressive functional decline, punctuated by exacerbations requiring hospitalizations[29]

Table 21.1 Advanced HF and Severe COPD Defined

Term	Definition	Manifestations
Advanced HF	Stage D	◆ Refractory HF with progressively worsening symptoms (i.e., edema, dyspnea with exertion, orthopnea) ◆ Complications of HF (i.e., rhythm complications, cardio-renal syndrome) ◆ Side effects associated with medical therapies (i.e., kidney injury with use of diuretics) ◆ Repeated hospitalizations, increased visits to outpatient providers
Severe COPD	GOLD Stage III or IV	◆ Airflow limitation measured with spirometry ◆ Stage III: FEV1 30%–49% predicted and FEV1/FVC less than 70% ◆ Stage IV: FEV1 less than 30% predicted or less than 50% predicted and FEV1/FVC less than 70%.

Note. HF = heart failure; COPD = chronic obstructive pulmonary disease.
Sources. Yancy CW, Jessup M, Bozkurt B, et al. 2013 ACCF/AHA Guideline for the management of heart failure: A Report of the American College of Cardiology Foundation/American Heart Association Task Force on Practice Guidelines. *J Am Coll Cardiol.* October 15, 2013;62(16):e147–e239; Abouezzeddine OF, Redfield MM. Who has advanced heart failure? Definition and epidemiology. Congest Heart Fail. 2011;17(4):160–168.

(see Figure 21.1). The hospitalizations for acute exacerbations often require aggressive interventions such as noninvasive mechanical ventilation, mechanical ventilation, or the use of inotropes and/or pressors. If patients leave the hospital alive, they often leave with a decrease in their functional status.[29] This unpredictable disease trajectory creates multiple downstream challenges, including difficulty with prognostication faced by healthcare providers, lack of clarity about disease course experienced by patients and their caregivers, and an unwillingness of providers to bring up the issues that are judged routine for cancer patients.

Across the board, predicting patients' prognosis is a difficult task, and healthcare providers are notoriously inaccurate.[30] This challenge is heightened by the unpredictable disease trajectories of HF and COPD and the difficulty of pinpointing where the individual patient is on the illness trajectory with each exacerbation. Although after an illness exacerbation patients may never fully return to their prior baseline, the expectation is they will survive the acute complication. This unpredictable disease course makes prognostication even more challenging in patients with these chronic, progressive, serious illnesses.

A topic that warrants more attention is goals of care discussions, which should include resuscitation preferences. Studies have shown that physicians are less likely to discuss resuscitation preferences with patients with advanced HF than other diseases with poor prognoses.[31] In fact, some patients even feel that their providers do not want to have these discussions so they avoid the topic.[32] Similarly in COPD, a study investigating attitudes of people with COPD in pulmonary rehabilitation program found that a mere 19% reported discussing resuscitation preferences with their healthcare provider, and only 14% were confident that their provider understood their wishes. Furthermore, 99% of these patients wanted to have this discussion with their provider.[33]

Another major hurdle in discussing advance care planning in these populations is patients' lack of knowledge regarding their illness trajectory. For instance, most patients with COPD are initially unaware that their disease is progressive and can result in death.[34] Additionally, COPD caregivers report receiving little information regarding what it means to have the disease in terms of what to expect for prognosis or symptoms that will arise.[7,34] A startling 44% of bereaved relatives of patients with severe COPD were not aware that their loved one might die from COPD.[9] Even at the stage when COPD severity necessitates home oxygen therapy, many patients remain unaware of the fact that they suffer from a life-limiting disease and cannot provide a correct name for their condition.[34,35] Similarly, most people living with HF are unaware that their illness is life-limiting.[36–38] HF patients were not able to connect an increase in symptoms with an exacerbation.[25,39] Given this lack of clarity on the part of healthcare providers, patients, and caregivers alike, we must undertake interventions to improve this knowledge gap; improved communication is a key to this effort.

Communication Strategies for Patients with Severe COPD or Advanced HF

In this section, we outline various communication tools that can be used to engage patients and families in discussions regarding their serious illness. These tools can be used to educate a patient about his or her condition or discuss patients' treatment preferences and their goals of care. The tools we review include "Ask-Tell-Ask,"

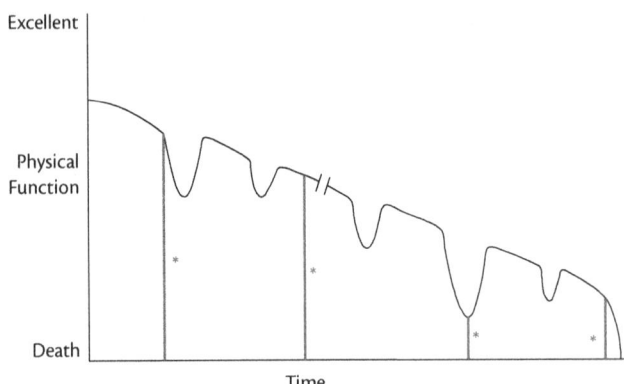

* Represents a potential sudden death event

Figure 21.1 This figure illustrates the trajectory of chronic diseases such as chronic obstructive pulmonary disease and heart failure, where there is general decline in function over time. These illnesses are punctuated by episodes of significant decreases in function, which represent disease exacerbations. The risk of sudden death (*) is present throughout the illness trajectory. Adapted from Murray SA, Kendall M, Boyd K, Sheikh A. Illness trajectories and palliative care. *BMJ.* 2005;330(7498):1007–1011; Goodlin SJ. Palliative care in congestive heart failure. *J Am Coll Cardiol.* 2009;54(5):386–396.

"hope for the best, and prepare for the worst," and "REMAP."[40–44] This section also includes approaches to address the use of medical technologies in HF and COPD, as well as prognostication.

Patients with either COPD or HF have frequent hospitalizations that result in recurring health status changes, which change treatment preferences and expectations. These fluctuations in clinical condition could serve as opportunities to reassess patients' understanding of their disease and their expectations for the future and directly address advance care planning.

Ask-Tell-Ask

The Ask-Tell-Ask tool has three components that allow healthcare providers to gauge patient or family readiness to engage in a conversation and their perception of the illness and to fill in any knowledge gaps[39–41] (Table 21.2). The first "Ask" enables providers to assess patients' readiness to discuss their health condition and to elicit patients' knowledge about their illness and perception about their current health status. Using open-ended questions such as, "What have doctors told you about your illness?" has been very effective.[45] This approach allows healthcare providers to gain insight into patients' perception of their illness and its burden.

Furthermore, it is important to learn how and in what context the patient prefers to receive the information and how much information the patient wants to hear. For instance, some patients want to know all of the details of their illness, while others prefer to hear the big picture, and others prefer that their surrogate hears the information.[46] In addition, a patient may prefer to be alone or have family or friends present. Curtis and colleagues conducted a study in COPD patients investigating how patients and families want and receive information from their healthcare providers.[46] Some patients and family members favored a more direct and explicit approach, while others preferred a discussion of prognosis in general terms.[46]

The second component of the Ask-Tell-Ask communication tool is the "Tell." This portion allows the provider to fill in knowledge gaps, correct misconceptions about the disease, or explain diagnosis/prognosis if needed. When providing information, it is important to use short sentences and pause to allow patient and family to respond or ask questions.[44] The final piece of this framework is the second "Ask," which allows healthcare providers to check-in with patients to see what they understood from the information that was just given. This final "Ask" allows a patient to ask questions or clarify their concerns (see Tables 21.2 and 21.3).

Another communication struggle that was highlighted earlier is the uncertainty that lies in the illness trajectory for patients with HF and patients with COPD (see Figure 21.1 for illness trajectory). In order to tackle this issue, healthcare providers need to communicate effectively about both the illness uncertainties and how to deal with the uncertainty, as well as make a plan for emergency situations. "Hope for the best, prepare for the worst" is a useful framework in this discussion.[39,42,47] This expression allows providers to explore both sides of the issues surrounding these diseases. On one hand, there is hope that patients will live long and fulfilling lives with infrequent hospitalizations. On the other hand, patients with these illnesses are likely to experience an early and sudden death and have a limited amount of time to live. When providers employ this phrase, they can structure the conversation to align themselves with the patient's hopes and goals. At the same time, the healthcare provider can educate the patient about the real possibility of sudden death or progressive functional decline with multiorgan failure.[39,42,47]

Eliciting Patient's Hopes, Goals, and Values

By eliciting patients' hopes, goals, and values, healthcare providers can better understand how patients would want to spend their time, which is often limited. When discussing this prognostic uncertainty with patients, the healthcare provider must acknowledge the patient's feelings of uneasiness and anxiety. Table 21.4 summarizes how to start these conversations and offers examples for how to respond to patients.

Table 21.2 Ask-Tell-Ask Tool

Steps	Purpose	Examples
Ask	Elicit patient's knowledge of health status Assess patient's readiness to continue the conversation or hear about his or her health status Elicit patient's values and preferences	♦ "What have the doctors told you about your condition?" ♦ "Is it okay if we talk about your disease and what to expect?" ♦ "Some patients like to hear all the details and some just want to know the big picture. How would you like to get your information?"
Tell	Provide information to the patient about his or her current health status, illness trajectory, prognosis Fill in any knowledge gaps Break bad news	♦ "Your illness can be very unpredictable . . ." ♦ "Unfortunately, I have some bad news about your condition . . ." ♦ "I want to clear up any confusion you have regarding your disease . . ."
Ask	Assess patient's understanding of the new information Check to see if patient/family has more questions Assess readiness to progress in conversation	♦ "I know I gave you a lot of information today; what are you going to tell your family when you get home?" ♦ "What are your questions?" ♦ "I want to make sure I did a good job giving the information; what did you understand from our discussion?" ♦ "Is it okay to move on to . . . ?"

Sources. Goodlin SJ. Palliative care in congestive heart failure. *J Am Coll Cardiol.* 2009;54(5):386–396; Back AL, Arnold RM, Baile WF, Tulsky JA, Fryer-Edwards K. Approaching difficult communication tasks in oncology. *CA: Cancer J Clin.* 2005;55(3):164–177; Whellan DJ, Goodlin SJ, Dickinson MG, et al. End-of-life care in patients with heart failure. *J Card Fail.* 2014;20(2):121–134.

176 TEXTBOOK OF PALLIATIVE CARE COMMUNICATION

Table 21.3 Some Examples of Medical Jargon to Avoid

Medical Term	Alternative Language
Acute	Suddenly—within a few days
Arrhythmia	An abnormal heart rhythm
BIPAP/CPAP	A special mask that provides pressure to allow lungs to expand
Chronic	Lasting a long time—usually 3 months or longer
Exacerbation	Worsening of disease or flare
Hypoxia/hypoxic	Not enough oxygen in the tissues, even though blood flow is adequate
MI	Heart attack
Intubation	When patients cannot breathe on their own, intubation is the use of a special breathing tube inserted into a patient's airway to do the work of breathing
Ventilator	Breathing machine
Pressors	Medications to increase blood pressure

[Handwritten note: Week 1: Assignment: Translate/Rewrite jargon from your practice — get to basics]

Table 21.4 Eliciting Hopes and Values

[Handwritten note: Assignment Rewrite]

Start Conversation	Patient	Provider Response	Goal
"I know you just got out of the hospital. What did the doctors tell you about your condition?"	"I was diagnosed with heart failure in the hospital. My legs got really swollen, but now I take a water pill and I'm back to normal. I'll be okay, right?"	1. "I hope that with the right management you can lead a long and fulfilling life. Have you ever thought about what you would want if this were not possible?" 2. "I hope that taking these new medications will get you back to feeling well. Unfortunately, knowing that your condition is getting worse, have you thought about the things that are important to you?"	◆ Align with patient and assure him or her that you will continue to provide support through the disease process ◆ Bring up the goals of treatment ◆ At the same time, educate the patient about the gravity of the illness and real possibility of death
"What are you hoping for with your treatments?"	"I want to do everything to stay out of the hospital, that's all."	"I also hope that we can work together to keep you out of the hospital. What are your other goals?"	◆ Align yourself with the patient ◆ Elicit the patient's goals ◆ Go back to the well to learn additional goals
"It sounds like you were told about risk of sudden death. What are your questions about the topic?"	"Do you know if that'll happen to me? How can you know?"	"It must be scary to hear this. Unfortunately, like many things in life, we don't know what will happen."	◆ Normalize feelings of anxiety ◆ Normalize the uncertainty
"Now that you've heard all of this information from the doctors in the hospital and me, what are you thinking?"	"I don't want to be negative and think about dying. I just want to focus on now and getting better."	"I respect that you want to focus on your current goals. But in case things don't go as we hope, what kinds of things would help prepare you or your family for an emergency situation?"	◆ Acknowledge patient's current emotion ◆ Structure the conversation to allow discussion of undesired possibilities ◆ Allow the patient to express concerns surrounding an emergency situation
"I understand that you just got back from the hospital. What are you thinking?"	"I know I've been in the hospital twice already, but I always get better."	"I understand that you've improved in the past; I think it is important to focus on how things are going now and prepare for emergencies."	◆ Recognize patient's perception of disease ◆ Structure the conversation so that emergencies or unexpected trajectories can be explored

[Handwritten note: Discuss patterns of illness & outcomes]

REMAP

In addition to eliciting hopes and values, the provider must build from these values to make treatment recommendations to patients and their families. REMAP[43] (Table 21.5) is a specific communication tool that allows providers to make recommendations to patients and families regarding the next steps in their care based on the stated values and goals. REMAP also allows providers to provide health status updates and address the uncertainty of a patient's situation. When providing health status updates, the Ask-Tell-Ask tool can be used within the larger REMAP framework. REMAP allows providers to move the conversation forward and translate patient values into action steps. For instance, for a patient with rapidly deteriorating health with imminent death who expresses that he values being comfortable and dying at home, the healthcare provider can recommend home hospice services.

Table 21.5 REMAP Tool

Steps	Purpose	Example
Reframe why current treatment plan is not working	Provide health status updates and role of current treatment	"Since you left the hospital the medications you used before are not working now because your disease has gotten worse." "What have your doctors told you about your last hospital stay?... Can I give you more information about what the new lung studies show?" (Ask-Tell-Ask format)
Expect emotion	Allow patient or family to express emotion and react to situation or news	"You seem upset about hearing that your lung function is declining..."
Map the goals	Explore patient/family values, goals, expectations	"After hearing this new information, what are you thinking? What is important to you?" "What are you hoping for with a ventricular assist device?"
Align with patient values	Demonstrate that you have heard the values of the patient/family	"It sounds like with a ventricular assist device you are hoping to live long enough to see your daughter's wedding..."
Plan medical treatment to match patient goals or values	Make treatment recommendations based on values/goals that were just discussed	"Based on what you are saying and knowing that your heart function is getting worse, I think we should implant a ventricular assist device..." "Since living comfortably and dying at home is important to you, I recommend..."

Source. Mahler DA, Wells CK. Evaluation of clinical methods for rating dyspnea. *Chest.* 1988;93(3):580–586.

Using REMAP, the provider can invite the conversation. For example, the healthcare provider must not assume that all patients will want to proceed when they are asked if they are ready to continue the conversation. For example, some patients may respond that they do not want to discuss their condition. By following the patient's lead, instead of completely abandoning the topic or barreling forward with the discussion, the provider can learn more about the patient's perception and, in particular, understand why the patient is choosing to not discuss the subject.[44]

Addressing Advanced Treatments and Technologies

Since severe COPD and advanced HF patients have innovative therapies available to them, providers face a unique set of topics that need to be addressed in regard to advance care planning. In the following sections, we discuss the communication challenges raised by most commonly used advanced therapies in both HF and COPD.

Disease-Specific Advanced Therapies in HF

Implantable Cardioverter Defibrillators

A specific therapy that deserves a tailored conversation is treatment with implantable cardioverter-defibrillator (ICD). There is a mortality benefit with ICD implantation.[48] In the SCD-HeFT trial, the mortality rate for patients with ICD after 5 years was 29% compared to 36% in patients with ICD.[49] There is limited evidence for placement of ICD in patients with very advanced HF, so this dialogue should be reserved for patients who meet ICD implantation criteria and patients who are expected to have good functional status for over 1 year.[48] The conversation should include the purpose of the ICD, the expected risks and benefits of the device, and the general risk of dying from HF. Generally patients have misconceptions about ICDs and overestimate the effectiveness.[48] An example of the framework of the conversation is as follows:

> If we put an ICD in 100 patients with heart disease like yours, over the next 5 years we would expect about 30 patients to die in spite of the ICD and 7 or 8 patients to be saved by ICD. As for complications, about 10 to 20 patients will receive a shock that is unnecessary and painful, and about 5 to 15 patients will have other complications. The rest of the patients with an ICD aren't affected by their device.[48]

Giving this information in short sentences and pausing for questions is a great way of beginning this conversation. Aside from misperceptions of the mortality benefit of ICDs, patients and their family members suffer from the psychological effects of ICDs.[50-52] Studies have demonstrated that patients are anxious about ICD shocks or misfirings.[53] More important, studies have shown that patients' families are more anxious than the patients themselves, thus it is crucial to involve family members in these discussions so that they can voice their concerns.[51] Interestingly, in a review of risks and benefits of ICDs, Atwater and Duabert described that implantation and shocks can reduce quality of life and increase anxiety, depression, and posttraumatic stress disorder.[54]

As important as deciding to implant an ICD device is the decision to deactivate the device. Patients should be informed, a priori, that there are burdens associated with the device that may outweigh any benefits. If patients are nearing the end of life, they may receive painful shocks if devices are not turned off.[55] Unfortunately, research shows that few patients have conversations regarding ICD deactivation.[56] A qualitative study specifically asking why providers have difficulty discussing deactivating ICDs found that healthcare providers often feel uneasy discussing device management at the end of life. In addition, they do not want their actions to be associated with withdrawing care.[57] The Ask-Tell-Ask tool allows healthcare providers to update patients and their families about the patient's health status and provide education about the risk of receiving defibrillator shocks at the end of life; this tool can also facilitate discussions about ICD deactivation.

Left Ventricular Assist Device

Left ventricular assist devices (LVADs) are an advanced therapy that can provide many benefits as well as present risks. This section outlines the current recommendations regarding candidacy for LVAD therapy, risks and benefits of this therapy and key discussions to have with patients and families.

The American Heart Association recommends LVAD implantation for patients with advanced HF, which is defined as HF with symptoms at rest, repeated hospitalizations for intensive management possibly including inotrope therapy, and life expectancy less than 2 years without heart transplant or mechanical circulatory support (i.e., a ventricular assist device).[58] An LVAD can be used in three settings: (a) as a bridge to recovery (i.e., following an intense surgical procedure with plan for removal after recovery); (b) as a bridge to transplant (i.e., to stabilize the patient until a donor heart can be procured for heart transplant, at which time LVAD is removed); and (c) as a destination therapy (i.e., a long-term therapy for patients who are ineligible for heart transplant).

The use of LVADs has increased since the results of the REMATCH trial were published in 2001.[43] The REMATCH trial was the first randomized study that evaluated the use of a LVAD as destination therapy compared with standard medical therapy alone.[26] In REMATCH, patients receiving the LVAD had a 48% reduction in the risk of death (from 52% to 25% at 1 year) from any cause, with improvement in quality of life. Since this study was published, there have been many advances to the devices, and recipients of devices in the United States are followed by the Interagency Registry for Mechanically Assisted Circulatory Support (INTERMACS) to document mortality, morbidity and quality of life outcomes.[43]

A recently published report by INTERMACS in 2014 revealed that patients with LVAD implantation as destination therapy had 75% survival rates at 1 year and 50% at 3 years.[59] Moreover, when compared to their baseline, LVAD patients had an improvement in functional status, as seen in the improvement in their six-minute walk test. Whereas pre-LVAD patients were able to walk 204 meters in six minutes, post-LVAD were able to walk 350 meters and 360 meters at 6 months and 24 months, respectively.[60] Furthermore, there was improvement in quality of life at both 6 months and 24 months.[60]

In spite of the survival and quality of life benefits, LVADs are considered high-risk therapies because there are a multitude of complications that are sometimes fatal, including infections, thrombosis and thromboembolic events including pulmonary emboli and strokes, bleeding (from anticoagulation therapy), hemolysis, aortic regurgitation, right HF, ventricular arrhythmias, and psychological distress.[61,62] The psychological burden after LVAD implantation includes depression, with particular concern for suicide, anxiety, difficulty coping with new therapy, and worries about burdening caregivers.[63–66] Because there are both benefits and risks associated with this intervention, it is vital for providers to engage patients in an open conversation about their values and goals; with this information, providers can recommend an LVAD when a patient's goals and values are in line with what LVAD can offer. The American Heart Association recommends that discussions regarding possible LVAD placement should include a frank discussion about a patient's health status and prognosis; specifically, these conversations should address that although LVADs improve quality of life and increase survival, the LVAD is not a curative therapy, and this treatment comes with high risks.[58]

LVAD therapy presents distinct challenges in end-of-life care, because providers may feel conflicted by the act of "turning off" the device. In order to address this situation and other unique scenarios that arise with LVAD therapy, Petrucci et al. crafted a three-phase model to serve as a guideline when caring for patients with LVADs.[67] The guidelines consist of 10 key points that highlight the importance of educating patients and caregivers about limitations of LVAD, discussing undesired outcomes, and the importance of having these conversations prior to LVAD implantation. Similarly, Swetz et al. created a more structured format called a "Preparedness Plan."[68] This outline allows physicians to explore advance care planning such as selecting healthcare proxy. It also delves into specific issues about living with a LVAD, including if LVAD can be discontinued if specific patient goals are no longer met, such as being unable to speak with family after a debilitating stroke. In addition, Swetz encourages the Preparedness Plan to be included as part of the medical chart.[68] By involving the patient and his or her caregiver in an open discussion, the entire healthcare team and the patient can mutually agree and understand the patient's expectations and values. Furthermore, these discussions can guide patient care in unforeseen outcomes.[67,68]

LVAD therapy is very complex and requires a multidisciplinary approach. With advances in LVAD therapy and increasing numbers of patients eligible for this therapy, it is important for healthcare providers to be able to communicate the benefits, burdens, and other issues (including end-of-life care) surrounding this treatment. Using the "hoping for the best and prepare for the worst" structure allows providers to explore patients' hopes, expectations, and worries regarding their care.

Disease-Specific Advanced Therapies in COPD

Mechanical Ventilation

Mechanical ventilation is a topic that must be discussed, because respiratory failure is inevitable in patients with advanced COPD. Unfortunately, this conversation seldom occurs; one study reported that only 14% of patients with advanced COPD discussed mechanical ventilation with their providers.[69] When discussions about mechanical ventilation do occur, it is often when the patient's disease is very advanced or the patient has impending respiratory failure.[70] By employing communication tools, such as Ask-Tell-Ask and "hope for the best, prepare for the worst," providers can elicit the patient's understanding of mechanical ventilation, inform the patient that respiratory failure is unavoidable, and discuss the patient's preferences.

Furthermore, it is important to educate patients about the purpose of mechanical ventilation and possible outcomes, including that mechanical ventilation does not always prevent death. In a retrospective study of 4,791 patients with COPD who were mechanically ventilated in a setting of acute respiratory failure,[51] 23% died in the hospital and 45% died within a year. In addition, 26.8% were discharged to either a nursing home or a skilled nursing facility. In this cohort, the majority were readmitted to the hospital, and 67% were readmitted at least once within 12 months following the initial hospitalization.[71] These data can offer patients realistic expectations of mechanical ventilation and prepare them for the unanticipated consequences of this treatment.

Noninvasive Positive Pressure Ventilation

Another commonly used therapy in advanced COPD is noninvasive positive pressure ventilation (NPPV). This mode of therapy decreases the work of breathing and allows respiratory muscles to rest during inspiratory phase. In a Cochrane review regarding utility and efficacy of NPPV in patients with COPD exacerbations, NPPV was found to decrease mortality rates, reduce need for intubation, and reduce hospital length of stay.[72] Nevertheless, this therapy can be cumbersome and burdensome and requires that the patient be alert enough to safely use it. In addition, the mask may interfere with patient communication and intimacy in patient–family interactions.

It is critical that the healthcare providers inform patients and family members of the therapy's benefits and burdens. Curtis and his colleagues, as part of the Society of Critical Care Medicine Palliative Noninvasive Positive Pressure Ventilation Task Force, summarized an NPPV discussion approach to use with patients.[73] This task force describes three separate patient clusters and their needs based on their treatment preferences. The first group is comprised of patients who want to seek all life-prolonging treatments regardless of prognosis; if they do not improve with NPPV, patients in this group are willing to accept mechanical ventilation. The second group includes patients who want to pursue life-prolonging therapies with some limitations (i.e., want all forms of treatment with exception of intubation, e.g., "do not intubate"). In this group, NPPV is used to reverse cause of respiratory failure or to support a patient's respiratory status while the reversible cause is being treated. If underlying respiratory failure etiology is not improving with treatment, then NPPV is discontinued. The third group includes patients who are dying of respiratory failure and have declined life-prolonging treatments with preference to focus exclusively on their comfort; these patients can use NPPV to palliate dyspnea and sometimes maintain wakefulness. The approach to all three groups is similar, in that each group needs to have realistic expectations and understand the NPPV therapeutic limitations. Specifically, NPPV can possibly defer the need for intubation, but it is not always effective at reversing acute respiratory failure.

For the last two groups, the healthcare provider should inform the patients of the NPPV burdens and offer other palliative options, such as opioids for dyspnea. In these groups, it is critical to define clearly a "time limited trial" of NPPV.[73] Providers need to explore and define what is considered an adequate trial of NPPV and, a priori, define what improvement would look like. Providers need to come to a consensus with patients and/or family members as to the "improvements" that will be seen during this trial period. Examples of clearly defined improvements include decreases in symptom burden, white blood cell count, or oxygen requirements in 48 hours. We recommend using Ask-Tell-Ask to facilitate these conversations about NPPV benefits and burdens. Furthermore, Ask-Tell-Ask enables providers to give health status updates, if patients are not responding to NPPV therapy, and then transition the conversation to planning the next steps for care.

Addressing Prognosis

The development of COPD and HF predictive models has become a research priority in order to assist providers when they have to face the question: "How long do I have?" The most commonly used COPD prognostication tool is the BODE Index (Table 21.6), which was developed to help calculate an individual's risk of death from COPD. The BODE Index takes four factors into account: **b**ody weight index (BMI), degree of airway **o**bstruction (%FEV1), **d**yspnea, and **e**xercise capacity, as measured by the six-minute walk distance.[74] When compared to the degree of airway obstruction alone (%FEV1), the BODE Index was a superior mortality prediction tool. For instance, an underweight patient (BMI = 19) with FEV1 of 40% who could walk 250 meters with shortness of breath when on level ground has a BODE index of 6, which correlates with 14% mortality at 2 years.

Similarly in HF patients, there have been numerous studies investigating which patient characteristics are associated with higher risk of death. The Seattle Heart Failure Model (SHFM) is the most widely used model for predicting prognosis.[41] The SHFM is the first risk assessment tool developed that uses commonly obtained clinical information, including commonly drawn lab markers, medications, and devices, to predict estimates of mean 1-, 2-, and 5-year survival.[75,76] The remarkable aspect of SHFM is that it factors in how different treatments can affect expected survival. An online calculator is accessible at www.SeattleHeartFailureModel.org, and smartphone versions are available as well.

Both the BODE Index and the SHFM are readily accessible by healthcare providers and only require information routinely available for patients with each respective illness. However, these disease-specific instruments do not take other comorbidities into account. To address this issue, e-Prognosis has been created.[77] e-Prognosis is an online prognostication tool based on prognostic indices from the literature used "to inform healthcare providers about possible mortality outcomes."[77] One of the advantages of this tool is that it combines a variety of prognostic indicators for community dwelling individuals to hospitalized patients. Based on the medical history that is entered in the calculator, an estimate of mortality is calculated. Mortality can be calculated at a variety of time points, ranging from 6 months to 10 years. Providers can input information that is more representative of a specific patient, rather than obtaining a general mortality estimate on a generic patient population. e-Prognosis is free and easy to use.[77]

All of the instruments mentioned are neither cumbersome nor necessitate special lab tests or imaging studies. Of course these tools do not individualize prognosis to each specific patient, so healthcare providers must be careful when interpreting the results. Nevertheless, these tools can provide valuable

Table 21.6. BODE Index

Variable	Points on BODE Index			
	0	1	2	3
FEV1 (% predicted)	≥65	50–64	36–49	<35
6-Minute Walk Test (meters)	≥350	250–349	150–249	< 149
MMRC Dyspnea Scale	0–1	2	3	4
Body Mass Index	>21	< 21	–	–

Source. Celli BR, Cote CG, Marin JM, et al. The body-mass index, airflow obstruction, dyspnea, and exercise capacity index in chronic obstructive pulmonary disease. *N Engl J Med.* 2004;350(10):1005–1012.

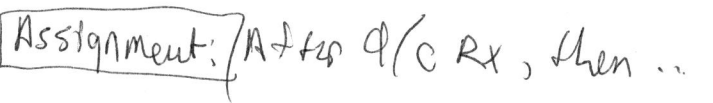

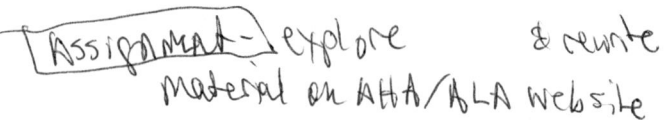

information for the healthcare team, patients, and families. Of course there is no substitute for sound clinical judgment, and the information provided predicts the average experience, not the individual patient experience with his or her illness. People want to know what is likely to happen to them, and these models give us averages to review.

Future Directions

The goal of this chapter is to empower providers with communication tools in order to improve patient-centered care. Future research needs to be conducted in numerous areas, including that regarding the ideal timing of these conversations, how to best deliver primary palliative education and communication training to healthcare providers who care for advanced HF and severe COPD patients, and the development of instruments to serve as decision aids to foster the shared decision-making process.

Current research suggests that cardiac or pulmonary rehabilitation programs may be a promising setting for these challenging conversations, especially those involving advance care planning in these serious illnesses. In one study, HF patients who were enrolled in a cardiac rehabilitation program received a survey inquiring about their preferences in advance planning, presence of advance care directives, and the need for more information.[33] The results showed that 86% desired more information on advance directives, 62% wanted to learn about life-sustaining care, and 96% were receptive to advance planning discussions with their physicians.[33] A similar study conducted in COPD patients enrolled in pulmonary rehabilitation programs found that 94% of rehabilitation participants had health worries and 88.6% wanted more information regarding advance care planning.[78] Since patients are asking for more information about their illness and advance care planning, healthcare providers who treat patients in these two populations need more education about how to have these conversations.

A few effective teaching models are available to educate physicians on these important skills. They include GeriTalk, OncoTalk, and Nephrotalk.[79–81] These intensive immersion courses are aimed at improving the communication skills of postgraduate medical trainees (fellows in geriatrics and palliative care, oncology, and nephrology, respectively). Using standardized patients to role-play various scenarios, the course introduces and builds on a variety of communication skills. The communication topics include delivering poor prognosis or serious or terminal diagnosis, providing health status updates, exploring emotional aspects of patients' responses, and discussing prognosis. The skills that are taught include Ask-Tell-Ask and REMAP, among others, and these courses have been well received by participants. Another resource is VITAL talk (available at www.vitaltalk.org).[82] The VITAL talk website also offers free provider resources that outline communication strategies on a variety of topics, including how to handle conflict and responding to patients' emotions. These new courses and online resources are promising; nonetheless, more work needs to be done to tailor communication skills training for the healthcare providers caring for patients with advanced HF or severe COPD.

Additionally, various sources of information, from the American Lung Association to the American College of Cardiology, include both printed material and material on their websites.[3,82,83] In order to aid patients and providers to engage in the shared decision-making process, a COPD patient decision aid has been created on mechanical ventilation. The tool can be used to educate the patient about the topic and fosters questions that patients can ask providers. An initial study found that this tool (available through Ottawa Hospital Research Institute at http://decisionaid.ohri.ca/docs/das/COPD.pdf) is a feasible and effective education tool.[70] Unfortunately, similar tools are not yet available for LVAD or ICDs at this time.

Conclusion

As the prevalence of patients with severe COPD or advanced HF continues to increase, and advanced therapies make it possible for patients to live longer with these chronic progressive illnesses, it is imperative that providers are able to effectively communicate with patients and their families. With more research on the timing of important conversations, the creation of more decision aids, and more primary palliative education including communication skills, providers will be able to engage in palliative communication with patients and families and, in turn, improve the quality of care for these populations and their families.

References

1. Hoyert D, Xu J. Deaths: Preliminary data for 2011. *National Vital Statistics Reports*. 2012;61(6):1–65.
2. American Lung Association. Chronic obstructive pulmonary disease (COPD) fact sheet. http://www.lung.org/lung-disease/copd/resources/facts-figures/COPD-Fact-Sheet.html#Sources. Published May 2014. Accessed June 1, 2014.
3. Go AS, Mozaffarian D, Roger VL, et al. Executive summary: Heart disease and stroke statistics—2013 update: A report from the American Heart Association. *Circulation*. January 1, 2013;127(1):143–152.
4. Lloyd-Jones DM, Larson MG, Leip EP, et al. Lifetime risk for developing congestive heart failure: The Framingham Heart Study. *Circulation*. December 10, 2002;106(24):3068–3072.
5. Hall M, DeFrances C, Williams S, Golosinskiy A, Schwartzman A. National Hospital Discharge Survey: 2007 summary. *National Health Statistics Reports*. 2010(29).
6. Jones I, Kirby A, Ormiston P, et al. The needs of patients dying of chronic obstructive pulmonary disease in the community. *Fam Pract*. June 1, 2004;21(3):310–313.
7. Gore JM, Brophy CJ, Greenstone MA. How well do we care for patients with end stage chronic obstructive pulmonary disease (COPD)? A comparison of palliative care and quality of life in COPD and lung cancer. *Thorax*. December 1, 2000;55(12):1000–1006.
8. Janssen DJ, Spruit MA, Wouters EF, Schols JM. Daily symptom burden in end-stage chronic organ failure: A systematic review. *Palliat Med*. December 2008;22(8):938–948.
9. Elkington H, White P, Addington-Hall J, Higgs R, Edmonds P. The healthcare needs of chronic obstructive pulmonary disease patients in the last year of life. *Palliat Med*. September 1, 2005;19(6):485–491.
10. Bergs D. "The hidden client"—women caring for husbands with COPD: Their experience of quality of life. *J Clin Nurs*. 2002;11(5):1365–2702.
11. Simpson AC, Young J, Donahue M, Rocker G. A day at a time: Caregiving on the edge in advanced COPD. *Int J Chron Obstruct Pulmon Dis*. 2010;5:141–151.
12. Bakas T, Pressler SJ, Johnson EA, Nauser JA, Shaneyfelt T. Family caregiving in heart failure. *Nurs Res*. May–June 2006;55(3):180–188.

13. Evangelista LS, Dracup K, Doering L, Westlake C, Fonarow GC, Hamilton M. Emotional well-being of heart failure patients and their caregivers. *J Card Fail*. October 2002;8(5):300–305.
14. Martensson J, Dracup K, Canary C, Fridlund B. Living with heart failure: Depression and quality of life in patients and spouses. *J Heart Lung Transplant*. April 2003;22(4):460–467.
15. Malik FA, Gysels M, Higginson IJ. Living with breathlessness: A survey of caregivers of breathless patients with lung cancer or heart failure. *Palliat Med*. July 2013;27(7):647–656.
16. Pressler SJ, Gradus-Pizlo I, Chubinski SD, et al. Family caregivers of patients with heart failure: A longitudinal study. *J Cardiovasc Nurs*. 2013;28(5):417–428.
17. Adler ED, Goldfinger JZ, Kalman J, Park ME, Meier DE. Palliative care in the treatment of advanced heart failure. *Circulation*. December 22, 2009;120(25):2597–2606.
18. Wouters EFM, Celis MPM, Breyer MK, Rutten EPA, Graat-Verboom L, Spruit MA. Co-morbid manifestations in COPD. *Respir Med: COPD Update*. 2007;3(4):135–151.
19. Hunt SA. ACC/AHA 2005 Guideline update for the diagnosis and management of chronic heart failure in the adult: A report of the American College of Cardiology/American Heart Association Task Force on Practice Guidelines (Writing Committee to Update the 2001 Guidelines for the Evaluation and Management of Heart Failure). *J Am Coll Cardiol*. September 20, 2005;46(6):e1–e82.
20. Bhullar S, Phillips B. Sleep in COPD patients. *COPD*. 2005;2(3):355–361.
21. Horne G, Payne S. Removing the boundaries: Palliative care for patients with heart failure. *Palliat Med*. June 1, 2004;18(4):291–296.
22. Bekelman D, Rumsfeld J, Havranek E, et al. Symptom burden, depression, and spiritual well-being: A comparison of heart failure and advanced cancer patients. *J Gen Intern Med*. May 1, 2009;24(5):592–598.
23. Connors AF, Dawson NV, Thomas C, et al. Outcomes following acute exacerbation of severe chronic obstructive lung disease. The SUPPORT investigators (Study to Understand Prognoses and Preferences for Outcomes and Risks of Treatments). *Am J Respir Crit Care Med*. 1996;154(4):959–967.
24. Curtis JR, Wenrich MD, Carline JD, Shannon SE, Ambrozy DM, Ramsey PG. Patients' perspectives on physician skill in end-of-life care: Differences between patients with copd, cancer, and aids. *Chest*. 2002;122(1):356–362.
25. Harding R, Selman L, Beynon T, et al. Meeting the communication and information needs of chronic heart failure patients. *J Pain Symptom Manage*. 2008;36(2):149–156.
26. Rose EA, Gelijns AC, Moskowitz AJ, et al. Long-term use of a left ventricular assist device for end-stage heart failure. *N Engl J Med*. 2001;345(20):1435–1443.
27. Lanken PN, Terry PB, DeLisser HM, et al. An official American Thoracic Society clinical policy statement: Palliative care for patients with respiratory diseases and critical illnesses. *Am J Respir Crit Care Med*. April 15, 2008;177(8):912–927.
28. Celli BR, MacNee W, Agusti A, et al. Standards for the diagnosis and treatment of patients with COPD: A summary of the ATS/ERS position paper. *Eur Respir J*. June 1, 2004;23(6):932–946.
29. Murray SA, Kendall M, Boyd K, Sheikh A. Illness trajectories and palliative care. *BMJ*. 2005;330(7498):1007–1011.
30. Poses RM, Smith WR, McClish DK, et al. Physicians' survival predictions for patients with acute congestive heart failure. *Arch Intern Med*. 1997;157(9):1001–1007.
31. Wachter RM, Luce JM, Hearst N, Lo B. Decisions about resuscitation: Inequities among patients with different diseases but similar prognoses. *Ann Intern Med*. September 15, 1989;111(6):525–532.
32. Rogers AE, Addington-Hall JM, Abery AJ, et al. Knowledge and communication difficulties for patients with chronic heart failure: qualitative study. *BMJ*. September 9, 2000;321(7261):605–607.
33. Heffner JE, Barbieri C. End-of-life care preferences of patients enrolled in cardiovascular rehabilitation programs. *Chest*. 2000;117(5):1474–1481.
34. Gott M, Gardiner C, Small N, et al. Barriers to advance care planning in chronic obstructive pulmonary disease. *Palliat Med*. October 1, 2009;23(7):642–648.
35. Gardiner C, Gott M, Payne S, et al. Exploring the care needs of patients with advanced COPD: An overview of the literature. *Respir Med*. 2010;104(2):159–165.
36. Zapka JG, Carter R, Carter CL, Hennessy W, Kurent JE, DesHarnais S. Care at the end of life: Focus on communication and race. *J Aging Health*. December 1, 2006;18(6):791–813.
37. Barnes S, Gott M, Payne S, et al. Communication in heart failure: Perspectives from older people and primary care professionals. *Health Soc Care Community*. 2006;14(6):482–490.
38. Remme WJ, McMurray JJV, Rauch B, et al. Public awareness of heart failure in Europe: First results from SHAPE. *Eur Heart J*. November 1, 2005;26(22):2413–2421.
39. Goodlin SJ. Palliative care in congestive heart failure. *J Am Coll Cardiol*. 2009;54(5):386–396.
40. Back AL, Arnold RM, Baile WF, Tulsky JA, Fryer-Edwards K. Approaching difficult communication tasks in oncology. *CA: Cancer J Clin*. May/June 2005;55(3):164–177.
41. Whellan DJ, Goodlin SJ, Dickinson MG, et al. End-of-life care in patients with heart failure. *J Card Fail*. 2014;20(2):121–134.
42. Back AL, Arnold RM, Quill TE. Hope for the best, and prepare for the worst. *Ann Intern Med*. 2003;138(5):439–443.
43. Kirklin JK, Naftel DC. Mechanical circulatory support: Registering a therapy in evolution. *Circulation*. September 1, 2008;1(3):200–205.
44. Back A AR, Tulsky J. *Mastering Communication with Seriously Ill Patients: Balancing Honesty with Empathy and Hope*. Cambridge, UK: Cambridge University Press; 2009.
45. Morris D, Johnson K, Ammarell N, Arnold R, Tulsky J, Steinhauser K. What is your understanding of your illness? A communication tool to explore patients' perspectives of living with advanced illness. *J Gen Intern Med*. November 1, 2012;27(11):1460–1466.
46. Curtis JR, Engelberg R, Young JP, et al. An approach to understanding the interaction of hope and desire for explicit prognostic information among individuals with severe chronic obstructive pulmonary disease or advanced cancer. *J Palliat Med*. May 2008;11(4):610–620.
47. Goodlin SJ, Quill TE, Arnold RM. Communication and decision-making about prognosis in heart failure care. *J Card Fail*. 2008;14(2):106–113.
48. Stevenson LW, Desai AS. Selecting patients for discussion of the ICD as primary prevention for sudden death in heart failure. *J Card Fail*. 2006;12(6):407–412.
49. Bardy GH, Lee KL, Mark DB, et al. Amiodarone or an implantable cardioverter-defibrillator for congestive heart failure. *N Engl J Med*. 2005;352(3):225–237.
50. Kamphuis HCM, de Leeuw JRJ, Derksen R, Hauer RNW, Winnubst JAM. Implantable cardioverter defibrillator recipients: Quality of life in recipients with and without ICD shock delivery: A prospective study. *Europace*. October 1, 2003;5(4):381–389.
51. Sowell LV, Sears SFJ, Walker RL, Kuhl EA, Conti JB. Anxiety and marital adjustment in patients with implantable cardioverter defibrillator and their spouses. *J Cardiopulm Rehabil Prev*. 2007;27(1):46–49.
52. Dunbar SB, Langberg JJ, Reilly CM, et al. Effect of a psychoeducational intervention on depression, anxiety, and health resource use in implantable cardioverter defibrillator patients. *Pacing Clin Electrophysiol*. 2009;32(10):1259–1271.
53. Pedersen SS, van Domburg RT, Theuns DAMJ, Jordaens L, Erdman RAM. Type D personality is associated with increased anxiety and depressive symptoms in patients with an implantable cardioverter defibrillator and their partners. *Psychosom Med*. 2004;66(5):714–719.

54. Atwater BD, Daubert JP. Implantable cardioverter defibrillators: Risks accompany the life-saving benefits. *Heart.* May 15, 2012;98(10):764–772.
55. Tanner CE, Fromme EK, Goodlin SJ. Ethics in the treatment of advanced heart failure: palliative care and end-of-life issues. *Congest Heart Fail.* 2011;17(5):235–240.
56. Goldstein NE, Lampert R, Bradley E, Lynn J, Krumholz HM. Management of implantable cardioverter defibrillators in end-of-life care. *Ann Intern Med.* 2004;141(11):835–838.
57. Goldstein N, Mehta D, Teitelbaum E, Bradley E, Morrison RS. "It's like crossing a bridge": Complexities preventing physicians from discussing deactivation of implantable defibrillators at the end of life. *J Gen Intern Med.* 2008;23(1):2–6.
58. Peura JL, Colvin-Adams M, Francis GS, et al. Recommendations for the use of mechanical circulatory support: Device strategies and patient selection: A scientific statement from the American Heart Association. *Circulation.* November 27, 2012;126(22):2648–2667.
59. Kirklin JK, Naftel DC, Pagani FD, et al. Sixth INTERMACS annual report: A 10,000-patient database. *J Heart Lung Transplant.* 2014;33(6):555–564.
60. Rogers JG, Aaronson KD, Boyle AJ, et al. Continuous flow left ventricular assist device improves functional capacity and quality of life of advanced heart failure patients. *J Am Coll Cardiol.* 2010;55(17):1826–1834.
61. Tsukui H, Abla A, Teuteberg JJ, et al. Cerebrovascular accidents in patients with a ventricular assist device. *J Thorac Cardiovasc Surg.* 2007;134(1):114–123.
62. Potapov EV, Stepanenko A, Krabatsch T, Hetzer R. Managing long-term complications of left ventricular assist device therapy. *Curr Opin Cardiol.* 2011;26(3):237–244.
63. Ben Gal T, Jaarsma T. Self-care and communication issues at the end of life of recipients of a left-ventricular assist device as destination therapy. *Curr Opin Support Palliat Care.* 2013;7(1):29–35.
64. Wray J, Hallas CN, Banner NR. Quality of life and psychological well-being during and after left ventricular assist device support. *Clin Transplant.* 2007;21(5):622–627.
65. Swetz K, Ottenberg A, Freeman M, Mueller P. Palliative care and end-of-life issues in patients treated with left ventricular assist devices as destination therapy. *Curr Heart Fail Rep.* 2011;8(3):212–218.
66. Tigges-Limmer K, Schönbrodt M, Roefe D, Arusoglu L, Morshuis M, Gummert JF. Suicide after ventricular assist device implantation. *J Heart Lung Transplant.* 2010;29(6):692–694.
67. Petrucci RJ, Benish LA, Carrow BL, et al. Ethical considerations for ventricular assist device support: A 10-point model. *ASAIO J.* 2011;57(4):268–273.
68. Swetz KM, Kamal AH, Matlock DD, et al. Preparedness planning before mechanical circulatory support: A "how-to" guide for palliative medicine clinicians. *J Pain Symptom Manage.* 2014;47(5):926–935.
69. Travaline JM, Silverman HJ. Discussions with outpatients with chronic obstructive pulmonary disease regarding mechanical ventilation as life-sustaining therapy. *South Med J.* 1995;88(10):1034–1038.
70. McNeely PD, Hebert PC, Dales RE, et al. Deciding about mechanical ventilation in end-stage chronic obstructive pulmonary disease: How respirologists perceive their role. *Can Med Assoc J.* January 15, 1997;156(2):177–183.
71. Hajizadeh N, Goldfeld K, Crothers K. What happens to patients with COPD with long-term oxygen treatment who receive mechanical ventilation for COPD exacerbation? A 1-year retrospective follow-up study. *Thorax.* 2015;70(3):294–296.
72. Lightowler JV, Wedzicha JA, Elliott MW, Ram FSF. Non-invasive positive pressure ventilation to treat respiratory failure resulting from exacerbations of chronic obstructive pulmonary disease: Cochrane systematic review and meta-analysis. *BMJ.* 2003;326(7382):185.
73. Curtis JR, Cook DJ, Sinuff T, et al. Noninvasive positive pressure ventilation in critical and palliative care settings: Understanding the goals of therapy. *Crit Care Med.* 2007;35(3):932–939.
74. Celli BR, Cote CG, Marin JM, et al. The body-mass index, airflow obstruction, dyspnea, and exercise capacity index in chronic obstructive pulmonary disease. *N Engl J Med.* 2004;350(10):1005–1012.
75. Levy WC, Mozaffarian D, Linker DT, et al. The Seattle Heart Failure Model: Prediction of survival in heart failure. *Circulation.* March 21, 2006;113(11):1424–1433.
76. Mozaffarian D, Anker SD, Anand I, et al. Prediction of mode of death in heart failure: The Seattle Heart Failure Model. *Circulation.* July 24, 2007;116(4):392–398.
77. Sei L, Smith A, Widera E, Yourman L, Schonberg M, Ahalt C. What is ePrognosis? http://eprognosis.ucsf.edu/about.php. Accessed June 24, 2014.
78. Heffner JE, Fahy B, Hilling L, Barbieri C. Attitudes regarding advance directives among patients in pulmonary rehabilitation. *Am J Respir Crit Care Med.* 1996;154(6):1735–1740.
79. Gelfman LP, Lindenberger E, Fernandez H, et al. The effectiveness of the Geritalk communication skills course: A real-time assessment of skill acquisition and deliberate practice. *J Pain Symptom Manage.* 2014;48(4):738–744.
80. Schell JO, Green JA, Tulsky JA, Arnold RM. Communication skills training for dialysis decision-making and end-of-life care in nephrology. *Clin J Am Soc Nephrol.* April 5, 2013;8(4):675–680.
81. Back AL, Arnold RM, Baile WF, et al. Efficacy of communication skills training for giving bad news and discussing transitions to palliative care. *Arch Gen Med.* 2007;167(5):453–460.
82. Back A AR, Tulsky J, Edwards K. VITAL talk. http://www.vitaltalk.org/about-us. Accessed June 24, 2014.
83. Au DH, Udris EM, Fihn SD, McDonell MB, Curtis JR. Differences in health care utilization at the end of life among patients with chronic obstructive pulmonary disease and patients with lung cancer. *Arch Intern Med.* February 13, 2006;166(3):326–331.

CHAPTER 22

Oncology Across the Trajectory

Lillie D. Shockney

Introduction

In 2014 the American Cancer Society estimated there would be approximately 1,665,540 new cancer cases diagnosed and 585,720 cancer deaths in the United States. Cancer remains the second most common cause of death in the United States, accounting for nearly one of every four deaths.[1] One in two men and one in three women will be diagnosed with a life-threatening cancer in their lifetime.[1] Improvements in earlier detection technology, increased cancer awareness via social media, and the increasing rate of baby boomers reaching midlife (the age group when most people are diagnosed with cancer) all contribute to a rise in the number of cancer incidences. Though there still are far too many people who die of their disease or its treatment, most individuals today become long-term cancer survivors. Even those diagnosed with metastatic disease are surviving longer than in the past. There are better care options than before due to innovative research at the molecular level, yielding less toxic treatment options and resulting in longer periods of survival. For example, 13.7 million individuals were breast cancer survivors in 2013. This number is anticipated to swell to 18 million by 2020 and climb as high as 22.2 million by 2030.[1,2]

Cancer, of course, is not a disease exclusive to the United States. Globally, the incidence is extraordinarily high, with the highest death rate occurring in developing countries, where access to care is limited. Table 22.1 summarizes the worldwide incidence of this disease, with lung cancer accounting for 13%, followed by breast cancer, at nearly 12% of all types of cancer diagnosed. The total incidence of cancer diagnoses for calendar year 2012 was more than 14.1 million people, with 7.4 million cases occurring in men and 6.7 million cases occurring in women. This worldwide number is expected to grow significantly, becoming 24 million by 2035.[3]

The World Health Organization reported that 8.2 million people died of cancer and/or its treatment in 2012. This makes cancer the leading cause of death globally. The most common cancer deaths were among people diagnosed with lung, liver, stomach, colorectal, and breast cancer. Significantly, 30% of cancer deaths are attributed to lifestyle behaviors; having a high body mass index, lack of physical activity, tobacco use, and alcohol use are the major contributing behaviors. Smoking is the most important risk factor for cancer, causing more than 20% of global deaths and approximately 70% of global lung cancer deaths. Viral infections that are known to be cancer-causing (i.e., HBV/HCV and HPV) are associated with up to 20% of cancer deaths, particularly in low- and middle-income countries. Geographically, 60% of worldwide cancer patients are in Africa, Asia, and Central and South America.[4,5] There still remains, however, a great number of people diagnosed with cancer for which its cause remains unknown.

The Palliative Care Needs of Oncology Patients and Families

For decades, no matter what organ site or hematologic malignancy, the goal of treatment for cancer was survival. This was the only goal. When oncologists looked at a graph of a survival curve and saw that over the past two decades more cancer patients survived to reach their fifth anniversary as a cancer survivor, they felt they had succeeded in treating their patients effectively and appropriately. However, cancer patients have different expectations of the outcome of their treatment today; they want survival with quality of life. Those with metastatic cancer want longevity, accompanied by quality of life. When the risks and benefits of treatment are discussed, initially out of fear of dying, patients may elect very toxic treatments and be accepting of whatever side effects may accompany that treatment. Once they realize they are likely going to live and beat their cancer, their tolerance for side effects, particularly those that impact quality of life, decreases. Every effort should be made to minimize and hopefully even prevent side effects from cancer treatment that inhibit patient quality of life.

Patients with metastatic disease may endure toxic treatments, believing that the next treatment will be the magic bullet that cures their cancer. When the healthcare provider says, "I hope your tumor responds to the next treatment," the patient may interpret the word "respond" as "cured."[6] One outcome of this travesty is patients' receiving toxic treatment with little or no benefit, causing them to be sicker, even requiring hospitalization shortly before their death. Healthcare providers need to provide more information regarding prognosis, choices, alternatives, and consequences, as well as how the patient might go about choosing what he or she wants to do. Therefore, the patient needs to receive realistic information about the various care options, along with the likelihood of successful treatment and adverse outcomes. The healthcare provider must supply honest, unbiased information along with decision aids, so the patient is better empowered with information to make an informed decision.[7]

Other metastatic cancer patients agree to endure another futile treatment that causes significant side effects and symptoms due to a desire to please the doctor, their family, or both. Oncologists are taught to treat the disease by considering the next line of treatment

Table 22.1 Worldwide Incidence of Cancer[5]

Rank	Cancer	New Cases Diagnosed in 2012 (1,000s)	Percent of All Cancers (excl. Non-melanoma Skin Cancer)
1	Lung	1,825	13.0
2	Breast	1,677	11.9
3	Colorectum	1,361	9.7
4	Prostate	1,112	7.9
5	Stomach	952	6.8
6	Liver	782	5.6
7	Cervix uteri	528	3.7
8	Oesophagus	456	3.2
9	Bladder	430	3.1
10	Non-Hodgkin lymphoma	386	2.7
11	Leukaemia	352	2.5
12	Pancreas	338	2.4
12	Kidney	338	2.4
14	Corpus uteri (endometrium)	320	2.3
15	Lip, oral cavity	300	2.1
16	Thyroid	298	2.1
17	Brain, nervous system	256	1.8
18	Ovary	239	1.7
19	Melanoma of skin	232	1.6
20	Gallbladder	178	1.3

Source. GLOBOCAN 2012 v1.0, Cancer Incidence and Mortality Worldwide: IARC CancerBase No. 11 [Internet]. Lyon, France: International Agency for Research on Cancer; 2013. http://globocan.iarc.fr, Accessed December 13, 2013.

options available for the patient. Family members do not want the doctor or the patient to give up and cannot always see or accept that the patient is ready for hospice and, in many cases, has been ready for some time. The end-of-life conversation, however, never happens; rather, patients discontinue treatment because complications prevent them from having anymore therapy. Their benefit from hospice care is short-lived. Shock, chaos, confusion, and stress are apparent among all of the individuals who loved the patient who is now gone. It makes it very difficult to ensure that such patients experience the "good death" they deserve.

Today, with methods available to minimize or even prevent certain side effects and symptoms, cancer patients need palliative care early in the oncology disease trajectory. For patients with a deadly form of cancer who will be able to live with their cancer diagnosis and treatment for an extended period of time, the historic practice has been to tell the patient to anticipate certain side effects and accept them as part of their treatment experience. Rather than telling the patient to expect (and accept) treatment side effects, which may linger for an extended period of time, palliative care provides, instead, methods to minimize the side effects. This helps put the patient on a patient-centered care path early in his or her treatment process and can minimize side effects' lingering during and after treatment completion. If 80% of cancer patients develop nausea and vomiting from specific chemotherapy regimens, it would make sense to provide anti-emetics in a preventative rather than a recovery manner. Patients who are receiving treatments with the hope of extending their lives can and do develop debilitating side effects. Chronic joint pain, fatigue, weakness, peripheral neuropathy, nausea, and other treatment side effects deemed common can be treated with the involvement of palliative care.

Patients who receive treatment with a curative intent, who see themselves as cancer survivors from diagnosis, are on a path of wellness from the journey's beginning. This includes asking the patients: What were your goals before diagnosis? Where do you see yourself in 1 year? 5 years? 10 years? perhaps starting a family or getting a work promotion, or planning for retirement? Whatever can be done to keep patients on track with their life goals should be part of their integrative treatment plan. In order to preserve these life goals, strategic decisions need to be made in selecting certain treatment regimens, as well as arranging, in a proactive manner, certain processes (such as fertility preservation prior to chemotherapy administration), which directly support the patients' remaining on track with the life goals they had before learning they had cancer. A patient's ability to remain active during treatment is beneficial from a psychosocial as well as a recovery perspective. Managing or preventing treatment side effects is thus necessary. Palliative care providers can offer great insight and expertise on symptom management by educating other oncology specialists about ways to diminish likely symptoms that can and do impact quality of life.

For patients with advanced cancer, however, life goals may need to be achieved in alternative ways. Unfulfilled hopes and long-term desires can drive the patient to continue treatment. The patient may want to be cured, to be present for an upcoming wedding or for the birth of a child. These milestones carry such significance that they overpower any understanding of the disease progression process. A discussion should occur about developing and implementing alternative ways to fulfill such hopes. What does a mother hope for her 10-year-old daughter when she grows up and weds? What would she want to tell her on that important day? This remains a treasured moment for them both, though this milestone moment will not happen for another decade or two. Having the patient write in a card, specially selected for that milestone event, can provide the solution needed to feel confident that this hope—this goal—is still going to be achieved. It may not necessarily be as important as seeing her daughter in her wedding gown as it is to feel that she can still convey her hopes, values, advice, and wishes for her daughter.

For patients with advanced cancer who are receiving noncurative treatments, palliative care needs to happen sooner rather than later. Intractable pain, severe fatigue, mucositis, nausea and vomiting, inability to concentrate, diarrhea, insomnia, dizziness, and other pronounced symptoms remain common for metastatic cancer patients enduring chemotherapy and other agents designed to try to control the disease. The healthcare provider should not wait for a patient to be in excruciating pain in the emergency department before ordering a palliative care consultation; rather, he or she should request a palliative care consultation as chemotherapy treatment gets underway. Using chemotherapy and other systemic or local treatments may be a more ideal way to integrate symptom management in a proactive way.

Patients' palliative care needs can change suddenly, depending on how the cancer progresses or the severity of side effects. This requires the provider to frequently touch base with the patient to see how effectively the current palliative care plan is working. As conditions and needs change, so must the palliative care plan. For those patients who reach a point when treatments directed at cancer control are no longer possible or practical, the healthcare provider needs to reassess with the patients what they value as important, what their goals of care are now, and how to accomplish these goals. The palliative care specialist engages in this thought-provoking and candid conversation to help the patient and his or her family members recognize the value of transitioning to a dedicated palliative care approach, hopefully with hospice care offered.

Palliative Care Communication Challenges in Oncology

Some oncologists believe that palliative care is unnecessary, because it is the oncologist's exclusive role to take care of all of the patient's needs. An oncologist may perceive that requesting a palliative care consultation represents a failure to take care of the patient, rather than an expansion of care services. Moreover, a provider may fear he or she is turning the patient over to someone else. Another challenge is the assumption that symptom management is limited to pain management and that pain management is best achieved with sedation through the use of narcotics. Patients are not experiencing quality of life if they are continuously sedated for pain control. Alternatives should always be considered, based on what patients want and respecting what they deem important and valuable. This includes helping to preserve or even restore the joys they experienced and valued before their disease progressed. Other debilitating symptoms can be far more disruptive to a patient's quality of life than pain, such as severe nausea or diarrhea.

When palliative care is recommended, patients may fear abandonment from their oncologist and choose to continue receiving treatment they likely do not want. Transitioning to palliative care is usually interpreted as getting bad news, which causes fear, anxiety, and sadness. A patient's uncertainty reaches a new heightened level. At this time, patients experience two very distinct needs: to know and understand and to feel known and understood. This is a challenging time because the healthcare provider must determine how much information patients want to know and then supply that information without overwhelming or escalating their anxiety more.[8] Life expectancy is the most pressing question patients commonly have. However, patients still need hope, to feel confident they will be guided in their care trajectory, and to know that the healthcare relationship they have built will remain intact.[8,9] When prognosis is discussed, patients expect to hear that their healthcare provider is committed to remaining involved in their care and that they will not be abandoned. Confusion results when palliative care is offered and associated only with hospice care.

Patients and family members formulate opinions about palliative care based on prior experiences with a similar situation. Lack of prior experience, knowledge, and miscommunication about the benefits of palliative care can become a barrier to a patient's and his or her family's embracing this needed specialty and the care it can provide. Additionally, the family may have a different set of goals than their ill loved one, and the treating oncologist may feel a sense of obligation to continue to try to treat the cancer, though a futile outcome is already anticipated. Oncologists do not want to imply they are "giving up," when the message needs to be that treatment for treatment's sake is bad treatment. Patients have been known to agree to treatments they have already refused in order to please their loved ones or healthcare provider.

Communicating with patients and their families about end of life is perhaps the most difficult and distressing part of a healthcare provider's role, primarily due to the lack of training on how to initiate end-of-life discussions. Due to lack of experience and lack of a good mentorship program to teach communication skills and help providers witness its success as part of that training process, healthcare providers avoid discussing end-of-life issues. This can be compounded by the patient's or his or her family's reluctance to talk about it as well. Barriers may include language, patient's age (especially those who are young), as well as a lack of an end-of-life protocol. Without such guidelines, there is great risk that only a selective few patients will be provided information about their condition and what to expect.[10] Table 22.2 summarizes oncologists' barriers to communication about end of life.[10]

Palliative Care Communication for Oncology Patients and Families

Patients do have specific preferences for how they desire information to be presented to them, especially when the information being bestowed is an explanation of poor prognosis. Table 22.3 outlines the specific patient preferences regarding the content of prognostic information based on work by Hagerty et al.[11] When explaining a poor prognosis, it is important that communication includes (a) content (what and how much information is going to

Table 22.2 Oncologists' Barriers to Communication about End of Life[10]

Physician Factors	Patient Factors	Institutional Factors
♦ Treating and palliation is difficult	♦ Family's reluctance	♦ Palliative care stigma
♦ Discomfort with death and dying	♦ Patient not ready	♦ Lack of protocol around end-of-life issues
♦ Team dynamics and responsibilities	♦ Language barriers	♦ Lack of tools/and or training
♦ The death-defying mode	♦ Younger patients more difficult	
♦ Lack of experience		
♦ Lack of good mentorship		

Table 22.3 Specific Prognostic Information Desired By Patients [11]

- Common side effects of treatment
- Treatment options
- Common symptoms from the cancer
- Chance that the treatment will improve symptoms
- Chances of treatment shrinking the cancer
- Likely time to be without symptoms

be revealed), (b) facilitation (setting and content variables), and (c) support (emotional support provided during the interaction).

Unfortunately, the majority of healthcare providers report that they lack a consistent plan or strategy when explaining prognosis to their patients. Among those taking a survey at an American Society of Clinical Oncology conference, 22% reported that they did not have a consistent approach to the task of breaking bad news to patients. Nearly 60% reported that they had several techniques or tactics but lacked an overall communication plan. Communicating to the patient regarding issues of importance to him or her in a manner the patient can comprehend is key.

When patients and their healthcare providers discuss life-threatening illness by focusing solely on hope, they may and commonly do miss important opportunities to improve pain and other symptom management, respond to underlying fears and concerns, explore life closure, and deepen the patient–physician relationship. However, by acknowledging all of the possible outcomes, patients and their providers can extend their discussion and medical focus to include symptomatic treatments as well as address psychological, spiritual, and existential issues.[12] Table 22.4 provides a summary of communication approaches for palliative care communication in oncology care.

One of the most important and profound things an oncology care provider can do for those patients who are likely to succumb to their disease and their families is to orchestrate a good death. The elements of a good death include

- Patients knowing they have purpose for having lived and that it was valued by others
- Leaving a legacy (which does not mean leaving money)
- Knowing they will be spoken of fondly after they are gone
- Leaving no financial debt for their family
- Giving forgiveness and receiving forgiveness
- Having the patient's affairs in order—financially and legally
- Being pain free
- Gaining a sense of closure

Table 22.4 Principles of Communication in Oncology Care[12]

Principle of Communication	Communication Approach
Always be honest	Open and honest communication is very important to patients. This is not meant to imply that giving a patient all of the information at once is wise, however. Communicating what is perceived to be important at that time should be the focus. Invite the patient and family to ask questions.
Communicate often	Caring for a seriously ill cancer patient and his or her family requires ongoing dialogue. Conversations about quality of life and end of life should begin early and happen often.
Discuss and agree upon a shared philosophy about optimism	Share with the patient and family the philosophy of being optimistic, for as long as it is realistic. This requires a careful balance between hope while still discussing the reality of poor prognosis.
Do more listening than speaking at specific times	When projecting a time frame regarding when end of life may come, listen—do not speak. Patients oftentimes knows how long they are going to live, based on how they feel. Listen to them.
Remove all physical barriers	Sit close to the patient. Remove barriers, such as a desk, computer, or medical chart. The patient being seen for the first time needs to develop a high level of trust with the healthcare provider. The key to relationship-building is trust. Being respectful, competent, reliable, and honest are critical features needed for successful relationship-building between a patient and his or her doctor.[13]
Start with just one question	Ask a leading question, then stop and listen, giving the patient time to respond. How much does the patient know about his or her cancer? How much does he or she want to know? Ask: What are you hoping for right now? What do you believe your family (caregiver) is hoping for? What are you most worried about? What are three things that give you joy, or gave you joy before your illness worsened?
Do no harm	Whenever engaging in a discussion about treatment options, remember the Hippocratic oath—do no harm. Weighing risks and benefits of treatment can end up being too sterile a conversation. Merely listing the probabilities of specific side effects does not focus on what is important. Consider: How will these side effects impact quality of life for my patient? Are the patient's goals in keeping with the anticipated outcomes of treatment?
Learn from patients how much information they want to be given	Elicit from the patient if he or she wants to hear all of the treatment option information, including non-cancer treatment options. Does the patient want to share in the decision-making process? A discussion about cancer treatment versus palliative treatment is a good place to start. Often treatment discussions include costs. This can add anxiety to patients who needs to be aware of the financial burden their cancer treatment may have on them and their loved ones. This is important information, because patients do not want to leave debt behind for their family to pay.

The timing of when to approach discussions about impending death vary depending on the patient's condition and the provider's experience and knowledge of the patient and family's coping style.

Communicating with family members after the patient has died is an important role for oncology care providers as well, and one that does not happen often. Post-death communication with family members should include an inquiry about how they are doing emotionally, physically, spiritually, and financially. Providers should ask family members who served as caregivers how they are doing now and what could be done better to support future caregivers, including questions such as: What are three things that you found most helpful? What are three things that you feel need improvement? This information can inform communication processes and approaches for future patients and their families.

Communication Education Needed for Oncology Care Providers

Integrating palliative care into oncology settings affords patients and families the opportunity to engage in quality discussions about treatment options and shared decision-making and enables patient and family communication at the end of life. Still, communication education is needed for oncology care providers in order to ensure that palliative care communication is a part of cancer care. Specifically, communication education is needed to teach providers how to engage patients and families in shared decision-making, establishing of goals of care concordant with the patient's goals, and ways to have thoughtful end-of-life discussions. Important considerations include the timing of these conversations, determining who among the family should be included, and the environment for where conversations should be held. Oncology care providers also need communication education about how to incorporate hope when introducing palliative care as a treatment option. Delayed introduction of palliative care oncology, as a segue to hospice care, perpetuates the notion that palliative care is end-of-life care. Instead, palliative care should be seen as an additional care service that can restore or improve quality of life.

There is a critical need to provide integrative palliative care instead of transitioning a patient to palliative care and, in doing so, improve the outcomes of the care experience for the patient through better symptom control, improved quality of life, and in some cases even prolonged survival. This requires teaching oncology care providers which patients are in particular need of specialty palliative care, when to make that referral to the palliative care team, and how to communicate this information to the patient and his or her family.[14] Promotion of the treating oncologist to remain involved with the patient after transference to hospice care can prevent feelings of abandonment (for the patient, family, and providers) as well as maintain better continuity of care. This also provides a mechanism for achieving closure.[15] Table 22.5 outlines the communication tasks in oncology care settings based on palliative care ambulatory guidelines used in the benchmark Temel study.[16] These guidelines should serve as a basis for communication curriculum development.

Table 22.5 Communication Tasks in Oncology Care Settings[16]

Ambulatory Palliative Care Guidelines[a]	Communication Tasks
Illness understanding/education Inquire about illness and prognostic understanding Offer clarification of treatment goals	Learn from patients how they view their illness and their understanding about what it means to them. Ask: "What do you think is currently going on regarding your cancer?"
Symptom management—Inquire about uncontrolled symptoms with a focus on: Pain Pulmonary symptoms (cough, dyspnea) Fatigue and sleep disturbance Mood (depression and anxiety) Gastrointestinal (anorexia and weight loss, nausea and vomiting, constipation)	When assessing for symptom management, get to know your patients beyond their pathology. Engage in a discussion that supports patient-centered care. Are they married? Have a family? What kind of work do they or did they do? How do they enjoy spending their time?
Decision-making Inquire about mode of decision-making Assist with treatment decision-making, if necessary	Though occasionally some patients may want to relinquish all decision-making to their healthcare provider, it is important promote shared decision-making about their care and treatment. Emphasize a partnership with the patient and family.
Coping with life-threatening illness Patient Family/family caregivers	Acknowledge that patients are more than their pathology. This means inquiring about them as real people, with lives and families before they were diagnosed. Emphasize that the intent is to improve the patient's quality of life and provide effective ways for symptom management.
Referrals/prescriptions Identify care plan for future appointments Indicate referrals to other care providers Note new medications prescribed	Check for support structure in place to facilitate medication management. With patient consent, involve the primary family caregiver in discussions about pain.

[a]Based on Temel JS, Greer JA, Muzikansy A, et al. Early palliative care for patients with metastatic non-small cell lung cancer. *N Engl J Med.* 2010;363:733–741.

Conclusion

To move oncology care forward, communication education is needed for oncology care providers to teach successful ways to engage in discussions about palliative care. The ultimate goal is to incorporate an integrative palliative care program into the plan of care for oncology patients and their families. Quality of life care and palliative care need to be seen as synonymous. Palliative care communication across the oncology trajectory will bring this closer together.

References

1. American Cancer Society. 2014. Cancer Facts & Figures 2014. Annual Report. http://www.cancer.org/research/cancerfactsstatistics/cancerfactsfigures2014/index. Accessed September 1, 2014.
2. Bray F, Jemal A, Grey N, et al. Global cancer transitions according to the human development index (2008–2030): A population-based study. *Lancet Oncol*. 2012;13:790–801.
3. World Cancer Research Fund International Website. www.wcrf.org/cancer_statistics/world_cancer_statistics.php. Accessed September, 1, 2014.
4. World Health Organization. Cancer Fact Sheet N297. www.who.int/mediacentre/factsheets/fs297/en/. Updated February 2014. Accessed September 1, 2014.
5. World Cancer Research Fund International. Worldwide data. http://www.wcrf.org/int/cancer-facts-figures/worldwide-data. Accessed December 13, 2013.
6. Van Roenn J., von Gunten C. Setting goals to maintain hope. *J Clin Onocol*. 2003;21(3):570–573.
7. Matsuyama R, Reddy S, Smith T. Why do patients choose chemotherapy near the end of life? A review of the perspective of those facing death from cancer. *J Clinic Oncol*. 2006;24(21):3490–3496.
8. Van Vliet LM, van der Wall E, Plum NM, Bensing JM. Explicit prognostic information and reassurance about nonabandonment when entering palliative breast cancer care: Findings from a scripted video-vignette study. *J Clin Oncol*. 2013;31(26):3242–3249.
9. Stajduhar KI, Thorne Se, McGuinness L, et al. Patient perceptions of helpful communication in the context of advanced cancer. *J Clin Nurs*. 2010;19:2039–2047.
10. Granek L, Krzyanowska MK, Tozer R, Mazzotta P. Oncologists' strategies and barriers to effective communication about the end of life. *J Oncol Pract*. 2014;9(4):131–135.
11. Hagerty RG, Butow PN, Ellis PA, et al. Cancer patient preferences for communication of prognosis in the metastatic setting. *J Clinic Oncol*. 2004;22(9):1721–1730.
12. Back AL, Arnold RM, Quill TE. Hope for the best, and prepare for the worst. *Ann Intern Med*; 2003;138:439–443.
13. De Haes H, Teunissen S. Communication in palliative care: A review of recent literature. *Curr Opin Oncol*. 2005;17:345–350.
14. Verg MT, Cullinan AM. Joining together to improve outcomes: Integrating specialty palliative care into the care of patients with cancer. *J Natl Compr Canc Netw*. September 2013;11(Suppl 4):S38–S46.
15. Back AL, Young JP, McCown E, et al. Abandonment at the end of life from patient, caregiver, nurse and physician perspectives: Loss of continuity and lack of cluster. *Arch Intern Med*. March 9, 2009;169(5):474–479.
16. Temel JS, Greer JA, Muzikansy A, et al. Early palliative care for patients with metastatic non-small cell lung cancer. *N Engl J Med*. 2010;363:733–741.

CHAPTER 23

Transplantation and Organ Donation

James D. Robinson and Teresa Thompson

Introduction

Transplantation presents several unique communication roles for the palliative care provider, including patient and family assistance with healthcare decision-making about transplant, coordination and communication between the transplant team and other healthcare providers, and assisting patient and family with legal issues such as the preparation of a living will or other advance directives. Typically, the family or next of kin discusses the patient's prognosis with the primary care physician and then works with a palliative care team to make decisions about end of life. This includes the decision to continue life-sustaining treatment, to add palliative care to life-sustaining treatment, and to discontinue life-sustaining treatment and transition to symptom management/palliative care. Once the decision has been made, healthcare providers (palliative care, intensive care, respiratory therapy, anesthesia, and, if donation is a possibility, a representative from the organ donation network) meet with the family to prepare them for end-of-life care vis-à-vis hospice and/or the withdrawal of life support interventions. Assistance in the decision to end life-sustaining treatment is one of the primary communication roles provided by the palliative care team.

In situations where transplantation or organ donation is possible, palliative communication also includes the identification and resolution of any concerns voiced by family members and appointment of a family spokesperson. In addition, the palliative care team describes what the family should expect as their loved one dies. This includes the physical setting in the operating room, the medical procedures involved during the process of harvesting organs, and an explanation of what will happen if the patient becomes an organ donor or a transplant recipient.

The palliative care team may also be involved in the care and symptom management of the organ donor patient. Such care occurs before and during withdrawal of life support, and it occurs afterward if the patient does not die within the institutional time frame for donation after cardiac death. The team's role is purely palliative, and they do not participate in the organ procurement process. The palliative care team is often involved in helping terminally ill patients decide the most appropriate time to choose for their death, before organ donation.[1,2]

Unfortunately, palliative care is sometimes viewed as the care of last resort, rather than as a component of care that should occur throughout the process. Even though it is becoming increasingly clear that patient choice is improved when patients have an appropriate level of information,[3] some providers do not realize that palliative care is not the same as hospice care,[4] and, regrettably, many transplant clinicians may perceive palliative care as a last resort measure that should only occur when "nothing more can be done."[5]

The purpose of this chapter is to remind providers and researchers that palliative care is a complex constellation of healthcare activities: palliative care professionals regard dying as a normal process, integrate the psychological and spiritual aspects of patient care, provide support to the patient and the family, utilize a team approach, and, of course, include pain relief. The recognition that, in palliative care, the emphasis is on care rather than cure is critical. Although the overall curative disease-directed approach of transplantation may seem to be at odds with the concept of palliative care, palliative care teams have much to offer patients and families facing transplantation. In fact, in all the studies to date,[6,7] survival has actually been the same or even longer when palliative care[8,9] or hospice[10,11] is involved, and sharing that data with transplant teams may be an eye-opener for them.

Transplantation and Palliative Care

The transplant team, patients, and their families are typically focused on a cure; if they did not have such a focus, they would not be pursuing a transplant. The failure of many healthcare providers, patients, and families to see the possibility of cure and care being simultaneously pursued can lead to the exclusion of palliative care. Patients expect providers to guide them in the healthcare system, with transplant providers serving as gatekeepers to palliative care access. Additionally, since most patients and families are focused on a cure, the need for palliative relief may seem contradictory or, at the very least, confusing. The fact remains, however, that, when studied,[12] the prevalence of symptoms (pain, anorexia, worry, fatigue, and dyspnea) are similar in non-cancer patients as cancer patients.

Bramstedt[13] argues that the best time to have conversations about healthcare—including diagnoses, symptoms, prognosis, treatment options, treatment preferences, and healthcare values—is early in the process and certainly before the patient's health is a full-blown crisis. As an ethicist, Bramstedt rightly argues that if a patient is unclear about the diagnosis and/or prognosis, he or she cannot make an informed decision about his or her healthcare. The ability to make an informed decision is further reduced in cases of diminished capacity and with the additional pressures or the exigencies of time and timing. There is no harm in discussing these difficult topics beforehand. In fact, many transplant patients may not even be aware that patients who undergo bone marrow or stem cell transplantation with an advance directive in place have *twice* the survival rates of those who have not completed advance directives.[14]

Solid Organ Donation

In the beginning, organs used for transplantation came from living relatives or brain-dead donors.[15] Donation after expected cardiac death was developed at the University of Pittsburgh and occurs when life-sustaining treatment is discontinued and consent for organ harvesting has been obtained from the patient's family. This is the most common type of organ donation,[16] and a variety of organs can be harvested, including liver, kidney, pancreas, lungs, and heart.[17] These types of organs are referred to as solid organs. A US Department of Health and Human Services report[18] indicated that, every day, 79 individuals receive a transplanted organ, yet 18 individuals die each day due to organ shortage. In 2012 28,051 individuals received a solid organ from a donor.[18]

As of May 2013, the population on the national transplantation waiting list was 44% Caucasian, 30% African American, 18% Hispanic/Latino, and 7% Asian, Native Hawaiian, and other Pacific Islander.[18] This is somewhat misleading, however, as each organ has a separate waiting list. In the United States, African Americans, Asians and Pacific Islanders, and Hispanics/Latinos are three times more likely than Caucasians to suffer from end-stage renal (kidney) disease, often as the result of high blood pressure and other conditions that can damage the kidneys. In fact, almost 35% of patients on the national waiting list for a kidney transplant are African American, while African Americans represent only 13% of the US population.[19] Of course this means that minority patients in need of an organ remain on the list much longer than their Caucasian counterparts.

Although organs are not matched according to race/ethnicity, and people of different races frequently match one another, all individuals waiting for an organ transplant have a better chance of receiving an organ if there are large numbers of donors from their racial/ethnic background. This is because compatible blood types and tissue markers—critical qualities for donor/recipient matching—are more likely to be found among members of the same ethnicity. A greater diversity of donors may potentially increase access to transplantation for everyone.

To understand organ donation, it is important to note that if a patient is not brain-dead but the family withdraws life support, the organs can be used only if the patient dies rather quickly. If the patient continues to live for 60 to 90 minutes, the organs cannot be used because they will have been deprived of oxygen for too long. Such a patient will be transferred to palliative care or hospice.

The Institute of Medicine has made clear that priority must be given to the dying patient and the family, not to the potential for organ donation. Palliative care providers take care of the patient once life support is withdrawn, no matter how long the patient continues to survive. Organ donation and palliative care are not mutually exclusive.[20] Many patients considered for transplantation die before receiving an organ, further emphasizing the importance of providing high-quality symptomatic relief and communication for all transplant patients.[21]

The pre- and peri-transplant patient experience is increasingly being recognized as having poor symptom management, lack of forthright communication, and major psychological stress,[22] in need of improvement.[21,23] Co-management with palliative care has been strongly recommended to correct some of these deficiencies,[24] but we lack randomized trial evidence of benefit.

Non-Solid Transplantation

Patients suffering from serious blood diseases (e.g., leukemia, multiple myeloma, thalassemias, sickle cell anemia, and aplastic anemia) often need bone marrow transplantation. Bone marrow is a spongy tissue inside some bones (e.g., hip and thigh) that consists of immature cells called stem cells. The term "bone marrow transplantation" refers to the replacement of the stem cells in bone marrow. In short, the patient is given a treatment that kills the cells in the cancer-laden bone marrow and is then given stem cells to replace that loss. Because stem cells are immature, they can develop into red blood cells for transporting oxygen throughout the body, white blood cells to fight infection, and platelets, which help blood to clot.[24] The most critical part of the transplant is the new graft immune system, such that a certain amount of "graft-versus-host" disease is desirable and crucial; without it, the chance of cancer relapse is much higher.

Approximately 130,000 Americans are diagnosed with a serious blood disease annually, and 44,000 of those diagnoses will be for leukemia (a blood cancer). About half of those adults and 700 of the 3,500 children diagnosed with leukemia will die from the disease. All of these patients need to receive a bone marrow transplant (BMT), but only 30% will find a matching donor within their family. The remaining 70% must find a donor from the National Donor Registry, where only about 2% of all Americans are registered.

Individuals in need of a blood marrow donor must find someone that matches their blood marrow. Generally, people of the same ethnic group are more likely to match, and this means that the number of people registered as potential donors is extremely important. Caucasian patients find a compatible donor about 75% of the time, but African Americans find a compatible donor only 25% of the time. This is a complicated issue, as there is more genetic heterogeneity within "African" and "Asian" populations due to the size of the continents and diversity of populations. In addition, more African Americans registered in the National Marrow Donor Registry are not "fit" donors when matched, and more refuse donation; efforts continue to enhance minority donor participation and donation.[25] Asians Americans and Hispanic Americans are more fortunate than African Americans, with successful donor availability occurring at 40% and 45%, respectively.

Estimates vary, but of the 6,000 people currently searching for a marrow match in the United States, only about 30% will find a match, and 70% will die before finding a match. Approximately 80% of the Caucasians on the list will find a match, while 70% or more of the ethnic minorities and people of mixed ethnicities will not find a match in time.[26] If an African American patient is successful at finding a matching donor on the national registry, there is an 80% chance that there is only one compatible donor on the entire national list. Finally, while bone marrow donation is potentially dangerous, more than 35,000 people have donated bone marrow to a stranger without a single donor death.

Kidney Disease

The organ most in demand at any point in time is the kidney. The kidney is essentially a filtering system containing millions of tiny blood vessels. The inability to process blood sugar effectively and the increased pressure on the small blood vessels tax the kidney; those small blood vessels begin to leak, and ultimately, the kidney fails. The first successful kidney transplant was performed in 1954 between identical twins. While there are no bridging treatments, dialysis and transplantation have literally been lifesaving for many patients. For others, their lot in life becomes an endless wait in a line longer than the patient's lifetime. Still, others find that their body rejects the transplanted organ, and they live through extremely unpleasant consequences that can negatively affect their quality of life.[27,28] Symptom control is a primary concern. Barriers to symptom control have been identified in three areas: (a) provider unawareness of symptoms, (b) provider's uncertainty as to whose responsibility it is to treat symptoms, and (c) inherent difficulty in symptom management.[29]

Currently there is little effort to incorporate palliative care into dialysis and transplantation programs—even though people in end-stage kidney failure are being ravaged by a chronic illness. Many programs have no clear protocol for providing support for patients who are either turned down for transplantation or elect not to undergo dialysis. Typically, success is measured by the success of the graft and not the quality of life of the patient, let alone the quality of life for the patient's family. As part of palliative care, psychiatrists have the opportunity to participate in the ongoing relationship between palliative care and nephrology. Compelling new data show concurrent palliative care and renal management improve healthcare outcomes such as compliance and unneeded emergency room visits.[30] Patience and older oral diuretics with a concurrent palliative approach can also lead to significant renal improvement.[31] Still, kidney patients who receive transplants do not have a life expectancy as high as the general population and most end-stage renal disease patients do not complete advance directives.[32,33] The decision not to begin dialysis is more common than is the decision to withdraw from it.

Liver Transplantation

The second most commonly transplanted organ is the liver. Currently, about 16,000 patients are on the liver waiting list, and only about 6,000 liver transplants are performed each year; the median wait-time for transplant was almost a year in 2007. More recent data from the UK National Health Service in 2014 indicates a median wait-time for adult patients of 145 days, while pediatric patients wait an average of 72 days. Research suggests that despite the long wait and the progressive nature of the underlying illness, palliative issues such as goals of care and end-of-life issues are seldom discussed before the actual transplant occurs.[34–36] The aim of liver transplantation is to cure the patient with acute or chronic liver disease. While this is often achieved, some patients will encounter continued acute rejection of their transplanted liver (graft), experiencing chronic rejection or disease recurrence.[34(p396)] Rossaro et al. argue quite vehemently for the use of palliative care in patients awaiting liver transplantation. Liver transplantation is, however, commonly perceived as an intervention with a curative aim. In such a setting, the incorporation of palliative care principles into treatment decisions may be compromised.[34(p396)]

Liver transplantation is an effective treatment for patients with acute or chronic liver failure.[37] Even though one-year patient survival rates approach 90% and 7- to 10-year survival rates are in the 60% to 80% range,[38,39] patient quality of life concerns post-transplant nonetheless necessitate palliative care. In a recent study of 313 consecutive transplant patients (excluding the patients who died within 6 months, which represent 10% to 15% of all liver transplantations), the 1-, 10-, and 20-year patient survival rates were 97.6%, 80.8%, and 58.8%, respectively.[39] This is in sharp contrast to the fact that the 10-year survival rate of advanced end stage liver disease patients who do not undergo transplantation is close to zero.[40] Unfortunately, 150 patients per 1,000 must be removed from the wait list because they have become too sick to receive a transplant or they have already died[38]—obviously skewing the success rate of the treatment.

However, it is important to remember that the patient population with end-stage liver disease often suffers from a high social, economic, physical, and emotional burden related to their chronic illness. They face multiple quality of life challenges such as fatigue resulting from malnutrition, mobility impairment from ascites, and depression and cognitive loss as a result of encephalopathy.[41] Thirteen percent of liver transplant recipients experience a hospital length of stay of more than 30 days. Prolonged length of stay is associated with postoperative infection, allograft rejection, gastrointestinal bleeding, renal failure, and decreased survival as well as higher cost and resource use.[42]

When evaluating a patient for potential transplant, an initial discussion of end-of-life issues should be included. This minimizes consequent surprise and emotional disturbance for both the patient and the family[43] and becomes part of the conversation. The patient must be prepared for the possibility that a donor will not arrive in time. Even if the patient has been approved for the transplant list, a donor may not become available for a variety of reasons, including substance abuse issues (which may have caused the liver problem), adherence concerns (as adherence is essential post-transplant and transplant teams must be convinced the individual will comply with adherence requirement), other health concerns, and/or psychiatric issues.

Noting that the majority of people who are eligible for organs never get one, Crone et al. argue[44] that all potential transplant patients should be offered palliative care. Unique patient characteristics of liver recipients may include associated cognitive loss from hepatic encephalopathy, the emotional experience of receiving an organ from another human, the fact that someone had to die for the procedure to happen, and guilt associated with the realization that a dangerous lifestyle is the most common reason for transplantation (e.g., the damage associated with alcoholism and hepatitis B or C).

Previous research suggests that some of the end-of-life needs identified by patients include pain management, the avoidance of inappropriate prolongation of dying, a sense of control over their situation and destiny, and the opportunity to strengthen their relationships with their loved ones before they die.[45,46] In addition, family members report the following: the desire to be with their loved one during the dying process, to be kept informed, to receive explanations regarding the process of what/why therapy is being done, to be assured of the patient's comfort, and to be supported in their medical and end-of-life decisions.[45–47]

The high level of success associated with liver transplantation has also produced elevated expectations among physicians, patients, and their families. This expectation exists despite the fact that the patient is suffering from a severe life-limiting underlying illness even after transplantation. This high level of anticipation can make the transition from curative to palliative care difficult for families and healthcare providers alike. Adam[34(p396)] further notes the principle of paternalism used by healthcare providers in advising patients that they should continue with transplantation

Table 23.1 Effect of PC Intervention for Liver Transplant Patients

	Baseline (n = 79)	After PC Intervention (n = 104)
Deaths	21	31 (p value NS)
Goals of care discussions	2%	38%
DNR status at the time of death	52%	81%
Withdrawal of life support when appropriate	35%	68%
SICU length of stay		3 fewer days

Note. PC = palliative care; NS = nonsignificant; DNR = do not resuscitate; SICU = surgical intensive care unit.
Source. Lamba S, Murphy P, McVicker S, Smith JH, Mosenthal AC. Changing end-of-life care practice for liver transplant service patients: Structured palliative care intervention in the surgical intensive care unit. J Pain Symptom Manage. 2012;44(4):508–519.

as a treatment because they view this as the best option. This compromises the patient's autonomy, and it is the provider's role to act as advocate and to facilitate an environment in which the patient has independence in decision-making.

Healthcare for liver transplant patients must include both disease-directed curative and palliative care.[37] The addition of palliative care increases patient–provider discussions about goals of care, decreases the amount of time for do-not-resuscitate (DNR) requests to be implemented, increases the amount of time between the DNR and patient death (allowing families to say goodbye to their loved one), decreases the decision time for withholding or withdrawal of life support, and increases the likelihood of families withholding or withdrawing life support.[24,48] Table 23.1 represents the first reported attempt to implement a liver transplant palliative care service for patients, their families, transplant surgeons, and surgical critical care nurses.[37] Findings are consistent with previous research suggesting that successful communication interventions improve goals-of-care discussions and end-of-life care in the critically ill.[49–53]

Lung Transplantation

The American College of Chest Physicians and the American Thoracic Society have gone on record emphasizing the importance of palliative care throughout the healthcare process. They recognize a clear distinction between hospice and palliative care and oppose the notion that palliative care should be limited to the terminal phase of an illness. This recommendation is predicated, in part, on the recognition that lung transplant patients are often required to wait 2 to 3 years, and palliative care provides hope and comfort to patients and their families, even though these patients are usually very symptomatic from their underlying disease.[54]

Lung transplantation is considered the most medically risky organ transplantation procedure, with a 5-year survival rate of 47.3%. While lung transplant patients typically see an improvement in their quality of life, it may not be apparent to the patient until a year after the surgery. Unfortunately, approximately 16.8% of lung transplant patients die waiting for a matching donor or within 1 year of the lung transplant taking place.[55] As lung transplant patients are forced to relocate to the vicinity of the lung transplant center, patients may be moved away from their homes and their loved ones. In addition, the strict body mass index measurements required of lung transplant patients means patients may be involved in a supervised exercise program (which can cause dyspnea or difficulty breathing) and require them to change their diet dramatically. This change may involve unpleasant dietary supplements or the use of feeding tubes and may deprive patients of their favorite foods.

Of the variety of barriers to palliative care for lung transplant patients,[56] the most commonly identified are (a) unrealistic expectations by the patient and his or her family about the likelihood of survival until a donor organ is available and (b) unrealistic expectations by the patient and his or her family about the likelihood of survival after the lung transplant. In addition, Colman et al. report that 57% of the physicians believed that patients and their families would feel abandoned if palliative care were initiated, and 61% of the physicians felt family disagreements about care goals were a significant barrier to palliative care.[56] Patients may be reassured by the data showing that concurrent care in cancer and non-cancer patients shows equal or even better survival and that involving another team to improve symptoms can only help.

For lung transplant patients, palliative care can be facilitated by (a) advance care planning for patients on the waiting list; (b) access to palliative care consultants; (c) regular meetings between transplant physicians, nurses, patients, and family members; and (d) communication between the transplant program and the referring physician. Additional training of transplant physicians in symptom management, end-of-life communication skills, the provision of experienced role models for transplant physician trainees, and supervision of transplant physician-trainees is helpful in improving palliative care.

Making this need even more apparent is a study of patients awaiting lung transplantation, which indicated that none had a DNR order at the time of hospital admission, and, when these orders were finally written, they were generally written on the same day the patient died.[43] These observations were based on the fact that many transplant patients desired to be full code in pursuit of a transplant,[57] and their physicians concurred.[35(p2168)]

Cardiac Transplantation

Heart failure in its chronic form is an irreversible and progressive disease. Unfortunately, transplant and cardiac assist programs do not include palliative care during treatment. Instead, palliative care is provided when the patient is no longer a candidate for transplantation or device therapy—or colloquially at the end of life. Heart failure patients are rarely referred to palliative care or hospice services early in the disease process. Recently, there has been a shift toward viewing treatment medicine and palliative medicine as "shared care" to optimize the patient's quality of life throughout illness.

Because of the extreme shortage of donor organs, the waiting time for a transplant can be significant—at times, several years. In addition to the psychological issues, the decline caused by the failing organ may produce a wide variety of symptoms, including shortness of breath, edema, dizziness, and nausea. These symptoms of physical decompensation can be relieved in some patients (e.g., paracentesis for ascites or diuretics for edema), but in other patients, these symptoms are intractable.[58,59] However, bridge treatments such as a left ventricular assist device are often given to aid patients until they can receive a new heart. These implanted devices often cause abdominal discomfort, appetite disruption, increased levels of anxiety, and sleep disturbance.[60,61]

Patients with heart problems often have questions about their prognosis and end-of-life issues but report being uncomfortable asking questions.[62] While many patients reported that they would welcome frank discussions about their prognoses, they believed that their physicians would not want to discuss end-of-life issues with them. Selman et al.[63] came to similar conclusions and found that heart failure patients live with fear and anxiety and are less than informed about their diagnosis or the implications of that diagnosis. Likewise, cardiac staff members rarely initiate discussion of such issues with their patients.

A more recent study by Schwarz et al.[64] tested the effectiveness of a palliative care program for cardiac patients. They found that palliative care consultation resulted in a decrease in the use of opioids and an increase in the levels of patient satisfaction. Patients and their family members generally reported improved holistic care, continuity of care, more focused goals of care, and improved planning of treatment courses. In addition, most patients reported increased levels of clarity about their goals of care and their treatment plans, particularly as their clinical condition changed. The topics of advance directives and goals of care were addressed with all patients by the palliative care team, and 30% of the patients completed advance care directives following palliative care involvement. (See chapter 21 in this volume on heart disease.)

Hematopoietic Stem Cell Transplantation Therapy/Bone Marrow Transplantation

Patients suffering from leukemia, lymphoma, multiple myeloma, multiple sclerosis, and sickle cell anemia are often treated by stem cell transplantation. This type of treatment is hematopoietic stem cell transplantation (HSCT). When the stem cells are taken from bone marrow, it is often referred to as a bone marrow transplant (BMT). When the stem cells are taken from other sources (e.g., the bloodstream or umbilical cord blood), the procedure is called a stem cell transplant. In both cases, stem cells damaged by illness and treatment are replaced with healthy stem cells.[65] There are approximately 20,000 hematopoietic stem cell transplants in the United States each year.

In roughly two-thirds of these transplants, the patient's own bone marrow or peripheral blood stem cells are removed and held in reserve for transplantation. In killing cancer cells, the radiation and/or chemotherapy also damage the stem cells and necessitates their replacement. When the patient receives his or her own stem cells, it is called autologous transplantation, and when the patient receives stem cells from a donor, it is called allogeneic transplantation.

Approximately 25% to 50% of BMT recipients develop long-term complications, and nearly 30% of patients receiving allogeneic transplants do not survive 5 years. Autologous transplants have a much better 100-day survival rate—nearly 90%—but are not appropriate for all types of ailments requiring a BMT.[66] Obviously, because the stem cells come from the patient, autologous transplantation is far less likely to result in rejection of the transplanted stem cells than allogenic transplantation.

Despite the high morbidity and mortality seen in this population, the focus of care in HSCT remains curative, and palliative care is likely to come late in the process or not at all.[4(p266)] To date, there is a lack of research on the incorporation of palliative care into BMT.[4] The palliative care and BMT teams rarely meet, except when a patient is dying, often after a long intensive care unit stay. Newly funded randomized trials of concurrent care are sorely needed and should tell us if palliative care is worthwhile in this population.[66] A yet unpublished trial at Virginia Commonwealth University suggests there is significant symptom burden, and it is unclear how much of that burden can be reduced by palliative care (Thomas Smith, personal communication).[67]

Many patients receiving HSCT are fighting cancer and, despite the severity of their illness, do not have advanced care directives. They continue to receive curative treatment without advanced care planning even during the last month of their lives.[68] Only a minority (20%–40%) use hospice care as they approach death. A study of 155 patients undergoing HSCT[70] determined that 69% of the patients had designated a healthcare proxy, 44% had a living will, 61% had an estate will, and 63% had discussed their wishes regarding life support with family and friends. Importantly, however, only 16% of the patients had discussed their wishes regarding life support with their provider, only 39% had actual written advance directives in their charts, and documentation of a discussion between patients and providers regarding advance care planning was unusual.

Younger patients, particularly those under age 40, are much less likely than older adult patients to have engaged in advance care planning, and many patients considering HSCT have neither discussed nor planned to talk about end-of-life contingencies with their provider.[69] For most patients considering HSCT, the procedure represents a last hope for long-term survival. In such cases, patients who decide to undergo the procedure may have strong psychological motivations to avoid dwelling on the substantial risks involved. The palliative care team, however, can help with symptom assessment and management (e.g., pain, mucositis, nausea and vomiting, nutrition, anorexia and weight loss, graft-versus-host disease, diarrhea, and transfusion dependence).[4] In fact, data show a high prevalence of symptoms in these types of patients: nine physical and two psychological ones severe enough to warrant treatment.[70]

The concept of palliative care for patients undergoing HSCT remains contentious to some healthcare providers. Barriers facing HSCT patients include illness trajectory variability, which requires disparate and at times highly technical therapies; care goals that are not clear to the patient; the complexities of the healthcare system; and a lack of understanding about palliative care by patients and providers alike.[71] Patients and family caregivers continue to hope that if a transplant is not successful, the patient may have quality care and symptom management at the end of life.[72] The multiple symptoms exhibited throughout transplant are frequently complex, and poor symptom control has been associated with higher levels of emotional distress for both patients and caregivers.[73]

Chung et al.[4] and Cheng et al.[31] provide detailed suggestions about communicating the prognosis and estimating cure rates to patients and their families. They conclude that written prognoses are rarely provided, and, generally, the worse the prognoses and curability numbers, the fewer specific numbers provided to the patient. This can be remedied, in part, by providing written prognoses, asking patients if they want to discuss their prognosis and curability numbers, and reviewing with the patient his or her situation at every inflection point and not only at the initial diagnosis. The authors recommend[4,31] standardized symptom and spiritual assessment along with advance care planning documentation.

Finally, they suggest[4, 31] that informational visits need to be conducted for all patients who might need hospice care within the next six months. Typically, this is not done until the last 6 to 9 days, and therefore many patients are not provided sufficient hospice care. These visits, when coupled with the opportunity to develop relationships with hospice providers before the care is needed, means that treatments such as transfusions and medications that do not fit in the $150/day requirements may be negotiated out. When providers create a form and utilize it for negotiating coverage of needed procedures, patients are 2% to 25% more likely to utilize hospice.[74]

It appears that the problems of providing palliative care to patients undergoing HSCT transplantation are frequently underestimated.[75] Patients undergoing HSCT need social support, positive reframing, information-seeking, problem-solving, and emotional expression.[76] The nurse plays a key role in advocating for the patient and the family to secure the necessary care. Introduction of palliative care and even hospice care early in the disease trajectory has been correlated with improved symptom management and care planning and has not been shown to decrease patient survival or detract from feelings of hope.[4(p265)] In fact, patients maintain hope even when a poor prognosis is disclosed, and hope seems to correlate directly with provider truthfulness and honesty.[77,78]

Symptom burden is frequently a significant problem for HSCT patients, and family caregiver burden is overwhelming.[65] BMT caregivers experience high levels of anxiety, distress, and depression, and yet these symptoms are often unrecognized and untreated.[77] The partners of those patients receiving stem cell transplantation report receiving less social support, self-report lower levels of spiritual well-being, and experience more loneliness than transplant survivors.[76(p179)] Having a family caregiver is nonetheless critical. The presence of a caregiver is associated with improved survival at 1 year after transplantation (75%) when compared with patients without a dedicated caregiver (26%).[78]

Referral to palliative care is especially important when the HSCT has failed.[65] Patients and family must be informed and begin coping with the effects of the malignancy combined with the effects of transplantation.[65] Pain is frequently the reason that a palliative care consultation is sought and provides an opportunity to form a relationship with the patient and the family as well as a chance to address other palliative care needs.[65(p7)] Relapse after HSCT is a distressing event for patients and families but provides an opportunity for education and psychosocial support.[79] Cooke et al. developed an end-of-life educational program for nurses, lay care providers, patients, and their families. This program includes a discussion with the patient and a complex family grief assessment and referral plan. In addition, the program includes a family teaching component and bereavement follow-up visits, as well as a discussion of the application of all of these to patient care.

Conclusion

Transplant recipients must wait for a considerable length of time before they are eligible for transplant and a suitable donor is located. During this time patients require intense symptom management, and family members often require counseling. Post-transplant needs also include considerable amounts of care and follow-up. Given these features of the disease trajectory for transplant patients, and the success of transplantation sciences in increasing the rates of survival and patient longevity, transplant patients live with a chronic illness condition and could benefit from palliative care. At the moment, there is no defined role for palliative care in the transplant setting, no structure for the incorporation of palliative care with transplant teams, and no guidelines available to outline palliative care for transplant patients. Palliative care teams are needed across all stages of the transplantation process to ensure that the patient and the family's search for a cure via transplantation includes discussing the possibility that transplantation will not occur in time and/or will not be effective, ensuring that advance care planning and the consideration of other legal, interpersonal, and economic decisions related to healthcare take place prior to an acute crisis or death.

References

1. Toossi S, Lomen-Hoerth C, Josephson SA, Gropper MA, Roberts J, Patton K, Smith WS. Organ donation after cardiac death in amyotrophic lateral sclerosis. *Ann Neurol.* 2012;71(2):154–156.
2. Smith TJ, Vota S, Patel S, Ford T, Lyckholm L, Bhushan A, Bobb B, Coyne P, Swainey C. Organ donation after cardiac death from withdrawal of life support in patients with amyotrophic lateral sclerosis. *J Palliat Med.* 2012;15(1):16–19.
3. Starzomski, R. Ethical issues in palliative care: The case of dialysis and organ transplantation. *J Palliat Care.* 1994;10(3):27–34.
4. Chung HM, Lyckholm LJ, Smith TJ. Palliative care in BMT. *Bone Marrow Transplant.* 2009;43(4):265–273.
5. Molmenti EP, Dunn GP. Transplantation and palliative care: The convergence of two seemingly opposite realities. *Surg Clin N Am.* 2005;85(2):373–382.
6. Parikh RB, Kirch RA, Smith TJ, Temel JS. Early specialty palliative care—translating data in oncology into practice. *N Engl J Med.* 2013;369(24):2347–2351.
7. Hughes MT1, Smith TJ. The growth of palliative care in the United States. *Annu Rev Public Health.* 2014;35:459–475.
8. Temel JS, Greer JA, Muzikansky A, et al. Early palliative care for patients with metastatic non-small-cell lung cancer. *N Engl J Med.* 2010;363(8):733–742.
9. Bakitas M, Lyons KD, Hegel MT, Balan S, Brokaw FC, Seville J, Hull JG, Li Z, Tosteson TD, Byock IR, Ahles TA. Effects of a palliative care intervention on clinical outcomes in patients with advanced cancer: The Project ENABLE II randomized controlled trial. *JAMA.* 2009;302(7):741–749.
10. Saito AM, Landrum MB, Neville BA, Ayanian JZ, Weeks JC, Earle CC. Hospice care and survival among elderly patients with lung cancer. *J Palliat Med.* 2011;14(8):929–939.
11. Connor SR, Pyenson B, Fitch K, Spence C, Iwasaki K. Comparing hospice and nonhospice patient survival among patients who die within a three-year window. *J Pain Symptom Manage.* 2007;33(3):238–246.
12. Moens K, Higginson IJ, Harding R, EURO IMPACT. Are there differences in the prevalence of palliative care-related problems in people living with advanced cancer and eight non-cancer conditions? A systematic review. *J Pain Symptom Manage.* 2014;48(4):660–677.
13. Bramstedt, K. A. Hoping for a miracle: Supporting patients in transplantation and cardiac assist programs. *Curr Opin Support Palliat Care.* 2008;2(4):252–255.
14. Ganti AK, Lee SJ, Vose JM, Devetten MP, Bociek RG, Armitage JO, Bierman PJ, Maness LJ, Reed EC, Loberiza FR Jr. Outcomes after hematopoietic stem-cell transplantation for hematologic malignancies in patients with or without advance care planning. *J Clin Oncol.* 2007;25(35):5643–5648.
15. Prommer E. Organ donation and palliative care: Can palliative care make a difference? *J Palliat Med.* 2014;17(3):368–371.

16. Bernat, JL, Capron, AM, Bleck, TP, et al. The circulatory respiratory determination of death in organ donation. *Crit Care Med.* 2010;38(3):963–970.
17. Port FL, Dykstra DM, Merion RM, et al. Organ donation and transplantation trends in the USA. *Am J Transpl.* 2003;4(S9):7–12.
18. Organ Procurement and Transplantation Network Website. United States Department of Human Services. http://optn.transplant.hrsa.gov/. Accessed June 19, 2015.
19. US Census Bureau. State & County QuickFacts. http://quickfacts.census.gov/qfd/states/00000.html. Accessed June 19, 2015.
20. Beach PR, Hallett AM, Zaruca K. Organ donation after circulatory death: A vital partnership. *Am J Nurs.* 2011;111(5):32–40.
21. Walling AM, Asch SM, Lorenz KA, et al. Impact of consideration of transplantation on end-of-life care for patients during a terminal hospitalization. *Transplant.* 2013;95(4):641–646.
22. Rosenberger EM1, Dew MA, DiMartini AF, DeVito Dabbs AJ, Yusen RD. Psychosocial issues facing lung transplant candidates, recipients and family caregivers. *Thorac Surg Clin.* 2012;22(4):517–529.
23. Colman RE, Curtis JR, Nelson JE, Efferen L, Hadjiliadis D, Levine DJ, Meyer KC, Padilla M, Strek M, Varkey B, Singer LG. Barriers to optimal palliative care of lung transplant candidates. *Chest.* 2013;143(3):736–743.
24. National Cancer Institute. Bone marrow transplantation and peripheral blood stem cell transplantation. http://www.cancer.gov/cancertopics/factsheet/Therapy/bone-marrow-transplant. Reviewed August 12, 2013.
25. Kollman C, Abella E, Baitty RL, et al. Assessment of optimal size and composition of the U.S. National Registry of hematopoietic stem cell donors. *Transplantation.* 2004;78(1):89–95.
26. Marrow Drives. Myths about marrow/stem cell donation. http://marrowdrives.org/bone_marrow_donor_myths_faqs.html.
27. Fox R, Swazey J. Leaving the field. *Hasting Cent Rep.* 1992;22(5):9–15.
28. Fox R, Swazey J. *Spare parts: Organ replacement in American society.* New York, NY: Oxford University Press; 1992.
29. Feldman R, Berman N, Reid C, et al. Improving symptom management in hemodialysis patients: Identifying barriers and future directions. *J Palliat Med.* 2013;16(12):1528–1533.
30. Chan KY, Benjamin Cheng HW, Yap DY, Yip T, Li CW, Sham MK, Wong YC, Vikki Lau WK. Reduction of acute hospital admissions and improvement in outpatient attendance by intensified renal palliative care clinic follow-up: The Hong Kong experience. *J Pain Symptom Manage.* 2015;49(1):144–149.
31. Cheng HW, Sham MK, Chan KY, Li CW, Au HY, Yip T. Combination therapy with low-dose metolazone and furosemide: A "needleless" approach in managing refractory fluid overload in elderly renal failure patients under palliative care. *Int Urol Nephrol.* 2014;46(9):1809–1813.
32. Cohen LM, Levy NB, Tessier EG, Germain, MJ. Renal disease. In Levenson, JL ed., *The American Psychiatric Association Textbook of Psychosomatic Medicine.* Washington, DC, American Psychiatric Association; 2001:483–493.
33. Meyer VA. Consult-liaison psychiatry. In Kupfer, D ed. *Oxford American Handbook of Psychiatry.* New York: Oxford University Press; 2008:941–985.
34. Adam SJ. Palliative care for patients with a failed liver transplant. *Inten Crit Care Nurs.* 2000;16(6):396–402.
35. Larson AM, Curtis JR. Integrating palliative care for liver transplant candidates "too well for transplant, too sick for life." *JAMA.* 2006;295(18):2168–2176.
36. Rossaro L, Troppmann C, McVicar JP, et al. A strategy for the simultaneous provision of pre-operative palliative care for patients awaiting liver transplantation. *Transpl Intl.* 2004;17(8):473–475.
37. Lamba S, Murphy P, McVicker S, Smith JH, Mosenthal AC. Changing end-of-life care practice for liver transplant service patients: Structured palliative care intervention in the surgical intensive care unit. *J Pain Symptom Manage.* 2012;44(4):508–519.
38. Organ Procurement and Transplantation Network. Annual report of the U.S. Scientific Registry for Transplant Recipients and the Organ Procurement and Transplantation Network: Transplant Data: 1999–2008. Rockville, MD and Richmond, VA: US Department of Health and Human Services, Health Resources and Services Administration, Office of Special Programs, Division of Transplantation; United Network for Organ Sharing; 2011. http://optn.transplant.hrsa.gov/ar2009/chapter_index.htm. Accessed July 22, 2011.
39. Schoening WN, Buescher N, Rademacher S, et al. Twenty-year longitudinal follow-up after orthotopic liver transplantation: A single-center experience of 313 consecutive cases. *Am J Transplant.* 2013;13(9):2384–2394.
40. Schafer D. Liver transplantation: Look back, looking forward. In Maddrey W, ed. *Transplantation of the Liver.* Philadelphia, PA: Lippincott Williams & Wilkins; 2001:1–3.
41. van der Plas SM, Hansen BE, de Boer JB, et al. Generic and disease-specific health related quality of life in non-cirrhotic, cirrhotic and transplanted liver patients: A cross-sectional study. *BMC Gastroenterol.* 2003;3(33):1–13.
42. Smith JO, Shiffman ML, Behnke M, et al. Incidence of prolonged length of stay after orthotopic liver transplantation and its influence on outcomes. *Liver Transpl.* 2009;15(3):273.
43. Crone CC, Marcangelo MJ, Shuster JL. An approach to the patient with organ failure: Transplantation and end-of-life treatment decisions. *Med Clin N Am.* 2010;94(6):1241–1254.
44. Crone CC, Marcangelo MJ, Shuster JL Jr. An approach to the patient with organ failure: Transplantation and end-of-life treatment decisions. *Med Clin North Am.* 2010;94(6):1241–1254
45. Thompson BT, Cox PN, Antonelli M, et al. Challenges in end-of-life care in the ICU: Statement of the 5th International Consensus Conference in Critical Care: Brussels, Belgium, April 2003: Executive summary. *Crit Care Med.* 2004;32(5):1781–1784.
46. Truog RD, Campbell ML, Curtis JR, et al. (2008). Recommendations for end-of-life care in the intensive care unit: A consensus statement by the American Academy of Critical Care Medicine. *Crit Care Med.* 2008;36(3):953–963.
47. The SUPPORT Principal Investigators. Perceptions by family members of the dying experience of older and seriously ill patients: Study to understand prognoses and preferences for outcomes and risks of treatment. *Ann Intern Med.* 1997;126(2):97–106.
48. Adam R, McMaster P, O'Grady JG, et al. Evolution of liver transplantation in Europe: Report of the European Liver Transplant Registry. *Liver Transpl.* 2003;9(12):1231–1243.
49. Campbell ML, Guzman JA. Impact of a proactive approach to improve end-of-life care in a medical ICU. *Chest.* 2003;123(1):266–271.
50. Curtis JR, Treece PD, Nielsen EL, et al. Integrating palliative and critical care: Evaluation of a quality-improvement intervention. *Am J Resp Crit Care Med.* 2008;178(3):269–275.
51. Curtis JR, White DB. Practical guidance for evidence-based ICU family conferences. *Chest.* 2008;134(4):835–843.
52. Lilly CM, De Meo DL, Sonna LA, et al. An intensive communication intervention for the critically ill. *Am J Med.* 2000;109(6):469–475.
53. Mosenthal AC, Murphy PA. Interdisciplinary model for palliative care in the trauma/surgical ICU. Robert Wood Johnson Foundation Demonstration Project for improving palliative care in the ICU. *Crit Care Med.* 2006;34(11):S399–S403.
54. Selecky PA, Eliasson CA, Hall RI, Schneider RF, Varkey B, McCaffree DR. American College of Chest Physicians. Palliative and end-of-life care for patients with cardiopulmonary diseases: American College of Chest Physicians position statement. *Chest.* 2005;128(5):3599–3610.
55. Scientific Registry of Transplant Recipients Website. Organ summary. http://srtr.org/csr/current/nationalViewer.aspx?organcode = LU.2010. Accessed July 10, 2014.
56. Colman RE, Curtis JR, Nelson JE, et al. Barriers to optimal palliative care of lung transplant candidates. *Chest* 2013;143(3):736–743.

57. Dellon EP, Leigh MW, Yankaskas JR, Noah TL. Effects of lung transplantation on inpatient end of life care in cystic fibrosis. *J Cyst Fibros*. 2007;6:396–402.
58. Gines P, Cardenas A. The management of ascites and hyponatremia in cirrhosis. *Semin Liv Dis*. 2008;28(1):43–58.
59. Licata G, Di Pasquale P, Parrinello G, et al. Effects of high-dose furosemide and small-volume hypertonic saline solution infusion in comparison with a high dose of furosemide as bolus in refractory congestive heart failure: Long-term effects. *Am Heart J*. 2003;145(3):459–466.
60. Dew MA, Kormos RL, Winowich S. Quality of life outcomes in left ventricular assist system inpatients and outpatients. *ASAIO J*. 1999;45(3):218–225.
61. el-Amir NG, Gardocki M, Levin HR, et al. Gastrointestinal consequences of left ventricular assist device placement. *ASAIO J*. 1996;42(3):150–153.
62. Rogers AE, Addington-Hall JM, Abery AJ, et al. Knowledge and communication difficulties for patients with chronic heart failure: qualitative study. *BMJ*. 2000;321:605–607.
63. Selman L, Harding R, Beynon T, et al. Improving end-of-life care for patients with chronic heart failure: "Let's hope it'll get better, when I know in my heart of hearts it won't." *Heart*. 2007;93(8):963–987.
64. Schwarz ER, Baraghoush A, Morrissey RP, et al. (2012). Pilot study of palliative care consultation in patients with advanced heart failure referred for cardiac transplantation. *J Palliat Med*. 2012;15(1):12–15.
65. Chow K, Coyle N. Providing palliative care to family caregivers throughout the bone marrow transplantation trajectory. *J Hosp Palliat Nurs*. 2011;13(1):7–13.
66. Cost of a hematopoietic stem cell transplant. http://biomed.brown.edu/Courses/BI108/BI108_2007_Groups/group03/cost.html
67. Personal Communication with Thomas Smith, MD, Director of Palliative Care, Johns Hopkins University.
68. Zhou G, Stoltzfus JC, Houldin AD, et al. (2010). Knowledge, attitudes, and practice behaviors of oncology advanced practice nurses regarding advanced care planning for patients with cancer. *Oncol Nurs Forum*. 2010;37: E400–E410. doi:10.1188/10.ONF.E400-E410
69. Joffee S, Mello MM, Cook EF, et al. Advance care planning in patients undergoing hematopoietic cell transplantation. *BioBMT*. 2007;13(1):65–73.
70. Tabbara I, Zimmerman K, Morgan C, Nahlah Z. Allogeneic hematopoietic stem cell transplantation: Complications and results. *Arch Intern Med*. 2002;162(14):1558–1566.
71. Manitta VJ, Philip JA, Cole-Sinclair MF. Palliative care and the hemato-oncological patient: Can we live together? A review of the literature. *J Palliat Med*. 2010;13(8):1021–1025.
72. Fife BL Fausel CA. Hematopoietic dyscrasias and stem cell/bone marrow transplantation. In Holland JC, ed. *Psycho-Oncology*. New York, NY: Oxford University Press; 2010:191–195.
73. Fife BL, Monahan PO, Abonour R, et al. Adaptation of family caregivers during the acute phase of adult BMT. *Bone Marrow Transp*. 2009;43(12):959–966.
74. Sexauer A, Cheng MJ, Knight L, Riley AW, King L, Smith TJ. Patterns of hospice use in patients dying from hematologic malignancies. *J Palliat Med*. 2014;17(2):195–199.
75. Tee ME, Balmaceda GZ, Granada MA, et al. End-of-life decision making in ematopoietic cell transplantation recipients. *Clin J Oncol Nurs*. 2013;17(6):640–646.
76. Roeland E, Mitchell W, Elia G, et al. Symptom control in stem cell transplantation: A multidisciplinary palliative care team approach. Part 2: Psychosocial concerns. *J Support Oncol*. 2010;8(4):179–183.
77. Bishop MM, Beaumont JL, Hahn EA, et al. Late effects of cancer and hematopoietic stem-cell transplantation on spouses or partners compared with survivors and survivor-matched controls. *J Clin Oncol*. 2007;25(11):1403–1411.
78. Foxall MJ, Gaston-Johansson F. Burden and health outcomes of family caregivers of hospitalized bone marrow transplant patients. *J Adv Nurs*. 1996;24(5):915–923.
79. Cooke LD, Gemmill R, Grant ML. (2011). Creating a palliative educational session for hematopoietic stem cell transplantation recipients at relapse. *Clin J Oncol Nurs*. 2011;15(4):411–417.

CHAPTER 24

Communication Challenges in Providing Advance Care Planning for People Living With HIV/AIDS

Maureen E. Lyon, Blaire Schembari, Brittney Lee, and Peter Selwyn

Introduction

In 2012 an estimated 35.3 million people were living with HIV worldwide.[1] Newly acquired HIV infections have decreased globally.[1] Much of this reduction can be attributed to medical care advances and global prevention programs.[2-5] However, despite HIV becoming a chronic illness,[6,7(p2)] deaths from AIDS and comorbidities continue. In the United States, HIV/AIDS deaths occur disproportionately among African Americans.[6-8] Yet, nationwide, African Americans are half as likely as whites to use any advance directive, even though, when surveyed, they indicate a desire to complete an advance care directive.[9-10] Advance care planning (ACP), which aims to relieve suffering and enhance quality of life, is perhaps the most important palliative care dimension with respect to family, provider, and patient communication. The negative consequences to the patient of poor or no ACP include unmet needs, inappropriate, or even unwanted care.[11,12] Conflicts with hospital staff about treatment choices or rejection of non-legally related caregivers such as unmarried partners,[13,14] loss of respect for autonomy in the spirit of the Patient Self-Determination Act (1990), may result from a lack of ACP while the patient is competent.[15]

Incorporating ACP during the "antecedent period of decision making"[16] is critical, because with AIDS timing of death is uncertain and decision-making capacity may be compromised by HIV-associated neurological disease or other cognitive impairment.[17,18] ACP can significantly reduce these negative consequences, promote excellence in HIV care, and yield better outcomes for patients, families, and providers.[16] Palliative care, which includes ACP, optimizes quality of life and addresses the physical, emotional, social, and spiritual needs[19-23] of people living with AIDS (PLWA) by facilitating autonomy, access to information, and choice.[24] Given the complex nature of caring for PLWA, palliative care is essential for supporting patients, their families, as well as their healthcare team, and should be implemented throughout the disease process. Thus it is recommended that palliative care be utilized alongside standard HIV treatment.[5] Moreover, both the World Health Organization[25] and UNAIDS[26] have suggested the appropriateness of incorporating palliative care throughout every stage of HIV disease and treatment.

Communication forms the foundation for quality ACP.[27] Communication creates a human connection, which not only transmits information but serves as the foundation for a relationship with the healthcare provider that unfolds over time.[28(p179)] Within the context of palliative care, research indicates that communication impacts treatment adherence, pain management, recovery rates, psychological functioning, and overall happiness with care.[29] This chapter reviews evidence-based models to increase patient–family communication and enhance provider–patient communication about palliative care for HIV patients who often have comorbid conditions. The chapter also discusses research in progress of models that can be adapted for PLWA.

Interpersonal Communication Theories

Communication is a basic tool in healthcare relationships that, under ideal circumstances, involves collaborative communication with the entire healthcare team, patient, and family.[30] ACP facilitation guides the practice of using interpersonal communication skills, including empathetic listening, to build a trusting relationship.[31,32] Interpersonal discussions about sensitive or difficult health topics, such as ACP, provide new information, guide patient decision-making, and promote behavioral change. Interpersonal communication can be defined as a selective, systemic, unique, and ongoing process of transactions that allow people to reflect and build personal knowledge of one another and create shared meanings.[33] Interpersonal communication messages are offered to initiate, define, maintain, or further a relationship; furthermore, interpersonal communication refers both to the content and quality of messages relayed. Research supports the notion that skillful interpersonal communication practice makes a positive difference to patients.[34] Patients feel they have been heard, supported, and understood and their concerns validated.[35,36]

The interpersonal communication transactional model most closely aligns with ACP principles. The transactional model emphasizes the dynamics of interpersonal communication and the multiple roles people assume during the process.[37] In ACP discussions, a trained/certified facilitator provides support for the patient and his or her surrogate decision-maker during sensitive discussions that may shape future clinical care to fit the patient's preferences and values. The Respecting Choices® model supports ACP discussions, clarifying communication as occurring within systems that affect "what and how people communicate and what meanings are created."[38]

Shared meaning is at the heart of interpersonal communication. We create meanings as we learn what each other's words and behaviors represent or imply.[34] Interpersonal communication involves two levels of meaning: content meaning and relationship meaning. ACP facilitators use content meaning to enhance the patient's and family's understanding of the medical condition, facilitate a discussion of the patient's key priorities in end-of-life care, and develop a care plan that reflects these priorities that the family can honor. Relationship-meaning is created when ACP facilitators explore the patient's and family's understanding, experiences, hopes, and goals for living well. Involving the patient's loved ones and/or surrogate decision-maker in ACP encourages discussion and increases agreement between the patient and his or her surrogate decision-maker, creating feelings of being better informed and supported.[35]

Person-Centered and Family-Focused Approach

For PLWA, the core philosophy of a person-centered[36] approach to palliative care, which focuses on patient preferences, is appropriate. Although HIV/AIDS is no longer a rapidly fatal illness, a great deal of stigma is still associated with the diagnosis. A patient being treated with respect, warmth, and empathy fosters a supportive and open patient–healthcare provider relationship. Research indicates that patients and their family members value healthcare providers' respect and that such positive regard impacts treatment outcomes.[37] Briggs and colleagues have consistently found that a person-based approach to ACP significantly changes healthcare professionals' beliefs and practices by increasing care and respect for patients' autonomy, families' experiences, and documentation of patients' wishes.[38] Family-focused palliative care takes into account patients' needs as well as the experiences and influences of family caregivers that may otherwise go unnoticed.[39] Qualitative research indicates the desire and importance of family involvement in palliative care.[40] The Institute for Family-Centered Care defines family-centered care as an approach to the planning, delivery, and evaluation of healthcare that is governed by mutually beneficial partnerships between healthcare providers, patients, and families.[41] Models of family-centered palliative HIV care initially emerged for pediatric populations as a way to better assist children and their caregivers with HIV treatment.[41] Family-centered care for PLWA aims to provide comprehensive health services for families' needs and promote communication among the patient, family, and healthcare providers. Empirical evidence supports both communication and decision-making as critical elements that impact dying youth and their families[42–55] (Table 24.1).

Respect for autonomy demands that healthcare providers afford PLWA the opportunity to make decisions about their own end-of-life care before a medical crisis impairs the ability to do so. Earlier in the epidemic, attention was given to ACP issues specific to HIV.[54,55] However, this clinical practice predated the current era of highly active antiretroviral therapy, which is characterized by longer survival, more uncertain prognoses, a growing range of comorbidities, and potential impaired decision-making for patients with advanced HIV or life-limiting comorbidities.[56–58] There is a growing consensus that palliative care and ACP should begin from the time of diagnosis, if not earlier.

Inappropriate scenarios often result in current ACP practice. For example, an ER clerk may hand a tonsillectomy patient an advance directive form to complete, or, alternatively, hospital systems may automatically mail an advance directive to patients with a chronic illness on their 18th birthday. Often patients expect their healthcare providers to initiate such discussions, but in the face of uncertain prognosis, lack of time, or individual comfort level the healthcare provider may not initiate this conversation. Sometimes, hospital or departmental policy designates a social worker or chaplain without ACP facilitation skills training to initiate this conversation during a medical crisis, often during an inpatient hospital stay.

Therefore, in direct response to this need, Lyon and colleagues[47–52] developed the FAmily CEntered Advance Care (FACE) planning model. This model, developed and adapted from Briggs and Hammes' Respecting Choices® model,[38] has been tested among adolescents and young adults with HIV[48–50] and cancer.[51,52] Currently, there are two ongoing longitudinal, multisite, randomized clinical trials to determine if the benefits of a patient-centered, family-focused approach for adolescents and adults with AIDS can be sustained over time (Pediatric Palliative Care: Quality of Life and Spiritual Struggle with adolescents with AIDS; Palliative Care in People Living with HIV/AIDS: Integrating into Standard of Care).[53] The following section details the FACE-HIV communication model and the tools used within the model and provides illustrative cases.

FACE-HIV Communication Model and Intervention

FACE-HIV is an evidence-based structured and individual model for facilitating communication between HIV/AIDS patients and their families.[48–50] The purpose of the FACE-HIV intervention program is to facilitate conversations about future healthcare decisions, including end-of-life care between patients living with HIV/AIDS (or other life-limiting illnesses) and their surrogate decision-makers. A specific FACE-HIV program goal is to train qualified professionals to deliver a standardized intervention, which opens communication channels, resulting in increased congruence in treatment preferences and decreased decisional conflict. This process supports the patient's and the family's psychological adjustment, improves quality of life, and documents the patient's goals of care and treatment preferences in his or her medical record (Table 24.1).

The FACE-HIV program consists of three 60- to 90-minute sessions in a face-to-face format with a trained/certified interviewer.

Table 24.1 Description of Family Centered Advance Care Planning (FACE) Intervention

Session 1 Foundation	Session 1 Goals	Session 1 Process
Lyon Family Centered Advance Care Planning Survey—Patient and Surrogate Versions,© which engages the participant in EOL questions. (30 minutes)	1. To assess the patients' and surrogates' values, spiritual and other beliefs and life experiences with illness and EOL care 2. To assess when to initiate EOL discussion and planning	1. Facilitator orients family to study and issues 2. Patient is surveyed separately from the surrogate 3. Surrogate is surveyed privately with regard to what he or she believes the patient prefers 4. Patient and surrogate are primed to think about and discuss issues they may not have considered before, prior to coming in for the structured conversation
Session 2 Foundation	**Session 2 Goals**	**Session 2 Process**
Disease-Specific Advance Care Planning Interview®[60] (60 minutes) See Gundersen Health System for training	1. To facilitate conversations and shared decision-making between the patient and surrogate about EOL care, providing an opportunity to express fears, values, spiritual, and other beliefs and goals with regard to death and dying 2. To prepare the surrogate to be able to fully represent the patient's wishes	*Stage 1* assesses the patient's understanding of current medical condition, prognosis, complications *Stage 2* explores patient's philosophy regarding EOL decision-making and his or her understanding of the facts *Stage 3* reviews rationale for future medical decisions the patient would want the surrogate to understand/act on *Stage 4* uses the Statement of Treatment Preferences to describe clinical situations common to AIDS and related treatment choices *Stage 5* summarizes the discussion/need for future discussions as situations/preferences change. Gaps in information are identified and referrals are made[a]
Session 3 Foundation	**Session 3 Goals**	**Session 3 Process**
The Five Wishes© is a legal document that helps people express how they want to be treated if they are seriously ill and unable to speak. It addresses all of a person's needs: medical, personal, emotional, spiritual (30 minutes)	**To determine** 1. Which person is to be the surrogate decision-maker 2. The kind of medical treatment the patient wants 3. How comfortable the patient wants to be 4. How the patient wants people to treat him or her 5. What the patient wants loved ones to know 6. Spiritual/religious concerns	For patients under the age of 18, the Five Wishes© must be signed by a legal guardian. Processes, such as labeling feelings and concerns, as well as finding solutions to any identified problem, are facilitated. Appropriate referrals are made to help resolve disagreements over decision-making (e.g., a hospital ethicist or their doctor) or spiritual issues (e.g., a hospital chaplain or their clergy).

Note: EOL = end-of-life.
[a] This session may include other family members or loved ones.

Three sessions are held 1 week apart to give families time to think over goals and values that inform end-of-life treatment preferences and to consult with family members, clergy, and others. A surrogate decision-maker must be chosen prior to the first meeting.

Session One Lyon Family Centered ACP Survey©—Patient and Surrogate versions.[59] This survey is used as a tool to engage participants in ACP and end of life decision-making.

Session Two Respecting Choices® Next Steps ACP Interview.[60] This patient-centered, structured interview is used to explore patients' understanding of their illness, open channels of communication between the patient and surrogate decision-maker, and discuss goals of care in "bad-outcome" situations. This in-depth conversation is facilitated by a trained/certified ACP facilitator to determine what goals of treatment should be followed, if complications occur. One end-product is the creation of a "disease-specific" advance directive. Facilitator certification is available. For more information see http://www.gundersen-health.org/respecting-choices.

Session Three The Five Wishes© advance directive document[61] was designed to reflect the patient's goals and values. A training video and the Five Wishes© document are available online at http://www.agingwithdignity.org/forms/5wishes.pdf. The completion of an advance directive document can be any document recognized in that state.

To ensure protocol fidelity and patient safety, each session is immediately followed by 15- to 30-minute assessment questionnaires. If the facilitator is also conducting research, the patient and family would separately complete the Quality of Patient-Facilitator and Surrogate-Facilitator End of Life Communication[62] and Satisfaction Questionnaire with a person other than the trained/certified interviewer. These participant ratings provide a quality assessment of the trained facilitator's

> **Box 24.1** Advance Care Planning: Selection of Surrogate Decision-Makers[60]
>
> 1. Is the person willing to be a surrogate? Sometimes even the most trusting and loving people find this role very difficult.
> 2. Do you trust the person to know your views and be willing to talk with you?
> 3. Is the person able to follow through and honor your wishes, even if he or she might not agree with your choices?
> 4. Can the person make decisions under stressful and difficult situations? Sometimes someone more removed from the situation is better suited emotionally for making tough choices.[38]

discussions and the program as a whole. The patient must first choose a surrogate decision-maker, also known as a healthcare proxy, to communicate his or her decisions in the event of the loss of the ability to make or communicate decisions. Patients often need help in designating a surrogate decision-maker or healthcare proxy. The patient is encouraged to select a surrogate using the guidelines in Box 24.1 for selecting a surrogate decision-maker for Disease-Specific ACP*.[60]

Disclosure of Diagnosis

One unique aspect of palliative care communication for PLWA is that the disease's stigma may inhibit the patient from disclosing the diagnosis to family, friends, or lovers, isolating the patient and cutting him or her off from possible social support. Stigma is not a problem reported for advance care planning or palliative care for patients with other diseases.[63–68] Many HIV patients experience slow decline and sudden complications and fail to make specific treatment plans, in part because they cannot identify someone they trust enough to make decisions for them or because they have not told anyone about their HIV diagnosis. This isolation is a barrier to the potential benefits of ACP, such as enabling a sense of control in a low control situation, strengthening families by moving them from a contractual agreement to a covenant to honor and respect the patient's preferences even when different from the families' own wishes, or providing opportunities to work in an ACP study using ACP as a process to disclose one's HIV diagnosis to a long-term friend and former lover.

Box 24.2 provides an example of how ACP can be used as a disclosure opportunity for PLWA. In our studies with adolescents and adults with HIV/AIDS, consistently 15% of the interested patients could not participate in the study because they had not disclosed to anyone outside their healthcare team or could not identify someone they trusted enough to make decisions for themselves. This marginalization and social stigmatization highlights the continuing gap in social support for PLWA. This is important, as a recent meta-analysis of more than 300,000 participants across all age groups demonstrated that adults have a 50% increased likelihood of survival with strong social relationships.[69] The association was strongest for complex measures of social integration.[69]

When disclosure does not occur, one possible approach is for the healthcare provider to offer to share the disclosure to the surrogate on behalf of the patient, informing the surrogate that the patient has an immune deficiency disorder and explaining the potential medical complications. In these instances, the patient should be advised that if the surrogate asks, "Does ___ have AIDS?", the provider would not lie. Knowing the patient's diagnosis offers the opportunity for a deep and authentic conversation between the patient and surrogate about the patient's understanding of his or her medical condition, illness complications, death and dying experience, and care goals and values in HIV-specific or other bad-outcome situations.

Box 24.3 depicts the important role providers have in encouraging disclosure as part of ACP and ensuring informed healthcare decision-making. There is potential for ethical dilemmas with regard to patient autonomy and the right to confidentiality versus the healthcare provider's values and the goals of ACP, which presume the surrogate decision-maker knows the patient's diagnosis as the first step in the process. Research is needed to find ways to support disclosure to families that will maximize the likelihood of family acceptance and minimize the patient's fear of abandonment.

> **Box 24.2** Advance Care Planning as a Disclosure Opportunity
>
> A 72-year-old Caucasian, self-identified gay man with HIV/AIDS who recently had a heart attack decided to participate in an advance care planning study for adults living with AIDS. After recruitment and enrollment at a neighboring hospital, he presented with his surrogate decision-maker, an old partner and friend, for study participation. As the trained facilitator began the Respecting Choices Interview®, it came to light that the surrogate knew of the patient's heart attack and other medical issues but not the HIV diagnosis. This was very confusing for the facilitator, as the consent form explicitly stated that the study was about advance care planning for HIV patients and the chosen surrogate should be fully aware of the patient's diagnosis. When the patient was asked, "What is your understanding of your illness?" He responded with an anxious smile, while looking at his surrogate, and said, "Which one?" Advance care planning for this patient was used as a disclosure opportunity.

> **Box 24.3** Disclosure and a Surrogate's Informed Decision-Making
>
> Dr. S's patient, DJ, a 52–year-old African American man, was in the final stages of kidney failure due to HIV/AIDS complications and treatment side effects, following years of dialysis. He contracted the virus, sexually, from another man but was not self-identified as gay. Dr. S noted in the electronic medical record that DJ's chosen surrogate decision-maker was his mother, but he had not disclosed his diagnosis to her. Each time Dr. S met with DJ he pressured him to disclose, arguing that DJ's mother could not make good decisions for him if she did not know his diagnosis or understand the potential complications. Dr. S offered to be present when DJ told his mother. The third time Dr. S asked if he had told his mother yet, DJ said, "Doc, I hate you." However, shortly afterward DJ did disclose to his mother, who surprised him by being very supportive. His mother knew the truth and did not reject him. DJ died shortly afterward.

Including Adolescents in ACP

While not every adolescent with a life-limiting illness is capable of or wants to participate in ACP, research demonstrates that adolescents have greater capacity for ACP participation than adults give them credit for.[47-52,70,71] Having families involved in ACP decision-making, even for older adolescents aged 18 to 21 years, makes sense on three fronts: (a) the ACP process sends a strong message to the patient that he or she will not be abandoned, (b) understanding the consequences of decisions is not fully formed until young adulthood,[72,73] and (c) the ACP process benefits adolescent patients and their families.[47-52,74,75] Consistent with research that young adolescents have a mature understanding of death,[75,76] ACP adolescent research (mean age 16 years; range 14–21 years) found no differences by age in analysis of outcome variables (congruence in treatment preferences, decisional conflict, quality of life, anxiety or depressive symptoms).[47-52] Healthcare providers should not underestimate the capacity children have to engage in conversations about very serious topics, such as end-of-life care, nor should we let healthcare providers' exaggerated fears that children cannot handle conversations about such serious topics become a barrier to ACP. Adolescents build the capacity to talk about death and dying through the process of ACP, within the context of family support and a protocol facilitated by a certified facilitator, as this gives them a voice in their own end-of-life care, if desired.

Cultural and Religious Sensitivity

The sacred teachings and writings of various religions provide a wealth of knowledge on how to face the critical moments of life: the beginning and the end. As technological and scientific advances in medicine have presented new possibilities for deciding about birth and death, we must acknowledge the different views religion, faith, and customs have on these issues, as illustrated in Box 24.4. Such differences inform health and healthcare providers on how to approach ACP conversations.

Patient–Family Provider Communication Models in Palliative Care

Ethnically sensitive programs have been developed for patient–family provider communication in end-of-life care. APPEAL (A Progressive Palliative Care Education Curriculum for the Care of African Americans at Life's End), developed by African American experts in palliative care, offers insights about providing palliative care to African American patients and their families. SPIRIT (Sharing Patients' Illness Representations to Increase Trust) is an evidence-based ACP intervention developed for African Americans with end-stage renal disease; it has been shown to be effective in promoting communication between patients and their surrogates.[76] As many African American adults with HIV/AIDS have end-stage renal disease at the end of life, this program may be adapted to meet their needs and was also adapted based on the Respecting Choices® model.

Box 24.5 outlines several benefits of using a structured ACP communication program. The case in Box 24.6 illustrates cultural and religious sensitivity and 24.7 summarizes the lessons learned from program implementation.

Comorbidities, Aging, and the Need for New Paradigms

One of the ironic developments in the advent of improved HIV infection therapeutics has been that prolonged survival has been accompanied by a growing list of comorbidities in patients who previously would not have lived long enough to experience them.[55-57]

Box 24.4 Out of the Mouths of Children

A 14-year-old male, AJ, came in for Session 3 of a three-session intervention to complete an advance directive with his mother, having had an in-depth conversation with her the week before about his understanding of his HIV disease, complications that could occur ("I'll die if I don't take my medicines"), and his values and goals for care in bad outcome situations. Unexpectedly, AJ's mother brought his 11-year-old brother to the session. The facilitator confirmed with the patient and mother that it was okay to have his brother present. When the patient was asked to respond to the item, "After my death, I would like my body to be (circle one): buried or cremated," it was discovered he did not know the meaning of cremation. The patient's younger brother, who had been quiet throughout the session, piped in with "That's when they burn your body and put your ashes in a jar." The family laughed anxiously but then continued without hesitation to complete the remainder of the advance directive form. On the satisfaction form administered by a research assistant, not the facilitator, AJ stated, "Yeah, I felt somewhat relieved. It's great to tell someone else what is going on with you. It's a great feeling to connect." His mother stated, "It's been extremely helpful. It's helped with my awareness and with how to think rationally and to think about what will happen in the long run and spares me and allows me to walk with him."

Box 24.5 Potential Benefits of Implementation of the FACE Program for a Healthcare System[60] for People Living With Aids

When used as a complement to the existing disease management and palliative care initiatives, the program includes the following:

- Documentation of specific patient goals for life-sustaining treatment, in advance of a medical crisis
- Strengthened surrogate's role as an effective substitute decision-maker by better understanding his or her loved one's goals for future medical care
- Greater patient and family satisfaction from patient-centered communication and end-of-life decision-making
- Focused/concentrated use of resources at the end of life due to patient-directed care plan (e.g., patient-chosen interventions)
- Increased use of comfort care services (e.g., palliative care consults, hospice referrals, hospice length of stay)

> **Box 24.6** Cultural and Religious Sensitivity of Advance Care Planning Communication
>
> An HIV-positive, 15-year-old adolescent and his father, immigrants from Pakistan and self-reported practicing Muslims, participated in an advance care planning (ACP) discussion. The conversation occurred in the family's home by two trained ACP facilitators. Throughout the conversations, the adolescent responded on a questionnaire that he felt as though his diagnosis was a punishment from God. While engaged in session 3, completing an advance directive, the father refused to be present, as his son completed the advance directive. At one point, he left the room altogether but asked us to continue. At the end of the session, the father expressed that he felt as though discussing your child's death was "disgusting and not allowed by Allah" and that it was morally offensive. Despite his father's anger with the idea of planning for his own son's death, he made it clear that he was not angry with the facilitators. After the session, the hospital chaplain was consulted. She in turn consulted with Imams in the community who explained that, in Islam, life is a gift of Allah and the sanctity of human life is ordained in the Quran. The chaplain further noted that Muslims are expected to seek Allah's help in a time of healthcare crisis and do everything one can to save a life. Moreover, she noted that death is never discussed with the children, and, most times, children are not present when caring for the very ill or dying. They also do not attend funeral services. "To speak of death before you're faced with it is like willing it to happen," noted the chaplain. This belief in divine destiny is what the young man's father tried to express. Expressing great regret for any potential harm to the family and as advised by the chaplain, a letter was written by the Principal Investigator to apologize for any unintentional offense the conversation may have caused the family. We also thanked him for helping us increase our sensitivity to religious beliefs, a purpose of the study.

> **Box 24.7** Lessons Learned in Advance Care Planning Program Implemenation[38,60]
>
> - *Leadership is critical.* It is important to have leaders who understand the short- and long-term goals of a comprehensive advance care planning (ACP) program. Leaders must be identified at multiple levels: administration, steering committee, project coordination, pilot areas, healthcare providers (physicians, nurses, social workers), and other communities as necessary.
> - *Administrative support is essential.* The time and resources needed to implement a successful ACP program must be recognized and supported by administrative representatives at multiple levels. Mechanisms to keep administration involved and supportive must be developed.
> - *Systems must be created or improved to honor written ACPs.* Many practices must be revised or developed to ensure individuals' preferences are honored. One of the key systems that must be improved is the consistent entry, retrieval, update, and transfer of ACPs that have been created. Trained facilitators can improve the quality of ACP discussions and create written plans that reflect an individual's preferences for future care. However, there are no guarantees that these preferences will be honored if community-wide systems are not created.
> - *Quality improvement activities are important to motivate and engage others.* Many teams miss opportunities to demonstrate success when organized efforts to collect baseline data and measure outcomes specific to identified goals are not conducted.
>
> Reprinted with permission.

In addition, the phenomenon of "accelerated aging," a term sometimes used to denote the increasing prevalence of frailty, cognitive decline, and general debility in long-surviving patients with AIDS, occurs at an earlier chronological age than one would otherwise expect.[4,77–79] As a result, ACP discussions need to focus on this changing clinical reality.

Conclusion

As research continues, healthcare providers should not hesitate to initiate ACP and end-of-life conversations; structured interventions, methods, and tools discussed in this chapter inform approach and evaluation of ACP with PLWA. Research also supports the referral of the patient/family dyad to trained/certified ACP facilitators who have the skills and time to implement this process. A thoughtful, methodological, and sensible approach to ACP can be implemented with sensitivity, even in youth with HIV/AIDS, with the goals of holistically minimizing suffering and enhancing quality of life in all dimensions. ACP represents one more level of support and ongoing communication for the treatment team. Initial ACP conversations with documented treatment preferences related to goals of care create opportunities for future conversations with the treatment team and establishes these conversations as a part of routine quality palliative care.

References

1. UNAIDS. *Global Report : UNAIDS Report on the Global AIDS Epidemic: 2013.* Geneva: UNAIDS; 2013.
2. Gallant JE, Adimora, AA, Carmichael, JK, et al. Essential components of effective HIV care: A policy paper of the HIV Medicine Association of the Infectious Diseases Society of America and the Ryan White Medical Providers Coalition. *Clin Infect Dis.* 2011;53(11):1043–1050.
3. Schwarcz, L, Chen, MJ, Vittinghoff, E, Hsu, L, Schwarcz, S. Declining incidence of AIDS-defining opportunistic illnesses: Results from 16 years of population-based AIDS surveillance. *AIDS.* 2013;27(4):597–605.
4. Mills, EJ, Barnighausen T, Negin, J. HIV and aging—preparing for the challenges ahead. *N Engl J Med.* 2012;366(14):1270–1273.
5. Selwyn PA, Forstein M. Overcoming the false dichotomy of curative vs. palliative care for late-stage HIV/AIDS. *JAMA.* 2003;290:806–814.
6. Kochanek KD, Xu JQ, Murphy SL, Miniño AM. Deaths: Preliminary data for 2009. *National Vital Statistics Reports* 59(4). Hyattsville, MD: National Center for Health Statistics; 2011.
7. District of Columbia HIV/AIDS, Hepatitis, STD and TB Annual Report 2010. Washington, DC: District of Columbia Department of Health; 2010.

8. James SA. Epidemiologic research on health disparities: Some thoughts on history and current developments. *Epidemiol Rev.* 2009;31:1–6.
9. Jones AL, Moss AJ, Harris-Kojetin LD. *Use of advance directives in long-term care populations.* NCHS Data Brief 54, Hyattsville, MD: National Center Health Statistics; 2011.
10. Johnson KS, Kuchibhatla M, Tulsky JA. What explains racial differences in the use of advance directives and attitudes toward hospice care? *J Am Geriatr Soc.* 2008;56(10):1953–1958.
11. Krug R, Karus D, Selwyn PA, Raveis VH. Late-stage HIV/AIDS patients' and their familial caregivers agreement on the palliative care outcome scale. *J Pain Symptom Manage.* 2010;39:23–32.
12. Sacajiu G, Raveis VH, Selwyn P. Patients and family care givers' experiences around highly active antiretroviral therapy (HAART). *AIDS Care.* 2009;21:1528–1536.
13. Chandan U. Strengthening families through early intervention in high HIV prevalence countries. *AIDS Care.* 2009;21:76–82.
14. Braun UK, Beyth RJ, Ford ME, McCullough LB. Voices of African Americans, Caucasian, and Hispanic surrogates on burdens of end of life decision making. *J Gen Intern Med.* 2008;23:267–274.
15. Woods SP, Moore DJ, Weber E, Grant I. Cognitive neuropsychology of HIV-associated neurocognitive disorders. *Neuropsych Rev.* 2009;19:152–168.
16. Robert Wood Johnson Foundation/Working Group on Palliative and End of life Care. Recommendations to the field—HIV care: An agenda for change. Promoting excellence in end of life care: A national program. www.promotingexcellence.org/downloads/hiv_report.pdf. Published 2008.
17. Allison S, Wolters PL, Brouwers P. Youth with HIV/AIDS: Neurobehavioral consequences. In: Paul RH, ed. *HIV and the Brain: New Challenges in the Modern Era.* New York, NY: Humana Press; 2009:187–211.
18. Lyon ME, McCarter R, D'Angelo L. Detecting HIV associated neurocognitive disorders in adolescents: What is the best screening tool? *J Adolesc Health.* 2009;44:133–135.
19. Skarupski KA, Fitchett G, Evans DA, Mendes de Leon CF. Daily spiritual experiences in a biracial, community-based population of older adults. *Aging Ment Health.* 2010;14:779–789.
20. Lee CC, Czaja SJ, Schulz R. The moderating influence of demographic characteristics, social support, and religious coping on the effectiveness of a multicomponent psychosocial caregiver intervention in three racial ethnic groups. *J Gerontol B Psychol Sci Soc Sci.* 2010;65B:185–194.
21. Ironson G, Stuetzle R, Ironson D, et al. View of God as benevolent and forgiving or punishing and judgmental predicts HIV disease progression. *J Behav Med.* 2011;34:414–425.
22. Pargament KI, McCarthy S, Shah P, et al. Religion and HIV: A review of the literature and clinical implications. *South Med J.* 2004;97:776–783.
23. Lyon ME, Garvie PA, Kao E, et al. Spirituality in HIV-infected adolescents and their families: FAmily CEntered (FACE) advance care planning and medication adherence. *J Adolesc Health.* 2011;48:633–636.
24. O'Neill JF, Selwyn PA, Schietinger H, eds. *A Clinical Guide to Supportive Palliative Care for HIV/AIDS.* Rockville, MD: Health Resources and Services Administration; 2003.
25. World Health Organization. *Palliative Care for People Living With HIV/AIDS: Clinical Protocol for the WHO European Region.* Geneva: World Health Organization; 2006.
26. UNAIDS, World Health Organization. *AIDS Epidemic Update.* Geneva: UNAIDS; 2009. http://data.unaids.org/pub/Report/2009/JC1700_Epi_Update_2009_en.pdf
27. Kasl-Godley JE, King DA, Quill TE. Opportunities for psychologists in palliative care: Working with patients and families across the disease continuum. *Am Psych.* 2014;69(4):364–376.
28. Mack JW, Hinds PS. Practical aspects of communication. In: Wolfe J, Hinds PS, Sourkes BM, eds. *Textbook of Interdisciplinary Pediatric Palliative Care.* Philadelphia, PA: Elsevier Saunders; 2011.
29. Epstein R, Street RL. *Patient-Centered Communication in Cancer Care: Promoting Healing and Reducing Suffering.* Bethesda, MD: National Institutes of Health: National Cancer Institute, US Department of Health and Human Services, National Institutes of Health; 2007.
30. Shen JM, Blank A, Selwyn PA. Predictors of mortality for patients with advanced disease in an HIV palliative care program. *J Acquir Immune Defic Syndr.* 2005;40(4):445–447.
31. Feudtner C. Collaborative communication in pediatric palliative care: A foundation for problem-solving and decision-making. *Pediatr Clin North Am.* 2007;54(5):583–607.
32. Briggs L. Shifting the focus of advance care planning: using an in-depth interview to build and strengthen relationships. *Journal of Palliative Medicine* 2004;7(2):341–349.
33. Wood CG, Whittet S, Bradbeer CS. ABC of palliative care: HIV infection and AIDS. *BMJ.* 1997;315(7120):1433–1436.
34. Hargie O. *Skilled Interpersonal Communication: Research, Theory and Practice.* 5th ed. New York, NY: Routledge; 2011.
35. Song MK, Kirchhoff KT, Douglas J, Ward S, Hammes B. A randomized, controlled trial to improve advance care planning among patients undergoing cardiac surgery. *Med Care.* 2005;43(10):1049–1053.
36. Rogers CR. Empathic: An unappreciated way of being. *Counseling Psych.* 1975;5(2):2–10.
37. Farber BA, Doolin EM. Positive regard. *Psychotherapy.* 2011;48(1):58–64.
38. Briggs L. Helping individuals make informed decisions: The role of the advance care planning facilitator. In: Hammes BJ, ed. *Having Your Own Say: Getting the Right Care When It Matters the Most.* Washington, DC: CHT Press; 2012:23–40.
39. Lavoie M, Blondeau D, Martineau I. The integration of a person-centered approach in palliative care. *Palliat Support Care.* 2013;11(6):453–464.
40. Vedel I, Ghadi V, Lapointe L, Routelous C, Aegerter P, Guirimand F. Patients', family caregivers', and professionals' perspectives on quality of palliative care: A qualitative study. *Palliat Med.* 2014;28(9):1128–1138.
41. Institute for Family-Centered Care. Family-Centered Care Website. www.familycenteredcare.org. Accessed June 18, 2014.
42. Luyirika E, Towle MS, Achan J, et al. Scaling up pediatric HIV care with an integrated, family-centered approach: An observational case study from Uganda. *PLoS One* 2013;8(8):e69548.
43. Hinds PS, Schum L, Baker JN, Wolfe J. Key factors affecting dying children and their families. *J Palliat Med.* 2005;8(Suppl 1):s70–s78.
44. Pessin H, Galietta M, Nelson CJ, Brescia R, Rosenfeld B, Breitbart W. Burden and benefit of psychosocial research at the end of life. *J Palliat Med.* 2008;11(4):627–632.
45. Walsh-Kelly CM, Lang KR, Chevako, J, et al. Advance directives in a pediatric emergency department. *Pediatrics.* 1999;103(4):826–830.
46. Hinds PS, Drew D, Oakes LL, et al. End of life care preferences of pediatric patients with cancer. *J Clinical Oncol.* 2005;23(36):9146–9154.
47. Lyon ME, McCabe MA, Patel KM, D'Angelo LJ. What do adolescents want? An exploratory study regarding end of life decision-making. *J Adolesc Health.* 2004;35:529 e1–e6.
48. Lyon ME, Garvie PA, Briggs L, He J, D'Angelo L, McCarter R. Development, feasibility and acceptability of the Family-Centered (FACE) advance care planning intervention for adolescents with HIV. *J Palliat Med.* 2009;12:363–372.
49. Lyon ME, Garvie PA, McCarter R, Briggs L, He J, D'Angelo L. Who will speak for me? Improving end of life decision-making for adolescents with HIV and their families. *Pediatrics.* 2009;123:e1–e8.

50. Lyon ME, Garvie PA, Briggs L, et al. Is it safe? Talking to teens about death and dying: A 3-month evaluation of FAmily CEntered (FACE) advance care planning—anxiety, depression, quality of life. *HIV/AIDS*. 2010;2:1–11.
51. Lyon ME, Jacobs J, Briggs L, Cheng YI, Wang J. A longitudinal randomized controlled trial of advance care planning for teens with cancer: Anxiety, depression, quality of life, advance directives, spirituality. *J Adolesc Health*. 2014;54(6):710–717.
52. Lyon ME, Jacobs S, Briggs L, Cheng YI, Wang J. Family centered advance care: Planning for teens with cancer. *JAMA Pediatr*. 2013;167(5):460–467.
53. Longitudinal Pediatric Palliative Care: Quality of Life & Spiritual Struggle http://clinicaltrials.gov/show/NCT01289444 and Palliative Care with Persons Living with AIDS: Integrating into Standard of Care http://clinicaltrials.gov/show/NCT01775436.
54. Wenger N, Kanouse D, Collins R, Liu H, Schuser M, Gifford A. End of life discussions and preferences among persons with HIV. *JAMA*. 2001;285:2880–2887.
55. Singer PA, Thiel EC, Salit I, Flanagan W, Naylor D. The HIV-specific advance directive. *J Gen Intern Med*. 1997;12(12):729–735.
56. Chu C, Selwyn PA. An epidemic in evolution: The need for new models of HIV care in the chronic disease era. *J Urban Health*. 2011;88(3):556–566.
57. Justice AC. HIV and aging: Time for a new paradigm. *Curr HIV/AIDS Rep*. 2010;7:69–76.
58. Rodriguez-Penney AT, Ludicello JE, Riggs PK, et al. Co-morbidities in persons infected with HIV: Increased burden with older age and negative effects on health-related quality of life. *AIDS Patient Care STDS*. 2013;27(1):5–16.
59. Lyon ME, Garvie PA, Briggs L, He J, McCarter R, D'Angelo L. Do families know what adolescents want? An end of life (EOL) survey of adolescents with HIV/AIDS and their families. *J Adolesc Health*. 2010;46:S4–S5.
60. Hammes BJ, Briggs L. *Respecting Choices: Palliative Care Facilitator Manual–Revised*. LaCrosse, WI: Gundersen Lutheran Medical Foundation; 2007.
61. Aging With Dignity. Five wishes. http://www.agingwithdignity.org/five-wishes.php. Accessed July 2, 2014.
62. Curtis JR, Patrick DL, Caldwell E, Greenlee H, Collier AC. The quality of patient-doctor communication about end of life care: A study of patients with advanced AIDS and their primary care clinicians. *AIDS*. 1999;13:1123–1131.
63. Wright AA, Zhang B, Ray A, et al. Associations between end of life discussions, patient mental health, medical care near death, and caregiver bereavement adjustment. *JAMA*. 2008;300(14):1665–1673.
64. Temel JS, Greer JA, Muzikansky A, et al. Early palliative care for patients with metastatic non-small-cell lung cancer. *N Engl J Med*. 2010;363:733–742.
65. Kirchhoff KT, Hammes BJ, Kehl KA, Briggs LA, Brown RL. Effect of a disease-specific planning intervention on surrogate understanding of patient goals for future medical treatment. *J Am Geriatr Soc*. 2010;58(7):1233–1240.
66. Song MK, Ward SE, Denne H, et al. Randomized controlled trial of SPIRIT: An effective approach to preparing African-American dialysis patients and families for end of life. *Res Nurs Health*. 2009;32(3):260–273.
67. Silveira MJ, Kim SY, Langa KM. Advance directives and outcomes of surrogate decision making before death. *N Engl J Med*. 2010;362(13):1211–1218.
68. Detering KM, Hancock AD, Reade MC, Silvester W. The impact of advance care planning on end of life care in elderly patients: Randomised controlled trial. *BMJ*. 2010;340:c1345.
69. Holt-Lunstad J, Smith TB, Layton JB. Social relationships and mortality risk: A meta-analytic review. *PLoS Med*. 2010;7(7):e1000316.
70. Weithorn LA, Campbell SB. The competency of children and adolescents to make informed treatment decisions. *Child Dev*. 1982;53:1589–1598.
71. Derish MT, Heuvel KV. Mature minors should have the right to refuse life-sustaining medical treatment. *J Law Med Ethics*. 2000;28:109–124.
72. Doig C, Burgess E. Withholding life-sustaining treatment: Are adolescents competent to make these decisions? *CMAJ*. 2000;162:1585–1588.
73. Wiener L, Ballard E, Brennan T, Battles H, Martinez P, Pao M. How I wish to be remembered. *J Palliat Med*. 2008;11:1309–1313.
74. Hinds PS, Drew D, Oakes LL, et al. End of life care preferences of pediatric patients with cancer. *J Clin Oncol*. 2005;23:9146–9154.
75. Field MJ, Behrman RE. *When Children Die: Improving Palliative and End-of-Life Care for Children and Their Families*. Washington, DC: National Academy Press; 2002.
76. Freyer DR. Care of the dying adolescent: Special considerations. *Peds*. 2004;113:381–388.
77. Onen N, Overton E. A review of premature frailty in HIV-infected persons: Another manifestation of HIV-related accelerated aging. *Curr Aging Sci*. 2011;4(1):33–41.
78. Mateen FJ, Mills EJ. Aging and HIV-related cognitive loss. *JAMA*. 2012;308(4):349–350.
79. Ances BM, Vaida F, Yeh Mj, et al. HIV infection and aging independently affect brain function as measured by functional magnetic resonance imaging. *J Infect Dis*. 2010;201:336–340.

CHAPTER 25

Homeless, Mentally Ill, and Drug-Addicted Patients

John D. Chovan

Introduction

Katie is a 55-year-old Caucasian woman who resides in a group home. When she was in college, she was the star of her college field hockey team. When she was 22 years old, she passed out at a party. When she was taken to the local emergency room, she had her stomach pumped and was also found to have high levels of several illegal substances in her urine. After she regained consciousness, she described feelings of paranoia, would not interact appropriately with her family or caregivers (at times screaming for them to leave her alone, particularly her maternal uncle), and would talk to herself when alone in her room. After a psychiatric consult, she was determined to have a new onset of schizophrenia, paranoid type, and was started on an atypical antipsychotic. As her symptoms were brought under control, she stopped talking to herself, but her affect was flattened, self-care suffered, and she began chain-smoking cigarettes. She was released to a group home where she has lived for most of the past 30 years. On the days she received her monthly paycheck, she would binge-drink an entire bottle of inexpensive vodka and pass out on the couch in her room in her own urine. Five years ago, she was diagnosed with chronic bronchitis and emphysema, along with coronary artery disease. She subsequently refused to see any healthcare professionals, saying, "Those bad doctors want to cut off my breasts." She stopped taking her psychiatric medications, became increasingly paranoid, and then disappeared from the group home. She was often seen living on the street and would refuse to go to a homeless shelter, repeating, "Those bad doctors want to cut off my breasts." She began using her monthly check to purchase oxycodone tablets on the street. One day, a police officer found her body in a secluded alley, where she had died several days before, under a flattened cardboard box and laying on a street grill, an empty prescription bottle for oxycodone in someone else's name in her hand.

Chronic homelessness, severe and persistent mental illness (SPMI), and drug addiction are stressors that have a major and long-lasting impact on every facet of a person's life. In all three situations, overall health is compromised, interpersonal relationships—particularly with family members—are difficult, culture shifts, self-care suffers, and life expectancy declines. As a result, chronic and life-threatening illnesses are common among these populations. The support of palliative care services, including hospice at the end of life, are highly appropriate.

Little is known about the use of palliative care services in these populations. Invariably, however, palliative and hospice teams will at one point or another care for someone from one or more of these populations. Individual abilities and challenges preclude applying the information in this chapter to any specific person. The astute healthcare provider who assesses and understands the patient through informed communication can improve the quality of care, and thus the quality of life, for the individual and his or her family.

This chapter focuses on palliative communication with persons who are particularly vulnerable and disenfranchised: those who are chronically homeless, those who are living with severe mental illness, and those who are drug addicted. Membership in one of these categories does not always imply membership in either of the other two or both. But, as in the case study at the beginning of the chapter, frequently two or all three can occur together. The theoretical framework that guides this chapter is summarized next, followed by an overview of these populations and a description of the health characteristics and challenges affecting them and their families. The chapter integrates a discussion of palliative communication with people in these populations and makes recommendations for communicating with them.

Theoretical Framework

The theoretical framework that guides this chapter is an amalgam of a few models and theories. The foundation of the framework is the midlevel theory set forward by Hildegard Peplau in the early 1950s. The theory of interpersonal relationships[1] brings the importance of the relationship between the nurse and the patient to healing. For this chapter, the relationship is also extended to the entire healthcare team and to the family of the patient, which can be the biological family, the patient's family of choice, or whomever the patient tells the healthcare team comprises his or her family. The primary roles of the healthcare provider in the therapeutic relationship are outlined in Table 25.1.

The diathesis-stress model of mental illness[2] is used to understand how stressors (both eustress and distress) confound the person's illness and also the communication with these particularly vulnerable people. The COMFORT model of communication[3] is summarized in Table 25.2 and is used to link population-specific communication issues to a known framework for palliative care communication.

Table 25.1 Roles of the Healthcare Provider in Therapeutic Communication

Role	Definition
Stranger	Unknown to the client, the nurse expects to be treated with the courtesy that one would expect when first meeting a new person
Resource	Answers questions or finds the answers to questions
Teacher	Provides a context in which the client can learn new things
Leader	Provides a role model for the client to adapt
Surrogate	Plays a role as needed that substitutes for one that the client needs
Counselor	Guides the client on a journey of self-discovery and healing

Note: Adapted from Peplau (1952).[1]

To facilitate the appropriate application, we use a case study to guide the reader through a fictional but realistic illustrative scenario, a tenet from adult learning theory.

Description of the Populations

The Centers for Disease Control and Prevention define vulnerable populations as those groups of people who are at risk for health disparities.[4] Health disparities are health outcomes that are seen in a greater or lesser extent in a target population than in persons who are not members of the target population.[5] This section presents information about these vulnerable populations and the health outcomes for which they are at a greater risk than persons who do not belong to the population.

Chronic Homelessness

According to the US Department of Housing and Urban Development (HUD),[6] more than 1 million persons receive housing assistance, either temporary or permanent, each year, and the actual number of homeless people in the United States may be 2 million or more. In 2013 more than 600,000 people in the United States availed themselves of the HUD Continuum of Care Housing Assistance Program at some point during the year.[7]

Table 25.2 COMFORT™ SM Model of Palliative Care Communication

Component	Explanation
Communication	Use clear and familiar language
Opportunity and options	Orient patients to the reality of their condition
Mindfulness	Avoid distractions, be present, make eye contact
Family	Include family
Openings	Provide ongoing care and ongoing communication; not alone
Relating	Restate messages over and over; change how it is said
Team	Consistency among the team

Note: Adapted from Wittenberg-Lyles (2012).[3]

HUD estimates that nearly 110,000 or about 17% were identified as chronically homeless, and about 72,000 people were unsheltered. Also in 2013, more than 124,000 participants were identified as living with a severe mental illness, and more than 134,000 participants were identified as substance abusers.

The National Health Care for the Homeless Council[8] lists the following tenets on its fact sheet about homelessness and health:

1. Poor health is a major cause of homelessness.
2. Homelessness creates new health problems and exacerbates existing ones.
3. Individuals experiencing homelessness have high rates of acute and chronic illness.
4. Recovery and healing are more difficult without housing.

Homeless women face major threats to their health, are predisposed to poor health, and have limited access to healthcare.[9] Housing instability significantly reduces use of acute care services by these women, and high levels of childhood victimization (such as physical and sexual abuse), poor self-esteem, and history of incarceration are common among homeless women. Access to other community resources is also limited.

People who are homeless are 3 to 4 times more likely to die than people who are not homeless. Deaths occur throughout the year and occur more frequently in younger people than the elderly. The causes of death are most often chronic medical conditions, but comorbid mental illness and/or substance abuse increases the risk of early death.[10] In Los Angeles County, for example, between January 1, 2000, and May 28, 2007 (or 2,708 days), about 1.05 million people experienced homelessness (more than 500 people on average every night).[11] During that time period, the Los Angeles County Coroner's office reported 2,815 homeless deaths (or about 0.3%), which is about one person every night for 7.5 years. The leading cause of death was cardiovascular issues (686, 24.4%), unknown (660, 23.4%), acute intoxication (619, 22%), and trauma (including suicide and homicide; 502, 17.8%). Other causes of significantly fewer proportion of deaths were: pneumonia (110, 3.9%), cirrhosis (102, 3.6%), infection or condition secondary to alcohol or IV drug use (90, 3.3%), cancer (31, 1.1%), hypothermia or environmental exposure (8, 0.3%), and tuberculosis (7, 0.2%). Some community-based clinics provide services for both physical and mental health, and mobile vans bring services to the homeless.[12]

Half of all persons who die while they are homeless die in a hospital. Of the other half of persons who die while they are homeless, one-third die outdoors and one-quarter die in a homeless shelter.[13] The following excerpt continues the case study introduced at the beginning of this chapter and is used throughout to illustrate the concepts discussed.

> Katie's homelessness appears to have been triggered by the stressful news that she had chronic obstructive pulmonary disease (COPD) and coronary artery disease (CAD). The interaction of Katie's homelessness and paranoia precluded any attempts by palliative care providers to care for her. She would not go to appointments or even go to a shelter, where she could be seen and treated for her COPD symptoms and supported to maximize her quality of life and a good death.

Severe and Persistent Mental Illness

Mental illness is not uncommon. The National Institute of Mental Health reports that in 2012, an estimated 43.7 million adults in the United States (18%) had some form of mental illness.[14] The US population of adults with SPMI, defined as mental disorders with serious functional impairment that substantially interferes with or limits one or more major life activities, was estimated at 9.6 million (4.1%). Examples of SPMI include some of the mood disorders (e.g., recurrent major depressive disorder, bipolar disorder), all of the thought disorders (e.g., schizophrenia-spectrum disorders, delusional disorder), and the personality disorders.

The characteristics of SPMIs that make them so debilitating include their cyclic nature (symptoms that change in severity and frequency with stress); symptoms so severe that they often result in a break with reality; poor insight about the illness; and changes in the ability to make choices based on consequences, to socialize appropriately, to access resources in the community, and to organize thoughts.

Several studies have confirmed that people with mental illness die earlier than people without mental illness and die from the same causes at a more frequent rate.[15,16] The modifiable risk factors that contribute to early mortality also have an earlier onset and are more common in people with SPMI, especially diet, tobacco use, and lack of exercise.[17] Side effects of psychiatric medications, particularly dyslipidemia and its sequela, lead to negative health consequences for persons living with SPMI. Persons living with SPMI in the United States are disproportionately affected by these conditions, and low rates of prevention, detection, and treatment result in substantial disease burden and premature mortality.[15,18,19] For example, the causes of death of the decedents in Ohio with mental illness between 2002 and 2007 were cardiovascular disease (3,853, 26.6%), other disease (2,229, 15.4%), unintentional injuries (2,069, 14.3%), cancer (1,982, 13.7%), respiratory disease (1,271, 8.8%), suicide (952, 6.6%), nervous system disease (865, 6%), diabetes mellitus (604, 4.2%), homicide (328, 2.3%), substance use disorder (198, 1.4%), injuries of undetermined intent (82, 0.6%), and the mental illness itself (67, 0.5%). When stratified by age, the leading cause of death in adults 35 years old or older in this population was cardiovascular disease, but for younger persons, the leading cause of death was injury and violence. When compared to persons without mental illness, 4 times as many people with mental illness died from injury than the general population. Nine in 10 persons without mental illness died from diseases, whereas only 3 of 4 persons with mental illness died from diseases.[20]

Effective approaches to these common conditions exist. However, evidence is sparse on how to bring these effective strategies to people with SPMI, who frequently experience cognitive impairment and motivational deficits.

Katie was diagnosed with COPD and CAD, which are not unusual for a smoker. Many persons with schizophrenia self-medicate with nicotine and will often present with tar stains on their fingers from chain smoking. Her psychiatric medications also have a side effect of dyslipidemia, contributing to her heart disease. But Katie could not comprehend all of this. The palliative care team would help communicate to her the severity of her illness and the negative consequences of her behaviors, if Katie would have allowed it. In this case, until the positive and negative symptoms of her schizophrenia were controlled, she did not have the resources to think clearly and rationally about her own health and well-being.

Drug Addiction

The Substance Abuse and Mental Health Services Administration reports annually the National Survey on Drug Use and Health. In 2012 nearly 60% of the US population aged 12 years and older had used dangerous substances in the past month. Illicit drugs (defined as marijuana, hashish, cocaine, crack cocaine, heroin, hallucinogens, inhalants, and nonmedical use of pain relievers, tranquilizers, stimulants, or sedatives) were used by 9.2%, tobacco (defined as cigarettes, smokeless tobacco, cigars, and pipe tobacco) was used by 26.7%, and alcohol was used to excess (five or more drinks at the same time or within a couple of hours of each other on at least 1 day [binge use] or on each of 5 or more days [heavy use] in the past 30 days) by 29.5%.[18]

The impact of substance abuse on health is well documented. Excessive use of alcohol can lead to liver disease, gastrointestinal disease, and negative effects of impaired judgment. The use of tobacco products has been linked to cancers (oral, lung, gastric), ulcers, upper respiratory infections, lower respiratory infections, and asthma. The use of illicit drugs can cause permanent organ damage, especially liver disease and kidney disease, lung diseases, and negative effects of impaired judgment.

More than 87,000 deaths occurred in the United States each year between 2006 and 2010 that were attributed to causes related to excessive alcohol use.[21] The top 10 causes of alcohol-attributable deaths during that time are listed in Table 25.3. Each year, more than 75% of alcohol-attributable deaths due to acute causes were caused by trauma (motor vehicle traffic crashes: 12,460, 25.15%; suicide: 8,179, 16.51%; homicide: 7,756, 15.65%; and fall injuries: 7,149, 15.22%). Nearly 60% of alcohol-attributable deaths caused by chronic causes each year were due to alcoholic liver disease (14,364, 38.23%) or liver cirrhosis unspecified (7,847, 20.88%).

Katie had a history of substance abuse from a very young age. She abused alcohol and illegal substances in college. She was a life-long user of alcohol to excess, which contributed to her irrationality and to her health problems. She was a long-time chain smoker, which enabled her symptoms of schizophrenia but also contributed to her heart and lung conditions. When she took her medications, she was more rational, although her affect was blunted and she "didn't feel like herself," making her want to stop taking her medications. She became irrational at the time of her COPD and CAD diagnoses, which may have been rooted in something that happened during her youth. She switched from alcohol to street-purchased oxycodone, using it until she died. She died alone and homeless on the street.

People who are homeless, living with SPMI, and/or addicted to drugs are at risk for chronic illness and premature death as a result of their membership in one or more of these vulnerable populations. Palliative care providers will encounter persons who are homeless, persons living with SPMI, and persons with drug addiction and will need to interact with them appropriately to determine their needs, to provide person-centered care, and to evaluate the outcomes of that care.

Trust

A major block to successful communication with persons who are homeless, mentally ill, or addicted to drugs is mistrust. Homeless people, mentally ill people, and drug-addicted people live in worlds where relationships can be transient and trust can be difficult, requiring an investment of a great deal of time and energy by all parties. Healthcare professionals need to understand their own beliefs about persons in these populations. Box 25.1 presents some questions to encourage reflections on thoughts, ideas, and biases about homeless,

Table 25.3 Alcohol-Attributable Deaths Due to Excessive Alcohol Use: Average for United States, 2006–2010[20]

Top 10 Causes—Overall	n	%
Alcoholic liver disease	14,364	16.49
Motor-vehicle traffic crashes	12,460	14.30
Poisoning (not alcohol)	8,404	9.65
Suicide	8,179	9.39
Liver cirrhosis unspecified	7,847	9.01
Homicide	7,756	8.90
Fall injuries	7,541	8.66
Alcohol dependence syndrome	3,728	4.28
Alcohol abuse	2,022	2.32
Stroke hemorrhagic	1,727	1.98
Other	1,309	15.03
Total	**87,119**	**100.00**

Top 10 Chronic Causes	n	%
Alcoholic liver disease	14,364	38.23
Liver cirrhosis unspecified	7,847	20.88
Alcohol dependence syndrome	3,728	9.92
Alcohol abuse	2,022	5.38
Stroke hemorrhagic	1,727	4.60
Hypertension	1,464	3.90
Liver cancer	974	2.59
Acute pancreatitis	724	1.93
Alcoholic psychosis	653	1.74
Alcohol cardiomyopathy	514	1.37
Other	3558	9.47
Total	**37,575**	**100.00**

Top 10 Acute Causes	n	%
Motor-vehicle traffic crashes	12,460	25.15
Poisoning (not alcohol)	8,404	16.96
Suicide	8,179	16.51
Homicide	7,756	15.65
Fall injuries	7,541	15.22
Alcohol poisoning	1,647	3.32
Fire injuries	1,089	2.20
Drowning	963	1.94
Hypothermia	265	0.53
Aspiration	220	0.44
Other	1020	2.06
Total	**49,544**	**100.00**

Box 25.1 Questions for Reflection

What are your preconceived notions about persons who are homeless?

Do you know anyone who is addicted to drugs? How has knowledge about it colored your perception of them as people?

You encountered psychiatric patients in your training. How did that go?

Once you understand your feelings and biases, are you able to check them so they do not interfere with communicating and caring for these individuals?

---

mentally ill, and drug-addicted individuals. Questions specific to the case study include the following:

> *How do you feel about Katie's life? Do you think she deserved the life she led? Do you think the system and mental health professionals failed her? Can you imagine living in her shoes for even one day?*

For palliative care professionals, building rapport and trust with persons in their care is the most important use of the professional self. Patients must be able to trust that the professional is not a threat to them or their well-being. They must trust that what the professional is telling them is in their best interests; likewise, professionals must trust that what the patients tell them is an accurate representation of what they are experiencing, what might have helped them in the past, and whether they will do what they agree to do. Professionals must trust themselves to accurately observe and record nonverbal communication that might impact on trust, particularly body language. Finally, professionals must trust that they are not sending nonverbal messages that countermand trust and thus the therapeutic relationship.

Building trust takes time, but breaking trust takes just an instant. Homeless persons, persons with mental illnesses, and persons addicted to drugs can have a world view that does not promote trust. Their need for constant vigilance often taxes their available resources. For example, homeless persons must keep a constant watch over their possessions, or they may be stolen. When faced with an actual or perceived breach in personal safety, their protective walls come up very quickly, and therapeutic communication shuts down.

> *Katie was paranoid from the time of her psychotic break when she was 22 years old. When her symptoms were under control, she could be reasoned with, within limits. But when she learned of her new health conditions, she immediately perceived a breach of trust with everyone, which spiraled out of control, and she completely cut herself off from the rest of the world, thwarting any chance of regaining a healthier life.*

Communication Characteristics and Homelessness

People who are homeless face major threats to their well-being and thus to their ability to trust. Basic needs that are unmet in homelessness include shelter, warmth, and safety. Other issues faced by homeless people include health and wellness; quiet; potential theft of possessions, including clothing, something to sleep on, and personal belongings; privacy, including personal hygiene, products, and facilities; keeping clothing clean; obtaining, acquiring, storing, and cooking food; staying in touch with family and friends; access to communication tools and technology; and potential charges for urban vagrancy.[22]

Thus homeless people face problems beyond lack of shelter. They are often faced with social discrimination as well. They can experience limited access to services or reduced access to services that enable their peaceful daily existence: health, dental, and vision care; education; bodily protection; banking services, communication technology, and the right to roam freely in public spaces.[23] Homeless people are also vulnerable to rejection and discrimination, the loss of personal relationships, employment discrimination, and victimization by others. Recognizing these vulnerabilities is the first step in developing trust and a therapeutic relationship with persons who are homeless and thus increasing the probability that communication will occur.

Access to communication technology, such as telephones and the Internet, can influence the ability of the homeless person or family to access telephone-based triage nurses or to schedule appointments with palliative care providers. The sometimes-transient nature of being homeless thwarts community outreach programs to find homeless persons, let alone provide needed services to them. Programs such as Reach Out Wireless[24] from Nexus Communications, Inc., and Assurance Wireless, which is a subsidiary of Virgin Mobile/Sprint,[25] offer free cell phones to homeless people in some states.

As a member of the interdisciplinary palliative care team, how would you have approached Katie? What would you do to keep track of her when she became homeless? Is there anything you could have done to get her back on track?

Communication Characteristics and Mental Illness

Communication with persons with SPMI is dependent on their cognitive abilities and their willingness to trust their healthcare provider. The issue of trust within the context of mental illness is related to the illness characteristics that the person is experiencing. Misplaced trust plays a role in several clinical conditions, including anxiety, paranoia, and personality disorders. The etiology of anxiety disorders is an irrational response to a perceived threat. Activation of the sympathetic nervous system in response to a threat is a nonpathological response. But when the limbic system triggers a fear response in the absence of a real threat, anxiety disorders can manifest. The triggers are not actual threats but perceived threats, although they can have their roots in a real threat that happened in the past. But whatever the etiology of the anxiety disorder, the ability to trust can be compromised.[2]

Persons with thought disorders have a difficult time distinguishing reality from their perception of the world, which instills fear and anxiety. This fear and anxiety can lead to a generalized mistrust of everything and everyone around them, or paranoia. Persons experiencing paranoia on a persistent basis are often unable to build trust and rapport, particularly with a stranger. Thus building a therapeutic relationship takes time. Challenging a paranoid person's irrational mistrust is destructive to the therapeutic relationship and/or communication and is a threat to any progress made.[2]

People with personality disorders are difficult to discuss as a group. These individuals, as a generalization, manipulate various components of their environment to reduce their experienced stressors, thus reducing anxiety. Personality disorders are commonly believed to have a developmental etiology and, as such, are highly ingrained in a person's behavior and belief system. Many persons living with personality disorders distrust others and attempt to manipulate their environments and the people in them to garner trust of others.[2]

The negative stigma toward persons with mental illness promotes the mistaken notion that they are all dangerous and unpredictable. The popular media tends to perpetuate this notion with sensationalism. The reality is that persons with mental illness are no more likely to be dangerous than persons without mental illness. The following guidelines can help palliative healthcare providers communicate with persons who are mentally ill.[26]

- Be respectful.
- Hallucinations and delusions are real to people experiencing them and can motivate the person experiencing them. Be honest in that you understand they are experiencing hallucinations or delusions, but do not pretend to be experiencing them yourself.
- If someone seems frightened, give them a bit more space than you would someone who is not frightened.
- Mental illness does not correlate with intelligence. Never assume that a person with a mental illness will believe anything you say.
- Refer to others only if there is a need to refer. Unnecessary referrals can aggravate anyone who is already upset.
- Engage the use of silence and active listening.
- Set limits and boundaries as needed.
- Keep a current list of community resources, like shelters, food programs, and mental health services to give people if they will accept help.
- If you feel threatened or need help with de-escalating a situation, call for help.

Katie was scared. How would you have helped her overcome her fears? What would you do to build trust and rapport with her when she was hallucinating?

Communication Characteristics and Drug Addiction

Substances that alter thought patterns, such as alcohol, cannabis, and hallucinogens, can instill poor decision-making and paranoia. Thus the drug-addicted person may be overly trusting of a person or a situation, leading him or her to harm, or be paranoid and untrusting. The need for a ready source of funds to support their addiction can cloud their judgment and influence their willingness to manipulate their environment to their advantage. The social taboos associated with drug addiction can also cause shame and thus negatively influence one's own sense of self-worth and feeling of being worthy to receive help from professionals and family members. Being sensitive to the individual's strengths and weaknesses will support therapeutic communication.

Why did Katie drink vodka every month? How did her drinking have an impact on her health and well-being? Why did she turn to street drugs? How did it influence her ability to communicate effectively? Could professional intervention and communication have been used to break this cycle?

A Word About Families

Communicating with family is paramount in palliative care to maximize their understanding and comfort and thus their quality of life. The term "family," as used in this chapter, can include biological or adopted relatives or families of choice. Biological links can be explored to learn about genetic influences on the patient's illness; communicating with the biological family can reveal this information. These links are harder to establish for persons who are adopted, particularly if court records are sealed. Thus any insights from genetics into the person's illness are compromised. Family of choice comprises persons who do not fit predefined family relationships but who are selected by the patient to be treated as if they are biological family. Family relationships are particularly important in understanding and determining the patient's legal healthcare proxy when the patient can no longer communicate his or her wishes. The legal healthcare proxy is often a family member. When the patient can no longer express his or her own wishes, family members often step up to speak for the patient and make expressed wishes known.

Family systems and interactions within families are complex. The palliative care professional understands that family members' needs and quality of life are as much a team concern as those of the patient. Sometimes, family members can help understand a patient's dysarthric speech because they have been living with them as the speech patterns developed. A family member can communicate a patient's wishes about food preferences, medical history, or medication allergies when he or she cannot make them known due to a clinical condition.

When working with persons in these vulnerable populations, communicating with family members can be challenging. Family members are often unavailable. Because homeless persons have no permanent home and limited resources, communication technology—cell phones, computers, the Internet—may be inaccessible. This can thwart their ability to maintain family connections. Many times, palliative patients who are members of one or more of these vulnerable populations have been disenfranchised from their families. The patient may have decided to separate from the family for one or more reason that include family dysfunction and abuse. Sometimes the patient has cultivated mistrust in the family, such as stealing from the household to support his or her drug habit. In a culture of addiction, family members take on specific roles. Palliative communication must take these roles into account and how the patient's addiction has affected family members and their assumed roles. Family members will often describe that they are "burned out" from trying for many years to help the patient, such as trying to help the patient "get back up on their feet" over and over again. In other situations, family members may have issues similar to the patient's and be unable to help because they are struggling with their own challenges.

Family members may blame the patient for how the homelessness, mental illness, or addiction has impacted on the family, particularly financially. Communication with angry family members should be met with the same therapeutic approach—not to alleviate their anger but to help the them understand the impact on the patient and the patient's quality of life. Additional resources, such as counselors, therapists, or chaplaincy, should be consulted, as appropriate, to assist with this communication.

One method for documenting family and understanding their communication pattern is to draw a genogram (Figure 25.1). Relationships between the patient and the family members can be visually indicated and include notes about an individual's

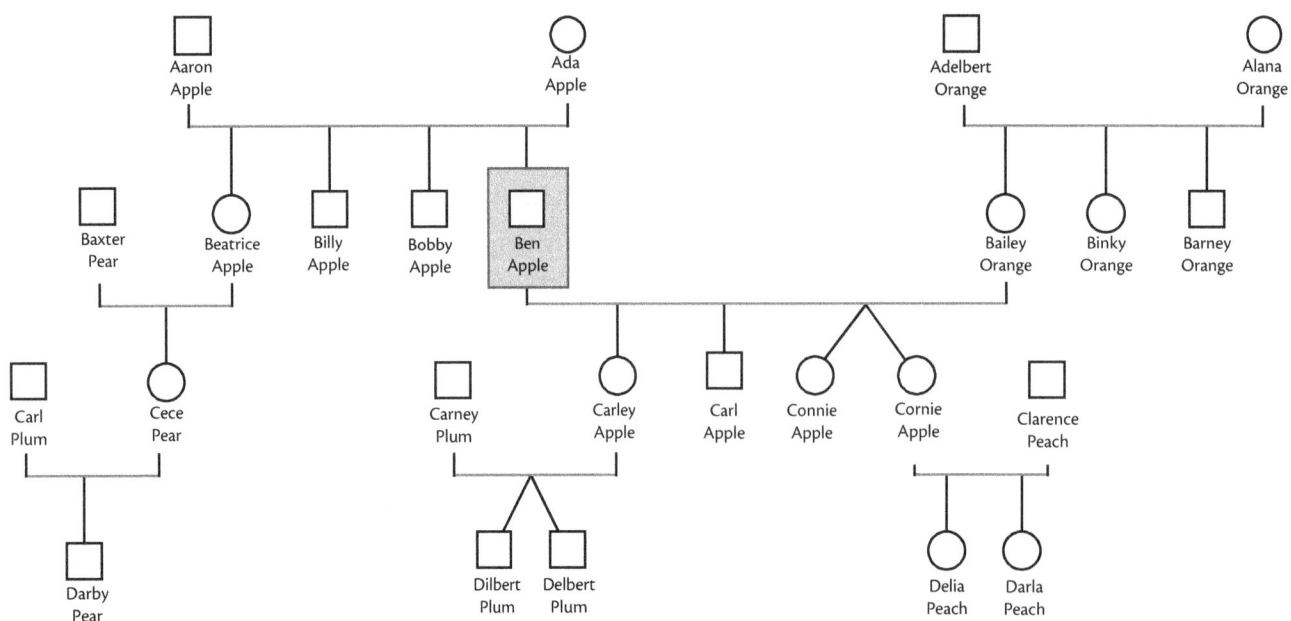

Figure 25.1 Example genogram to document family relationships to assist with palliative communication. Courtesy of John D Chovan.

communication needs. Sharing this document with the interdisciplinary team will also facilitate the delivery of a consistent message.

Recommendations

Meeting the individual and the family where they are at (in terms of understanding of disease/prognosis) will instill a sense of trust and facilitate communication for assessment, diagnosing, planning, implementing, and evaluating the outcomes to provide excellent palliative care. Adding additional stressors to an already stressful situation should be avoided; this could include asking sensitive questions that are obviously uncomfortable, asking family members to take time away from their jobs in the middle of a work shift to attend a family meeting, or interrupting family visitation to perform tasks that can wait. One goal is to prevent exacerbating the factors that contribute to homelessness, mental illness, and/or drug addiction. Consistent with the COMFORT Model of Communication,[3] recommendations from the literature,[26] and my professional clinical experience, when working with persons who are homeless, mentally ill, or addicted to drugs, the palliative care team should

- Deliver a consistent message across time and from all members of the team. Care providers may not be able to contact homeless persons frequently, so with every interaction, a consistent message must be delivered. Persons with mental illness or who are substance users may not have the capacity to understand what they are being told, so a consistent message each time is imperative. Do not use jargon, but keep the language simple and consistent. If you can, develop a genogram of the family and share it with the team.

- At every interaction, explain in simple language what is happening with the patient and what decisions will need to be made. Write things down for the patient to take with him or her to show to others. Recommend to caretakers and family they keep a list of questions for the next time you meet with them.

- Meet with individuals and their families in a location where the distractions are minimized. Depressed and anxious persons, for example, are easily distracted and have difficulty concentrating. Make good eye contact with them and pay attention to nonverbal cues indicating their discomfort. Assess a person with schizophrenia for active hallucinations, particularly command hallucinations, to assist them to focus.

- Reassure the individuals that you and your team will be taking care of them throughout the trajectory of their illness. Make sure they know the members of the team and, if the team members change, have the former team member introduce to the patient and family the new person who is replacing that role.

- Make efforts to ensure the message was communicated correctly. Ask the patient to repeat the message and to restate it in different terms. If the patient has a cognitive deficit, use extremely simple language. Diagrams may be helpful.

- Expect setbacks. Mentally ill patients will often stop taking their medications for their mental illness and for their other chronic physical illnesses. Admonish such behavior, but assist the patient to understand the need to take their medication as prescribed to maximize their quality of life. Drug-addicted patients who have experienced a steady state of sobriety may fall back into alcohol. This should not be viewed as a failure but as a temporary setback. Families may express disdain, and can be helped by refocusing their energies or making the decision not to participate in the care of their loved one.

- Persons with personality disorders need strong boundaries around their behaviors. Do not enable their dysfunction; set boundaries. Consistency is critical from every member of the palliative care team.

Katie died alone and on the streets. It did not have to happen this way. How could things have been handled differently? What would you have done to help maximize her quality of life? How would you have communicated with her, and at what points, to ensure she received the best quality of care possible?

The Palliative Care Team Communication

The interdisciplinary nature of the palliative care team is a rich setting for communicating perspectives that are shared among the disciplines at the table and those that might be different from one another. Physicians, nurses, social workers, and chaplains are trained in their specialties and come together to serve palliative care patients and their families, bringing their unique perspectives. Medicine, for example, brings the perspective of intervening to repair the physiological process that is causing distress in a patient, whereas nursing is focused on the process of caring for patients in their unique responses to their illness. The disciplines do overlap, which brings the team together to achieve a common goal: maximize quality of life. But the philosophies underlying their actions are distinct, and their language often does not overlap to a great extent. When working with patients who are members of one or more of the populations discussed in this section, the work of the interdisciplinary team, however, is greater than the sum of its parts. Healthcare team members must be aware of their own discipline-specific philosophies, language, and practices, as well as that of the other disciplines on the team, to allow the most appropriate patient outcome for each individual and family to emerge.

Future Research

The current understanding of the palliative care needs of the homeless is beginning to unfold. More research into caring for this population, particularly the unsheltered homeless, is needed, and thus how to reach these people and keep them engaged in palliative care is necessary. Working together with government agencies, such as the Department of Health and Human Services and state and local agencies, as well as grassroots, consumer-driven groups such as the National Health Care for the Homeless Commission, to develop new knowledge and translate evidence-based practice about the palliative care needs of the homeless population is necessary.

Substance abusers and those who are addicted to drugs are often misunderstood within the healthcare system in general. This misunderstanding spills over to palliative care, particularly palliative care that involves a primary team rather than palliative care specialists. The stigma of drug addiction and the impact of increased levels of tolerance to pain medicine are still rampant in hospitals and clinics. Palliative care communication with this population is based on trust: trusting patients to report their substance issues and carefully titrating pain medication to keep ahead of their pain. To minimize abuse, the prescriber can take some precautions to minimize the potential for abuse and diversion of these medications. Drugs with lower street values (such as morphine, as of the writing of this chapter) have a lower potential for abuse than drugs with higher street value (such as oxycodone and the fast-acting benzodiazepines) and as such are less likely to be diverted and abused. Similarly, long-acting drugs (such as clonazepam) are slower to build up tolerance, so they have a lower potential for abuse than short-acting drugs in the same class (such as alprazolam and lorazepam).

Finally, little is known about the palliative care needs of persons living with severe mental illness, but communication techniques are very well known within the psychiatric and mental health arena. Professionals who are not specialists in psychiatry and mental health who encounter these patients in the hospital or health clinic need to understand their communication needs. One size does not fit all. Although we know quite a lot about how people with mental illness die, there is still much work to be done to help them understand their illness and trajectory, and their wishes, so we may maximize their quality of life until the very end.

Both the mentally ill and drug-addicted populations would benefit from collaboration between local, state, and federal governmental agencies such as the National Institutes of Health's National Institute on Drug Addiction and the Department of Health and Human Services' Substance Abuse and Mental Health Services Agency, grassroots organizations, and the palliative care community to develop strategies, tools, and techniques for achieving the aforementioned goals. Funding for substance abuse and mental health are typically directed from the federal level, to state agencies, to the county alcohol, drug, and mental health boards for dissemination to the service providers. National and local chapters of organizations such as the National Alliance for the Mentally Ill, Mothers Against Drunk Driving, and Rockers in Recovery should partner with the research community to identify the issues and challenges and solve them for the benefit of these underserved populations.

Conclusion

Working with persons who are experiencing chronic, life-threatening illnesses and the end of life is full of challenges and opportunities. When working in this arena with persons who are homeless, mentally ill, or addicted to drugs presents additional challenges, particularly in communication. The goal is to maximize the quality of life. But doing so relies on dedicated, focused efforts to understand the special circumstances, strengths, and weaknesses of the individual who is ill and of the people who care about him or her. One way to build bridges between members of interdisciplinary teams is to provide opportunities for specialists to learn together. Cross-training opportunities and joint fellowships across disciplines would give individuals and teams time to immerse themselves in each other's specialty areas. The learning opportunities through the Palliative Care Leadership Centers,[27] a program coordinated by the Center to Advance Palliative Care, bring entire teams together to share about not only the similarities and differences between the professions of social work, medicine, nursing, and chaplaincy but also how each profession approaches issues of addiction, mental illness, and homelessness. At the heart of the team is the patient and the family. As a healthcare team, we owe it to our homeless patients, our patients with mental illness, and our patients who abuse drugs to meet them more than halfway through skillful palliative communication.

References

1. Peplau, H. *Interpersonal Relations in Nursing*. New York, NY: G.P. Putnam and Sons; 1952.
2. Salomon K, Jin A. Diathesis-stress model. In Geellman M, Turner J, eds., *Encyclopedia of Behavioral Medicine*. New York, NY: Springer; 2013:591–592.
3. Wittenberg-Lyles E, Goldsmith J, Ferrell B, Ragan S. *Communication in Palliative Nursing*. New York, NY: Oxford University Press; 2012.
4. Centers for Disease Control and Prevention. Other populations. http://www.cdc.gov/minorityhealth/populations/atrisk.html#Other. Accessed July 1, 2014.
5. HealthyPeople.gov. Disparities. http://healthypeople.gov/2020/about/disparitiesAbout.aspx. Accessed July 1, 2014.
6. US Department of Housing and Urban Development. Homelessness assistance. http://portal.hud.gov/hudportal/HUD?src=/program_offices/comm_planning/homeless. Accessed July 1, 2014.
7. US Department of Housing and Urban Development. HUD continuum of care housing assistance programs. https://www.onecpd.info/reports/CoC_PopSub_NatlTerrDC_2013.pdf. Accessed July 1, 2014.
8. National Health Care for the Homeless Council. Homelessness & health: What's the connection? http://www.nhchc.org/wp-content/uploads/2011/09/Hln_health_factsheet_Jan10.pdf. Accessed July 1, 2014.
9. Teruya C, Longshore D, Andersen RM, et al. Health and health care disparities among homeless women. *Women Health*. 2010 December; 2010;50(8):719–736.
10. O'Connell JJ. *Premature Mortality in Homeless Populations: A Review of the Literature* [White Paper.] Nashville, TN: National Healthcare for the Homeless Council; 2005.
11. Hawke W, Davis M, Erlenbusch D. *Dying without Dignity: Homeless Deaths in Los Angeles County: 2000-2007*. Los Angeles, CA: Los Angeles Coalition to End Hunger & Homelessness; 2007.
12. Families First. Mobile health care. http://www.familiesfirstseacoast.org/health_care_for_homeless.html. Accessed September 14, 2014.
13. Department of Health and Mental Hygiene, Bureau of Vital Statistics. Sixth Annual Report on Homeless Deaths New York City. http://www.nyc.gov/html/records/pdf/govpub/62826th_annual_report_final.pdf. Accessed July 1, 2014.
14. National Institute of Mental Health. Any mental illness. http://www.nimh.nih.gov/statistics/1ANYDIS_ADULT.shtml. Accessed July 1, 2014.
15. Druss BG, Zhao L, Von Esenwein S, Morrato EH, Marcus SC. Understanding excess mortality in persons with mental illness: 17-Year follow up of a nationally representative US survey. *Med Care*. 2011;49(6):599–604.
16. Colton CW, Manderscheid RW. Congruencies in increased mortality rates, years of potential life lost, and causes of death among public mental health clients in eight states. *Prev Chronic Dis*. 2006;3(2):A42.
17. De Hert M, Correll CU, Bobes J, et al. Physical illness in patients with severe mental disorders: I. Prevalence, impact of medications and disparities in health care. *World Psychiatry*. 2011;10(1):52–77.
18. Substance Abuse and Mental Health Services Administration. *Results from the 2012 National Survey on Drug Use and Health: Summary of National Findings*, NSDUH Series H-46, HHS Publication No. (SMA) 13-4795. Rockville, MD: Substance Abuse and Mental Health Services Administration; 2013.
19. Nasrallah HA, Meyer JM, Goff DC, et al. Low rates of treatment for hypertension, dyslipidemia and diabetes in schizophrenia: Data from

19. ... the CATIE schizophrenia trial sample at baseline. *Schizophr Res*. 2006;86(1–3):15–22.
20. Sherman ME, Knudsen KJ, Sweeney HA. Analysis of causes of death for all decedents in Ohio with and without mental illness, 2004–2007. *Psychiatr Serv*. 2013;64:245–251.
21. Centers for Disease Control and Prevention. Alcohol Related Disease Impact (ARDI) application. http://apps.nccd.cdc.gov/DACH_ARDI/Default.aspx. Accessed July 1, 2014.
22. Amster R. *Lost in Space: The Criminalization, Globalization, and Urban Ecology of Homelessness*. El Paso, TX: LFB Scholarly Publishing; 2008.
23. Roark, ML. Homelessness at the cathedral. *Miss Law Rev*. 2014;80(1):53–130.
24. Reach Out Mobile Website. http://www.reachoutmobile.com/ Accessed July 1, 2014.
25. Assurance Wireless Website. http://www.assurancewireless.com/Public/Welcome.aspx Accessed July 1, 2014.
26. Swink DF. Communicating with people with mental illness: The public's guide: Strategies for communicating effectively with people with mental illness. [Blog Posting] *Psychol Today*. October 19, 2010. http://www.psychologytoday.com/blog/threat-management/201010/communicating-people-mental-illness-the-publics-guide. Accessed July 1, 2014.
27. Center for the Advancement of Palliative Care. Palliative Care Leadership Centers. https://www.capc.org/palliative-care-leadership-centers/ Accessed September 14, 2014.

CHAPTER 26

Seriously Ill Veterans

VJ Periyakoil

Introduction

The Veteran's Administration (VA) provides care to a large aging population of veterans with various chronic illnesses. The veteran population is older and sicker than the population at large. Historically, recognizing the care needs of the growing population of older veterans with serious illnesses, the VA has implemented innovative models of care to address their specific needs. Beginning in 1978, the VA developed and supported policies and structures for providing quality hospice care for veterans. Over the past 15 years, the VA has implemented nationwide efforts to grow palliative care services. In 2002, the VA Office of Academic Affiliations established several interprofessional fellowship programs in palliative care. In 2008 a VA mandate required all VA facilities to have a palliative care consult team.

In order to provide high-quality care to seriously ill veterans and their families, it is important that interdisciplinary providers have a good understanding of the unique culture and experiences of veterans and the associated health risks and coping strategies that may be common in this population. This chapter includes a summary profile of each of the major military conflicts in the last eight decades that have produced the largest cohorts of veterans. Each cohort possesses comorbid patterns, which are featured in brief introductory case studies (please note that these cases are based on real patient experiences and have been altered significantly to protect patient confidentiality). Specific challenges and strategies in communicating with seriously ill veterans are addressed and a selective review of communication interventions for patients, families, as well as healthcare personnel is provided.

US Veterans

The major cohorts of Veterans include World War II (WWII), Korean War, Vietnam War, and Gulf War veterans. The Department of Veterans Affairs[1] estimates that in 2010 approximately 22,658,000 Americans were veterans, including those who live outside the United States. Of this number, an estimated 37% of veterans are enrolled in the Department of Veterans Affairs healthcare system.[2] Currently, it is estimated that 1,840,000 are women and 9,166,000 are older adults (65 years or older). The number of WWII veterans is estimated to be 1,901,000; they are the oldest cohort and are dying quickly (more than 550 WWII veterans die every day). The Korean War veterans are estimated at 2,448,000, and most are older adults. The Vietnam War veterans are the largest cohort, estimated at 7,526,000, followed by Gulf War veterans, who are the youngest cohort and number approximately 5,737,000 Americans.[2] An estimated 997,000 veterans served both during both WWII and the Korean War; approximately 347,000 Korean War Veterans served during the Vietnam War; and 291,000 veterans served during all three wars. Previous to the Gulf War, the veteran population was predominantly non-Hispanic white, male, and married. Recently, more women and ethnic minorities have joined the US Armed Forces. About one-third of all veterans have been in combat and exposed to experiences related to death and dying during their tour of duty.

World War II Veterans

Mr. O is an older WWII veteran who saw intense combat in France. He never thought he would live through the series of conflicts he encountered on Omaha Beach. But he did live. Nearly all of his battalion did not. He remembered mortars going off to the side and the back of him and seeing his brothers sent in countless directions as metal fragments tore through them. He remembered seeing this and then losing consciousness. Mr. O woke up in a hospital. He stayed there for 1 year. His family did not know about his year-long hospital stay on a mental ward until this week—over 70 years later; this week he entered hospice care provided by the VA. After his time in France, he came home to east Tennessee and never left his house, unless he was gardening. He missed his children's graduations, weddings, and ball games that took place just a mile or two from his home. He missed the same for his grandchildren. Home was the only safe place. He was never treated for posttraumatic stress disorder (PTSD) and was not diagnosed with the illness until he also learned he had advanced liver cancer 2 months ago.

WWII veterans have fought on the continents of Europe, Asia, and Africa and have worked in extreme weather conditions, in very hot and very cold areas. Approximately 200,000 US service personnel performed occupation duties in Hiroshima and Nagasaki following the atomic bombing of Japan, and a similar number participated in atmospheric nuclear weapons tests from 1945 to 1962. Veterans who were stationed in Nagasaki and Hiroshima, Japan, during WWII before 1946 and those who participated in nuclear tests from 1945 to 1962 are known as "atomic veterans." The Department of Veterans Affairs identifies 195,000 servicemen who were involved in the occupation of Hiroshima and Nagasaki, with an additional 210,000 personnel participating in 200 postwar nuclear tests. Studies[3-9] of Japanese atomic bomb survivors have shown that exposure to radiation has been associated with leukemia, various cancers, and cataracts. Exposure to asbestos is seen in this cohort and may be associated with mesotheliomas. WWII veterans are predominantly men.

Korean War Veterans

Mr. P's first assignment was with a fighter-bomber squadron in Japan, but the Air Force decided to make a medical corpsman out of him. Shortly after the United States went to war in Korea in 1950, Mr. P was on active duty, loading casualties onto transport planes bound for Japan. He spent time with a MASH unit, claiming it was hardly like what was depicted in the famed TV show. Returning home from the war, he remained sensitive to those who would diminish his service because he was not an infantry soldier. Within days after he returned home, he detached from the armed services and started a new career. As the years passed, he experienced more and more difficulty with his mental health issues due to recurrent bouts of depression. Never marrying or having children, Mr. P relied for years on an older brother who was also a veteran, but now he finds himself completely dependent on the VA for his care as he ages and his physical health diminishes.

According to the 1990 US Census, 92% of the 4.9 million Korean War veterans are white. Korean War veterans are rapidly aging and dying. By the 2010 census, the number of Korean War veterans was estimated to be just under 2.5 million. Approximately 5% percent of Korean War veterans are women. The median age of these veterans is 78.5 years. Most Korean War veterans are mid-old (75 to 84) or old-old (over 85). The Korean War hostilities (fighting) occurred from June 27, 1950, to July 27, 1953, and the official Korean War era dates from June 27, 1950, to January 31, 1955 (all veterans who served on active duty during this period are deemed to be Korean War veterans).

A total of 5,720,000 persons served in the US Armed Forces during the Korean War, with 33,741 battle deaths and 103,284 wounded. Injuries from cold weather conditions were common during this era; many veterans have delayed squeal, including peripheral neuropathy, skin cancer in frostbite scars (in such locations as the heels and earlobes), arthritis, collapsed foot arches, stiff toes, nocturnal pain, and cold sensitization. These cold-related problems may worsen as they grow older and develop complicating conditions such as diabetes and peripheral vascular disease, placing them at higher risk for late amputations. The Korean War was initially deemed to be a police action and a conflict, rather than a war. This may be a sensitive issue for Korean War veterans, who may not feel their service was appropriately acknowledged.

Vietnam War Veterans

In 1965 Ms. B was a nurse on a mission. Inspired by her brothers' service in the Vietnam War, and having earned a master's degree in psychiatric nursing and graduated from Officer Candidate School, she enlisted in the Air Force. She knew the need for psychiatric care was exigent and insisted that she be assigned to the front line to take care of infantry combat soldiers, not officers. Her concern included wounded servicemen as well as local civilians. In her 2 years in the field she was unwavering in her commitment not only to American soldiers but also wounded Viet Cong combatants. Upon her return to the states, Ms. B entered private nursing practice. In her early 50s she retired and was soon diagnosed with Parkinson's disease. She opted to receive care outside of the VA (as she felt that she needed specialized women healthcare programs, which were not available through her local VA) but missed the camaraderie of others who served and could relate to women's war experiences.

The Vietnam War (aka the Second Indochina War) occurred from 1954 to 1973. The United States and other members of the Southeast Asia Treaty Organization fought in support of the Republic of South Vietnam against the Viet Cong (Communist forces of South Vietnamese guerrillas, also known as the National Liberation Front) and the North Vietnamese Army. Direct U.S. military involvement ended on August 15, 1973. The North Vietnamese Army captured Saigon in April 1975, and North and South Vietnam were reunified under the Communist regime. More than 47,000 US service members were killed in battle, and another 11,000 suffered noncombat deaths. The Vietnam War is known as "the only war America ever lost." This perceived failure, in addition to the extensive US antiwar protests, had a significant negative impact on Vietnam War veterans.

US citizens did not welcome the returning veterans as war heroes. Instead, these veterans, who had suffered tremendous physical and emotional harm (during the extreme war conditions) defending their country in a war they did not instigate, were subjected to public anger and protests, provoking in them a sense of guilt and shame. Many experts feel that this suboptimal reception is a primary etiological factor in some of the psychological aftermath these veterans report.

Vietnam veterans suffer high rates of chronic mental illnesses, including major depression, suicide, PTSD, and substance abuse as well as the consequences of chemical warfare. Chemical warfare was used to destroy bushes, crops, and trees to prevent Communist insurgents from having the cover they needed to ambush passing convoys. Americans sprayed millions of tons of defoliant herbicide ("Agent Orange"),[9-12] which contained the toxic byproduct dioxin. According to the VA, diseases associated with Agent Orange exposure include amyloidosis, chronic b-cell leukemias, chloracne (or similar acne-type diseases), diabetes mellitus type 2, Hodgkin's disease, ischemic heart disease, multiple myeloma, non-Hodgkin's lymphoma, Parkinson's disease, peripheral neuropathy, porphyria cutanea tarda, prostate cancer, respiratory cancers (including cancers of the lung, larynx, trachea, and bronchus), and soft tissue sarcomas (other than osteosarcoma, chondrosarcoma, Kaposi's sarcoma, or mesothelioma). Of note, the VA presumes that Lou Gehrig's disease (amyotrophic lateral sclerosis [ALS]) diagnosed in all veterans who had 90 days or more continuous active military service is related to their service, although ALS is not (so far) thought to be related directly to Agent Orange exposure. There are no specific tests to detect Agent Orange exposure or to demonstrate that the herbicides caused individual medical problems. As a result, veterans who served in Vietnam or the Korean demilitarized zone are presumed to have been exposed to Agent Orange.[13] Hepatitis C infection is more common in this population as compared to the general population. Sixty-three percent of veterans enrolled in the VA who test positive for hepatitis C virus are Vietnam Era veterans.[12] Chronic hepatitis C infection can result in hepato-cellular cancer, which is a serious life-limiting and eventually fatal illness.

Gulf War, Afghanistan, and Iraq War Veterans

Mr. J joined the army at age 17. Within the next 3 years he was a trained paratrooper preparing for deployment to the Gulf. He was also a trained Spanish linguist as tensions were high in areas of Central America. However, his battalion was posted to the Saudi desert region. At 21, he had lost part of four toes due to frostbite. Many years later, Mr. J was diagnosed with gout, arthritis, depression, and PTSD and was a heavy drinker. He had persistent pain and was on high doses of prescription analgesics. Due to his multiple chronic illnesses and pain, he had difficulty working and no steady income, thereby making his housing situation tenuous.

Fibromyalgia and chronic fatigue syndrome are common in Gulf War (Desert Storm) veterans. Afghanistan War (Operation Enduring Freedom) and Iraq War (Operation Iraqi Freedom) veterans exhibit infectious disease (multidrug-resistant acinetobacter Leishmaniasis, a sand fly–transmitted infection of the skin) and problems caused by exposure to depleted uranium, contaminants and toxins from pollution (e.g., sewage-polluted water, air pollution, food and water affected by agricultural and industrial contamination), cold weather, high altitudes, and severe sand and dust storms. Additionally, these veterans are at higher risk for depression, suicide,[14,15] PTSD, substance abuse, and other chronic mental illnesses.[16,17]

Palliative Care Needs of Seriously Ill Veterans

The burden of chronic illness is higher in veterans compared to the general population, and most veterans die of chronic illness. Veterans' palliative care needs are similar to those of the general population in that they need high-quality palliative care early in the trajectory of serious illness. In addition, veterans have some unique palliative care needs due to their combat exposure, including prisoner of war experiences and the unique risks specific to each war (as described previously). Veterans also exhibit the unique characteristics of battlemind and stoicism when facing serious illness, behaviors secondary to their training and work in the armed forces.

"Battlemind"[18-25] is defined as a soldier's inner strength to face fear and adversity during combat with courage. It is the will to persevere and win in circumstances of grave danger. When on a tour of duty, a member of the US Armed Forces is expected to be strong and fully operational at all times. There is a significant stigma associated with any show of weakness or retreat from the warfront. The armed forces are expected to meet challenges head on and maintain mental toughness during times of great stress, adversity, and challenge. For example, the US Navy Sea Air and Land personnel often quote the phrase, "The only easy day was yesterday." They know and expect to encounter adversity and train in teams to overcome extremely challenging battle-related circumstances, while being fully cognizant that they may be gravely injured or die in service to their country. This battlemind comes from the ongoing rigorous training they receive when on active duty and often becomes an integral part of their identity.

Thus veterans, when faced with serious illness, demonstrate tremendous courage and resilience and work hard to maintain a stoic approach. While this can certainly be a strength and help veterans cope with serious illness, this stoicism may also prevent them from openly discussing their illness-related fears and concerns with their family and healthcare team, leaving them to suffer in isolation. Data also shows that veterans are at a higher risk for PTSD, depression, and substance abuse.[16,17,26] Veterans who are reluctant to openly discuss the consequences of serious illness with their family members may use suboptimal coping strategies, including alcohol and recreational drugs, further isolating themselves from their loved ones.

Unique Stresses Veterans Experience That Influence Their Responses to Serious Illness

Life Threat

About 30% to 40% of veterans have been exposed to combat, which includes death and dying, during their tours of duty. Some have survived being prisoners of war. Medics in combat zones are at high risk for loss of life. Even those who are not directly involved in fighting are at high risk for fatalities, including drivers of supply trucks and convoys in war zones. When encountering serious illness at the end of life, veterans may have a sense of *déjà vu*—of being back on the warfront—and feel the same sense of threat, helplessness, and lack of control. This is one of the reasons why veterans who receive healthcare in the community may choose to return to VA for end-of-life care, as they may feel safer in the familiar surroundings of the VA among their fellow veterans when facing potential loss of life. This is also the reason that veterans on home hospice care continue to seek care at the VA, as they are reluctant to sever ties with a familiar and trusted environment. Likely a related finding is that families of veterans who have died experienced higher satisfaction with end-of-life care than those veterans who died in non-VA facilities.[27] Veteran desire to stay connected to the VA and its people becomes a source of conflict when home hospice personnel tell the veterans to cancel all VA appointments and not to contact the VA.

Loss of Colleagues and Friends/Relationships and Loss of Limbs

Loss is a pervasive experience for many members of the armed forces. Armed forces personnel often miss important life events and milestones of their loved ones when on a tour of duty and feel a sense of guilt about missing these events. They lose friends and colleagues in the line of duty. Many will put their own lives at risk without a second thought in an effort to rescue fellow team members on the warfront. While this past experience with grief and loss gives veterans tremendous courage to deal with serious illness, it also puts them at risk for suffering in silence and not adequately communicating with their care team or seeking the help they need.

Warrior Culture and Moral Injury

Men and women on active duty may be forced to commit actions that may be in direct conflict with their fundamental values and beliefs. For example, they have to deploy force, wound, and even kill enemy soldiers. They may also witness collateral harm that befalls civilians, women, and children who are at the battlefront and become war casualties, all in the line of duty. Hoge[28] surveyed US soldiers and Marines and found that 52% of soldiers and Marines reported shooting or directing fire at the enemy; 32% reported being directly responsible for the death of an enemy combatant; 65% reported seeing dead bodies or human remains; 31% reported handling or uncovering human remains; and 60% reported having seen ill/wounded women and children whom they were unable to help.

Many of these experiences and actions may conflict with their personal and religious/spiritual beliefs, causing tremendous guilt and shame. Veterans may not fully grasp the impact of violence or the warrior culture during active duty. However, there may be delayed consequences that take a big toll on long-term physical, emotional, and spiritual health. When they separate from the armed forces culture and context and return home to lead civilian lives with family, veterans may ponder their past experiences and actions and suffer tremendous distress. These issues come to the forefront at the end of life, when they are in the process of doing a life review and confronting imminent death. During these vulnerable times, they may lack the defenses to cope with their guilt and shame, and, depending on their religious/spiritual beliefs, they may fear after-life consequences of their actions in the line of duty.

These experiences can skew how veterans interpret pain due to serious illness. Some may feel that the disease-triggered pain is retribution for the pain they have inflicted on others during wartime. Others may believe in redemptive suffering and choose not to treat their pain but instead suffer to atone for their "sins." In a study[31] of pain and coping conducted on a group of 109 veterans with chronic pain, researchers studied nine specific pain-related adaptive and maladaptive coping and belief domains: guarding, exercise/stretch, resting, catastrophizing, control, disability, harm, medication, and pacing. Each of the pain-related coping responses and beliefs were classified as adaptive (exercise/stretch, control, and pacing) or maladaptive (guarding, resting, catastrophizing, disability, harm, and medication). The study results showed that maladaptive coping and beliefs played a more powerful role than adaptive coping and beliefs in predicting pain interference and depression. Further, adaptive responses may be more important than maladaptive responses in predicting patient-reported pain intensity.

Posttraumatic Stress Disorder

Prior to 1980, PTSD did not appear in the *Diagnostic and Statistical Manual of Mental Disorders*. It was included in the third edition of the manual and became a common diagnosis for Vietnam veterans.[32] Over time, the illness was recognized in all classes and generations of military members. PTSD is an anxiety disorder that can develop when a person has experienced, has witnessed, or has been confronted with an event (s) that involved actual or threatened death or serious injury or a threat to the physical integrity of self or others. The *Diagnostic and Statistical Manual of Mental Disorders* classifies PTSD as an anxiety disorder characterized by a triggering trauma, followed by a series of intense negative emotional responses to the trauma. PTSD[23] is more common in war veterans, especially in combat veterans, and is extremely common in prisoners of war. According to the National Center for PTSD, one in three veterans who survived combat in WWII, Korea, or Vietnam developed chronic PTSD, and more developed some PTSD symptoms. The estimated prevalence of PTSD is about 30% in Vietnam War veterans, 10% in Gulf War veterans, 6% to 11% in Afghanistan War veterans, and 12% to 20% in Iraq War veterans.

It is important to note that trauma-related memory can be triggered by somatosensory triggers such as pain or nausea. For example, a veteran who was a prisoner of war and experienced pain and torment in the enemy camp may have recurrent flashbacks and related agitation when he or she is experiencing pain at the end of life as a part of serious illness. Alternatively, a veteran who has coped with PTSD by repressing related memories may become vulnerable due to serious illness and have a resurgence of intrusive memories. Some veterans, when treated with opioids for pain related to serious illness, may have nightmares and flashbacks due to the mind-altering properties of these drugs. In such situations, they may prefer to forego the medication and bear the physical pain rather than experience the extreme suffering triggered by PTSD. Finally, PTSD patients have a higher prevalence of depression and recreational substance abuse. Colored by their negative war experiences, they may be mistrustful of government-related services, including the Veterans Health Administration.

The multifaceted nature of PTSD as a mental illness presents compounding effects for healthcare teams as well as family caregivers once a veteran is facing a chronic or terminal period of illness. Avoidance is a common coping mechanism for individuals with PTSD.[31] This, in addition to distrust of the healthcare system, can create a dynamic in which the patient is viewed as difficult—causing healthcare professionals to respond in kind with avoidance. A patient-centered approach is suggested by experts as an effective way of caring for veterans with PTSD.[32] A series of behavioral health interventions have been systematically introduced by the VA to offer caregiver counseling and support. These interventions include emotionally focused couples therapy for trauma, lifestyle management courses, conjoint cognitive behavioral therapy for couples, strategic approach therapy for couples (targeting spousal anxiety), and many others.[33]

Communication Challenges for Seriously Ill Veterans

As described previously, veterans have unique life experiences and are at risk for certain illnesses, which influence their worldview and how they choose to interact with healthcare providers. Stoicism is common in veterans, who tend to be particularly reticent about their war experiences. It is also common for a veteran's spouse and family members to be completely unaware of the details of the veteran's war experiences and consequences. For example, a veteran may have significant PTSD or be in the throes of moral injury–related distress without their loved ones even knowing. Thus it is important to talk directly to the patient, document his or her branch of service, and routinely and gently explore whether he or she experienced or witnessed combat, as well as to screen him or her for PTSD and moral injury. Box 26.1 offers several example questions that providers can use to learn more about veteran experiences.

Box 26.1 Sample Questions to Promote Sensitivity to Veteran Experiences

- What kind of feelings have you had about your deployment experience?
- How have you been feeling about yourself since returning home?
- What would help you come to terms with your deployment experiences?
- Can you tell me about some of the workplace challenges you have faced recently?
- As a service member, you already have many skills prospective employers may be interested in. Can you tell me some of the skills you cultivated in the military?
- Who are you spending time with after returning home?
- How have you felt that your friends or family relationships have changed while you were deployed?
- Can you identify one person whom you can talk to about your deployment experiences?

Source: Koenig CJ, Maguen S, Monroy JD, Mayott L, Seal KH. Facilitating culture-centered communication between health care providers and veterans transitioning from military deployment to civilian life. *Patient Educ Couns*. June 2014;95(3):414–420.

In order to mitigate distrust, it is best to first elicit the patient's preferred communication style (direct vs. indirect) and information-seeking preferences and tailor the communication to the specific needs of the individual patient. Veterans from ethnic minorities who are socioeconomically disadvantaged may be wary of discussing limiting high-intensity care due to fear of racial prejudice. Fortunately, most veterans tend to prefer a direct style of communication and value honesty very highly. An open approach about the benefits and burdens of each aspect of the care plan usually alleviates any mistrust. If asked, providers should be willing to refer the patient for a second opinion and not be defensive about this request. One study found that telephone communication for primary care needs is the preferred strategy among veterans, as only slightly half of those surveyed were regular computer users and had ever used the Internet.[34]

Communication Interventions for Improved Care

The majority of veterans receive care in the community. Many veterans may be concurrently receiving care through Medicare, Medicaid, or private insurance but also enroll to receive care at the VA. Sometimes veterans may be receiving medications and other interventions both in a VA facility as well as through the community-based healthcare system. Currently there are no coordinated communication systems that seamlessly integrate electronic medical records across systems of healthcare. Thus veterans may be at risk for receiving medications concurrently from the VA and from community providers. More than one-third of veterans in one study reported never discussing non-VA medications with their VA physicians.[35] To facilitate care coordination and communication between VA and non-VA providers, Shi et al. suggest five best practices for both VA and non-VA sites[36] (see Box 26.2). Furthermore, there is a great need to educate community-based healthcare personnel about veterans' unique needs. This is especially true for end-of-life care, as home hospice care received by veterans is provided through Medicare-certified community hospices.

Currently the VA provides home-based primary care but does not provide home hospice care because it is funded by the Medicare Hospice Benefit. The VA contracts with Medicare-certified community-based home hospices and will pay for home-hospice services for seriously ill veterans who are not eligible for the Medicare Hospice Benefit (as hospice care is a fundamental entitlement for all veterans). Thus all community-based palliative care personnel should familiarize themselves with the unique health risks, communication preferences, and needs of veterans and their families. It is important to ask all patients about their veteran status and document this carefully. Veterans with ALS or Agent Orange-exposure and other service-connected conditions may be eligible for special benefits both for themselves as well as their families. Most veterans receive also some funeral benefits from the VA.

In 2003 the VA was the first system to introduce a Web-based Personal Health Record (PHR) to its patients and their families. The intervention was designed to complement face-to-face services and empower patients and their caregivers, as well as create an extended sense of community for sick veterans. The PHR includes features that make a medical health record available to patients/caregivers and most recently secure messaging with the entire healthcare team. A recent study[37] of usability for the VA's PHR showed that the majority of users wanted family caregivers to have access to and use the system to schedule appointments, help manage prescription medications, and communicate with healthcare team members. Additionally, veterans indicated a desire to share access of the PHR to care providers outside of the VA system. Other programs are under examination at VA facilities across the country.

Conclusion

In summary, veterans who served their country have an increased prevalence of chronic illnesses, have unique approaches to pain and illness based on military training, and are likely to have PTSD. Special attention is required to identify illnesses that are specific to each war era. It behooves all providers to gain a deeper understanding of how veterans' past training and experiences in the armed services influence how they cope with serious illness. A gentle and open communication approach bolstered by knowledge of the key issues more common in war experiences will help us better support and enable veterans to live and die with dignity.[38–40]

Box 26.2 Recommended Best Practices for Veterans Administration and non-Veterans Administration Care Coordination and Communication[38]

- Educate veteran patients about possible risks and challenges of dual care
- Request veteran patient records from the counterpart in a timely manner
- Identify the list and doses of medications prescribed by VA and non-VA physicians
- Update the counterpart about health conditions of veteran patients frequently
- Contact patients frequently by phone to obtain information

References

1. US Department of Veteran Affairs. Veteran population. http://www.va.gov/vetdata/Veteran_Population.asp. Accessed October 2, 2014.
2. National Center for Veterans Analyses and Statistics http://www.va.gov/vetdata/Veteran_Population.asp. Accessed October 2, 2013.
3. Hansen D, Schriner C. Unanswered questions: The legacy of atomic veterans. *Health Physics*. August 2005;89(2):155–163.
4. Dalager NA, Kang HK, Mahan CM. Cancer mortality among the highest exposed US atmospheric nuclear test participants. *J Occup Environ Med*. 2000;42:798–805.
5. Department of Veterans Affairs. *Veterans and Radiation: Independent Study Course*. Birmingham, AL: Veterans Health Initiative Employee Education System; 2001.
6. Finch SC. Leukemia: Lessons from the Japanese experience. *Stem Cells* 1997;15(Suppl 2):135–139.
7. Institute of Medicine. *Adverse Reproductive Outcomes in Families of Atomic Veterans: The Feasibility of Epidemiologic Studies*. Washington, DC: National Academy Press; 1995.
8. Veterans' Claims for Disabilities from Nuclear Weapons Testing. *Hearing Before the Committee on Veterans Affairs*. 96th Congress, 1st session. Washington DC: Government Printing Office; 1979.

9. Schull WJ, Otake M, Neel JV. Hiroshima and Nagasaki: A reassessment of the mutagenic effect of exposure to ionizing radiation. In: Hook EB, Porter IH, eds. *Populations and Biological Aspects of Human Mutation*. New York, NY: Academic Press; 1981:277-303.
10. Institute of Medicine. *Update on Veterans and Agent Orange: Hearing Before the Subcommittees on Hospitals and Health Care of the Committee on Veterans' Affairs, House of Representatives, 104th Congress, 2nd session*. Washington, DC: Government Printing Office; 16 April 1996
11. Institute of Medicine Committee to Review the Health Effects in Vietnam *Veterans of Exposure to Herbicides: Veterans and Agent Orange. Update 2000*. Washington DC: National Academy Press; 2001.
12. National Hospice and Palliative Care Organization. Vietnam War health risks. http://www.wehonorveterans.org/vietnam-war-health-risks. Accessed October 2, 2014.
13. Young A, Cecil P. Agent Orange exposure and attributed health effects in Vietnam veterans. *Milit Med*. 2011;176(7 Suppl):29-34.
14. Kaplan MS, Huguet N, McFarland BH, Newsom JT. Suicide among male veterans: A prospective population-based study. *J Epidemiol Commun Health*. 2007;61(7):619-624.
15. US Department of Veterans Affairs Mental Health Services Suicide Prevention Program. Suicide data report, 2012. http://www.va.gov/opa/docs/suicide-data-report-2012-final.pdf
16. Brooks MS, Fulton L. Evidence of poorer life-course mental health outcomes among veterans of the Korean War cohort. *Aging Mental Health*. 2010;14(2):177-183.
17. Hoge C, Terakopian A, Castro C, Messer S, Engel C. Association of PTSD with somatic symptoms, health care visits, and absenteeism among Iraq War veterans. *Am J Pschiatr*. 2007;164:150-153.
18. Zamorski MA, Guest K, Bailey S, Garber BG. Beyond battlemind: Evaluation of a new mental health training program for Canadian forces personnel participating in third-location decompression. *Mil Med*. 2012;177(11):1245-1253.
19. Foran HM, Adler AB, McGurk D, Bliese PD. Soldiers' perceptions of resilience training and postdeployment adjustment: Validation of a measure of resilience training content and training process. *Psychol Serv*. 2012;9(4):390-403.
20. Castro CA, Adler AB, McGurk D, Bliese PD. Mental health training with soldiers four months after returning from Iraq: Randomization by platoon. *J Trauma Stress*. 2012;25(4):376-383.
21. Mulligan K, Fear NT, Jones N, et al. Postdeployment battlemind training for the U.K. armed forces: A cluster randomized controlled trial. *J Consult Clin Psychol*. 2012;80(3):331-341.
22. McNally RJ. Are we winning the war against posttraumatic stress disorder? *Science*. 2012;336(6083):872-874.
23. Lew HL, Amick MM, Kraft M, Stein MB, Cifu DX. Potential driving issues in combat returnees. *NeuroRehabilitation*. 2010;26(3):271-278.
24. Adler AB, Bliese PD, McGurk D, Hoge CW, Castro CA. Battlemind debriefing and battlemind training as early interventions with soldiers returning from Iraq: Randomization by platoon. *J Consult Clin Psychol*. 2009;77(5):928-940.
25. Orsingher JM, Lopez AT, Rinehart ME. Battlemind training system: "Armor for your mind." *US Army Med Dep J*. July-September 2008;66-71.
26. Seal K, Bertenthal D, Miner C, Saunak S, Marmar C. Bringing the war back home: Mental health disorders among 103,788 US veterans returning from Iraq and Afghanistan seen at Department of Veterans Affairs facilities. *JAMA Intern Med*. 2007;167(5):476-482.
27. Lu H, Trancik E, Bailey A, Ritchie C, Rosenfeld K, Shreve S, Furman C, Smith D, Wolff C, Casarett D. Families' perceptions of end-of-life care in Veterans Affairs versus non-Veterans Affairs facilities. *J Palliat Med*. 2010;13(8):991-996.
28. Hoge CW, Castro CA, Messer SC, McGurk D, Cotting DI, Koffman RL. Combat duty in Iraq and Afghanistan, mental health problems, and barriers to care. *N Engl J Med*. 2004;351:13-22.
29. Tan G, Teo I, Anderson KO, Jensen MP. Adaptive versus maladaptive coping and beliefs and their relation to chronic pain adjustment. *Clin J Pain*. November-December 2011;27(9):769-774.
30. Wilbur S. PTSD in DSM-III: A case in the politics of diagnosis and disease. *Soc Probl*. 1990;37(3):294-310.
31. Amir M, Kaplan Z, Efroni R, Levine Y, Benjamin J, Kotler M. Coping styles in post-traumatic stress disorder (PTSD) patients. *Pers Individ Differ*. 1997;23:399-405.
32. Feldman DB, Periyakoil VS. Posttraumatic stress disorder at the end of life. *J Palliat Med*. February 2006;9(1):213-218.
33. Schumm J, Fredman S, Monson C, Chard K. Cognitive-behavioral conjoint therapy for PTSD: Initial findings for Operations Enduring and Iraqi Freedom male combat veterans and their partners. *Am J Fam Ther*. 2013;41(4):277-287.
34. LaVela SL, Schectman G, Gering J, Locatelli SM, Gawron A, Weaver FM. Understanding health care communication preferences of veteran primary care users. *Patient Educ Couns*. September 2012;88(3):420-426.
35. Stroupe KT, Smith BM, Hogan TP, et al. Medication acquisition across systems of care and patient-provider communication among older veterans. *Am J Health Syst Pharm*. May 2013;70(9):804-813.
36. Shi J, Peng Y, Erdem E, Woodbridge P, Fetrick A. Communication enhancement and best practices for co-managing dual care rural veteran patients by VA and non-VA providers: a survey study. *J Community Health*. June 2014;39(3):552-561.
37. Zulma D, Zazi KM, Turvey C, Wagner T, Woods SS, An LC. Patient interest in sharing personal health record information: A web-based survey. *Ann Intern Med*. 2011;155(12):804-810.
38. Periyakoil VS, Stevens M, Kraemer H. Multicultural long-term care nurses' perceptions of factors influencing patient dignity at the end of life. *J Am Geriatr Soc*. March 2013;61(3):440-446.
39. Periyakoil VS, Noda AM, Kraemer HC. Assessment of factors influencing preservation of dignity at life's end: Creation and the cross-cultural validation of the preservation of dignity card-sort tool. *J Palliat Med*. May 2010;13(5):495-500.
40. Periyakoil VS, Kraemer HC, Noda A. Creation and the empirical validation of the dignity card-sort tool to assess factors influencing erosion of dignity at life's end. *J Palliat Med*. December 2009;12(12):1125-1130.

CHAPTER 27

Neonatal and Pediatrics

Barbara L. Jones and Kendra D. Koch

Introduction

Like adult palliative care, pediatric palliative care is not one service but an approach to care that may be offered at different facilities and by different providers. Used in both inpatient and outpatient settings, pediatric palliative care seeks to prevent and relieve suffering in children with life-threatening illness. It offers culturally sensitive social, emotional, and spiritual interventions and appropriate medical treatments to optimize quality of life during the child's illness and to extend emotional care and social support to the patient and his or her family.[1,2] The World Health Organization (WHO) expounds on this definition, explaining that

> Palliative care for children represents a special, albeit closely related field to adult palliative care. WHO's definition of palliative care appropriate for children and their families is as follows; the principles apply to other paediatric chronic disorders (WHO; 1998a):

- Palliative care for children is the active total care of the child's body, mind and spirit, and also involves giving support to the family.
- It begins when illness is diagnosed, and continues regardless of whether or not a child receives treatment directed at the disease.
- Health providers must evaluate and alleviate a child's physical, psychological, and social distress.
- Effective palliative care requires a broad multidisciplinary approach that includes the family and makes use of available community resources; it can be successfully implemented even if resources are limited. It can be provided in tertiary care facilities, in community health centers, and even in children's homes.[3]

These echo the American Academy of Pediatrics' Core Principles of Patient- and Family-Centered Care, which encourage healthcare providers to listen to and respect "each child and his or her family"[4] while promoting the confidence of patients and families as they "participate in making choices and decisions about their health care."[4]

Why Is Communication Important to Children and Families?

Without communication in the form of honest, clear, and accessible dialogue, parents may not have the information they need to make decisions or the education and support they need to care for their children. This makes communication not only an issue of quality care but of ethical care.[5,6] Often, parents are asked to make decisions for their ill child based on information and options communicated to them by members of the child's palliative care team. If this communication is ambiguous or unclear, the parent is unfairly limited in the quality of the decision that he or she can make. At the end of a child's life especially, parents want adequate information and supportive communication so they can make the best decisions for their child and so those decisions will be less likely to lead to regret.[7,8] Parents express that good communication in pediatric palliative care leads to better social and emotional outcomes for the child and family[9,10] and, inversely, bad communication results in negative social and emotional outcomes for the family.[9,10]

Note that the word "child" is used in this chapter to refer to the patient's status as a minor. Unless otherwise noted in context, it refers to patients from birth to adulthood (i.e., infancy, childhood, and adolescence).

Identifying the Population

The population that receives pediatric palliative care is comprised of children diagnosed with life-threatening illnesses who are not expected to reach adulthood due to the illness or symptoms caused by it. Cancer is the most common illness associated with pediatric palliative care in developed countries and is the leading cause of nonaccidental or traumatic death in children ages 1 to 19. According to the latest data from the Centers for Disease Control and Prevention, 45,068 children died in 2010. Almost half of those deaths occurred before the age of 1 because of congenital anomalies or sudden infant death syndrome. Of the remaining deaths due to natural causes (not unintentional injuries, suicides, or homicides), the majority occurred because of congenital anomalies (6,114 deaths), followed by cancer (2,160 deaths).[11,12] Other children who may benefit from palliative care may be diagnosed with a range of neurological, metabolic, and pulmonary diseases. Cardiac, respiratory, renal, and gastrointestinal diseases are also common along with immunodeficiency and other congenital anomalies.[13,14] These medically complex diseases account for most cases in which a child needs palliative care.[14]

The need for palliative care can stem from either the disease itself or the symptoms produced by the disease. The *Oxford Textbook of Palliative Care* groups children with palliative needs into four categories:[13]

Category 1 includes children who have diseases for which a cure exists, but the cure has not been successful for the specific child patient. Cancer is an example of such a disease.

Category 2 encompasses children with a disease for which no cure exists; however, medication and therapy can be used for symptom management and to prolong life. Examples of diseases in this category are cystic fibrosis and Duchenne's muscular dystrophy.[13]

Category 3 contains children with diseases that cannot be cured or without a direct approach to cure. Here, symptom management is the main goal. Metabolic diseases are often seen in this category.[13]

Category 4 presents providers and clinicians with special challenges. This category consists of children with static diseases that do not directly progress to a stage where death is imminent. Instead, the symptoms and secondary effects of the disease are the life-threatening aspects. An example is a child with encephalopathy caused by an anoxic brain injury, such as a near-drowning event.[13] The disease or injury is not continuing, but the disruptions caused by the disease or injury are.

Symptoms that may arise because of the diseases in each of these categories include seizures, cognitive impairments, speech difficulty, problems with external intake, fatigue, somatic pain, dyspnea, appetite disturbances, weight changes, constipation, anxiety or depression, urinary problems, irritability, and diarrhea.[14] For many of these diseases, developments in treatment and technology have led to prolonged lifespans for children who, in the not-so-distant past, would likely have died in infancy or childhood. Survival rates of infants born prematurely[15] or with various congenital anomalies have increased as well.[16,17] This in turn has led to increased usage of life-extending medical technologies including feeding tubes (gastrostrostomy tubes, nasogastric tubes, jejunostomy tubes), central venous catheters, tracheostomy, noninvasive ventilation, and ventriculoperitoneal or ventriculo-jugularshunts shunts.[14]

Pediatric Needs Differ From Adult Needs

Although pediatric palliative care shares many of the same aims and interventions as adult palliative care, it differs from adult palliative care in several ways that directly affect communication:

1. Children live much longer than adults after initiating palliative care,[14] making communication in care coordination and continuity of care an integral feature of pediatric palliative care.

2. Palliative care for children is often used concurrently with curative care.[18] This means that conversations about decision-making and goal-setting may be more complex and require information and options that consider the patient's and family's goals for cure *and* comfort.

3. Different life-limiting diagnoses are found in children than in adults,[13,14,19] requiring pediatric healthcare providers to discuss with families different trajectories of illness, treatments, and potential outcomes than they might with adult populations. Because many of these diseases are rare or undiagnosed, trajectories of illness and prognosis become especially difficult for healthcare providers, adding complexity to communication about areas of anticipatory guidance, including medical decision-making and symptom management.

4. At one time, physicians were the primary decision-makers in pediatric medical care (patriarchal model). More recently, shared decision-making has become most often viewed as ideal.[20] This model encourages parents to consider the wishes of their child and to receive the guidance of their child's palliative care team to make the most optimal decision for the care of their child.[4,21,22] Shared decision-making requires appropriate and concise communication with parents and patients to achieve the most effective patient care.[21]

5. The ill child's developmental age requires medical providers and psychosocial practitioners to employ communication, interventions, and treatments that are age appropriate.[22,23]

6. Because children who use palliative care services live in the context of a family, addressing the family's needs helps support and care for the ill child.[6,23] Communication is the mechanism used to maintain dialogue and intervene with families.

7. The death of an adult, especially in the last third of life, is "expected" and, although painful to families, is generally more accepted than the death of a child.[24] When the time comes that purely palliative measures are the best options for ill children, communication becomes a key part of allowing families to make meaning of what for many seems tragic and "unnatural."[23]

8. Children cannot legally consent to treatment or make binding medical decisions; their parents and caregivers become their surrogate decision-makers. This can create complex communication and ethical challenges.[25]

Understanding these differences is foundational to being able to offer comprehensive and effective care to children with life-threatening illnesses and their families. Although pediatric palliative care and adult palliative care have many commonalities, ill children and their families truly do need specialized treatments, care, and communication.

Pediatric Palliative Care Needs

Family Support Needs

As noted, pediatric palliative care should not be limited to the patient alone but should promote a patient- and family-centered approach that provides assessment and care for parents, siblings, and the ill child.[4,6] Families of children with serious illness face unique challenges, including reorganization of family roles, coping with the trauma of their child's diagnosis, and both anticipatory and actual losses.[26] Family is impacted when care for the child affects marital/partnered relationships[27] and emotionally impacts siblings.[27,28] Cost of medical care and wages lost to care (time off work, reducing work hours) cause financial stress on families,[29] while the physical demands of care-giving and stress itself take a negative toll on parents' (especially mothers') physical and mental health.[27,30] In addition to caring for their ill children, families whose children are at the end of their lives have the added tasks of making the most difficult decisions about artificial hydration and feeding, life-prolonging treatments, and whether or not to allow for natural death[21] at a time that may feel anything but natural. In order to provide good and effective palliative care to the child, the interdisciplinary team must include both medical and behavioral healthcare providers who can support and care for the family and child.[6,26]

Providing this type of care requires pediatric palliative care providers to attend to three consensus-based principles: (a) respect for the child and the family, (b) understanding the family as part of the care team, and (c) effectively and compassionately caring for the child and his or her family from diagnosis through death and bereavement. Quality communication allows members of healthcare teams, including physicians, social workers, nurses, chaplains, child life specialists, psychologists, and others, to address these aims most effectively.[31]

Communication Needs

Parents voice that good communication is integral to good care.[6,10] Exchange of information, treatment and symptom management options, end-of-life decisions, caring, patient improvement, and patient decline are all conveyed through communication. The informational content exchanged between parent and healthcare provider composes the *what* of communication. In addition, the tone, language, style, and cultural sensitivity of the communication compose the *how*, and both aspects are important to quality communication. Based on research and consensus, Feudtner organizes the tasks that need to be achieved by the palliative care team into three groups:[31]

1. Problem-solving and decision-making activities such as identifying and describing the problems that confront the patient and family. This includes clarifying the goals and hopes that motivate and guide care and evaluating the pros and cons of a variety of options.

2. Interventions typically used to improve the quality of life and minimize suffering for patients, family members, and clinical staff. They address the physical, mental, emotional, social cultural, spiritual, and existential needs of the individual.

3. Logistical efforts that aim to provide high-quality services in various settings, including the hospital and home, the coordination of these services, and the arrangement of appropriate payment.

Using these three domains, we can frame the communication needs of healthcare providers and children with life-threatening illnesses and their families. The remainder of this chapter focuses primarily on providing communication information, challenges, and strategies from the perspectives of parents, clinicians, and patients to address these three areas:

- Problem-solving and decision-making
- Assessing for and implementing interventions
- Managing logistical efforts

Bringing Children and Adolescents Into Conversations

Although evidence has existed for some time that children and adolescents benefit socially and emotionally from being invited into discussions about their medical prognoses, diagnoses, trajectories of illness, and treatments, some parents and some healthcare providers still hesitate to give them a primary role in the management of their health or a meaningful voice in decision-making. Healthcare providers highly rate family opinions as impacting their clinical decision-making; however, the child is often seen as part of the familial aggregate and not a separate or predominant voice, potentially leading children and adolescents to be marginalized in their own care.[32] Reasons given by parents and healthcare providers for excluding children and adolescents from discussion include fear of destroying the child's hope or damaging the child psychologically; not wanting to burden the child with medical information, prognosis, medical decisions, or diagnosis;[33] the child not having the cognitive ability to understand medical concepts and options for treatment;[34] and being concerned that the child would make "wrong" choices about his or her care.[34]

Research offers evidence that ameliorates many of the concerns expressed by parents and healthcare providers. Studies indicate that children with serious illness desire involvement in decision-making and conversations about their health.[32,35] Even more, children and adolescents who take part in discussions about their care, including diagnosis, prognosis, treatments, and decision-making, have better social and emotional outcomes, especially related to anxiety and depression, than those for whom engagement has been limited.[34]

Logistical issues (such as time constraints), parents' concern with the appropriateness of a child's presence in meetings (e.g., a child being in a care conference with several specialists) or the parents' desire to "protect" the child from information that they may deem too burdensome may compel parents to take on the role of "communication broker," acting as the mediator of information between the healthcare provider and the child.[36,37] Research shows that parents acting in this role both facilitate and inhibit communication between the child and the healthcare provider.[36] For their part, children do value aspects of this arrangement, knowing that parents can act as buffers for information that is indeed too cumbersome or that they feel does not specifically involve them.[36] This outlook corresponds with several other studies in non-US or Western Europe contexts, which reveal that, for particular parts of communication, family filters may be culturally expected and desired by healthcare providers, patients, and family.[38] Although many parents value direct, developmentally appropriate communications between healthcare providers and child,[37] in some cases of communication brokering, parents may want to limit communication to minors for personal or cultural reasons.[38] In these scenarios, the parents' authority should be respected, and they should be permitted to filter communication in ways they feel are most fitting to their family's cultural beliefs and practices. The palliative care team may also employ strategies to negotiate with parents, encourage truth-telling, and encourage future communications with the child.[39] These strategies include

1. Ally with the parent in expressing the desire for what is best for the child.[22]

2. Educate the parents about research that shows that children often know of the bad news, including if they are dying, even when they are not explicitly told, and anxiety in children may increase when they are left without information, leaving them to imagine what is wrong.[34]

3. Encourage parents by telling them that the team will help share news with the child, be present when the news is discussed, and help them choose the best words to tell their child difficult news.[39]

4. Devise a plan with the parents that allows the child to be told the diagnosis, prognosis, and other information as the treatment proceeds or the illness progresses. This should be customized according to the child's questions or at signs of increased stress in the child.[22,39]

5. Reassure the parent that he or she is a "good parent" who obviously cares deeply for his or her child.[40]

Efforts to communicate with children about their illness honors the ethical principles of truth-telling and respecting patient autonomy. Children often know more about their illness and prognosis than adults realize. Children have a right and a desire to make sense or find meaning in their living, their suffering, and their potential death. If families and healthcare providers do not communicate with children in compassionate, developmentally appropriate, and honest ways, then they inhibit children from being a part of their own journey. Far from protecting them, preventing children from engaging in information, discussion, and meaning-making actually isolates them.

Talking with Children and Adolescents

Communication with children depends on understanding the social, relational, cultural, developmental, and emotional factors that may affect each child's understanding and beliefs about his or her illness.[41] It is important to remember that the appropriateness of communication is based on developmental (not chronological) age. When talking about illness, the *Oxford Textbook of Palliative Care for Children* makes several suggestions, as outlined in Table 27.1.[41]

The interdisciplinary team members can be very helpful in communicating with children in developmentally appropriate ways. Social workers, child life specialists, and psychologists all have specific training and skills in communicating with children directly about their illness and helping them understand what is happening to their bodies and their lives.

Problem-Solving and Decision-Making

Parents and guardians of children with serious illness are their children's surrogate medical decision-makers. Types of decisions that family members of children with life-threatening illness may be asked to assist in making include whether to continue chemotherapy or other potentially curative treatments when there is little hope of successful outcome, whether to intubate or whether to extubate a child who has already been put on ventilation, whether to begin or discontinue artificial hydration and nutrition, whether to allow a child to undergo surgery for placement of a tracheostomy or feeding tube, and whether to allow the child to undergo other invasive surgical interventions.

Parents are asked to make these decisions at the same time they are potentially grieving, trying to cope with the everyday tasks of caring for their ill child, working, attending to the normal concerns of living, and accounting for incremental losses in their child's function or prognosis. This medical decision-making role affects parents in many ways, including increasing stress, worry, and decisional regret. However, greater parent participation in decision-making also affects good outcomes for the child, including potentially improved care.[25] Shared decision-making that encourages meaningful participation by healthcare providers and parents can decrease uncertainty and allow for greater expression of parent and child preferences.

Parent Communication in Decision-Making

Research suggests that parents may make decisions based on several factors. Previous experience with disease,[42] growing understanding of the disease trajectory combined with ambiguity around the success of the treatment options presented,[25] and provider recommendations all influence the decision that parents will make regarding the comfort and care of their ill child.[42] In addition, parents place high importance on the child's quality of

Table 27.1 Recommendations for Talking About Illness

Dos	Don'ts
♦ Listen first	♦ Do not equate age with understanding
♦ Take cues from the child	♦ Do not regard the concepts of disease or death as fixed
♦ Take stock of your own beliefs and anxieties	♦ Do not assume that children do not know about death/are not aware of the signs just because they do not verbalize their knowledge or awareness
♦ Talk in terms that the child can understand	
♦ Be concrete	♦ Do not use euphemisms or overly complicated explanations
♦ Pace your explanation	♦ Do not make explanations about what the child is asking
♦ Elicit clarifying information before responding to the child's questions	♦ Do not assume that one conversation will be enough
♦ Ask the child to repeat back what has been said, in order to make sure that he or she has understood it	♦ Do not say what you do not believe
	♦ Do not be afraid to say "I don't know."
♦ Share literature for children appropriate to the situation at hand	
♦ Consider using creative activities such as drawing, painting, storytelling, and puppet shows to help to facilitate discussions	
♦ Reassure the child that he or she is loved, will be cared for, and will not be abandoned	
♦ Be honest	

Source: Oxford Textbook of Palliative Care for Children.[13]

life, his or her neurologic prognosis, and their perception of the child's pain and suffering.[43]

The type of language used by parents can give clues as to the decisions that they will make. In one study, heuristic features in a parent's speech supported decision-making by offering greater understanding, clarity, ease of communication, a decision-making compass, and choice selection.[44] Examples of heuristic devices used by parents in palliative conversations could include "We need to fight," "I want to give my child a chance," or "It's in God's hands." These phrases should not be viewed as contrived expressions but as opportunities to extend conversations and to explore and problem-solve difficult situations and decision-making scenarios. Providers should listen for the language that parents use and reflect that back in their communication but not impose their own definitions on the situation.

As professionals, members of palliative care teams may favor a "rational" discussion of burdens versus benefits of any one particular treatment or intervention (or the cessation of these) to the child. However, parents may not make decisions based on belief or thought alone. Parents may employ more complex decision-making pathways, including emotions and feelings.[45] In particular, expression of "hopes," may serve as a helpful synthesis for thoughts and feelings about current and future scenarios in the lives of their children,[46] allowing for hopeful thinking to be a pathway of decision-making for parents of children with life-threatening illness. Healthcare providers can make use of these influences by providing space for emotional content in conversations and by asking about and affirming feelings and emotions within the context of decision-making and problem-solving.[45]

Pediatric Palliative Care Team Communication: Facilitating Parent Decision-Making

Parents in decision-making roles find three aspects of communication with healthcare providers to be especially helpful: *affirmation, information, and discussion*. Healthcare providers' acknowledging the reasonableness of the parent's choice and offering verbal reassurances communicates affirmation that helps parents not only to make decisions but to cope afterward with the decisions they have made. Access to clear and accurate information is often mentioned in studies as affecting parents in their decision-making. In one study, healthcare professionals' verbal reassurance and providing adequate information predicted overall satisfaction of parents with the decision-making experience.[47] Inversely, in another study, too little information was negatively associated with parents' decision-making competence.[48] Parents are helped (or expressed that they *will* be helped) by choices or options being communicated to them,[9,48–50] and parents expect that healthcare providers will be available to engage in discussions about the decision(s) to be made.[5,51]

Decision-making tools may be used to assist the family and team in framing specific questions about social needs and context, burdens versus benefits of interventions, goals of care, family hopes, and the child's wishes. Ross Hays, a physician at Seattle Children's Hospital has developed the Decision-Making Tools)[52] to be used by general pediatric providers, as well as those on palliative care teams. The protocols for its use and a pdf of the tool can be found at http://www.promotingexcellence.org/tools/pe4824.html.

Assessing For and Implementing Interventions

Anticipatory Guidance

Anticipatory guidance may mean different things based on the illness of the child and the communication needs of the family. For some, this guidance may include describing future conditions that may develop as part of the trajectory of the child's illness and the treatments or intervention options that might be used in the eventuality that those conditions develop. For instance, a child with severe cerebral palsy, who is nonambulatory, may be at risk of developing recurrent aspiration pneumonia.[41] As the child progresses in age and in his or her disease, information regarding potential risks to the child developing infection should be communicated to the parent, and choices that may become an option during that time should be explored. In this instance, the parents might be told that their child is at risk of recurrent infection from aspiration. This could lead to discussions about the use of feeding tubes, tracheostomy, and ventilation, as needed, depending on where the child is in the course of illness.

In the same way, a child who is at a later stage of respiratory illness may already be facing end-stage illness and may have already utilized normal treatment courses, including frequent antibiotics, supplemental oxygen, and numerous hospitalizations.[41] Anticipatory guidance, in this case, may include describing the likelihood of the development of further respiratory symptoms, such as further dyspnoea, pain, noisy secretions, psychosocial issues,[41] and the discussion of burdens versus benefits, goals of care, and wishes of the child for end of life.

Each of these conversations, although different in content, requires that the healthcare provider use a team approach, enlisting the expertise of child life specialists, nurses, social workers, psychologists, physicians, and others to comprehensively address the different facets of living that are impacted for the child and family. As with all of pediatric palliative care, anticipatory guidance is more than a medical issue; it encompasses social, emotional, and spiritual domains of care as well.

Information, Information, Information: Delivering What Parents Need and Want

Whether it is news of first diagnosis, prognosis, discharge orders, or possible side effects, parents of children with life-threatening illness are asked to hear, digest, and retain masses of information. The way that information is delivered is incredibly important to parental outlook and to supporting a therapeutic relationship between parents and healthcare providers.[37,53] People want their information in different ways. Some people find that more information in illness allows them to exert more control, reducing the uncertainty in a situation. For these people, information may act as an instrument for coping. However, others want no information or limited information.[54] Although some parents find certain types of information upsetting and may even seek to limit it, most parents want more medical information[55] about their child's illness. In addition, parents want information that is timely and linguistically and culturally accessible.

Specific Communication Strategies

Because of the difficult decisions that parents need to make and because difficult news must be delivered, parents want to be able to trust the communication and information they are receiving from their healthcare providers. Part of that trust comes when the provider is able to communicate information and promote discussion in ways that are most accessible and useful to the parent. This may include presenting the information at a particular time, in a particular language, or using a particular style (i.e., directive versus nondirective). Subtleties in communication such as showing respect (calling an infant by name) or cultural humility (avoiding the use of culturally bound metaphors when giving descriptions or information) allow parents to participate in the decision-making process more fully and with greater feelings of competence[9,50] and allows for clearer communication between all members of the palliative care team.

Managing Logistical Efforts

Continuity of care is essential to caring for children with life-threatening conditions. According to a study undertaken by Heller and Solomon, assuring continuity of care requires that healthcare providers attend to three areas of care and communication.[56]

1. *Informational continuity* guarantees that a medical history and history of prior events, along with the patient's and family's values, preferences, and social context, are clearly and consistently related to all providers involved in patient care.

2. *Relational continuity* promotes knowing the patient and family as people and as a system by acknowledging that the well-being of each individual in the family has the potential to affect every other individual in the family system.

3. *Management continuity* ensures that care is planned, timely, and complementary. This requires that healthcare providers communicate not only with child and family but with other specialists, as they create plans of care that are seamless, disease-appropriate, and implementable.

Care Conferences and Rounding With Families

Care conferences may contribute to continuity of care and clarification of the care plan and treatment options. In some studies, parents do not prefer care conferences to other routine communication that they have with healthcare providers, but they do recognize that care conferences offer a venue for achieving particular decision-making goals, including "discussing treatment limitations" and "discussing repercussions of decisions made."[51] In a different study about families "rounding" with medical teams, the communication that is regarded as most beneficial is that which most engages parents in dialogue. As the care team learns more about the needs and routines of the child through family-centered, multidisciplinary rounds, decisions on care and plans were affected by parent communication and engagement in 90% of interactions.[57] These studies offer evidence that care conferences and rounding with medical teams offer parents venues for conversation that positively affect and support communication between families and healthcare providers.[51,57]

Specific Populations and Communication Needs

Palliative Care in Neonatal and Perinatal Care

Palliative care in perinatal and neonatal care is distinct from pediatric care in several notable ways. Perinatal palliative care is often delivered at a time when families were expecting a "healthy" or "normal" birth and can be incongruent with the typical expectations of a joyful arrival of a newborn.[58] The birth of a child with a congenital anomaly or life-limiting condition may come as a shock to the family and cause an immediate sense of fear and confusion. High-tech interventions exist that help sustain and continue life in the neonate population, but this raises many ethical dilemmas and opportunities for communication with families. Family-centered care in neonatal care is increasingly important due to the growth in diversity of this population, their extended needs for complex care, and the intricate decision-making required. Familial distress and lack of confidence and support in caring for their children during this time are additional reasons necessitating family-centered care.[59] Perinatal palliative care may be delivered after the prenatal diagnosis of a lethal or life-limiting condition or may occur after diagnosis at birth. Palliative care can also be provided following unsuccessful attempts at curative treatment of a severe medical problem. Palliative care in this setting may last a few hours, weeks, or potentially years, depending on the condition. Providing neonatal palliative care involves working closely with families to understand their unique needs and helping them find meaning in their child's life, even if it is brief.

Despite recent medical advances, deaths in the first year of life are still the leading number of childhood deaths in the United States.[11,12] Neonatal and perinatal healthcare practitioners must become adept at working with families to honor their child's life, reduce suffering, and collaboratively make decisions. Integrating palliative care principles into this care involves true partnership with families. As with older children, the goals of care include helping the family make the best possible decision in a supported environment while minimizing distress in the child.

In a recent survey of pediatric palliative care programs in the United States, Feudtner et al. found that 90% of programs surveyed reported covering neonates and 53.5% provided prenatal consultation.[60] However, there was a wide variety of models and staffing levels in these programs. While there have been increasing efforts toward family-centered care in neonatal intensive care units (NICU), many parents express dissatisfaction with healthcare provider–parent communication, parent involvement, availability of information, and transitions of care.[61,62] Parents of babies in the NICU demonstrate high levels of psychological distress.[63] Clearly, communication and family-centered care are necessary for supporting parents and children in the NICU.[59]

Healthcare practitioners have an ethical duty to care for the family in pediatric palliative care, including during the perinatal and neonatal period.[6] Members of the interdisciplinary team, including physicians, nurses, and social workers, can be trained in effective and compassionate communication strategies to reduce suffering in families as they face these difficult decisions.[59]

Recommendations for improving family support in the NICU include communication training for NICU staff, parental participation in decision-making, parent presence and participation in caregiving, parent-to-parent connection, psychological support when an infant dies, and transition to home support.[59] Parents report that the most important aspects of care are open and honest communication, sharing of information and the meaning of this information, involvement in decision-making, healthcare provider–parent partnerships, and policies and programs that promote parenting skills and family involvement.[59] Various studies have shown the benefits of family-centered care, including communication, in neonatal care. Family-centered communication strategies appear to improve parental well-being, parental satisfaction, and staff satisfaction.[59]

Palliative Care for Adolescents and Their Families

Providing palliative care to adolescents and their families also requires healthcare practitioners to use communication strategies that respond to the needs of this population.[64] Adolescence is a time of growing maturity, capacity, identity development, personal growth, and exploration.[64] Adolescents are old enough developmentally to make their own decisions and to contemplate the spiritual and psychological aspects of their illness and impending death but do not have the legal status to make their own decisions.[22,64] Even though parents and guardians are the legal decision-makers in adolescent care, healthcare practitioners are ethically obligated to include adolescents in their care decisions. This can create communication challenges for the healthcare team as they try to help adolescents and families facing end of life.

In order to support adolescents, practitioners must communicate with both the young person and his or her family and assess for any points of disagreement or discomfort.[65] Specifically, when working with adolescents, healthcare practitioners must earn and maintain trust in order to best elicit feelings and support their concerns.[66] According to the American Academy of Pediatrics, pediatric palliative care providers should "facilitate clear, compassionate, and forthright discussions with (pediatric) patients and families about therapeutic goals and concerns, the benefits and burdens of specific therapies, and the value of advance care planning."[67] (p. 966) Parents are sometimes concerned about "being honest" with their child at the end of life. Typically, adolescents have very strong opinions about their treatment and palliative care and need to be included in all decision-making. They may, however, attempt to protect their parents or providers and be reticent to share their true wishes. Conversely, they may openly disagree with either their parents or their healthcare providers. Providers should create opportunities for the adolescent to voice his or her desires. Based on their growing autonomy and independence, adolescents express that they want and need: informed control in decisions about their care, structured dialogues with their family and healthcare team about medical decisions, and opportunities for expression of psychological and spiritual concerns.[68,69]

When adolescents are facing end of life, they need communication strategies that elicit and honor their wishes and values.[64,65] It is critical to ask questions such as: "What is most important to you?" "What do you hope to be able to do?" "How can we best support you in meeting these goals?" "What is the hardest part about this treatment?" "Is there some part of care or treatment that is simply too much for you right now?" "What do you want most?" Specific tools, such as Voicing my Choices©, have been developed to assist adolescents and their families communicate their preferences.[68,70] All of these strategies can facilitate communication with adolescents about their end-of-life care preferences.

Areas in Need of Improvement

Despite many advances in family-centered care and collaborative communication in pediatric palliative care, there are still areas for improvement.

- Palliative care can and should be introduced early in the diagnosis of a perinatal or childhood illness. Palliative care can occur simultaneously with curative treatments and offers opportunities for decision-making and preparation before a crisis.
- Perinatal and neonatal palliative care initiatives must continue to be developed that recognize the trauma of receiving a lethal or life-limiting diagnosis before, during, or after birth. The incongruence of expectations of birth and the reality of severe illness or death create unique challenges for these families.
- Adolescents need to be involved and informed in their medical decision-making. Healthcare providers should strive to have private and exhaustive conversations with adolescents and their families about their palliative care needs.
- Interdisciplinary teams that include both medical and behavioral healthcare providers should be used to assist children and families in palliative care. Social workers, child life specialists, psychologists, psychiatrists, and art therapists can all help the interprofessional team facilitate communication.
- All providers need training and ongoing education in family-centered communication strategies.
- Healthcare teams should work from a stance of cultural humility and awareness and pay specific attention to the differing meanings of illness, childhood, death, and bereavement across cultures.
- Funding streams should support healthcare providers in having meaningful conversations with children and family.

Conclusion

Pediatric palliative care providers offer comprehensive care for the child and family within their cultural and familial context. Communication is a key to relationship-building that will allow the child and family to be heard, supported, and helped throughout their care. Palliative care practitioners must listen to the child's and family's needs, support and partner with children and families in problem-solving and decision-making, assess child and family needs moment to moment, implement culturally relevant and child- and family-focused interventions, and be prepared to have multiple conversations in order to ultimately reduce suffering and enhance quality of life. Healthcare providers are encouraged to communicate with humility, effectively share information in the way the family has requested, and co-create care and treatment plans through conversation and dialogue. Communication is greater than a collaborative exercise. It is the means to good pediatric palliative care. It is the foundation upon which parents build trust and the ability to act as decision-maker with and on their child's behalf during the incredibly difficult time of their child's illness and death.

References

1. Bogetz JF, Ullrich CK, Berry JG. Pediatric hospital care for children with life-threatening illness and the role of palliative care. *Pediatr Clin N Am*. 2014;61(4):719–733.
2. Zhukovsky DS, Herzog CE, Kaur G, Palmer JL, Bruera E. The impact of palliative care consultation on symptom assessment, communication needs, and palliative interventions in pediatric patients with cancer. *J Palliat Med*. 2009;12(4):343–349.

3. World Health Organization. WHO definition of palliative care for children. http://www.who.int/cancer/palliative/definition/en/. Accessed June 19, 2014.
4. Committee on Hospital Care and Institute for Patient- and Family-Centered Care. Patient-and family-centered care and the pediatrician's role. *Pediatrics.* 2012;129(2):394–404.
5. Carnevale FA. Understanding the private worlds of physicians, nurses, and parents: A study of life-sustaining treatment decision in Italian paediatric critical care. *J Child Health Care.* 2011;15(4):334–349.
6. Jones B, Contro N, Koch K. The duty of physicians to care for the family in pediatric palliative care: Context, communication, and caring. *Pediatrics.* 2014;133(Suppl 1):S8–S15.
7. Mack JW, Wolfe J, Cook EF, Grier HE, Cleary PD, Weeks JC. Parents' roles in decision making for children with cancer in the first year of cancer treatment. *J Clin Oncol.* 2011;29(15):2085–2090.
8. Kassam A, Skiadaresis J, Habib S, Alexander S, Wolfe J. Moving toward quality palliative cancer care: Parent and clinician perspectives on gaps between what matters and what is accessible. *J Clin Oncol.* 2013;31(7):910–915.
9. Caeymaex L, Speranza M, Vasilescu C, et al. Living with a crucial decision: A qualitative study of parental narratives three years after the loss of their newborn in the NICU. *PLoS One.* 2011;6(12):e28633.
10. Nelson JE. In their own words: Patients and families define high-quality palliative care in the intensive care unit. *Crit Care Med.* 2010;38(3):808–818.
11. Centers for Disease Control and Prevention. US Child Mortality Data, 2010. Injury Prevention & Control: Data & Statistics (WISQARS™). http://www.cdc.gov/injury/wisqars/.
12. Murphy S, Xu J, Kochanek K. *Deaths: Final data for 2010.* Washington, DC: US Department of Health and Human Services; 2013.
13. Davies B. Siden H, Children in Palliative Medicine. In: Hanks G, Cherny N, Christakis N, Fallon M, Kaasa S, Portenoy R, eds. *Oxford Textbook of Palliative Medicine.* 4th ed. Oxford: Oxford University Press; 2010:1301–1317.
14. Feudtner C, Kang T, Hexem K, et al. Pediatric palliative care patients: A prospective multicenter cohort study. *Pediatrics.* 2011;127(6):1094–1101.
15. Blencowe H, Say L, Lawn JE, et al. National, regional, and worldwide estimates of preterm birth rates in the year 2010 with time trends since 1990 for selected countries: A systematic analysis and implications. *Lancet.* 2012;379(9832):2162–2172.
16. Tennant P, Pearce M, Bythell M, Rankin J. 20-year survival of children born with congenital anomalies: A population-based study. *Lancet.* 2010;375:649–656.
17. Cohen E, Kuo D, Agrawal R, et al. Children with medical complexity: An emerging population for clinical research initiatives. *Pediatrics.* 2011;127(3):529–538.
18. Lindley LC. Healthcare reform and concurrent curative care for terminally ill children: A policy analysis. *J Hosp Palliat Nurs.* 2011;13(2):81–88.
19. Knapp CA. Research in pediatric palliative care: Closing the gap between what is and is not known. *Am J Hospice Palliat Med.* 2009;26(5):392–398.
20. Feuz C. Shared decision making in palliative cancer care: A literature review. *J Radiother Pract.* 2014;13(3):340–349.
21. Fiks AG, Jimenez ME. The promise of shared decision-making in paediatrics. *Acta Paediatr.* October 2010;99(10):1464–1466.
22. Bluebond-Langner M, Belasco J, Wander M. "I want to live, until I don't want to live anymore": Involving children with life-threatening and life-shortening illnesses in decision making about care and treatment. *Nurs Clin N Am.* 2010;45:329–343.
23. Papadatou D. Training health professionals in caring for dying children and grieving families. *Death Studies.* 1997;21(6):575–600.
24. Hendrickson KC. Morbidity, mortality, and parental grief: A review of the literature on the relationship between the death of a child and the subsequent health of parents. *Palliat Support Care.* 2009;7(1):109–119.
25. Nelson KE, Mahant S. Shared decision-making about assistive technology for the child with severe neurologic impairment. *Pediatr Clin N Am.* 2014;61(4):641–652.
26. Jones B. The challenge of quality care for family caregivers in pediatric cancer care. *Semin Oncol. Nurs.* 2012;28(4):213–220.
27. Whiting M. Impact, meaning and need for help and support: The experience of parents caring for children with disabilities, life limiting/life-threatening illness or technology dependence. *J Child Health Care.* 2012;17(1):92–108.
28. Knapp C, Contro N. Family support services in pediatric palliative card. *Am J Hosp Palliat Care.* 2009;26(6):476–482.
29. Bona K, Dussel V, Orellana L, et al. Economic impact of advanced pediatric cancer on families. *J Pain Symptom Manage.* 2014;47(3):594–603.
30. Brehaut JC, Kohen DE, Garner RE, et al. Health among caregivers of children with health problems: Findings from a Canadian population-based study. *Am J Public Health.* 2009;99(7):1254–1262.
31. Feudtner C. Collaborative communication in pediatric palliative care: A foundation for problem-solving and decision making. *Pediatr Clin N Am.* 2007;54:583–607.
32. Wicks L, Mitchell A. The adolescent cancer experience: Loss of control and benefit finding. *Eur J Cancer Care.* 2010;19(6):778–785.
33. Anderzén-Carlsson A, Kihlgren M, Svantesson M, Sorlie V, Institutionen för kliniskt m, Örebro u. Parental handling of fear in children with cancer: Caring in the best interests of the child. *J Petriatr Nurs.* 2010;25(5):317–326.
34. Coyne I, Amory A, Kiernan G, Gibson F. Children's participation in shared decision-making: Children, adolescents, parents and healthcare professionals' perspectives and experiences. *Eur J Oncol Nurs.* 2014;18(3):273–280.
35. Stegenga K, Ward-Smith P. On receiving the diagnosis of cancer: The adolescent perspective. *J Pediatr Oncol Nurs.* 2009;26(2):75–80.
36. Coyne I, Harder M. Children's participation in decision-making: Balancing protection with shared decision-making using a situational perspective. *J Child Health Care.* 2011;15(4):312–319.
37. Zwaanswijk M, Tates K, van Dulmen S, et al. Communicating with child patients in pediatric oncology consultations: A vignette study on child patients', parents', and survivors' communication preferences. *Psycho-Oncology.* 2011;20(3):269–277.
38. Wiener L, Mcconnell D, Latella L, Ludi E. Cultural and religious considerations in pediatric palliative care. *Palliat Support Care.* 2013;11:47–67.
39. Gupta VB, Willert J, Pian M, Stein MT. When disclosing a serious diagnosis to a minor conflicts with family values. *J Dev Behav Pediatr.* 2010;31(3 Suppl):S100–S102.
40. Hinds P, Oakes L, Hicks J, et al. "Trying to be a good parent" as defined by interviews with parents who made phase I, terminal care, and resuscitation decisions for their children. *J Clin Oncol.* 2009;27(35):5979–5985.
41. *Oxford Textbook of Palliative Care for Children.* 2nd ed. New York, NY: Oxford University Press; 2012.
42. Lipstein EA, Brinkman WB, Britto MT. What is known about parents' treatment decisions? A narrative review of pediatric decision making. *Med Decis Making.* March-April 2012;32(2):246–258.
43. Michelson K, Koogler T, Sullivan C, Ortega M, Hall E, Frader J. Parental views on withdrawing life-sustaining therapies in critically ill children. *Arch Pediatr Adolesc Med.* 2009;163(11):986–992.
44. Renjilian CB, Womer JW, Carroll KW, Kang TI, Feudtner C. Parental explicit heuristics in decision-making for children with life-threatening illnesses. *Pediatrics.* 2013;131(2):e566–e542.
45. Feudtner C, Carroll KW, Hexem KR, Silberman J, Kang TI, Kazak AE. Parental hopeful patterns of thinking, emotions, and pediatric palliative care decision making: A prospective cohort study. *Arch Pediatr Adolesc Med.* 2010;164(9):831–839.

46. Reder E, Serwint J. Until the last breath: Exploring the concept of hope for parents and health care professionals during a child's serious illness. *Arch Pediatr Adolesc Med*. 2009;163(7):653–657.
47. McKenna K, Collier J, Hewitt M, Blake H. Parental involvement in paediatric cancer treatment decisions. *Eur J Cancer Care (Engl)*. September 2010;19(5):621–630.
48. Miller V, Nelson R. Factors related to voluntary parental decision-making in pediatric oncology. *Pediatrics*. 2012;129:903–908.
49. Brooten D, Youngblut JM, Seagrave L, et al. Parent's perceptions of health care providers actions around child ICU death: What helped, what did not. *Am J Hosp Palliat Care*. February 2013;30(1):40–49.
50. Lee S-Y, Weiss S. When East meets West: Intensive care unit experiences among first0generation Chinese American parents. *J Nurs Scholarsh*. 2009;41(3):268–275.
51. Michelson KN, Emanuel L, Carter A, Brinkman P, Clayman ML, Frader J. Pediatric intensive care unit family conferences: One mode of communication for discussing end-of-life care decisions. *Pediatr Crit Care Med*. November 2011;12(6):e336–e343.
52. Hays R, Team P. *Promoting Excellence: Decision-Making Tool and Care Plan*. Seattle, WA: Children's Hospital and Regional Medical Center, Pediatric Palliative Care Project.
53. Pantilat S. Communicating with seriously ill patients: Better words to say. *JAMA*. 2009;301(12):1279–1281.
54. Eheman C, Berkowitz Z, Lee J, et al. Information-seeking styles among cancer patients before and after treatment by demographics and use of information sources. *J Health Commun*. 2009;14(5):487–502.
55. Lyon M, Garvie P, McCarter R, Briggs L, He J, D'Angelo L. Who will speak for me? Improving end-of-life decision-making for adolescents with HIV and their families. *Pediatrics*. 2009;123:e199–e206.
56. Heller K, Solomon M. Continuity of care and caring: What matters to parents of children with life-threatening conditions. *J Pediatr Nurs*. 2005;20(5):335–346.
57. Rosen P, Stenger E, Bochkoris M, Hannon M, Kwoh K. Family-centered multidisciplinary rounds enhance the team approach in pediatrics. *Pediatrics*. 2009;123:e603–e608.
58. Toce S, Leuthner S, Dokken D, Catlin A, Brown J, Carter B. Palliative care in the neonatal-perinatal period In: Levetown M, Carter B, Friebert S, eds. *Palliative Care for Infants, Children, and Adolescents—A Practical Handbook*. Baltimore, MD: John's Hopkins University Press; 2011:345–386.
59. JS G, Cooper L, Blaine A, Franck L, Howse J, Berns S. Family support and family-centered care in the neonatal intensive care unit: Origins, advances, impact. *Semin Perinatol*. 2011;35:20–28.
60. Feudtner C, Womer R, Augustin R, et al. Pediatric palliative care programs in children's hospitals: A cross sectional national survey. *Pediatrics*. 2013;132(6):1063–1070.
61. Reis MD, Rempel GR, Scott SD, Brady-Fryer BA, Van Aerde J. Developing nurse/parent relationships in the NICU through negotiated partnership. *J Obstet Gynecol Neonatal Nurs*. 2010;39(6):675–683.
62. Franck L, Axelin A. Differences in parents', nurses', and physicians', views of NICU parent support. *Acta Paediatr*. 2013;102:590–596.
63. Forcada-Guex M, Borghini A, Pierrehumbert B, Ansermet F, Muller-Nix C. Prematurity, maternal posttraumatic stress and consequences on the mother–infant relationship. *Early Hum Dev*. 2011;87(1):21–26.
64. Ajayi T, Linebarger J, Jones B. Transitions in care for adolescents and young adults in palliative care. *Pediatr Clin N Am*. in press.
65. Pritchard S, Cuvelier G, Harlos M, Barr R. Palliative care in adolescents and young adults with cancer. *Cancer*. 2011;117(Suppl 10):2323–2328.
66. Wien S, Pery S, Zer A. Role of palliative care in adolescent and young adult oncology. *J Clin Oncol*. 2010;28:4819–4824.
67. American Academy of Pediatrics Section on Hospice and Palliative Medicine and Committee on Hospital Care. Pediatric palliative care and hospice care commitments, guidelines, and recommendations. *Pediatrics* 2013;132(5):966–972.
68. Wiener Z, Battles B, Ballard O, Pao. Allowing adolescents and young adults to plan their end of life care. *Pediatrics*. 2012;130:897–905.
69. Jones BL. Companionship, control, and compassion: A social work perspective on the needs of children with cancer and their families at the end of life. *J Palliat Med*. 2006;9(3):774–788.
70. Jones B. Palliative Care Needs of Older Children and their Families. In Conversations in Perinatal, Neonatal and Pediatric Palliative Care. Hospice and Palliative Nurses Association. 2012.

CHAPTER 28

Lesbian, Gay, Bisexual, and Transgender Communication

Carey Candrian and Hillary Lum

Introduction

When I was eleven years of age, spending the summer on my grandparents' estate, I used, as often as I could do it unobserved, to steal into the stable and gently stroke the neck of my darling, a broad dapple-gray horse. It was not a casual delight but a great, certainly friendly, but also deeply stirring happening. If I am to explain it now, beginning from the still very fresh memory of my hand, I must say what I experienced in touch with the animal was the Other, the immense otherness of the Other, which, however, did not remain strange like the otherness of the ox and the ram, but rather let me draw near and touch it. When I stroked the mighty mane, sometimes marvelously smooth-combed, at other times just as astonishingly wild, and felt the life beneath my hand, it was as though the element of vitality itself bordered on my skin, something that was not I, was certainly not akin to me, palpably the other, not just the another, really the Other itself; and yet it let me approach, confided itself to me, placed itself elementally in the relation of Thou and Thou with me.[1(pp26-27)]

For Buber, the famous philosopher, the "I-Thou" connectedness described in this quote is a product of interaction, created mutually among individuals in relation to one another.[2] In short, it is a feeling of unity or oneness achieved when attending to the other. Moreover, Buber is not suggesting by "thouness" that every relationship should move toward intimacy and the disclosure or realization of the other's real self but that "realness" of the other resists fixation of meaning that is often prescribed through the act of labeling.[3] When we label someone or something, it is no longer the same. The very act of defining causes clear distinctions in what someone is and is not, how they behave, how we should behave, and even what someone looks like. From a communication perspective, the moment language is used to define an "other" is often the critical moment that precludes authentic conversation and understanding.[3]

This chapter is titled "Lesbian, Gay, Bisexual, Transgender Communication," otherwise known as LGBT. The labels, and the accompanying initials, draw attention to genuine difference and "otherness." We must remember that homosexuality was included in the *Diagnostic and Statistical Manual of Mental Disorders* until 1973.[4] Like Buber and his philosophy on dialogue that is relational and responsive, we share an appreciation of difference and a deep respect of the singularity of the other and his or her unique struggles beyond categories. We also believe that every clinical interaction holds the possibility of either closure or growth, including new meaning, shared understanding, and improved partnership. Dialogue is a process by which patients, families, and physicians engage from their individual perspectives. In so doing, they have the opportunity to communicate productively, to create something new together, rather than reinforce what either one already has or is. The goal of this chapter is to improve communication between LGBT adults living with serious illness, their family of choice, and their healthcare providers with the goal of creating conversations that are inclusive of difference and responsive to the individual's values, goals, and informed choices.

Overview of Nonheterosexual Populations

Although the abbreviation LGBT is commonly used as an umbrella term for identifying the health needs of this community, we cannot overemphasize that within the diverse, larger group of nonheterosexual individuals are several unique populations, each with their own health concerns.[4,5] In this discussion, we draw from available studies and advocacy literature, focusing on palliative care communication needs and strategies and recognizing that current information has limits in its generalizability.

Global population estimates of LGBT persons range between 4% and 10%.[6] According to the American Community Survey of the 2010 US Census, there are over 152,000 same-sex married-couple households among a total of 594,000 same-sex couple households in the United States.[7] Nationally, about 1% of all couple households were same-sex couples. It is estimated that by 2050, LGBT people, ages 65 years and older, will account for 1 of every 13 elders in the United States.[8] Since a majority of health issues appear later in life, the experience and burden of disease faced by older LGBT people will likely be considerably worse, given that they often face ageism, long-term effects of negative social attitudes, sexual stigmatization, overt discrimination, and homophobia when they access the healthcare system.[9] These issues are exemplified through the critically acclaimed documentary film *Gen Silent*, in which filmmaker Stu Maddux follows six LGBT elders who must decide whether to hide their sexuality in order to survive the healthcare system.[10]

Nonheterosexual individuals have the same basic health needs as the general population, although they experience significant health disparities and barriers related to sexual orientation and/or gender identity or expression.[5,11] Many individuals avoid, delay, or receive inappropriate/inferior care, which often translates into a lack of genuine understanding. Furthermore, nonheterosexual individuals have increased substance use and dependence,[12] often attributed to stress from stigmatization, marginalization, or fear of discrimination when disclosing sexual identity. Although healthcare needs are similar across populations, the means of understanding them are different.

To assist nonheterosexual patients, LGBT families of choice, and healthcare providers with meeting the communication needs of these individuals when they face serious illnesses, this chapter (a) summarizes the palliative care needs of this population, (b) describes the communication challenges, (c) highlights communication strategies, and (d) concludes with practical clinical approaches and areas in need of improvement.

Palliative Care Needs of Nonheterosexual Individuals

The goal of this section is to provide an overview of the palliative care needs of sexual minorities who are living with serious illnesses and their families of choice. As already described, these individuals have unique needs and circumstances. In this context, given that the goals of palliative care are to deliver person-centered and family-focused care that assists patients and their significant others in meeting physical, intellectual, emotional, social, and spiritual needs, it is essential that healthcare providers effectively communicate and engage individuals in patient–provider relationships that recognize and accept sexual orientation and identity.

In the context of increased burden of serious illnesses, LGBT persons face significant unmet palliative and end-of-life care needs.[13] A recent systematic review of the palliative care needs, experiences, and preferences of LGBT populations found that the majority of current literature focused on the cancer experience of gay men and lesbian women.[14] Only a few papers had evidence for the bisexual population, and there were no studies on transgender people. In the context of health disparities relating to serious illness, the palliative and end-of-life care needs of sexual minorities and their families of choice include unique considerations relating to advance care planning and decision-making, partner and family caregiver support, and end-of-life care and closure.[15]

Health Disparities Related to Serious Illnesses

LGBT persons experience higher incidences of life-limiting and life-threatening diseases. Disparities in cancer and other life-limiting illnesses have been identified. Lesbians experience a higher risk of obesity and associated secondary outcomes of these conditions, such as type 2 diabetes, coronary heart disease, stroke, osteoarthritis, and breast and colon cancer.[16,17] Furthermore, lesbians have a higher lifetime risk of breast, cervical, and ovarian cancer than heterosexual women.[18,19] HIV infection rates are disproportionately higher among gay, bisexual, and other men who have sex with men; African American and Hispanic men appear to be at particularly high risk.[20] Both HIV infection and long-term antiretroviral therapy have been associated with increased risk of cardiovascular disease, including coronary artery disease, myocardial infarction, peripheral arterial disease, and chronic heart failure.[21] Additionally, gay men with HIV infection or AIDS are also at a higher risk for hepatitis B and hepatitis C coinfection.[22] Gay men have a much higher risk of anal cancer, in addition to the burden of HIV-related cancers.[23,24]

In addition to disparities in chronic medical conditions, including malignancies, there is a growing emphasis on the need to minimize discrimination and increase awareness of the high baseline prevalence and burden of mental health issues among nonheterosexual individuals.[25,26] Existing health disparities may reflect the historical and social context that LGBT persons have experienced. Victimization and discrimination create significant risks in the aging and health of LGBT older adults and their caregiver partners. Over the course of their lifetime, most LGBT older adult participants have faced serious adversity: 82% have been victimized at least once because of their perceived sexual orientation or gender identity, and 64% have been victimized three or more times.[27] Many LGBT adults have encountered discrimination in employment and housing, impacting their economic security. Discrimination experiences are linked with poor health outcomes. Nearly 4 out of 10 LGBT adults have contemplated suicide at some point during their lives.[27]

Of note, there are very few studies regarding the specific experiences of bisexual or transgendered persons and their experience of life-limiting illnesses, though concern for health disparities exists.[5] In fact, there is a greater risk of HIV, breast, and prostate cancer for male-to-female transgender people and higher risk of ovarian, breast, and cervical cancer for female-to-male transgender people.[28-30]

Advance Care Planning and Advance Directives

Nonheterosexual individuals face challenges in developing future medical care plans and including the people whose input would make a difference in decision-making and advance care planning. The inclusion of same-sex partners in decision-making and treatment planning has been shown repeatedly to be a priority for LGBT patients facing life-limiting illness.[14] Those who desire their same-sex partner to be their healthcare representative ("healthcare power of attorney" or "healthcare agent/proxy") must complete an advance directive (AD) formally making such a designation. Without such documentation, a same-sex partner may have limited or no rights regarding the medical decision-making and treatment planning for her or his partner, especially if there has been a history of nonacceptance of the same-sex relationship by the patient's biological family members.[13,31]

One study suggests that while a majority of LGBT patients are knowledgeable about ADs and the identification of healthcare proxies, only 49% of those who desire a same-sex partner to be their surrogate decision-maker have completed the necessary documentation.[31] Providers are encouraged to educate patients about the importance of completing such documentation so that their medical and end-of-life wishes may be met. State-specific legal recognition of same-sex marriage is expanding in the United States. However, even legally married LGBT individuals who want their partner to be their surrogate decision-maker are still advised to complete legal ADs to provide clear documentation.

For instance, a legal AD may help promote the recognition of the surrogate decision-maker partner, especially if the individual is hospitalized while traveling in a state that does not recognize the legality of their marriage. Additional ethical considerations relating to palliative and end-of-life care for LGBT individuals have been described elsewhere.[32]

Effective advance care planning should include an open and inclusive medical decision-making process. In a qualitative study involving gay men and lesbian women with cancer, partners were important to the patients' decision-making, with a preference for involvement from the time of diagnosis.[33] Additionally, lesbian women with cancer experienced a heterosexually biased environment and desired their partners to be included in decision-making and treatment planning. This study highlighted the importance of open communication between patients, families of choice, and healthcare providers for more holistic, patient-centered care.[34] Providers who are involved in assisting with decision-making may consider inquiring about whether a patient's biological family knows that a patient's legally designated surrogate decision-maker is the patient's LGBT partner. Strategizing with the patient on how to proactively communicate this may help avoid conflicts, especially when it is not clear that sexual orientation is known among family members. For instance, as discussed in chapter 35, advance care planning conversations in the context of HIV/AIDS may involve a first-time disclosure of sexual orientation.

An emphasis on the location and nature of care in the context of advance care planning has been reported. In a study of older gay and lesbian caregivers, the majority of patients had completed ADs mainly to protect themselves and their caregiver partner from biological family members and professionals who might otherwise disregard their advance care planning and care preferences.[35] For instance, because care in a long-term care facility is often associated with fear of stigmatization and harassment, LGBT persons may specifically discuss and document their wishes to avoid care in certain healthcare settings.

Partner and Family Involvement and Support

LGBT persons with serious illnesses may have a different definition of "family" compared to heterosexual persons. LGBT families of choice are more likely to include same-sex partners and friends rather than biological family members.[36] LGBT elders are less likely to have had children than their heterosexual peers; those who do are less likely to receive care from their adult children.[5] Moreover, LGBT patients may receive support from unique social circles, sometimes referred to as "lavender families" or "families of choice," with whom they find acceptance.[37] These LGBT families of choice may be comprised of heterosexual friends, other members of the LGBT community, coworkers, and biological relatives, all of whom may provide support at the end of life.[13] The United Kingdom's National End of Life Care Strategy discussed potential consequences of lack of openness and discussion of death and dying. Specifically, where same-sex partners have not discussed their relationship status, healthcare professionals may subsequently exclude the partner's involvement in the patient's care.[38] The challenges that LGBT persons face in disclosure of sexual identity and recognition of same-sex partners, including the healthcare providers' responses to the presence of same-sex partners, is discussed in the next section.

Looking beyond the individual's support system, there is also a lack of formal support groups for gay and lesbian individuals, which are often a mainstay of patient and family-focused support in malignancy and other chronic illnesses (i.e., progressive neurologic diseases). In a qualitative study of gay and lesbian individuals with cancer, participants highlighted the lack of support groups for lesbian/gay people and the difficulty of disclosing their personal life experiences in heterosexual support groups.[33] Moreover, a study of lesbian and heterosexual women with newly diagnosed breast cancer found that lesbian women were more likely to receive support from their partners and friends.[39]

End-of-Life Care and Closure

In working with terminal patients, providers should be able to assist patients in activities such as reflecting on their life and events. Thus palliative care providers should be aware of potential experiences of hostility and discrimination during the patient's life and be willing to provide direct support and connection to counseling if requested. The end-of-life period can be a time of reunion and reconciliation with estranged family and friends; this may be especially true for LGBT patients who may have experienced isolation from these individuals in the past due to their sexual orientation.[13] Providers should be sensitive to potentially complex family and social dynamics that reunions can create for both the patient and his or her partner. For instance, a patient's biological family may initiate some reconciliation with a patient but in a way that denies the role of the same-sex partner or LGBT family of choice. Additionally, when such reunions do not occur, feelings of grief, loss, and abandonment experienced by an LGBT individual at the end of life may be magnified.

Not surprisingly, partners facing the loss of their same-sex loved one may experience disenfranchised grief—grief that is not acknowledged or viewed as legitimate, owing to the relationship not being fully recognized by the patient's biological family or community.[40,41] Such disenfranchisement may limit the partner's ability to grieve openly, resulting in a lack of bereavement support from healthcare professionals and worsening feelings of isolation.[13,42] Palliative care, hospice, and primary care providers should be attuned to this when monitoring the grief reaction of a newly widowed partner and proactively offer bereavement support services as indicated.

Communication Challenges

When caring for nonheterosexual persons, it is important to explore sexual preferences, avoid heterosexist assumptions, recognize the importance of partners in decision-making, and foster genuine understanding and opportunities for relationships.[14] There is a significant need for palliative care providers to acknowledge the patient's identity and provide an open, nonjudgmental environment. To accomplish this, palliative care providers need to acknowledge potential discrimination in staff, address and ensure sensitive assessment, and recognize that meaningful relationships in healthcare are not just founded on technically appropriate transactions but on what providers say (content skills), how providers communicate and relate to patients (process skills), and what providers are thinking, including the feelings, attitudes, biases, assumptions, and intentions (perceptual skills) that enter into and structure the interaction.[41] If providers fail to have an open discussion with the patient about sexuality, patients are less likely to reveal their sexuality, and care of the whole person is compromised.

Past negative reactions or instances of discrimination may affect an LGBT patient's decision to disclose and discuss his or her sexual orientation with healthcare providers. For example, a study of gay and lesbian caregivers of persons with dementia revealed three strategies related to disclosure communication: active disclosure, passive disclosure, and passive nondisclosure (i.e., patients neither revealed their sexuality nor claimed a heterosexual identity).[43] According to a comprehensive 2011 survey conducted in partnership with Services and Advocacy for GLBT Elders and funded by the National Institutes of Health and the National Institute on Aging, more than one-fifth of LGBT older adults surveyed said they had not reported their sexual orientation or gender identity to their primary physician.[44] Given that sexual orientation is an important part of an individual's personhood and social history, its recognition and acceptance by healthcare providers is essential to the provision of holistic and patient-centered palliative care. Additionally, an appreciation of a patient's sexuality and sexual orientation is especially pertinent to end-of-life care, given the importance of assisting patients in reviewing and reflecting on their life.[13]

Communication Strategies

Consider the following case scenario that introduces the palliative care needs, communication challenges, and strategies relevant to nonheterosexual individuals who face serious illnesses:

Julie, a 72-year-old white male-to-female transgender woman who had a history of congestive heart failure, suffered a hip fracture after falling at home. Surgical repair of the hip fracture was complicated by postoperative respiratory failure requiring several days of mechanical ventilation, Clostridium difficile infection, and delirium. Prior to admission, Julie had lived alone and used a walker for ambulation, and her partner of 15 years, Mark, lived a few miles away. Julie had four adult children including a local daughter whom Mark described as "being in an elevator that only goes down," suggesting the daughter had her own challenges.

During her hospitalization, Julie was transferred to the medical floor where she was assessed by physical therapy and occupational therapy and recommended for subacute rehabilitation. However, she clearly expressed a desire for comfort-oriented care with hospice and asked to speak with the palliative care consult team. Initially, Mark continued to urge Julie to participate in therapy. The palliative care team met with Julie and facilitated completion of an advance directive, where Julie chose Mark as her healthcare power of attorney because she didn't want her daughter to be overwhelmed. Julie planned to speak with Mark fully about her end-of-life care preferences but was hesitant to include her daughter in those conversations because their relationship had been strained over the years.

Julie chose a nursing home that she was familiar with, since she had been previously admitted to the same facility for subacute rehabilitation one year prior. The palliative care team assisted with the transition, including transmitting the advance directive and documenting that Julie's preference was to be referred to using female pronouns. Julie's preferences and desire to be treated with dignity and respect were primarily evident through Mark's discussion, requests, and advocacy on Julie's behalf. The nursing home multidisciplinary team discussed the appropriateness of assigning Julie to a single room with its own bathroom both related to C. difficile infection and to provide her with privacy. Members of the hospice team met with Julie and Mark, both individually and separately, to provide support. Julie expressed that she was ready to die, desired to be alone at the time of death, and was still deciding how involved she wanted her daughter to be with after-death arrangements. Mark described Julie's very difficult life, including harsh interactions from members of her biological family. He was pleased with the care she was receiving in the facility, feeling that the staff was able to provide care and support that she had not received from others close to her. Mark visited Julie daily in the nursing home and recognized that Julie was becoming increasingly less responsive. He described fond memories including her broad smile after she woke up from her transgender surgery 9 years previously. Julie died almost 3 weeks after admission. Mark was able to be present with her; however, her daughter remained distant and struggled with the burial arrangements.

Improving the quality of communication for LGBT individuals often has more to do with understanding how to engage others in language choices than giving language advice.[45] In Julie's case, this meant being intentionally available to Julie and Mark to hear their story and concerns in the moment. For members of the LGBT community, which includes individuals from diverse cultural, ethnic, and religious backgrounds, palliative care providers can employ key communication skills to promote relationship-centered, authentic, and open communication (Table 28.1). Like the case illustrated with Julie preferring female pronouns only, a core communication strategy is to incorporate language choices as directed by the patient, using her or his words to understand and safely discuss the individual's sexual orientation and/or gender identity and related concerns. A necessary initial step is to make sure that the patient is encouraged to be open about his or her identity, including but not limited to sexual orientation and gender identity—without fear of discrimination or inferior treatment. In Julie's case, this was achieved by openness to engage Julie's partner, Mark, even before formal ADs had been completed. To reduce the barriers that LGBT individuals face, the US National Resource Center on LGBT Aging and the Joint Commission advise healthcare providers to offer all clients the option and opportunity to disclose their sexual orientation or gender identity (both in person and on paper) but never force such disclosure.[44,46] When talking with Julie and Mark, for instance, it was important to provide space for them to share about what their relationship meant to them, including their struggles with acceptance over the years. In the following sections, communication strategies are described to facilitate opportunities for LGBT patients to discuss their sexual orientation and/or gender identity using their preferred language. Table 28.1 offers a set of communication skills for engaging nonheterosexual patients and their families of choice using open and inclusive language that cultivates relationship-centered communication.

Language Makes a Difference

It is important that LGBT community members are part of the healthcare organization's vocabulary. For example, terms such as "husband," "wife," or "spouse" should be expanded to reflect the scope of significant relationships that nonheterosexual people

Table 28.1 Communication Skills: Inclusive of Nonheterosexual Patient Populations

Skill	Description of Skill	Example of Skill
Initiating the Session		
Establishing initial rapport	♦ Greet patient and obtain name ♦ Introduce self and role ♦ Demonstrate respect and interest ♦ Use patient's preferred terms (if patient does not explicitly state, the words "partner" or "significant other" are favored over "husband/wife/spouse" because they are gender neutral)[11,47]	Convey respect through eye contact, supportive gestures (e.g., uncross arms, refrain from using the computer while talking)
Identifying reason(s) for visit	♦ Identify problems/issues/needs ♦ Provide openness for disclosure ♦ Negotiate agenda, include needs of patient, families of choice, and providers	The Patient Dignity Question can provide an early expression of openness: "What do I need to know about you as a person to give you the best care possible?"[53]
Gathering Information		
Exploring needs	♦ Encourage patient to tell story free of judgment ♦ Listen attentively without interrupting ♦ Facilitate patient's responses verbally and nonverbally ♦ Clarify patient's statements that are unclear ♦ Refrain from speculating about sexual orientation or gender identity	"It sounds like you have someone in your life who you really care about. Are you open to telling me about them?" To elicit more information try asking, "Is there anything else you think is important for me to know so I can better support you during this journey?"
Understanding the patient's perspective	Determine, acknowledge, and explore ♦ patient's ideas ♦ patient's concerns regarding each problem ♦ patient's expectations ♦ effect on patient's quality of life Encourage patient to express feelings: ♦ listen with supportive gestures including eye contact ♦ express support by seeking to understand first, not simply saying the next thing ♦ acknowledge that your own beliefs and values influence what you say and what you hear Summarize to verify interpretation and express that patient is heard	I would love to ask you a few questions about your support system. Who do you consider family? Who do you rely on for support? Who would you like to have here with us when we are discussing your care?
Building Relationship		
Developing rapport	♦ Accept patient's views and feelings nonjudgmentally ♦ Empathize with patient, including overtly acknowledging past hardships ♦ Provide support and describe partnership by the palliative care team ♦ Deal sensitively with embarrassment or distressing topics	When patient discloses information, acknowledge before moving on, "How long ago was the surgery?" or "I really appreciate you sharing this information with me. If there is anything I, or the team, can do to make you feel more supported during this time, please let us know."
Involving the patient and other desired individual(s)	♦ Ask permission to discuss personal questions ♦ Share your own thinking as appropriate ♦ Explain rationale regarding questions that may be surprising to patient	"Thank you for sharing this aspect of your life with me. Would you like to invite your partner to join us? How would you like other people to be involved?"
Explaining and Planning		
Incorporating the patient's preferences	♦ Elicit patient's beliefs, concerns, and expectations ♦ Encourage patient to ask questions and express doubts ♦ Observe patient's verbal and nonverbal cues ♦ Elicit patient's beliefs and feelings about medical information, options, and decisions	"I noticed when I mentioned having a family meeting your body posture changed and you took a few deep breaths. Is there anything you want me to know before we all talk?"

(continued)

Table 28.1 Continued

Skill	Description of Skill	Example of Skill
Planning: shared decision-making	♦ Ascertain patient's desired level of involvement in decision-making ♦ Explore patient preferences on care options ♦ Offer suggestions and choices, incorporating patient input ♦ Share own thought processes, recommendations, and dilemmas ♦ Check with patient (i.e., if plan is acceptable and if concerns have been addressed)	"If time is limited because of your illness, what is important to you? Who would you like to be involved? Are there things that you want to discuss?"
Closing the Session		
Forward planning	Connect with patient about next steps: ♦ explain possible unexpected outcomes ♦ what to do if plan is not working ♦ when and how to seek help	"What gives you strength or help during this challenging time? There are many different ways of coping. Are you interested in a support group? Are there LGBT community resources that you would like us to help you explore?"
Ensuring appropriate closure	Summarize visit ♦ ask for corrections or additions ♦ check if patient is comfortable with the plan or has questions	"I learned from you today that it is very important that you feel safe and in control. Do our next steps feel okay to you?"

Note: Adapted from *Teaching and Learning Communication Skills in Medicine* (2nd ed.)[54] and *Skills for Communicating with Patients* (2nd ed.).[41]

may have, such as "significant other," "life partner," or "domestic partner." Unfortunately, many traditional intake forms only ask for "male or female," which fails to capture information on gender nonconforming or transgender individuals. The National Resource Center on LGBT Aging has identified several ways to incorporate inclusive language into forms and conversations to foster diversity and inclusivity:[44]

♦ Avoid making assumptions about sexual orientation and gender identity by using inclusive language when asking about sexuality.

♦ Use forms that include relationship options such as "partner" or "significant other."

♦ Create opportunities for LGBT persons to talk about families of choice by asking, "Who do you consider family?," "Who in your life is especially important?," and "Are you currently in an intimate relationship?"[47]

♦ Let the person or members of the families of choice guide how to address the individual; consider asking, "Am I using the term or pronoun you prefer?" or "How do you self-identify?"

Cultivate Relationship-Centered Interaction Skills

Unlike other communication skills that focus on guiding patients to elicit and strengthen motivation for *changing* behavior, relationship-centered interaction skills provide a communication strategy for *understanding* behavior in order to meet LGBT individuals' palliative care needs. Relationship-centered communication starts with the premise that forging a relationship, however short or long, is essential for making decisions and acting together. Palliative care providers need to foster open communication where individuals feel they are genuinely understood and respected. To accomplish this, palliative care providers need to create opportunities for people to feel heard, connected, and engaged in on-going medical care. Table 28.1 provides tangible examples of palliative care communication specific to LGBT persons within a clinical visit, including key aspects of initiating the visit, gathering relevant information, building the relationship, explaining and planning medical care, and closing the visit.

Create a Welcoming Environment

Beyond specific verbal communication strategies as outlined previously, the need for welcoming and inclusive environments is also critical. As a group of people who have been historically marginalized, LGBT persons tend to "scan the room" when they first enter a new facility, looking for visible signs that it is welcoming. The National Resource Center on LBGT Aging has developed a helpful checklist[44] (Table 28.2) of nonverbal visibility strategies for individuals and healthcare organizations, including palliative care and hospice agencies, to consider as part of a comprehensive plan to create environments and settings that are welcoming and show positive signs of inclusion and respect. Organizations can utilize local or regional visual signs and SafeZone Programs designed to convey respect for all people regardless of race, ethnicity, gender expression, gender identity, sexual orientation, socioeconomic background, age, religion, body shape, size, and ability.[48,49]

Future Needs and Areas of Improvement

Given the extensive periods of discrimination, stigmatization, and resulting health disparities, consistent relationship-centered and family-focused care for members of the LGBT community requires a commitment to improving communication on multiple levels. First is the need for professional education for clinical team members (including medicine, nursing, and allied health professionals) to promote comfort and acceptance, identify and diminish bias, facilitate disclosure of sexuality, and minimize heterosexual assumptions within assessment and care and thus

Table 28.2 Communication Environment: Creating Welcoming and Inclusive Palliative Care Agencies

Material Visibility
Hang images of LGBT adults in welcome areas and high-traffic common spaces.
♦ Include representations from multiple racial and ethnic groups, aging generations, sexual orientations, and gender identities.
♦ Hang Safe Zone signs around the agency to signify LGBT solidarity and acceptance.[48] Safe Zone Trainings help provide participants with the skills to create a safer space for nonheterosexual individuals.[49]
♦ Display copies of LGBT-relevant magazines, publications, and information about local LGBT resources.
Policy Visibility
Post the agency's nondiscrimination policy on the website and in the lobby.
♦ The policy should specifically state the agency's commitment to inclusion and protection of all people, as well as their caregivers, family members, and friends, regardless of sexual orientation and gender identity and regardless of whether the state specifically protects against sexual orientation and/or gender identity discrimination.
Structural Visibility
If possible, have single-stall, gender-neutral bathrooms available for staff members, patients, and visitors.
♦ All individuals should be allowed to use the restroom they feel most aligns with their gender.
Community Visibility
Highlight or display agency partnerships with, or outreach to, the LGBT community.
♦ Consider regularly hosting LGBT programming.
♦ Hang banners or advertisements displaying local LGBT community center events and partnerships.

Note: Adapted from *Inclusive Services for LGBT Older Adults: A Practical Guide To Creating Welcoming Agencies.*[44]

Table 28.3 Palliative Care Team Communication: Improving Partnership

Visiting Policies
Review visiting policies to ensure it includes the patient's right to review visitors that the patient has designated, such as a partner, domestic partner, spouse, or friend.
♦ Policies for accepting visitors should be the same for both same-sex and opposite-sex partners.
Defining Family
Review definitions for "family" to ensure they include a patient's "family of choice"—friends, partners, and other people close to the individual—as well as "family of origin"—biological family members or those related by marriage.
Intake Forms
Review intake forms and provide options to include nonheterosexual relationships, not defined through "husband" and "wife" categories.
♦ Single, Married, Widowed, or Partnered should be included.
Team Liaison
Select at least one team member to be responsible for continually improving services and care welcoming toward LGBT and other diverse older adults.
♦ This individual could also serve as a direct liaison between patients, their friends, partners, and families to receive input and suggestions about improving care for LGBT patients.
Team Recognition
Highlight and honor staff members who demonstrate exceptional care or a commitment to serving LGBT adults and their families of choice.
♦ Use exemplary staff members as mentors or guides for other staff members who are less familiar with engaging LGBT patients.
Accountability and Monitoring
Create ongoing monitoring mechanisms for patients to report and address biased behavior from fellow patients and staff, and for staff to report discriminatory or biased behavior.
♦ Be sure to outline process for handling and learning from potential complaints.

Note: Adapted *Inclusive Services for LGBT Older Adults: A Practical Guide to Creating Welcoming Agencies. National Resource Center on LBGT Aging*[4] and *Advancing Effective Communication, Cultural Competence, and Patient- and Family-Centered Care for the Lesbian, Gay, Bisexual, and Transgender (LGBT) Community: A Field Guide.*[46]

strengthen communication and disclosure.[14] Second is the need to recognize the importance of respecting the patient's wishes and involving the partner in decision-making and treatment discussions. Providers should be aware of the legal situation for same-sex couples in their state and establish mechanisms to ensure that patient and partner preferences can be met. Third is to ensure that palliative care teams can respectfully identify the needs of this patient population and are equipped to make appropriate referrals for services and resources. Specific ways to ensure that organizational care policies and procedures are inclusive of nonheterosexual patient populations and focused on improving partnership with LGBT persons are described in Table 28.3.

Conclusion

At its core, communication between nonheterosexual individuals, their families of choice, and their healthcare providers should be relationship-centered, grounded in four underlying principles of patient-provider relationships that are well known to the palliative care team:[50,51]

♦ Each patient is a unique individual with her or his own set of experiences, values, and perspectives.

♦ Communicating genuine emotion is fundamental to developing and maintaining relationships.

♦ Allowing an equal opportunity to express all relevant positions and opportunity to make a choice based on these positions emphasizes respect within the clinical relationships.

♦ Genuine and authentic relationships improve satisfaction for patients, families of choice, and healthcare providers.

Thus, for palliative care providers, the goal is to build open and authentic relationships, so that patients feel comfortable disclosing their experiences, allowing exploration of their physical, intellectual, emotional, social, and spiritual needs. To consistently strive for relationship-centered care, we must remember that every person, message, and choice is important. Any idea should not be dismissed and, when possible, should be written down, even if the idea does not seem clinically relevant in the moment.[52]

Nonheterosexual individuals face a number of challenges when accessing healthcare and interacting with their caregivers and healthcare providers. Although caring for the whole person at the end of life is a familiar concept to palliative care providers, a greater emphasis on aspects of communication and care relating to sexual orientation and lifestyle choices must be consistently integrated into healthcare interactions. If unaddressed, many of the issues nonheterosexual individuals face at the end of life can ultimately lead to increased health disparities. Identifying communication strategies that facilitate conversations that are inclusive of difference and responsive to the individual's values, goals, and informed choices is one way to improve the healthcare environment and healthcare experience of LGBT individuals.

References

1. Buber M, Friedman MS. *Meetings*. La Salle, IL: Open Court; 1973.
2. Buber M. *I and Thou*. Smith RG, trans. Edinburgh, UK: T&T Clark; 1937.
3. Deetz S, NetLibrary Inc. *Democracy in an Age of Corporate Colonization: Developments in Communication and the Politics of Everyday Life*. SUNY Series in Speech Communication. Albany: State University of New York; 1992.
4. Institute of Medicine. *The Health of Lesbian, Gay, Bisexual, and Transgender People: Building a Foundation for Better Understanding*. Washington, DC: National Academy Press; 2011.
5. Lim FA, Brown DV, Justin Kim SM. Addressing health care disparities in the lesbian, gay, bisexual, and transgender population: A review of best practices. *Am J Nurs*. June 2014;114(6):24–34; quiz 35, 45.
6. Meyer IH, Wilson PA. Sampling lesbian, gay, and bisexual populations. *J Couns Psych*. 2009;56(1):23–31.
7. US Census Bureau. Same-sex couple households. Report from the American Community Survey. http://www.census.gov/prod/2011pubs/acsbr10-03.pdf Published September 2011. Accessed November 1, 2014.
8. Lim FA, Bernstein I. Promoting awareness of LGBT issues in aging in a baccalaureate nursing program. *Nurs Educ Perspect*. 2012;33(3):170–175.
9. Grant JM. *Outing Age 2010: Public Policy Issues Affecting Lesbian, Gay, Bisexual, and Transgender Elders*. Washington, DC: National Gay and Lesbian Task Force Policy Institute; 2010. http://www.thetaskforce.org/downloads/reports/reports/outingage_final.pdf. Accessed November 1, 2014.
10. Maddux S, dir. 2011. *Gen Silent: A Documentary Film About LGBT Aging*. Boston: Interrobang Productions.
11. Gay and Lesbian Medical Association. Guidelines for care of lesbian, gay, bisexual and transgender patients. http://safezone.sdes.ucf.edu/docs/glma-guidelines.pdf. Accessed September 26, 2014.
12. Ryan H, Wortley PM, Easton A, Pederson L, Greenwood G. Smoking among lesbians, gays, and bisexuals: A review of the literature. *Am J Prev Med*. August 2001;21(2):142–149.
13. Rawlings D. End-of-life care considerations for gay, lesbian, bisexual, and transgender individuals. *Int J Palliat Nurs*. January 2012;18(1):29–34.
14. Harding R, Epiphaniou E, Chidgey-Clark J. Needs, experiences, and preferences of sexual minorities for end-of-life care and palliative care: A systematic review. *J Palliat Med*. May 2012;15(5):602–611.
15. Lawton A, White J, Fromme EK. End-of-life and advance care planning considerations for lesbian, gay, bisexual, and transgender patients #275. *J Palliat Med*. January 2014;17(1):106–108.
16. Boehmer U, Bowen DJ, Bauer GR. Overweight and obesity in sexual-minority women: Evidence from population-based data. *Am J Public Health*. June 2007;97(6):1134–1140.
17. Cochran SD, Mays VM. Risk of breast cancer mortality among women cohabiting with same sex partners: Findings from the National Health Interview Survey, 1997–2003. *J Womens Health*. May 2012;21(5):528–533.
18. Dibble SL, Roberts SA, Nussey B. Comparing breast cancer risk between lesbians and their heterosexual sisters. *Womens Health Issues*. March-April 2004;14(2):60–68.
19. Brown JP, Tracy JK. Lesbians and cancer: An overlooked health disparity. *Cancer Causes Control*. December 2008;19(10):1009–1020.
20. Centers for Disease Control and Prevention. HIV in the United States: At a glance. http://www.cdc.gov/hiv/pdf/statistics_basics_factsheet.pdf. Published November 2013. Accessed November 1, 2014.
21. Esser S, Gelbrich G, Brockmeyer N, et al. Prevalence of cardiovascular diseases in HIV-infected outpatients: Results from a prospective, multicenter cohort study. *Clin Res Cardiol*. March 2013;102(3):203–213.
22. Sanchez MA, Scheer S, Shallow S, Pipkin S, Huang S. Epidemiology of the viral hepatitis-HIV syndemic in San Francisco: A collaborative surveillance approach. *Public Health Rep*. January-February 2014;129(Suppl 1):95–101.
23. Anderson JS, Vajdic C, Grulich AE. Is screening for anal cancer warranted in homosexual men? *Sex Health*. 2004;1(3):137–140.
24. Lyter DW, Bryant J, Thackeray R, Rinaldo CR, Kingsley LA. Incidence of human immunodeficiency virus-related and nonrelated malignancies in a large cohort of homosexual men. *J Clin Oncol*. October 1995;13(10):2540–2546.
25. King M, Semlyen J, Tai SS, et al. A systematic review of mental disorder, suicide, and deliberate self harm in lesbian, gay and bisexual people. *BMC Psychiatry*. 2008;8:70.
26. Warner J, McKeown E, Griffin M, et al. Rates and predictors of mental illness in gay men, lesbians and bisexual men and women: Results from a survey based in England and Wales. *Br J Psychiatry*. December 2004;185:479–485.
27. Fredriksen-Goldsen, KI et al. *The Aging and Health Report: Disparties and Resilience among Lesbian, Gay, Bisexual, and Transgender Older Adults*. Seattle: Institute for Multigenerational Health.
28. Feldman J, Romine RS, Bockting WO. HIV risk behaviors in the U.S. transgender population: Prevalence and predictors in a large internet sample. *J Homosex*. 2014;61(11):1558–1588.
29. O'Hanlan KA. Health policy considerations for our sexual minority patients. *Obstet Gynecol*. March 2006;107(3):709–714.
30. Clements-Nolle K, Marx R, Guzman R, Katz M. HIV prevalence, risk behaviors, health care use, and mental health status of transgender persons: Implications for public health intervention. *Am J Public Health*. June 2001;91(6):915–921.
31. Stein GL, Bonuck KA. Attitudes on end-of-life care and advance care planning in the lesbian and gay community. *J Palliat Med*. 2001;4(2):173–190.
32. Cartwright C. Ethical challenges in end-of-life care for GLBTI individuals. *J Bioeth Inq*. March 2012;9(1):113–114.
33. Katz A. Gay and lesbian patients with cancer. *Oncol Nurs Forum*. March 2009;36(2):203–207.
34. Matthews AK. Lesbians and cancer support: Clinical issues for cancer patients. *Health Care Women Int*. May-June 1998;19(3):193–203.
35. Hash KM, Netting FE. Long-term planning and decision-making among midlife and older gay men and lesbians. *J Soc Work End Life Palliat Care*. 2007;3(2):59–77.
36. Croghan CF, Moone RP, Olson AM. Friends, family, and caregiving among midlife and older lesbian, gay, bisexual, and transgender adults. *J Homosex*. 2014;61(1):79–102.
37. Neville S, Henrickson M. The constitution of "lavender families": A LGB perspective. *J Clin Nurs*. March 2009;18(6):849–856.
38. US Department of Health. 2008. End of life care strategy: Promoting high quality care for all adults at the end of life. https://www.gov.uk/government/uploads/system/uploads/attachment_data/file/136431/End_of_life_strategy.pdf. Accessed November 1, 2014.

39. Fobair P, O'Hanlan K, Koopman C, et al. Comparison of lesbian and heterosexual women's response to newly diagnosed breast cancer. *Psycho-Oncology.* January-February 2001;10(1):40–51.
40. Almack K, Seymour J, Bellamy G. Exploring the impact of sexual orientation on experiences and concerns about end-of-life care and on bereavement for lesbian, gay and bisexual older people. *Sociology.* 2010; 44(5):908–924.
41. Silverman J, Kurtz S, Draper J. *Skills for Communicating with Patients.* 2nd ed. Oxford: Radcliffe; 2005.
42. Cartwright C, Hughes M, Lienert T. End-of-life care for gay, lesbian, bisexual and transgender people. *Cult Health Sex.* 2012;14(5):537–548.
43. Price E. Coming out to care: Gay and lesbian carers' experiences of dementia services. *Health Soc Care Community.* March 2010;18(2):160–168.
44. Services & Advocacy for GLBT Elders (SAGE), National Resource Center on LGBT Aging. Inclusive services for LGBT older adults: A practical guide to creating welcoming agencies. http://www.sageusa.org/resources/publications.cfm?ID=107. Published March 14, 2012. Accessed October 4, 2014.
45. Deetz S, Radford G. *Communication Theory at the Crossroads: Responding to Globalization, Pluralism and Collaborative Needs.* Oxford: Blackwell; 2008.
46. Joint Commission. Advancing effective communication, cultural competence, and patient- and family-centered care for the lesbian, gay, bisexual, and transgender (LGBT) community: A field guide. http://www.jointcommission.org/assets/1/18/LGBTFieldGuide.pdf. Accessed June 19, 2015.
47. Group for the Advancement of Psychiatry. LGBT mental health syllabus: Taking a sexual history with LGBT patients. http://www.aglp.org/gap/. Published 2012. Accessed November 25, 2104.
48. Boulder County Public Health. Safe Zone. http://www.bouldercounty.org/family/youth/pages/phfreeposters.aspx. Accessed November 25, 2014.
49. Gay Alliance of the Genesee Valley. SafeZone Training Programs. http://www.gayalliance.org/safezonet.html. Accessed November 25, 2014.
50. Beach MC, Inui T, Network R-CCR. Relationship-centered care. A constructive reframing. *J Gen Intern Med.* January 2006;21(Suppl 1):S3–S8.
51. Broadfoot KJ, Candrian C. Relationship-centered care and clinical dialogue: Towards new forms of "care-full" communication. *Nat Med J* 2009;1(4):1–2.
52. Gawande A. *Better: A Surgeon's Notes on Performance.* New York, NY: Picador; 2007.
53. Dignity in Care. Toolkit: Patient Dignity Question. http://dignityincare.ca/en/toolkit.html#The_Patient_Dignity_Question. Accessed November 25, 2014.
54. Kurtz SM, Silverman JD, Draper J. *Teaching and Learning Communication Skills in Medicine.* Oxford: Radcliffe; 1998.

CHAPTER 29

Patient-Centered Communication

Marleah Dean and Richard L. Street Jr.

Introduction

Mrs. Cohen is a 72-year-old, African American patient who was diagnosed with stage III breast cancer less than a year ago. Since her diagnosis, she has undergone a double mastectomy, radiation, and several rounds of chemotherapy. Healthcare providers have been monitoring her health, and, so far, her recovery has been going well. However, yesterday she presented to the emergency department with chest pain, difficulty breathing, and persistent coughing. Mrs. Cohen does not have any other medical conditions or issues that might complicate this event (e.g., heart problems, asthma, diabetes, or psychological problems). Based on these symptoms and her medical history, the emergency department physician on duty is concerned if it is a distant (metastatic) recurrence of the breast cancer that has now traveled to her lungs. The physician refers Mrs. Cohen to her oncologist who confirms it is indeed cancer.

Mrs. Cohen is devastated, as is her family. She has three children and nine grandchildren. She is frustrated and overwhelmed with the information provided by her emergency department physician and oncologist. Due to the progression of the cancer, the oncologist says she has anywhere from 3 to 6 months to live.

This news means Mrs. Cohen will now receive palliative care—care focused on improving the patient's and family's quality of life through pain management and psychosocial support. Mrs. Cohen wants to return home and live out her remaining months with her children and grandchildren; however, her children want her to stay in the hospital so she can receive the best care and management for her pain. *If you were Mrs. Cohen's healthcare provider, how would you take care of her? What could you do to improve her physical health but also her emotional well-being and quality of life, as well as address the family's requests?*

One answer is to engage in patient-centered communication. According to the Institute of Medicine's report "Crossing the Quality Chasm," patient-centered care was identified as one of the six aims for improving the quality of the US healthcare system.[1] Patient-centered communication is vital to patient and family-centered care.[2,3] Recent research has identified seven pathways through which patient-centered communication can lead to better patient health outcomes, such as greater knowledge and understanding, quality health decisions, heightened social support, increased patient empowerment, enhanced therapeutic relationships, and better emotional management.[4,5] Following this framework and extending this research to palliative care, this chapter (a) summarizes the components of patient-centered communication and (b) discusses the challenges of patient-centered communication in palliative care and communication skills to address those challenges.

Overview of Patient-Centered Communication

The term "patient-centeredness" originated based on the limitations of the biomedical approach to medicine.[6] There are two dominant medicine models—the biomedical model and the biopsychosocial model. The biomedical model focuses on the patient's disease pathophysiology, whereas the biopsychosocial model of medicine accounts for the ways in which an illness's behavioral, psychological, and social dimensions can influence a patient's disease.[7]

Healthcare communication from a biomedical model perspective extracts a disease's symptoms and isolates a biological cause for the abnormality. In contrast, patient-centered care involves communication that not only recognizes patients' expressions of symptoms but also their emotions, concerns, and feelings. In other words, it is not enough for a healthcare provider to simply treat a patient's disease; the provider must also address the person who has the illness.

The biopsychosocial model is reflected in the various definitions of patient-centeredness. Consider, for instance, the following paraphrased definitions:

- Seeking to understand the patient as unique[8]
- Trying to enter and see the patient's illness from their eyes[9]
- Performing care that is close to the patients' wants, needs, and preferences[10]
- Exploring the illness and disease experience; understanding the individual as a whole; discovering "common ground" for treatment management; incorporating prevention and health promotion into care; enhancing the clinician-patient relationship; "being realistic" about personal limitations and issues[11]

Several important dimensions of patient-centeredness are portrayed here. The first dimension extends the practice of medicine from the absence of disease to the inclusion of "dysfunctional states."[12] At the root of patient-centered care is the belief that effective healthcare does not simply encompass healing the physical body but also attending to the emotional, psychological, and social aspects of being human. The second dimension includes the patient's nonmedical issues in clinical encounters (e.g., emotional, psychological, and social issues) in the healthcare provider's responsibilities, because such issues can affect health problems.[6,11] The last dimension is the provider's ability to view and perceive health from the patient's world.[13] To use the common phrase, providers must be able to "walk in their patients' shoes."

Although patient-centered communication has been conceptualized and measured in various ways, this chapter adopts the patient-centered communication framework Epstein and Street[4] advocate. Accordingly, patient-centered communication should focus on the key communication goals inherent to patient-centered care, including

- eliciting, understanding, and validating the patient's perspective (e.g., concerns, feelings, expectations)
- understanding the patient within his or her own psychological and social context
- reaching a shared understanding of the patient's problem and its treatment
- helping a patient share power by offering him or her meaningful involvement in choices relating to his or her health.[4(p2)]

It is clear from this definition that treating the "whole" patient and being responsive to his or her medical and psychosocial needs is central to patient-centered care.[14] Being patient-centered means caring for patients based on the patients' own experiences as well as listening, respecting, and honoring their perspectives throughout the healthcare journey.[15] Patient-centered communication means balancing between "the art of generalizations and the science of particulars"[9(p100),15] Furthermore, patient-centered care requires patient-centered healthcare systems,[16] families, and patients. In other words, healthcare providers, patients, families, and healthcare services create the relationships through which patient-centered care is achieved.[4,17] Figure 29.1 depicts the collaborative nature of patient-centered care.

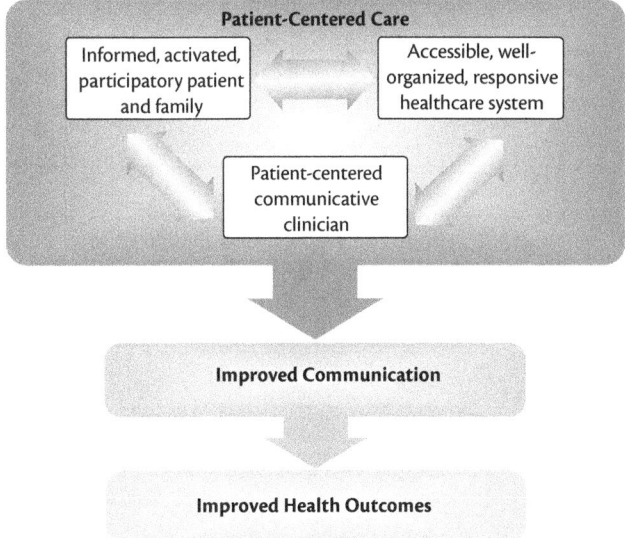

Figure 29.1 Patient-centered care, communication, and health outcomes.[4]

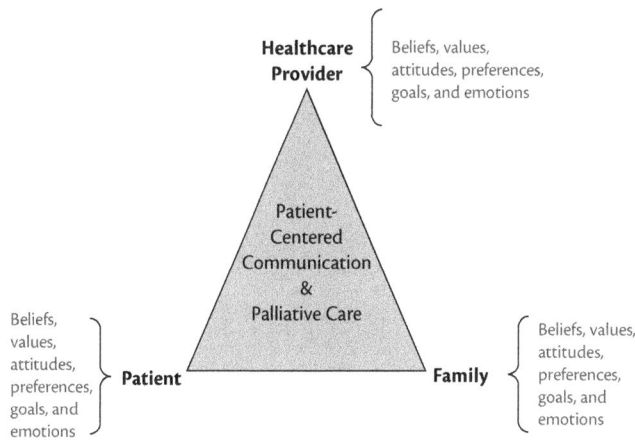

Figure 29.2 Patient-centered communication and palliative care.

Yet challenges exist for patient-centered communication in palliative care. One of the deeply rooted characteristics of palliative care is the involvement and support of the patient and his or her family.[18] The very involvement of families in palliative care encounters—especially with patients who have advanced diseases and illnesses—can be problematic. Indeed, palliative care encounters are fundamentally different from other care contexts (e.g., primary care, dermatology, emergency care, etc.), because there are usually three parties in every clinical encounter. The healthcare provider, the patient, and the family come to the interaction with their own beliefs, values, attitudes, preferences, goals, and emotions, which ultimately influence communication and care. Figure 29.2 provides a visual representation of this dynamic interaction and how it affects patient-centered communication and care.

Patient-Centered Communication Functions

To accomplish the key goals of patient-centered care and overcome challenges to palliative care, Epstein and Street propose a functional perspective, emphasizing the "work" that must be done to achieve patient-centered communication.[4] In order to communicate effectively in a patient-centered manner, providers, patients, and families—as appropriate—should focus on the following six main functions: (a) fostering the patient–provider relationship, (b) providing and receiving information, (c) responding to emotions, (d) managing uncertainty, (e) making decisions, and (f) enabling patient self-management.

While these functions are not independent from one another and often overlap, they do represent key communication tasks to accomplishing patient-centered care. These functions are not communicative actions that one person (e.g., the healthcare provider) does or is responsible for; rather, they are accomplished interactively as healthcare providers and patients and families work collaboratively to achieve these communication goals inherent in these functions. Figure 29.3 provides a visual of this model.[4]

Important here is how these functions are used effectively and under what circumstances, which will depend on the palliative care situation and the unique clinical, personal, and familial attributes in play.[19] While palliative clinicians should be versatile in all six functions of patient-centered communication, specific

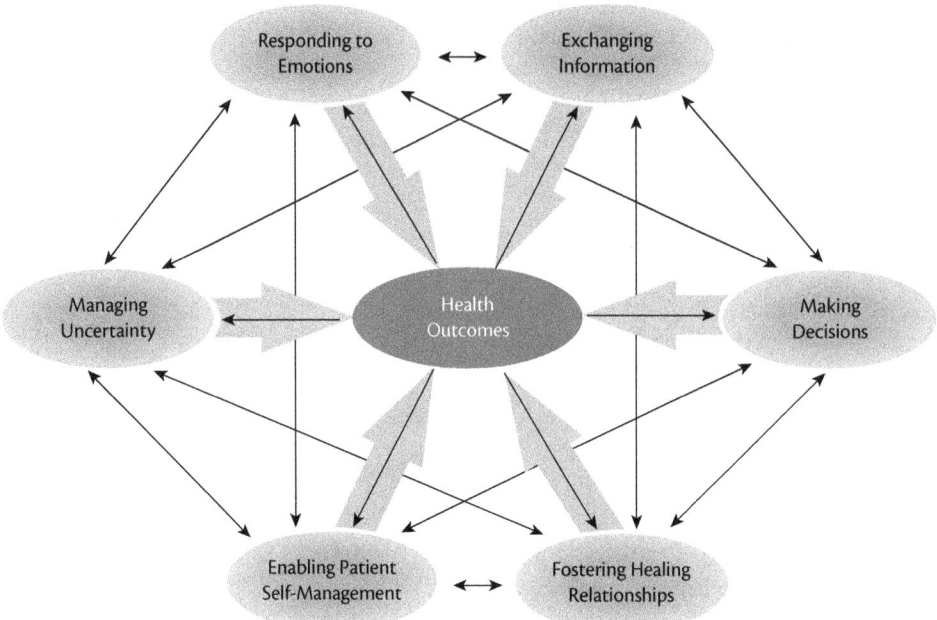

Figure 29.3 Patient-centered communication: Six core functions.[4]

communication skills are discussed throughout and serve as good resources for clinicians. Table 29.1 provides a summary of these communication skills.

Fostering the Patient/Family–Provider Relationship

The first function is fostering the patient/family–provider relationship. This relationship is important for palliative care because, often, healthcare providers are responsible for patient care leading up to death, and these final months can be unpredictable.[20] Pivotal characteristics of this patient-centered communication function are trust, rapport, and shared understanding of responsibilities and roles.[21,22] These characteristics help build strong relationships between providers and patients and their families.[4]

First, patients trust healthcare providers who are informative, include them in the decision-making process, and are sensitive to their concerns.[23,24] Second, building rapport—or connecting with patients through verbal and nonverbal communication—leads to satisfactory relationships.[25] Third, healthcare providers and

Table 29.1 Patient-Centered Communication Skills

Patient-Centered Communication Function	Communication Skill	Definition	Conversational Example
Fostering the patient/family–provider relationship	Name the problem or issue	Articulate each person's perspective in the encounter and come to agreement on the main issue	"From our discussion thus far, it is evident we all have different opinions. Let's specifically point out what those are and then decide how we should proceed."
Providing and receiving information	Clarify the facts	Check understanding by asking verbal questions	"Please repeat back what I explained to you to make sure we are on the same page."
Responding to emotions	Address negative emotions	Identify, acknowledge, and validate each person's emotions	"It seems like you feel overwhelmed and frustrated. That is completely understandable. Is there anything I can do to help you?"
Managing uncertainty	Frame an uncertain prognosis	Determine the source of uncertainty and frame information based on what is known and unknown	"The future is uncertain. How about we discuss what information we do know?"
Making decisions	Encourage participation	Provide opportunities and prompt each person's preferences	"Your opinion is important as we make these last decisions. What would you like to do?"
Enabling patient self-management	Teach self-activation	Represent and advocate for one's interests and desires	"Let's discuss specific issues you and your family can look for at home that might signal a need for clinical treatment. I will also teach you what you can do to help treat these possible issues."

patients must understand each other's roles and responsibilities by learning and comprehending each other's preferences.[26] Last, providers should build partnerships, listen actively, ensure patient understanding, display empathetic nonverbal behaviors, and engage in joint agenda-setting with the patient.[27-29]

One challenge to fostering relationships in palliative care is discovering the patient's and family's health preferences, developing shared goals, and creating a plan to accomplish those goals. Because there are multiple parties involved in palliative care encounters, healthcare providers must manage a variety of beliefs, values, attitudes, preferences, goals, and emotions. The patient enters the clinical encounter with a particular perspective; the family may enter with a different perspective,[30] and often the patient and family have not discussed each of their perspectives. This adds an additional level of complexity to a difficult situation, requiring the healthcare provider to navigate relational dynamics.[31]

To address the challenge of multiple perspectives, providers can *name the problem or issue* (see Table 29.1). Doing so helps paint a clear, overarching picture for the patient and his or her family. First, healthcare providers cannot assume everyone has the same perspective or shared understanding of what the situation is and how it should be addressed.[4] In fact, research regarding patient and healthcare provider goal concordance is often poor, except when goals are explicitly discussed.[32] Second, providers must discover and learn about each person's perspectives and preferences and then try to accomplish a consensus through negotiation and discussion.[4] While determining family preferences is important, the healthcare provider is caring for the patient and must adhere to the patient's wishes.[30] Likewise, providers must also express their own perspectives, as they are the healthcare experts.

For example, suppose a female patient has lymphoma cancer that normally would be treated with chemotherapy. If she receives this treatment, the cancer is potentially controllable; however, the patient recently had bowel surgery, resulting in several complications and infections as well as significant weight loss. As such, the cancer progressed. Now the patient's body is not responsive to chemotherapy, which would have saved her life. During a clinical encounter, the healthcare provider explains this situation to the patient and her husband. Each seems to understand, but at the end of the conversation, the husband says, "But we are, of course, working toward a cure, right?" The husband clearly does not understand a cure is not possible because of the problems from surgery; he does not make the connection that these issues have influenced his wife's ability to survive the cancer. Thus, healthcare providers need to work on establishing common understanding and achievable goals. Here the husband's uncertainty about the prognosis and treatment produced goal confusion.[33] Naming the problem or issue at hand decreases the likelihood of confusion.

Providing and Receiving Information

The second function is providing and receiving information. Information is essential to palliative care, because patients experience life-threatening illnesses and must cope with disease progression, symptom management, and treatment options.[34] Information exchange entails three main components: information-seeking (e.g., asking questions, eliciting beliefs), information-giving (e.g., explanation, reports, beliefs), and information-verifying (e.g., checking for understanding and accuracy).[35]

Healthcare providers, patients, and families must present and manage information with each other in order to reach a shared understanding of patients' health.[4] However, many times there is lack of agreement and misunderstanding. For instance, Bruera et al. found providers and palliative care cancer patients only agreed 38% on treatment options.[32] Furthermore, due to the nature and magnitude of the information, palliative care patients commonly do not understand their disease, its extent, and even the likelihood of a cure.[36] So in order to effectively exchange information, healthcare providers must learn patients' information needs, understand their health beliefs and values, and present clinical information in comprehendible ways.[4] Overall, providing information enhances patient satisfaction, facilitates participation, decreases anxiety, and increases coping abilities.[37,38]

A challenge to exchanging and managing information in palliative care is achieving a balance between providing enough information to the patient and the family for them to make an informed health decision while also not overwhelming them with the information. Because patients must make quality of life and end-of-life care decisions, they need information on diagnosis, prognosis, treatment, symptom management, and hospice services. At the same time, receiving this information can be devastating and distressing.[39,40]

In order to address this challenge, providers should *clarify the facts* (see Table 29.1). Healthcare providers can provide small amounts of information in increments and check understanding about that information. Providers should repeat this process until the patient has the information he or she needs or wants or there is saturation and giving more information will be counterproductive. Engaging in this process reduces the likelihood the patient and his or her family will become overwhelmed with the amount of information provided.

Also, questions such as "Do you understand what is going on?" and "Can you describe the current situation and what that means for the patient's health?" are helpful. This strategy, called the "teach-back" approach (providing information and then asking the patient to repeat the information back to ensure comprehension)[41,42] enables healthcare providers to better identify when information becomes distressing and when to stop providing information. Additionally, by occasionally assessing comprehension of information, providers can gain an idea of how much information the patient or family needs/wants and specifically evaluate where the information provision is lacking. Finally, this technique is particularly helpful for making decisions. Clarifying facts enables the provider to determine if all persons (e.g., provider, patient, and family) are on the same page about the course of treatment and health trajectory.

Responding to Emotions

The third function is responding to emotions. Because palliative care includes care at the end of life, patients and their families commonly manifest emotional distress.[43] The patient may feel anxiety and fear, while the family members may experience sadness and depression. For instance, fear is a common emotion experienced by palliative care patients and caregivers. Penman and Ellis found patients and caregivers experienced different types of fear, such falling and getting hurt and not being able to help, dying alone and being alone, not being comfortable, and confronting the process of death.[43] Unfortunately, palliative care often fails to provide needed emotional support to address these fears.[44]

Recognizing negative emotions, both providers' own emotions and those of their patients and families, is a challenge. Previous research reveals that providers have a difficult time recognizing the patient's or family's emotions for several reasons. Healthcare providers may lack the skills to identify and deal with emotional issues; they may believe that attending to emotional subjects will take too much time, that discussing emotions will cause further patient distress, or that it is not their responsibility.[45–48] However, healthcare providers must address and deal with these emotions, since it is part of their social role as providers.[48]

Furthermore, responding to emotions in palliative care can be challenging because there are multiple perspectives among providers, patients, and family members. On one hand, patients and their families experience emotions such as fear, anxiety, and sadness, which can have psychosocial effects on individuals' health.[46] On the other hand, healthcare providers can experience overwhelming emotions too, which can result in their feeling uncomfortable, burnt out, fatigued, or distressed and ultimately making it difficult to care for the patients.[49,50] In fact, providers engaged in end-of-life care are more likely to experience significant burnout due to feelings of frustration, failure, and powerlessness.[51,52] Such burnout and being overwhelmed may be why providers often engage in avoidance behaviors in clinical encounters.[53] Yet, because caring for patients who are approaching death inevitably means responding to emotions, healthcare providers must learn how to process with their own emotions in order to assist patients.

To address this challenge, providers can *address the negative emotions* (see Table 29.1). Healthcare providers must identify the type of emotion the patient or family is experiencing, then acknowledge and validate the emotion while constantly checking to see if the emotional distress is distressing and requires a referral.[48] Also, healthcare providers must acknowledge their own negative emotions as well as their patients', without letting the negative emotions overwhelm them. By doing so, providers can maintain emotional stability.

Dean and Street's three-stage model of patient-centered communication for addressing emotional distress can be an effective tool in palliative care.[48] A thorough description of this model is beyond the scope of this chapter, but the model's three stages are recognition, exploration, and therapeutic action. First, a healthcare provider should seek to recognize negative emotions. To enhance the likelihood of recognizing patients' emotions, providers can enact mindfulness (e.g., being conscious of people, interactions, and situations), self-situational awareness (e.g., self-reflexivity), active listening (e.g., verbal and nonverbal behaviors to learn a perspective), and facilitative communication (e.g., supportive communication, rapport building). After identifying a negative emotion, the healthcare provider should explore that emotion with the patient. This way, providers can acknowledge and validate negative emotions as well as be empathetic. However, sometimes engaging in these patient-centered behaviors is not enough to mitigate patients' negative emotions; when this is the case, the model's therapeutic action stage calls providers to offer referrals and interventions to reduce emotional distress. In fact, two-thirds of the referrals in palliative care are for emotional care and support.[54] Overall, the model's stages impact health outcomes through direct (e.g., responding empathetically reduces alleviate distress to some degree) and indirect pathways (e.g., helping the patient feel known may offer comfort and produce greater emotional well-being).[48]

Managing Uncertainty

The fourth function is managing uncertainty. Uncertainty is inherent in all health experiences but especially in palliative care. An individual experiences uncertainty when he or she believes aspects of health or illness are unclear, inconsistent, unknown, or unpredictable.[55] Unfortunately, managing uncertainty is one of the most understudied and problematic elements of patient-centered communication,[4,56,57] and the specific strategies with which to manage uncertainties are poorly understood.[55] Providers can assist patients and their families by acknowledging that uncertainty exists, framing information based on what is known and unknown, being empathetic and engaging in active listening, and teaching patients coping techniques to personally assist them in their day-to-day lives.[4,58]

Uncertain prognoses and treatment discrepancies are common barriers to effective palliative communication and care.[33] Healthcare providers must frequently explain poor prognosis, treatment failure, and end-of-life estimates. A challenge to managing a patient's and family's uncertainty is that the ambiguity of diagnosis, prognosis, and treatment can produce confusion. Also, patients and their families do not know when the patient might die, and not knowing can produce anxiety, fear, and stress.[20] As such, uncertainty cannot always be eliminated and therefore must be managed.[4]

To address the challenge of managing uncertainty, providers can *frame an uncertain prognosis* to the patient and their family members (see Table 29.1). The amount of information and the way in which the information is provided is based on a patient's and family's preferences and can influence health outcomes. For example, some patients may want to know the prognosis. In this case, the healthcare provider should first determine how many details the patient wants to know (e.g., statistics, future plans, success rates); provide the information, including the negative and positive aspects; assess, acknowledge, and respond to the patient's emotional reactions; and evaluate the patient's understanding of the information.[59]

Other patients may not want to know the prognosis. In this case, the provider should learn why the patient holds this preference, acknowledge his or her emotional and informational needs, and provide enough information for the patient to make an informed health decision while respecting the patient's preferences. Last, some patients may want to know their prognosis but are afraid of the information. In these cases, the provider should acknowledge the ambivalence, work with the patient to discuss the pros and cons of knowing versus not knowing, and provide a variety of ways the information can be presented in order to reduce the concerns and fears.[59]

Making Decisions

The fifth function is making decisions. Decision-making is essential to any patient–provider interaction, including palliative care. Decision-making includes three main steps: information exchange, deliberation, and the final decision.[60] Exchanging information involves seeking and providing perspectives on the health condition, while deliberation encompasses discussing clinical findings and recommendations based on patients' and family's preferences in order to make a final decision.

Decision-making becomes especially relevant during end-of-life care.[61] Patients and their families must make decisions about treatment, life support, and hospice care. A patient might want to spend their last few months at home, while family members may prefer hospital-based palliative care—revealing a fundamental difference in what the patient and family value and consider important to the best quality of life and death. Decision-making at end of life is also important because decisions about life and death are often made based on personal and spiritual beliefs.[62] For example, palliative care patients' perceptions regarding patient–provider communication about psychosocial/spiritual needs and decision-making are strongly correlated to distress about death.[63]

A challenge to making a high-quality decision is discovering and understanding patients' preferences. Healthcare providers often do not know their patients' needs and values, and patients may not know or understand all treatment options.[4] Patients vary on their desired degree of participation in clinical encounters,[64] in part based on their preferences for decision-making involvement[65,66] and in part based on functional capacity (e.g., illness), where family members become the decision-makers.[61,67] In other words, patient participation in decision-making ranges on a continuum from paternalistic (e.g., provider decides) to shared (e.g., provider and patient decide together) to informed (e.g., patient decides based on provider's information).[60]

Generally, to address this challenge and enact patient-centered decision-making, providers can engage in a variety of communication strategies such as active listening, setting an agenda, checking understanding, accommodating preferences, and communicating empathy and warmth.[4] Yet, more specifically, providers can *encourage patient participation* (see Table 29.1). This means not only providing opportunities for patients to be involved throughout the decision-making process (e.g., pausing and utilizing silence) but also prompting and soliciting patients' opinions about treatment and care as well as telling patients their opinion is important to making decisions (e.g., open-ended verbal questions).

Enabling Patient Self-Management

The final patient-centered communication function is enabling patient self-management. Self-management is the perceived ability to self-manage one's illness by navigating the healthcare system, seeking information, coping with side effects, and finding help when needed.[4,68] Such ability is crucial to palliative care patients and their families. Management encompasses tasks that providers can perform for their patients (e.g., creating contingency action plans) that may eliminate barriers to self-management and strategies providers can engage in to assist patients in caring for themselves outside of the clinical encounter (e.g., teaching and encouraging meditation, positive thinking, and journaling). In palliative care, providers may need to act or advocate on the patients' behalf in order to help them navigate the healthcare system (e.g., coordinate care, arrange referrals), support patient autonomy to enhance patient self-efficacy and motivation,[69] and provide guidance and skills as well as resource access (e.g., Internet, health educators, or interactive media).[4]

The challenge to enabling patient self-management is the patient's ability to be autonomous. Because palliative care often encompasses healthcare outside of clinical environments, patients must learn how to effectively care for themselves, and family members must learn how to care for their ill loved one. Pain and symptom management requires patient autonomy in palliative care. Providers must assist patients with managing their pain in order to increase a patient's quality of life and well-being.[70,71] Autonomy-supportive behaviors include investigating patients' ambivalence about autonomy, giving various options to achieve the same objective, and providing patients with ample time to make a decision.[4] Such behaviors cultivate patient motivation (e.g., the desire and willingness to perform a behavior) and self-efficacy (e.g., a patient's belief that he or she can indeed perform that behavior), which are essential to enacting patient autonomy.[4,69]

In order to address this challenge, providers can *teach patients self-activation* (see Table 29.1). Activation refers to self-advocacy—the ability to represent oneself. By teaching patients and their families how to navigate the healthcare system, locate providers who best fit their needs, and recognize potential health problems,[72] providers can help patients become active in their decision-making and overall care.[4]

In sum, patient-centered communication includes fostering patient/family–provider relationships, providing and receiving information, responding to emotions, managing uncertainty, making quality decisions, and enabling self-management. These communication functions overlap and work together in order to meet needs, overcome challenges, and impact health outcomes. However, it is important to note that these functions of patient-centered communication are only a guide for communication. At a certain point, healthcare providers must improvise, be creative, and adapt to the environment[19]—in other words, be willing and able to communicate competently.[73]

Patient-Centered Communication Competence

Traditionally, communication competence has been conceptualized two ways: as an individual outcome and as a process.[73,74] As an outcome, communication competence is defined in relation to the communicator's success (e.g.: Is the individual able to accomplish both relational and personal goals during communicative interactions?).[73,75–77] As a process, the communicator learns how to communicate competently by being motivated, gaining knowledge, and practicing skills.[76,78] Taken together, communicating competently is a collaborative and constitutive process[19] whereby "communication focuses on the key tasks or 'work' communication must do well in order to achieve the interaction's goals."[58(p11)] In other words, communicating competently is a contextual, goal-specific process in order to accomplish particular outcomes.[19] This perspective is helpful for examining patient-centered communication, because it acknowledges that the success of the encounter is jointly achieved through the communicative exchange of the participants.[79]

In short, palliative care providers need to be what Ronald Epstein (personal communication) calls, a "skilled communicator." A skilled communicator is someone who not only learns how to engage in effective patient-centered communication but also knows how to adapt communication and knows when to use communication in order to achieve particular goals (e.g., mutual understanding and shared decision-making). Researchers and healthcare providers must work hard to create programs and trainings to teach providers how to be skilled communicators by enacting patient-centered communication.

Conclusion

Reflecting back to Mrs. Cohen's health experience, patient-centered communication provides the means to overcome her palliative care challenges. In order to overcome Mrs. Cohen's negative emotions, her providers can address her emotions by acknowledging, validating, and managing them. To address her information overload and assist her in making health decisions, Mrs. Cohen's palliative care providers could clarify the facts and check her understanding throughout the clinical encounter. To assist her family and future decisions, her providers can name the problem, frame the prognoses, and discuss the health options with Mrs. Cohen and her children.

Overall, patient-centered communication addresses both the patient's and the family's health and psychosocial needs by treating the patient as a "whole" person; respecting all parties' preferences; and actively listening, effectively informing, and checking understanding. In essence, patient-centered care puts into practice an idea of Sir Williams Osler's: "The good physician treats the disease; the great physician treats the patient who has the disease."

Acknowledgments

The authors would like to express their gratitude to Dr. Ronald Epstein for his willingness to share his insight regarding the clinical practice of patient-centered palliative care and communication.

References

1. Committee on Quality of Health Care in America, Institute of Medicine. *Crossing the Quality Chasm: A New Health System for the 21st Century.* Washington, DC: National Academies Press; 2001.
2. Levinson W, Lesser CS, Epstein RM. Developing physician communication skills for patient-centered care. *Health Aff.* 2010;29(7):1310–1318.
3. Mazor KM, Beard RL, Alexander GL, et al. Patients' and family members' views on patient-centered communication during cancer care. *Psycho-Oncol.* 2013;22(11):2487–2495.
4. Epstein RM, Street RL Jr. *Patient-Centered Communication in Cancer Care: Promoting Healing and Reducing Suffering.* Bethesda, MD. National Cancer Institute; 2007.
5. Street RL Jr., Makoul G, Arora NK et al. How does communication heal? Pathways linking clinician-patient communication to health outcomes. *Patient Educ Couns.* 2009;74(3):295–301.
6. Mead N, Bower P. Patient-centredness: A conceptual framework and review of the empirical literature. *Soc Sci Med.* 2000;51:1087–1110.
7. Fortin AH, Dwamena FC, Frankel RM, et al. *Smith's Patient-Centered Interviewing: An Evidence-Based Method.* New York, NY. McGraw-Hill; 2012.
8. Balint E. The possibilities of patient-centred medicine. *Br J Gen Pract.* 1969;17:269–276.
9. McWhinney I. The need for a transformed clinical method. In: Stewart M, Roter D, eds. *Communicating with Medical Patients.* London: SAGE; 1989.
10. Laine C, Davido F. Patient-centered medicine: A professional evolution. *JAMA.* 1996;275:152–156.
11. Stewart M, Brown J, Weston W, et al. *Patient-Centered Medicine: Transforming the Clinical Method.* London: SAGE; 1995.
12. Silverman D. *Communication and Medical Practice: Social Relations in the Clinic.* London: SAGE; 1987.
13. Grol R, deMaeseneer J, Whitfield M, et al. Disease-centred versus patient-centred attitudes: Comparison of general practitioners in Belgium, Britain, and the Netherlands. *Fam Pract.* 1990;7(2):100–104.
14. Institute of Medicine. *Cancer Care for the Whole Patient: Meeting Psychosocial Health Needs.* Washington, DC. National Academy Press; 2007.
15. Epstein RM, Street RL Jr. The values and value of patient-centered care. *Ann Fam Med.* 2011;9(2):100–103.
16. Institute of Medicine. *Crossing the Quality Chasm: A New Health System for the 21st Century.* Washington, DC. National Academy Press; 2001.
17. Epstein RM, Fiscella K, Lesser CS, et al. Analysis & commentary: Why the nation needs a policy push on patient-centered health care. *Health Aff.* 2010;29(8):1489–1495.
18. Davies B. Family functioning and its implications for palliative care. *J Palliat Care.* 1994;10:29–36.
19. Street RL, De Haes HCJM. Designing a curriculum for communication skills training from a theory and evidence-based perspective. *Patient Educ Couns.* 2013;93(1):27–33.
20. Teno JM, Fisher ES, Hamel MB, et al. Medical care inconsistent with patients' treatment goals: Association with 1-year Medicare resource use and survival. *J Am Geriatr Soc.* 2002;50(3):496–500.
21. Mok E, Chiu PC. Nurse-patient relationships in palliative care. *J Adv Nurs.* 2004;48(5):475–483.
22. Spross J. Coaching and suffering: The role of the nurse in helping people face illness. In: Ferrell B, ed. *Suffering.* Boston: Jones and Bartlett; 1996:173–208.
23. Gordon HS, Street RL Jr, Sharf BF, et al. Racial differences in trust and lung cancer patients' perceptions of physician communication. *J Clin Oncol.* 2006;24:904–909.
24. Salkeld G, Solomon M, Short L, et al. A matter of trust—patient's views on decision-making in colorectal cancer. *Health Expect.* 2004;7:104–114.
25. Tickle-Degnen L, Rosenthal R. The nature of rapport and its nonverbal correlates. *Psychol Inq.* 1990;1:285–293.
26. Krupat E, Yeager CM, Putnam S. Patient role orientations, doctor-patient fit, and visit satisfaction. *Psychol Health.* 2000;15:707–719.
27. Street RL Jr, Gordon HS, Ward MM, et al. Patient participation in medical consultations: Why some patients are more involved than others. *Med Care.* 2005;43:960–969.
28. Street RL Jr, Voigt B, Geyer C Jr, et al. Increasing patient involvement in choosing treatment for early breast cancer. *Cancer.* 1995;76:2275–2285.
29. Williams GC, Deci EL. Activating patients for smoking cessation through physician autonomy support. *Med Care.* 2001;39:813–823.
30. Shields CG, Epstein RM, Fiscella K, et al. Influence of accompanied encounters on patient-centeredness with older patients. *J Am Board Fam Pract.* 2005;18(5):344–354.
31. Willard C. Caring for patient and relatives: An appraisal of palliative care philosophy. *European J Oncol Nurs.* 1999;3:38–43.
32. Bruera E, Sweeney C, Calder K, et al. Patient preferences versus physician perceptions of treatment decisions in cancer care. *J Clinical Oncol.* 2001;19(11):2883–2885.
33. Davies B, Sehring SA, Partridge JC, et al. Barriers to palliative care for children: Perceptions of pediatric health care providers. *Pediatrics.* 2008;121(2):282–288.

34. Schofield P, Carey M, Love A, et al. "Would you like to talk about your future treatment options?" Discussing the transition from curative cancer treatment to palliative care. *Palliat Med.* 2006;20(4):397–406.
35. Cegala DJ, Coleman MT, Turner JW. The development and partial assessment of the medical communication competence scale. *Health Comm.* 1998;10(3):261–288.
36. Gattellari M, Butow PN, Tattersall MHN, et al. Misunderstanding in cancer patients: Why shoot the messenger? *Ann Oncol.* 1999;10(1):39–46.
37. Davidson R, Mills ME. Cancer patients' satisfaction with communication, information and quality of care in a UK region. *Eur J Cancer Care.* 2005;14:83–90.
38. Arraras JI, Wright S, Greimel E, et al. Development of a questionnaire to evaluate the information needs of cancer patients: The EORTC questionnaire. *Patient Educ Couns.* 2004;54:235–241.
39. Morita T, Akechi T, Ikenaga M, et al. Communication about the ending of anticancer treatment and transition to palliative care. *Ann Oncol.* 2004;15(10):1551–1557.
40. Chang VT and Sambamoorthi N. Decision-making in palliative care. In: Werth JL and Blevins D, eds. *Decision Making Near the End of Life: Issues, Development, and Future Directions*. London, New York: Brunner-Routledge; 2008:143–168.
41. Dean M, Oetzel J, Sklar D. Communication in acute ambulatory care. *Acad Med.* 2014;89(12):1617–1622.
42. Schillinger D, Piette J, Grumbach K, et al. Closing the loop: Physician communication with diabetic patients who have low health literacy. *Arch Intern Med.* 2003;163(1):83–90.
43. Penman J, Ellis B. Palliative care clients' and caregivers' notion of fear and their strategies for overcoming it. *Palliat Support Care.* 2015;13(3):777–785.
44. Teno JM, Clarridge BR, Casey V, et al. Family perspectives on end-of-life care at the last place of care. *JAMA.* 2004;291(1):88–93.
45. Butow PN, Brown RF, Cogar S, et al. Oncologists' reactions to cancer patients' verbal cues. *Psycho-Oncology.* 2002;11(1):47–58.
46. Ryan H, Schofield P, Cockburn J, et al. How to recognize and manage psychological distress in cancer patients. *Eur J Cancer Care.* 2005;14(1):7–15.
47. Zimmermann C, Del Piccolo L, Finset A. Cues and concerns by patients in medical consultations: A literature review. *Psychol Bull.* 2007;133(3):438–463.
48. Dean M, Street RL Jr. A three-stage model of patient-centered communication for addressing cancer patients' emotional distress. *Patient Educ Couns.* 2014;94:143–148.
49. Gleichgerrcht E, Decety J. The costs of empathy among health professionals. In: Decety J, ed. *Empathy: From Bench to Bedside*. Cambridge, MA: MIT Press; 2012:245–2611.
50. Halpern J. Clinical empathy in medical care. In: Decety J, ed. *Empathy: From Bench to Bedside*. Cambridge, MA: MIT Press; 2012:229–244.
51. Meier DE, Back AL, Morrison RS. The inner life of physicians and care of the seriously ill. *JAMA.* 2001;286(23):3007–3014.
52. Whippen DA, Canellos GP. Burnout syndrome in the practice of oncology: Results of a random survey of 1,000 oncologists. *J Clinical Oncol.* 1991;9(10):1916–1920.
53. Galushko M, Romotzky V, Voltz R. Challenges in end-of-life communication. *Curr Opin Support Palliat Care.* 2012;6(3):355–364.
54. Skilbeck J, Payne S. Emotional support and the role of clinical nurse specialists in palliative care. *J Adv Nurs.* 2003;43(5):521–530.
55. Mishel MH. Uncertainty in chronic illness. *Ann Review Nursing Res.* 1999;17:269–294.
56. Decker CL, Haase JE, Bell CJ. Uncertainty in adolescents and young adults with cancer. *Oncol Nurs Forum.* 2007;34:681–688.
57. Politi MC, Street RL Jr. The importance of communication in collaborative decision making: Facilitating shared mind and the management of uncertainty. *J Eval Clinical Pract.* 2011;17:579–584.
58. Dean M, Street RL Jr. Managing uncertainty in clinical encounters. In Spritzberg, B. & Hannawa, A. Mouton de Gruter Publishing. Berlin 2015. Handbook of Communication Competence.
59. Ngo-Metzger Q, August KJ, Srinivasan M, et al. End-of-life care: Guidelines for patient-centered communication. *Am Fam Physician.* 2008;77(2):167–174.
60. Charles C, Gafni A, Whelan T. Decision-making in the physician-patient encounter: Revisiting the shared treatment decision-making model. *Soc Sci Med.* 1999;49:651–661.
61. Sudore RL, Casarett D, Smith D, et al. Family involvement at the end-of-life and receipt of quality care. *J Pain Symptom Manage.* 2014;48(6):1108–1016.
62. Jenkins C, Lapelle N, Zapka JG, Kurent JE. End-of-life care and African Americans: Voices from the community. *J Palliat Med.* 2005;8:585–592.
63. Chibnall JT, Videen SD, Duckro PN et al. Psychosocial-spiritual correlates of death distress in patients with life-threatening medical conditions. *Palliat Med.* 2002;16:331–338.
64. Janz NK, Wren PA, Copeland LA, et al. Patient-physician concordance: Preferences, perceptions, and factors influencing the breast cancer surgical decision. *J Clin Oncol.* 2004;22(15):3091–3098.
65. Degner LF, Kristjanson LJ, Bowman D, et al. Information needs and decisional preferences in women with breast cancer. *JAMA.* 1997;277(18):1485–1492.
66. Street RL Jr., Elwyn G, Epstein RM. Patient preferences and healthcare outcomes: An ecological perspective. *Expert Review Pharma Outcomes Res.* 2012;12(2):167–180.
67. Van Eechoud IJ, Piers RD, Van Camp S, et al. Perspectives of family members on planning end-of-life care for terminally ill and frail older people. *J Pain Symptom Manage.* 2014;47(5):876–886.
68. Bodenheimer T, Wagner EH, Grumbach K. Improving primary care for patients with chronic illness: The chronic care model, part 2. *JAMA.* 2002;288(15):1909–1914.
69. Deci EL, Ryan RM. *Intrinsic Motivation and Self-Determination in Human Behavior*. New York, NY: Plenum Press; 1985.
70. Oliver DP, Wittenberg-Lyles E, Demiris G, et al. Barriers to pain management: Caregiver perceptions and pain talk by hospice interdisciplinary teams. *J Pain Symptom Manage.* 2008;36(4):374–382.
71. Kelley M, Demiris G, Nguyen H, et al. Informal hospice caregiver pain management concerns: A qualitative study. *Palliat Med.* 2013;27(7):673–682.
72. Kaplan SH, Greenfield S, Ware JE Jr. Assessing the effects of physician-patient interactions on the outcomes of chronic disease. *Med Care.* 1989;27:S110–S127.
73. Street RL Jr. Communication in medical encounters: An ecological perspective. In: Thompson TL, Dorsey A, Miller KL, Parrott R, eds. *Handbook of Health Communication*. New York, NY: Routledge; 2003:63–93.
74. Street RL.Interpersonal communication skills in healthcare contexts. In: Greene JO, Burleson BR, eds. *Handbook of Communication and Social Interaction Skills*. New York, NY: Psychology Press; 2003:909–933.
75. Parks MR. Communication competence and interpersonal control. In: Knapp ML, Miller GR. *Handbook of Interpersonal Communication*. 2nd ed. Thousand Oaks, CA: SAGE; 1994:589–620.
76. Spitzberg BH, Cupach WR. *Interpersonal Communication Competence*. Beverly Hills, CA: SAGE; 1984.
77. Wiemann JM. Explication and test of a model of communicative competence. *Human Commun Res.* 1977;3(3):195–213.
78. Greene JO. A cognitive approach to human communication: An action assembly theory. *Comm Monog.* 1984;51:289–306.
79. Salmon P, Young B. Creativity in clinical communication: From communication skills to skilled communication. *Med Edu.* 2011;45(3):217–226.

CHAPTER 30

Care Coordination and Transitions in Care

Finly Zachariah, Brenda Thomson, Matthew Loscalzo, and Laura Crocitto

Introduction

Healthcare today consumes nearly 18% of the gross domestic product, and this is expected to increase to 25% by 2037.[1] It is projected that the aging population will drive this increase in spending. Between the years 2011 to 2030, nearly 10,000 people will turn 65 each day.[2] By 2030, nearly one in five US residents will be 65 and older, with an increasing percentage of adults being over the age of 85.[3] Elderly patients have higher healthcare costs, often due to multiple, coexisting comorbidities, more complex care needs, heavy reliance on social support systems to meet their needs, and a higher incidence of cancer and cancer-related mortality. Costs of care are also expected to increase with the growth of molecular-targeted treatments, genome-based diagnostics, new technologies, and coverage expansions as mandated by the Affordable Care Act in the United States.

While implementation of the Affordable Care Act is expected to result in an additional 34 million citizens being insured by 2019,[4] this sudden increase in demand for healthcare services will occur amidst a national shortage of healthcare providers. An estimated shortage of 20,400 primary care providers is expected by 2020, with a projected shortage of 200,000 physicians within the next 20 years.[5] By 2020, the number of registered nurses is expected to fall 29% below predicted requirements.[6] Similarly, social workers, typically arriving at their profession later in life, have shorter career lengths and are more likely to live in metropolitan areas, leaving unfilled needs in many rural areas.[4,7] In addition, the expanded role of spiritual care with Joint Commission palliative care standards along with the aging population and workforce will lead to a shortage of chaplains.

As a result of increasing demand and small workforces, healthcare delivery systems are transitioning from "volume to value" by implementing new models of healthcare delivery.[8] Some new models include team-based care approaches, shifting toward population health management, the development of medical homes, and accountable care organizations. Consequently, team member roles will need to change and provider partnerships will need to improve.[9–14] Better care coordination and transitions to community care settings are necessary, as patients will increasingly rely on family caregivers.[15–17] This chapter provides an overview of care coordination and transitions in care by highlighting shared decision-making (SDM) with patients and families that requires the efforts of an interprofessional team. A model care coordination pathway for cystectomy patients at City of Hope National Medical Center is described.

Care Coordination and Provider Communication

The Agency for Healthcare Research and Quality defines care coordination as

> deliberately organizing patient care activities and sharing information among all of the participants concerned with a patient's care to achieve safer and more effective care. This means that patient's needs and preferences are known ahead of time and communicated at the right time to the right people, and that this information is used to provide safe, appropriate, and effective care to the patient.[18]

Collaboration, knowledge sharing, transitional planning, patient/caregiver engagement, and alignment of resources are crucial to all care coordination efforts.[19]

In 2011 poorly managed care transitions were responsible for $25 billion to $45 billion in unnecessary spending, partly due to unnecessary readmissions and avoidable complications.[20] It is estimated that $17.5 billion is spent on the 2 million Medicare beneficiaries who are readmitted each year.[21] When care is not coordinated well, fragmentation and inefficiencies ensue,[22] causing negative outcomes such as treatment delays, dangerous errors, and increased mortality.

Care coordination relies on SDM between patient, family, and the healthcare team to determine care plans that address quality of life priorities. SDM involves facilitating a patient's right to self-determination, and it helps patients and families integrate values, evidence-based medicine, and a provider's expertise to make informed decisions.[23] The utilization of decision aids during SDM has been shown to improve engagement, knowledge, confidence, and decision-making quality and reduce uncertainty, often resulting in patients choosing more conservative therapies.[24] Most patient-centered communication and SDM models have focused on communication between patient and physician, and only recently are promising models being taught and implemented that incorporate the entire healthcare team.[25–28]

Within the context of cancer care, a functional, patient-centered communication model includes the following six domains: exchanging information, fostering healing relationships, managing uncertainty, recognizing and responding to emotions, making decisions, and enabling self-management and patient navigation.[29] Elements of patient-centered communication include (a) understanding a patient within his or her psychosocial context, (b) addressing the patient's fears and goals, (c) involving patient and family to the level desired, (d) developing a shared understanding of problems and prognosis, (e) exploring perspectives on trade-offs and impaired function, and (f) creating a mutually agreed-on best-practice, feasible treatment plan consistent with patient values.[23,29,30] Unfortunately, patient-centered communication is still not commonplace due to lack of familiarity, time, and applicability, as well as the presence of specialty-driven biases toward certain treatments.[25,31–36]

In addition to patient-centered communication and SDM, care coordination requires that providers from all disciplines work together as an interprofessional team. An Institute of Medicine workgroup designed to evaluate team-based, patient-centered healthcare identified the following key values and principals of highly functioning healthcare teams: honesty and transparency about decisions and mistakes, discipline in carrying out roles even when inconvenient, creativity in tackling problems, using all outcomes as opportunities to learn, humility in respecting each member's role, and curiosity in using daily lessons for continuous improvement.[37] Five key principals identified were shared goals reflecting patient and family priorities, clear roles and accountabilities for each member's functions, effective communication skills, measurable processes and outcomes with timely feedback on results, and mutual trust.[38]

In the absence of care coordination among providers, patients and families can receive conflicting, mixed messages rather than clearly focused information that enables decision-making. Two studies analyzing interprofessional primary healthcare teams attributed conflict to a lack of clarity on role boundaries and scope of practice, providers' failure to trust and act on other professional team members' recommendations, and a lack of accountability.[39,40] Barriers to resolving conflict stem from provider time constraints and workload, the hierarchical nature of healthcare settings, the inclination to avoid confrontation for fear of causing anxiety, and a lack of recognition or motivation to address conflict.[40] Table 30.1 outlines provider roles and responsibilities for collaborative transitions in care. The table sets forth the team roles ideally performed and the implications for patient, staff, and the healthcare system when team roles are performed well.

Communicating Transitions in Care

A core tenet of palliative care is to treat patient and family as a unit, exploring who they are and what they value and then offering medical therapies that fit their goals.[41] The involvement of patients and families in making decisions about goals of care and transitions of care should happen at the start of diagnosis and at key time points throughout the illness.[42] Studies indicate that discussions occurring too early or too late may not allow appropriate reflection or capture a patient's values for his or her present medical care.[43] A prospective study of more than 1,200

Table 30.1 Provider Roles and Responsibilities for Collaborative Transitions in Care

Provider	Role and Responsibilities	Implications for Patient, Staff, and Healthcare System
Inpatient RNs	♦ Conduct assessment of patient that includes but is not limited to risk factors, educational level and health literacy, coping, pain, activity level, beliefs, sexuality, quality of life, advanced directives ♦ Medication reconciliation ♦ Provide education regarding disease process, self-care, and medications ♦ Synthesize findings and develop care plan in collaboration with medical team and patient/caregiver ♦ Referrals to social services as appropriate ♦ Carry out medical treatments and assesses responses ♦ Document interventions and outcomes ♦ Maximize patient autonomy	Patient: Secure and confident in healthcare team, knows needs are being addressed Staff: Less burnout because of decreased distress and empowerment System: Engaged patient and family
Outpatient RNs	♦ Education/medication teaching ♦ Triage for medical needs and psychosocial barriers, referring to medical team, clinical social worker, or case manager as appropriate ♦ Nursing assessment and medical reconciliation at each encounter Home Health Nurses: ♦ Home safety evaluation, transportation, nutrition, ability to perform activities of daily living, symptom and side effect control ♦ Home medication reconciliation, compliance, and education ♦ Prepare and reinforce education to patients and families for their roles at home, link to resources as appropriate	Patient: Comfort in being cared for as an individual, satisfaction, safety, trust in staff Staff: Satisfaction, empowered healthcare team member System: Holistic approach, patient centered

(continued)

Table 30.1 Continued

Provider	Role and Responsibilities	Implications for Patient, Staff, and Healthcare System
Primary MD	♦ Decisions around and communication of disease directed care ♦ Diagnose, provide treatment options, assess patients' preferences and goals of care, develop individualized plan of care, monitor disease status and modify treatment plan as indicated, educate patient and family on disease ♦ Communicate in an open, honest, and timely manner; document clearly and effectively ♦ Facilitate coordination of care with other providers and consultants	Patient: Patient and family actively engaged and partners in care, individual values identified and respected, adherence to care plans increased, patient anxiety decreased, improved patient satisfaction Staff: Reduced staff distress, reduced turnover and sick time and increased communication, coordination, and job-related satisfaction Systems: Patient-centered, quality, cost-efficient care delivered
Consultants	♦ Assessing, recommending, ultimately providing guidance or co-management assistance to colleagues for optimal management ♦ Effective communication to care team and patient regarding treatment plan and follow-up	Patient: Coordinated, safe care Staff: Team building, respect as an important team member Systems: Efficient and effective use of resources; improved patient safety
Nurse Practitioners, Physician Assistants	♦ Proactively assess and manage signs and symptoms within scope of license ♦ Implement plan as outlined by physician or pathway/protocol. ♦ Facilitate consults, communicate discharge needs to case manager, obtain medication authorizations, refills for medications and supplies, and communicate test results to patients in timely fashion ♦ Interface and liaison between physician and patient	Patient: Coordinated care across the continuum including at transitions Staff: Extension of physician respected and valued healthcare team member System: Efficient and effective use of staff resources; coordinated and safe patient care
Social Workers	♦ Screen, identify, address psychosocial problems and barriers ♦ Manage high-risk patient populations facilitating adherence to complex treatment protocols ♦ Problem-based supportive counseling ♦ Prepsychiatry/psychology assessments ♦ Second-line advance care planning ♦ Facilitate goals of care conversations/family meetings ♦ Support and guide end-of-life transitions. ♦ Bereavement counseling for family members and caregivers	Patient: Prospective identification and management of problems and barriers to maximizing the benefits of medical care, adjustment to illness and finding meaning Staff: Support medical and nursing staff in patient and family management System: Patient, family, staff enhanced satisfaction; ensure beneficial use of resources; goal-directed patient-centered care delivered
Nurse Coordinators	♦ Evaluation and preparation of patient for treatment ♦ Provide patient education at key points throughout care tailored to cultural and literacy needs; refer to ancillary specialists as appropriate ♦ Direct patients along trajectory of care ♦ Contact/point person for patient ♦ Liaison for interdisciplinary team ♦ Provide medical guidance—highest level of coordination ♦ Assessment at follow-up visit ♦ Provide continuity through transitions ♦ Identify and address system barriers to care	Patient: Informed, confident, and compassionately cared for Staff: Valuable and respected team member System: Patient-centered compassionate, holistic care delivered
Child Life Specialists	♦ Age-appropriate education/interventions ♦ Play therapy ♦ Coping strategies ♦ Assess and recommend appropriate referrals ♦ End-of-life rituals ♦ Use cultural/age-appropriate language	Patient: Consistency and continuity with home life, family supported, coping tools provided and increased adherence to treatment plans; connected to community resources Staff: Engagement in normalizing processes to manage stress System: Patient-centered care; patient and family needs addressed; staff empowered through education
Patient Navigators	♦ Assist patient in navigating care needs within a complex medical system. ♦ Provide a single point of contact for the patient. ♦ Assist in the coordination of care, managing multiple appointments, consults and follows up through transitions of care	Patients: Patients and families feel welcome and safe in new, complex environment from the beginning Staff: Increased adherence and compliance from patients System: Patient-centered coordinated and compassionate care delivered; efficient use of institutional resources

(continued)

Table 30.1 Continued

Provider	Role and Responsibilities	Implications for Patient, Staff, and Healthcare System
PT/OT/Rehab Providers	♦ Functional assessments ♦ Recommend equipment needs to improve mobility and maximize safety ♦ Maximize physical functioning in rapidly changing environment ♦ Provide education on exercises to be done at home ♦ Adapt care plans based on progress	Patient: Patient, family and community resources prospectively activated to maximize function, rehabilitation, and satisfaction Staff: Increased functional status, which maximizes therapeutic options, increases patient safety (decreased falls) System: Provides safe methods of transitioning to lower level of care, increases patient safety, enhances functional status, thus improving quality of life
Patient Educators	♦ Assist with creation of education incorporating literacy level, cultural, and linguistic needs of patients/families	Patient: Actively engaged and informed about all aspects of care leading to increased shared decision-making; apply knowledge to maximize benefits of medical care and positive outcomes Staff: Improved patient adherence to complex protocols System: Patient, family, staff enhanced satisfaction; efficient use of institutional resources; improved independence with home care
Pharmacy Personnel	♦ Passive drug monitoring ♦ Monitor utilization in complex care ♦ Reconcile discharge medications with home meds ♦ Identify and report interactions (in highly complex patients, need to round with team, ICU rounds, BMT, etc., for active engagement in clinician consultation) ♦ Active management in protocol-driven care (renal dosing, coumadin/diabetes/cholesterol clinics)	Patient: Informed, more confident and adherent; pharmacist is a trusted resource available to patients Staff: Increased knowledge; knowledgeable expert consultation available 24 hours a day System: Increased safety, decreased cost
Case Managers[a]	♦ Screen patients for factors that affect progression of care ♦ Develop safe and effective discharge plan in collaboration with interdisciplinary teams and patient/caregiver ♦ Anticipate, develop, and coordinate for successful transitions in care across the trajectory and settings communicating unmet goals ♦ Ensure appropriate level of care ♦ Facilitate timely and efficient delivery of care ♦ Collaborate and build relationships with community partners. ♦ Ensure compliance with regulatory requirements related to utilization review and discharge planning ♦ Proactively prevent unnecessary readmissions ♦ Demonstrate patient advocacy ♦ Prevent medical necessity denials ♦ Track avoidable delays ♦ Knowledgeable of coverage limitations and financial responsibilities of organization and patient balancing cost and quality	Patient: Less stress and anxiety, more satisfaction Staff: Empowered, valuable/knowledgeable team member System: Compliant with regulations; patient safety is priority; fiscally sound

[a] Utilization review and discharge planning.

patients examining discussions about end-of-life care and the care received showed that having discussions with patients and families was most effective anytime (31–60, 61–90, and >90 days) before the last 30 days of life and resulted in less aggressive care (e.g., chemotherapy in the last 14 days of life, acute care and ICU care in the last 30 days of life) and greater utilization of hospice.[44] When physicians wait until a patient medically declines to have these discussions, patients are often already in the hospital under situations of higher stress. The study also found that only patient- or family-recognized end-of-life discussions had an impact on aggressiveness of care as compared to provider-recognized/documented end-of-life discussions, highlighting the need to continually assess patient and family perceptions in active goals of care discussions.[44] One study examining family perspectives around SDM at the end of life recommended the healthcare team maintain hope while preparing for death, discuss achievable goals and preparing for the future, pace their explanations, remain open to discussing alternative medicine, maximize the patient's physical strength, and avoid statements that the healthcare team can do nothing for the patient.[45]

Decision-Making Involving Possible Transitions From the Acute Care Hospital

A critical decision-making juncture occurs in discharge planning from hospitals. Any decisions should be made in the context of a person's overall values and goals. Many resources detail the communication framework of appropriate goals of care conversations and elements of the conversation patients and families find most important.[46–50] One review looked at outcomes of goals of care discussions and found six goals: to be cured, live longer, improve or maintain function/quality of life/independence, be comfortable, achieve life goals, and provide support for family/caregiver.[51] The first three goals may indicate a patient is not yet hospice-ready, but all six goals would be supported by palliative care. When a patient is ready to leave the acute care setting, transitions can be made to home with or without additional services, or to an intermediate location, as listed in Table 30.2.

Numerous transitions occur throughout a patient's care trajectory both within hospital units and between settings, and all require a formal relay of patient/family information between providers (called a handover). As team members collaborate regarding care planning, they too should ensure that the next healthcare provider has a clear understanding of unmet goals of care and necessary follow-up. Failure to provide details related to the patients' ongoing needs leads to adverse consequences.[52] Communication between the sending and receiving providers should follow a common plan of care and include a discharge summary with a problem list, baseline physical and cognitive functional status, documentation of patient goals and preferences (including advance directives), allergies, a medication list

Table 30.2 Patient Goals, Medical Criteria, and Resources Needed to Transition to Post-Acute Care Settings[56]

Setting	Description of Services	Patient Goals	Medical Criteria	Resources
Home Health[a]	Skilled nursing, rehabilitation services, social work, home health aide performed by certified home health providers	• Desire to be cured/live longer • Desire to be home	Interventions can safely be provided in the home either by teaching patient/caregiver as taught and supported by a licensed, skilled home care agency. If interventions are custodial in nature, a licensed agency may not be required	• Caregivers capable and available, either family or hired. • Resources to support
Hospice[b]	Services are provided to terminally ill patients in any care setting. Includes bereavement and support services for caregivers.	• Desire to support highest quality of life possible over quantity • Desire for comfort and support for self and loved ones • Curative therapies are a greater burden than benefit	Terminal illness with prognosis of six months or less to live.	• Covered by insurance • May be paid privately • May qualify for services through charity directly from the agency
Rehabilitation and Therapy	Services are provided in any setting, but typically in an acute rehabilitation facility or a skilled nursing facility	• Desire to improve or restore functional status	Medically assessed functional improvement possible	• Covered by insurance
Long-Term Acute Care	Care for the medically complex patients who require 25 days or more of inpatient care	• Acceptance that care is not possible in alternative level of care • Desire or necessity to be outside of home at end of life	Serious medical conditions that require extended inpatient hospital stays. Complicated interventions such as dialysis, ventilator care, complex wounds, pain management, multiple intravenous medications	• Covered by insurance
Skilled Nursing	Less intensity of care providing 24-hour a day skilled nursing care, rehabilitation services, and medical management	• Acceptance that care is not possible in alternative level of care • Desire or necessity to be outside of home at end of life	Requires 24-hour skilled nursing care	• Covered by most insurances • If custodial in nature only, limited coverage options unless Medicaid or long-term care insurance
Subacute Care	Specialize in care for the medically complicated, stable patients who have medical needs that cannot be managed in a less intensive setting	• Acceptance that care is not possible in alternative level of care • Desire or necessity to be outside of home at end of life	Frequently more stable than long-term acute. Requires complex needs such as ventilator weaning or extensive therapy prior to going home	• Covered by insurance

[a] Service is provided at home. [b] Service can be provided at home or in a facility.

that reconciles home medications with present regimen, clear follow-up instructions for labs and appointments, and clear guidance on warning signs and symptoms with appropriate contact information.[53] Especially important, and often overlooked, is the capacity and willingness of the family to care for the patient at home.

An intervention engaging patients to take a more active role in their care, facilitating communication between settings with the assistance of a "transition coach," was found to be effective in improving patient care and decreasing hospital admissions.[54] More significant transitions occur where the primary provider can change, such as when a patient enrolls in hospice. One study examining perceptions noted that patients and families felt abandoned from the loss of continuity with their providers and also felt a lack of closure. Nurses and healthcare providers did not feel abandoned but did note a lack of closure.[55] Decision making for an ideal transition incorporates medical criteria and required resources, but in addition involves patients and families as part of the team and fundamentally uses patient goals to drive the level of care delivered.

Piloting a Care Coordination Pathway

Communication engagement among healthcare providers and the patient and family is the foundation for true patient- and family-centered care. What is less obvious and appreciated is that, taken together, competence, communication, connection, and coordination create the trust that is essential for the level of biopsychosocial complexity that is endemic to excellence in healthcare. In reviewing more than 700 case reports in which formal complaints were lodged at City of Hope National Medical Center (where we are employed), virtually all of the problems listed by patients or their families related to perceptions of inadequate communication, coordination, and connection. We describe here the development of a pilot project of a care coordination pathway, a method of patient-care management of a group of patients during a defined period of time.

The aim of the project was to develop an evidence-based pathway that fostered collaboration of the disciplines with the patient on a regular basis to stimulate an interprofessional level of team interaction, decrease care variation among providers, engage and empower the patient, and improve the quality of care delivered. First, two previous years of cystectomy patients at City of Hope National Medical Center were reviewed and compared to that of other cancer centers. The length of stay, readmission rate, reasons for readmission, and utilization of services and resources were analyzed. Patients who undergo cystectomy, similar to national figures, typically have a greater than 60% complication rate and greater than 30% readmission rate. Upon presentation of the statistics analyzed, the urology group discussed and agreed to the development of a care coordination pathway. An interdisciplinary team was convened with nursing, social work, patient education, case management, medical oncology, supportive care medicine, chaplaincy, pharmacy, nutrition, and urology representatives, with input from former patients, to develop a care pathway. The baseline challenges were lack of expertise in team-based models of care, initial resistance to change, lack of infrastructure for a nurse care coordinator, disciplinary silos with an interdisciplinary approach to care, and urologist rounding time of 7 AM.

The pathway begins with identification of a newly diagnosed bladder cancer patient (see Figure 30.1). The patient is screened prior to surgery for biopsychosocial issues that may impact his or her health. Next, patient communication preferences are elicited and the patient is screened for initial goals of care involving advance directives. Problem-based biopsychosocial screening is performed utilizing a tablet-based platform (SupportScreen), which allows for real-time identification and triaging of the patient concerns, whether it is the desire for educational information in written or electronic formats, the desire for providers to know of symptoms that may need to be addressed, or perhaps an endorsement of suicidal ideation where the system would page a social worker to come up immediately to assess the veracity of the concern. Utilizing information from the SupportScreen and National Comprehensive Cancer Network criteria, the patient, caregiver, and urologist have a detailed conversation integrating the information preferences and advance care planning concerns identified on SupportScreen as well as goals of care. The patient, family, and healthcare provider then decide on the best value-based treatment course for the patient (often the patient then proceeds to cystectomy or adjuvant chemotherapy followed by cystectomy).

Preoperatively, the patient and family attend a new patient orientation class and meet the care coordinator. The care coordinator performs the stoma marking (identification of the site on the skin where the surgeon creates an opening) and educates the patient and family on the pathway and procedure. In addition, the coordinator meets with the social worker regarding completion of an advance directive, further goals of care, and any barriers to treatment. With the case manager, the coordinator discusses a discharge plan, including caregiver assistance, discharge medications and supplies, and a standard medical workup with appropriate medical clearances, labs, and X-rays. A lay patient navigator is available throughout the continuum of care to answer questions, remind patients of appointments, coordinate appointments, triage for any specific needs, and guide the patient through the system.

The patient is then admitted the day of surgery, follows a standardized care plan with deviations documented in a progress note. Daily multidisciplinary rounds occur at the bedside with the urology and palliative medicine attendings, a case manager, nurse coordinator, social worker, urology fellow, urology mid-level provider, and bedside nurse. When the model was originally implemented, each team member had clearly delineated roles and responsibilities and reported during bedside rounds. Over time, the daily discussion on rounds has led to an increased understanding of each of the other disciplines' roles and an increased awareness by all members of the team of what must occur for the patient. With the urologist's continued daily encouragement to the team, while in the patient's room, to raise any issues of concern, team confidence has been built, and team members increasingly discuss concerns within and even outside their discipline, indicating they are starting to operate in an interprofessional fashion. Medical, psychosocial, nutritional, and educational needs are discussed with the patient during rounds along with daily patient goals, goal progress, and discharge plan. A whiteboard in the patient's room is updated to reflect the outcomes of daily rounds and is used to communicate the information to all team members, including the patient and family. Upon discharge, patients are monitored closely, as they are at high risk for readmission. The care coordinator calls

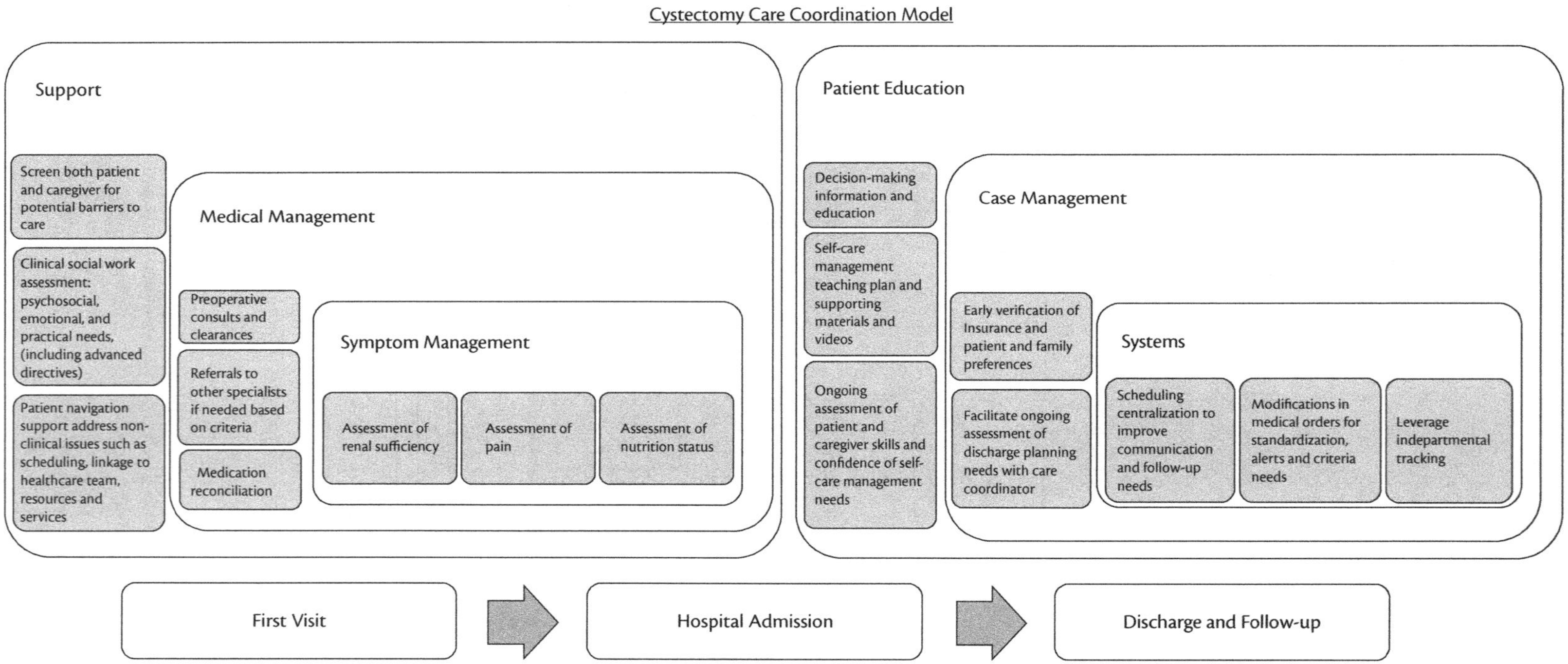

Cystectomy Care Coordination Model

Support
- Screen both patient and caregiver for potential barriers to care
- Clinical social work assessment: psychosocial, emotional, and practical needs, (including advanced directives)
- Patient navigation support address non-clinical issues such as scheduling, linkage to healthcare team, resources and services

Medical Management
- Preoperative consults and clearances
- Referrals to other specialists if needed based on criteria
- Medication reconciliation

Symptom Management
- Assessment of renal sufficiency
- Assessment of pain
- Assessment of nutrition status

Patient Education
- Decision-making information and education
- Self-care management teaching plan and supporting materials and videos
- Ongoing assessment of patient and caregiver skills and confidence of self-care management needs

Case Management
- Early verification of insurance and patient and family preferences
- Facilitate ongoing assessment of discharge planning needs with care coordinator

Systems
- Scheduling centralization to improve communication and follow-up needs
- Modifications in medical orders for standardization, alerts and criteria needs
- Leverage indepartmental tracking

First Visit → Hospital Admission → Discharge and Follow-up

Figure 30.1 Pilot Care Coordination Pathway Project at City of Hope

each patient 24 hours after discharge, and patients return to the clinic 3 and 7 days following discharge, and then again at 3 weeks, where the family is screened to assess whether there are developing or existing concerns that may impact the support the patient needs in the postdischarge period.

In addition to the assistance rendered by the nurse care coordinator and healthcare team, patients often have home health needs. The major home health agencies caring for cystectomy patients are engaged and provided specific hands-on training in urostomy care. They are notified to observe for potential red flags and are provided with direct lines of communication with the urology healthcare team to ensure optimal collaboration and the ability to quickly convey any concerns while caring for the patient. Similar training is done with the triage nurses. Quality metrics including length of stay, postoperative complications, readmissions, pathway adherence, and patient satisfaction are tracked and regularly assessed. Team huddles with team members occur weekly and, when needed, to address issues, concerns, modify practice, and build cohesiveness.

City of Hope has been successful in obtaining hospital and provider support, developing a collaborative multidisciplinary team for cystectomy patients. The triage nurses indicate that the volume of calls since pathway inception has decreased and that patient education and communication has been much more effective, as patients have a much better understanding of the procedure, type of diversion, and care techniques. Early analysis also shows a trend toward decreased readmissions and increased patient satisfaction. Furthermore, advance directive completion rate has increased from a baseline of 38% to 68% in the 6 months of the pathway. In addition, there has been post-pathway implementation of direct referrals from the urology service to hospice. Historically, patients would first transition to medical oncology and then proceed with hospice. The direct referral from urology indicates an enhanced level of communication and patient-centric care. The biggest challenge has been establishing and maintaining a high functioning team. This entails changing the current way of practice and the current culture and remembering that competent, caring, connected professionals can coordinate activities on the basis of clear communication, which allows delivery of the best care possible to patients.

Conclusion

Communication is a key component to delivering quality healthcare. A patient-centered communication model insures that the patient, family, and provider share in the decision-making; an interprofessional team coordinates care to treat the whole person from diagnosis throughout the transitions in care that follow. Both tenets are key to insuring the best possible healthcare for the patient and the family in an increasingly complex and overly burdened healthcare environment.

References

1. Cuckler GA, Sisko AM, Keehan SP, et al. National health expenditure projections, 2012–22: Slow growth until coverage expands and economy improves. *Health Affairs (Project Hope)*. October 2013;32(10):1820–1831.
2. Cohn D, Taylor P. Baby boomers approach 65—glumly. http://www.pewsocialtrends.org/2010/12/20/baby-boomers-approach-65-glumly/. Published December 20, 2010. Accessed November 16, 2014.
3. Medicine Io. *Delivering High-Quality Cancer Care: Charting a New Course for a System in Crisis.* Washington, DC: National Academies Press; 2013.
4. Messner C. Impending oncology social worker shortage? Brain drain, retention, and recruitment. *Oncol Issues*. September-October 2010:46–47.
5. Kirkwood MK, Bruinooge SS, Goldstein MA, Bajorin DF, Kosty MP. Enhancing the American Society of Clinical Oncology Workforce Information System with geographic distribution of oncologists and comparison of data sources for the number of practicing oncologists. *J Oncol. Pract.* January 1, 2014;10(1):32–38.
6. National Center for Health Workforce Analysis. *The Impact of the Aging Population on the Health Workforce in the United States: Summary of Key Findings*. Rensselaer, NY: Center for Heath Workforce Studies; 2006.
7. Nadelhaft A, Rene D. Landmark study warns of impending labor force shortages for social work profession. http://www.socialworkers.org/pressroom/2006/030806.asp. Published March 8, 2006. Accessed March 18, 2008.
8. Porter ME, Teisberg EO. *Redefining Health Care: Creating Value-Based Competition on Results.* Boston, MA: Harvard Business School Press; 2006.
9. Fairman JA, Rowe JW, Hassmiller S, Shalala DE. Broadening the scope of nursing practice. *N Engl J Med*. 2011;364(3):193–196.
10. Coates SM. Upholding the patient narrative in palliative care: The role of the healthcare chaplain in the multidisciplinary team. *Health Soc Care Chaplain*. 2013;13(1):17–21.
11. Dranove D. In ACO era, physicians will still play a leading—but changing—role. *Mod Healthcare*. 2014;44(28):39–39.
12. Baker C. Keynote speech. Presented at Boston College Graduate School Forum, February 27, 2014. http://www.eurekalert.org/pub_releases/2014-02/bc-swr022714.php. Accessed November 16, 2014.
13. George VM, Shocksnider J. Leaders: Are you ready for change? The clinical nurse as care coordinator in the new health care system. *Nurs Admin Q*. 2014;38(1):78–85.
14. Bookman A, Harrington M. Family caregivers: A shadow workforce in the geriatric health care system? *J Health Politics Policy Law*. December 1, 2007;32(6):1005–1041.
15. Levine C, Reinhard S, Feinberg LF, Albert S, Hart A. Family caregivers on the job: Moving beyond ADLs and IADLs. *Generations*. 2003;27(4):17–23.
16. Given BA, Given CW, Kozachik S. Family support in advanced cancer. *CA: Cancer J Clin*. 2001;51(4):213–231.
17. Agency for Healthcare Research and Quality. Care coordination. http://www.ahrq.gov/professionals/prevention-chronic-care/improve/coordination/index.html. Accessed June 20, 2015.
18. McDonald KM, Sundaram V, Bravata DM, et al. *Closing the Quality Gap: A Critical Analysis of Quality Improvement Strategies.* Vol. 7: *Care Coordination*. Rockville, MD: Agency for Healthcare Research and Quality; 2007.
19. Medicine Io. *Crossing the Quality Chasm: A New Health System for the 21st Century*. Washington, DC: National Academies Press; 2001.
20. Rau, J. Medicare to penalize 2,217 hospitals for excess readmissions. http://www.kaisernews.org/Stories/2012/August/13/medicare-hospitals-readmissions-penalties.aspx. Accessed August 13, 2014.
21. National Transitions of Care Coalition. Improving care transitions: Findings and considerations of the "Vision of the National Transitions of Care Coalition" http://www.ntocc.org/Portals/0/PDF/Resources/NTOCCIssueBriefs.pdf. Published September 2010.
22. US Department of Health and Human Services. 2012 annual progress report to Congress. National strategy for quality improvement in health care. http://ahrq.gov/workingforquality/nqs/nqs2012annlrpt.pdf. Published April 2012.
23. Ferrer RL, Gill JM. Shared decision making, contextualized. *Ann Fam Med*. July-August 2013;11:303–305.

24. Elwyn G, Frosch D, Thomson R, et al. Shared decision making: A model for clinical practice. *J Gen Intern Med.* 2010;27(10):1361–1367.
25. Légaré F, Stacey D. An interprofessional approach to shared decision making: What it means and where next. In: Woodruff TK, Clayman ML, Waimey KE, eds. *Oncofertility Communication*: New York, NY: Springer; 2014:131–139.
26. Legare F, Stacey D, Briere N, et al. Healthcare providers' intentions to engage in an interprofessional approach to shared decision-making in home care programs: A mixed methods study. *J Interprof Care.* May 2013;27(3):214–222.
27. Korner M, Ehrhardt H, Steger AK, Bengel J. Interprofessional SDM train-the-trainer program "Fit for SDM": Provider satisfaction and impact on participation. *Patient Educ Couns.* October 2012;89(1):122–128.
28. Legare F, Stacey D, Briere N, et al. An interprofessional approach to shared decision making: An exploratory case study with family caregivers of one IP home care team. *BMC Geriatrics.* 2014;14(1):83.
29. McCormack LA, Treiman K, Rupert D, et al. Measuring patient-centered communication in cancer care: A literature review and the development of a systematic approach. *Soc Sci Med.* April 2011;72(7):1085–1095.
30. Clark K, Bardwell WA, Arsenault T, DeTeresa R, Loscalzo M. Implementing touch-screen technology to enhance recognition of distress. *Psycho-Oncology.* August 2009;18(8):822–830.
31. Hoffman RM, Elmore JG, Fairfield KM, Gerstein BS, Levin CA, Pignone MP. Lack of shared decision making in cancer screening discussions: Results from a national survey. *Am J Prevent Med.* September 2014;47(3):251–259.
32. Han PKJ, Kobrin S, Breen N, et al. National evidence on the use of shared decision making in prostate-specific antigen screening. *Ann Fam Med.* 2013;11(4):306–314.
33. Bouma AB, Tiedje K, Poplau S, et al. Shared decision making in the safety net: Where do we go from here? *J Am Board Fam Med.* March-April 2014;27(2):292–294.
34. King VJ, Davis MM, Gorman PN, Rugge JB, Fagnan LJ. Perceptions of shared decision making and decision aids among rural primary care clinicians. *Med Decis Making.* July-August 2012;32(4):636–644.
35. Knight RQ, Waddimba AC, Foster F, Alberts B, Sorensen J. "Big pros and big cons": Factors Influencing utilization of shared decision-making in low back pain from a surgeon's perspective. *J Spine.* 2013;2(5):146.
36. Gravel K, Legare F, Graham ID. Barriers and facilitators to implementing shared decision-making in clinical practice: A systematic review of health professionals' perceptions. *Implement Sci.* 2006;1:16.
37. Mitchell P, Wynia M, Golden R, McNellis B, Okun S, Webb CE, Rohrbach V, Von Kohorn, I. Core principles & values of effective team-based health care. Washington, DC: Institute of Medicine. https://www.nationalahec.org/pdfs/VSRT-Team-Based-Care-Principles-values.pdf. Published October 2012.
38. Hui D, Kim SH, Roquemore J, Dev R, Chisholm G, Bruera E. Impact of timing and setting of palliative care referral on quality of end-of-life care in cancer patients. *Cancer.* 2014;120(11):1743–1749.
39. Lingard L, Vanstone M, Durrant M, et al. Conflicting messages: Examining the dynamics of leadership on interprofessional teams. *Acad Med.* 2012;87(12):1762–1767.
40. Brown J, Lewis L, Ellis K, Stewart M, Freeman TR, Kasperski MJ. Conflict on interprofessional primary health care teams—can it be resolved? *J Interprof Care.* 2011;25(1):4–10.
41. Morrison RS, Meier DE. Palliative care. *N Engl J Med.* 2004;350(25):2582–2590.
42. Hui D, Kim SH, Roquemore J, Dev R, Chisholm G, Bruera E. Impact of timing and setting of palliative care referral on quality of end-of-life care in cancer patients. *Cancer.* 2014;120(11):1743–1749.
43. Billings JA, Bernacki R. Strategic targeting of advance care planning interventions: The Goldilocks phenomenon. *JAMA Intern Med.* April 2014;174(4):620–624.
44. Mack JW, Cronin A, Keating NL, et al. Associations between end-of-life discussion characteristics and care received near death: A prospective cohort study. *J Clin Oncol.* December 10, 2012;30(35):4387–4395.
45. Shirado A, Morita T, Akazawa T, et al. Both maintaining hope and preparing for death: effects of physicians' and nurses' behaviors from bereaved family members' perspectives. *J Pain Symptom Manage.* May 2013;45(5):848–858.
46. Boyd K, Murray SA. Recognising and managing key transitions in end of life care. *BMJ.* 2010;341:c4863.
47. von Gunten CF, Ferris FD, Emanuel LL. Ensuring competency in end-of-life care: Communication and relational skills. *JAMA.* 2000;284(23):3051–3057.
48. Bruera E, Hui D. Integrating supportive and palliative care in the trajectory of cancer: Establishing goals and models of Care. *J Clin Oncol.* September 1, 2010;28(25):4013–4017.
49. Goldstein NE, Back AL, Morrison R. Titrating guidance: A model to guide physicians in assisting patients and family members who are facing complex decisions. *Arch Intern Med.* 2008;168(16):1733–1739.
50. You JJ, Dodek P, Lamontagne F, et al. What really matters in end-of-life discussions? Perspectives of patients in hospital with serious illness and their families. *Can Med Assoc J.* December 9, 2014;186(18):E679–E687.
51. Kaldjian LC, Curtis AE, Shinkunas LA, Cannon KT. Review article: Goals of care toward the end of life: A structured literature review. *Am J Hospice Palliat Med.* December 1, 2009;25(6):501–511.
52. Kripalani, S. What have we learned about safe inpatient handovers? http://webmmahrq.gov/perspective.aspx?perspectiveID=100 Published March 2011
53. Coleman EA. Falling through the cracks: Challenges and opportunities for improving transitional care for persons with continuous complex care needs. *J Am Geriatr Soc.* 2003;51(4):549–555.
54. Coleman EA, Smith JD, Frank JC, Min S-J, Parry C, Kramer AM. Preparing patients and caregivers to participate in care delivered across settings: The Care Transitions Intervention. *J Am Geriatr Soc.* 2004;52(11):1817–1825.
55. Back AL, Young JP, McCown E, et al. Abandonment at the end of life from patient, caregiver, nurse, and physician perspectives: Loss of continuity and lack of closure. *Arch Intern Med.* March 9 2009;169(5):474–479.

CHAPTER 31

Trust, Hope, and Miracles

Rhonda S. Cooper, Louise Knight, and Anna Ferguson

Introduction

The oncologist requested that the palliative consult team see a 41-year-old leukemia patient whose disease had recurred after numerous rounds of chemotherapy and only a brief period of remission. During a lengthy consult with the oncologist, the patient and her longtime partner had been advised that all available treatment options had been exhausted, except for the possibility of a Phase I trial. The oncologist also had spoken to the patient about hospice service availability. With little hesitation, the patient and her partner replied, "We will consider the trial, although frankly, we are hoping for a miracle."

No scenario occasions the discussion of miracles like that in which a healthcare provider presents to a patient the choice of either hospice services or a Phase I trial. While the offer of the trial extends the active treatment options beyond additional standard protocols, it offers the least certainty of success of all the clinical trials. Offering some reassurance and hope for many patients, in Phase I trials the drug is being tested for the first time in humans to find a safe dose and explore toxicity.[1] For the informed patient, therefore, the hope for a miracle is a poignant, reality-based response to the situation since the expected outcome is that the trial will not extend the patient's life and may even shorten it.

Regardless of the clinical decision in this scenario, the healthcare provider is, in essence, advising the patient and her family of the probable terminal nature of the patient's disease. In this instance, the palliative team should further explore the range of options (hospice care or clinical trial) with the patient and her partner. In the process, the team needs to encourage them to talk about their feelings, including their hopes and fears, as well as encourage them to plan for the future should the leukemia prove fatal.

Fortunately, in this case, the physician, palliative nurse, and social worker had met previously with the patient for symptom management concerns, and the palliative chaplain had met the patient and her family during a previous admission. The entire team was well aware of the patient's need to be heard and understood and had built an empathic relationship that had given attention to the patient's affective needs as well as her need for objective information. A relationship of trust had been established, so that the patient felt confident that the healthcare team would respect both her decisions and her religious beliefs. "We know God can do this," the patient said with conviction, "and we just need the doctors not to give up hope. We fully expect a miracle to happen."

Many people, including healthcare providers, believe that miracles can and do happen, even in the most traumatic of injuries.[2,3,4] Some writers note that the belief in miracles is based in irrationality, meaning that something will occur despite the laws of science.[5] Others frame the belief in a miracle as a statement of faith or piety, since the holy texts and traditional writings of many religions contain reports and stories of miraculous occurrences. Daniel Sulmasy, a practicing physician and former Franciscan friar, has contributed notably to this discussion on the role of religious faith.[6,7,8] For many people, medical interventions are conduits of divine and otherworldly healing energy; and medical practitioners are a "heaven-sent" instrument of divinely empowered healing.

While most patients enter treatment with hearts full of hope, the hope for a miracle may also be the *cri de coeur* in the face of uncertainty and existential distress. In other words, a miracle becomes the ultimate treatment option when all others have failed. For the distraught parent, child, spouse, or partner who cannot imagine life without his or her loved one, the hope for a miracle is a reasonable option. Besides, who can positively assert that miracle cures never happen? Patients intuitively understand that healthcare providers "have no particular ability to determine the actual chances that a miracle will occur."[9(p582)] In fact, for a patient who may be facing the threat of losing his or her life, or a caregiver losing a beloved family member or friend, the hope for a miracle may come from a place of grief and distress as well as sincere religious faith.

The related topics of trust, hope, and the expectation of a miracle, whether rooted in a sincere belief in divine intervention or as a visceral response to the anxiety of uncertainty, is explored in this chapter, along with palliative team response strategies. Indeed, some have pointed out that an archaic definition of hope is trust, or reliance, as in the expectation that something will happen for the good and that there is something or someone who may be able to help.[10] Further, hope in relation to illness or infirmity is considered to be a commonly utilized, if not a primary, coping strategy.[11–13]

While the equation of hope with trust may be relevant in certain cases, we contend that trust is a "preexisting condition" and that hope is much more than a coping strategy. The capacity for trust is a psychological reality that all parties bring to the relationship from the outset. This trust baseline, which is rooted in the attachment bonds developed in a child's early life experiences with his or her primary caregiver,[14] likely sets the stage for the entire trajectory of the patient–caregiver–provider relationship. That said, trustworthiness may be fostered and built over time as the care relationship itself develops.

In this process of relationship-building, hope holds great promise as a reliable and fitting way for healthcare providers to frame the palliative conversation, from the very beginning of treatment to the conclusion of the patient–family–provider relationship. Rather than being a flashpoint for conflict, the hope for a miracle has the potential to engender a deeper provider–patient/family discussion about their hope. Indeed, the introduction of the possibility of a miracle cure, despite all medical evidence to the contrary, may be embraced by the healthcare provider as an invitation to initiate or advance the conversation about hope in the context of a trustworthy relationship. The provider's willingness to enter into such a discussion takes courage, sensitivity, and a commitment to patient partnership, components upon which palliative communication inarguably is built.

As the case is built for these contentions, this chapter explores the notable challenges presented to the palliative care provider: namely, issues of trust occasioned by psychosocial and/or cultural predispositions, as well as issues of power inherent in the patient–healthcare provider relationship. This chapter acknowledges the possible reasons for the patient or family's belief in a miracle in the dialectical framework of hope and denial, while the case of the African American community is explored as an example of the delicate interplay of trust, power, and religious sensibilities. The healthcare provider's strategies for responding in ways that continue the palliative conversation, rather than forestall it, are discussed, notably through the conversational AMEN protocol. Finally, the conversation framed by hope is exemplified as a worthy endeavor for the palliative care provider who is committed to person-centered and family-focused care.

Trust as a "Preexisting Condition": The Psychosocial Reality

Healthcare providers, when working with a patient and his or her family, must remember that they are working within the positive and negative experiences of the patient's lifetime. The provider may represent to the patient or family all past healthcare providers, all in authority, or all who control some aspect of the patient's/family's lives. When a person seeks healthcare, he or she brings to the relationship each and every life experience, his or her premorbid health behaviors and emotions, and other individual character traits. Likewise, healthcare providers contribute the same to this newly formed relationship. The healthcare provider must recognize this reality, a critical component of self-awareness and the development of skills to monitor one's level of engagement with the patient and family.

Unrecognized feelings and emotions, including those around trusting or being trusted, may distort how the healthcare provider interprets a clinical encounter as well as adversely affect patient–provider communication.[15] In the case of the hope for a miracle, providers can personalize the perception that the patient/family has lost faith in their ability to prognosticate or provide appropriate treatment and set off a chain reaction of negative responses. While the content of the discussion is about the disease and treatment, the healthcare provider may internalize the discussion as a personal failure. Internal and external pressures within the healthcare system can drive this perceived internal failure as can the provider's lifelong experiences that are brought to the relationship.

In the formation of the healthcare relationship, each party tests the other on varying trust levels starting with the simplest, for example, the return of a phone call, to the most complex, including treatment planning and outcome discussions. In this context, trustworthiness is built as an emotional and intellectual joining within a relationship. Behaviors, language, attitude, tone, and nonverbal communication play a role in the development of trust within the patient/family and healthcare provider relationship. Within this fragile dynamic, demonstrated behaviors of trustworthiness by the healthcare provider solidify the relational foundation. In turn, these behaviors set the stage for the conversational exchange around treatment planning, disease prognosis, and healthcare goals, which will occur within the provider–patient trust framework.

The use of self is an important concept in all healthcare providers' practices, whether as chaplain, social worker, nurse, or physician. Every discipline has its own knowledge base and competence measure, and all healthcare providers practice the art of healing. Indeed, every healthcare provider, to be most effective, uses his or her emotional resources and personal life experiences to connect with patients, learn their stories, formulate assessments, and support them throughout their illness trajectory. Self-awareness, therefore, enhances a provider's effectiveness, regardless of his or her team role, especially when caring for people who have significant disease burden, physical or emotional distress brought about by symptoms, and/or anxiety as a result of facing end-of-life issues.

The way a person responds to an illness or provider is not determined solely by the illness or the personalities involved but instead by the entirety of who the patient is. Everyone, including the healthcare provider, has an outlook, values, or worldview that impacts the way he or she experiences and makes meaning of his or her illness.[16] The palliative care provider should be aware of the patient's capacity (or lack thereof) to trust the providers. Accordingly, the healthcare provider can resist the tendency to personalize the emotional issues unconsciously brought to the relationship. However, the provider also must be aware of the trust issues he or she brings to the relationship. All parties in the patient–family–provider triad (or dyad, as the case may be) play a role that may well be influenced by psychosocial realities beyond the immediate encounter.

If the healthcare provider is not aware of his or her own core beliefs, values, family of origin influences, gender issues, sociocultural influences, especially around trust, he or she may be nonplussed by the unconscious redirection or shift of emotions from a person in the patient's life to the provider. Similarly, the healthcare provider may unconsciously redirect some of his or her feelings toward the patient and become emotionally entangled in ways that do not benefit the caregiving relationship. These transference and countertransference issues are part and parcel of the intense caring relationship occasioned by life-threatening or chronic illness, and only through self-awareness can the provider understand and manage these dynamics in a helpful way.

As an example, the difficult patient may be so labeled more as a result of the healthcare provider's unrecognized/unacknowledged issues than as a result of the patient's issues.[17] While some patients clearly have psychiatric or psychological issues that affect the patient–provider relationship, healthcare providers may have emotional reactions to certain patients because of their own biases. Similarly, a healthcare provider of any discipline may label as religious ideation a person's hope for a miracle in the face of seemingly incontrovertible evidence, thus preventing his or her own ability to communicate an empathetic acknowledgement and response to a patient's hopes and fears.

By being self-aware, providers understand how they impact the relational dynamics, thereby setting the stage for the patient–family–provider relationship trajectory from beginning to end. For example, if a healthcare provider has unresolved feelings about death, dependency, vulnerability, or loss of control or a hesitancy to give bad news for fear of the response, he or she may unknowingly fail to be empathetic. The provider's response will depend on his or her personal history of responding to difficult situations. Based on a person's life experience and unresolved personal issues, he or she may create distance between himself/herself and the patient or may become overinvolved and foster an unhealthy emotional dependency between himself/herself and the patient. Lack of self-awareness will impact a healthcare provider's ability to foster trustworthiness by his or her presence or demonstrate sincere concern for the well-being of the whole person, a hallmark of good palliative care.[5]

Issues of Power

Quality palliative care is resolutely person-centered as well as family-focused and prizes communication and patient involvement, even partnership, in care discussions and decisions.[18] In the medical context, regardless of the provider's affability or openheartedness, the provider generally sets the relationship tone and parameters. Past research suggests that, in general, patients speak less than healthcare providers during meetings or consults and mainly in response to provider questions.[19] Indeed, one study found that in professional conversations with physicians, parents of pediatric patients under the age of 13 asked questions or gave their opinions in an assertive manner, as in disagreement with the physician or making a recommendation, in less than 10% of their utterances.[20]

During challenging conversations that are part of the care of patients with chronic, incurable, or terminal diseases, the "miracle question" often arises. Experience shows that the healthcare provider rarely welcomes this as part of the discussion about end-of-life matters. The authors contend that the healthcare provider's power, both of status and interaction, is a factor in communication with the patient or family, including that of the palliative intervention, since "power relations are always relations of struggle."[21(p72)] Therefore, a rudimentary understanding of language and power may be instructive in terms of palliative care communication, especially when the conjoined subjects of hope and miracles emerge or become problematic from the healthcare provider perspective.

Status-based power refers to that of the person who is in control of the destiny of another by virtue of position or role. The provider's uniform or white coat, along with his or her title, signifies this type of power in the healthcare setting and is undeniably connected to the healthcare provider's interactional power as well. Generally the provider not only has more to say but also controls the content being discussed, topics introduced and developed, and is the one whose opinions take precedence.[22] Even with the best of intentions, the healthcare provider *controls the floor*, while the "difficult patient" is one who often is described as "talking too much," "always changing the subject," or "in denial" about some aspect of the information being discussed.

In relation to the hope for a miracle, we suggest that on a conscious or unconscious level, some patients/family members attempt to shift the balance of power in a difficult conversation by introducing assertions that presumably are outside the healthcare provider's comfort zone, including the belief in miracle healing or other similar statement of faith. This shift may be a clue that the patient does not feel involved or engaged, that shared decision-making is not felt,[23] or that the patient is simply resistant to the information being presented as it relates to disease progression or the lack of treatment options available. Regardless, it behooves healthcare providers to recognize the power dynamics at play, so that they will not unknowingly marginalize or minimize the patient's contribution to the conversation or take personally the miracle comments as a statement of distrust in their competence.[17]

The Miracle Hope in the Context of Hope and Denial

Whether as a conscious or unconscious attempt on the part of the patient/family to shift the balance of power, or as a sincere expression of religious piety, or simply as an existential "gut response" to uncertainty and distress, the patient/family often introduces the hope for a miracle into discussions with providers. In the opening case scenario about the leukemia patient whose disease had relapsed, the patient/family member raised the hope for a miracle at a point at which continuing treatment was being offered. The miracle discussion becomes more problematic for the healthcare provider when a challenging conversation is taking place about end-of-life decisions such as discontinuing aggressive treatment, allowing a natural death, or using extraordinary means to extend life.

At these poignant times, the provider often interprets the patient or family's hope for a miracle as a way to "prolong the inevitable" or as denial that further medical treatment will not be effective or life-enhancing. The healthcare provider faces the contradictory pressures to treat the patient both as an "object" to be fixed, in terms of his or her disease, and as a "subject," a person with feelings, beliefs, hopes, and fears.[24,21] Hope and denial remain in play, alongside each other, during every interaction along the trajectory of both the disease progression and, as this chapter suggests, the patient–provider relationship itself.

Oftentimes, the healthcare provider uses the phrase "false hope" to dismiss or diminish the patient's or family's hope for a miraculous cure in the face of insurmountable medical challenges. A belief in miracles may result in the continuation of nonbeneficial treatments that prolong death rather than uphold life;[25] however, the person who sincerely trusts in a higher power or divine interventionist possesses a worldview that believes there is more to life than meets the eye. If healthcare providers diminish or discount this belief, they may be setting themselves in opposition to, or competition with, the higher truth or supernatural reality that the patient embraces and trusts.

False hope must be considered in light of who judges what is true and false. In terms of the aforementioned power dynamics, generally the one in power is the one naming or defining the falsity or trueness of the specific hope, which rarely advances either the conversation or the relationship of trust. For instance, the patient who hopes for a miracle may respond to the healthcare provider: "You have to understand, we are people of faith," as the healthcare provider communicates skepticism or impatience. For whether the healthcare provider grasps it or not, a person's belief is generally based in logic, whether that belief is in a divine presence with power over the natural world or in the possibility of divine intervention leading to a miraculous outcome that defies science. In other words, the patient believes not in the miracle per se but in the power of the subject/object of his or her faith to intervene.

The patient's or family's insistence on a miraculous cure also may be a "necessary rest-stop" on the road to acceptance of what is to be.[26] Mental health professionals have long known that denial may be an adaptive coping strategy, if it gives a person time to adjust to a distressing life change or painful issue, such as that occasioned by a serious illness. Indeed, denial is common in the face of life-limiting or incurable disease.[27] The idea of the rest-stop on the way to acceptance is one way to imagine this, in that the image is congruent with the idea of denial as a coping strategy. Without respite a person may be unable to persevere in the face of what may appear to be insurmountable physical or emotional challenge. Without a pause, some people are not able to reflect meaningfully on the implications of their circumstances.

A particularly vexing situation arose in a critical care unit in which the husband of an intubated patient who was dying from a lung infection insisted, based on his religious faith, that the extraordinary measures medically supporting his wife not be withdrawn. His reason was, in part, because he and his faith community were trusting God for a miracle healing. He was convinced that it was not time for his wife to die, for she had recently been elevated to a position of authority within their community, and her heart's desire was to fulfill that responsibility and role. The healthcare team explained the medical situation to this man many times and threw up their hands figuratively and literally in rounds, repeatedly asserting that this patient's spouse was "in deep denial."

Interestingly, the patient's husband was having a parallel discussion with the hospital chaplain about such practical items as how to choose a funeral home and when to notify the patient's family, who lived several time zones away, to come to the bedside to say their good-byes. He was processing his feelings of anticipatory grief with the chaplain as well as exploring his religious commitments in light of the circumstances. His greatest concern clearly was to advocate faithfully for his wife with the healthcare team and at the same time practically prepare for the loss of his beloved spouse. The chaplain assessed that the man was not deeply in denial, although he did express seemingly contradictory expectations about the outcome of his wife's illness. On the one hand, he said he believed that God could "work a miracle" and heal his wife; on the other, he believed that this outcome was not likely given her medical condition.

Sometimes a patient or family member maintains two perspectives that appear to the healthcare team to conflict.[28] The family member, for instance, in fulfilling his or her role as the patient's advocate with the healthcare team, will insist on the best care possible or "everything that can be done," so that a miracle might have the time and space to occur. The family is attempting to live out their core religious belief in a divine power that has the ability to intervene for the good. At the same time, the family member, in his or her role as a practical family caregiver, is considering how to accept what he or she innately fears will happen and how the unknown future will unfold for himself/herself and other family members.

This creative tension between hope and denial is explored in the work of Steve Nolan, a palliative care chaplain.[29] Chaplain Nolan builds on a model of hope development espoused by Rumbold,[30] who earlier incorporated psychiatrist Avery Weisman's review of the defenses that dying persons use to ameliorate the anxiety aroused by their impending death.[31] Drawing on these two theorists, Nolan explores the interplay between hope and denial and joins Weisman in his suggestion that each instance or level of denial has a corresponding acceptance level. In other words, each level of denial yields, when impossible to sustain, to an acceptance of a new reality in which the individual is living. With respect to Rumbold, he continues, "hope is, by definition, always associated with, and sustained by, denial and acceptance."[29(p24)]

With this in mind, Nolan concludes that "stealing denial is a maleficent act that healthcare providers should resist, no matter how much they feel that the person for whom they are caring needs to face up to reality."[29(p25)] This insight is relevant in the case of the patient who is religiously grounded, as well as the one who does not have a specific faith preference. For just as denial may yield to acceptance, so also patient and provider hopes alike may evolve and change along with the understanding of cure and healing.

A Case in Point: The African American Community

A fact well known to the hospice and palliative care community is the general underutilization of palliative and hospice services by the African American population, including both Christian and Muslim adherents.[32] Barriers have been explored, including history and heritage, religion and spirituality, education, bioethical issues, breach of trust, and health policy; and work groups have been formed to address the situation. The issues of trust and spiritual/religious hopes, including for a divine intervention such as a miracle, are inextricably related. The person-centered, family-focused healthcare team should be aware of these.

Some studies have concluded that cultural mistrust of medical care appears to have significant influence on the attitudes and decisions of African American patients in the case of advance directives and other end-of-life matters.[33] In urban areas of the United States, where the majority of population may be non-Caucasian, the Caucasian minority will likely comprise the dominant culture. In other words, the segment of the population that holds most of the decision-making power and exerts the greater economic weight will be Caucasian. In healthcare settings, the fact that the majority of the administrators are not persons of color or female—rather, are primarily Caucasian and male—demonstrates who holds the power both in the management and delivery of services. These factors give us clues as to why African Americans may mistrust healthcare providers.

Add to this dynamic that of the aforementioned provider–patient power struggles. Whether valid or not, many providers will intuit or feel African American patients' or families' distrust—especially healthcare providers new to the family. A relationship formed in distrust will quickly fail or be minimally productive. At the medical center where we serve, the case is well known in the community of Henrietta Lacks, an African American woman of humble means who died of cancer in 1951. Healthcare providers harvested samples of Lacks's tissue without her permission. Thereafter, these providers cultured the samples in a laboratory and then bought and sold them for research purposes; they survive as the HeLa cell line to this day in medical scientists' laboratories around the world.[34]

African Americans' experiences with the US healthcare system, which includes segregated hospitals, breaches in trust such as mentioned, and a legacy of poor access, may explain why many African Americans do not take a healthcare provider's pronouncement at face value, especially regarding the use of extraordinary measures to extend a critically ill person's life.[35] Our checkered history in the United States may lead the patient and/or family to insist that "everything be done" regardless of the medical facts of the case. In this and other situations, distrust (by the patient and/or family) as a "preexisting condition" is a lived reality for many healthcare providers, in particular the feeling that palliative and hospice care will be of a "second order" or less than would be provided for non-African American patients.

The African American community is also, by and large, more religiously oriented than other cultural groups in the United States, including Asian Americans and Caucasian Americans.[33,36] An interesting study that characterizes the physician as "God's mechanic" reviews spiritual practice and beliefs in rural southeastern states, including a significant African American population. The results show that 80% of respondents to a telephone survey said that they believed God acts through physicians to cure illness, and 40% believe God's will is the most important factor in recovery. Most people (87.5%) expressed belief in religious miracles, including healing of illness.[37] This predisposition to view healthcare providers through the lens of a theocentric faith, along with a belief in God's ability to perform miracles, may well set the stage for palliative care resistance that seemingly diminishes the care level or "gives up on God."

A notable exception may be found among African Americans who belong to the Jehovah Witness faith, comprising between 20% to 30% of the church's membership in the United States. Although Jehovah Witnesses are known in healthcare settings for their refusal of most blood products on religious grounds, less well known is the church's emphasis on completing and regularly reviewing advance directives. The document is often reduced to a wallet-sized card and attached to the back of the driver's license, in the hope that instructions will be found in a medical emergency about the person's end-of-life decisions, medical proxy, and preferences regarding blood products. Jehovah Witness theology also teaches that God does not perform miracles in the present day, medical or otherwise, so a devout, informed Witness would not express this hope.[38]

Healthcare providers who may be confounded or frustrated by an African American patient's or family's perceived mistrust in them, or their deep resistance to palliative and hospice discussions, should resist personalizing the distrust. Palliative care providers also must resist the temptation to minimize the resistance by attributing it solely to denial or false hope or communicate a less than respectful attitude toward an individual's cultural or religious beliefs. A mindfulness of a patient's or family's religious sensibilities, including the belief that only God gives or takes away life, will help healthcare providers resist putting themselves in competition with the God of the patient's understanding. Why? Because everyone knows who will win that contest, at least in the patient's or family's mind.

Communication Strategies: The AMEN Protocol

Adherents of many religions in various cultural settings believe in miraculous medical recoveries or cures, including Islam, Judaism, Buddhism, and Christianity. Even within these religions, a spectrum of belief exists in the probability of miracles occurring. The cultural preferences and setting, as well as the depth of adherent's religious practice, may all affect a patient's hope for a miracle in the face of serious illness. Healthcare providers who are nonplused by the patient or family who expresses hope for a miracle in response to bad news about the prognosis or treatment outcome may do well to consider a communication strategy called AMEN[39] (see Box 31.1).

The goal of person-centered palliative communication is staying engaged, especially in the midst of challenging conversations about terminal, chronic, or life-limiting illness, during which patients' religious beliefs are discussed, namely, those that involve the hope for a miracle. As mentioned earlier, there is a difference between trust and trustworthiness. While trust is a "preexisting condition," the provider who has created a safe space of hearing the patient and family and their concerns also has created a trustworthy space. Tolerance is not enough in this case, since tolerance is merely a passive response to a difference. More critical than tolerance are the tools of humility and respect for the patient's/family's lived experience and background.

In light of the goal of remaining engaged with patients and families, a conversational protocol called AMEN may be helpful. The tool can help normalize what is often viewed as solely religious by framing it in the concept of hope. When the patient or family and healthcare provider do not share the same religious beliefs and attempt to engage in a theological discussion or disputation, they disrupt the provider–patient communication and compromise the

---

Box 31.1 AMEN Protocol[39]

♦ **Affirm** the patient's belief. Validate his or her position: "Ms. X, I am hopeful, too."

♦ **Meet** the patient or family member where they are: "I join you in hoping (or praying) for a miracle."

♦ **Educate** from your role as a healthcare provider: "And I want to speak to you about some medical issues."

♦ **No matter what**; assure the patient and family you are committed to them: "No matter what happens, I will be with you every step of the way."

Cooper RS, Ferguson A, Bodurtha JN, Smith TJ. AMEN in challenging conversations: Bridging the gaps between faith, hope, and medicine. *J Oncol Pract*. July 2014;10(4):e191–e195.

relationship—possibly to the detriment of the patient's well-being and comfort.

The heart of the AMEN protocol is the commitment to joining rather than placing more distance between patient and provider. Note the emphasis on the use of the word "and" rather than "but" in the response of the provider. Even a "yes, but" is a token join, in that the "but" expresses a contradictory opinion that fails to address the person's ideas who has just spoken their opinion or hope.[40] The word "but" dismisses the patient or family member who has spoken of his or her hope for a miracle. Furthermore, the protocol and its movement toward joining and assuring patients of remaining with them "every step of the way" abrogates the responsibility of the healthcare provider to engage on a theological or religious level.

The concept of nonabandonment of the patient by the healthcare provider has been shown to provide hope for patients entering palliative breast cancer care.[41] How physicians communicate is often as important, or more important, than what they communicate.[5,42] Providers' communication should reassure patients that they will not be alone as their disease progresses or distressing symptoms persist and provide reassurance and the certainty of continuing care. The challenge for healthcare providers, of course, is in the realistic ability to meet their own goal of nonabandonment, especially in the case of the patient who transitions to hospice care. With this in mind, providers may prefer to speak of the healthcare team's commitment: "*We* will be with you, every step of the way," thereby symbolically enlarging the circle of care for the patient.

An experienced palliative care nurse shared that the subject of divine intervention often became an issue in the cardiac center where she cared for patients. She also confessed that she quickly changed the subject when it did, even though she was a religious person herself. After a presentation on the AMEN protocol, she reported that the very next day a patient responded to news of his disease progression with the assertion, "I hear what you are saying, but I believe I will be cured by a miracle." This time, however, the nurse felt empowered by the protocol to say, "I join you in your hope for healing, and I respect your faith. I also want to be faithful to my role as a nurse and share some information as we make some decisions about your care. Remember, we are in this together, all the way."

With the AMEN protocol, the palliative care provider steps out of the provider role for a moment and responds as a human being, whether he or she is a religious person or not. The use of "and" signifies two people in conversation and signals a momentary suspension of the power dynamic. After all, healthcare providers also are hoping for cure, remission, and relief from suffering for their patients, are they not? Providers also are able to clarify their role, as did the palliative care nurse in the aforementioned scenario, and speak from that perspective. The reassuring statement of nonabandonment will, in fact, facilitate hope, albeit an evolving or changing set of specific hopes. When healthcare providers join the patient or family as a person, they do not give false hope—on the contrary, they recognize that hope is real, hope is energizing, and hope is at the center of healing.

Hope Reimagined

Sometimes the palliative care provider may best respond to the expectation for a miracle healing with the simple invitation, "Tell me more about the miracle." This allows the healthcare provider to accept the invitation to engage in a deeper conversation about hope, since the courageous palliative care provider is the one who will walk through the portal provided by the "miracle conversation" and continue the conversation about hope. Challenging conversations will always be challenging conversations, yet the self-aware provider will not be thwarted by his or her own biases, anxieties (e.g., about loss of health or death), or issues.

A patient with refractory leukemia had endured months of grueling, life-limiting treatments and lengthy hospital admissions. As a person with a well-known religious commitment, from the first consultation with his physician the man had shared his belief that God would heal him. "God is in control," he would say, "and my family and I are claiming a miracle, no matter what the doctors say." Although all the healthcare providers patiently listened and were tolerant of his evangelistic fervor, the healthcare team shared an unspoken understanding that the treatment options had become wholly ineffective, even as the patient's level of physical suffering was increasing.

One day, the chaplain was informed that this patient was expressing a high level of diffused anger at every healthcare provider who entered the room, including his nurses, the dietary staff, and the primary care team. When the chaplain engaged the patient and asked him why he was angry, he was clear: "I'm angry because I have hoped and prayed for a miracle, and it is just not happening. I am not getting better. I am getting worse." After a time of respectful silence, the chaplain quietly asked, "Bob, what is your back-up hope?"

Almost reflexively, the patient responded with a list of hopes—for discharge from the hospital to the hospice near his home, for food that he enjoyed, for the opportunity to make his own funeral plans. He spoke as if he had been freed from the burden of the hoping for a miracle and empowered to express and bring to fulfillment the more mundane, realizable hopes. He related to the idea of the back-up hope in a way that surprised the entire healthcare team, and indeed he soon was transferred to a hospice facility where he was surrounded by loved ones and caring staff. He died peacefully three days later, after making his own funeral plans and leaving his two sons with his parting wisdom.

A reimagining of the concept of hope, as a present-oriented endeavor rather than solely future oriented, may help the palliative care provider navigate the conversation as well as assist the patient to stay grounded in the present. Hope as an essential attribute of being is that which may energize and motivate a person to live as well as possible in the present day. Hope for the person with an incurable and life-limiting disease may be allowed to transform from a hope for recovery to a hope beyond recovery,[29] thus allowing sadness, as well as resolve, to coexist with hope. As the family of the aforementioned patient said at the memorial service, "Bob trusted God with his life and with his death. God is always in control. The miracle happened. Bob truly was healed."

Sometimes healthcare providers are concerned that a person will lose their faith when the hoped-for miracle cure does not occur. Similarly, they are reluctant to fully disclose to the patient the terminality of his or her disease, because the healthcare provider is fearful that the patient will lose hope or be unable to cope.[43] Smith et al. found the inverse to be true: that the more honest and clear information patients received, the more hopeful they were able to be. The authors attributed this to the patients' ability to plan their daily life intentionally in the context of knowing their time may be limited.[44]

Individuals often prove to be more spiritually resilient than one might think. The negative predictions, or fears, on the part of healthcare providers, that a patient or family will lose their faith, hope, or ability to cope when a miracle healing does not occur do not take into account this resiliency. For one thing, "expectation is not based solely on some objectively demonstrable external reality, but on what persons believe the reality to be."[27(p236)] In addition, faithful people, those who are devout in their religious faith, generally find a way to make meaning of their circumstances, as in the case of patient Bob. Consciously or intuitively, they are able to reframe their healing and hope understanding, as patient and provider alike are challenged by hope to expand their understanding/definition of healing.

The Conversation Framed by Hope

In light of the understanding of hope as both future- and present-oriented, the Hope Project has been introduced at the comprehensive cancer center where we work. A goal of the project is to encourage physicians, nurses, social workers, chaplains, and other members of the healthcare team to ask from the beginning of their relationship with a patient the open-ended question: "What are you hoping for?" This simple yet thought-provoking query then can serve as a cornerstone for current decision-making, future conversations, and the patient–provider relationship as a whole. Hope can become the common ground and the place where everyone has an equal voice.

The world of oncology, for better or worse, tends to be suffused with military metaphors. This language is heard at all levels—from patients, to staff, to families. Cancer is spoken of as an enemy, patients as warriors or fighters, chemotherapy as "the big guns," t-cells as generals, and treatment as the fight or battle. At the time of diagnosis, most people share the same hope that the battle can be won and the cancer cured. Then, when patients feel they are at war, which many do, discussing hope with them can be like bringing in the Red Cross. Discussing hope is humanitarian aid: the box of rescue supplies that arrives in a war-ravaged place.

The contents of that box alone may not cure or solve a single problem people have, but its very arrival brings a life-sustaining message—and that message is that we as providers know that the war has taken so much from the patient, but it has not taken his or her humanness, and that humanness has not been forsaken or forgotten. Further, it is an opportunity to humanize the conversations that are to follow, whether about treatment protocols, prognosis, or progress. For even when the "big hope" for cure is not realizable, healthcare providers can simultaneously allow patients and families the space to grieve that loss and help them trust that hope is not reserved only for the curable. This is rooted in the belief that hope can shift, evolve, and change, as curative possibilities begin to fade.[45]

The Hope Project's exploratory study of the patients' and providers' hope perceptions concluded that hope is essential to good quality of life and also very individualized in terms of its content. These findings may be utilized by using interview techniques established in other areas of subjective assessment. For example, just as pain is what the patient says it is, so too is hope. As a provider would not treat patients' pain without first asking them to describe it, neither can providers get very far in a hope discussion without first asking what it is that hope means to the individual. By virtue of taking care of patients at the most vulnerable moments of their lives, healthcare providers influence a patient's hope experience, whether or not they intend to, for better or worse.

A conversation framed by hope allows healthcare providers to efficiently and compassionately talk about what is probable versus what is possible. It allows palliative care providers to put words on the paradoxes that are part and parcel of end-of-life care, namely that fear and peace can coexist, as can disappointment and hope. The gift to patients and families is the reminder that they do not need to choose one or the other. Patients can hope for a miracle drug while at the same time prepare their family for life without them. They can grieve the loss of moving toward a cure and yet, at the same time, celebrate the way they feel in the present day (see Box 31.2).

As patients with cancer and other chronic conditions live even longer, it becomes necessary to have strong yet dynamic threads that can tie together years' worth of remissions, relapses, side effects, setbacks, decisions, new therapies, anxiety, and research. Hope can be one of these threads, for it is likely the unacknowledged undercurrent in many patient–provider conversations. In this case, there is power when the unspoken is spoken. For it may be that identifying what we hope for this week, this month, from this treatment—whether there is a "this time next year" or not—these are the hopes that drive people, that sustain them during difficult treatments, that get them out of bed in the morning and into their daily lives. These seemingly "lesser" hopes often may be those that bring the most joy and meaning to life.

Conclusion

A modern-day sage, Oprah Winfrey, has observed that every person shares the common desire to be seen and heard. As commonsensical as it may sound, a patient's or family member's expression of the hope for a miracle, particularly during a difficult conversation about a poor medical outcome, may be, in part, a plea to be "seen and heard" by not only the God of their understanding but the healthcare provider team as well.

> Understanding that one principle, that everybody wants to be heard, has allowed me to hold the microphone for you all these years with the least amount of judgment. Now I can't say I wasn't judging *some* days. Some days, I had to judge just a little bit. But it's helped me to stand and to try to do that with an open mind and to do it with an open heart. It has worked for this platform, and I guarantee you it will work for yours. Try it with your children, your husband, your wife, your boss, your friends. Validate them. "I see you. I hear you. And what you say matters to me."[46]

Box 31.2 Talking about Hope

For healthcare providers, the hope question is a tool. The next time a patient says, "They told me there was no hope left, so I came to you," or "You're not giving up hope on me are you?" or "Please tell me there's still hope," the provider can respond, "I'm really glad you mentioned hope—we know how important hope is. I want to make sure it's part of our conversations. So tell me more about what hope means to you." The conversation about hope can evolve and change, in stages, just as the relationship itself is built incrementally, as trustworthiness is demonstrated by the healthcare provider.

The courageous palliative care provider is the one who will walk through the door provided by the miracle conversation, hear what the patient or family has to say, value and affirm it, and continue the conversation about their hopes—and fears. The healthcare team members who set the stage from the outset of the relationship by asking the patient and family what they are hoping for set the expectation that they will be heard and seen, no matter what the future holds.

References

1. Olver IN. Bioethical implications of hope. In: Eliott J, ed. *Interdisciplinary Perspectives on Hope.* Hauppauge, NY: Nova Science; 2005:241–254.
2. Widera EW, Rosenfled KE, Fromme EK, Sulmasy DP, Arnold RM. Approaching patients and family members who hope for a miracle. *J Pain Symptom Manage.* 2011;42:119–125.
3. Jacobs LM, Burns K, Bennett Jacobs B. Trauma death: Views of the public and trauma professionals on death and dying from injuries. *Arch Surg.* 2008;143:730–735.
4. Orr RD. Responding to patient beliefs in miracles. *South Med J.* 2007;100(12):1263–1267.
5. Tulsky JA. Hope and hubris. *J Palliat Med.* 2002;5(3):339–341.
6. Sulmasy DP. Distinguishing denial from authentic faith in miracles: A clinical-pastoral approach. *South Med J.* 2007;100(12):1268–1272.
7. Sulmasy DP. What is a miracle? *South Med J.* 2007;100(12):1223–1228.
8. Pawlikowski J. The history of thinking about miracles in the West. *South Med J.* 2007;100(12):1229–1235.
9. Clarke, S. When they believe in miracles. *J Med Ethics.* 2013;39:582–583.
10. Hope. In: *Merriam Webster Dictionary.* http://www.merriam-webster.com/dictionary/hope Accessed September 1, 2014.
11. Gum A, Snyder CR. Coping with terminal illness: The role of hopeful thinking. *J Palliat Med.* 2002;5(6):883–894.
12. Lazarus SR. Hope: An emotion and a vital coping resource against despair. *Soc Res.* 1999;66(2):653.
13. Maden S, Pakenham KI. The stress-buffering effects of hope on adjustment to multiple sclerosis. *Int J Behav Med.* 2014;21(6):877–890.
14. Bowlby J. *Attachment: Attachment and Loss, Vol. 1* (2nd ed.). New York, NY: Basic Books; 1983.
15. Novack DH, Suchman AL, Clark, W, Epstein RM, Najberg E, Kapland C. Calibrating the physician: Personal awareness and effective patient care. *JAMA.* 1997;278(6):502–509.
16. Chochinov, HM. *Dignity Therapy: Final Words for Final Days.* New York, NY: Oxford University Press; 2012.
17. Alfandre DJ. Do all physicians need to recognize countertransference? *Am J Bioeth.* 2009;9(10):38–39.
18. Street RL, Millay B. Analyzing patient participation in medical encounters. *Health Commun.* 2001;13(1):61–73.
19. Roter DL, Hall JA, Katz NR. Patient-physician communication: A descriptive summary of the literature. *Patient Educ Couns.* 1988;12:99–119.
20. Street RL Jr. Communicative styles and adaptations in physician-parent consultations. *Soc Sci Med.* 1992;34:1155–1163.
21. Fairclough N. *Language and Power.* Hoboken, NJ: Taylor & Francis; 2013.
22. Puckett A. Language and power. In: Clark AD, Hayward NM, eds. *Talking Appalachian: Voice, Identity, and Community.* Lexington: University Press of Kentucky; 2013:141–161.
23. Legare F, Ratte S, Stacy D et al. Interventions for improving the adoption of shared decision making by healthcare professionals. *Cochrane Database Syst Rev.* 2010;5:CD006732.
24. Fairclough N. *Critical Discourse Analysis: The Critical Study of Language.* New York, NY: Routledge; 2013.
25. Wagner JT, Higdon TL. Spiritual issues and bioethics in the intensive care unit: The role of the chaplain. *Med Ethics.* 1996;12(1):15–27.
26. Lisagor M. The chaplain's ears and the alchemy of instinct. *PlainViews* 2014;11(5).
27. Brooksbank MA, Cassell EJ. The place of hope in clinical medicine. In: Eliott J, ed. *Interdisciplinary Perspectives on Hope.* Hauppauge, NY: Nova Science; 2005:231–239.
28. Keene Reder EA, Serwint, JR. Until the last breath. *Arch Pediatr Adolesc Med.* 2009;163(7):653–657.
29. Nolan S. *Spiritual Care at the End of Life.* London: Jessica Kingsley; 2012.
30. Rumbold BD. *Hopelessness and Hope: Pastoral Care in Terminal Illness.* London: SCM Press; 1986. Cited in Nolan, 2012.
31. Weisman A. *On Dying and Denying: A Psychiatric Study of Terminality.* New York: Behavioural Publications; 1972. Cited by Nolan, 2012
32. National Hospice and Palliative Care Organization. NHPCO's Facts and Figures: Hospice Care in America 2013. http://www.nhpco.org/sites/default/files/public/Statistics_Research/2013_Facts_Figures.pdf Accessed September 1, 2014.
33. Crawley L, Payne R, Bolden J, Payne T, Washington P, Williams S. Palliative and end-of-life care in the African American community. *JAMA* 2000;284(19):2518–2521.
34. Skloot R. *The Immortal Life of Henrietta Lacks.* New York, NY: Crown; 2010.
35. Blackhall LJ, Frank G, Murphy ST, Michel V, Palmer JM, Azen SP. Ethnicity and attitudes towards life sustaining technology. *Soc Sci Med.* 1999;48:1779–1789.
36. Johnson KS, Elbert-Avila KI, Tulsky JA. The influence of spiritual beliefs and practices on the treatment preferences for African Americans: A review of the literature. *J Am Geriatr Soc.* 2005;53:711–719.
37. Mansfield CJ, Mitchell J, King DE. The doctor as God's mechanic? Beliefs in the southeastern United States. *Soc Sci Med.* 2002;54:399–409.
38. Watchtower Online Library. Miracles. *Insight* 2:411–414. http://wol.jw.org/en/wol/d/r1/lp-e/1200003073. Accessed June 20, 2015.
39. Cooper RS, Ferguson A, Bodurtha JN, Smith TJ. AMEN in challenging conversations: Bridging the gaps between faith, hope, and medicine. *J Oncol Pract.* July 2014;10(4):e191–e195.
40. Gantt SP, Agazarian YM. Systems-centered emotional intelligence: Beyond individual systems to organizational systems. *Organizational Analysis* 2004;12(2):147–169.
41. van Vliet, LM, van der Wall E, Plum NM, Bensing JM. Explicit prognostic information and reassurance about nonabandonment when entering palliative breast cancer care: Findings from a scripted video-vignette study. *J Clin Oncol.* 2013;31(26):3242–3246.
42. Mast MS, Kindlimann A, Langewitz W. Recipients' perspective on breaking bad news: How you put it really makes a difference. *Patient Educ Couns.* 2005;58:244–251.
43. Collis E, Sleeman KE. Do patients need to know that they are terminally ill? *BMJ* April 24, 2013;346:f2589.
44. Smith TJ, Dow LA, Virago EA, Khatcheressian J, Matsuyama R, Lyckholm LJ. A pilot trial of decision aids to give truthful prognostic and treatment information to chemotherapy patients with advanced cancer. *J Support Oncol.* March-April 2011;9(2):79–86.
45. Eliott JA, Olver IN. Hope, life, and death: A qualitative analysis of dying cancer patients' talk about hope. *Death Stud.* 2009;33:609–638.
46. The Oprah Winfrey Show Final. http://www.oprah.com/oprahshow/The-Oprah-Winfrey-Show-Finale_1/7. Published May 25, 2011. Accessed 31 June 2014.

CHAPTER 32

Physical Pain and Symptoms

Danielle Noreika, Barton Bobb, and Patrick Coyne

Introduction

Symptom assessment and treatment is a crucial component of managing most disease processes. Optimal symptom management includes assessment of the state of the disease process and comorbid disorders, technical skill and experience in choosing among various therapeutic options, and healthcare system utilization. Although these and many other features are important, one of the most vital aspects is the thoroughness of discussion about pain. In order for healthcare providers to successfully treat pain, they must consider the many facets of communication about symptom management. In many disease processes, the most predominant symptom a patient encounters is pain. Communication about pain is necessary to address the symptom but also to properly diagnose and assess, evaluate therapy success, and manage complications of some pain treatments (such as addiction disorders).[1]

Pain assessment, in particular, includes verbal and nonverbal pain score reporting, cultural influences on pain reporting, and patient history to fully characterize pain prior to selecting an optimum therapeutic regimen.[2] There are also special patient populations, such as geriatrics and pediatrics, that may require additional considerations for communication about pain. In the absence of objective data to measure pain, the provider's communication skills become quintessential in pain assessment and symptom management. Communication may occur with the patient themselves (e.g., nausea) or with the patient's family (e.g., in the case of delirium). Communication about pain and physical symptoms, as discussed more closely in this chapter, is integral to successful evaluation and management.

Obtaining a Complete Pain History

Obtaining a complete pain history requires a thorough discussion about the many variables that impact pain. First is the pain score that is generally rated on a scale of 10 (zero being no pain, 10 being the most severe). The pain score relies on subjective patient experience and clearly cannot be validated by laboratory or physiologic data.[3] A highly personal report, the pain score varies greatly between patients in similar disease scenarios. The healthcare provider utilizes the pain score not only to guide initial treatment plans but also to reassess efficacy of therapy over time. Providers place much emphasis on the pain score from the patient's pain history but also must consider a multitude of other items for effective pain management.

As providers try to determine the pain etiology in order to direct the therapy course, many times, they view pain location as the most crucial piece of the equation. Some pain providers use a diagram and ask patients to indicate the areas of the body where they are experiencing pain.[4] Pain quality is also generally necessary to create a differential. Neuropathic pain, for instance, may be described by patients as a "burning" or "shooting" pain, whereas somatic pain may be described as "dull" or "aching."[5] Radiating pain also may be concordant with a neuropathic pain origin. Alleviating and exacerbating factors should be reviewed, especially in light of previously successful pain therapies. The healthcare provider may potentially discover in this portion of the history medication or nonmedication options that can be further explored based on prior use, as well as therapies already tried and not tolerated. This information should be condensed into an area that is easy to reference in the electronic medical record for other providers to access. Taking a thorough pain history also involves discussing a number of variables and consideration of the patient's nonverbal values.

Assessment of Pain Severity in Special Populations

Nonverbal assessment of pain severity is at times necessary for patients who cannot give a score, such as nonresponsive patients and pediatric patients. Certainly teenage patients can utilize numerical rating scales as well as accurately describe pain history, but younger children may not possess the language skills to do so. A number of nonverbal pain severity scales have been developed and validated for use in young children including Faces and Faces–Revised (R), Oucher, and the Wong Baker Faces Pain Rating Scale (WBFPRS).[6] Faces-R updates the Faces scale by allowing scoring from 1 to 10, instead of 1 to 6; both scales are easy to use, require little to no training to administer, and are available in a multitude of languages. The Oucher uses a numerical pain rating scale out of 100 that can be utilized by older children and has different culturally specific pictures available for younger children. Like the other two scales, the WBFPRS is easily administered and available in multiple languages. All of these scales are appropriate for use in children ages 4 and up.

However, in patients under 4 years old, behavioral observational scales are often utilized. For this age group, CRIES, the Neonatal Infant Pain Scale (NIPS), and the Face, Legs, Activity, Cry, Consolability (FLACC) scale have been validated. These scales assess different cry, facial expression, leg movement combinations, and other observable characteristics.[2] CRIES stands for "Crying, Requiring oxygen, Increased vital signs (blood pressure and heart rate), Expression, Sleepless" and is scored on a 10-point scale by provider observation for infants 6 months or less in age. Six indicators (facial expression, cry, breathing patterns, arms, legs, and state of arousal) are assessed in the NIPS scale for children up to 1 year of age. The FLACC scale can be used for patients who are between 2 months and 7 years of age.[2] The use of specific tools vary across institutions, and it should be noted that the use of any one tool should be used with the appropriate patient population consistently.

In addition to differences in pain severity assessment, younger patients may be able to provide only a limited pain history or none at all, challenging the healthcare provider to design appropriate treatment plans. A parent or caregiver must be involved in communication aimed at describing pain in pediatrics, especially in the age range where changes in observable behaviors are perhaps the only pain indicator. Pain assessment in pediatrics potentially differs from that of the standard adult encounter, but effective tools may be similar to those utilized in the assessment of selected populations of adults.

For elderly patients, especially those with cognitive disorders, healthcare providers may be challenged to discern the pain level the patient is experiencing. Elderly patients commonly experience persistent pain related to increase in chronic medical conditions, as well as the higher frequency of musculoskeletal disorders such as arthritis. Older patients should be carefully assessed and frequently screened because pain reporting may differ from that of younger patients or may manifest in other ways such as agitation or declining functional status. The healthcare provider should consider setting aside more time for pain assessments in the elderly, as history-taking may be somewhat more challenging, involving the use of nonverbal scales and family or other caregiver discussions.[7] Families may be asked to share their perception of the patient's pain, information about periods of agitation, previous history of pain and pain behaviors, withdrawal from touch, avoidance of movement, or other indicators that pain may be an issue for the elderly patient who is unable to report a history.

Prompt diagnosis and appropriate treatment for pain is essential, as uncontrolled pain can lead to multiple consequences, including functional impairment, falls, decreased socialization, mood changes, sleep disturbances, and greater healthcare utilization. Discussion of potential evaluation and management strategies are time consuming if done correctly, as elderly patients are more likely to experience side effects or complications, and this requires thorough explanation to patients (if they have the capacity) and caregivers. Caregivers need to be assessed carefully, as persistent pain can be a strain on family as well as the patient.[8] Successful pain management in elderly patients generally necessitates precise communication and observation as well as potential caregiver support for treatment planning.

Chronic Pain Assessment Scales

Healthcare providers utilize several scales to help patients communicate salient aspects of their pain history in order to guide treatment courses. The Brief Pain Inventory (BPI) and the McGill Pain Questionnaire are the most utilized. The BPI is a short instrument that helps gauge the severity and impact of pain on patients and can be used at serial visits over time to assess improvement on therapy. It was originally validated in cancer patients, but evidence now also exists for non-cancer chronic pain, and it is available in multiple languages. This questionnaire includes a body diagram for patients to indicate areas of pain, multiple ratings for pain scores over the week prior to presentation (highest, lowest, average, etc.), and scoring related to function and quality of life factors (sleep, interactions with other people, work, mood, etc.). It can be filled out by patients and quickly reviewed at visits to document pain trends over time, as well as the effect of pain management on patient function to help gauge treatment success.[4] The McGill Pain Questionnaire was developed to as a quantitative pain measure. It is an in-depth measurement of pain descriptors, activities, or environmental factors that affect pain, and it rates pain severity at multiple points prior to the visit. The final score is a summation of the present pain score, the number of words chosen to describe the pain, and a pain-rating index that can be assigned to pain descriptors. The patient can complete this, although the short form is likely most easily utilized for pain assessment. In contrast to the BPI, it does not give any assessment of function in relation to pain.[9]

Although the BPI and the McGill Pain Questionnaire are likely the most commonly cited multidimensional tools, healthcare providers employ others, including the Massachusetts General Hospital Pain Center's Pain Assessment Form; the Initiative on Methods, Measurement, and Pain Assessment in Clinical Trials; the Memorial Pain Assessment Card, and others.[10] Additionally, specific scales exist in order to further explore certain types of pain, such as the Neuropathic Pain Scale, Leeds Assessment of Neuropathic Symptoms and Signs, the Neuropathic Pain Questionnaire, and others.[11] In-depth rating scales such as the BPI and McGill Pain Questionnaire may aid healthcare providers in better evaluating patient pain histories and allow for more accurate assessment of pain management courses over time.

The Role of Culture in Communication About Pain

A patient's cultural background may affect the solicitation of a pain history and discussion of pain. Pain perception and reporting varies widely based on the patient's ethnic or cultural background. Also, pain expression can differ cross-culturally ranging from stoic to consistent outward displays of pain. Similarly, misunderstanding or misinterpreting verbal and nonverbal expressions can skew the pain score. Descriptions of pain may change the interpretation of the patient's pain history. For patients who speak another language, translation variations can cause pain descriptions to be misinterpreted or misconstrued. Some cultures believe that patients should be able to manage pain to a certain degree on their own, as a measure of self-control over life, or that "complaining" of pain to a healthcare professional represents inappropriate behavior.

Religion may also impact the interpretation of pain. For instance, patients of a Buddhist background may believe enduring pain is a path toward spiritual growth.[12] Healthcare providers need to be aware of cultural differences in pain expression. Many assessment scales, including the BPI and the McGill Pain Questionnaire, have been translated into multiple languages and validated in a variety of cultural backgrounds.[12] Once the healthcare provider takes a complete history, continued detailed communication may be necessary for a successful pain management plan.

Pain management goals and acceptable treatment plans may also vary by culture and background. In general, many Western civilization patients find medications to be an appropriate initial step to pain therapy, while patients in Eastern civilizations may be more comfortable with complementary or alternative treatments prior to considering medications. In addition, for some patients there is a discomfort with the use of opioids for pain management because of cultural taboos. Providers must often take extra time in these instances to ensure that pain histories are not underreported because of discomfort with the treatment plans or medications being offered.

Situations in which there is a language barrier in addition to a cultural barrier may be especially challenging. Ideally, in such instances, a healthcare provider would carefully discuss with the patient and family members (using a translator, if needed) a summary of the relevant symptoms and potential treatment plans, including culturally-based therapy options.[13] If language is a barrier, interpreters should be offered at the initial and subsequent visits to allow patients and family members to express treatment plan side effects, intolerances, or other issues. Failure to do so may cause patients to stop medications or other therapeutic agents, allowing uncontrolled symptoms to continue because the patient could not fully communicate his or her concerns.[12] Consideration should be made to investigating nonpharmacological measures that may be culturally preferable to use of medications. Culture may play a significant role in pain evaluation and management, and healthcare providers should consider culture as a factor in pain communication. Team members who have expertise in these therapies as well as their culture should be consulted.

Communicating Treatment Goals and Evaluating Therapeutic Response

Once a management plan is selected, ongoing, open communication between provider, patient, and family gives the highest chance of success. Nonjudgmental, supportive communication and shared decision-making with a common goal may allow the best chance for the patient to accurately follow the management plan.[14] It is also necessary to define clear outcomes for the patient who might have the impossible goal of being pain free. Discussing with the patient, from the outset of therapy and intermittently throughout the course, that the goal is general improvement over time to a tolerable level of pain on average may help prevent treatment failures. Patients should expect days where their pain is worse, even if the average is improved over previous levels.[15] Although these concepts are most commonly found in chronic nonmalignant pain, they are important tenants when communicating about pain with patients and families.

Patients with malignancy-related pain share several contextual factors that impact communication and can result in treatment plans that do not lead to anticipated results. Time constraints influence the provider's ability to engage in pain communication with the patient and may preclude a thorough exploration of all concerns. Time may be limited at the provider visit or may exist in the inability to reach a nurse or provider after the encounter when an issue arises. The healthcare provider must have a supportive staff available to the patient when questions or concerns about pain occur. Delays in communication about pain may impact the patient's ability and willingness to uphold the pain management agreement from the beginning of the therapeutic relationship. For example, a patient may call to discuss an emergency department visit that resulted in an opioid prescription. Another contextual factor impacting communication about pain is patient/family fear of addiction to pain medications. Some patients with pain may avoid utilizing opioid pain medications because of addiction fears as well as side effects; these patients may have improved success in therapy when their concerns are fully addressed. The involvement of family caregivers also impacts adherence to treatment plans. Caregivers often play a critical role in pain and symptom management and should be involved in education to manage the patient's discomfort.[16] Communicating about patient pain with family caregivers is an opportunity to determine if they have concerns regarding pain management. Communication with other team members as well as other healthcare providers will help solidify pain treatment planning.

Pain treatment plans that are supported by an interdisciplinary palliative care team as well as the other providers caring for the patient are potentially more likely to achieve success. Although time-consuming, constant communication between healthcare providers is vital to pain management. If the healthcare provider has in-depth knowledge of the treatment plan, this allows for more patient support and helps prevent the addition of medications or other therapies that may pose patient risk. Healthcare provider collaboration may also result in new ways to address pain such as radiation therapy, physical therapy, psychology, and so on. Patients benefit from a multifaceted approach to therapy by a healthcare team, continued communication regarding the care plan, and assistance in achieving the treatment goals.[17] Active communication with patients, families, team members, and other healthcare providers assures the pain management plan has the highest chance for success.

Communication About Complications of Pain Management

One of the most feared risks of chronic pain management is addiction. According to the American Society of Addiction Medicine, addiction is "a chronic disease of brain reward, motivation, memory and related circuitry leading to characteristic biological, psychological, social and spiritual manifestations reflected in an individual pathologically pursuing reward and/or relief by substance use and other behaviors."[18] The National Institute on Drug Abuse estimates that illicit drug and alcohol abuse contributes to the death of more than 100,000 Americans per year. In 2011 a survey estimated that 52 million Americans over age 12 have used prescription medications (pain medications, sedatives, and stimulants) nonmedically in their lifetime.[19] Given the overwhelming prevalence of addiction disorders, it is imperative that communication about pain with patients and families include screening and provision of treatment of additive behaviors.

Healthcare providers should screen patients who are at high risk of opioid abuse, especially in the prescription of controlled substances to treat chronic nonmalignant pain. Available validated screening tools are the Opioid Risk Tool, the Diagnosis, Intractability, Risk, Efficacy score, the Current Opioid Misuse Measure, and the Screener and Opioid Assessment for Patients with Pain–Revised.[20] Positive screens do not indicate that the patient cannot be prescribed opioids; rather, the healthcare provider must develop a careful safety plan prior to institution. In addition to these scales, in every initial patient encounter, the healthcare provider should discuss mental health disorders, social factors, personal or family history of substance abuse, employment, and any legal issues related to substance use or distribution.[1] At therapy introduction, the provider must communicate the safety standards that will be utilized. Various safeguard tools that many practitioners employ include controlled substance informed consent or agreements, random urine drug screening, pill counting, and review of state prescription monitoring data. Careful review of controlled substance informed consent agreements, if utilized, is necessary to develop a trusting relationship between patient and healthcare provider. Many of these agreements include sole provider status for controlled substances prescription, restriction of replacement of lost or stolen medication, submission to random drug screening, compliance with pill counting, review of state prescription monitoring data, and (likely most important to highlight with patients) instances where controlled substance prescriptions will be tapered or discontinued.[21] It is important to explain to patients, in terms they can easily understand, the importance of chosen outlined safeguards and potential consequences of any noted behaviors at the first visit, prior to prescribing any controlled substance. Patients should also understand that this tool is utilized to promote safety not only for the prescribing provider but also for the patients. After an initial therapy plan is chosen, adherence to delineated safety agreements and periodic screening for substance abuse issues is a necessary part of continued treatment.

Continued communication throughout a pain management treatment course is a safe prescribing expectation. The Federation of State Medical Boards has highlighted multiple areas of recurrent communication in appropriate management including repeated assessment of changes in pain reports, ongoing discussion of nonopioid therapy for pain (coanalgesic pain medications, physical therapy, etc.), and investigation into function. Assessment of function, which includes activities of daily living, employment, and interaction with other people, is an important monitoring tool in the prescription of pain medication in chronic nonmalignant pain. Lack of improvement or function decline with appropriate titration and rotation of pain medication over time may indicate the potential for underlying addiction.[20] Patients may also display aberrant behavior, including asking for repeat prescriptions between visits, self-escalation of medication, or visiting multiple providers for prescriptions. Careful provider–patient communication should occur in all of these instances, as well as a thorough investigation, which may indicate an undertreated medical or addiction issue. The screening tools may also be utilized periodically during the course of treatment to identify substance abuse disorders.[1] If an addiction disorder is identified, treatment should commence as soon as possible.

If a patient appears to have behaviors consistent with addiction or meets criteria for substance dependence or abuse, the healthcare provider will need to address multiple issues. First and foremost, the patient will need treatment for his or her substance abuse disorder, with mental health providers engaged for this process. Supportive therapy is often crucial for successful treatment, and many patients will benefit from programs such as Alcoholic Anonymous and Narcotics Anonymous, in addition to treatment of any mental health disorders.

Although the cornerstone of substance dependence treatment or abuse is referral to mental health specialists, there is certainly a continued role for the primary healthcare or palliative care provider. Supportive techniques such as brief motivational interviewing have been shown to be effective in helping to develop rapport even with patients with challenging situations or personality conflicts. Brief motivational interviewing includes the use of open-ended questions, affirmation, and reflective listening and requires that the healthcare provider avoid any hostile or judgmental behavior.[22] If possible, patients who have pain disorders and have been diagnosed with substance abuse or dependence should be titrated down on the opioids dose or have their opioids discontinued. There is evidence to suggest that decreases, even significant ones, in opioid dosages may not produce a notable change in pain scores, and, after taper, the risk inherent in continued opioid therapy (i.e., side effects such as constipation or risk of harm such as overdose) will be minimized.[23] In a retrospective study performed at Massachusetts General Hospital over a 7-year period, a chart review of 109 patients with chronic pain revealed that both increases and decreases in opioid dose did not produce a significant change in pain score over time.[23] The healthcare provider should undertake a very careful pain management strategy preferably in consultation with a mental health professional caring for the patient. Management plans may range from use of long-acting basal opioids (such as methadone) without any short-acting opioid for breakthrough with small prescriptions (1 to 2 weeks at a time) and frequent follow-up to the use of buprenorphine/naloxone for treatment of the co-occurring disorders.[24] Treatment of concurrent pain and substance abuse disorders is challenging and will require careful communication with patients, mental health professionals, and the healthcare team caring for the patient. Table 32.1 summarizes considerations for patients with high-risk behaviors.

Communication About Pain Management at End of Life

A patient's final moments are a lasting memory for loved ones, and uncontrolled pain or discomfort at the time of death can be a significant stressor for the bereaved. Pain histories at the end of life can be difficult or impossible to obtain, and information about patient pain must often be sought from patient observation over time as well as nursing staff, family, and other provider reports. Nonverbal scales, as noted previously in this chapter, are frequently utilized, as many patients at this stage are unable to report pain scores. Healthcare providers, including nursing staff, must be attuned to any change in the patient status as a potential indicator of pain, especially the onset of delirium or agitation. Input of close family members who are spending time with the patient is important to incorporate into management plans, as they are often able to identify the presence of pain in the patient.[25] Close communication regarding treatment plans, that often include opioids, should be conducted with family members to ensure complete understanding of the medication rationale. Some family members develop the erroneous assumption that carefully titrated pain medications are being utilized for the purpose of sedation. Since many loved ones are highly focused on interactions with the patient when time is short, this may be a great burden that would potentially improve with thorough discussion. Families

Table 32.1 Considerations in Patients with High-Risk Behavior

Suspicious or Red Flag Behaviors	Screening for Red Flag Behaviors	Measures to Take With Red Flag Behaviors
1. Requesting early refills	1. Review state prescription monitoring program data	1. Clear documentation of behaviors
2. Filling prescriptions from multiple providers	2. Random urine/serum drug screening	2. Repeated explanations of controlled substances agreements
3. Finding of illicit substances on urine drug screening	3. Pill counts at each visit	3. More frequent urine drug screening
4. Absence of prescribed medication on urine drug screening	4. Controlled substance agreement discussed and signed	4. Prescriptions for shorter intervals (1 to 2 weeks)
5. Personal or family history of substance misuse	5. Complete substance use, family, legal, and occupational history	5. Avoidance of immediate-release medications
6. Decline in functional status with increasing medication doses	6. Obtaining records from prior providers	6. Avoidance of medications with higher abuse potential or street value
7. Self-titration of opioids	7. Screening tools (CAGE, ORT, SOAPP)	7. Evaluation by substance abuse trained professional
8. Reluctance to pursue non opioid therapies for pain		8. Requirement that prescriptions are only filled at one pharmacy

Note: CAGE = Cut down, Annoyed, Guilty, Eye-Opener; ORT = Opioid Risk Tool; SOAPP = Screener and Opioid Assessment for Patients with Pain.

may also benefit from reinforcement that medications used are intended for the sole purpose of pain control, and, when given in this way, they are very unlikely to shorten the time until death.[26] Communication about pain at the end of life with families may be challenging but has direct impact on their understanding of the experience and their bereavement.

The Role of Culture and Religion in Communication About Symptom Management

Palliative care providers need to be prepared to engage patients and family members about questions and concerns related to culture and religion when they arise. These types of situations can be particularly challenging when the patient and family's religious beliefs prevent healthcare providers from giving patients the care they need. How does this affect providers' ability to discuss pain in a nonjudgmental manner? If healthcare providers have a difficult time identifying with the religious beliefs espoused in the first place, could their ability to communicate become compromised even further? Even if healthcare providers try to hide their negative feelings, they may still unconsciously send messages of disapproval that can negatively impact their interactions with patients/their families. The palliative care chaplain or other available spiritual care provider should be consulted to provide a thorough assessment of the patient's and family's beliefs and to mediate the communication with the healthcare team. In some cases, when possible, a provider may ask a colleague to take over primary care for this particular patient and his or her family if they fear their level of discomfort will prevent them from communicating with and caring for the patient and family.

Cultural and religious differences can become particularly important when the healthcare provider raises the topic of palliative sedation for intractable symptoms. How does the family's culture/worldview/religion conceptualize the process of artificially sedating their loved one, potentially until death? The family may already view this method of managing refractory symptoms, such as terminal delirium or dyspnea, as hastening death/euthanasia. In discussing this issue, it may therefore be necessary for the provider to be aware of and explore the family's beliefs in more detail.

As in any conversation with patients/families from other cultures or religions, providers should not assume to know or understand a family's beliefs just because they are from a certain cultural/religious background. Religious beliefs may potentially affect the patient's care when intractable symptoms are present and palliative sedation is suggested. A patient scenario is offered to demonstrate the importance of the team approach in communication about culture and pain:

> A palliative care team caring for an African American female with terminal delirium hears from the patient's bedside nurse that the family is arguing over whether to continue palliative sedation or not. The nurse reports that the family's biggest concern is over the patient's spiritual beliefs and how that may affect her after death. Some family members are devout Muslims, making the situation even more complicated. The bedside nurse notifies the advanced practice nurse on the team who in turn spends some time talking to the family about their concerns. She then calls in the chaplain and social worker to help assess the situation further and to provide support to the family. The social worker, who has established a good rapport with the family, further assesses family dynamics and explores how she can help ensure continued peaceful relationships among family members. The chaplain spends time with both Christian and Muslim family members to explore their concerns in more depth. Finally, the entire palliative care interdisciplinary team discusses how to best care for this patient and her family during their next semiweekly team meeting.

In addition to having a different culture and/or religion, patients and their families may also speak in a different native tongue. When treating intractable nausea or dyspnea, for example, a healthcare provider may need to discuss the potential advantages and side effects of a variety of medications (e.g., steroids, metoclopramide, or haloperidol) and complex interventions (e.g., stenting, draining gastrostomy tube, peritoneal or pleural fluid drainage catheter placement). It is imperative that patients and their families have a good grasp of the potential benefits versus risks/burdens to the patient and family prior to treating these symptoms as aggressively as possible. More important, providers should use lay language to discuss pain medications and symptoms with patients and families to enable understanding of pain processes and how pain medications work. The Plain Language Planner for Palliative Care is one tool that can be used to help translate routine medical language into plain language for patients and families (see Table 32.2).

Table 32.2 Plain Language Planner for Palliative Care

Medicine	Recommended Use in Palliative Care (Symptom)	Plain Language Explanation
Amitriptyline	Nerve pain	Nerve pain can feel like "tingling," "burning," or "electrical" zaps. This medicine helps that kind of pain.
Dexamethasone	Anorexia Fatigue Pain Nausea	Decadron can help with a queasy stomach and also create an appetite. It also gives energy and helps reduce pain.
Diazepam	Anxiety	The feeling of dread or worry goes hand in hand with the challenges of this illness. Valium is a short-acting medicine that can help with those feelings of worry that are so strong they distract from you enjoying things.
Docusate Sodium	Constipation	A lot of the medicines you are using to help with pain can also slow down your gut. And this is common. So we have to keep your poop moving. This drug is good in helping with that.
Fluoxetine	Depression	Feelings of sadness and loss are really normal for someone dealing with all you are dealing with. Prozac is an antidepressant medicine that can make those feelings less painful.
Haloperidol	Delirium	Confusion can be improved with this medicine called Haldol. It will help clear your thoughts.
Hyoscine Butylbromide	Nausea Respiratory tract secretions	An uneasy stomach is common. Being in a car can make it worse. Also, this medicine can help dry up the fluid that gets stuck in your breathing tubes.
Ibuprofen	Pain	Your bones can hurt. And your joints. Ibuprofen gets at that kind of pain.
Loperamide	Diarrhea	Really loose poop, or diarrhea, can get better quickly with Immodium.
Lorazepam	Anxiety	Feeling nervous or dreading things is a common thing. And we want you to feel better and less nervous. Ativan can make the anxiety and worry less intense.
Metoclopramide	Nausea and vomiting	Nausea can include the feeling of being full or even queasy after eating just a few bites of food. Reglan can make this feeling go away.
Morphine	Pain Dyspnea	Morphine relieves many different types of pain. It can also help you breathe easier.
Senna	Constipation	A lot of the medicines you are using to help with pain can also slow down your gut. And this is common. So we have to keep your poop moving. This drug is good in helping with that.

©Palliative Care Communication Institute.
Note: Available for free download/print at www.pccinstitute.com and fully integrated into the free iOS app Health Communication.

Ideally, a professional third-party medical translator is available to translate, either in person or over a special translator phone or computer. The use of a translator can help ensure that the message is conveyed accurately and without any potential mistranslation. If friends or family members are tasked with the translation, information may not be communicated in the manner intended, whether accidentally or subconsciously/intentionally, especially when discussing bodily functions may be a cultural taboo considered embarrassing and cause translation to be inaccurate. Communication about pain may also involve sharing poor prognosis and cultural customs may inhibit a family member or friend from accurately translating the information. In some countries/cultures—Saudi Arabia for example—family members may try to withhold bad news from patients, especially women, usually in an effort to protect them.[27] Yet another Saudi Arabian study found that all cancer patients interviewed wanted to know their prognosis and almost all of them wanted detailed information about potential risks versus benefits of treatment.[28]

From one our own clinical experiences, similar behavior was exhibited in a family from Yemen who initially did not want to disclose information about diagnosis and prognosis to their 20-year-old daughter with end-stage liver disease and poor overall prognosis. The patient was often minimally communicative with healthcare staff, apparently by choice, but she was not confused and had the ability to understand information presented to her and make her own decisions. When the patient was interviewed with help of a translator and expressed the desire to receive information, her family reluctantly agreed to allow the healthcare provider to provide it. The healthcare provider must be able to maintain the proper balance of person-centered communication and family-focused care.

Family/Caregiver Communication in the Absence of Patient Communication

One of the more challenging aspects of communication regarding symptom management for palliative patients occurs when the patients themselves are unable to participate in the discussion and decision-making. Terminal delirium, brain damage/coma, and end-stage dementia commonly cause such incapacitation. When patients are unable to communicate their symptoms, providers have to rely on family members to report and discuss treatment plans and options. Since symptom ratings are usually based on a subjective patient rating, it is particularly important for all healthcare providers and family members at the bedside to discuss how symptoms will be assessed (e.g., respiratory rate greater than 24 per minute, increased work of breathing for dyspnea) while also devising a treatment strategy.

Sometimes, as previously mentioned, patients require palliative sedation for intractable symptoms at the end of life, and they are frequently unable to discuss symptom management either before or after treatment initiation. There are no universally accepted guidelines on what communication needs to take place prior to implementing palliative sedation, but a variety of organizations have issued position statements, including the National Hospice and Palliative Care Organization.[29] This organization's statement indicates that part of the process involves ensuring that patients/families understand the reasoning behind and goals for the therapy and obtaining detailed informed consent from them prior to starting it.[29] It should also be established what other potentially life-sustaining therapies should or should not be continued (e.g., artificial hydration) and whether attempts should be made to lighten or even stop sedation periodically to reassess symptoms without it.[29]

Throughout the process of caring for patients who are unable to rate their symptoms themselves, it is essential that an inpatient primary care team in charge maintains close communication among the various providers involved in the care, including the bedside nurses and nurses' aides who are able to watch closely for signs of worsening symptom control throughout the day and night and are also usually speaking to family members at the bedside more frequently. Keeping close contact with family members and making sure they receive the support and information they need is also crucial. If the patient's dying process and/or, even worse, perceived suffering is prolonged beyond what was expected, family members will need increased levels of support, communication, and reassurance on a continual basis. In an outpatient setting (e.g., a home hospice situation), nurses will need to make more frequent home visits and phone calls for closer patient monitoring and family support. For further information, see the chapters on acute care and outpatient care settings in this volume.

Role of the Interdisciplinary Team

Several members of the interdisciplinary team play a critical role in talking to patients and families about symptom management. For example, a palliative psychologist can assist with depression and/or anxiety. Psychologists can not only help patients with the assessment and treatment of their depression and anxiety through therapeutic communication visits but may also be able to help reinforce the potential role of medications used to treat their symptoms, especially if patients are reluctant to receive treatment. If a patient has insomnia, a psychologist can discuss this symptom, offer sleep hygiene measures, and review potential mental health causes for the symptom. Social workers can also play a significant role for these patients and their families with their expertise in counseling.

Chaplains may also play an important part in helping patients and family members talk about symptoms, especially spiritual distress and existential suffering that may occur alongside depression and anxiety. Patients may be willing to talk about depression and anxiety in more depth with a chaplain than they would with other healthcare providers, especially if the patient is spiritual and thus does not feel threatened by the chaplain yet may attach stigma to speaking with a mental health specialist about his or her symptoms. Chaplains may discuss and assess the patient's spiritual health in-depth and its potential bearing on overall mental health. They can assist in talking to both patients and family about how to manage symptoms, especially at the end of life, when spiritual/existential suffering may become more prevalent. As patients and their families face impending death, chaplains may be helpful in assisting in the exploration of this time and its implications from a spiritual standpoint (e.g., relating to the belief of an afterlife postdeath that may induce fear and uncertainty).

Another member of the interdisciplinary team who can help significantly in communicating with patients and families about certain symptoms is the dietitian. When patients complain of anorexia, the dietitian can talk to them about this symptom and how to find the right kinds of food to provide the best nutritional value and meet their caloric requirements. Dietitians can also reinforce to both patients and families the importance of not forcing food intake when the patient is simply not hungry or even actively dying and the question of artificial feeding or hydration is raised. If patients are complaining about nausea, dietitians can talk to them about this symptom in more detail and what kinds of foods to avoid triggering further nausea.

Conclusion

Clinical communication skills are essential in achieving success in facilitating physical pain and symptom management. Physical pain and symptoms are common among palliative patients who experience life-limiting diseases, and special patient populations offer unique communication challenges for assessing and providing pain management. Ongoing communication requires focusing on ensuring that patients and their families are well informed and that their needs are heard and addressed. Further research is needed to help define better symptom assessment of nonverbal patients, more uniform symptom assessment across cultures, and management strategies for patients with substance abuse disorders and life-limiting illnesses.

References

1. Jackman R, Purvis J, Mallett B. Chronic nonmalignant pain in primary care. *Am Fam Physician*. 2008;78(10):1155–1162.
2. Herr K, Coyne P, McCaffery M, Manworren R, Merkel S. Pain assessment in the patient unable to self-report: Position statement with clinical practice recommendations. *Pain Manage Nurs*. 2011;12(4):230–250.
3. Hjermstad M, Fayers P, Haugen D, et al. Studies comparing numerical rating scales, verbal rating scales, and visual analogue scales for assessment of pain intensity in adults: A systematic literature review. *J Pain Symptom Manage*. 2011;41(6):1073–1093.
4. Keller S, Bann C, Dodd S, Schein J, Mendoza T, Cleeland S. Validity of the Brief Pain Inventory for use in documenting the outcomes of patients with noncancer pain. *Clin J Pain*. 2004;20(5):309–318.
5. Haanpaa M, Backonja M, Bennett, M, et al. Assessment of neuropathic pain in primary care. *Am J Med*. 2009;122:S13–S21.
6. Tomlinson D, von Baeyer CL, Stinson JN, Sung L. A systematic review of Faces scales for the self-report of pain intensity in children. *Pediatrics*. 2010;126(5):1168–1198.

7. Kaye A, Baluch A, Scott J. Pain management in the elderly population: A review. *Ochsner J.* 2010;10(3):179–187.
8. American Geriatrics Society Panel on the Pharmacological Management of Persistent Pain in Older Persons. Pharmacological management of persistent pain in older persons. *J Am Geriatr Soc.* 2009;57(8):1331–1346.
9. Melzack R. The McGill Pain Questionnaire: Major properties and scoring methods. *Pain.* 1975;1(3):277–299.
10. Breivik H, Borchgrevink P, Allen S, et al. Assessment of pain. *Br J Anaesth.* 2008;101(1):17–24.
11. Jones RC III, Backonja M. Review of neuropathic pain screening and assessment tools. *Curr Pain Headache Rep.* 2013;17:363–370.
12. Narayan M. Culture's effects on pain assessment and management. *Am J Nurs.* 2010;110(4):38–47.
13. Lasch K. Culture, pain, and culturally sensitive pain care. *Pain Manage Nurs.* 2000;1(3 Suppl 1):16–22.
14. Butow P, Sharpe L. The impact of communication on adherence in pain management. *Pain.* 2013;154(1):S101–S107.
15. Whitten C, Evans C, Cristobal K. Pain management doesn't have to be a pain: Working and communicating effectively with patients who have chronic pain. *Perm J.* 2005;9(2):41–48.
16. Kimberlin C, Brushwood D, Allen W, Radson E, Wilson D. Cancer patient and caregiver experiences: Communication and pain management issues. *J Pain Symptom Manage.* 2004;28(6):566–578.
17. Turk D, Paice J, Cowan P, et al. Interdisciplinary pain management. http://americanpainsociety.org/uploads/about/position-statements/interdisciplinary-white-paper.pdf. Accessed June 6, 2014.
18. American Society of Addiction Medicine. Public policy statement definition of addiction. http://www.asam.org/for-the-public/definition-of-addiction. Adopted April 2011. Accessed June 12, 2014.
19. National Institute on Drug Abuse. The science of drug abuse and addiction. http://www.drugabuse.gov/publications/drugs-brains-behavior-science-addiction/introduction. Revised August 2010. Accessed June 7, 2014.
20. Sehgal N, Manchikanti L, Smith H. Prescription opioid abuse in chronic pain: A review of opioid abuse predictors and strategies to curb opioid abuse. *Pain Physician.* 2012;15:ES67–ES92.
21. Collen M. Analysis of controlled substance agreements from private practice physicians. *J Pain Palliat Care Pharmacother.* 2009;23(4):357–364.
22. Bowman S, Eiserman M, Beletsky L, Stancliff S, Bruce D. Reducing the health consequences of opioid addiction in primary care. *Am J Med.* 2013;126:565–571.
23. Chen L, Vo T, Seefeld L, et al. Lack of correlation between opioid dose adjustment and pain score change in a group of chronic pain patients. *J Pain.* 2013;14(4):384–392.
24. Pade P, Cardon K, Hoffman R, Geppert C. Prescription opioid abuse, chronic pain and primary care: A co-occurring disorders clinic in the chronic disease model. *J Sub Abuse Treat.* 2012;43:446–450.
25. Desbiens NA, Mueller-Rizner N. How well do surrogates assess the pain of seriously ill patients? *Crit Care Med.* 2000;28:1347–1352.
26. Mularski R, Puntillo K, Varkey B, et al. Pain management within the palliative and end of life care experience in the ICU. *Chest.* 2009;135(5):1360–1369.
27. Ajubran, AH. The attitude towards disclosure of bad news to cancer patients in Saudi Arabia. *Ann Saudi Med.* 2010;30(2):141–144.
28. Al-Amri, AM. Cancer patients' desire for information: A study in a teaching hospital in Saudi Arabia. *East Mediterr Health J.* 2009;15(1):19–24.
29. Kirk TW, Mahon MM. National Hospice and Palliative Care Organization (NHPCO) position statement and commentary on the use of palliative sedation in imminently dying terminally ill patients. *J Pain Symptom Manage.* 2010;39(5):914–923.

CHAPTER 33

Complementary and Alternative Medicine

Paul Posadzki and Fiona Poland

Introduction

In the United States, the National Center for Complementary and Alternative Medicine defines complementary and alternative medicine as non-mainstream approaches that go together with or in place of conventional medicine.[1] Complementary and alternative medicine (CAM) includes (a) natural products such as herbal medicines; (b) mind–body practices such as yoga, guided imagery, and tai chi; and (c) manipulative body-based practices that include chiropractic and massage therapy. In the context of palliative care, people often use CAM to palliate their symptoms or alleviate the side effects of conventional treatments, detoxify their bodies, boost immunity, and enhance their overall quality of life, or to cope better physically, emotionally, and spiritually.[2] A national survey on home and hospice care in the United States found that 4 out of 10 Americans use some type of CAM, primarily for pain and cancer care, and 42% of hospice providers offer CAM services, primarily message therapy, support group, music therapy, and pet therapy.[3] CAM practitioners include acupuncturists, aromatherapists, chiropractors, naturopaths, osteopaths, reflexologists, nutritional advisors, spiritual/energy healers, and massage practitioners. These practitioners are widely seen by patients as more compassionate, respectful, and empathic than their allopathic counterparts.

CAM practitioners are perceived as optimal providers of patient-centered care.[4] The CAM conceptual terrain clearly stresses the importance of compassionate patient–provider communication in pedagogy and practice.[5] The ontological and epistemological values and rationale underlying communication skills are emphasized in the education of CAM practitioners. Although the dichotomous construct of mind and body (underpinning medical curriculum and research) has been suggested as an obstacle to health professional–patient interactions,[6] most CAM practitioners are taught that there is no mind–body dualism, only a holistic (somatic–psychosocial–spiritual) human being.[7] As a result, CAM practitioners often have a more comfortable relationship with their patients than conventional healthcare providers, as they do not have to communicate distressing information such as prognosis rate or survival statistics. The aims of this chapter are to summarize the role of communication in using CAM therapies, identify the features of communication about CAM therapies, and summarize the communication approach for CAM conversations in palliative care.

Role of Communication in CAM

Since the 1980s, qualitative and quantitative researchers have shed light on the communication process in healthcare consultations.[8] Communication between healthcare provider and patient has been shown to positively impact a number of health outcomes, including reductions in emotional distress, levels of discomfort, concerns, fear, hopelessness, aggression, grief, depression, resignation, or utilization of health services such as fewer diagnostic tests and referrals. Quality communication also leads to better emotional and physical health, higher symptom resolution, enhanced pain control, better treatment regimen compliance, and improved patient satisfaction.[9]

Communication between a patient and a CAM practitioner is of paramount importance, especially within the context of palliative care[10] where an individual explores the unknown environment of one's own death and suffering.[11] The CAM practitioner's interpersonal and communication skills greatly influence how the "therapeutic alliance" or partnership is established.[12,13] In palliative care, respecting the patient's inherent worth, dignity, integrity, and autonomy is essential for establishing a therapeutic alliance. CAM practitioners have professional and, more important, moral obligations to understand and meet the patient's needs and challenges, fears, and anxieties. A patient-centered communication style involves an ability to explore and discuss patients' expectations, needs, or wishes; a warm and friendly approach; and an ability to gain the patient's trust and influence patient behavior.[14] Talking about CAM modalities requires building a patient relationship, in addition to strictly supplying information to the patient.

In clinical practice, communication requires honesty and open disclosure,[15] two communication features needed for effective symptom control. For a CAM practitioner, communication means accurately understanding patients' psychological challenges (anger, resignation), physical symptoms (pain), and their needs or concerns. While communicating with patients, CAM practitioners screen for signs of physical, emotional, and spiritual discomfort and offer knowledge, guidance, support, and a nonjudgmental approach. The CAM practitioner and patient primarily use interpersonal communication (both verbal and nonverbal) to exchange vital and emotionally charged information. Both verbal and nonverbal communication are equally important in building the practitioner–patient relationship, and both parties can contribute to the patient's feelings of vulnerability, hope, abandonment, and being seen as a person (holistically).[16]

Communication About CAM

There are different ways to talk about CAM modalities, and cultural setting influences the manner in which a particular modality's purpose and desired or/and expected outcomes are explained.[17] A traditional Korean medicine practitioner prescribing herbals or doing acupuncture in Korea might use a different terminology (e.g., "damp phlegm") compared to one practicing in the West who might not use such terms. A spiritual healer or Reiki master might explain the importance of mindfulness or acceptance in coping with cancer-related nausea and vomiting. A mind–body practitioner or yoga teacher may want to explain the role of meditating or clearing one's mind in managing insomnia. Such diverse modes/ways of communication can enhance patients' understanding of CAM modalities, improve satisfaction, and assist with health decision-making. Hence, most CAM professionals realize the huge potential for patient benefit from lifestyle modifications. These modifications might include enhanced self-agency, sense of coherence, self-efficacy, and empowerment, boosting psychosocial and spiritual resources.

A CAM practitioner must constantly work to understand how patients communicate and find ways to respond effectively and efficiently. Patients associate the use of metaphors in positive ratings of healthcare provider communication skills.[18–20] So, for instance, a herbalist wanting to improve communication skills might employ metaphors adjusted to patient age, gender, needs, beliefs, or knowledge, while remaining aware that some patients prefer qualitative information (values, metaphors) to quantitative (numbers, facts) or a combination of the two. Several examples of such metaphors might include

- This herb (*Echinacea spp.*) will cause flooding of your self-defense cells.
- Acupuncture will slowly extinguish your pain.
- Meditation structurally alters the brain and builds your mental resources.
- Relaxation creates an inner sanctuary.
- Aromatherapy delicately touches your senses.
- Osteopathy sets your bones and muscles in a perfect alignment.

Furthermore, the use of adjectives will necessarily differ from one another according to the CAM modalities themselves. For instance, it would be perfectly reasonable to describe lavender essential oil with such adjectives as "beautiful," "delicate," "soft/delicate," whereas the same phrasing would sound trivial if used in an acupuncture session, for instance in talking about a "beautiful" needle. Therefore, when interpreting a particular CAM modality, the practitioner must use words related to the essence of that particular practice.

A CAM practitioner is also responsible for providing reliable evidence of effectiveness. The practitioner's communication should (and often does) include understanding a patient's (and family members') experience and expectations of a given treatment. CAM practitioners should mention risks associated with the practice they pursue and conduct a balanced discussion of the uncertainties and safety of a given modality. For instance, a herbalist should openly and honestly discuss the possibilities of potential interactions of antiemetic drugs with St. John's Wort. An acupuncturist should clearly mention the risks of pneumothorax or infections following a session. In both examples, however, CAM practitioners must remain balanced in communicating the risk–benefit ratio (positive in these examples) of the therapies without scaring their patients unnecessarily. Communication should include the CAM practitioner's recommendations as informed by clinical judgment and patient preferences, while insuring the patient understands and agrees to the recommendations.[21,22] It has been reported that patients express a strong preference for some modes of communicating treatment benefits over others, for example, preferring pictures to words.[18] Therefore, CAM therapists might consider using more graphs and charts. The CAM practitioner's role is to balance information, for example, by explaining acupuncture and the emotional support associated with the treatment, which are both likely to be relevant to decision-making and clinical outcomes.

Because so much information is now available on the Internet, CAM practitioners must also be aware of both the strengths and limitations of patient and family knowledge when discussing CAM. Practitioners should be able to effectively discuss poor prognosis, adverse medical outcomes, as well as limitations of so-called miracle medicines without giving the patient false hopes or unrealistic expectations. Inability to do so breaches moral and ethical standards of care. Table 33.1 provides a list of websites of evidence-based CAM practices where patients and families can access reliable information on CAM and cancer.

CAM practitioners must also be able to clearly communicate with patients of all age groups, taking into account various cognitive abilities such as perception/reception, logical thinking and reasoning, ability to memorize facts, and attention span. Often, the growing population of elderly patients receives little attention.[23] In addition, in certain types of diseases, cognitive problems can complicate treatment decision-making. For example, dementia may affect a patient's competence to express treatment preferences,[24] making practitioner communication even more important. Ultimately, such communication will help the practitioner accomplish the fundamental duty of conveying the information necessary to enable the patient to make an informed and appropriate decision.[25]

Communicating about CAM options and patient values and beliefs, and openly discussing the benefits of CAM with patients and families, are part of the holistic services provided by palliative care providers. Discussions should convey support, provide education, and review the potential role of CAM in the relief of suffering and potential improvement to a patient's quality of life. CAM practitioners must also discuss life expectancy with sensitivity and honesty while deciding whether or not to encourage hope.[26] If needed, practitioners should provide information on palliative care planning, treatment decision-making, effect on family, symptom management, and mode of death.

Communication Approach for Conversations About CAM

In their training or professional practice relating to palliative care, CAM practitioners may need a specific strategy to ensure respect for patients' autonomy and to recognize their needs and wishes.

Table 33.1 Websites of Evidence-Based CAM Practices for Patients and Families

Organization	Description	Website
CAM-Cancer	Concerted Action for Complementary and Alternative Medicine Assessment in the Cancer Field. Originally funded by the European Commission within the Framework 5 Programme, it is now hosted by the National Information Center for Complementary and Alternative Medicine at the University of Tromsø, Norway	www.cam-cancer.org
National Center for Complementary and Alternative Medicine	Conducts and supports research and provides information about complementary health products and practices	www.nccam.nih.gov
NHS Choices	NHS Choices offers a wide range of resources that can support healthcare professionals in their work with patients and clients	www.nhs.uk
The Royal Marsden	Information and education services for doctors, nurses, allied health professionals, and health service managers	www.royalmarsden.nhs.uk
We Are MacMillan Cancer Support	Independent, expert, up-to-date information to meet the information needs of people affected by cancer	www.macmillan.org.uk
Cancer Research UK	A number of bodies work together to ensure the best use of funds received and continue to carry out world-class cancer research	www.cancerresearchuk.org
NCI at the National Institutes of Health	The NCI coordinates the National Cancer Program, which conducts and supports research, training, health information dissemination, and other programs with respect to the cause, diagnosis, prevention, and treatment of cancer, rehabilitation from cancer, and the continuing care of cancer patients and their families	www.cancer.gov
Physician Data Query	The NCI's comprehensive cancer database. It contains summaries on a wide range of cancer topics, a registry of clinical trials from around the world, and a directory of professionals who provide genetics services. Contains the NCI Dictionary of Cancer Terms, with definitions for medical terms, and the NCI Drug Dictionary, with information on agents used in the treatment of cancer or cancer-related conditions	www.cancer.gov/cancertopics/pdq/cancerdatabase
National Hospice and Palliative Care Organization	The largest nonprofit membership organization representing hospice and palliative care programs and professionals in the United States	www.nhpco.org

Note: CAM = complementary and alternative medicine; NCI = National Cancer Institute.

With the goal of strengthening the therapeutic alliance between practitioner and patient, communication about CAM should be embedded in the humanist moral values of empathy and compassion. The following guidelines are suggested for those communicating about CAM:

♦ Convey compassion and empathy and acknowledge the patient's dignity and autonomy.
♦ Recognize the patient's biopsychosocial-spiritual (holistic) needs and wishes.
♦ Ensure sensitivity to, and respect for, the patient's concerns and values.
♦ Be aware of or taking cues from a patient's emotional and psychological responses.
♦ Adopt humanistic and ethical principles of care.
♦ Intend healing and provide relief for the patient's symptoms.
♦ Transmit positive emotions.
♦ Enact a trustworthy, open, and clear approach.
♦ Be sensitive and understanding.
♦ Be responsible for the patient.
♦ Actively engaging with the process of care.
♦ Support the patient's quality of life.

The importance of interpersonal relationships and the social environment of care to the overall perception of potential CAM benefits have frequently been stressed in the literature.[27–32] The power of meaningful conversation is seen as a core component of CAM practitioners' patient approach;[28,29,32–34] in other words, some patients mainly want to be listened to. The desire to have a meaningful dialogue, including a CAM practitioner's focus on patient needs and wants, is often discussed in qualitative studies.[33] "Chatting" and bringing a nonjudgmental approach are central to this process, often exposing seemingly irrelevant but diagnostically important details.[32] Palliative care patients should be encouraged to talk and given enough time for discussion. Communication, in itself, is an effective way of alleviating patient symptoms and is associated with the social interactive support that CAM practitioners offer their patients. However, a lack of appropriate dialogue may, in turn, result in a patient's loss of confidence in CAM practitioners;[28] one study found that there were instances where older patients had either not been fully informed about their condition or their treatment requests had been ignored. Patient anger, lack of trust, and a "broken patient–practitioner therapeutic alliance" resulted.

Conclusion

Quality palliative care communication includes creating a relaxing CAM treatment environment and enabling patients to be more at ease talking about CAM therapy. Open conversations about CAM therapies facilitate patient coping and psychological and social wellness. The CAM practitioner who shows interest, pays attention and gets involved, identifies and explores the patient's health concerns, and exercises quality communication can improve patient satisfaction, outcome, and healing as well as meet patient expectations/preferences, and establish a therapeutic alliance. Discussions about CAM empower patients by encouraging them to take an active part in managing symptoms, which, in turn, can lead to broader lifestyle changes.

Drawing on concepts in humanistic values and ethical principles such as respect for patients' autonomy and integrity and recognition of their needs and wishes, we have outlined a communication approach to discussions about CAM. Cultivating these values and principles should inform a CAM practitioners' code of practice. Such an approach may reflect and address patients' needs for sharing experiences and facilitate delivery of patient-centered care during CAM consultations. The power of individualized care, a compassionate attitude, and open environment can be seen as a catalyst for more quality communication in the palliative care setting.

References

1. National Center for Complementary and Alternative Medicine. What is complementary and alternative medicine (CAM)? nccam.nih.gov/health/whatiscam/. Accessed September 12, 2014.
2. Correa-Velez I, Clavarino A, Eastwood H. Surviving, relieving, repairing, and boosting up: Reasons for using complementary/alternative medicine among patients with advanced cancer: a thematic analysis. *J Palliat Med*. October 2005;8(5):953–961.
3. Nahim RL, Barnes PM, Stussman FJ, Bloom B. *Costs of Complementary and Alternative Medicine (CAM) and Frequency of Visits to CAM Practitioners: United States, 2007.* National Center of Health Statistics Reports 18. Hyattsville, MD: National Center for Health Statistics; 2009. nccam.nih.gov/about/plans/2011/introduction.htm. Accessed September 12, 2014.
4. Victoria Maizes, David Rakel, and Catherine Niemiec, American Medical Association. Integrative Medicine and Patient-Centered Care. EXPLORE September/October 2009;5(5):277. doi:10.1016/j.explore.2009.06.008.
5. Martin C. Perspective: To what end communication? Developing a conceptual framework for communication in medical education. *Acad Med*. December 2011;86(12):1566–1570.
6. Grace VM. Mind/body dualism in medicine: The case of chronic pelvic pain without organic pathology—A critical review of the literature. *Int J Health Serv*. 1998;28(1):127–151.
7. Posadzki P, Glass N. Mind-body medicine: A conceptual (re)synthesis? *Adv Mind-Body Med*. Fall 2009;24(3):8–14.
8. Brown B, Crawford, P., Carter, R. *Evidence-Based Health Communication*. Maidenhead, UK: Open University Press; 2006.
9. Wong SY, Lee, A. Communication skills and doctor patient relationship. *Hong Kong Med Diary*. 2006;11(3):7–9.
10. Turner M, Payne S, O'Brien T. Mandatory communication skills training for cancer and palliative care staff: Does one size fit all? *Eur J Oncol Nurs*. December 2011;15(5):398–403.
11. Loetz C, Muller J, Frick E, Petersen Y, Hvidt NC, Mauer C. Attachment theory and spirituality: Two threads converging in palliative care? *Evid Based Complement Alternat Med*. 2013:740291.
12. Torke AM, Petronio S, Sachs GA, Helft PR, Purnell C. A conceptual model of the role of communication in surrogate decision making for hospitalized adults. *Patient Educ Couns*. April 2012;87(1):54–61.
13. Luckett T, Davidson PM, Green A, Boyle F, Stubbs J, Lovell M. Assessment and management of adult cancer pain: A systematic review and synthesis of recent qualitative studies aimed at developing insights for managing barriers and optimizing facilitators within a comprehensive framework of patient care. *J Pain Symptom Manage*. August 2013;46(2):229–253.
14. Maeland JG. [Changing patients' health behavior—consultation and physician-patient relationship]. *Tidsskr Nor laegeforen*. January 10, 1993;113(1):47–50.
15. Bradley CT, Brasel KJ. Core competencies in palliative care for surgeons: Interpersonal and communication skills. *Am J Hospice Palliat Care*. December 2007-January 2008;24(6):499–507.
16. Coyle N, Sculco L. Communication and the patient/physician relationship: A phenomenological inquiry. *J Support Oncol*. September-October 2003;1(3):206–215.
17. Claramita M, Utarini A, Soebono H, Van Dalen J, Van der Vleuten C. Doctor-patient communication in a Southeast Asian setting: The conflict between ideal and reality. *Adv Health Sci Educ*. March 2011;16(1):69–80.
18. Goodyear-Smith F, Arroll B, Chan L, Jackson R, Wells S, Kenealy T. Patients prefer pictures to numbers to express cardiovascular benefit from treatment. *Ann Fam Med*. May-June 2008;6(3):213–217.
19. Casarett D, Pickard A, Fishman JM, et al. Can metaphors and analogies improve communication with seriously ill patients? *J Palliat Med*. March 2010;13(3):255–260.
20. Cable DG. Caring for the terminally ill: Communicating with patients and family. *Henry Ford Hospital Med J*. 1991;39(2):85–88.
21. Epstein RM, Alper BS, Quill TE. Communicating evidence for participatory decision making. *JAMA*. May 19, 2004;291(19):2359–2366.
22. Torke AM, Petronio S, Purnell CE, Sachs GA, Helft PR, Callahan CM. Communicating with clinicians: The experiences of surrogate decision-makers for hospitalized older adults. *J Amer Geriatr Soc*. August 2012;60(8):1401–1407.
23. de Haes H, Teunissen S. Communication in palliative care: A review of recent literature. *Curr Opin Oncol*. July 2005;17(4):345–350.
24. Yamanaka R, Koga H, Yamamoto Y, Yamada S, Sano T, Fukushige T. Characteristics of patients with brain metastases from lung cancer in a palliative care center. *Support Care Cancer*. April 2011;19(4):467–473.
25. Bogardus ST, Jr., Holmboe E, Jekel JF. Perils, pitfalls, and possibilities in talking about medical risk. *JAMA*. March 17 1999;281(11):1037–1041.
26. Hagerty RG, Butow PN, Ellis PM, Dimitry S, Tattersall MH. Communicating prognosis in cancer care: A systematic review of the literature. *Ann Oncol*. July 2005;16(7):1005–1053.
27. Bishop FL, Yardley L, Lewith GT. Why consumers maintain complementary and alternative medicine use: A qualitative study. *J Altern Complem Med*. February 2010;16(2):175–182.
28. Cartwright T. "Getting on with life": The experiences of older people using complementary health care. *Soc Sci Med*. April 2007;64(8):1692–1703.
29. Gambles M, Crooke M, Wilkinson S. Evaluation of a hospice based reflexology service: A qualitative audit of patient perceptions. *Eur J Oncol*. March 2002;6(1):37–44.
30. Golischewski S, Kitto S, Anderson D, Lyons-Wall P. Women's perceptions and beliefs about the use of complementary and alternative medicines during menopause. *Complement Ther Med*. June 2008;16(3):163–168.
31. Hughes JG. "When I first started going I was going in on my knees, but I came out and I was skipping": Exploring rheumatoid arthritis patients' perceptions of receiving treatment with acupuncture. *Complement Ther Med*. October-December 2009;17(5–6):269–273.

32. Little CV. Simply because it works better: Exploring motives for the use of medical herbalism in contemporary UK health care. *Complement Ther Med.* October-December 2009;17(5-6):300-308.
33. Andrews GJ. Private complementary medicine and older people: Service use and user empowerment. *Ageing Soc.* May 2002;22:343-368.
34. Shaw A, Thompson EA, Sharp D. Complementary therapy use by patients and parents of children with asthma and the implications for NHS care: A qualitative study. *BMC Health Serv Res.* June 15, 2006;6:76

CHAPTER 34

Redefining Comfort Measures:
Communicating About Life Support, Artificial Hydration, and Nutrition

Dawn M. Gross, Nancy Clifton-Hawkins, and Mariela Gallo

Introduction

Based on recent National Vital Statistics, over 2.5 million people die per year from illness.[1] Of these deaths, the leading causes are heart disease, malignant neoplasms, cerebrovascular diseases, Alzheimer's disease, and kidney disease. The age-adjusted death rate increased for six leading causes of death: chronic lower respiratory diseases, diabetes mellitus, influenza and pneumonia, chronic liver disease and cirrhosis, Parkinson's disease, and pneumonitis due to aspiration of solids and liquids.[1] Every day, healthcare providers ask families and friends if it is time to end their loved one's life support, artificial nutrition, and hydration. In our complicated world, neither families nor healthcare providers want to make such decisions.[2] Many factors hinder decision-making when patient and healthcare providers come to this crossroad in care. Studies have found that healthcare providers have little or no training in conducting these difficult conversations with patients and families.[3] To make these life transition points as seamless as possible, a provider must be a skilled communicator.

Being aware that a healthcare provider's individual moral and ethical standards also influence his or her ability to communicate about end-of-life plans with patients and family members is critical to developing competency in these areas of communication. Researchers often infer that moral and ethical issues affect the healthcare provider's "comfort level" with end-of-life care. Advances in medical care may affect this comfort level further, in that such advances have blurred the decision of how far to go in treating a terminally ill patient.[4] Because we *can* is not that same as we *should*.

This chapter examines the important factors that influence how providers can successfully facilitate conversations about goals of care related to life support, artificial hydration, and nutrition so they align with transitions in care delivery. We define what providing care actually means as it pertains to life-sustaining treatments. Beginning with the science behind the physiological responses of a terminal patient receiving life support, artificial nutrition, and hydration, the discussion then moves to the communication process between the healthcare provider and patient, emphasizing that honesty and truthfulness are key components in initiating a conversation about end-of-life care. Finally, vignettes detail these complex conversations and tools and strategies are discussed that assist the healthcare provider and the patient as they embark on this journey together.

Fundamental Science of Life Support, Artificial Hydration, and Nutrition at the End of Life

Guiding patients and families through the transitions of the body at the end of life sets the foundation for informed decision-making.[5] As healthcare professionals, we recognize that discussing care details with patients and families is a complex conversation that can be daunting for all involved. However, giving vague or incomplete information about the end of life can increase distress.[6]

Communication with patients and families about advanced disease and end of life is often referred to as "breaking of bad news."[6] Instead of instilling a sense of loss, healthcare professionals can begin to refocus this communication by acknowledging and discovering the unique needs of patients and families, with attention to providing comfort rather than withdrawing care. The Education for Physicians on End-of-Life Care project from the Institute for Ethics at the American Medical Association provides an eight-step protocol to discuss end-of-life treatment options. The underlying goal of this protocol is to seek clarity from both the patient/family and healthcare provider. The protocol states: (1) be familiar with policies and statutes, (2) arrange and use an appropriate setting for the discussion, (3) ask the patient and family what they understand, (4) discuss the general goals of care, (5) establish context for the discussion, (6) discuss specific treatment preferences, (7) respond to emotions, and (8) establish and implement the plan.[7] The healthcare provider has an ethical and legal obligation to appropriately discuss end-of-life treatments with patients and families. This can only be achieved with timely, respectful, and honest discussion.

In a study based on qualitative secondary data, patients were asked to describe examples of helpful communication as they entered advanced care. Four key elements were described: respecting the importance of time, demonstrating caring, acknowledging fear, and balancing hope and honesty in the provision of information.[6] These elements, in the context of information-giving and education, become essential for making life-altering decisions about healthcare. Using the four elements provided from this study, a framework is created for walking patients and families through the details of the dying process and understanding the roles of life support, artificial hydration, and nutrition.

Discussing Illness Prognosis With Patients and Families

Healthcare professionals are responsible for informing and preparing patients as illness progresses. Throughout the continuum of care, this involves providing information and education related to the patient's health status and prognosis. Over the past decade, extensive research has been conducted on the type of information that should be shared when discussing a person's health status. Findings reveal that healthcare providers should offer information on prognosis that includes a potential timeline for death, signs and symptoms of the dying process, and potential management of the patient's comfort.[8] While prognosis is crucial, clinical guidelines rarely include when to inform patients and families of prognosis and initiate end-of-life decision-making. Timing is critical for informing and educating in accordance with the patient's and family's readiness to process the information. Is there a point in terminal illness when patients and families are "ready" to hear that death is near?

Results from studies exploring timing and location of such conversations vary, yet they trend toward favoring nonacute settings, early in the illness trajectory.[9] Earlier communication takes preparation on behalf of the provider to establish the appropriate environment, ensure there is enough time to communicate, and take into account whom the patient wants to be present when information is given.[9] Whenever prognosis is discussed, the patient should be encouraged to have a supportive companion such as a spouse, immediate family member, or close friend present. The setting for the conversation is important as well. Turning off electronic devices to prevent interruptions and eliminating other potential distractions may permit both healthcare professionals and patients and their families to fully engage in the conversation. The healthcare provider should allot sufficient time for the conversation, so that he or she can present as many facts as possible, while giving patients and families the opportunity to pause, process, and question. Healthcare providers need to invite questions as well, even if patients and families convey a good understanding of the information.

Studies have found that patients and families have little to no understanding of the benefits and risks related to life support, artificial nutrition, and hydration.[10] Discussions about benefits and risks related to these kinds of treatments are often weighed on the basis of improving the quality of life for the patient. However, in a recent study researchers found the decision to remove or sustain life support, artificial nutrition, and hydration continues to be significantly misunderstood as a "life-prolonging" measure.[10] This is a clear indication of the need to better inform and educate patients and families about the benefits and risks related to these forms of care for terminally ill patients.

Table 34.1 Discussion Points, Possible Misunderstandings, and Alternative Statements

Discussion Point	Patient/Family Possible Misunderstanding	Alternative
"It may be time to think about withdrawal of care."	Removal of care to induce death	"It may be time to think of other ways to provide care and comfort."
"At this point, hospice is the next step to take."	There is no more hope/reason to keep patient alive	"At this time, I want to make sure special care and attention is given to the patient's comfort."
"The treatment failed to work."	There is nothing more that can be done	"The cancer did not respond to the treatment, as we had hoped."

Using simple language is the best way to educate and communicate sensitive information. Table 34.1 describes sensitive discussion points, potential misunderstandings, and alternative statements using simple language for end-of-life discussions. Using simple terms also helps invite patients and families to reveal important cultural and religious beliefs that may greatly impact their decision to use or forego artificial nutrition and hydration. For example, studies have found that religious beliefs such as Jewish principles of prioritizing the sanctity of life can influence decisions related to the use of artificial nutrition and hydration.[10] Also, different ethnic groups treat food and fluids as culturally significant.

In some cultures, the symbolic nature of food in relation to the provision of nutrition and hydration for a terminally ill patient can be viewed as a vital necessity. A study in Taiwan found that a patient's loved one worries that the terminally ill patient will become a "starving soul" after death if nutrition and hydration is removed.[11] Such a concern can drive a family's decision to continue artificial nutrition and hydration, which may cause greater discomfort for the patient. In Western society an overarching principle of autonomy guides decisions in clinical ethics. This speaks to the autonomy of the patient's or authorized surrogate's right to self-determine end-of-life care related to sustaining or removing life support, artificial nutrition, and hydration.[12] However, it is important to realize that this definition of autonomy does not translate to more communal cultures where individual autonomy is not a prevailing principle. Acknowledging this reality augments the need for healthcare providers to continuously refocus communication about end-of-life care. Beginning with clearly discussing the specific signs and symptoms that will occur in the dying process will help everyone involved understand what comfort measures optimally align with the patient's and family's values.

Discussing Signs and Symptoms

Although each person approaches death in a unique way, there are expected physical changes the body endures at the end of life. Most people experience some or a combination of symptoms related to the body's shutting down as death approaches. The body begins to transition from a living to a dying state. Beginning with loss of appetite, the body no longer needs the energy to stay alive. There is a gradual disinterest in food, followed by loss of desire to drink fluids, which is natural and normal. Loss of appetite and desire to drink will become apparent to families, as the patient begins to have difficulty swallowing and experiences dry mouth. This can be one of the hardest experiences for families if not understood. As the body becomes weaker, the body's system progressively slows down. A dying person will begin to sleep more, become disoriented, and progressively lose bladder and bowel control. As the body continues to lose its ability to maintain itself, the person's pulse rate begins to slow down, body temperature fluctuates from hot to cold, perspiration may increase, and breathing takes on new patterns.

Educating patients and families to anticipate these physical changes can help them remain calm so they can be fully present and empowered to provide care that is intuitively comforting based on their relationship with their loved ones. By partnering with the patient and family, healthcare providers can support patient and family wishes by exploring traditions, values, and ways of coping. For example, in a survey of individuals from many different cultural and faith traditions, a recurrent theme of comfort was family members' wish to keep their loved ones warm near the end of life by the act of applying blankets. As a healthcare provider, taking time to describe and explain typical changes in body temperature and skin color at the end of life is critical. By doing this, we can ensure that family/friends are not misinterpreting their own intuitive acts of providing comfort as unhelpful or harmful, if the physiologic response to these actions (i.e., regaining of normal skin temperature or color) is not achieved.

Discussing Removal of Life Support, Artificial Nutrition, and Hydration

Even when patients and families understand the common signs and symptoms of the normal dying process, many issues can still arise. A very common fear is that the patient will suffer from thirst and hunger if artificial nutrition and hydration is removed. It is essential to help the patient and family understand that the loss of appetite and reduced fluid intake is normal and that aggressive attempts to counteract this process could lead to discomfort and create more symptoms such as bloating, swelling, cramps, diarrhea, and shortness of breath, without improving the outcome. Important points for education include that the body no longer needs large amounts of energy and the patient's digestive system is progressively slowing down. At this stage, the patient is no longer interested in food or in need of it. The same is true for fluids, and, when drinking tapers off, the body naturally becomes dehydrated. Dry mouth can appear to be a sign of thirst to the family. However, if the patient is close to dying, the family should be informed that dry mouth is best relieved by providing mouth care, such as keeping the patient's lips moist using a swab, rather than by providing artificial hydration.

Removing other forms of life-sustaining treatment is another area of concern for patients and families. Initiating and/or discontinuing cardiopulmonary support is often based on the preferences stated in the patient's advance directive. Healthcare providers should never assume that family members were involved in this decision or that they understand what will follow. If the patient has no advance directive or is unable to decide what he or she wants, the healthcare provider must conduct a more extensive discussion and, at times, engage in a process of negotiation with the family. Prior to transitioning modalities of care, the healthcare provider must explain to patients and families what will happen after life-sustaining treatment is removed. Equally important, the healthcare provider must demonstrate empathy by inviting families to show support to the patient in as many ways as they wish.

The cultural and religious aspects of comfort for the patient and family become the center for the provision of care. As part of a qualitative survey, participants were asked to state their ethnicity and answer 10 questions about end-of-life care decisions.[13] When asked to describe comfort measures, a Chinese participant replied that "music, touch, anything that would enhance the individual's sense of well-being and physical, psychological, emotional, and spiritual ease."[13] Participants were also asked how their healthcare team could support their needs while discontinuing artificial nutrition and hydration. A respondent shared, "Loving care on their last days and allow for cultural practice in the healthcare setting, if requested."[13] The results of the survey demonstrate the importance of redirecting care, so that patients and families feel comforted in ways that are valuable to them.

Holistic Approach to Care

Many providers are drawn to healthcare to save lives, alleviate suffering, provide assistance to patients and families, and assist with the spiritual journey that can accompany illness and disease. Even when a cure is no longer possible, our duty to provide care does not end. Such care may, in fact, include the removal of life-sustaining treatment. As healthcare professionals, the way that we approach care is based on the training we received. How we interact with our patients is influenced by our focus on a Western medical model that can be detached and fragmented.

Healthcare, from a traditional perspective, is primarily about saving lives. It is about finding causes for an illness and offering a cure. Much of the time, this emphasis separates a person from his or her body, as healthcare providers focus solely on a singular body part and neglect the person as a whole.[14] Feelings and emotions fall to the more scientifically bound discussions and findings, and patient-centeredness is lost to a universe of large, incomprehensible scientific words. In his 2002 article, Little defined "humanistic medicine" as a reminder to healthcare providers that they need to be more compassionate and empathetic toward their patients. Little believes that healthcare should be more of a balance between the traditional view of medical care and the humanistic view.[15] He suggests that practitioners use the term "value-based" medicine. Per Little, this phrase "reminds clinicians of the sustaining values that underpin the whole health endeavor. These values include an acceptance of the value of individual human life in quality and quantity. Both individuals and communities hold a place of importance that contributes to human security and flourishing."[15(p319)]

Terminally ill patients often experience emotional distress from distorted thinking.[16] When providers are able to connect the emotional to the cognitive functions of an individual, they will be able to help the patient gain insight, change behavior, and regain control.[16] By effectively incorporating the emotional and cognitive aspects of each individual involved in the end-of-life experience, namely, the terminally ill patient, healthcare provider, family, and community as defined by the patient, we can see the entire picture and better understand the overarching "human" needs that a patient and family are facing. The 2014 study of patient and physician relationships from the Empathy and Relational Science Program at Massachusetts General Hospital found that "relationship factors really do make a difference in patients' health outcomes."[17(e94207)] While the care we provide at the end of life does not cure, it is still care. It is what allows for the healing of patients and their families. It is up to us as healthcare providers to recognize the needs, beyond cure, and provide care that meets these needs.

Provider-Driven Versus Patient-Directed Healthcare

Part of recognizing patients' and their family's needs is to understand where each person is emotionally and cognitively. A person's ability to cope will determine his or her ability to take in the information that is presented. Roeland and colleagues advise that providers determine the family's and/or patient's coping level prior to engaging in difficult medical discussions and develop a pathway to determine a person's coping capacity and how this influences modes of communication during end-of-life care decision-making[2] (see Figure 34.1). They suggest that as a patient approaches death, knowing where he or she is emotionally and cognitively can help the healthcare provider play a larger role in identifying viable options, such as helping to facilitate the process of moving from artificial nutrition and hydration to other forms of care and comfort.

Understanding where patients are along the illness continuum is key—as any misinterpretation of where they are could have disastrous effects on trust and future relationship-building. Roeland and colleagues have devised a communication assessment model that can help frame patient/healthcare provider discussions. Any member of the healthcare team would benefit from ascertaining the coping mode of the patient and adjust his or her communication approach accordingly. For example, open-ended or patient-directed communication works when the patient is adaptively coping. If we were to approach such a patient with a "clinician-driven" mode, he or she would consider us "condescending and patronizing."[2] Conversely, if we were to use a patient-directed modality with a patient who is engaging in maladaptive coping, "you can increase patient suffering, provide poor medical care and set the stage for a complicated bereavement process with the family."[2(417)] Both misinterpretations will damage trust and all levels of communication from this point forward.

A 19-year-old woman with long-standing cystic fibrosis is readmitted for pseudomonas pneumonia. The primary team is frustrated and consults the palliative care team to assist with her "noncompliance" in the respiratory therapy plan of care. When the team enters the patient's room at 4 PM, she is lying in bed, looking quite fatigued, attempting to dry her hair with a towel. The team introduces themselves. One of the members acknowledges that she appears quite tired. She looks up at them and says, "Yes. I finally was able to get help to the shower," she nods at the nurse. "So at least now, I finally feel half-human after feeling so terrible and exhausted all day. What do you want?" The physician responds, "We're glad you have finally been able to shower." The chaplain adds, "It sounds like you have had quite a frustrating day." The social worker asks, "Would you like us to visit now, or would you prefer we come back at another time?" "Yes, tomorrow afternoon," the patient replies. The team returns the next day to find the young woman, still exhausted but ready to talk.

In this patient-directed approach, the team discovers how an illness is interfering with what matters most in this patient's life (i.e., showering and feeling "human again"). The healthcare team takes the first steps toward developing trust with this patient by conveying empathy and acknowledging the patient's frustration. Patient-directed care is enacted by returning the next day to discuss her care as requested, rather than prioritizing the team's goal of discussing her care on their initial visit.

Fang's Story

An 86-year-old, Cantonese-speaking woman, previously well and living independently, is now on her fourteenth day of ventilator dependence in the ICU. She developed an aspiration pneumonia that became complicated by sepsis and renal failure. The family is adamant that they continue to "do everything" possible to save her. The ICU team is trepidatious about discussing placement of a tracheostomy and PEG tube.

The opportunity to educate patients and family on possible conflicts that might arise between healthcare and cultural practices becomes possible once the foundation of trust has been laid. The more open to dialogue and discovery a provider is, the more nimble a conversation can be. In other words, if providers notice themselves becoming uncomfortable in a conversation, the first place to consider looking is internally. What is making them frustrated, anxious, angry, or despondent? What a healthcare provider might consider "futile care" may have significant meaning to the patient and family. Consider the goals of any given intervention and explore other actions that could ultimately achieve the same desired outcome. Often, the impasse we think we are facing when exploring a refocus of care from life-sustaining measures to comfort-focused care are not as different as we think. Those actions are merely misperceptions about how the action can or cannot achieve what someone actually wants.

Fang's Story, Continued

A family meeting is called with the support of the palliative care team and interpreter services. A pre-meeting occurs to understand any cultural preferences in communication practices (e.g., being in the presence of the patient, the first-born son acts as decision-maker, etc.). The meeting begins by thanking the family for meeting (trust-building with acknowledgment of time and effort taken to be present) and by asking the family their understanding of their mother's illness (trust-building by being curious). The son states, "We want you to just keep doing what you are doing." This is an opening to ask what it is he thinks is being done and what the anticipated outcome will be. "You can cure her so she can be at my wedding next month," the son replies. A member of the healthcare team responds, "I wish we could make your mother well again, so she could breathe on her own and attend your wedding. Unfortunately, that is not what we see as possible." At this point, another family member speaks, "She cannot die this month. The wedding has been set on this date for its auspiciousness and cannot be changed. If she dies in the same month, it will be very bad luck."

This last statement is an opening for the healthcare team to align their care efforts in support of the family's wishes on behalf of the patient. Negotiations can now move toward how to attempt to achieve the newly discovered goal (i.e., to not have the patient die the same month as her child is married) in a way that allows for the uncertainty of life and death to be openly discussed, so that if the goal is not met, it is not out of lack of respect or understanding.

By providing open and honest communication, providers maintain trust even in the face of potential disappointment and loss. This "turning toward" what might likely be an uncomfortable conversation is key to maintaining trust. So how can we engage in these types of conversations? John Gottman, renowned researcher and author of *The Science of Trust*, describes any interaction as a trust-building opportunity.[18] Each interaction holds the possibility of turning toward or turning away from a person. These "sliding door moment[s]" are points in time when one can choose to make a difference by choosing to connect with another person and be present versus choosing to turn away and be alone. Gottman notes that trust erodes gradually over time, if we continually turn away. He created the ATTUNE acronym (Box 34.1) to support actions of engagement: A: Awareness, T: Turning Toward, T: Tolerance, U: Understanding, N: Nondefensive responding, and E: Empathy.[20]

Healthcare providers build trust by uncovering and discovering aspects of the patient, the family, and even themselves. Trust-building involves an attitude that throws out assumptions and embraces the present moment. Taking advantage of John Gottman's "sliding door moments," where we can honestly engage

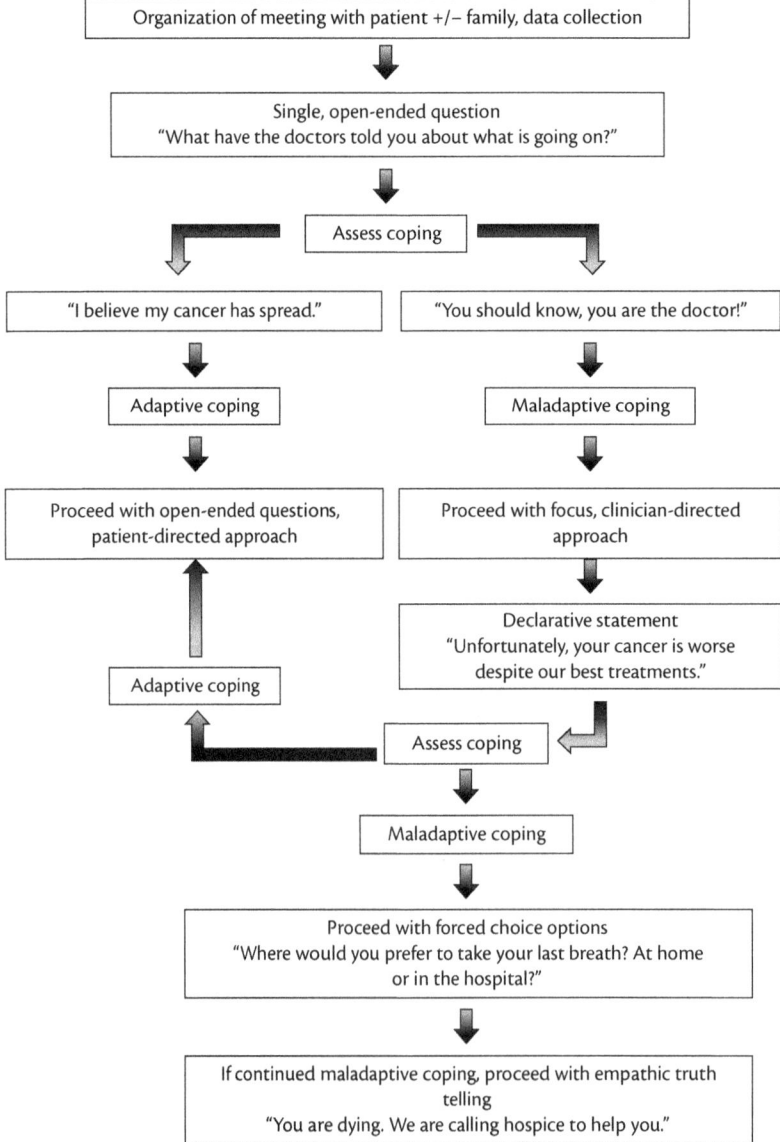

Figure 34.1 Approach to medical discussions based on assessment of patient coping
From: Roeland E, Cain J, Onderdonk C, Kerr K, Mitchell W, Thornberry K. When open-ended questions don't work: The role of palliative paternalism in difficult medical decisions. *J Palliat Med.* 2014;17(4):415–420.

> **Box 34.1** ATTUNE Acronym to Support Engagement With Patients and Family Members
>
> - **A**wareness of your partner's emotion
> - **T**urning toward the emotion
> - **T**olerance of two different viewpoints
> - trying to **U**nderstand your partner
> - **N**ondefensive responses to your partner
> - responding with **E**mpathy
>
> Source: http://greatergood.berkeley.edu/article/item/john_gottman_on_trust_and_betrayal

with the patient, it becomes possible to develop a strong trusting relationship that will be a bridge to having the conversation about providing other forms of comfort care at the end of life.[18] Now we are in a position to engage in the following conversation as Fang's story continues:

The primary physician offers, "I wish I had a different answer. We have simply reached the extent of what medical science has to offer." The chaplain adds, "This has nothing to do with the desire or effort on your part." Time is given to allow the family to hear this news and respond with words or emotions. The social worker then continues, "The questions ahead of us that we really need your guidance on is how can we now best support her and your family in honoring what is most important to her. You have stated that it is very bad luck if she were to die during the same month as your wedding. When any person is as sick as your mother, it is important to know that they can die at anytime." Another pause is offered to allow family to respond. The nurse on the team then suggests, "We would like talk with you about some things we can do together to best honor her and your wishes."

The relationship has been grounded in empathy, by hearing the family's concerns and needs, and trust, by articulating the truth in what is and is not possible. The conversation can now focus on what is possible moving forward and supporting the patient and family each step of the way despite the heightened uncertainty of Fang's care.

Principles of Communication for Building End-of-Life Plans

Diverse patient populations require healthcare professionals to be mindful of the various values, beliefs, and existing knowledge that patients bring to discussions about palliative care. Building trust and moving toward the discovery of patient goals requires a hybrid approach that removes the provider's personal assumptions and recenters the conversation around the patient's own culture and belief system. This allows the patient to make decisions that best meets his or her needs.[19] Much like the pathway for building trust, there are several communication principles that providers need to be aware of when building end of life plans with patients and families (Table 34.2).

Case Study: Mr. and Mrs. Burton

Mr. and Mrs. Burton, a 99- and 95-year-old husband and wife, were both hospitalized for aspiration pneumonia and urinary tract infections. Family had recently moved from out of state to be with them. Their son is suffering from a chronic illness and can no longer take them home. Mr. and Mrs. Burton have some mild to moderate dementia, have had other recent admissions, and are now looking at long-term placement.

Prior to meeting the patients or family, the palliative care team considers the best, most comprehensive discharge plan based on the information they have already gathered. They begin to identify an inpatient hospice unit with space in a double room as an option to present to the family should their goals be consistent with this plan.

The team enters Mrs. Burton's room. No family is present at the moment. Mrs. Burton is able to easily communicate the longtime suffering she has experienced in her legs after sustaining a hip fracture and undergoing repair. She also is able to tell the team with equal clarity that she wants to eat macaroni and cheese. With this information in hand, the team heads to her husband's room. Mr. Burton's designated power of attorney, his son Daniel, and his wife are positioned on opposite sides of his bed. Daniel's sister is in a chair, toward the foot of the bed.

The team shares their experience visiting with Mrs. Burton before they began speaking directly to Mr. Burton. Knowing about Daniel and the family disposition, the team had decided not to suggest that either parent go "home" to Daniel's house. Regardless, the team also wants to provide an opportunity for Mr. Burton to express his goals and priorities to see if they are aligned with his family's. Daniel does not appreciate this line of questioning, as noted by his frequent interruptions and cold stares.

The team offers to meet with the family in a separate room as tension seems to be mounting. Being very conscious of body language and making certain no table or physical object is in between Daniel and the team, the lead physician maintains an open posture with arms and legs relaxed, leaning into the family while she asks, "So, how can I help you?" Daniel quickly launches into why it is impossible for him to take his parents home and how angry he is at the team's questioning. The physician acknowledges this and gently offers a provider-driven response, "I have no intention of having your parents go home with you." This immediately allows Daniel to relax. She continues, "I am aware of your own health struggles and want to do everything in my power to support you, while ensuring your parents receive the most impeccable care in the setting they would feel most comfortable." Daniel's sister and spouse then began to communicate their support of identifying alternate care settings with maximal support focusing on comfort so as to alleviate further stress on Daniel.

This natural and powerful transition in a conversation occurs, more often than not, when families are allowed to and aided in hearing each other speak. Having assessed a maladaptive coping environment, provider-driven communication may be the best initial approach to establish a trusting relationship.

The Burden of Decision-Making

Making the decision to discontinue artificial hydration and nutrition and refocus care at the end of life is easier said than done.

Table 34.2 Principles of Communication for Building End-of-Life Plans

Communication Principles	Explanation/Examples
Be reliable. Do what you say.	If you make an appointment with a patient and family, be present for the appointment.
Honor your promise.	If you are unable to come back at the agreed-on time, then acknowledge this as quickly as possible and agree on an alternate time. Failure to acknowledge a broken promise dissolves any formation of trust.
Do not belittle a promise.	The seemingly most trivial of promises may hold great significance to a patient (e.g., you notice a patient appears thirsty during your visit. If you say, "I will go get you some water," *you* need to do this). *Your* doing this demonstrates follow-through and builds an experience of commitment and integrity. Failure to follow through erodes trust.
Recognize if you cannot keep a potential promise.	Quickly renegotiate the promise and deliver on it.
Be honest. Tell the truth.	If you believe a patient is dying, say so (e.g., "This is difficult for me to say, but I am concerned your father is dying. I hope I am wrong about this. In case I am not, it is important for me to be sure I am doing all that you believe matters most to your father.").
Admit if you are uncomfortable.	It is okay to have emotions and share them (e.g., the pathology report is pending but, in your clinical experience, your gut tells you this person has cancer. Instead of avoiding the subject (or the patient's room altogether), state what your concerns are, why, and the possibility that you might be wrong—which is why the pathology is being studied. The person is thinking about it whether you speak it out loud or not, so validating their concerns and unease allows for compassion and empathy to develop in both directions.
Speak from the heart.	Be vulnerable. Speak to what will make a difference and to what you are committed to, for the patient and family (e.g., "I am here to discover what you wish, so we can provide the care you want").
Speak your feelings.	We are part of health*care*; it is okay to show we care. If moved to cry, allow yourself to cry; if moved to laugh, allow yourself to laugh, but be moved.
Be open—volunteer information.	If asked how you are, challenge yourself to go beyond "fine" or "great" and answer honestly. Share some of your thoughts and feelings with the patient. This demonstrates you are not afraid to express and to hear the truth. In fact, you are actually keenly interested and open.
Do not omit important details.	If we fail to speak clearly, such as saying someone is *dying*, we fail to support people in preparing for death, which then sets up a legacy of complicated grief instead of hope, healing, and gratitude.
Do not mask truths.	By sharing your truth (e.g., that the pathology results may not be what we are hoping for), you foster trust and partnership, so if difficult decisions need to be made later, you have laid a foundation of compassion and honesty from which to work.
Establish rapport.	Exchange information. Invite patients and families to articulate their needs and wants. Ask questions to identify interests and values. Find opportunities to demonstrate your understanding of their strengths, expectations, and expertise.
Express gratitude.	Acknowledge the willingness of the patient and family to engage in these difficult conversations.

When viewing the decision-making process, the practice of shared decision-making (decisions made with healthcare team, patients, and their family) may benefit from re-examination. Why is it that a surgeon, for example, can assess a situation as being too risky and refuse to do a surgery, but when it comes to deciding whether or not to offer or stop artificial food and hydration at the end of life, providers abdicate and direct the decision-making process to the patient and family? For patients, the reasons can be founded in cultural, filial, and religious beliefs. Healthcare providers, while trained to be involved in decision-making, may be challenged to make decisions related to end-of-life care. The questions for the provider are: "How do we move through this? How can we acknowledge that we are very uncomfortable with making this end-of-life decision?" Maybe the answer lies in our ability to acknowledge the fact that we have reached the end of what science and technology can do for us. Maybe, if we can recognize that life has a beginning and an end, we can begin to escort the patient and their family into the next phase of their life. The decision then shifts from what we should do to how we can best support the process.

Providers are often reluctant to approach the subject of changing care from life support, artificial nutrition, and hydration to comfort care because they do not know what the family and patient may be thinking. A survey by, Clifton-Hawkins and Gallo asked individuals what other forms of comfort care they would want to give them if they knew that providing food and water to their loved one was actually hurting them.[13] Box 34.2 and 34.3 summarize family definitions of comfort care and goals for end-of-life care. Understanding what a patient and family really wants aids the decision on how to shift the paradigm of comfort care.

Healthcare Providers' Previous Experiences Frame Their Ability to Make Decisions

When having a challenging end-of-life conversation about removing some forms of medical support, healthcare providers may be confronted with their own feelings. If a nurse has experienced a patient improving after the removal of artificial nutrition and/

Box 34.2 Family Definitions of Comfort Care
♦ Physical affection to convey love (e.g., hugs, holding patient's hand, massaging)
♦ Medication to manage patient discomfort
♦ Medication to stop patient pain
♦ Presence of relaxing fragrances
♦ Soothing music
♦ Sharing memories
♦ Reading to patient

or hydration, he or she may hesitate weighing in on the decisions surrounding end-of-life planning.[20] Other times, providers may internalize their feelings to protect themselves, thereby stifling patient interactions. Healthcare providers such as social workers recognize that individual attitudes and self-awareness can influence their role in the provision of palliative and end-of-life care.[21] It is vital that the provider identifies where past experiences may influence his or her patient interactions. The key is to recognize how to set aside personal preferences and assumptions in favor of discovering another's preferences, goals, and values.

Case Study: Ms. William

For several days, Ms. William, a 75-year-old with a terminal lung disease, had been complaining of increasing abdominal discomfort. She was receiving nutrition via a tube running from her nose into her stomach, so she had not been able to taste food for several days. She really wanted to have the tube removed, but so long as she was on the ventilator she had no ability to eat on her own. The following day, as the palliative care team walked in to visit, she grabbed a pen and journal and wrote, "I vomited head-to-toe last night." The team was shocked by her jovial mood as she wrote and they read: "My stomach feels much better." She patted her stomach and kept writing. "It was the first time anyone had thought to let me try and brush my teeth since I have been in here!"

Listening closely to our patients, we allow our own assumptions of what comfort may look like to fade away in favor of an alternate, individualized view. Ms. William's story is a stark reminder that patients, not providers, define comfort.

Box 34.3 Family Goals for End-of-Life Care
♦ Patient is pain-free.
♦ Patient is clean.
♦ Patient is able to be with loved ones.
♦ Environment is beautiful, peaceful.
♦ There is a comfortable place to lie down.
♦ Lights are gentle.
♦ The patient's wishes are respected.
♦ Medication is available to manage pain.

Ms. William, Continued

At her request, Ms. William was able to be taken off the ventilator for what was predicted to be just a few hours before her respiratory status would decompensate again, requiring mechanical support or natural death. These few hours without the ventilator placed her in a rare position to answer the question, "If your lungs were to fail again, would you want the tube put back down your throat and be placed back on the breathing machine?" "If that's what it takes to keep me alive, so be it. I am not ready to pull the plug yet, if I don't have to."

The following morning, Ms. William was reintubated. When the palliative care team entered her room, they found her alert and writing in her journal, "I still want to live." The team spoke with Ms. William's attending physician who had earlier been frustrated and confused by the palliative care team's support of Ms. William's request to be re-intubated, despite being terminal. He shared that he was confronted by his own discomfort and not Ms. William's.

Perhaps what makes medicine a frontier of endless discovery has less to do with the scientific advances pushing the envelope on our medical know-how and more to do with how our patients challenge what we believe we know about ourselves. Pema Chodren, in her book *Taking the Leap: Freeing Ourselves from Old Habits and Fears*, suggests the reason behind our inability to tackle difficult situations is the existence of a negative back story that fuels our reluctance.[22] She suggests taking the opportunity to step back before having difficult conversations with patients and reflecting on what is making it hard to begin the conversation. Healthcare providers should aks themselves: Is there an unresolved experience preventing me from having this conversation? Did I suffer emotional harm? How is holding onto that experience going to help me in the present moment or keep me from being honest with my patient? Once providers are able to free themselves from past experiences, they open the door to more truthful and trustworthy relations with patients and their families.

Conclusion

Maura Schlairet and Richard Cohen state in their article, "Allow-Natural-Death (AND) and Other Orders: Legal, Ethical, and Practical Considerations," that conversations with patients ought to begin with a different way of viewing end of life.[23] Rather than looking at the process as one in which care is removed, we need to look at this time in life as one in which care is redefined. Borrowing from the work of Salladay, it has been suggested that this redefining of care be referred to as decision-making that allows for a natural death.[4] This language communicates to patients and family members that comfort measures are being provided. Planning end-of-life care that supports a natural death will require the healthcare provider to develop a foundational relationship of trust, compassion, empathy, and honesty. This foundation will allow the ongoing provision of patient and family care, according to how the patient and family define the care and the comfort they want and need.

References

1. Donna L, Hoyert PD, Jiaquan Xu MD. Deaths: Preliminary data for 2011. *Natl Vital Stat Rep*. 2012;61(6):1–51.
2. Roeland E, Cain J, Onderdonk C, Kerr K, Mitchell W, Thornberry K. When open-ended questions don't work: The role of palliative

paternalism in difficult medical decisions. *J Palliat Med.* 2014;17(4):415–420.
3. Harris LL, Placencia FX, Arnold JL, Minard CG, Harris TB, Haidet PM. A structured end of life curriculum for neonatoal-perinatal postdocotral fellows. *Am J Hosp Palliat Care.* 2015;32(3):253–261.
4. Salladay A. DNR alternative: Making plans to "allow natural death." *Nursing.* 2002;32(5):24–25.
5. McSteen K, Peden-McAlpine C. The role of the nurse as advocate in ethically difficult care situations with dying patients. *J Hosp Palliat Nurs.* 2006;8(5):259–269.
6. Stajduhar, KI, Thorne SE, McGuinness L, Charmaine KS. Patient perceptions of helpful communication in the context of advanced cancer. *J Clin Nurs.* 2010;19(13–14):2039–2047.
7. Robinson K, Sutton S, Von Gunten CF, Ferris FD, Molodyko N, Martinez J, Emanual LL. Assessment of the Education for Physicians on End-of-Life Care (EPEC) project. *J Palliat Med.* 2014;7(5):637–645.
8. Lamont EB, Christakis NA. Complexities in prognostication in advanced cancer: "To help them live their lives the way they want to." *JAMA.* 2003;290(1):98–104.
9. Von Gunten CF, Ferris FD, Emanuel AL. Ensuring competency in end of life care-communication and relational skills. *JAMA.* 2005;284(23):3051–3057.
10. Malia C, Bennett M. What influences patients' decisions on artificial hydration at the end of life? A Q-methodology study. *J Pain Symptom Manage.* 2011;42(2):192–200.
11. Chui TY, Hu WY, Chuang RB, Cheng YR, Chen CY. Terminal cancer patients' wishes and influencing factors toward provision of artificial nutrition and hydration in Taiwan. *J Pain Symptom Manage.* 2004;27(3):206–214.
12. Geppert C, Andrews MR, Druyan ME. Ethical issues in artificial nutrition and hydration: A review. *J Parenter Enteral Nutr.* 2010;34(1):79–89.
13. Clifton-Hawkin N, Gallo M. *Food and Nutrition at the End of Life Survey.* Durate, CA: City of Hope Department of Supportive Care Medicine; 2014.
14. Miles A. Person-centered medicine—at the intersection of science, ethics and humanism. *Int J Pers Cent Med.* 2012;3(2):329–333.
15. Little JM. Humanistic medicine or values-based medicine . . . what's in a name? *Med J Aust.* 2002;177:319–321.
16. Mannix KA, Blackburn IM, Garland A, Gracie J, Moorey S, Reid B, Standart S, Scott J. Effectiveness of brief training in cognitive behaviour therapy techniques for palliative care practitioners. *J Palliat Med.* 2006;20:579–584.
17. Kelley JM, Kraft-Todd G, Schapira L, Kossowsky J, Riess H. The influence of the patient-clinician relationship on healthcare outcomes: A systematic review and meta-analysis of randomized controlled trials. *PLoS One.* 2014;9(4):e94207.
18. Gottman JM. *The Science of Trust.* New York, NY: W.W. Norton; 2011.
19. Nielson LS, Angus, JE, Howell D, Husain A, Gastaldo D. Patient-centered care or cultural competence: Negotiating palliative care at home for Chinese Canadian immigrants. *Am J Hosp Palliat Care.* 2015;32(4):372–379.
20. McMillen RE. End of life decisions: Nurses perceptions, feelings and experiences. *Intensive Crit Care Nurs.* 2008;24:251–259.
21. Gwyther LP, Altilio T, Blacker S, Christ G, Csikai EL, Hooyman N. Social work competencies in palliative and end-of-life care. *J Soc Work End Life Palliat Care.* 2005;7:87–120.
22. Chodren, P. *Taking the Leap: Freeing Ourselves from Old Habit and Fears.* Boston, MA: Shambala; 2010.
23. Schlairet MC, Cohen RW. Allow-natural-death (AND) orders: Legal, ethical, and practical considerations. *HEC Forum.* 2013;25:161–171.

CHAPTER 35

Advance Care Planning

Jeanine Blackford and Annette F. Street

Introduction

Conversations about end-of-life planning are increasing in complexity and scope. Advance care planning (ACP) is a process that has developed internationally to facilitate communication between individuals and healthcare providers to identify and document medical and personal care preferences consistent with personal values in the event that a patient becomes too ill in the future to express his or her wishes.[1] In this process, patients also identify a person (or persons) whom they trust to insure that their healthcare wishes are respected should they lose decision-making capacity. The ACP conversation is designed to address two key questions:[2]

1. If you are unable or do not want to take part in your healthcare decision-making, what do we need to think about when making decisions about your care?
2. If you are unable or do not want to take part in your healthcare decision-making, to whom should we speak?

Based on the ethical principle of patient autonomy and the legal doctrine of patient consent, ACP helps to insure that the concept of consent is respected if a person becomes incapable of participating in his or her treatment decisions. It allows a commitment to person-centered care, where personal values can be respected.

These conversations occur in a context where medical technology advances have given healthcare providers the ability to prolong life by artificial and mechanical means. These advances have created their own ethical dilemmas that need careful consideration, especially when treatments may be of limited benefit to the patient. People may live longer but with increasing disabilities or comorbidities. Aside from lengthening the illness trajectory, these technological advances have also increased palliative care options. The boundaries between active medical management for cure and palliative care for symptom control are now blurred, and patients are offered more choices, some of which may be unwanted or unwarranted.[3] Irrespective of the reason for palliative care admission, patients have the right to make decisions about their healthcare, now and for the future. Informed decision-making about treatment requires that patients with life-limiting illnesses, and others making decisions on the patient's behalf, understand the consequences of potential treatments. However, many patients are too ill at the end of life to make treatment decisions or discuss their preferences for place of death, family involvement, or spiritual care.

This chapter explores the role of communication in ACP, discussion points in an ACP conversation, and communication strategies for initiating and maintaining ongoing dialogue about ACP with patients and family members.

Conversation Through the ACP Process

The ACP process has three key components: (a) a guided discussion to provide information and explore healthcare options and treatment preferences; (b) appointment of a proxy or substitute decision-maker; and (c) expression of a person's wishes for care, preferably in writing. A guided ACP discussion(s) has a number of key elements to assist patients in clarifying their end-of-life healthcare preferences. Discussions are designed to assist individuals to understand their medical condition and potential future complications; consider the benefits and burdens of current and future treatments; reflect on their goals, values, and personal beliefs to guide future care; discuss choices with family and/or important others and healthcare providers; decide on a decision-maker in the event that the person is unable to make decisions or communicate; and document these choices.

To participate in ACP, patients need to have knowledge about their life-limiting illness and possible outcomes so they can determine their healthcare preferences. In a person-centered approach, information is not merely a biomedical description of the disease; patients need to explore the illness in terms of their experience and its potential impact and consequences of living with the disease.[4] The palliative care provider's role is to ascertain what the patient and family understands of the diagnosis and prognosis and to facilitate a discussion that explores what matters to them. The discussion can simply begin with: "Tell me what you understand about your illness."

Patients need information about their illness trajectory, cardiopulmonary resuscitation; potential treatment options such as ventilation, artificial nutrition, and hydration; and, more specifically, comfort care. Patients can easily become confused between treatments they received in the curative phase of their illness and those offered as palliation—as treatment may be the same but for different purposes. A key element of ACP discussions must include decisions about when to have treatment and when to stop treatment, and an overview of acceptable alternatives should be discussed. Patient decision-making relies on the thoroughness of discussion about current and future benefits and burdens of treatment. Healthcare providers need to help patients understand the likeliness of treatment outcomes and to consider how long treatment should continue and what symptoms and side effects are acceptable.

Religion, spirituality, and culture interplay to influence future care decisions.[5] Different religions with their specific values, beliefs, and practices can shape a person's illness meaning and influence future treatment options.[6] More broadly, spirituality is a part of how we think about the world and ourselves. As palliative care providers help individuals explore their values and beliefs, they address patients' dimensions of spirituality; the meaning they attribute to their life, their sense of purpose, and their relationship with themselves and others are a part of how they make sense of their world.[5,7]

Culture can influence who participates in the discussion, who makes the decisions, what types of decisions are made, and what rituals are important in end-of-life care. In this exploration, the decisions the patient and/or family (and/or community) make can challenge palliative care providers' beliefs about what constitutes good end-of-life care. ACP is based on Western values and can be contrary to a family's own cultural beliefs.[8] A family's decision to withhold prognostic information can be difficult in a Western medical culture that values and promotes truth-telling in healthcare. Cultural humility can assist palliative care providers to understand their own cultural positioning, both personally and professionally.[9,10] It is in the process of critical reflection that our own cultural complexities become evident. In ACP, cultural humility also requires palliative care providers to engage in ACP themselves to be truly self-aware.

Family members and significant others form an important part of the ACP process. Choices about who participates in the discussion are influenced by personal preferences as well as religious and cultural influences. Before treatment options are fully explored, the patient must decide, if able, about how he or she wants the process to proceed. The sequence in which these discussions occur can vary. Some may prefer to talk with palliative care team members first to become clear about their goals and future treatment preferences; others may prefer the discussion to occur in consultation with the family and health providers; while some may be present at the conversation but expect the family to lead. Finally some, particularly older people, may even prefer that the doctor make the decisions.

The Appointment of a Decision-Maker

With the involvement of the family and/or significant others, patients may choose to nominate and legally identify a person(s) to make decisions on their behalf in the event they become unable to make decisions. The appointment of a decision-maker is done informally in some countries or states; in other places, it is a legal process with powers of attorney or guardianship to make decisions on the behalf of the person who is not competent or able to do so. Choice of a substitute decision-maker or proxy is based on trust, but there are other factors that also need to be considered, including whether the chosen person is willing, available, and capable. Increasingly, families are scattered geographically, so it is hard for family members to remain informed and have an understanding of the context in which the patient is living/dying. It is not a unique scenario where a son returns home to insist his mother be treated, whereas those who have lived locally have witnessed the deterioration and recognize her declining health. Alternatively, the proxy may actually be sicker than the person for whom he or she is making decisions.

A Written Plan

Internationally and nationally, the forms of documentation vary that detail healthcare wishes such as living wills, advance directives, and statements of choices. Although there are inconsistencies within and between countries regarding the terminology and legislative procedures used in the ACP process, there is general agreement in the literature and in practice that facilitated discussion is at the heart of the process.[11-15]

The ACP process may be different over the illness trajectory, but the need for open and ongoing communication between all parties remains the same. Palliative care providers, irrespective of their location in the healthcare system, have a responsibility to be able to initiate, facilitate, and document ACP conversations with their patients and families. ACP is only possible when there is quality communication throughout the process and that communication is clearly documented and available for future use.

Communication Strategies

Serious illness provides patients with an opportunity to prepare for a future, while possibly limited, that focuses on quality of life—a fundamental principle of palliative care. For the majority of patients, ACP concerns are not so much about treatment options as they are questions of pain and symptom management, reduced burden on their loved ones, and a desire to die in familiar surroundings.[16-18] ACP and the provision of palliative care are intimately linked, as they provide opportunity to achieve person-centered care. A number of palliative care national associations and organizations recognize this importance and provide resources and tools for palliative care health providers to enable them to facilitate ACP in their practice (see Table 35.1).

With the palliative care team appropriately prepared and equipped with information and decision-support tools, the next steps of ACP are to assess competence, appoint a proxy or substitute decision-maker, clarify values, and find opportunities along the illness trajectory to facilitate discussion. This chapter includes a set of original conversation starters (Table 35.2) that draws on a previously published framework[19] and follows transition points in palliative care practice.

ACP Discussion Points

In any admission to a healthcare service, there are routine practices. Patients expect healthcare providers to ask questions, take vital signs, conduct an examination, and collect information. ACP information could form part of this "routine" collection. Useful information may already be evident in the referral information. Information about competence level, appointment of a substitute decision-maker, and advance directives or plans may be absent from a referral, partly because those who designed such documents did not consider requesting such information. As part of the admission process, the palliative care provider needs to know what the patient understands about his or her diagnosis and prognosis.[20,21] This understanding may also extend to the family and/or significant others.

In addition to assessing understanding, patient competence needs to be assessed. An assessment of competence in any detail is beyond the scope of this chapter. Briefly, before a patient is

Table 35.1 National Associations and Organization Resources and Tools for Palliative Care Health Providers

Country	Organizations/ Resources	Description / Website	Web Address
United States	The Conversation Project	Tools to assist people formulate their healthcare preferences and introduce the topic with family and health professionals. Health professionals education programs available.	http://theconversationproject.org/
	Elder Guru: Keeping Professionals Informed	Website designed for aged care. Provides ACP information. Direct links to all US state-based Attorney General's Office to obtain specific ACP details.	http://www.elderguru.com/resources/
	Gunderson Health System	Respecting Choices program commenced La Crosse, Wisconsin. Model used in a number of US states and internationally. Tools, resources, and training for health professionals available. Tools are also available for community. (Note there is some cost involved with some of these tools.)	http://www.gundersenhealth.org/respecting-choices
	Physicians Orders for Life-Sustaining Treatment	POLST model begun in Oregon adopted in a number of states. Each site complies a variety of resources for health professionals and patients and families.	http://www.or.polst.org/
		Everplans website provides access to each state to access POLST specific documents.	https://www.everplans.com/tools-and-resources/state-by-state-polst-forms
		Coalition for Compassionate Care of California	http://capolst.org/
Mexico	Hospice Mazatlan	Although advance care planning is not legally recognized in Mexico, some information is available for palliative care patients.	http://www.hospicemazatlan.org/index.php?option=com_content&view=article&id=51&Itemid=55&lang=en
Canada	Canadian Hospice Palliative Care Association	ACP documents and tools for health professionals; patients, and families.	http://advancecareplanning.ca/making-your-plan.aspx
		Provincial and territorial specific resources.	http://advancecareplanning.ca/making-your-plan/how-to-make-your-plan/provincialresources.aspx
	Canadian Virtual Hospice	A variety of "Tools for Practice" compiled by clinical experts to facilitate ACP and end-of-life decision-making. Includes assessment and evaluation tools as well as videos to demonstrate different aspects of ACP.	http://www.virtualhospice.ca/en_US/Main+Site+Navigation/Home/For+Professionals/For+Professionals/Tools+for+Practice/Advanced+care+planning+_+Decision+making.aspx?page=1#id_357bb8eb26753c8037c723f34d1a834e
	Educating Future Physicians in Palliative and End-of-Life Care	ACP education program designed for health professionals; specific emphasis on physicians. For use in undergraduate, postgraduate, and continuing education. Includes useful information about how to have "the conversation," explain life-sustaining therapy, and explore own values, which can influence ACP.	http://www.virtualhospice.ca/en_US/Main+Site+Navigation/Home/For+Professionals/For+Professionals/Tools+for+Practice/Education/Facilitating+Advance+Care+Planning_+An+Interprofessional+Education+Program+(Curriculum+Materials).aspx
Australia	Palliative Care Australia	Provides an overview of Australian ACP with links to state-specific information.	http://www.palliativecare.org.au/AdvanceCarePlanning.aspx
	Respecting Patient Choices	Based on US Respecting Choices model commenced in Melbourne and expanded to other states and territories. Provides state-specific information and documents and training for health professionals.	http://www.rpctraining.com.au/
	Advance Care Planning Australia	Provides information for health professionals, patients, and families. Access to state/territory-specific information is available. Training for health professionals also provided.	http://advancecareplanning.org.au/
	Clinical Practice Guidelines	Clinical practice guidelines for communicating prognosis and end-of-life issues with adults in the advanced stages of a life-limiting illness, and their caregivers[a]. These guidelines include useful phrases to assist doctors facilitate ACP.	https://www.mja.com.au/journal/2007/186/12/clinical-practice-guidelines-communicating-prognosis-and-end-life-issues-adults?0=ip_login_no_cache%3Dd1e88addd541a563c573fb749f2f5357

(continued)

Table 35.1 Continued

Country	Organizations/Resources	Description / Website	Web Address
United Kingdom	National Council for Palliative Care	Information and booklets to assist health professionals facilitate ACP. Also pamphlets for the general public. Also a series of booklets that address "Difficult conversation for disease specific conditions."	http://www.ncpc.org.uk/sites/default/files/
		Advance care planning: A guide for health and social care staff	http://www.ncpc.org.uk/sites/default/files/AdvanceCarePlanning.pdf
		Difficult conversations (note these require a small fee):	http://www.ncpc.org.uk/difficult_conversations
	National Gold Standards Framework	National initiative developed to improve the quality of end-of-life care provide information for health professionals and general public about ACP.	http://www.goldstandardsframework.org.uk/advance-care-planning
	UK General Medical Council	Guidelines and tips for doctors about what to address in facilitating an ACP conversation.	http://www.gmc-uk.org/guidance/ethical_guidance/end_of_life_advance_care_planning.asp
New Zealand	National Advance Care Planning Cooperative	Includes online learning; tools and booklets that address all aspects of ACP. Designed for use in the community and by health professionals.	http://www.advancecareplanning.org.nz/

Note: ACP = advance care planning.
[a] Clayton JM, Hancock KM, Butow PN, Tattersall MNH, Currow DC. *Med J Aust.* 2007;186(12):77.

Table 35.2 Conversation Starters for Discussions about ACP

Transition Points	Potential Prompts in Practice	Sample of Conversation Starters
Referral to palliative care	Referral indicates • appointment of substitute decision maker • written healthcare wishes • not for resuscitation order • evidence of future care preferences • planned treatments	*Clarification with the referrer about ACP information provided including:* "Has Joan received any advance care planning information?" "Have you discussed advance care planning with her? Is there any reason why this has not occurred?" "Has Joan appointed anyone as her (proxy/substitute decision maker)?" "Your referral has indicated that there is an NFR order; has this been discussed with her?"
Admission to palliative care	Use of evidence in referral to confirm situation at first meeting: • understanding of diagnosis/prognosis • planned or refused treatments • ACP status recorded	*To the patient:* "Simon, the information I received from the hospital tells me that you are . . . Can you tell me a bit more about that so I can better understand what you want?" "Jack, I see that you have decided not to proceed with the surgery. Can you tell me about this so we can work with you on what care you do want?"
	Routine palliative care practice to verify ACP status. • yes/no advance directive/plan • yes/no copy of documents in file • yes/no proxy appointed; "no" responses leads to provision of written ACP information	"Simon in this admission I need to ask whether you have done any advance care planning. It is routine we ask this of everyone we admit to our service" "You're not sure about advance care planning. It is . . . Here I will leave some information for you to read and we can talk about it next time I visit." "You know about advance care planning. Have you made any decisions? Are they written down?"
	Routine provision of ACP information	We provide all our clients with advance care planning information. You and your wife can read it and we'll talk about it next time. It is really important as it will help us ensure that the care we provide is what you want (or: what your future healthcare wishes might be)." "I have done ACP myself and with my family. Would it help if I talk about my experiences first?"

(continued)

Table 35.2 Continued

Transition Points	Potential Prompts in Practice	Sample of Conversation Starters
	Identification of ♦ primary carer ♦ next of kin ♦ family relationships	"I'd like to know a little bit more about you and your family. Can we work on this together? I'd like to draw a family tree/ecomap so I can understand them better. This is what it looks like." "Now that I have a better picture of who is important in your life, if you become too sick at any time to make your own healthcare decisions, who would you trust to make them for you?" "I see that you have nominated your daughter to make these decisions. Does she know that you want her to do this? Does she know what decisions you would like her to make?"
	Insight into illness	"Can you tell me about your illness? What has the doctor told you is going to happen?" "Jenny, what can you tell me about your future treatment plans? I notice that . . . "
	Preferred site of care	"Mrs. Smyth, where do you prefer to be cared for if you get sicker?" "Okay, so you would really like to stay at home. I'd like to talk about the sort of care that you want . . . "
	Discussion of ACP information provided	"Last time I visited I asked you to read this pamphlet. I'd like to take the opportunity to sit down with you and discuss it a little further."
Ongoing palliative care management	A visit to the doctor	"I see you have been to visit your doctor again. Did he have any news to report? . . . He said that you weren't getting any better. I wish the news had been better too. If we cannot make the disease stay in remission then maybe we can work on some short-term goals that you can achieve."
	A significant event	"John, it is good news that your grandson is getting married. Have you thought about . . . ?"
	Recovery from an acute episode of the chronic illness	"John, it is good to see you home again after that bowel obstruction. You were in hospital for a very long time. Have you thought about what you want to do if you get sick again and it doesn't go as well next time? Sometimes having a plan that prepares you for the worse makes it easier to focus on what you hope most for."
	Past caregiver experiences	"Have you or any of your friends had to care for a person and make decisions for them?" "Have you or anyone that you know had to make decisions about treatments that might prolong life but wondered if it was the right thing to do?"
Discharge from palliative care or terminal care	Resuscitation	"I notice in the documents I received that you want to be resuscitated if your heart stops beating. Can you tell me what you expect will happen?"
	Discharge planning	"Hi, Mrs. Clarke, I am here today to finalize your discharge from our service. It is good you are better now. What do you understand will happen in the future with your illness? Have you thought about . . . ?"

Note: ACP = advance care planning.

able to make an advance care plan, his or her competence must be assessed. To be considered competent, patients must be able to understand and reflect on their illness in accordance with their own values and belief systems.

During serious illness, a patient's competence may fluctuate. If possible, providers should delay decisions until they can establish if the patient is able to make his or her own wishes known. It is also important to remember that despite diminished competence, a patient may still be able to participate in the decision-making process. The patient may lack capacity to make medical decisions but still be able to contribute meaningfully to a discussion about care and choose a proxy for more complex care decisions. If a patient is assessed as mentally incompetent, then decision-making responsibility rests with the appointed proxy. If a proxy has not been appointed, some jurisdictions identify who has decision-making responsibility.

Following affirmation of mental competence, the palliative care provider must establish whether a substitute decision-maker(s), sometimes called a proxy, has been appointed. If this has already been achieved, then the proxy should participate in the discussion. It remains, however, the patient's choice whether to have the proxy present in the initial conversations as he or she clarifies what is important. A patient may choose to have the first conversation before involving the proxy.

An important aspect for all those involved in palliative care is the person's preferred place of care and place of death. There are number of reports that identify that patients prefer to die at home,[16-18] but this is not often achieved due to high symptom burden, caregiver exhaustion, or failure to ask. When it is clear that a patient has indicated the preferred place of care, then the question follows: "Given that you have indicated you would like to be cared for at home, can you talk about the care that you want?"

Decision-Support Tools

Increasingly, a range of decision support tools are being used to assist individuals and their families to make choices between different treatment options. These aids include structured interviews, scenario-based decisions, value clarification, interactive CDs/DVDs, and self-directed online choices (see Box 35.1).

Box 35.1 Sample of Advance Care Planning Decision Support Tools

Target Audience	Decision Aid Tool	Website
General public	ACP (downloadable application for mobile users)	http://www.acpdecisions.org/about/.
	Five Wishes	https://fivewishesonline.agingwithdignity.org
	My Voice—Planning Ahead	http://www.calgaryhealthregion.ca/programs/advancecareplanning/
	Making your Wishes known: Planning Your Medical Future	http://pennstatehershey.org/web/humanities/home/resources/advancedirectives
	PREPARE	https://www.prepareforyourcare.org/
	Your life, Your Choices. Planning for Future Medical Decisions: How to Prepare a Personalized Living Will (available on a variety of websites)	http://www.elderguru.com/download-the-your-life-your-choices-planning-for-future-medical-decisions-workbook/
Palliative care focus	When you need extra care, should you receive it at home or in a facility? A decision aid to prepare you to discuss the options	http://decisionaid.ohri.ca/decaids.html#poc
	"Thinking Ahead" Gold Standard Framework Advance Care Planning Discussion	http://www.goldstandardsframework.org.uk

Barriers to and Enablers of Effective ACP Discussions

Despite the World Health Organization's endorsement and widespread government support for ACP in developed and developing countries, as well as community support, utilization of ACP across all countries remains low. Multiple interconnected barriers contribute to the lack of presence. These barriers are discussed in detail next, with consideration of potential ways to overcome these barriers.

Lack of Knowledge of ACP

Reluctance for patients to engage in ACP may simply be due to a lack of knowledge about the process. Despite the increasing global spread since its inception in the United States in the 1990s, ACP still remains an unfamiliar concept in public discourse. Palliative care increasingly includes patients with non-cancer-related diseases such as dementia,[22] lung disease,[23–25] renal disease,[26,27] and heart failure,[28] where ACP discussions are less common than among patients with cancer.[29]

The crisis response to sudden deterioration in health status is created when loved ones and healthcare providers are not clear about the range and scope of care wanted. The concept of palliative care advocates having end-of-life conversations early in the illness trajectory.[30] These conversations focus on elucidating personal values, which can be used to inform healthcare decision-making.[31] Patients can reflect and consider their future healthcare decisions[32] before the onset of a crisis that can occur over the illness trajectory.

Public health initiatives to promote and educate about ACP are important. In a number of countries, federal and state governments and palliative care organizations have developed public campaigns to inform the general public about ACP. These strategies include government-sponsored websites with information about ACP and guidance on how to proceed to develop a plan, distribution of ACP pamphlets in plain language,[33] training volunteers to talk through end-of-life issues in their community,[34] and providing access to tools and documents to assist people to begin ACP. In the United States, "The Conversation Project," designed to help people talk about their end-of-life care, include in the tool kit a guide called "How to talk to your doctor (or any member of your healthcare team)."

Who Is Responsible for Facilitating ACP?

Confusion exists about who is responsible for initiating and facilitating ongoing ACP discussions.[24] This leads to the problem that ACP is always "someone else's" responsibility. Despite promotion by governments and recognition of ACP in palliative care guidelines,[35–37] many healthcare providers remain reluctant to have an ACP conversation. Two recent UK surveys,[38,39] consisting of 2,055 members of the general public and 1,003 general practitioners (GPs), found that 25% of GPs had never initiated a conversation about end-of-life care wishes. However, 40% of GPs indicated they were prepared personally for the end of life, but only 8% had documented their end-of-life wishes. For physicians, reluctance to engage in ACP with patients is often linked to difficulties in prognostication in some disease groups,[40] whereas other healthcare providers report they are waiting for the patient to raise the issue.[41] A consequence of providers' inability or reluctance means that many people with life-limiting illnesses, who have been in the care of generalist and specialist healthcare providers over their protracted disease trajectory, reach the palliative phase of their illness without ever having had "the conversation." A recent US survey of healthcare providers about ACP and end-of-life care suggested that palliative healthcare providers have an important role in facilitating ACP.[42]

Provider discomfort in talking about end-of-life matters is not matched by discomfort in patients who benefit from ACP. Interestingly, despite 83% of the general public stating they were uncomfortable talking about death, 90% of the general public surveyed stated that health professionals should receive compulsory training to learn how to talk about end-of-life matters sensitively. There is a clear difference between "death talk" with the general public and the clientele of palliative care.

Research demonstrates that provision of ACP information alone is insufficient to motivate the majority of people to proceed with the ACP process and formally document their wishes.[43,44] People with life-limiting illness expect healthcare providers to raise the issue,[15,45,46] and interactions with such providers are known to increase ACP completions.[44] Palliative care providers need to be confident and comfortable facilitating these conversations. A variety of communication workshops have been developed to prepare healthcare providers to facilitate ACP. These vary in focus and intensity, from a generalist approach to disease-specific workshops that can extend from 1 to 3 days. The difficulty with such workshops is that they may increase healthcare provider knowledge, but the skills do not necessarily translate into practice.[47,48] An important component of the educational process is effective mentoring and opportunity to practice and assess competencies that will encourage incorporation of ACP into routine practice. More important, palliative care providers, working toward cultural humility, need to engage in their own ACP.

"I'm Not Ready to Talk About It"

Lack of acceptance of a terminal prognosis[49] or death preparedness[50] is seen as a major barrier to ACP. If patients remain focused on cure or survival, they may be unwilling to accept the reality that they are dying.[46] As a result of this failure to engage in ACP conversations, it could be assumed that the default position is to treat at all costs. These costs are not only financial but, more important, are an emotional cost to family and staff. The reverse may also be true, where family members or significant others are "not ready" to discuss future healthcare decisions, as they expect their loved one will get better. In this case scenario, the dying person may acquiesce to unwanted treatment at the behest of the family. Some cultural groups believe that discussing death will hasten it, create a bad omen for possible health outcomes, or encourage the dying person to give up.

Reluctance to prepare for end-of-life care is not limited to the individual with advanced disease or the family; healthcare providers may also find such conversations stressful, with patients choosing to avoid end-of-life discussions to protect the doctor.[40] Healthcare providers' perception that a person is "not ready" to discuss can also be an excuse for family and providers not to begin ACP discussions.

High Symptom Burden

A fundamental principle of palliative care is early involvement of the palliative care team in a patient's illness trajectory.[51] However, referrals are not a common occurrence due to organizational barriers, healthcare provider reluctance to refer early to palliative care, and health insurance structures that restrict palliative care access. Patients admitted to palliative care services late in the illness trajectory usually have high symptom burden, which may limit their capacity to engage in an ACP conversation. Understandably, patients with severe pain or other intractable symptoms often associated with severe emotional distress find it difficult to focus on end-of-life discussions.[52,53] Research confirms that patients admitted to palliative care experiencing high levels of pain and nausea tend to refuse do-not-resuscitate orders,[53] as they are too uncomfortable to consider their options. In person-centered care, symptom management becomes the primary concern before initiating an ACP discussion. Yet ACP can guide symptom management by providing information such as whether the person prefers to be pain-free or trade off some pain to retain a clearer mind.

If a palliative healthcare provider is not able to engage in an ACP discussion, he or she needs to set up another time or refer the patient to another member of the palliative care team. The size and scope of the palliative care team and its administering body will influence this decision. Roles and responsibilities may be distributed equally across the team or quite focused for different discipline areas. For example, the physician's role might be to discuss treatment options, while the social worker addresses appointment of a substitute decision-maker and the nurse discusses location and type of care. Alternatively, the strength of relationships between specific palliative care team members and the person with the life-limiting illness may dictate who is best suited to facilitate ACP.[4,54]

Interpersonal Relationships

The quality of the relationships within the family and/or significant others and with healthcare providers can affect ACP.[55] Individual family circumstances and their history can be complex and layered with emotional, psychological, and financial issues. Palliative care team members often find the most complex and difficult family relationships would benefit from ACP discussion, but they require expert providers to facilitate such conversations.

Difficulties may begin with choosing the right person to be the substitute decision-maker. A patient may perceive the family has expectations as to who would be selected as a substitute decision-maker. In one situation, an elderly woman was fearful her daughter "would bully her way into having to be that person because she'd just expect that." A palliative healthcare provider encouraged her to talk with her daughter. It became clear that the daughter did not want the role, and the family reached agreement about the most suitable person to be nominated as proxy.[56]

Some healthcare providers perceive that such a discussion will impair therapeutic relationships. Community palliative care nurses report a concern that introduction of ACP may affect their relationship with the patient and limit access to the home. Yet GPs report that open discussion strengthens their relationship with patients.[57] It is clear when families are harmonious, open to discussion, and able to support their loved one, formal documentation may be considered unnecessary. In complex family relationships with disharmony and potential misunderstanding, however, ACP may help resolve conflicts and build trust with healthcare providers.[57] In such situations, written directives or plans become an important goal to achieve person-centered care.

Cultural Barriers

The dominance of a white-centric healthcare system[58] has meant that minority groups have suffered from discrimination in their care.[15,59,60] This has created a long-standing cultural mistrust of a healthcare system that has for generations failed to respect cultural needs and often delivered suboptimal care. Much US research in ACP with different cultural groups has highlighted this mistrust and shown that there is low ACP utilization within these groups and a tendency to request medical interventions. US-based research also shows that higher educated and white people are more likely to engage with ACP.[59,60] Failure to provide ACP information at an appropriate literacy level, as well as in a culturally acceptable form, may limit ACP to people located within a particular culture and class.[15,61]

In addition to cultural barriers created through different values and practices, there are also language barriers for people who have English as a second language. People may be able to speak some English, but engaging in an ACP conversation is unfair and unjust to the person and family. Healthcare providers need interpreters working alongside them to facilitate a discussion. Although there is written ACP information available in different languages, some patients and families will have limited or no literacy. More recently, Web-based videos and YouTube clips have appeared that explain ACP in different languages. These communication means, if reliable, open up the potential to ensure ACP equity.

Time

Time is an ongoing problem for all parties trying to achieve successful ACP. Yet time can also be a convenient excuse to avoid a sensitive and delicate topic. Medical appointments are often taken up dealing with the current health situation with no time left for the patient to raise questions about the future. Physicians report they have no time to have such discussions.[24,62,63] Realistically, given the limited uptake of ACP internationally, palliative care providers often find that they are required to initiate the ACP conversation. Late referrals to palliative care services also means truncated time to establish rapport to the level required to discuss sensitive issues and less opportunity to conduct an in-depth discussion.

Conclusion

ACP conversations provide individuals and their families with opportunities to make choices and express their preferences for medical treatment, social, and spiritual support in advance of their death. The communication approach undertaken in ACP needs to encourage a conversation with a focus on elucidating the desired place of care and of death, personal values to inform healthcare decision-making, and identification and/or confirmation of substitute decision-maker(s) and may include specific, time-limited treatment preferences. Before the palliative care team can realistically facilitate ACP, certain conditions must be present. These include the palliative care team understanding their ACP roles and responsibilities, appropriate healthcare provider ACP education, and the provision of useful decision-making tools and legislatively appropriate documents.

An understanding of the barriers to and enablers of ACP, along with the strategic use of conversation starters, can facilitate effective person-centered palliative care. ACP can help reduce family tensions and bewilderment concerning the individual's preferences and equip healthcare providers to meet the desired care needs and goals of person-centered palliative care.

References

1. Mullick A, Martin J, Sallnow L. An introduction to advance care planning in practice. *BMJ*. 2013;347:f6064.
2. Mahon MM. An advance directive in two questions. *J Pain Symptom Manage*. 2011;41(4):801–807.
3. Teno JM, Gozalo PL, Bynum JP, et al. Change in end-of-life care for Medicare beneficiaries: Site of death, place of care, and health care transitions in 2000, 2005, and 2009. *JAMA*. 2013;309(5):470–477.
4. Simpson AC. An opportunity to care? Preliminary insights from a qualitative study on advance care planning in advanced COPD. *Prog Palliat Care*. 2011;19(5):243–253.
5. Lunsford B. Religion, spirituality, culture in advance care planning. In: Rogne L, McCune SL, eds. *Advance Care Planning: Communicating About Matters of Life and Death*. New York, NY: Springer; 2014:89–103.
6. Lo B, Ruston D, Kates L, et al. Discussing religious and spiritual issues at the end of life: A practical guide for physicians. *JAMA*. 2002 287(6):749–754.
7. Chrash M, Mulich B, Patton CM. The APN role in holistic assessment and integration of spiritual assessment for advance care planning. *J Am Acad Nurse Pract*. 2011;23(10):530–536.
8. Mei Ching L, Hinderer KA, Kehl KA. A systematic review of advance directives and advance care planning in Chinese people from Eastern and Western cultures. *J Hosp Palliat Nurs*. 2014;16(2):75–85.
9. Tervalon M, Murray-Garcia J. Cultural humility versus cultural competence: A critical distinction in defining physician training outcomes in multicultural education. *J Health Care Poor Underserved*. 1998;9(2):117–125.
10. Yeager KA, Bauer-Wu S. Cultural humility: Essential foundation for clinical researchers. *Appl Nurs Res*. 2013;26(4):251–256.
11. Tulsky JA. Beyond advance directives: Importance of communication skills at the end of life. *JAMA*. 2005;294(3):359–365.
12. Turner M, Payne S, O'Brien T. Mandatory communication skills training for cancer and palliative care staff: Does one size fit all? *Eur J Oncol Nurs*. 2011;15(5):398–403.
13. Black K. Advance directive communication: nurses' and social workers' perceptions of roles. *Am J Hosp Palliat Care*. 2006;23(2):175–184.
14. Back AL, Anderson WG, Bunch L, et al. Communication about cancer near the end of life. *Cancer*. 2008;113(7 Suppl):1897–1910.
15. Wagner GJ, Riopelle D, Steckart J, Lorenz KA, Rosenfeld KE. Provider communication and patient understanding of life-limiting illness and their relationship to patient communication of treatment preferences. *J Pain Symptom Manage*. 2010;39(3):527–534.
16. Gomes B, Higginson IJ, Calanzani N, et al. Preferences for place of death if faced with advanced cancer: A population survey in England, Flanders, Germany, Italy, the Netherlands, Portugal and Spain. *Ann Oncol*. August 1, 2012;23(8):2006–2015.
17. Wilson DM, Cohen J, Deliens L, Hewitt JA, Houttekier D. The preferred place of last days: Results of a representative population-based public survey. *J Palliat Med*. 2013;16(5):502–508.
18. Higginson IJ, Gomes B, Calanzani N, et al. Priorities for treatment, care and information if faced with serious illness: A comparative population-based survey in seven European countries. *Palliat Med*. February 2014;28(2):101–110.
19. Blackford J, Street AF. Facilitating advance care planning in community palliative care: Conversation starters across the client journey. *Int J Palliat Nurs*. 2013;19(3):132–139.
20. Blackford J, Street AF. Tracking the route to sustainability: A service evaluation tool for an advance care planning model developed for community palliative care services *J Clin Nurs*. 2012;21:2136–2148.
21. Robinson CA. "Our best hope is a cure": Hope in the context of advance care planning. *Palliat Support Care*. 2012;10(02):75–82.
22. Dempsey D. Advance care planning for people with dementia: Benefits and challenges. *Int J Palliat Nurs*. 2013;19(5):227–234.
23. Colman RE, Curtis JR, Nelson JE, et al. Barriers to optimal palliative care of lung transplant candidates. *Chest*. 2013;143(3):736–743.
24. Gott M, Gardiner C, Small N, et al. Barriers to advance care planning in chronic obstructive pulmonary disease. *Palliat Med*. 2009;23(7):642–648.
25. Heffner JE. Advance care planning in chronic obstructive pulmonary disease: Barriers and opportunities. *Curr Opin Pulm Med*. 2011;17(2):103–109.

26. Janssen DJA, Spruit MA, Schols JMGA, van der Sande FM, Frenken LA, Wouters EFM. Insight into advance care planning for patients on dialysis. *J Pain Symptom Manage.* 2013;45(1):104–113.
27. Luckett T, Sellars M, Tieman J, et al. Advance care planning for adults with CKD: A systematic integrative review. *Am J Kidney Dis.* 2014;63(5):761–770.
28. Sarkar U, Schillinger D, Bibbins-Domingo K, Nápoles A, Karliner L, Pérez-Stable EJ. Patient–physicians' information exchange in outpatient cardiac care: Time for a heart to heart? *Patient Educ Couns.* 2011;85(2):173–179.
29. Barnes S, Gardiner C, Gott M, et al. Enhancing patient-professional communication about end-of-life issues in life-limiting conditions: A critical review of the literature. *J Pain Symptom Manage.* December 2012;44(6):866–879.
30. Kellehear A. Advance care planning as a public health issue. In: Rogne L, McCune SL, eds. *Advance Care Planning: Communicating About Matters of Life and Death.* New York, NY: Springer; 2014:333–345.
31. Clarke A, Seymour J. "At the foot of a very long ladder": Discussing the end of life with older people and informal caregivers. *J Pain Symptom Manage.* 2010;40(6):857–869.
32. Bomba PA, Vermilyea D. Integrating POLST into palliative care guidelines: A paradigm shift in advance care planning in oncology. *J Natl Compr Cancer.* 2006;4(8):819–829.
33. Nielson A, Baxter S. Advance care planning in Canada: Past experience and current strategies. In: Thomas K, Lobo B, eds. *Advance Care Planning in End of Life Care.* Oxford: Oxford University Press; 2011:219–228.
34. Sanders C, Seymour J, Clarke A, Gott M, Welton M. Development of a peer education programme for advance end-of-life care planning. *Int J Palliat Nurs.* 2006;12(5):214–223.
35. Ferris FD, Balfour HM, Bowen K, et al. A model to guide patient and family care: Based on nationally accepted principles and norms of practice. *J Pain Symptom Manage.* 2002;24(2):106–123.
36. National Hospice and Palliative Care Organisation. Standards of practice for hospice programs. http://www.nhpco.org/i4a/pages/index.cfm?pageid=5308. Accessed July 20, 2011.
37. Dahlin C, ed. *Clinical Practice Guidelines for Quality Palliative Care.* 3rd ed. Brooklyn, NY: National Consensus Project for Quality Palliative Care; 2013.
38. ComRes. Poll digest—Social—NCPC: Dying matters survey. http://www.comres.co.uk/polls/ncpc-dying-matters-survey/. 2014.
39. Smith R, Kelly N. Global attempts to avoid talking directly about death and dying. http://blogs.bmj.com/bmj/2012/08/16/richard-smith-and-nataly-kelly-global-attempts-to-avoid-talking-about-death-and-dying/. Published August 12, 2012.
40. Hancock K, Clayton JM, Parker SM, et al. Truth-telling in discussing prognosis in advanced life-limiting illnesses: A systematic review. *Palliat Med.* 2007;21(6):507–517.
41. De Vleminck A, Houttekier D, Pardon K, et al. Barriers and facilitators for general practitioners to engage in advance care planning: A systematic review. *Scand J Prim Health Care.* 2013;31(4):215–226.
42. Mattes MD, Tung K, Baum R, Parikh K, Ashamalla H. Understanding the views of those who care for patients with cancer on advance care planning and end-of-life care. *Am J Hosp Palliat Care.* June 2014;16:1–8.
43. Brunnhuber K, Nash S, Meier DE, Weissman DE, Woodcock J. *Putting Evidence Into Practice: Palliative Care.* Hoboken, NJ: BMJ Publishing Group; 2008.
44. Ramsaroop SD, Reid MC, Adelman RD. Completing an advance directive in the primary care setting: What do we need for success? *J Am Geriatr Soc.* 2007;55(2):277–283.
45. Davison SN, Simpson C. Hope and advance care planning in patients with end stage renal disease: Qualitative interview study. *BMJ.* 2006;333(7574):886–890.
46. Barnes KA, Barlow CA, Harrington J, et al. Advance care planning discussions in advanced cancer: Analysis of dialogues between patients and care planning mediators. *Palliat Support Care.* March 2011;9(1):73–79.
47. Gysels M, Richardson A, Higginson IJ. Communication training for health professionals who care for patients with cancer: A systematic review of effectiveness. *Support Care Cancer.* 2004;12(10):692–700.
48. Moore PM, Wilkinson SSM, Rivera Mercado S. Communication skills training for health professionals working with cancer patients, their families and/or carers. *Cochrane Database Syst Rev.* 2004;2:CD003751.
49. Zimmermann C. Acceptance of dying: A discourse analysis of palliative care literature. *Soc Sci Med.* 2012;75(1):217–224.
50. McLeod-Sordjan R. Death preparedness: A concept analysis. *J Adv Nurs.* 2014;70(5):1008–1019.
51. World Health Organization Executive Board. Report by the Secretariat: Strengthening of palliative care as a component of integrated treatment throughout the life course. Vol EB134/282013. January 23, 2014.
52. Delgado-Guay MO, Parsons HA, Li Z, Palmer LJ, Bruera E. Symptom distress, interventions, and outcomes of intensive care unit cancer patients referred to a palliative care consult team. *Cancer.* 2009;115(2):437–445.
53. Parsons HA, de la Cruz MJ, Zhukovsky DS, et al. Characteristics of patients who refuse do-not-resuscitate orders upon admission to an acute palliative care unit in a comprehensive cancer center. *Cancer.* 2010;116(12):3061–3070.
54. Educating Future Physicians in Palliative and End-of-Life Care. Facilitating advance care planning: An interprofessional educational program [Curriculum Materials]. http://market-marche.chpca.net/Educating-Future-Physicians-in-Palliative-and-End-of-Life-Care-Curriculum-Materials-and-Training-Guide. 2008.
55. Bibby R. "I hope he goes first": Exploring determinants of engagement in future planning for adults with a learning disability living with ageing parents. What are the issues? *Br J Learn Disabil.* 2013;41(2):94–105.
56. Street A, Blackford J, Threlkeld G, Bidstrup B, Downing J. *Entrust-U: Evaluative Life Review and Advance Care Planning. The Entrust-U Final Report to the Palliative Care Program of the Department of Health.* Melbourne: La Trobe University; 2011.
57. Rhee JJ, Zwar NA, Kemp LA. Advance care planning and interpersonal relationships: A two way street. *Fam Pract.* 2012;30(2):219–226.
58. Blackford J. Cultural frameworks of nursing practice: Exposing a whitecentric health care culture. *Nurs Inq.* 2003;10(4):236–244.
59. Dow LA, Matsuyama RK, Ramakrishnan V, et al. Paradoxes in advance care planning: The complex relationship of oncology patients, their physicians, and advance medical directives. *J Clin Oncol.* 2010;28(2):299–304.
60. Guo Y, Palmer JL, Bianty J, Konzen B, Shin KR, Bruera E. Advance directives and do-not-resuscitate orders in patients with cancer with metastatic spinal cord compression: Advanced care planning implications. *J Palliat Med.* 2010;13:513–517.
61. Sudore RL, Landefeld CS, Barnes DE, et al. An advance directive redesigned to meet the literacy level of most adults: A randomized trial. *Patient Educ Couns.* 2007;69(1–3):165–195.
62. DuBenske LL, Chih M-Y, Dinauer S, Gustafson DH, Cleary JF. Development and implementation of a clinician reporting system for advanced stage cancer: Initial lessons learned. *J Am Med Inform Assoc.* September 1, 2008;15(5):679–686.
63. Knauft E, Nielsen EL, Engelberg RA, Patrick DL, Curtis JR. Barriers and facilitators to end-of-life care communication for patients with COPD. *Chest.* June 2005;127(6):2188–2196.

CHAPTER 36

Palliative Care Communication and Sexuality

Les Gallo-Silver

Introduction

To be touched can communicate affection, comforting, agreement, appreciation, encouragement, and support and is one of the pleasures and blessings of the human condition.[1] Our first associations with touch begin in infancy and continue to develop as we mature. Our physical contacts with extended family and friends contribute to our touch history, which also includes our experiences with romantic and sexual relationships. Our touch histories can be complicated, but the overall importance of touch in the human experience and the benefits when a person is ill behoove healthcare professionals to emphasize the importance of touch for each patient.

Illness, whether acute or chronic, increases our needs for the physical communication of love.[2] Sexual expression in its many forms supports a patient's overall mental and physical health.[3] In this way, the touch of others is part of preserving and enhancing the quality of life for people receiving palliative care. Palliative care communication of human sexuality focuses on our need for being held, stroked, and soothed by another's touch.[4] Culture and faith-based struggles have negatively impacted the concepts of sex and sexuality, in part from the conflation of sexuality with nudity, genitals, and sexual intercourse.[5] Unfortunately, this is a very narrow and inaccurate understanding of the human need for physical closeness and the touch of others. The need to touch and be touched includes the skin covering our entire bodies, not just the genitals.[1] Physical affection, comforting, and encouragement are not erotic in nature but are sensual experiences. Eroticism includes the sexual thoughts we associate with certain sensations, while sensuality is the physical enjoyment of various forms of touch, including but not limited to the erotic.[5-7]

Freud's stages of psychosexual development have had a long-lasting influence on our culture's conceptions of human sexuality. It is important to go beyond Freud's theory based on the idea that primitive sexual drive is devoid of an interpersonal context.[8] The other person involved in the expression of sexual drives does not seem to exist in Freud's formulation. Fairburn did not agree with Freud's drive theory and based his understanding of infantile sexuality on the need for intimacy and emotional connection to another human being, providing a broader understanding of sexual development.[9,10] Viewing human sexuality as a vehicle for the physical expression of connection and closeness provides the context for palliative care communication about sexuality and the power of touch.[11]

The Touch Continuum

Touch is an integral part of caretaking and love. Touch is essential for helping an infant organize his or her budding abilities to relate to others. Infants sense the emotional state of their caregivers by the way they are held.[6,7] The Touch Continuum captures the development of the infant's body awareness[12,13] (see Figure 36.1).

While infants communicate nonverbally, their caretakers communicate verbally and nonverbally. The infant responds to vocal tone rather than to words. Instinctively caretakers hold, rock, and stroke infants to comfort them.[12-14] Holding is the infant's primary experience of touch. Touch becomes associated with communication, as the infant cries his or her request for closeness and then ceases crying when comforted. An infant's crying communicates a myriad of needs. As the caregiver attempts to interpret the infant's needs, the caregiver's soothing touch in the form of holding, rocking, and stroking comforts the infant. When the caregiver changes the infant's diaper and makes sounds to soothe the infant, the infant associates the touch with comfort. Bathing, drying, swaddling, rubbing, and tickling the infant add to the infant's touch experiences.[6] To this, the caregiver adds kissing, paying particular attention to the top of the infant's head, face, belly, and feet. These are highly sensitive body parts with multiple nerve endings and well nourished by blood vessels. The infant responds by smiling or giggling at the touch of the caregiver's hands, fingers, and lips. The caregiver enjoys the infant's response and repeats the touching that elicits the wanted response from the infant. The mutual positive reinforcement of touch cements the attachment of caregiver and child.[6,7] The intimate connection between caregiver and infant, founded on touch and response to touch, is a consistent model for intimate relationships between partners, family members, and close friends.[6,7] Touch is the physical "language" of love, affection, support, comfort, encouragement, affirmation, and validation.[6,7]

The Sensuality of Touch

Sensual feelings are a misunderstood aspect of the human condition. Sensuality is not necessarily a prelude to sexual arousal. Rather, sensual responses are a series of visceral, pleasurable, physical sensations that can involve any part of the body. Our skin is our largest organ and is highly attuned to the sensuality of touch, texture, temperature, and moisture.[1] For instance, many

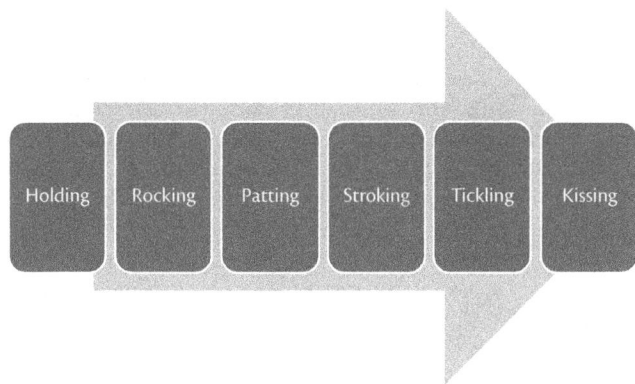

Figure 36.1 Touch Continuum.
(Based on Maltz W. *The Sexual Healing Journey: A Guide for Survivors of Sexual Abuse*. 3rd ed. New York, NY: HarperCollins; 2012; Maltz W. Healing the sexual repercussions of sexual abuse. In: Kleinplatz PJ, ed. *New Directions in Sex Therapy*. New York, NY: Routledge Taylor & Francis; 2012:267–284).

people enjoy having someone else wash their hair. One is typically not sexually interested in the hair washer, and may not even know his or her name, but may find the sensation of the water and soap massaged into the scalp a bodily sensation that frequently relaxes.[6] Our infantile response to touch and its relationship to sensuality remain with us as we develop into adults.[7] The enjoyment of hair washing and scalp massaging is an extension of our enjoyment of being bathed, dried, and swaddled. The physical communication of caring, which is inherently nonverbal, is not limited to providing personal care or assistance with activities of daily living. Typical acts of affection communicate connection and caring, long after verbal communication ceases to be effective.[15]

Example: Carlos and His Father, Tomas

Carlos, the 60-year-old son of 88-year-old Tomas, who is receiving palliative care for end-stage dementia in a nursing home, kisses his father noisily on the top of his baldhead. Tomas, who has not spoken in months, responds to his son that he no longer recognizes by saying "thank you." If we persist in conflating human sexuality with sexual intercourse, then the beauty of this emotionally moving moment between father and son is missed. For Tomas, the kiss on the bald head is an imprint from childhood, the softness of the lips, their warmth and moistness, as well as the noise of the kiss continue to have meaning for Tomas even in his much-compromised state. The sensuality of the kiss cuts through the haze of dementia. Carlos did not know if his father would respond, or if his father would become angry or frightened. Carlos did not think about it; he acted in the only way that was natural to him and to his father. His father's "thank you" became a treasured memory that is a counterpoint to the heartbreak and powerlessness experienced by families of people with dementia. Tomas died in his sleep 4 days later.

Expressive and Procedural Touch

Palliative care communication, in the context of a more expansive definition of sexuality proposed by this chapter, seeks to honor, encourage, and facilitate comforting experiences for patients and their families by using expressive touch.[16] In terms of the palliative care practitioner, touch can take two forms: procedural and expressive.[1,2] Procedural touch is part of examinations, tests, and physical examinations.[1,2] The acutely and chronically ill suffer through a myriad of tests, treatment, blood draws, and body repositioning that are so much a part of modern curative medical care. The patient's anticipation of these sensations, and their association with pain, discomfort, and related distress, may contaminate the patient's perception of another's touch. Patients may categorize all touch as procedural touch and potentially unpleasant and distressing.[6,7] Families and friends, fearful of adding to their loved ones' suffering, may hesitate to touch the patient for fear of causing additional suffering.[7] The palliative care provider, as all healthcare providers, is taught to touch patients when necessary and in ways that do not stimulate the patient. Distracting the patient with unrelated conversation and ignoring any sign of the patient's enjoyment of the process are some of the skills of managing the potential stimulation of touch. The palliative care provider teaches the same management skills to partner/caregivers when teaching them how to bathe, dress, change, or catheterize their loved one using procedural touch.[6,7,16–18] Partners, family members, and friends may eliminate expressive touch without specific permission and instruction from the patient's healthcare team.[6,7,19]

Expressive touch in palliative care communicates concern and affection but most importantly communicates respect and recognition of the patient's humanity. This type of nonverbal communication is more effective if the palliative care provider is eye level with the patient. Standing over the patient's bed or wheelchair creates social distance by emphasizing the power differential that is typical of relationships in healthcare.[6,7,16] While there are wide cultural variations in permissible touch, for the most part it is acceptable to create an empathic environment by touching the patient's bed or wheelchair with permission.[1,2,16] In situations where there is a more established, long-term relationship with the patient, touching the patient's hand or lower arm establishes a powerful empathic connection.[1,2,16]

Example: Keisha and Her Mother, Odette

Odette receives hospice care for her progressive post-polio syndrome. She is now bedbound and living with her daughter, Keisha. Odette's hospice nurse instructs Keisha on how to change her mother's bed sheets. The nurse uses procedural touch to help Odette reposition herself during the process. She also uses expressive touch, reassuring Odette with comforting pats on her hands and touching her shoulder, as the bed sheet changing process causes Odette considerable anxiety and discomfort. The nurse models the way Keisha can change the sheets in a professional way but also encourages her to use touch to communicate love and caring. The nurse gives Keisha permission to kiss her mother's hands as she grips the bedrails during the process.

Without this type of encouragement, caregivers learn the correct care procedures, safety, and sterile techniques, yet patients, family, and especially partners can experience mounting disconnection and isolation.[20,21] Couples often grieve the loss of connection, spontaneity, fun, and reciprocity of their pre-illness relationship.[22,23]

Example: Alexi and His Wife, Sonia, Part 1

Alexi and Sonia survived a horrific car accident. Alexi's injuries healed. Sonia, paralyzed from the chest down, learned various skills in acute rehabilitation. The inpatient rehabilitation program taught Alexi, her husband of 35 years, how to catheterize her so she could urinate. Sonia told her occupational therapist: "It used to be when he touched me there, he would stroke it and kiss it; now he is a plumber, and I am just a clogged sewer system." Using procedural touch, Alexi followed the instructions and accomplished this important task with the same efficiency as Sonia's nurses. Alexi is not Sonia's nurse, but the man that used to enjoy making love to Sonia.

Increasingly, the jobs of family members and friends include helping with daily living activities, personal care, feeding-tube management, suctioning, nebulizer treatments, ordering durable medical equipment, and wound care, among other responsibilities. Nurses and other healthcare providers teach family and friends to accomplish these tasks safely and effectively, using the correct techniques for more complex care plans. Palliative care providers teach these activities preserving professional boundaries with patients using procedural touch. Yet Sonia and Alexi's relationship is not that of patient and nurse. Is there a way for Alexi to catheterize his wife in a way that better reflects the nature of their relationship? Can it be more loving, romantic, and sensual and still use sterile technique? The answers to these questions are yes, by using the concept of expressive touch that recognizes their relationship as inclusive of love, romance, and sex.[24] Communicating sexuality through touch enables the discussion and exploration of these issues. While there are always concerns about the need for training in human sexuality, respecting patient's privacy, and maintaining appropriate boundaries, many times a palliative care provider's professional discomfort with the issues of physical intimacy may cause him or her to avoid addressing them.[23,25–27]

Example: Alexi and His Wife, Sonia, Part 2

Sonia needed reassurance from her husband that she was attractive and that helping her urinate did not disgust him. A psychologist's intervention at the acute rehabilitation center helped Sonia discuss her concerns and fears with her husband. The psychologist sat with her hand on the bed rail and leaned slightly forward, diminishing the space between their faces appropriate for people having a private conversation. When Sonia cried about her loneliness, the psychologist gently touched Sonia's shoulder, and Sonia put her hand over hers. The psychologist asked Sonia if there was a way Alexi could comfort her as well. Through her tears, Sonia shared how much she enjoyed it when Alexi used to kiss her neck.

In response to the psychologist's intervention, Sonia and Alexi developed a new first step to catheterizing her that was not part of his original instruction: Alexi kissed his wife's neck and fondled her earlobes. The simple act of expressive touch (nonverbal communication) facilitated Sonia's realization that she became sexually aroused when Alexi catheterized her. Her physiatrist reassured Sonia that this was normal and suggested she share this with her husband. Sonia's occupational therapist suggested she obtain a leather-bolstered wedge pillow designed to help a woman with spinal cord injury get into a safe position for vaginal intercourse.

Assessment of the Patient's Touch Experiences

The foundation of human sexuality is touch, and therefore the element of a previously sexual relationship requires assessment and intervention before a palliative patient and partner restore sexual intimacy to their relationship.[28] The most commonly used assessment tool in this area is Ex-PLISSIT.[19] The Ex stands for the extended version of this model of practice over several meetings with a patient and her or his partner. The P is for giving permission for discussion of the topic of sexuality. This is a proactive stance for any healthcare professional, instead of putting the burden of raising the topic of sexuality on the patient.[6,7,19,28] LI stands for providing some information of how the patient's specific condition may affect sexual functioning. Limiting information to the central facts is less overwhelming to patients and partners.[19,28] SS addresses the need to make some basic suggestions about addressing changes in sexual functioning, and IT encompasses referring the couple to a specialist in the field of sexual rehabilitation.[19]

Although Ex-PLISSIT offers an assessment of touch as sexual communication, this does not always match the patient's medical and health realities or personal interests. This chapter's expanded definition of sexuality includes all forms of pleasurable touch whether or not erotic in nature. Fatigue, pain, unstable heart functioning, shortness of breath, low white counts, low platelets, and any number of physical obstacles may render sexual activity a long-term, rather than a short-term, goal or may not be a realistic goal at all. Therefore, prior to the use of Ex-PLISSIT, attention must first be made to expressive touch as a form of nonverbal communication. The TOUCH intervention and assessment tool can serve as the primary intervention for palliative care patients (see Box 36.1).

T: *Taking* a history is the natural first step of any assessment and intervention. A typical level and type of pre-illness touch accompanies the nature of the patient's relationship with the primary caregiver. This is the touch "baseline" for this relationship and gives the healthcare provider the type of information needed to assess the physical affection and comforting changes in the relationship.

O: As some patients' histories reveal, not all touch experiences are positive. In addition, medical issues make certain areas of the body off limits to touch because of pain and/or unpleasant sensitivity. Body mapping enables the healthcare provider to *organize* the patient's touch responses as positive, negative, or neutral.[12,13]

Box 36.1 TOUCH Assessment and Intervention Tool for Communication About Sexuality

- Take a history of touch and its place within the relationships with caregivers
- Organize touch responses using body mapping to help the patient identify where he or she likes and does not like to be touched
- Unify physical touch with emotional feelings and the resulting connection with another person
- Co-create, with patient, partner or loved one, and the professional, opportunities for the patient to be touched by the partner or loved one
- Honor, with patient, partner or loved one, and the professional, the effort and risk-taking required by the patient/partner or loved one to reinvest in and make gains with touch

U: Touch without emotional intent is easily misunderstood and misperceived, as is the withdrawal of touch. *Unifying* the touch's emotional intent with the accompanying physical sensation enables the patient and caregiver to communicate clearly and mutually benefit from touch.

C: Healthcare providers, patients, and caregivers *co-create* positive touch opportunities and practices based on the pre-illness natural rhythms of physical affection and support.[6,12,13]

H: It often causes anxiety to stretch one's self emotionally and physically while also feeling ill. Likewise, caregivers are often fearful and reluctant to make any demands on an ill loved one. Healthcare providers *honor* this difficult process through normalization and praise.[6,7]

The following extensive case study demonstrates the use of the TOUCH assessment as an interdisciplinary tool. Team meetings enable palliative care practitioners to share information and contribute their specialized skills to the patient, thereby facilitating use of the TOUCH assessment tool.[11,23,27]

Example: Mary-Ellen and Her Husband, Gavin

Gavin, at 57 years old, struggled with progressive congestive heart failure (CHF) and chronic pulmonary obstructive disease (COPD) and required increasing amounts of oxygen support. Mary-Ellen, his wife of 30 years, no longer slept in the same bed as Gavin; he slept in a reclining chair in the living room. Multiple visits to the emergency room, bouts of pneumonia, and the painful water retention in her husband's feet and ankles left Mary-Ellen emotionally exhausted. The visiting nurse noticed they both were irritable with each other. He asked them to describe their relationship before the CHF and COPD symptoms worsened. Mary-Ellen described Gavin as playful and affectionate. Gavin described Mary-Ellen as ticklish and a "good kisser." Clearly, the physical communication between them deteriorated in direct relationship with the disease progression.

The visiting nurse asked if she could see the couple's photo album, which had many playful and "goofy" pictures of the couple.[6,7,12,13] The nurse was able to point out the couple's physicality and wondered if they missed this part of their relationship. The touch assessment (T) continued with the couple's description of the changes in their relationship. The couple explained that many of their arguments often focused on her tending to the skin breakdown on his feet. Gavin disclosed to his nurse that when he was an altar boy, the parish priest would masturbate by rubbing against Gavin's feet. Mary-Ellen's putting the antibacterial salve on his feet reminded him of the abuse. The nurse used body mapping to help Gavin organize (O) his responses to touch.[12,13] The nurse drew a simple stick figure and asked Gavin where he liked being touched. Gavin pointed to his shoulders. He explained they always felt sore and tense. He indicated he wanted this area massaged but felt unable to request this of Mary-Ellen because he felt "ugly and useless."

Mary-Ellen told the social worker that Gavin did not appreciate all she did for him and treated her "like a servant." She missed how Gavin used sneak-up on her to touch her breasts. To her, this was a sign Gavin loved her and found her attractive. Gavin, though, told the hospice social worker he perceived the same touch as a prelude to making love and certainly was not mobile enough to sneak up on her. As he felt incapable of this type of sexual activity, he withdrew from physical displays of affection.[6,7] He did not want Mary-Ellen "to get the wrong idea"; he failed to realize that he was sending a message that he did not love her anymore. Gavin and Mary-Ellen's pre-illness physical affection was playful and comforting. The social worker suggested that Gavin and Mary-Ellen discuss this exact issue with her assistance. The social worker encouraged and facilitated the couple's sharing of their thoughts and feelings about their relationship. Gavin disclosed his sexual abuse for the first time. Mary-Ellen's response was tearful and loving. The social worker validated and praised Gavin's brave disclosure and Mary-Ellen's empathic response.[6,7] The social worker asked Gavin if Mary-Ellen could touch one of his feet. He placed a foot in her lap. Mary-Ellen continued to weep while caressing her husband's foot. In this way Mary-Ellen's emotion unified (U) with her loving touch helped Gavin reinterpret the sensations he felt.[6,7,12,13]

The occupational therapist suggested that the couple "practice" being affectionate when Mary-Ellen helped Gavin bathe, co-creating (C) a positive touch opportunity.[6,7,12,13] She indicated that if Gavin kept his hands below his shoulders, he would use less energy than if he reached up for Mary-Ellen, while he sat on the shower chair. It was Mary-Ellen's idea to bathe Gavin while she was topless. Although shocked, Gavin soon enjoyed touching his wife's breasts while being bathed. The couple resumed kissing, and Mary-Ellen enjoyed the pleasure Gavin felt when she massaged his shoulders and neck.

The nurse, social worker, and occupational therapist all provided the couple with positive reinforcement and affirmed their progress, which honored (H) their efforts as a couple. Gavin's nurse using the Ex-PLISSIT intervention process helped the couple meet with an occupational therapist that specialized in sexual issues. The occupational therapist, at the couple's request, helped the couple learn how to accomplish and enjoy mutual masturbation. Following her husband's death, Mary-Ellen told the team that their "special help" allowed her to feel closer and more loved by her husband. Even in her grief, Mary-Ellen was able to picture with a smile Gavin's face when she first bathed him topless.

The TOUCH intervention teaches that it is not sufficient to merely accept or assume patient sexuality within the palliative care treatment plan. Rather, healthcare providers need to suggest opportunities for patients and their partners to enjoy affectionate, romantic, and erotic touch as well as affectionate, comforting, and encouraging touch with other family members and friends. Encouraging the patient's loved ones to touch the patient begins with giving them positive reinforcement when observing touch between them.[29]

Example: Tina and Her Grandmother, Sarah

Sarah's amyotrophic lateral sclerosis (ALS) progressed to the point where she had to suction out her saliva from her mouth on a frequent basis. She retained full mobility of her arms and hands, so the mechanics of self-suctioning were not difficult for her. Yet, suctioning in front of her family repulsed her, and she feared it disgusted her family. The special ALS nurse visited Sarah weekly. One day when the nurse visited, Sarah's 5-year-old granddaughter, Tina, was visiting her as well. The little girl watched with great interest as her grandmother suctioned herself. She told Tina, "Don't watch me when I do this; it is disgusting to watch." Tina took her hand and lovingly kissed it. The nurse commented, "She loves you, and she doesn't care about the suctioning." Sarah, with tears in her eyes, asked Tina, "You love Grandma?" Tina replied, "And I love Grandma's mouth vacuum cleaner!" The nurse laughed and added, "I love her mouth vacuum too." From then on, Tina kissed her grandmother whenever she saw her suctioning. They made it a game and counted the number of kisses each visit.

Unlearning Negative Touch Associations

Some patients experience arduous aggressive medical care that ultimately cures the underlying illness but leaves them struggling with numerous health problems caused by the treatment's side effects. While palliative care improves the patient's quality of life by managing his or her physical symptoms, the vicissitudes of procedural touch require specific intervention as well.[6,7,30] These interventions use behavioral techniques to help patients acclimate to expressive touch.[1,2,16] For instance, finger writing involves "writing" a word on the patient's hand or arm with a fingertip as the patient looks away, with the goal of the patient guessing the word based on the sensation. This requires the patient to concentrate on the sensations to determine the letters of the word.[6,7,12,13]

Example: Rafaela and Her Wife, Louisa

Louisa's first treatment for leukemia was not successful. At 60 years of age, Louisa required a bone marrow transplant, and her closest match was her adult son. The transplant experience was long and difficult for Louisa but her wife, Rafaela, was always there caring for and supporting her. Going home cancer-free was a "dream come true" for the whole family, but mounting graft-versus-host disease (GVHD) symptoms indicated her body was rejecting the transplanted cells. GVHD soon made Louise's posttransplant life a "nightmare." Louise's skin deteriorated due to GVHD, and she did not want anyone, especially Rafaela, to touch her. Her skin problems, which once covered almost 50% of her body, slowly resolved with treatment, but her reluctance to be touched remained. Rafaela presented as increasingly sad and withdrawn during her wife's outpatient appointments. The nurse practitioner met with the couple and learned of their physical relationship deterioration. The nurse suggested that the couple practice a touch exercise called "finger writing" on the palm of Louisa's hand and provided them with simple instructions. The couple enjoyed the game and experimented with finger writing on other parts of the body. Six months later, Louisa reported that she and Rafaela were sexually active. Rafaela described feeling more normal, as she was a "real wife" again.

Using the Ex-PLISSIT process, the nurse made a referral to a sex therapist who gave the couple specialized help to reawaken sexual responsiveness for both women by adding a variety of sex toys.[6,7,19] While Louisa needed to become reacquainted with her body following her lengthy illness, likewise, Rafaela needed to address her feelings of "being rusty" after the long absence of their sexual relationship. From this point, they were able to sexually experiment with how to give each other pleasure while protecting Louisa's still fragile health. Ultimately, Rafaela and Louisa united their affection, need, and desire for each other in ways more satisfying than before Louisa's illness.

Professional Barriers and Obstacles

Sadly, there are continued and consistent professional barriers to addressing patient sexuality and communicating about touch in healthcare and homecare settings. Anecdotally, the most frequently cited barriers and obstacles include a lack of specific training and the fear of being inappropriate by being the first to raise sexuality issues with patients.[3,27,28,31,32] Healthcare providers across a variety of disciplines persist in requiring patients to raise the issue of sexuality first before addressing it at all.[33-36] The healthcare provider, who waits for the patient or family member's questions on sex, communicates that sex is not an appropriate discussion topic and is unrelated to their healthcare.[28,31,32]

Despite the perceived awkwardness and in appropriateness of communicating about sexuality with patients, healthcare providers report that they desire additional training in this area.[31-36] At times, a specific provider within the healthcare team helps patients with sexuality issues, presenting team members the opportunity to make direct referrals. In other instances, there is a trained rehabilitation counselor in the community.[6,7,19] Patients benefit from the availability of specially trained human sexuality and sexual rehabilitation professionals.[37] Nonetheless, the multidisciplinary team, as first-line palliative care providers, remains professionally responsible for proactively addressing sexuality and communicating about touch as an integrated part of the patient's life.[21-23,27] To begin this process, a palliative care provider may decide to practice with a patient age group and or gender with which they feel most comfortable.[21-23,27] The strength of interdisciplinary practice is that team members may have a comfort level with different patient populations. The entire team can practice using simulated patients and a variety of typical scenarios that involve discussions of sexuality.[21,27,37-40] Palliative care providers can use any of the case examples in this chapter as the basis for scenarios with simulated patients.

Sex Affirmative Healthcare Environments

Skilled nursing facilities, residential hospice programs, subacute care units, and acute rehabilitation programs may have patients living in them for several weeks to months or longer. Most institutions did not consider the sexual needs of residents in their design plans.[38] Rooms are gender segregated except for married couples who require the same level of care. In addition, all patients are deemed heterosexual unless they self-identify otherwise.[7] Establishing a sex-affirmative environment within healthcare is the result of the multidisciplinary teams' acceptance of sexuality as typical part of the patient's normal daily activities.[7,38,42] Sexual expression requires privacy, and such privacy must be made available to patients in medical, nursing, and rehabilitative environments.[7]

Example: Vimesh and His Partner, Rama

Vimesh visited his partner Rama in the subacute nursing facility, where he had lived since his stroke. Both in their 70s and separated from their wives, who lived in India, they had been lovers for 40 years. For the first time since meeting each other, they slept in separate beds, in separate rooms, and in separate buildings. Because Rama was aphasic, could no longer speak, and was paralyzed to an extent preventing him from using the call bell, he was placed in a room closest to the nursing station. The multidisciplinary staff was accustomed to checking in on Rama if he was not sitting in a special wheelchair outside of his room. In the afternoons, on more than one occasion, staff found Vimesh in bed with Rama. Vimesh would be asleep, snoring, and spooning Rama under the covers. Rama would be awake with a lopsided smile on his face. Finally, the nursing home closed Rama's door with his permission when Vimesh visited. The nurse manager told Rama that the staff wanted to give him and Vimesh the privacy they "deserved." A simple and respectful solution gave the couple the privacy without putting Rama at increased risk but improving his quality of his life.

Conclusion

Sexuality is an essential element of the human experience. It is part of a continuum of the human need for contact, connection, and love. There is a primitive drive for sexual release, as well as a primitive need to connect to another person emotionally and physically through touch. The TOUCH assessment and intervention tool offers a method for palliative care professionals to communicate about patients' and their partners' sexual needs. However, the TOUCH tool requires additional qualitative research to determine its effectiveness in palliative care settings. Some patients receiving palliative care may want to retain the erotic elements of their relationships. Others may want to focus more on their needs for affection and physical comforting through expressive touch. Palliative care communication on the issue of sexuality encompasses the entire variety of sensual experiences that help patients retain feelings of acceptance, respect, belonging, and desirability. Maximizing the ability to communicate love and to accept the love of others prevents loneliness and isolation.[42]

References

1. Elkiss ML, Jerome JA. Touch—more than basic science. *J Am Osteopath Assoc*. 2012;112(8):512–517.
2. Cocksedge S, George B, Renwick S, Chew-Graham CA. Touch in primary care consultations: Qualitative investigation of doctors' and patients' perceptions. *Br J Gen Pract*. 2013;63(609):283–290.
3. Cagle JG, Bolte S. Sexuality and life-threatening illness: Implications for social work and palliative care. *Health Soc Work*. 2009;34(3):223–232.
4. Woodhouse J, Baldwin M.A. Dealing sensitively with sexuality in a palliative care context. *Br J Community Nurs*. 2008;13(3):20–25.
5. Nyatanga B. Sexuality in palliative care: More than sex. *Br J Community Nurs. Nursing*, 2014;19(3):151.
6. Gallo-Silver L. Sexuality, sensuality, and intimacy in palliative care. In: Altilio S, Otis-Green S, eds. *Oxford Textbook of Palliative Social Work*. New York, NY; Oxford University Press; 2011:261–270.
7. Gallo-Silver L, Bimbi DS. Human sexual health. In Gehlert S, Browne TA, eds. *Handbook of Health Social Work*. 2nd ed. Hoboken, NJ: John Wiley; 2012:343–370.
8. Freud S. *Beyond the Pleasure Principle*. London: International Psycho-Analytic Press; 1922.
9. Fairbairn WRD. Object relations and dynamic structure. *Int J Psycho-Anal*. 1946;27(1–2):429–440.
10. Fairbairn WRD. *Psychological Studies of the Personality*. London: Routledge & Kegan Paul; 1952.
11. Steinke EE. Sexuality and chronic illness. *J Gerontol Nurs*. 2013;39(11):18–27.
12. Maltz W. *The Sexual Healing Journey: A Guide for Survivors of Sexual Abuse*. 3rd ed. New York, NY: HarperCollins; 2012.
13. Maltz W. Healing the sexual repercussions of sexual abuse. In Kleinplatz PJ, ed. *New Directions in Sex Therapy*. New York, NY: Routledge Taylor & Francis Group; 2012:267–284.
14. Mlodinow L. *Subliminal: How Your Unconscious Mind Rules Your Behavior*. New York, NY: Pantheon Books; 2012.
15. Silverman M. Sighs, smiles, and worried glances: How the body reveals women caregivers' lived experiences of care to older adults. *J Aging Stud*. 2013;27(3):288–297.
16. Connor A, Howett MA. Conceptual model of intentional touch. *J Holist Nurs*. 2009;27(2):127–135.
17. Kaufman M, Silverberg C, Odette F. *The Ultimate Guide to Sex and Disability*. San Francisco, CA: Cleis Press; 2007.
18. McRuer R, Mollow A. *Sex and Disability*. Durham, NC: Duke University Press; 2012.
19. Taylor B, Davies S. Using the Extended PLISSIT model to address sexual healthcare needs. *Nurs Stand*. 2006;21(11):35–40.
20. Pilon N, Bouti C, Bouffart L, Mallet D. [Sexuality between couples in palliative care, from taboo to the possible]. *Soins*. 2012;762:22–25.
21. Verschuren JE, Zhdanova MA, Geertzen JH, Enzlin P, Dijkstra PU, Dekker R. Let's talk about sex: Lower limb amputation, sexual functioning and sexual well-being: A qualitative study of the partner's perspective. *J Clin Nurs*. 2013;22(23):3557–3567.
22. Taylor B. Experiences of sexuality and intimacy in terminal illness: A phenomenological study. *Palliat Med*. 2014;28(5):438–447.
23. Blagbrough J. Importance of sexual needs assessment in palliative care. *Nurs Stand*. 2010;24(52):35–39.
24. Bach LE, Motimer JA, VandeWeerd C, Corvin J. The association of physical and mental health with sexual activity in older adults in a retirement community. *J Sex Med*. 2013;10(11):2671–2673.
25. Horden AJ, Street AF. Let's talk about sex: Risky business for cancer and palliative care clinicians. *Contemp Nurse*. 2007;27(1):49–60.
26. Nyatanga B. From bowel habits to sexuality: The taboos of caring in palliative care. *Br J Community Nurs*. 2012;17(5):210–211.
27. de Vocht H, Horden A, Notter J, van de Wiel H. Stepped Skills: A team approach towards communication about sexuality and intimacy in cancer and palliative care. *Australas Med J*. 2011;4(11):610–619.
28. Sargent NN, Smallwood N, Finlay F. Sexual history taking: A dying skill? *J Palliat Med*. 2014;17(7): 829–831.
29. Dune T.M. Sexuality and physical disability: Exploring the barriers and solutions in healthcare. *Sex Disabil*. 2008;26(4):1–9.
30. Kedde H, Van De Wiel HBM, Weijmar Schultz WCM, Vanwesenbeek WMA, Bender JL. Efficacy of sexological healthcare for people with chronic diseases and physical disabilities. *J Sex Marit Ther*. 2010;36:282–294.
31. Saunamaki N, Engstrom M. Registered nurses' reflections on discussing sexuality with patients: Responsibilities, doubts and fears. *J Clin Nurs*. 2014;23(3–4):531–540.
32. Fitch M.I, Beaudoin G, Johnson B. Challenges having conversations about sexuality in ambulatory settings: Part II—health care provider perspectives. *Can Oncol Nurs J*. 2013;23(3):182–196.
33. McGrath M, Lynch E. Occupational therapist' perspectives on addressing sexual concerns of older adults in the context of rehabilitation. *Disabil Rehabil*. 2014;36(8):651–657.
34. Helland Y, Garratt A, Kjeker I, Kvien TK, Dagfinrud H. Current practice and barriers to the management of sexual issues in rheumatology: Results of a survey of health professionals. *Scand J Rheumatol*. 2013;42(1):20–26.
35. Sobecki JN, Curlin FA, Rasinski KA, Lindau ST. What we don't talk about when we don't talk about sex: Results of a national survey of U.S. obstetrician/gynecologists. *J. Sex Med*. 2012;9(5):1285–1294.
36. Rosenbaum T, Vadas D, Kalichman L. Sexual function in post-stroke patients: Considerations for rehabilitation. *J Sex Med*. 2014;11(1):15–21.
37. Hattjar B, ed. *Sexuality and Occupational Therapy*. Bethesda, MD: American Occupational Therapy Association; 2012.
38. Chan ZC. A qualitative study on non-verbal sensitivity in nursing students. *J Clin Nurs*. 2013;22(13–14):1941–1950.

39. Sleeper J.A, Thompson C. The use of high fidelity simulation to enhance nursing students' therapeutic communication skills. *Int J Nurs Edu Scholarsh*. 2008;5(1):1–12.
40. Nehring W, Lashley F. *High Fidelity Patient Simulation in Nursing Education*. Sudbury, MA: Jones and Bartlett; 2010.
41. Rosenberg S, Gallo-Silver L. Therapeutic communication skills and student nurses in the clinical setting. *Teach Learn Nurs*. 2011;6(1):2–8.
42. Appel JM. Sex rights for the disabled. *J Med Ethics*. 2010;36(3):152–154.

CHAPTER 37

Spiritual Communication

Shane Sinclair

Introduction

Communicating about spiritual issues is both a unique aim and a challenge of palliative care. Addressing spiritual issues is identified as a core component of both the World Health Organization's definition of palliative care[1] and the National Consensus Project for Quality Palliative Care.[2] The centrality of spiritual care to palliative care was so vital that Cicely Saunders, the founder of the modern hospice and palliative care movement, suggested that one way to measure the quality of end-of-life care was the degree to which spiritual care was being practiced.[3] While the spiritual care imperative is advocated by policymakers and healthcare providers alike, the greatest advocates for addressing spiritual needs at the end of life are patients themselves, who consistently identify their spiritual needs as an integral yet underaddressed aspect of palliative care.[4] While the importance of addressing spiritual needs at the end of life is extolled, implementing theory and a growing evidence base into clinical practice remains a persistent challenge. In this chapter the importance of communicating with patients and their family members about spiritual issues is discussed, providing the foundation for a clinical framework to assist in addressing this essential domain of comprehensive palliative care.

Conceptualizing Spirituality

Defining Spirituality

A fundamental and persistent challenge in communicating with patients about their spiritual needs is the lack of specificity surrounding the concept of spirituality and its relationship with religion. The lack of specificity is evident in a recent review of the palliative care literature that identified 92 definitions of spirituality,[5] within a field of inquiry that has emerged from relative obscurity to a burgeoning field of research over the past 30 years.[6] Within palliative care, spirituality is conceived as a universal domain of human health that is informed by and expressed through both secular and religious means. While a universal approach has been criticized as "generic,"[7] it embodies a person-centered approach that recognizes both the diverse patient populations healthcare providers serve and an underlying assumption that the search for meaning and purpose traverses and transcends religion, culture, and humanity. The need for a shared vocabulary to better address these conceptual issues has been recognized[8] and recently resulted in the formulation of consensus definitions of spirituality, based on the expert opinion of leaders from diverse spiritual, religious, and cultural backgrounds.[9-11] The culmination of this work resulted in the following interdisciplinary global consensus definition of spirituality:

> Spirituality is a dynamic and intrinsic aspect of humanity through which persons seek ultimate meaning, purpose, and transcendence, and experience relationship to self, family, others, community, society, nature, and the significant or sacred. Spirituality is expressed through beliefs, values, traditions, and practices.[9(p5)]

While representing a broad conceptualization of spirituality, this consensus definition acknowledges that the form and content of a patient's spirituality may vary significantly from patient to patient. For the purposes of this chapter, spirituality is defined as "an individual's beliefs, values, behaviors, and experiences related to ultimate meaning."[12(p260)]

The Relationship Between Spirituality and Religion

While most scholars recognize spirituality and religion as distinct yet interrelated concepts,[6] the nature of their relationship is an additional source of debate among patients and scholars alike. For many patients and the majority of healthcare researchers, religion is subsumed under the broad and more inclusive rubric of spirituality, whereas for some patients and scholars, spirituality is subsumed under the construct of religion. On the one hand, spirituality is inextricably linked to religion, resulting in spirituality being defined as a "conversation between the classics of various religious traditions and contemporary human experience."[13(p90)] In contrast, the view espoused by many healthcare researchers conceptualizes spirituality as an overarching construct, conceiving "religion as codified, institutionalized, and a relatively narrow expression of spirituality."[14(p135)]

These contrasting and often dichotomous perspectives have unfortunately led to a disparaging debate whereby religion has been dismissed by many healthcare researchers as a human construct, archaic and disappearing from Western society,[15,16] causing some religious studies scholars to suggest that "'religion is alternatively demonized and dismissed in favour of 'spirituality' within the hospice literature.'"[17(p13)] While recognizing that for many patients spirituality and religion are interrelated terms, increasingly patients and the general public identify themselves primarily with spirituality, with religion taking an important but secondary role.[18-22] For the purposes of this chapter, religion is defined as "an individual's beliefs, values, behaviors, and experiences related to ultimate meaning, often involving deities and dogma, formulated by faith groups or institutions over time."[12(p260)]

Distinguishing and subsuming religion under the broad rubric of spirituality is supported by survey data and clinical evidence that demonstrates that individuals, whether their spirituality is expressed through religious or more secular means, increasingly identify spirituality as an overarching universal construct that includes religious and nonreligious forms.[15] As Sulmasy summates, "While not everyone has a religion, spiritual issues, in this wider sense, arise for almost all dying persons."[23(p1386)] While the number of individuals identifying no religious affiliation has increased marginally over the past 25 years in both Canada (12% to 17%)[21] and the United States (7% to 14%),[24] when religious affiliation is combined with other factors of religiosity (attendance, importance, and personal practice) there is an apparent shift from a primarily religious orientation to a spiritual orientation across contemporary society. A US Gallup survey, for example, indicated that only 13% of Americans strongly endorsed all nine items of a spiritual commitment scale; however, 47% considered themselves to be spiritually commited.[25] These results are similar in Canada, where a national survey reported that 78% of Canadians believed that God or a Higher Power exists,[20] despite only 29% of the population being characterized as highly religious.[21] The broad identification with the term "spirituality" has even been reported among atheists—25% of whom acknowledge having spiritual needs.[20]

In hindsight it seems that Karl Rahner's prediction 50 years ago that "the committed believer of tomorrow will be either a 'mystic'—someone who has 'experienced' something—or will not exist anymore,"[26(p15)] served as a clarion call that has come to fruition within contemporary Western society. Individual spirituality remains strong, despite a gradual decline in religiosity. Clinical research identifies a similar trend toward a universal conceptualization of spirituality that is inclusive of religious and more secular forms. Astrow and colleagues conducted a modest (n = 369) US-based study of cancer patients and found that while 94% of the sample reported a religious affiliation, 66% identified themselves as spiritual but not religious.[27] A separate study of advanced cancer patients reported a similar trend, as 56% of patients identified themselves as moderately or highly religious, while 72% considered themselves to be moderately or highly spiritual.[28] Healthcare providers communicating with patients about spiritual issues at the end of life are therefore encouraged to adopt a broad and inclusive person-centered approach to spiritual discussions, an approach that honors and reflects the deeply personal, dynamic, and eclectic understandings and experiences of spirituality at the end of life.

Patients' Perspectives on Addressing Spiritual Needs

While conceptualizing spirituality is an ongoing challenge for healthcare providers and researchers alike, the importance that patients and their family members attribute to addressing spiritual needs is unequivocally endorsed.[23,29,30] A Canadian study (n = 361) identifying patient priorities for end-of-life care identified the need for improved spiritual support as one of its highest priorities.[31] In a separate study,[32] Heyland reported that 70% of patients considered having their spiritual and religious needs met an important component of comprehensive end-of-life care. Still, when other interrelated study items were taken into consideration—such as receiving healthcare that is respectful and compassionate, being treated in a manner that preserves dignity, and having an opportunity to discuss fears of dying—the salience of spirituality to communication at the end of life becomes more apparent. In the United States, similar results have been reported, as 78% of advanced patients stated that religion and/or spirituality had been an important component of their cancer experience.[28] When compared with other dimensions of quality of life as measured by the McGill Quality of Life Questionnaire, spiritual issues are consistently ranked as being as important, and in some instances more important, than other domains of quality of life.[33] Likewise in a US study of palliative care patients (n = 332), patients ranked coming to peace with God and pain control as the most important items among 44 factors of quality end-of-life care.[34] While addressing spiritual needs are particularly important at the end of life, US survey data indicates that the majority of nonpalliative patients also desire their healthcare provider to inquire about their spiritual needs.[23,25]

Sadly, there is discordance related to the perceived importance of addressing spiritual needs by patients and their healthcare providers. While 92% of palliative patients identified "being at peace with God" as a very important factor in their end-of-life care, only 65% of palliative care physicians considered this to be a very important factor.[34] Similar results were reported in a study on the benefits of addressing spirituality at the end of life among advanced cancer patients (n = 75) and oncologists and oncology nurses (n = 339).[35] While the majority of patients, physicians, and nurses felt that routine spiritual care was at least slightly beneficial to patients, only 25% of patient participants reported ever receiving spiritual care during their illness trajectory. Balboni et al. reported a similar trend, as 72% of advanced cancer patients felt that their spiritual needs were minimally or not at all supported by the healthcare system.[36] A similar disparity between patient needs and healthcare providers' abilities to assess spiritual care needs was reported in a study of cancer outpatients where the majority of patients felt that it was appropriate for physicians to communicate with them about their spiritual needs, yet only 18% reported that these needs were met, with only 6% recalling a single instance, across their entire cancer trajectory, in which a staff member had inquired about their spiritual needs.[27] In a separate study, while oncologists and oncology nurses felt responsible for addressing spiritual issues, the importance of addressing spiritual concerns was ranked considerably lower by participants in comparison to addressing other psychosocial issues.[37] Patients and healthcare providers agree that communicating about spiritual issues is a vital component of quality palliative care; however, there is a significant gap between theory and practice, as healthcare providers lack the necessary communication tools to effectively address this vital domain.

The Impact of Addressing Spiritual Issues

A growing evidence base suggests that addressing spiritual needs has serious ramifications beyond simply the patient experience.[38] In a study at a large Canadian cancer center, patients identified prayer as both the single most utilized and the most effective coping strategy in their cancer experience.[39] Similar findings have been reported in US studies where 74% of patients reported that religion and spirituality played a central role in their ability to cope with cancer and 56% of families identified religion as the most important factor in helping them cope with their loved one's illness.[40] While spirituality provides patients and families with an important resource in coping with end-of-life distress, spirituality has also been shown to have an important modifying effect on many prominent and problematic issues at the end of life.

Spiritual well-being ameliorates pain,[41] anxiety,[42] depression,[42,43] and desire for a hastened death[44–46] and also enhances dignity[47] and quality of life.[48] Research has shown a significant negative correlation between spiritual well-being and a desire for hastened death, hopelessness, and suicidal ideation.[49] In the state of Oregon, where physician-assisted suicide has been legal for more than 15 years, patients who have exercised this right have done so for largely spiritual and/or existential reasons. Patients identified loss of autonomy, loss of dignity, and inability to participate in activities that make life enjoyable as the most prominent reasons for choosing to end their life through physician-assisted suicide.[45,50] While spiritual well-being is a complex and multifaceted construct that is influenced by other factors beyond clinical communication, failing to communicate with patients about their spiritual needs has also been shown to have a significant negative impact on ratings of satisfaction with care,[27] increased preferences for aggressive treatments at the end of life,[36] and increased healthcare costs at the end of life.[51]

What Do Patients Want?

A significant issue pertaining to spiritual communication with patients and families is the ephemeral nature of spiritual needs and the lack of clinical guidance provided to healthcare providers on how to effectively address and assess spiritual concerns. A lack of formal training in spiritual care has been identified by healthcare providers as the primary barrier to spiritual communication.[52] Spiritual needs by their very nature are complex, multifaceted, ill-defined, and typically evade a script-based approach, having a more narrative tone that often challenges the clinical acumen of the traditional biomedical model. Patients spiritual needs include overcoming fears, finding hope, discovering meaning in life, and a desire to talk to someone about finding peace, meaning in life, and death and dying.[53] In a separate study investigating the spiritual concerns of cancer patients, the most common spiritual struggles included wondering why God allowed illness to occur and questioning abandonment from God. Still, patients reported that they sought a closer connection to God and reflected on the meaning of life.[48]

Research shows that spiritual distress is a prevalent issue among palliative care patients,[54,55] raising a number of clinical questions: How do healthcare providers engage in spiritual communication? How is spiritual distress similar or different from psychosocial distress? How can healthcare providers help patients and families in their search for meaning? Which member of the palliative care team is best suited to address spiritual needs and deliver the spiritual care plan? Finally, how do palliative care team members determine which aspects of the spiritual care plan require the expertise of a spiritual care professional (chaplain)?

The Role of Healthcare Providers in Spiritual Communication

Communicating with patients and families about basic spiritual needs falls within the purview of a number of palliative care team members including, but not limited to, spiritual care professionals, physicians, nurses, social workers, psychologists, as well as community faith leaders. In one study, dying patients and their family caregivers reported primarily talking with family or friends about spiritual concerns, followed by clergy and healthcare providers.[56] However, other studies have reported that the provision of spiritual care comes from within the religious community, followed by healthcare providers and chaplains.[57]

While community faith resources are an important source of support for those patients whose spirituality is expressed through religious means, these supplemental supports should not preclude healthcare providers from addressing spiritual needs. In a study investigating the utilization of community clergy, few patients reported that they had talked to clergy about their hospitalization.[58] Patients with high spiritual support from their religious community are less likely to receive hospice care and more likely to receive aggressive measures at the end of life.[59] In contrast, patients with high spiritual support from their religious community who also received spiritual support from their healthcare team had higher rates of hospice utilization, fewer aggressive end-of-life interventions, and fewer intensive care unit deaths.[59] While spiritual support from the healthcare team does not replace community-based resources, it does augment them and often serves an important mediatory function between healthcare and faith communities.

The Essential Skills for Spiritual Communication

A persistent challenge facing healthcare providers is how to adequately address and effectively intervene regarding patients' and families' important but deeply human spiritual concerns. In contrast to biomedical needs, spiritual care does not attempt to provide answers to life's questions but rather aims to promote healing by acknowledging, listening to, and providing a compassionate presence to deeply spiritual questions. Technical skills and knowledge are important components to spiritual communication; however, equally important is the intrinsic and tacit qualities of healthcare providers. The mnemonic SACR-D (see Table 37.1) provides healthcare providers with a framework of essential skills for spiritual communication.[60]

Self-Awareness

Provider self-awareness is recognized as a hallmark of therapeutic communication in general[61,62] and seems to play a particularly important role when addressing the sensitive domain of spirituality. The importance of self-awareness to both healthcare providers' well-being and quality patient care was recently recognized in an Institute of Medicine report that recommended the inclusion of curricula focused on the recognition of how one's beliefs and personal history impact clinical communication.[63] While healthcare providers' own spiritual and religious beliefs should never usurp the spirituality of their patient, their own self-exploration of spirituality can create a foundation of shared understanding and relatedness whereby the ephemeral and sensitive nature of spiritual issues can be honored and appreciated. The importance of self-awareness in communicating about spiritual issues is underscored by research findings that healthcare providers' spiritual and religious beliefs often differ significantly from those of their patients, with the former being less religious, less likely to

Table 37.1 SACR-D

Concept	Definition	Sample Questions/Clinical Strategies
S—Self-awareness	Conscious knowledge of how one's own spirituality or beliefs, practices, behaviors, and experiences related to ultimate meaning[12] impact clinical communication	• What are my spiritual beliefs and how do they impact my clinical practice? • How can I express spiritual sensitivity in my clinical communication? • What is the impact of frequent exposure to death and dying on me as a person and as a healthcare provider?[67]
A—Assessment	Extrinsic and intrinsic means that enable healthcare providers to determine the role and importance of spirituality in a patient or family member's life and healthcare	• FICA (see Box 37.1)[70] • Are there visual cues available to me that can help me understand this person's spirituality? • As I listen to this person, what are the sources of meaning and purpose in his or her life?
C—Compassionate presence	The use of healthcare providers whole self when engaging a person in suffering, coupled by a desire and action aimed at alleviation	• How is my presence impacting the clinical encounter? • Who is the person behind the disease?[29] • How can I actively engage in and alleviate this person's suffering? • How does this person best receive compassion?
R—Refer to additional spiritual supports	The act of referring to a spiritual care professional (chaplain), healthcare team member, or community spiritual/religious resource for additional support	• Which member of the healthcare team is best suited to address this person's spiritual needs? • Are they a part of a religious or spiritual community? • Is there a spiritual care professional/chaplain I can refer to?

D—Dialogue	Clinical conversations intended to understand and/or address a person's spirituality in a language that is accessible to them	• How can I communicate about clinical matters in a language that honors this person's sense of meaning and purpose?
		• Dialect of dignity:
		  · What do you feel most proud of?[112]
		  · Are there things that you are still needing to say to your loved ones?[112]
		  · What are your hopes and dreams for them in the future?[112]
		  · Are there issues that you feel are affecting your sense of dignity?
		• Dialect of meaning:
		  · What gives your life meaning?
		  · Where have you found meaning when you have faced challenges in the past?
		  · What meaning do your current health challenges have in your life?
		• Dialect of hope:
		  · What is your hope for the future?
		  · How might hope change for you if you knew you had 6 years to live? 6 months to live? 6 weeks to live? 6 days to live?
		  · How do I personally conceptualize hope and how is my understanding similar or different to this person?
		  · How can I enhance this person's hope, beyond a hope for a cure?

Source: Sinclair S, Chochinov HM. Communicating with patients about existential and spiritual issues: SACR-D work. *Prog Palliat Care.* 2012;20(2):72–78.

rely on God when dealing with a major problem, and more likely to identify themselves as spiritual but not religious.[34,35,64]

While spiritual backgrounds may differ between patient and healthcare provider, the clinical implications associated with patient-reported attunement between their spirituality and that of their healthcare provider cannot be easily dismissed. Attunement, the degree to which patients feel that their healthcare provider are open to and can relate on a spiritual level, has been identified by patients as a very important factor in clinical communication[22] and a facilitator in the identification of spiritual needs.[65] Provider spirituality is often an invisible and an involuntary ingredient in the provision of spiritual care that can have both a positive and/or negative effect in the clinical encounter.[29] Healthcare providers are therefore implored to cultivate self-awareness regarding their own spirituality and its impact in clinical communication, recognizing that self-awareness related to spirituality seems to be more associated with qualities such as openness, tolerance, and curiosity rather than self-assessed spirituality, religiosity, or technical competence on the part of healthcare providers.[29,56,60]

Spiritual self-awareness has also been shown to have a positive impact on providers' personal and professional lives. The landscape of death and dying, where spiritual issues are prevalent, permeate the clinical encounter, challenging healthcare providers to reflect on their own mortality and spirituality. A study of interdisciplinary palliative care team members identified healthcare provider spirituality as an important factor that informed spiritual communication with patients.[66] The reciprocal nature of spiritual communication between patient and palliative care provider has also been shown to have a positive impact on providers' personal and professional lives, including the cultivation of their own spirituality.[67] Similar research has also found enhanced work satisfaction, effective patient care, and buffering against workplace burnout as provider benefits of healthcare provider spirituality.[67-69]

Assessment

Communicating with patients about their spirituality can also occur through more extrinsic means, utilizing a variety of tools aimed at measuring aspects of spirituality. A spiritual history, such as FICA (Box 37.1) provides healthcare providers with a validated and efficient tool for spiritual communication and can be easily incorporated into existing comprehensive assessment during intake or at an initial clinical visit.[70,71] The FICA tool and spiritual assessments[72,73] contain standardized questions that have been validated and are intended to facilitate a conversation rather than being utilized in a formulaic fashion. Two of the inherent challenges of spiritual assessments are their utility and validity in applying broad constructs to measure the deeply personal and culturally embedded domain of spirituality. As Selman et al. observed in a systematic review of spiritual measures in palliative care, of the 85 tools identified, only 38 had been validated in palliative care populations and only 9 were validated in one or more ethnically diverse populations.[74] Since the evidence base for the evaluation of spiritual assessment remains nascent, healthcare professionals should be cautious in adopting a "one-size-fits-all" approach to assessing the spirituality of their patients.

An essential seemingly self-intuitive yet often overlooked modality in assessing patients spirituality is listening. Active listening has been identified as a core component of optimal therapeutic effectives.[75] Intuitive listening, focused on both the subtext of the patient's story while also being attuned to the guidance of a spiritual source (God, higher power, life force, etc.) is one of five essential skills in the provision of spiritual care.[29] Having someone listen is one of the most frequently identified spiritual needs of palliative care patients.[76] Listening is a foundational and often forgotten component of the clinical dialogue in general.[77-80]

Compassionate Presence

The presence of the healthcare provider involves the externalization of the provider's intrinsic qualities into the relational space created with the patient.[29] While technical skills are consistently ranked higher by providers than intrinsic qualities, the opposite is revealed in patient responses.[81-84] Patients who feel connected to their healthcare provider and feel that there is a care partnership are more motivated to manage their illness and have a greater sense of well-being.[85] Healthcare providers who are identified as warm and friendly and have developed reassuring relationships with their patients are more likely to be considered effective healthcare providers then those who adopt a more objective and formal approach.[86]

An important component of Chochinov's dignity-conserving care is the healthcare provider's presence or the tone of care, conveyed through body language and attitude, and how it impacts the patient's sense of dignity.[87] The positive attributes of a healthcare provider's presence can facilitate healing, and the impact of negative healthcare intrinsic qualities such as apathy, disregard, and despair seem to have an equally powerful adverse affect. Kuhl coined the term "iatrogenic suffering" to describe the suffering inflicted on patients through negative aspects of healthcare providers' presence in the clinical encounter.[88] Applying the concept of iatrogenic suffering to spiritual care refers to the negative impact that healthcare professionals' own spirituality, ranging from overt religious beliefs to unresolved spiritual issues, has on their patient's spiritual well-being.

Presence is a poignant modifier of clinical communication, particularly as it relates to psychosocial and spiritual communication. Presence was identified as a foundational element that all spiritual interventions are predicated on and delivered through.[29] Exemplary spiritual care providers are characterized as being present, recognizing shared humanity, and having the ability to integrate a patient's spiritual concerns into the care plan.[56] The paramount role that presence plays in the provision of spiritual care is evident in the words of Puchalski, who summates, "Which word [God, divine energy, oneness] is not as important as what happens between people and living beings. Spiritual care is the practice of compassionate presence."[89(p40)]

Imbuing healthcare provider presence with compassion is of particular relevance in spiritual communication. Compassion has been defined as "a deep awareness of the suffering of another coupled with the wish to relieve it,"[90] finding its ethos from the "golden rule" and thus serving as both the quintessential indicator and the outcome of spiritual care.[91] Compassion, along with dignity, have

---

Box 37.1 FICA: Spiritual History Tool

F—Faith, belief, meaning

"Do you consider yourself spiritual or religious?" or "Do you have spiritual beliefs that help you cope with stress?"

If the patient responds "No," the physician might ask, "What gives your life meaning?" Sometimes patients respond with answers such as family, career, or nature.

I—Importance and influence

"What importance does your faith or belief have in your life? Have your beliefs influenced how you take care of yourself in this illness? What role do your beliefs play in regaining your health?"

C—Community

"Are you part of a spiritual or religious community? Is this of support to you and how? Is there a group of people you really love or are important to you?"

Communities such as churches, temples, and mosques or a group of like-minded friends can serve as strong support systems for some patients.

A—Address/action in care

"How would you like me, your healthcare provider, to address these issues in your health care?"

Adapted by C. Puchalski with permission from Puchalski CM, Romer AL. Taking a spiritual history allows clinicians to understand patients more fully. *J Palliat Med.* 2000;3:129–137.

been conceptualized as twin pillars of spiritual care.[92] Compassion's universality traverses faith traditions where it is considered to be the marker of authentic faith,[93] while also extending to secularist expressions of spirituality where it is considered a cardinal virtue of humanity.[94,95] Healthcare providers who are perceived as compassionate by patients and families are less likely to have malpractice suits filed against them and are more likely to have their caregiving perceived in a positive manner.[96–98] Vulnerability, the ability of healthcare providers to not only acknowledge the suffering of another but to proactively position themselves alongside patient suffering, is an essential factor in the development of compassionate presence.[29]

Referral to Additional Spiritual Supports

Spiritual communication is a standard of care across palliative care disciplines, with spiritual care professionals possessing specialized knowledge and skills in assessing and addressing acute spiritual issues.[12] Historically, spiritual care was synonymous with religious care delivered by denominational chaplains who were commissioned and employed by their faith communities.[99] In contrast, spiritual care professionals address and/or coordinate the spiritual needs of patients from diverse religious and spiritual backgrounds, are members of an interdisciplinary healthcare team, and are accountable to the healthcare instution.[99] The recognition and integration of spiritual care within comprehensive palliative care, along with the development of the discipline of spiritual care, has led to an integrated model where spiritual care professionals are recognized as core members of interdisciplinary palliative care teams.[12,100,101]

Interdisciplinary palliative care team members report that spiritual care is understood as a function of the healthcare team, while recognizing the spiritual care professional/chaplain possesses advance knowledge and skills to meet spiritual needs of a more acute nature.[66] Similarly, oncology interdisciplinary team members report that spiritual communication falls within their scope of practice, yet they recognize that a spiritual care professional is best suited to address spiritual issues.[37] While there is broad recognition of the role of spiritual care professionals in interdisciplinary healthcare teams by patients, healthcare providers, and policymakers, a significant theory–practice gap exists, as spiritual care services continue to be treated as an ancillary,[12] often being relegated to the periphery of so-called core healthcare services.[101]

In general, spiritual care professionals are certified by a professional spiritual care organization, are master's degree prepared, have completed a clinical residency program, are bound by a common code of ethics and standards of practice, and must be recertified through a peer review process every 5 years.[9,12] In addition to specialized spiritual care, spiritual care professionals are also skilled in the provision of supportive psychosocial care. In a study of colorectal cancer patients, chaplains were the primary source of psychosocial support, followed by social workers and psychologists.[102] Referrals to chaplaincy services are often for emotional support, with nurses and patients being the greatest referral sources.[103–105] The impact of spiritual care visitations are associated with lower rates of aggressive end-of-life care and hospital deaths and higher rates of hospice enrollment.[106]

Dialogue

The problem of language in spiritual communication is a well-recognized issue within the literature and at the bedside.[6,8] This is due, in large part, to the ephemeral nature of spirituality and the limitations of language in the articulation of spiritual understanding, meaning, and appropriate, comforting responses. As patients and family members struggle to describe spiritual distress and concerns, healthcare providers are equally challenged to engage in conversations that address them. This has caused some clinical researchers to advocate that spiritual communication should be based on a standardized, universal, and codified vocabulary,[107] as "the language of spirituality is often an obstacle to communication rather than an aid to understanding."[8(p303)] While the problematic nature of language in spiritual communication seems to largely be reflective of the nature of the topic, critics note that the field of spirituality and health has perpetuated a discourse of ambiguity which is "rich in narcissm"[108(p439)] and employs terminology that everyone uses but no one understands.[109] While the lack of conceptual specificity has led to a number of broad and inclusive definitions of spirituality[9,10] these do not preclude the need for providers to tailor their communication about spiritual issues in the vernacular of each patient and to develop literacy within the following construct-based dialects of spirituality that traverse the sacred and the secular.[60]

The Dialect of Dignity

Dignity, while not being a uniquely spiritual construct, provides a language for eliciting the spiritual landscape of patients facing the end of life.[110] The Patient Dignity Inventory (PDI) is a validated 25-item measure of dignity-related distress.[111] There is a significant correlation between the PDI Peace of Mind factor and the Functional Assessment of Chronic Illness Therapy-Spiritual Well Being Inner Peace Factor.[111] While the PDI contains questions specifically focused on spiritual and existential issues, it also addresses broader issues such as continuity of self, worth, unfinished business, and control in life that, while not representing overtly spiritual issues, may be rooted in spiritual concerns or alleviated through spiritual resources. Dignity therapy, a one-session intervention that allows patients to reflect on their legacy and any unfinished issues, utilizes a nine-item protocol and can be administered in 1 to 1.5 hours.[112] Patients responses are audio-recorded, transcribed, and edited, creating a legacy document that can provide comfort to bereft family members after the patient is deceased. Clinical trials of dignity therapy have reported a high satisfaction rate and a heighted sense of personal dignity among patients,[112] with 78% of family members reporting that the legacy document helped them in their grief, with 95% indicating they would recommend dignity therapy to patients and family members.[113]

The Dialect of Meaning

The construct of meaning provides healthcare providers with another dialect to communicate with patients about spiritual issues. Psychotherapist and existential thinker Viktor Frankl identified meaning as a primary drive of humanity that could be both derived from and ameliorate suffering.[114] The relevance of meaning at the end of life, where suffering is prevalent, and its relationship to spirituality has been investigated by Breitbart and colleagues.[115,116] In a US-based survey reporting on the prevalence of spiritual needs at the end of life, issues of meaning and purpose were the most frequently identified spiritual needs.[117] In spiritual communication, meaning-making is an important buffer against end-of-life distress, depression, and hopelessness.[43,37,118] A "loss of meaning life" is one of the greatest predictors of patient's desire for a hastened death.[119] Meaning-centered group psychotherapy, a manualized eight-session psychotherapeutic intervention focusing on particular meaning-based themes, is reported to significantly improve patient spiritual well-being, sense of meaning, anxiety, and desire for death.[120] Addressing spiritual issues through the framework of meaning can occur through more pragmatic means such as asking patients, "What gives your life meaning?"; "Where have you found meaning when you have faced challenges in the past?"; and "What meaning do your current health challenges have in your life?"

The Dialect of Hope

A final dialect for communicating about spiritual issues is hope. The nature of hope in palliative care extends beyond the hope for a cure[121] and instead id defined as "a multidimensional dynamic life force characterized by a confident yet uncertain expectation of achieving a future good which, to the hoping person, is realistically possible and personally significant."[122(p380)] Olsman et al. identified three perspectives on hope in palliative care: a realistic perspective that involves titrating patients' hope with prognostic information; a functional perspective that calls for emphasis on hope as a way of coping with the impact of disease; and a narrative perspective wherein hope is used as a way to find and maintain meaning.[123] Palliative care providers need to oscillate between these perspectives in accordance with a patient's own perspective on hope, recognizing that this may fluctuate over the palliative trajectory. Duggelby developed a living with hope program consisting of a short video with various hope activities such as journaling and letter writing, which resulted in significantly higher scores on the McGill Quality of Life Existential subscale for patient participants versus those in the control group.[124] Broaching the topic of hope in palliative care may involve asking focused questions of patients such as: "What is your hope for the future?"; "How might hope change for you if you knew that you had 6 years to live, 6 months to live, 6 weeks to live, or 6 days to live?" Communicating about hope also involves healthcare providers' reflection of their own clinical practice in order to determine their own perspectives on hope and its effect on patients' hope. Reflective questions may include: "How do I conceptualize hope?"; "How is my understanding of hope similar and/or different from my patient?"; "How can I provide truthful information to this person without destroying all hope?";[121] "What is this person's tolerance for uncertainty?";[121] "How can I enhance this persons' hope, beyond a hope for a cure?"[121,123]

Conclusion

Communicating with palliative care patients about spiritual issues is an essential component of comprehensive palliative care. While both patients and healthcare providers struggle to express the deeply personal nature of their spirituality and engage in spiritual communication, the inherent difficulties associated with this domain do not preclude the necessity and importance of entering into these therapeutic conversations. The mnemonic SACR-D provides healthcare providers with a clinical framework for spiritual communication, providing a means for alleviating patient distress as well as promoting professional and personal growth for healthcare providers working in palliative settings.

References

1. World Health Organization. http://www.who.int/cancer/palliative/definition/en/. Accessed June 20, 2015.
2. National Quality Forum. National framework and preferred practices for palliative and hospice care. http://www.qualityforum.org/publications/2006/12/A_National_Framework_and_Preferred_Practices_for_Palliative_and_Hospice_Care_Quality.aspx. Published December 2006. Accessed June 21, 2014.
3. O'Connor P, Kaplan M. The role of the interdisciplinary team in providing spiritual care: An attitudinal study of hospice workers. In: Wald F, ed. *In Quest of the Spiritual Component of Care for the Terminally Ill*. New Haven, CT: Yale University Press; 1986:51–62.
4. Ferrell B, Otis-Green S, Economou D. Spirituality in cancer care at the end of life. *Cancer J*. 2013;19(5):431–437.
5. Unruh AM, Versnel J, Kerr N. Spirituality unplugged: A review of commonalities and contentions, and a resolution. *Can J Occup Ther*. 2002;69(1):5–19.
6. Sinclair S, Pereira J, Raffin S. A thematic review of the spirituality literature within palliative care. *J Palliat Med*. 2006;9(2):464–479.
7. Paley J. Spirituality and nursing: A reductionist approach. *Nurs Philos*. 2008;9(1):3–18.
8. Mount BM, Lawlor W, Casell EJ. Spirituality and health: Developing a shared vocabulary. *Ann R Coll Physicians Surg Can*. 2002;35(5):303–307.
9. Puchalski CM, Vitillo R, Hull SK, Reller N. Improving the spiritual dimension of whole person care: Reaching national and international consensus. *J Pain Symptom Manage*. 2014;17(6):1–15.
10. Puchalski CM, Ferrell B, Otis-Green S, et al. Improving the quality of spiritual care as a dimension of palliative care: The report of the Consensus Conference. *J Palliat Med*. 2009;12(10):885–904.
11. Nolan S, Saltmarsh, Leget C. Spiritual care in palliative care: Working toward an EAPC Task Force. *Eur J Palliat Care*. 2011;18(2):86–89.
12. Sinclair S, Chochinov HM. The role of chaplains within oncology interdisciplinary teams. *Curr Opin Support Palliat Care*. 2012;6(2):259–268.
13. McGinn B. Spirituality confronts its future. *Spiritus*. 2005:5(1):88–96.
14. Walter T. Spirituality in palliative care: Opportunity or burden? *Palliat Med*. 2002;16(2):133–139.
15. Grant L, Murray SA, Sheikh A. Spiritual dimensions of dying in pluralist societies. *BMJ*. 2002;34:659–662.
16. Kearney M, Mount B. Spiritual care of the dying patient. In: Chochinov HM, Breitbart W, eds. *Handbook of Psychiatry in Palliative Medicine*. Oxford: Oxford University Press; 2000:357–373.
17. Garces-Foley K. Hospice and the politics of spirituality. In: Bramadat P, Coward H, Stajduhar KI, eds. *Spirituality in Hospice and Palliative Care*. Albany, NY: SUNY Press; 2013:13–40.
18. Marler PL, Hadaway CK. "Being religious" or "being spiritual" in America: A zero-sum proposition? *J Sci Study Relig*. 2002:4(2):289–300.
19. Bibby R. *The Emerging Millennials: How Canada's Newest Generation is Responding to Change and Choice*. Lethbridge, AB: Project Canada Books; 2009.
20. Bibby R. *The Boomer Factor: What Canada's Most Famous Generation Is Leaving Behind*. Toronto: Bastian Books; 2006.
21. Clark W, Schellenberg G. Who's religious? *Can Soc Trends*. 2006;81:2–9.
22. Gallup G. The George H. Gallup International Institute: Spiritual beliefs and the dying process: A report on a national survey. Princeton, NJ: Princeton Religion and Research Center; 1997.
23. Sulmasy D. Spiritual issues in the care of dying patients. *JAMA*. 2006;296(11):1385–1392.

24. *American Religious Identification Survey*. New York, NY: Graduate Center of the City University of New York; 2000.
25. Gallup. Americans' spiritual searches turn inward. http://www.gallup.com/poll/7759/americans-spiritual-searches-turn-inward.aspx. Published February 11, 2003. Accessed June 21, 2014.
26. Rahner, K. *Theological Investigations*, Vol. 7. London: Darton, Longman and Todd; 1971.
27. Astrow AB, Wexler A, Texeira K, Kai He MK, Sulmasy DP. Is failure to meet spiritual needs associated with cancer patients' perceptions of quality of care and satisfaction with care? *J Clin Oncol*. 2007;25(36):5753–5757.
28. Alcorn S, Balboni MJ, Prigerson HG, et al. "If God wanted me yesterday, I wouldn't be here today": Religious and spiritual these in patients' experiences of advanced cancer. *J Palliat Med*. 2010;13(5):581–588.
29. Sinclair S, Raffin S, Chochinov HM, Hagen NH, McClement S. Spiritual care: How to do it. *BMJ Support Palliat Care*. 2012;2:319–328.
30. Ehman J, Ott B, Short T, Ciampa R, Hansen-Flaschen J. Do patients want physicians to inquire about their spiritual or religious beliefs if they become gravely ill? *Arch Intern Med*. 1999;159(15):1803–1806.
31. Heyland DK, Cook DJ, Rocker GM, et al. Defining priorities for improving end-of-life care in Canada. *CMAJ*. 2010;182(16):E747–E752.
32. Heyland DK, Dodek P, Rocker G, et al. What matters most in end-of-life care: Perceptions of seriously ill patients and their family members. *CMAJ*. 2006;174(5):627–633.
33. Cohen SR, Mount BM, Tomas JJ, Mount LF. Existential well-being is an important determinant of quality of life: Evidence from the McGill Quality of Life Questionnaire. *Palliat Med*. 1996;77(3):576–586.
34. Steinhauser KE, Christakis NA, Clipp EC, McNeilly M, McIntyre L, Tulsky J. Factors considered important at the end of life by patients, family, physicians, and other care providers. *JAMA*. 2000;284(19):2476–2482.
35. Phelps AC, Lauderdale KE, Alcorn S, et al. Addressing spirituality within the care of patients at the end of life: Perspective of patients with advanced cancer, oncologists, and oncology nurses. *J Clin Oncol*. 2012;30(20):2538–2544.
36. Balboni T, Vanderwerker LC, Block SD, et al. Religiousness and spiritual support among advanced cancer patients and associations with end-of-life treatment preferences and quality of life. *J Clin Oncol*. 2007;25(5):555–560.
37. Kristeller JL, Zumbrun CS, Schilling RF. "I would if I could": How oncologists and oncology nurses address spiritual distress in cancer patients. *Psycho-Oncology*. 1999;8(5):451–458.
38. Lin HR, Bauer-Wu SM. Psycho-spiritual well being in patients with advanced cancer: An integrative review of the literature. *J Adv Nurs*. 2003;44(1):69–80.
39. Zaza C, Sellick SM, Hillier LM. Coping with cancer: What do patients do? *J Psychosoc Oncol*. 2005;23(1):55–73.
40. Koenig HG, Hover M, Bearon LB, Travis JL. Religious perspectives of doctors, nurses, patients, and families. *J Pastoral Care*. 1991;45(3):254–267.
41. Brady MJ, Peterman AH, Fitchett G, Mo M, Cella D. A case for including spirituality in quality of life measurement in oncology. *Psycho-Oncology*. 1999;8(5):417–428.
42. Johnson KS, Tulsky JA, Hays JC, et al. Which domains of spirituality are associated with anxiety and depression in patients with advanced illness? *J Gen Intern Med*. 2011;26(7):751–758.
43. Nelson C, Rosenfield B, Breitbart W. Spirituality, religion, and depression in the terminally ill. *Psychosomatics*. 2002;43(3):213–220.
44. Wilson K, Chochinov HM, McPherson C, et al. Desire for euthanasia or physician-assisted suicide in palliative cancer care. *Health Psychol*. 2007;26(3):314–323.
45. Sullivan A, Hedberg K, Fleming D. Legalized physician-assisted suicide in Oregon: The second year. *N Engl J Med*. 2000;342(8):598–604.
46. Chochinov HM, Hack T, Hassard T, Kristjanosn L, McClement S, Harlos M. Dignity in the terminally ill: A cross-sectional cohort study. *Lancet*. 2002;360(9350):2026–2030.
47. Chochinov HM, Hassard T, McClement S, et al. The landscape of distress in the terminally ill. *J Pain Symptom Manage*. 2009;38(5):641–649.
48. Winkelman WD, Lauderdale K, Balboni MJ, et al. The relationship of spiritual concerns to the quality of life of advanced cancer patients: Preliminary findings. *J Palliat Med*. 2011;14(9):1022–1028.
49. McClain CS, Rosenfield B, Breitbart W. Effect of spiritual well-being on end-of-life despair in terminally ill patients. *Lancet*. 2003;361:1603–1607.
50. Department of Human Services. Summary of the state of Oregon's Death with Dignity Act. http://public.health.oregon.gov/ProviderPartnerResources/EvaluationResearch/DeathwithDignityAct/Pages/ar-index.aspx. Published March 2009. Accessed June 21, 2014.
51. Balboni T, Balboni M, Paulk ME, et al. Support of cancer patients' spiritual needs and associations with medical care costs at the end of life. *Cancer*. 2011;117(23):5383–5391.
52. Rasinski KA, Kalad YG, Yoon JD, Curlin FA. An assessment of US physicians' training in religion, spirituality, and medicine. *Med Teach*. 2011;33(11):944–945.
53. Moadel A, Morgan C, Fatone A, et al. Seeking meaning and hope: Self-reported spiritual and existential needs among an ethnically-diverse cancer patient population. *Psycho-Oncology*. 1999;8(5):378–385.
54. Mako C, Galek K, Poppito S. Spiritual pain among patients with advanced cancer in palliative care. *J Palliat Med*. 2009;9(5):1106–1113.
55. Hui D, de la Cruz M, Thorney S, Parsons HA, Delgago-Guay M, Bruera E. The frequency and correlates of spiritual distress among patients with advanced cancer admitted to an acute palliative care unit. *Am J Hosp Palliat Care*. 2011;28(4):264–270.
56. Daaleman T, Usher B, Williams S, Rawlings J, Hanson LC. An exploratory study of spiritual care at the end of life. *Ann Fam Med*. 2008;6(5):406–411.
57. Pearce MJ, Coan Ad, Herndon JE, Koenig HD. Unmet spiritual care needs impact emotional and spiritual well-being in advanced cancer patients. *Support Care Cancer*. 2012;20(10):2269–2276.
58. Sivan A, Fitchett G, Burton L. Hospitalized psychiatric and medical patients and the clergy. *J Religion Health*. 1996;35(1):11–19.
59. Balboni TA, Balboni M, Enzinger AC, Gallivan K, Paulk ME, Wright. Provision of spiritual support to patients with advanced cancer by religious communities and associations with medical care at the end of life. *JAMA Intern Med*. 2013;173(12):1109–1117.
60. Sinclair S, Chochinov HM. Communicating with patients about existential and spiritual issues: SACR-D work. *Prog Palliat Care*. 2012;20(2):72–78.
61. Wachtel PH. *Therapeutic Communication: Knowing What to Say When*. New York, NY: Guildford Press; 2011.
62. Stein H. What is therapeutic in clinical relationships? *Fam Med*. 1985;17:188–194.
63. Institute of Medicine. *Improving Medical Education: Enhancing the Behavioral and Social Science Content of Medical School Curricula*. Washington DC: National Academies Press; 2004.
64. Shafranske EP. Religious beliefs, affiliations, and practices of clinical psychologists. In: Shafranske EP, ed. *Religion and the Clinical Practice of Psychology*. Washington, DC: American Psychological Association; 1996:149–162.
65. Curlin FA, Selleergren SA, Lantos JD, Chin MH. Physicians' observations and interpretation of the influence of religion and spirituality on health. *Arch Intern Med*. 2007;167(7):649–654.

66. Sinclair S, Raffin S, Pereira J, Guebert N. Collective soul: The spirituality of an interdisciplinary team. *Palliat Support Care.* 2006;4(1):13–24.
67. Sinclair S. Impact of death and dying on the personal lives and practices of palliative and hospice care professionals. *CMAJ.* 2011;183(2):180–187.
68. Holland J, Neimeyer R. Reducing the risk of burnout in end-of-life care settings: The role of daily spiritual experiences and training. *Palliat Support Care.* 2005;3(3):173–181.
69. Wasner M, Longaker C, Fegg M, Boarasio G. Effects of spiritual care training for palliative care professionals. *Palliat Med.* 2005;19(2):99–104.
70. Puchalski C, Romer AL. Taking a spiritual history allows clinicians to understand patients more fully. *J Palliat Med.* 2000;3(1):129–137.
71. Borneman T, Ferrell B, Puchalski CM. Evaluation of the FICA tool for spiritual assessment. *J Pain Symptom Manage.* 2010;40(2):163–173.
72. Pruyser PW. *The Minister as Diagnostician.* Philadelphia, PA: Westminster Press; 1976.
73. Fitchett G. *Assessing Spiritual Needs: A Guide for Caregivers.* Lima, OH: Academic Renewal Press; 2002.
74. Selman L, Harding R, Gysels M, Speck P, Higginson IJ. The measurement of spirituality in palliative care and the content of tools validated cross-culturally: A systematic review. *J Pain Symptom Manage.* 2011;41(4):728–753.
75. Chochinov HM, McClement SE, Hack TF, et al. Health care provider communication: An empirical model of therapeutic effectiveness. *Cancer.* 2013;119(9):1706–1713.
76. Wright M. Chaplaincy in hospice and hospital: Findings from a survey in England and Wales. *Palliat Med.* 2001;15(3):229–242.
77. Matthew DA, Sledge WH, Lieberman PB. Evaluation of intern performance by medical inpatients. *Am J Med.* 1987;83(5):938–944.
78. Harris, SR, Templeton E. Who's listening? Experiences of women with breast cancer in communicating with physicians. *Breast J.* 2001;7(6):444–449.
79. McDonagh JR, Elliott TB, Engelberg RA, et al. Family satisfaction with family conferences about end-of-life care in the intensive care unit: Increased proportion of family speech is associated with increased satisfaction. *Crit Care Med.* 2004;32(7):1484–1488.
80. Beckman HB, Frankel RM. The effect of physician behavior on the collection of data. *Ann Intern Med.* 1984;101(5):692–696.
81. Flocke S, Miller W, Crabtree B. Relationships between physician practice style, patient satisfaction, and attributes of primary care. *J Fam Pract.* 2002;51(10):835–840.
82. Attree M. Patients' and relatives' experiences and perspectives of "good" and "not so good" quality care. *J Adv Nurs.* 2001;33(4):456–466.
83. Thorne S, Kuo M, Armstrong E, McPherson G, Harris SR, Hislop TG. Being known: Patient perspectives of the dynamics of human connection in cancer care. *Psycho-Oncology.* 2005;14(10):887–898.
84. Sanghavi D. Beyond the white coat and the johnny: What makes for a compassionate patient-caregiver relationship? Findings from a national conversation sponsored by the Kenneth B. Schwartz Centre. *Jt Comm J Q and Patient Saf.* 2006;32:293–292.
85. Fox S, Chesla C. Living with chronic illness: A phenomenological study of the health effects of the patient-provider relationship. *J Am Acad Nurse Pract.* 2008;20(3):109–117.
86. Stewart M. Effective physician-patient communications and health outcomes: A review. *CMAJ.* 1995;152(9):1423–1433.
87. Chochinov H. Dying, dignity, and new horizons in palliative end-of-life care. *CA Cancer J Clin.* 2006;56(2):84–103.
88. Kuhl, D. *What Dying People Want.* Toronto: Anchor; 2001.
89. Puchalski, C. *A Time for Listening and Caring: Spirituality and the Care of the Chronically Ill and Dying.* New York, NY: Oxford; 2006.
90. *The American Heritage Dictionary of the English Language.* Compassion. http://www.thefreedictionary.com/compassion. Published 2011. Accessed June 21, 2014.
91. Armstrong K. *A History of God.* New York, NY: Ballatine Books; 1993.
92. Mowat H, O'Neill M. Insights: Spirituality and ageing: Implications for the care and support of older people. *IRISS Insights.* 2013;19:1–15.
93. Armstrong K. *Jerusalem: One City Three Faiths.* New York, NY: Ballantine Books; 1997.
94. Oveis C, Horberg E, Keltner D. Compassion, pride, and social intuitions of self-other similarity. *J Pers Soc Psychol.* 2010;98(4):618–630.
95. Sprecher S, Fehr B. Compassionate love for close others and humanity. *J Soc Pers Relat.* 2005;22(5):629–651.
96. Gilbert P, ed. *Compassion: Conceptualisations, Research and Use in Psychotherapy.* East Sussex, UK: Routledge; 2005.
97. Stewart M, Brown J, Donner A, et al. The impact of patient-centered care on outcomes. *J Fam Pract.* 2000;49(9):796–804.
98. Levinson W, Roter D, Mullooly J, Dull V, Frankel RM. Physician-patient communication: The relationship with malpractice claims among primary care physicians and surgeons. *JAMA.* 1997;277(7):553–559.
99. Handzo GF, Cobb M, Holmes C, Kelly E, Sinclair S. Outcomes for professional health care chaplaincy: An international call to action. *J Health Care Chaplain.* 2014;20(2):43–53.
100. National Comprehensive Cancer Network. NCCN clinical practice guidelines in oncology: Palliative care. http://www.nccn.org/professionals/physician_gls/pdf/palliative.pdf. Published 2011. Accessed on June 21, 2014.
101. Sinclair S, Mysak M, Hagen NA. What are the core elements of oncology spiritual care programs? *Palliat Support Care.* 2009;7(4):315–322.
102. Hamilton NS, Jackson GL, Abbott DH, Zullig LL, Provenzale D. Use of psychosocial support services among male veterans affairs colorectal cancer patients. *J Psychosoc Oncol.* 2011;29(3):242–253.
103. Vanderwerker LC, Ranney KJ, Galek KJ, et al. What do chaplains really do? III. Referrals in the New York Chaplaincy Study. *J Health Care Chaplain.* 2008;14(1):57–73.
104. Glombicki JS, Jeuland J. Exploring the importance of chaplain visits in a palliative care clinic for patients and companions. *J Palliat Med.* 2014;17(2):1–2.
105. Piderman KM, Marek DV, Jenkins SM, et al. Patients' expectations of hospital chaplains. *Mayo Clin Proc.* 2008;83(1):58–65.
106. Flannelly KJ, Emanuel LL, Handzo GF, Galek K, Silton NR, Carlson M. A national study of chaplaincy services and end-of-life outcomes. *BMC Palliat Care.* 2012;11(10):1–6.
107. Candy B, Jones CB, Varagunam M, Speck P, Tookman, King M. Spiritual and religious interventions for well-being of adults in the terminal phase of disease. *Cochrane Database Syst Rev.* 2012;5:1–52.
108. Marty M. Getting organized. *ChrCent.* 1996;113(13):439.
109. Rose S. Is the term "spirituality" a word that everyone uses, but nobody knows what anyone means by it? *J Contemp Relig.* 2001;16(2):193–207.
110. Sinclair S, Chochinov HM. Dignity: A novel path into the spiritual landscape of the human heart. In: Cobb M, Puchalski CM, Rumbold B, eds. *Oxford Textbook of Spirituality in Healthcare.* New York, NY: Oxford University Press; 2012:145–149.
111. Chochinov HM, Hassard T, McClement S, et al. The patient dignity inventory: A novel way of measuring dignity-related distress in palliative care. *J Pain Symptom Manage.* 2008;36(6):559–571.
112. Chochinov HM, Hack T, Hassard T, Kristjanson L, McClement S, Harlos M. Dignity therapy: A novel psychotherapeutic intervention for patients near the end of life. *J Clin Oncol.* 2005;23(24):5520–5525.
113. McClement S, Chochinov H, Hack T, Hassard T, Kristjanson LJ, Harlos M. Dignity therapy: Family member perspectives. *J Palliat Med.* 2007;10(5):1076–1082.
114. Frankl V. *Man's Search for Ultimate Meaning.* New York, NY: Plenum; 1997.

115. Breitbart W. Spirituality and meaning in supportive care: Spirituality and meaning centered group psychotherapy interventions in advanced cancer. *Support Care Cancer.* 2002;10(4):272–280.
116. Breitbart W, Gibson C, Poppito SR, Berg A. Psychotherapeutic interventions at the end of life: A focus on meaning and spirituality. *Can J Psychiatry.* 2004;49(6):366–372.
117. Flannelly KJ, Galek K, Bucchino J, Vane A. The relative prevalence of various spiritual needs. *Scot J Healthcare Chaplain.* 2006;9(2):25–30.
118. Breitbart W, Rosenfeld B, Pessin H, et al. Depression, hopelessness, and desire for hastened death in terminally ill patients with cancer. *JAMA.* 2000;284(22):2907–2911.
119. Meier DE, Emmons CA, Wallersten S, Quill T, Morrison S, Cassel CK. A national survey of physician-assisted suicide and euthanasia in the United States. *N Engl J Med.* 1998;338(17):1193–1201.
120. Breitbart W, Rosenfeld B, Gibson C, et al. Meaning-centered group psychotherapy for patients with advanced cancer: A pilot randomized controlled trial. *Psycho-Oncology.* 2010;19(1):21–28.
121. Nekolaichuk CL, Bruera E. On the nature of hope in palliative care. *J Palliat Care.* 1998;14(1):36–42.
122. Dufault K, Martocchio BC. Hope: Its spheres and dimensions. *Nurs Clin North Am.* 1985;20(2):379–391.
123. Olsman E, Leget C, Onwuteaka-Philipsen B, Wellems D. Should palliative care patients' hope be truthful, helpful or valuable? An interpretative synthesis of literature describing healthcare professionals' perspectives on hope of palliative care patients. *Palliat Med.* 2014;28(1):59–70.
124. Duggelby W, Degner L, Williams A, et al. Living with hope: Initial evaluation of a psychosocial hope intervention for older palliative home care patients. *J Pain Symptom Manage.* 2007;33:247–257.

CHAPTER 38

Grief Reactions

E. Alessandra Strada

Introduction

An experience of significant loss creates a wide range of emotional, cognitive, and physical responses that can be described as grief. Grief represents a complex component of the illness experience for patients and family caregivers from the time of diagnosis through treatment and transitions of care, in advanced illness, during the death and dying process, and in bereavement. "Bereavement" is defined as the state of having experienced the death of someone close. It is virtually impossible to fully understand the complex needs of a patient and a family without a deep understanding of how they conceptualize, experience, and express grief.

The Clinical Practice Guidelines for Quality Palliative Care identifies grief and bereavement care as a mandate for palliative care providers.[1] Thus developing expertise in understanding and addressing the experience and manifestation of grief reactions in patients and family caregivers is an essential component of person-centered and family-centered palliative care. It is important that palliative care providers of various disciplines—medicine, nursing, social work, psychology, spiritual care, music therapy, and others—develop assessment skills to allow a deep understanding of grief reactions within their discipline. Sharing their assessments will then allow palliative care providers to work collaboratively for the development of interdisciplinary care plans. It is evident that the ability to effectively and compassionately communicate with patients and family caregivers, as well as with members of the care team, about grief reactions underscores quality care.

Every palliative care patient and family caregiver experiences loss, and therefore grief, in a profoundly personal manner, shaped and modulated by a multitude of psychosocial variables, including personal history, cultural practices and values, and spiritual and religious beliefs and affiliations.[2,3] While grief reactions are a common and probably universal component of human experience, the grieving process affects the fundamental domains of an individual's existence and significantly impacts his or her cognitive, psychological, social, behavioral, spiritual, and physical functioning. And yet, it is not an illness or a disease to treat. The experience of grief in the context of serious and advanced illness can be a powerful catalyst for psycho-spiritual growth and allow for deepening of relationships and mutual support between patients and their caregivers. Similarly, while distressing and painful, the grieving process after the death of a loved person can slowly be integrated into a meaningful life narrative for the griever.

On the other hand, the physical and emotional distress elicited by grief can become unmanageable and seriously threaten the psychological well-being of those affected. The varieties and intensity of grief reactions that can be observed in the palliative care setting can range from contained sadness to overt despair; they can include distressing physical manifestations and trigger major depressive episodes, anxiety disorders, and even transient psychotic reactions. Therefore, while grief is not a disease, it may develop into one if the pain of loss cannot be managed and integrated.

Caring for patients and families during their grief reactions can be challenging. Confusion exists about what grief is and how it is experienced and expressed. The question of what manifestations represent pathology and what types of interventions are best suited to assist grievers are still being actively debated in the scholarly literature. Patients and family caregivers often describe manifestations and "symptoms" that are confusing or concerning to them, because they do not appear directly related to their grieving process, nor are symptoms characteristic of that individual's range of response. For example, a transient period of even significant difficulty in the areas of memory, concentration, focus, and overall functioning can be completely normal and adaptive in bereavement. However, these experiences may trigger a sense of loss of control that may be profoundly alien and distressing. Thus palliative care providers' ability to sensitively and competently communicate with patients and families is of critical importance at all stages of illness. While palliative care providers should never pathologize a grieving process that is following a normal course, they also should never trivialize the presence of severe distress by labeling it "normal grieving." Providers need to identify and address risk factors and other contributing variables to the development of pathological grief reactions. Care plans can then be implemented to adequately minimize the impact of risk factors and facilitate access to professional support for patients and families when needed.

This chapter reviews key concepts and aspects of grief reactions common in the palliative care setting, with a focus on anticipatory (preparatory) grief and bereavement. Current conceptualizations of grief are discussed to help palliative care providers understand grief reactions. In addition, elements of clinical assessment, differential diagnosis, and care planning are presented to help healthcare providers integrate and translate clinical information into care planning. The overall goal is to emphasize the importance of developing skillful communication in these areas.

Theoretical Frameworks for Understanding Grief Reactions

The understanding and conceptualization of grief reactions has evolved significantly over the years. Early grief studies focused nearly exclusively on bereavement and differentiating nonpathological from pathological forms. Frameworks were focused on identifying the right way to grieve and on the role of detaching emotionally from the deceased as a path to effective mourning.[4] Additionally, it was believed that a significant amount of expressed emotional distress, termed "grief work," was necessary to the grieving process.[5] Otherwise, "absent grief" would remain symbolically lodged in the body and psyche, with the potential of creating significant health and emotional disruption later on.[6] Furthermore, the grieving process was conceptualized as a series of stages or phases, each defined by a predominant emotional state.[7,8] Finally, researchers studied the difference between pathological and nonpathological forms of bereavement, emphasizing the difference between mourning and the development of melancholia, which indicated a depressive syndrome.[4]

Large empirical studies have provided data on bereaved individuals in different population groups and have assisted in the development of recent theoretical frameworks, such as the Dual Process Model, used to conceptualize the nature, manifestations, and course of grief reactions. Perhaps the most important contribution to the current conceptualization of grief reactions is the recognition of the uniqueness of the grieving process to each individual and family. The empirical literature has not supported the concept of linear stages or phases in mourning. Bereaved individuals often experience contrasting emotions at the same time and oscillate between them. Instead of focusing on ensuring individuals are grieving the "correct" way, the emphasis is now on recognizing the multiple variables that affect the grieving process, as well as the particular individual style of expressing grief. Thus the main goal of grief and bereavement care is to support the individual's unique and personal grieving process without a preconceived notion of how that process should present or develop.

With this new appreciation of how personal, unique, and unpredictable grief reactions are, studies have focused on identifying risk factors for developing bereavement complications,[9,10] such as bereavement-related depression[11] and persistent complex bereavement disorder.[12] While early grief conceptualizations emphasized the importance of emotionally detaching from the deceased, recent conceptualizations, such as the Continuing Bonds model, have highlighted the value of maintaining an emotional connection with the memory of the deceased.[13] Additionally, as described in the Dual Process Model, the grieving process is now generally understood as a process of fluctuating between moments of restorative grief, with engagement in life-enhancing activities, and loss-oriented grief, with significant distress.[14,15] For example, after the death of a spouse, a griever may experience frequent pangs of pain resulting in crying spells lasting for several hours. However, even after a distressing crying spell, the same griever may experience a change in emotional state and be able to get dressed to attend a grandson's graduation, connecting with loved ones with genuine feelings of contentment, perhaps even sharing positive stories about the deceased spouse.

In contrast with the early belief that every bereaved individual should experience significant distress as a necessary part of mourning, recent research has emphasized the role of resilience.[17,18] Research has indicated that some bereaved individuals who have had a close relationship with the deceased will be able to return to a good functioning level relatively soon after the loss, without experiencing disabling distress.

Palliative care providers have several important communication tasks in this area (Box 38.1 and Box 38.2). For example, some patients and families are not familiar with the manifestations of grief and will benefit from psycho-education in this area. Others may have misconceptions and old beliefs about the

---

Box 38.1 Basic Communication Skills in Grief and Bereavement

- Elicit descriptions of patient's and caregiver's personal experience of loss
  - "What has it been like for you since you received the diagnosis?"
- Explain that the grieving process affects every thought and emotion in a person's life
- Provide information and facilitate access to professional and community resources
- Normalize through education by explaining normal range of experiences
  - Emphasize that others experience similar symptoms
  - Acknowledge that although it doesn't feel normal, grief is normal
- Use simple language and avoid technical terms
- Listen carefully for any metaphors used by the patient/caregiver and explore meaning

---

Box 38.2 Team Communication for Grief and Bereavement Care

- Identify and monitor patient's and family caregiver's existing risk factors for complications of grief reactions (i.e., depression, complicated grief)
- Discuss ongoing team support needed for patients and caregivers with high-risk factors
- Educate team members that an individual recently bereaved can be diagnosed with major depression
- Develop and implement care plans for delivery of evidence-based interventions
- Make a team decision on what terms will be used to discuss grief
  - Complicated grief or prolonged grief disorder
- Provide education so that team members are able to recognize signs of disenfranchised grief
- Encourage team members to reflect on their own loss and grief history in order to recognize patient's/family member's grieving process and their needs. Explore the following areas:
  - Self-awareness in the area of emotional experience and expression of grief
  - Personal loss and grief history
  - Personal grieving style
  - Countertransference reactions when witnessing others' grieving process

grieving process. Bereaved caregivers may express concern about whether they are "grieving the right way" or "the healthy way," whether the distress they are experiencing is normal, or whether their apparent lack of distress is normal. Because of the old belief that all bereaved persons should experience great distress during their grieving process, those who appear to be adjusting relatively well to the loss relatively soon may feel guilty about "not suffering enough." Others may become concerned about the degree of distress they are experiencing. Thus supportive psycho-education, normalization of symptoms whenever possible, and ongoing assessment to recognize complications of grief and bereavement are necessary elements of competent care.

Classification of Grief Reactions in Palliative Care

Grief is a multidimensional construct that can be divided into subtypes, depending on the setting, phenomenology, and manifestations. Furthermore, grief-related terms describing separate processes are often used interchangeably, creating confusion for providers. Some providers might feel that focusing on constructs and terminology is somewhat artificial and does not help us better appreciate the grieving experience. Nonetheless, while the essence of grief experiences may appear to be substantially similar person to person, they raise different concerns and risk factors for grievers that need to be appropriately addressed. In fact, the growing body of research literature has prompted the creation of new terminology considered more adequate to describe particular grief reactions. Knowledge of the accurate and recent terminology commonly used in the context of grief reactions is of considerable use for palliative care providers, both for patient care and for communication between members of the care team. Academic knowledge in this area should be used in synergy with the emotional and personal experiences of patients and caregivers. For this reason, one of the main communication challenges for providers is to translate academic knowledge into information that is clinically and practically meaningful and can be communicated to patients and caregivers to help them put their experiences in context and process the pain of loss.

Grief-related terms indicating the same type of grief reaction are frequently used interchangeably in the grief and bereavement literature. For example, "anticipatory grief" and "preparatory grief" both describe the grieving process occurring prior to the patient's death. In this chapter, the term "anticipatory grief" is used, specifying whether it applies to the patient or to the family caregiver. Similarly, "complicated grief," "prolonged grief disorder," and the newly proposed term "complex persistent bereavement disorder" all indicate a bereavement process marked by severe morbidity representing a clinical disorder. Because it is frequently used in the professional literature and it is familiar to most providers, the term "complicated grief" is used in this chapter.

Loss and Grief

Grief represents the normal reaction to loss, which can be generally defined as the experience of being deprived of something or someone important.[19] While each individual responds to loss differently, in most cases a certain degree of distress for variable periods of time is to be expected. Even though bereaved caregivers have been studied most, palliative care patients who are grieving their own loss of health and decline or approaching death may experience intense preparatory grief resulting in significant overall distress.[20,21]

Every patient and family will grieve in unique ways, because their response to loss is personal and unique. Within a family, there may be different perceptions about what represents a loss and how its impact is experienced. Healthcare providers should not assume that all family members will experience, process, and express grief in the same way. In many cases, differences in these areas can, if not recognized and addressed, create conflict within a family. The ability to grieve together as a family and support one another during a difficult time of loss and grief may require skillful and sensitive psycho-education about grief to clarify expectations, assumptions, and misunderstandings.

Losses are commonly divided into two general categories: physical losses and symbolic or psychosocial losses.[22,23] The experience of palliative care patients and their families is characterized by numerous losses, starting at the time of diagnosis. There may be physical losses, such as the loss of body parts and disfigurement due to surgical treatments and worsening of illness. There may also be several and often ongoing symbolic or psychosocial losses, such as loss of a sense of identity, loss of a particular role in the family due to the illness, loss of meaning and purpose, or loss of a sense of hope. While physical losses are easily recognized by external observers, symbolic losses may not be obvious, but they can have even a stronger impact on patients and families.

Grief and bereavement care starts with providers' ability to understand the types of losses experienced by a particular patient and family and their impact on everyone's well-being. It is helpful to note whether they are making a connection between the experience of loss and the pain of grief. People who are grieving may not recognize their distressing physical and emotional experiences as part of a natural grieving process. This is because, while it is emphasized that "grief is normal," it actually does not feel normal. Therefore, patients and family caregivers may not notice the connection between their grief and a sudden decrease in the ability to concentrate, altered emotional responses, a decline in short-term memory, or the presence of pain, aches, and gastrointestinal distress.

It is helpful to use neutral and gentle language and open questions to elicit descriptions of patients' and caregivers' personal experiences of loss; for example, the question, "What has it been like for you since you received the diagnosis?" is an open question that allows answers at different levels of depth. Carefully noticing both the content expressed and the affect, tone of voice, and nonverbal communication provides a wealth of information about the patient's and family's internal experience. Nonverbal communication becomes an even more critical source of information when the patient and the family are not fully fluent in the language spoken by the provider or when there are significant cultural differences. In this case, it would not be appropriate to rely primarily on the spoken language as a source of nuanced communication.

The metaphor of a *journey* is sometimes used to explore patients' and families' experiences (i.e., "What has this journey been like for you?") While some patients may resonate with the metaphor of the journey, others will not and may find it irritating, because they associate positive images and emotions to the word "journey" and do not feel that the disease with which they were diagnosed carries any positive association. It is also important to recognize potential problems with the use of possessive adjectives when talking to patients. For example, referring to "your diagnosis [cancer, pain, loss]" may be perceived by the patient as creating an uncomfortable sense of intimacy with the disease and its consequences. In these circumstances, a subtle resentment may be created. Other patients will intentionally use the expression "my cancer," especially when they want to emphasize a sort of negotiated relationship with the disease that feels empowering to them.

In essence, it is important to use neutral language when exploring patients' and families' history of loss. Over time, metaphors often come directly from them, as well as particular interpretations about their situation. And it must be recognized that as a conversation organically unfolds and reaches different depths, a synergy is created where healthcare provider and patient and/or family exchange perceptions in a more personal and less neutral manner. However, initial communication in the clinical setting about grief reactions should not cloud the core experience of the patient and the family as it is developing.

Anticipatory Grief

This term refers to the grieving process experienced by patients and their family caregivers that occurs prior to the actual death.[24] The experience and manifestation of anticipatory grief can have significantly different presentations in patients and caregivers, even in members of the same family. Anticipatory grief in palliative care patients specifically indicates their personal grief, as the unique psychological adaptation process they experience in the context of transitions of care, worsening illness, and approaching death.[25] While it may cause significant distress, it generally does not represent pathology. However, it may become severe and trigger depressive episodes, especially in patients who have a prior history of depression. While preparatory grief and depression can coexist, it is important to differentiate between the two conditions. In preparatory grief, patients' moods generally fluctuate, and they retain the ability to enjoy the company of loved ones and look forward to special occasions. Their self-esteem is generally intact and, while they may feel guilt related to behaviors that may have had a negative impact on their health (e.g., smoking, IV drug use), they do not generally feel irrational guilt.

In depression, patients feel low or sad most of the time and may experience a sense of worthlessness. Additionally, they may develop the belief that no one cares about them or that they do not deserve the care they are receiving. In depression, these beliefs are very hard to modify, even in the presence of evidence to the contrary. As a result, the patient may withdraw emotionally from family and/or become less talkative and engaged in what used to be a source of pleasure, meaning, and comfort.[26-28]

Anticipatory grief in family caregivers should be monitored carefully. While it indicates a normal process, it may also become unmanageable. The early belief that experiencing significant grief before the death of a loved one could facilitate integration of the loss and ease the bereavement process has not been supported by empirical and clinical evidence. High levels of anticipatory grief in caregivers may become a risk factor for increased morbidity during bereavement. Palliative care team members should provide more intense support to caregivers who present risk factors and whose behaviors raise concern. Significant risk factors for complications of bereavement in family caregivers are previous psychiatric history, high levels of ambivalence in the relationship with the patient, inability to accept or process the patient's prognosis, financial stressors, history of domestic abuse, substance abuse, and current health problems.[29-31]

Characteristics of Noncomplicated Bereavement

Bereavement indicates the state of having experienced the death of someone close and involves a grieving process of variable duration and intensity.[32] It is characterized by a constellation of physical, cognitive, emotional, and spiritual manifestations varying in duration and severity. Physical symptoms of loss may include shortness of breath, tightness in the throat, feeling of emptiness and heaviness, physical numbness, feeling outside one's body, body aches, headaches, dizziness, nausea, gastrointestinal problems, and heart palpitations. Commonly experienced somatic symptoms are similar to those present in depression. They are crying spells, fatigue, disturbances in sleeping and eating patterns, anorexia, weight loss, lack of strength, and loss of sexual desire or hypersexualiy.[33,34] Noncomplicated bereavement can also include transient perceptual disturbances, such as visual and auditory hallucinations, impaired short-term memory, and constant worry, slowed and disorganized thinking, passive suicidal ideation, and constant preoccupation with the deceased. The content of the perceptual disturbances may be focused on difficult circumstances surrounding the death or on unresolved relationship issues that may elicit guilt, anger, or shame. While a grieving process may enhance and deepen one's connection with a faith or spiritual community, it may also result in conflicts in faith beliefs or loss of meaning and purpose.[35] Studies have shown that noncomplicated bereavement can have a significant impact on cardiac function and immune and neuroendocrine function.[36,37]

While the effects of bereavement can create significant distress for variable periods of time, with adequate psycho-social and spiritual support, the majority of bereaved individuals are able to slowly integrate the loss, process the pain of grief, maintain or regain the ability to function adequately for their life demands, and maintain acceptable physical and emotional health. The length of time necessary for the loss to be processed and integrated is variable, unique to the individual, and often unpredictable. For some individuals, highly distressing manifestations of grief may be experienced immediately after the death. In other cases, bereavement involves an initial period of shock, disbelief, or denial, often followed by a phase characterized by distressing physical and emotional symptoms. And, for some, grief may be suppressed for weeks or months.

Complications of Bereavement

Complicated Grief

The past decade has seen a significant amount of research aimed at understanding the nature of grief and its manifestations, distinguishing what is commonly referred to as normal bereavement from pathological forms. Even though the majority of bereaved individuals are able to integrate the loss of a loved one after a variable period of time, 15% to 25% of bereaved individuals continue to experience maladaptive reactions and psychiatric symptoms that significantly impair their level of functioning. Complicated grief has been associated with increased risk for major depressive disorder, anxiety disorders (posttraumatic stress disorder, generalized anxiety disorder, panic disorder), hypertension, cardiac events, and overall significantly reduced quality of life.[39] The symptoms overlap with other psychiatric disorders, making diagnosis challenging. The terms "complicated grief," "prolonged grief disorder," and, more recently, "persistent complex bereavement" all refer to the morbidity caused by grief that is not effectively processed and integrated by the individual. As a result, the distressing symptoms continue to cause severe and disabling impairment long after the loss has occurred.

While complicated grief and prolonged grief disorder were proposed for inclusion as formal diagnoses in the *Diagnostic and Statistical Manual of Mental Disorders* (5th ed.; *DSM-5*), the DSM-5 Task Force concluded that insufficient evidence exists to support inclusion. Instead, persistent complex bereavement disorder was included as a condition warranting further study. The criteria include features of complicated grief and prolonged grief disorder; however, they should not be used clinically as they are intended for research purposes.[40] While the creation of additional terminology may help standardize future research, the terms "complicated grief" or "prolonged grief disorder" are familiar to the majority of palliative care providers.

It is important to recognize that palliative care patients may also be experiencing complicated grief from unprocessed past deaths of loved ones, especially if they have sustained multiple losses over a short period of time. Therefore, assessment of current condition and risk factors for developing pathological grief reactions should be carefully considered for both patients and families.

Bereavement-Related Depression

Major depression can become a complication of bereavement. Because of the significant overlap in physical, emotional, and cognitive manifestations, differentiating between the two can be challenging, especially in the early phases of bereavement. In some cases, bereavement and depression may coexist, which may further impair the individual's ability to integrate the loss and process grief. In the past decade, the question of whether bereavement-related depression is substantially different from depression developing in the context of other factors and circumstances has been debated in the research and scholarly literature.[41] As a result, the new edition of the *DSM* (*DSM-5*) has eliminated the bereavement exclusion criterion from the diagnostic criteria of major depressive episode. This change implies that an individual who is recently bereaved can also be diagnosed with major depression. Differentiating depression from bereavement in the acute stages of grief can be challenging. Generally speaking, in bereavement, the individual maintains the ability to emotionally connect with others and be consoled by loved ones; suicidal ideation is rare, and, when present, it is focused on joining the loved one; the pain of loss is mixed with good memories about the relationship; grieving is often experienced as moments of profound distress, alternating with the ability to feel connection to others.[42–44] Recognizing depression in the bereaved will allow providers to develop an appropriate bereavement care plan. Generally speaking, while grief is characterized by mood fluctuation with an ability to experience positive emotions, albeit briefly, clinical depression often presents with constantly depressed mood that often does not respond to emotional support. Additionally, basic self-esteem is generally maintained in grief; however, clinical depression is often characterized by a sense of profound worthlessness and guilt.[20]

Disenfranchised Grief

This term refers to grief reactions for losses that are not supported or recognized as such by community or societal norms. Here the grieving person feels less social permission to express grief and is at risk for not receiving adequate support.[45] Examples of disenfranchised grief are grieving a miscarriage, the death of a pet, or the death of a family member in prison. Grieving the death of someone close who died by suicide is also an example, due to feelings of shame and guilt often present in survivors. Bereavement of older lesbians also has the potential for being disenfranchised.[46] When the grieving process is not recognized or supported by their community, bereaved individuals are forced to grieve privately, as if their grief needs to be a secret, with their emotions suppressed when in the presence of others. Disenfranchised grievers may feel as if they do not have "the right" to express their emotions, or they may feel embarrassed about their grief and may remain caught in a vicious cycle that impairs their ability to allow the grieving process to occur. Palliative care providers should be able to recognize when individuals are at risk for experiencing disenfranchised grief. For example, former spouses or partners who still feel emotionally connected to the patient but are not welcomed by the current family may have difficulty receiving support during their grieving process. There may also be family members who had a conflictual relationship with the patient and are now attempting to reconnect. Reconciliations and reconnections after years of alienation among family members are not always possible, or even desirable, and palliative care providers should never force this agenda on the patient or the family. However, it must be recognized that this situation may leave some survivors without the necessary support network to facilitate a normal grieving process.

The Importance of Self-Awareness for Palliative Care Providers

Because loss is such a common part of the human experience, palliative care providers commonly have experienced grief, both in their personal and their professional lives. However, while familiarity with loss and grief will help providers feel compassion and empathy for their patients and families, it will not automatically translate into needed communication skills. Grief is a highly personal, unique experience for healthcare providers as well as patients and family caregivers. It is important that providers be able to reflect on their own grief in order to recognize another's grieving process and address their needs.

Self-awareness involves providers' ability to engage in a personal reflective dialogue that allows exploration and recognition of their own core values, belief systems, and behaviors that characterize their own experience of grief reactions to loss. Knowledge of one's own relationship with loss and grief and the ability to recognize the impact of personal, social, and cultural variables on how grief is processed is of crucial importance to recognize and manage countertransference reactions. It allows palliative care providers to preserve important personal and professional boundaries without imposing their own countertransference or even ongoing grieving process on patients and families. Then it becomes possible to establish a bond with patients and families based on a compassionate recognition of their grief and an ability to honor it, support it, and provide professional guidance and intervention when necessary.[47] In essence, self-awareness can be framed as an ability to connect or communicate with one's self by engaging in exploration of the following areas:

Self-awareness in the area of emotional experience and expression of grief

Personal loss and grief history

Personal grieving style

Countertransference reactions when witnessing others' grieving process

Awareness of personal values, belief systems, and emotional responses in these areas will prove of significant value for providers' development. Perhaps most important, it allows them to lay aside any personal agenda or countertransference reaction in their work with patients and families.

Developing an Anticipatory Grief and Bereavement Plan of Care

The third domain of palliative care under the National Quality Project guidelines, the psychological and psychiatric domain of care, includes specific guidelines and best-practice models for the delivery of grief and bereavement care. This care begins at the time of diagnosis and continues throughout the illness, during the dying process, and in bereavement. It is offered to the patient and caregivers, with the recognition that each individual's unique responses need to be recognized and supported. Grief reactions are part of the fabric of interactions and relationships between patients, family caregivers, and all palliative care team members during all phases of care. And while palliative care's intensive approach is to relieve suffering and improve quality of life, it can also become the stage for emotionally difficult conversations about goals of care in advanced illness.

Communication with patients and family caregivers about grief reactions involves conveying information in a manner that is clear, supportive, and nonjudgmental. It also involves an ongoing collaborative exchange that includes delivering information; checking for understanding; calibrating the delivery; and eliciting questions, comments, and reflections. Ultimately, communication with patients and caregivers allows all parties to move toward a reasonable plan that is believed to be realistic, beneficial, and, most important, agreed upon.

Grief and bereavement care begins at the initial contact with the palliative care team and continues during the death and dying process and in bereavement. Before the patient's death, attention should be focused on providing anticipatory grief assessment and treatment to both the patient and the family; after the death, the plan should focus on facilitating normal grieving in bereaved caregivers. The areas of assessment and care planning are summarized in the following.

Current Concerns and Sources of Grief

The palliative care team should explore patients' and caregivers' concerns and sources of grief. Team members should facilitate expression of beliefs, thoughts, and emotions related to the experience of loss and grief, as well as patients' and caregivers' questions and concerns. It is important that providers not base their assessments and care plans merely on assumptions or impressions. It is best to gently ask if the patients' and/or family members' understanding is accurate, so that the care plan will provide personalized care.

Risk Factors and Comorbid Conditions

The palliative care team should evaluate the impact of the grieving process on the individual, risk factors, presence of comorbid-conditions, development of complications (i.e., depression, exacerbation of prior psychiatry illness). Additionally, team members need to evaluate the effectiveness of current coping strategies. Before the death, level of function and risk level should be monitored on a regular basis in both patients and caregivers, especially when they are vulnerable, socially isolated, or have a history of psychiatric illness. Providers should remember that every assessment is valid at the point in time when it is performed, and there is no guarantee that it will not change. Sudden health crises or unexpected psychosocial stressors may intensify grief reactions and cause the distress to become unmanageable. For example, patients described as "coping well" may have believed that somehow the illness would not continue to worsen and may experience profound and disabling grief reactions as they begin noticing a significant decline in function. Similarly, family caregivers who had been described as "prepared for the death" may begin experiencing significant distress months after the death and become overwhelmed by it.

Psycho-Education and Emotional Support Needs

Patients and their family members must be educated, separately or together, about the range and uniqueness of grief reactions, and unsupportive beliefs need to be clarified (e.g., I am not grieving the right way; I should not be feeling these emotions; I should not be thinking these thoughts, etc.). When providing supportive psycho-education to patients and caregivers, it is important to explain the normal range of manifestations of distress in anticipatory grief and in bereavement. The provider should listen carefully to the individual's experience and normalize whenever possible by educating and emphasizing that many experience similar symptoms when grieving. They should acknowledge that, while grief is normal, it does not feel normal, and it is only natural to have concerns about what one is experiencing. Describing the most common manifestations can be helpful, especially in the areas that are concerning to them. For example, if a bereaved caregiver reports difficulty with short-term memory, it is useful to clarify that this is, though unwelcome, a normal component of bereavement. The provider can also explain that several tasks the bereaved person used to perform without any difficulty, such as reading a book, may now require special effort; they may find it necessary to read the same page several times. They may lose objects more frequently or have significant difficulty remembering appointments, or even people's names. It is helpful to explain that the grieving process affects every thought and emotion and that, for some time, it may seem the mind does not have space for anything other than the pain of grief.

Plan and Recommend Referrals

The healthcare provider can expand patients' and families' possibilities for healing during the grieving process by providing information about or facilitating access to professional and community resources. If depression develops in the context of anticipatory grief, the provider should consider a combined and integrated approach that includes psychotherapy and medication. Treatment decisions will be made based on the patient's current level of functioning, ability to engage in psychotherapy, and burden versus benefit of including antidepressant medication. Integrative approaches, such as music therapy, and art therapy should always be considered, if acceptable and indicated, for their potential to bring well-being and facilitate connection.[48-50] If the patient or family is raising issues that indicate spiritual distress, referral to a professional chaplain or other community religious resource may be indicated.

When working with bereaved caregivers, it may be necessary to provide referrals to primary care physicians and/or bereavement services. As part of this task, palliative team members should explain the relevance of the referral and why it is important to follow up. For example, if the bereaved caregiver reports that his or her sleep is persistently disrupted, it is important to explain that rest is important to support the grieving process. Similarly, if they report using maladaptive strategies to disconnect from the pain of grief, such as binging on alcohol, using drugs, or taking more of certain prescribed medication such as opioids or benzodiazepines, a physician and, ideally, a mental health professional, should be involved in the bereavement care plan. Bereaved caregivers may resist the suggestion to reach out for professional support due to a lack of physical and emotional energy, lack of motivation, and difficulty imagining that their suffering can be relieved. In this case, healthcare providers can reframe the referral as a way of expanding opportunities to facilitate the mourning process. Providers should never minimize or underestimate the impact of maladaptive coping strategies developed in the bereavement context.

Case Example: Jack and Millie

Consider the following case scenario to illustrate the aspects previously described.

Jack and Millie have been referred to the palliative care outpatient clinic for pain management by Jack's oncologist. Jack is a 67-year-old African American man who was diagnosed 3 months ago with pancreas cancer metastatic to the liver. After the diagnosis, chemotherapy was started, with the goal to slow progression. Jack is a widower; his wife died 2 years ago of colon cancer. He has no children. Jack used to teach math in high school, but he retired following his wife's death. He met Millie in church 1 year ago. She is 65 years old and also a widow. Jack and Millie live separately but are close. Millie would like to live with him, but Jack feels he does not have enough energy to be with someone for prolonged periods of time.

Jack's pain has increased significantly and is less controlled with the medication regimen prescribed by his oncologist. He also experiences more nausea. He has difficulty sleeping at night, is fatigued, and has been losing weight. He reports that his mood has been very low since his wife's death. He still cries when he thinks about her and has difficulty stopping. When Millie is with him, she attempts to comfort him, and he appears to respond to her attention. Jack describes himself as a devout Catholic who felt strongly supported by his faith until his wife's death. He now wonders if God cares about him and if anything that he believes in is true.

Jack is aware that his prognosis is poor, and he may have only a few more months to live. He tearfully explains that when he looks in the mirror he no longer recognizes himself, but he does not elaborate. Millie explains that lately Jack has become more withdrawn, and he will spend hours on the couch watching TV without interacting with her. She feels lonely and sometimes hopeless, because she would like to help Jack but does not know how. Millie describes herself as an extrovert who likes being around people, and she would like Jack to be more social. As Millie describes her feelings, Jack becomes tearful and shakes his head, complaining of pain in his abdomen.

Anticipatory Grief Assessment and Plan
Concerns and Sources of Grief

Jack is still actively grieving his wife's death, which is a source of sadness. His life has changed drastically since her death; he has stopped working and has become increasingly socially isolated. In addition, while he still goes to church, he has developed doubts and is indirectly questioning his faith. This situation also represents a significant loss because Jack used to rely on his faith as an important source of meaning and purpose.

Additionally, as Jack stated, he no longer recognizes himself in the mirror; he is grieving the change in his personal appearance. It is important to explore how this loss is affecting him and if it is affecting the relationship with Millie. Jack's expression of sadness about the progressive change in personal appearance should be approached with deep listening and supportive presence. Attempting to bypass his grief would be clinically contraindicated. Instead, the palliative care provider should allow Jack to openly grieve, while at the same time reassuring him that the team will support him every step of the way.

The provider should also gently explore if Jack's sense of self and personal identity have been affected. One approach is to ask Jack how he has defined himself in the past in terms of personality and core values and explore if he would still describe himself that way. The steps of this intervention could be described as (a) allow Jack to openly express his grief, providing a calming and empathic presence; (b) reassure Jack that the team will be with him through all the changes and challenges that the disease may cause; (c) gently ask about the aspects of his personality that he values the most or that other people value the most about him (Millie can be asked, if she is present, whether the aspects of Jack's personality that she appreciates the most are still present, in spite of the disease); and (d) gently refocus Jack's attention, helping him also notice that the essence of who he is has not changed and then exploring how this awareness is affecting him.

Risk Factors and Comorbid Conditions

Given his current symptoms, it is important to evaluate Jack for depression and complicated grief. His mood is low most of the time; he is often tearful. Some of the somatic symptoms he is experiencing, such as fatigue and weight loss, are also typical of advanced illness. Thus the palliative care provider should focus on the psychological rather than somatic symptoms of depression, which overlap with symptoms of advanced illness. Additionally, the provider should be aware that pancreatic cancer and depression are often comorbid.

Psycho-Educational and Emotional Support

A caregiver support group may be appropriate for Millie, considering her extrovert personality and desire to connect with other people. Just because Jack values his faith and religious affiliation and he and Millie met in church, it should not be assumed that Millie shares his beliefs at this time or that she still feels supported by her faith community. Therefore, her personal relationship with spirituality and/or religion should be explored. Also, she should be asked about her health status and whether she is facing any challenges in that area.

Plan and Recommend Referrals

The following is a sample plan for dealing with Jack and Millie's situation.

- Conduct a throughout evaluation for depression and complicated grief on Jack and, if positive, consider appropriateness of a pharmacological approach, individual psychotherapy, or both. A combined approach, if indicated, seems feasible in this case as Jack's prognosis is in the order of months.

- Explore with Jack whether he would like to see a professional chaplain or be more connected to a priest from his church to restore his ability to use his faith as a source of strength and support. Jack may also wish to discuss his spiritual distress and concerns with a medical or psychosocial provider he feels close to, sharing his deepest and most meaningful beliefs and thoughts. Palliative care providers of all disciplines should develop a level of comfort exploring the spiritual and existential domain with patients and caregivers and providing emphatic and reflective listening. This ability certainly does not replace the need for a professional spiritual care provider, but it represents an example of integrated interdisciplinary care.

- Provide Millie with psycho-education and encouragement. Explore her sense of hopelessness and reframe it as a strong desire to help Jack. A provider may say, "The situation is very challenging right now, and you are so committed to helping Jack. It's only normal to feel overwhelmed or even hopeless sometimes, not knowing exactly what to do. Perhaps we could talk about this together for a while and see how we can develop a practical plan to support you both." Help her focus on the positive impact of her presence on Jack's grief.

- Evaluate Millie's risk factors for complicated grief.

The palliative care team should coordinate care so that Jack's dying process will reflect his wishes (dying at home perhaps with hospice care versus dying at the hospital) and that Millie will receive optimal support during that time. The team should ensure that Jack's pain and symptoms are adequately managed during the dying process. This will not only prevent and relieve Jack's suffering but will also protect Millie from being exposed to traumatic images and lasting memories of distress in her loved one.

After Jack's death, the palliative team should facilitate Millie's connection with the bereavement team, since she will be the primary bereaved caregiver. It is important to note that bereaved caregivers may decline bereavement care initially and seek it later on. Furthermore, bereavement care can take many forms and should be individualized to meet the individual's needs. Similar to the anticipatory grief plan, the bereavement care plan includes an assessment component and a plan component. The assessment component is a gentle exploration of the bereaved individual's current challenges in the physical and psycho-social-spiritual domains. The plan lists the therapeutic interventions recommended in each case. In this particular case, a bereavement coordinator phoned Millie 1 month after Jack's death; the bereavement coordinator assessed and discussed Millie's grieving process and concerns. The following indicates areas that should be explored; this bereavement assessment and care plan is detailed in Table 38.1.

Bereavement Assessment and Care Plan

Physical Domain

How does Millie feel overall? Has she lost or gained weight? Is she taking her medication as prescribed? How is she sleeping? What

Table 38.1 Bereavement Care Assessment and Plan: Areas for Exploration

Physical Domain	Emotional Domain	Cognitive Domain	Spiritual Domain
♦ Sleep	♦ Anxiety	♦ Memory	♦ Currently Supported by faith or spiritual community?
♦ Eating patterns	♦ Depression	♦ Focus	
♦ Physical Symptoms	♦ Panic	♦ Concentration	♦ Spiritual distress?
♦ Medication compliance	♦ Suicidal ideation		♦ Sense of alienation?
♦ Substance use			
Level of Support	**Overall Risk**	**Plan**	
♦ Adequate?	♦ Risk factors for complicated grief?	♦ Bereavement groups?	
♦ Unstable family situation?	♦ Depression?	♦ Individual counseling?	
♦ Social stressors?	♦ Suicide risk	♦ Bereavement phone calls?	
		♦ Referral to mental health professionals?	
		♦ Coordination with other medical providers?	

are her sleeping patterns? Does she have nightmares or wake up in the middle of the night with severe anxiety?

As mentioned previously, while difficulty sleeping and severe anxiety is often to be expected, sleep that is persistently disrupted will interfere with the bereaved person's ability to integrate the loss.

Emotional Domain
Is Millie tearful during the encounter or phone call? If yes, is she able to stop crying? Does she feel even minimally better after crying, or does she feel even more distressed? Is she experiencing severe anxiety, panic attacks, or shortness of breath? Can she catch her breath while talking? Is she concerned about how she is feeling? Does she express anger, guilt, or regrets? Is there a sense that she is feeling overwhelmed by these emotions? Does she describe suicidal thoughts?

Cognitive Domain
Is Millie experiencing significant memory and concentration impairment? How is this affecting her ability to take care of herself? If memory problems are present, are they interfering with her ability to take medication appropriately or go to medical appointments?

Spiritual Domain
If Millie belongs to a church or other spiritual community, is she still connected to it and receiving the level of support from it that she desires? Is she expressing spiritual and existential distress? Does she describe feeling disconnected from a sense of meaning and purpose in life?

Level of Support
Does Millie have family members or neighbors, friends who are helpful to her? Is she able to accept help, or is she isolating herself, refusing social contact? Does she feel that other family members and friends are allowing her to express grief in a manner that feels helpful to her? For example, is she allowed to cry when she needs to, or does she feel she must suppress her emotions, so that others will not worry about her? If she feels the need to suppress her reactions for periods of time during the day, does she find opportunities to be openly expressive about her grief?

Overall Risk
What is Millie's risk for developing complicated grief? The palliative team member should list all the elements that may represent risk factors for the bereaved individual. The presence of risk factors does not necessarily imply that complications will occur. However, risk factors may create higher vulnerability for the bereaved. Thus team members will need to monitor them and follow up more closely, so that assistance can be provided if needed.

What strategies is Millie using to deal with her current challenges? What does she think about her grieving process? Is she hopeful that things will improve for her? Is she able to imagine being able to continue living her life? Does she have any concerns about the intensity and severity of her grieving process? Would she benefit from supportive psycho-education? Would she benefit from more formal and structured support in the form of grief counseling or grief therapy? Does she need referrals to primary care physicians to discuss possible short-term use of pharmacotherapy to help with severe and constant anxiety or persistently disrupted sleep?

Considerations of the Plan

When making a plan for the griever, the information gathered during the assessment portion should be integrated into clinically meaningful and behavioral action. Elements of the care plan should be specific and goal-oriented, even when the goals are present-focused. General psycho-social terminology is not particularly useful. For example, "support" is a term that is often used in the context of bereavement care plans. It is important that healthcare providers describe what "support" means to a particular griever. Does the griever need more practical help with activities of daily living (e.g., in the case of an older individual)? Or does he or she need help processing traumatic memories related to the death (e.g., witnessing a loved one with poorly managed pain or uncontrolled hyperactive delirium)? Could the griever benefit from reassurance and education about the grieving process? Or does he or she need assistance setting healthy boundaries with other family members and friends who would like to talk about the loved one who died when the griever cannot tolerate it? In some cases, the griever may need assistance communicating with family members without creating alienation.

Conclusion

Grief and bereavement care are an essential component of patient- and family-centered palliative care. This care begins at the first contact with patients and families; it continues during transitions of care and during end-of-life care; and it refocuses on bereaved caregivers after the death of the patient. Grief and bereavement care can be challenging due to the uniqueness and unpredictability of the grieving process. Palliative care providers should be knowledgeable about current conceptualizations of grief that more accurately describe the grieving process. It is important that each palliative care patient and family member is supported in his or her experience and expression of grief. Furthermore, palliative care team members should closely monitor grief reactions and recognize possible complications, such as depression and complex persistent bereavement disorder. When these occur, it is crucial that the treatment plan include referrals to mental health professionals and pharmacological approaches be considered to decrease morbidity and assist the griever to slowly integrate the loss and process the pain of grief.

References

1. National Consensus Project for Quality Palliative Care. *Clinical Practice Guidelines for Quality Palliative Care*. Brooklyn, NY: National Consensus Project for Quality Palliative Care; 2013.
2. Attig T. *How We Grieve: Relearning the World*. New York, NY: Oxford University Press; 2011.
3. Stroebe M, Stroebe W, Hansson R, eds. Handbook of Bereavement. Cambridge, UK: Cambridge University Press; 1993.
4. Freud S. Mourning and melancholia. In: Strachey J, ed. and trans. *The Standard Edition of the Complete Psychological Works of Sigmund Freud*, Vol. 14. London: Hogarth; 1957:237–259.
5. Lindemann E. The symptomatology and management of acute grief. *Am J Psychiatry*. 1944; 101:141–148.
6. Deutch H. Absence of grief. *Psychoanal Q*. 1937;6:12–22.
7. Kubler-Ross E. *On Death and Dying*. New York, NY: Touchstone; 1969.

8. Kessler DA, Kubler-Ross E. *On Grief and Grieving: Finding the Meaning of Grief Through the Five Stages of Loss.* New York, NY: Scribner; 2007.
9. Shear MK, Shair H. Attachment, loss, and complicated grief. *Dev Psychobiol.* 2005;47(3):253–267.
10. Shear MK, Scritskaya NA. Bereavement and anxiety. *Curr Psychiatry Rep.* 2012;14(3):169–175.
11. Kendler KS, Myers J, Zisook S. Does bereavement-related major depression differ from major depression associated with other stressful life events? *Am J Psychiatry.* 2008;165(11):1449–1455.
12. American Psychiatric Association. *Diagnostic and Statistical Manual of Mental Disorders.* 5th ed. Washington, DC: American Psychiatric Association; 2013.
13. Klass D, Silverman PR, Nickman SL, eds. *Continuing Bonds: New Understandings of Grief.* Philadelphia, PA: Taylor & Francis; 1996.
14. Stroebe MS, Shut H. The dual process model of coping with bereavement: Rational and description. *Death Stud.* 1999;23:197–224.
15. Stroebe MS, Hansson RO, Stroebe W, Shut H, eds. *Handbook of Bereavement Research: Consequences, Coping, and Care.* Washington, DC: American Psychological Association.
16. Stroebe M, Shut H. The dual process model of coping with bereavement: A decade on. *Omega.* 2010;61(4):273–289.
17. Bonanno GA. Loss, trauma, and human resilience: Have we underestimated the human capacity to thrive after extremely adverse events? *Am Psychol.* 2004;59:20–28.
18. Bonanno GA. *The Other Side of Sadness: What the New Science of Bereavement Tells Us About Life After a Loss.* New York, NY: Basic Books; 2009.
19. Clieren M. *Bereavement and Adaptation: A Comparative Study of the Aftermath of Death.* Washington, DC: Hemisphere; 1993.
20. Strada EA. *The Helping Professional's Guide to End of Life Care.* Oakland, CA: New Harbinger; 2013.
21. Evans AJ. Anticipatory grief: A theoretical challenge. *Palliat Med.* 1994;8(2):159–165.
22. Pomeroy EC, Garcia RB. *The Grief Assessment and Intervention Workbook: A Strength-Based Perspective.* Belmont, CA; Brooks/Cole; 2009.
23. Parkes CM. *Love and Loss: The Roots of Love and Its Complications.* New York, NY: Routledge; 2006.
24. Rando TA, ed. *Clinical Dimensions of Anticipatory Mourning.* Champaign, IL: Research Press; 2000.
25. Cheng JO, Lo RS, Chan FM, Kwan BH, Woo J. An exploration of anticipatory grief in advanced cancer patients. *Psycho-Oncology* 2010;19(7):693–700.
26. Strada EA. Grief, demoralization, and depression: Diagnostic challenges and treatment modalities. *Prim Psychiatry.* 2009;16(5):49–55.
27. Endicott J. Measurement of depression in patients with cancer. *Cancer.* 1984;53:2243–2248.
28. Bennet J, Berndt N, Hunter L. Issues in bereavement: Preparatory grief vs. depression. *S D Med.* 2008;Spec:41–42.
29. Allen JY, Haley WE, Small BJ, et al. Bereavement among hospice caregivers of hospice caregivers of hospice patients one year following loss: Predictors of grief, complicated grief, and symptoms of depression. *J Pall Med.* 2013:16(7):745–751.
30. de Groot M, Kollen BJ. Course of bereavement over 8–10 years in first degree relatives and spouses of people who committed suicide: A longitudinal community based cohort study. *BMJ.* 2013;347:f5519.
31. Shear MK, Ghesquiere A, Glickman K. Bereavement and complicated grief. *Curr Psychiatry Rep.* 2013;15(11):406.
32. Raphael B, Dobson M. Bereavement. In: Harvey JH, Miller ED, eds. *Loss and Trauma.* Philadelphia, PA: Brunner Routledge; 2000:45–61.
33. Hensley PL, Clayton PJ. Bereavement: Signs, symptoms, and course. *Psychiatr Ann.* 2008;38:649–654.
34. Parkes C. *Bereavement: Studies of Grief in Adult Life.* 3rd ed. Madison, WI: International Universities Press; 1998.
35. Rosik CH. The impact of religious orientation in conjugal bereavement among older adults. *Int J Aging Human Devel.* 1989;28:251–260.
36. Hall M, Baum A, Buysse D, et al. Sleep as a mediator of the stress-immune relationship. *Psychosom Med.* 1998;60:48–51.
37. Lindstrom TC. Immunity and health after bereavement in relation to coping. *Scand J Psych.* 1997;38:253–259.
38. Miller MD. Complicated grief in late life. *Dialogues Clin Neurosci.* 2012;14(3):195–202.
39. Shear MK, Shair H. Attachment, loss, and complicated grief. *Dev Psychobiol.* 2005;47(3):253–267.
40. Boelen PA, Prigerson HG. The influence of prolonged grief disorder, depression, and anxiety on quality of life among bereaved adults. *Eur Arch Psychiatry Clin Neurosci.* 2007;257:444–452.
41. Shah SN, Meeks S. Late-life bereavement and complicated grief: A proposed comprehensive framework. *Aging Mental Health.* 2012;16(1):39–56.
42. Zisook S, Shear K. Grief and bereavement: What psychiatrists need to know. *World Psychiatry.* 2009;8(2):67–74.
43. Kessing LV, Bukh JD, Bock C, et al. Does bereavement-related first episode depression differ from other kinds of depression? *Soc Psychiatr Epidemiol.* 2010;45(8):801–808.
44. Ogrodniczuck J, Piper W, Joyce AS, et al. Differentiating symptoms of complicated grief and depression among psychiatry outpatients. *Can J Psychiatry.* 2003;48(2):87–93.
45. Doka K. Disenfranchised grief. In Doka K, ed. *Disenfranchised Grief: Recognizing Hidden Sorrow.* Lexington, MA: Lexington Books; 1998:3–11.
46. Jenkins CL, Edmindson A, Averett P, Yoon I. Older lesbians and bereavement: Experiencing the loss of a partner. *J Gerontol Soc Work.* 2014;57(2–4):273–287.
47. Fenge LA. Developing understanding of same-sex partner bereavement for older lesbians and gay people: Implications for social work practice. *J Gerontol Soc Work.* 2014;57(2–4):288–304.
48. Gallagher LM. The role of music therapy in palliative medicine and supportive care. *Semin Oncol.* 2011;38(3):403–406.
49. Magill L. The spiritual meaning of pre-loss music therapy to bereaved caregivers of advanced cancer patients. *Palliat Support Care.* 2009;7(1):97–108.
50. O'Callaghan CC, Mcdermott F, Hudson P, Zalcberg JR. Sound continuing bonds with the deceased: The relevance of music, including pre-loss music therapy, for eight bereaved caregivers. *Death Stud.* 2013;37(2):101–125.

CHAPTER 39

Team Communication in the Acute Care Setting

Andrew Thurston, Lyle Fettig, and Robert Arnold

Introduction

The prevalence of hospital-based palliative care has increased dramatically in the 21st century. In 2011 67% of hospitals in the United States with more than 50 beds had a palliative care team, compared to only 25% of hospitals in 2000.[1] Palliative care benefits patients, families, and hospitals in a number of ways, including the improved identification and management of symptoms, timely clarification of patient-centered goals of care, and coordination of care across settings.[2] These interventions result in improved outcomes for patients and their loved ones, improved satisfaction with healthcare providers, and cost savings.[3]

This chapter highlights the role of the interdisciplinary palliative care team in various acute care settings, the challenges faced in these settings, and the crucial role of communication in overcoming these challenges. With the use of a specific case example, we illustrate strategies and skills for provider–patient and provider–provider communication, describing methods by which individual providers and teams can improve communication skills. The acute care setting represents a complex cog in the care of patients with serious illness, involving many providers and multiple transitions of care between inpatient and outpatient environments. This chapter demonstrates how well-planned, timely, and skillful communication in the acute care setting impacts the care of patients and their families and leads to more effective identification of patient goals and values across all spectrums of care.

Acute Care Setting

Three acute care settings are discussed in this chapter: the emergency department (ED), the general inpatient non-intensive care unit setting, and the intensive care unit (ICU). The ED is an important location of care for patients with serious illness. Most patients with serious illness enter the ED at some point during their disease course, and many have multiple visits.[4] ED providers encounter seriously ill patients at a time of crisis when patients and families are particularly vulnerable: sudden changes in functional status and the interplay of multiple symptoms result in a high stress and emotionally charged atmosphere. Often, patients and their families first learn about a life-limiting diagnosis in the ED, with subsequent clinical evaluation providing clearer, and often unexpected, insight into prognosis.[5] In addition to providing rapid evaluation of the patient's condition, ED staff manage evolving symptoms and triage post-ED care. Providers help patients and families decide whether care should transition back to the pre-ED setting, to an alternative outpatient setting, or to the hospital for an inpatient admission. ED providers who thoughtfully consider goals of care and prognosis are more likely to identify a plan that best meets the needs of the patient and family.[6]

The palliative care team provides a number of benefits to patients, families, and healthcare professionals in the ED.[7] Palliative care partners with ED providers in determining the significance of new tests as they relate to the patient's illness, helps deliver this information to patients while further exploring goals of care with empathy, aids in the evaluation and management of acute symptoms, and helps determine the next steps in post-ED care. Given the mission and pace of many EDs, providers are sometimes biased toward aggressive, life-prolonging management that is inconsistent with a patient's goals and values. The palliative care team helps overcome this bias and, if appropriate, assists with transitions to alternative care settings often with additional resources such as hospice.

The palliative care team also provides continuity for patients previously evaluated by palliative care in another setting (e.g., inpatient, clinic, skilled nursing facility, home). When this occurs, the palliative care team often accelerates the evaluation process in the ED because of prior knowledge of the patient's condition, prognosis, goals, and psychosocial/spiritual factors. The team acts as a resource for ED staff, helping to clarify how hospice and other non-hospital-based services operate, and serves as a liaison between the ED and those services.[8]

Additionally, the palliative care team helps ED staff develop plans to provide primary palliative care for seriously ill patients. Such plans typically include routine screening of patients for palliative care needs, development of management protocols, and identification of patients appropriate for a formal palliative care consultation. Clinical practice guidelines exist for palliative care in the ED,[9] and the team may direct ED staff to resources for improving the quality of palliative care such as symptom management protocols and training programs (e.g., End-of-Life Nursing Education Consortium for nurses and Education in Palliative and End-of-life Care–Emergency Medicine for physicians).

While communication in the ED follows many of the same principles discussed later in this chapter, the clarification of expectations is crucial. Asking the consulting ED provider about specific reasons for consultation and ways in which the palliative team can be most helpful often clarifies expectations and efficiently streamlines the plan of care. Other expectations to clarify include hours of availability for direct patient evaluation, anticipated timeframe for evaluation, and after-hours availability.

Another acute care setting for palliative care is the general inpatient non-intensive care unit. The general inpatient setting provides an opportunity for the palliative care team to assist with the management of a wide variety of acute and chronic serious illnesses. Illnesses commonly encountered include cancer, congestive heart failure, chronic obstructive pulmonary disease, cirrhosis, end-stage renal disease, dementia, stroke, and HIV/AIDS. Palliative care teams work alongside hospitalists, surgeons, and numerous physician subspecialists in addition to disciplines such as nursing, physical therapy, speech and language pathology, medical nutrition, medical ethics, and hospital chaplaincy.

The inpatient palliative care team provides either primary care of hospitalized patients or acts as a consultant (in some instances, a team serves both roles). When the palliative team provides primary care, the patient is admitted to a hospice/palliative care unit or interspersed with other general inpatients. The model of care depends on a number of institutional factors, such as patient volume, hospital culture, availability of specialist palliative care providers, and preference of the palliative care team.[10]

Consultative palliative care is the most common model of care in hospitals in the United States. When the palliative care team provides consultation for a hospitalized patient, each palliative care discipline (e.g., physician, nursing, social work, and chaplaincy) may have a hospital counterpart already involved in the patient's care. To avoid confusion, palliative teams often develop procedures to determine how each team discipline works with their counterpart to provide care without duplication of services. For example, a palliative care social worker may collaborate with a primary medicine social worker to develop a procedure to clarify, at the time of consultation, their respective roles. The procedure includes a "pre-briefing" at the beginning of consultation to assess patient and team needs (e.g., assessment of living arrangement, transportation needs, financial resources). The palliative care social worker's expertise in some areas (e.g., counseling family members who have anticipatory grief or initiating hospice referrals) leads to management of these needs while the primary social worker continues to manage general needs (e.g., skilled nursing referrals, assistance with Family Medical Leave Act paperwork). Because of the numerous social needs of many seriously ill patients, the palliative care social worker may, after discussion with the primary social worker, assume sole responsibility for managing the social needs of the patient. Routine communication at the onset of palliative care consultation can help social workers negotiate task-sharing.

A comprehensive inpatient palliative care evaluation typically includes the assessment of a patient's goals of care and personal values. In some cases, the assessment determines that the current plan of care is not consistent with the goals of the patient. This leads to discontinuation of some interventions (e.g., antibiotics) and implementation of others (e.g., aggressive analgesia). Additionally, the palliative care team helps anticipate how post-hospital care may contribute to or detract from the patient's goals, broadening the focus of care planning from the acute illness to the overall trajectory of the life-limiting illness.

Involving outpatient providers in the coordination and planning of care is often helpful. Consider the following example: a hospitalist consulting palliative care assumes that a chemotherapy plan for advanced lung cancer still meets the patient's goals after an admission for postobstructive pneumonia and a decline in performance status. The palliative care physician recognizes the low likelihood of functional improvement and senses that the patient is shifting goals toward comfort and contacts the outpatient oncologist. The outpatient oncologist shares valuable insight on the patient's overall trajectory and feels that hospice is appropriate. The palliative care team arranges a family meeting where the goals of care are reviewed, and the oncologist recommends hospice and discontinuation of chemotherapy. Afterward, the palliative care team remains with the patient and family to further develop the plan of care and address concerns about the end of life.

Finally, a third acute care setting for palliative care is the ICU. The ICU is an appropriate setting for primary palliative care interventions embedded within the unit. Early family meetings conducted by the ICU team improve the timeliness of shifts in goals of care as well as reduce conflict,[11] and structured communication interventions conducted by ICU clinicians reduce symptoms of posttraumatic stress disorder, anxiety, and depression in bereaved family members.[12] While many patients continue to receive life-prolonging ICU therapies after palliative care evaluation, evidence suggests that palliative care consultation reduces average ICU length of stay, increases the chance of transition to a less acute setting of care, and reduces the cost of care without an increase in mortality.[13]

Communication is central to any palliative care consultation, and the ICU highlights this concept. As patients often lack decision-making capacity, substituted judgment is the gold standard for surrogate decision-making, but surrogates often lack a clear understanding of the patient's wishes.[14] A palliative care consultation in the ICU helps clarify these wishes and often contributes to the resolution of conflict. Consider this example: a nephrology consultant feels strongly that continuing chronic dialysis for a patient with end-stage renal disease who suffered an anoxic brain injury is futile. The patient's family resists the withdrawal of dialysis. In a conversation with the patient's wife, the palliative care nurse explores the wife's perceptions of how the patient might view his situation. The patient's wife believes he would want more time to solidify the prognostic assessment by the neurologist. The palliative care nurse speaks with the ICU team and nephrologist and proposes a 72-hour time-limited trial of therapy that allows for more time to confirm the prognosis while establishing a plan to stop dialysis if the patient does not clinically improve.

Acute Care Team Communication Strategies

Communication Within the Team

Communication in the acute care setting is a challenging and constantly evolving issue affected not only by the different environments within the hospital but also by the interplay of different teams with different agendas.[15] Before discussing specific communication strategies and techniques, it is important to first reflect on how palliative care team members communicate and then address ways for improving team communication. Table 39.1 identifies some signs and symptoms of a dysfunctional team compared to an effective team.

Table 39.1 Comparison of Team Dynamics

Dysfunctional Team Dynamics	Effective Team Dynamics
Unclear responsibilities of team members	Team members have clear roles
Unclear care plans for patients	Care plans are clear
Disorganized family meetings	Family meetings are organized and well planned
Confusion among patients/family	Patient/family member information received is consistent
Confusion among other medical services	Other medical services are on the same page, aware of changes
Avoidable delays in discharge	Smooth discharge planning
Lack of debriefing/communication during the work day	Continued communication/debriefing during the work day
Unilateral decision-making	Collaborative decision-making
Lack of constructive feedback or defensive handling of constructive criticism	Constructive feedback appreciated
Signs of burnout	Continued support for team members/acknowledgment of self-care
Lack of support/self-care for team members	

Strategies to improve team dynamics, and consequently team communication, include the following:

1. Understand each other's roles. Understanding the roles and responsibilities of different team members is key to effective communication.[16,17] For example, assessing the team social worker's perception of his or her responsibilities and comparing this to the rest of the team's perception helps clarify any confusion in expectation. One way to clarify roles is to ask: "Could you help me better understand your responsibilities when someone wants to enroll in hospice?"

2. Identify shared goals and values. Remembering that care in the acute hospital setting is fundamentally patient-centered helps reframe the team's focus and shifts priority away from interpersonal differences.[18] One way to do this is to say: "I'm sensing that we each have strong feelings about this case; it might be helpful to take a step back and get a better sense of what Mr. X would want in this situation."

3. Address disagreements. Openly discuss disagreements as they occur in a nonjudgmental fashion. It helps to acknowledge the other person's perspective, the value of the perspective, and uncertainty when there is no clear "right answer."[15] One way to do this is to say: "I'm sensing we're on different pages regarding Mr. X's plan. I appreciate your insight into the situation—tell me a little more about what you are thinking and why."

4. Communicate frequently. Touching base with your team frequently during the day helps minimize redundancy and ensure that goals and expectations for patient care are consistent. It is also useful to recognize how different team members communicate. The DiSC personal assessment tool is helpful in identifying different communication styles.[19] For example, a type D (Dominance) personality tends to make quick decisions and seek immediate results, whereas a type S (Steadiness) personality tends to listen more and avoid conflict in a stressful situation. Presenting information in a way that best fits a colleague's communication style helps improve comprehension while minimizing conflict.

5. Provide constructive feedback. Give feedback immediately, and focus comments on specific observations while suggesting ways for improvement or acknowledging a job well done.[20] Any member of the interdisciplinary team should feel comfortable providing constructive feedback to any other member of the team.

Communication Between Teams

Once the palliative care team establishes solid communication, communication between the team and other medical services warrants attention. As mentioned, many palliative care services act as consultants in the acute care setting: as such, certain guidelines exist for communication with the primary consulting service.[21,22] Communication generally acknowledges the following principles:

1. Recognize the duality of the consultant's role. The focus of the consultation is the patient or family, but failure to recognize the role and responsibilities of the primary service leads to more work and confusion for the primary team and potentially fewer consults for the palliative care service. This concept applies to every member of the interdisciplinary palliative care team, including but not limited to the physicians, social workers, chaplains, and nurses. For example, a primary service may want to discharge a medically stable patient with metastatic lung cancer who is thinking about hospice. Recognizing the primary team's role in facilitating a safe and timely discharge, and continuing hospice discussions as an outpatient rather than delaying the discharge, is an effective way for the social worker to balance these roles.

2. Speak to the primary service before seeing the patient. Clarify the reason for consultation. Sometimes it is useful to ask: "How can we be of most help to you?" or "Can you tell me a little more about what is going on?" Assuming that the medical record tells the whole story is dangerous: direct communication with the primary team before seeing a patient not only prepares the palliative care team; it also clarifies expectations for the consult and identifies undocumented concerns.[23] Ask if there are things the team should avoid discussing, explore background information and any reports of "challenging" family dynamics, and negotiate your role in the management of the patient by identifying the team's needs.

3. Close the loop after seeing the patient. Speak with the primary service providers again and talk to them about your thoughts and findings. Be concise, and try not to give more than three to five recommendation while detailing specific action plans (e.g., "morphine 2mg IV every 1 hour as needed for pain" instead of "morphine as needed"). In addition to your documentation, convey recommendations in person and see if there are any follow-up questions or needs from the team. Try to anticipate issues before they arise, and help the primary team prepare for any challenges to the plan of care.

Managing Conflict Between Teams

One frequent source of conflict in the acute care setting is the difference between a primary team's expectation for the consult and the end result of the palliative care consult.[15] For example, the primary team may think a patient should not be resuscitated, but the healthcare power of attorney feels otherwise. The palliative care team is then consulted with the hope of obtaining a DNR/DNI order, but after speaking with the family the patient remains full code. The primary team considers the palliative care team ineffective as their expectation was not met. The physician on the primary team wonders if she should consult palliative care in the future for this issue.

One solution to this problem is to involve the primary team in any palliative care meetings with their patients and families.[24,25] There are several benefits to this approach: it decreases the risk of miscommunication by ensuring that all necessary medical services are present; it indicates to the patient that his or her healthcare team is all on the same page; and it provides an opportunity for the primary team to hear firsthand the logic and rationale behind a patient's decision as elicited by the palliative care consultant. Other strategies for managing conflict between teams include:

1. Acknowledge the conflict in a timely manner. Meet with the other team in a comfortable setting to discuss the difference of opinion as the difference is made known. Do not wait until the patient is discharged. Say something like, "I was hoping we could chat briefly about Mrs. X; I think we might be on slightly different pages regarding her goals."

2. Identify missing pieces of information. Sometimes the palliative care team identifies an important part of the patient's story unknown to the primary team, or vice versa. Sharing this information may resolve the conflict while focusing on the patient's goals and values.

3. Discuss any individual/team emotions affecting perception. Sometimes an oncologist, nurse, or social worker has developed a long, trusting, emotional relationship with a patient that makes discussing end-of-life planning difficult. There is nothing fundamentally unhealthy about this type of relationship, but it warrants recognition and exploration.[26] Sometimes discussing emotion in the work environment is viewed as condescending or inappropriate and requires a gentle, tactful approach with colleagues. Saying something general such as "This is a devastating situation" helps normalize the emotion by focusing on the situation rather than the person.

4. Arrive at a consensus moving forward. Disagreement or confusion between various teams in the acute care setting is often a major source of stress and confusion for patients and can damage a patient's trust in the primary or palliative care team.

5. Remember the consultant's role. At the end of the day, the primary team is in charge of the care plan. The role of the palliative care team as consultants is to provide recommendations based on expertise rather than creating and implementing a new care plan.

Communication on Hospital Discharge

The acute care setting is unique in that it is often a transition point between chronic, long-term environments. Patient care is greatly impacted by poor communication in this transition.[27,28] Discharge instructions and summaries often help clarify appointments and medication lists, but speaking directly with an accepting physician or primary care physician to communicate the events of the hospitalization is important—particularly if end-of-life decisions were made.

Helpful written tools for improving communication include the Out of Hospital DNR form and the Physician Order for Life Sustaining Therapy (POLST), both of which convey a patient's end-of-life wishes to family members, paramedics, nursing home personnel, and others.[29] Living wills and advance directives such as the Five Wishes form also help identify particular end-of-life wishes as well as individual goals and values often in the patient's own words.[30,31] When appropriately completed and witnessed, advance directives are considered legal documents and are particularly helpful in situations in which the patient lacks decision-making capacity or there is disagreement among family members.

Communication Strategies With Patients and Families

While much of palliative care in the acute care setting is done in multidisciplinary teams, patients and families remain the primary focus. There are strong parallels between the techniques used in team-to-team communication and communication with patients. As communication between healthcare providers often benefits from team meetings, so too does communication with patients often benefit from family meetings.[12,32] Family meetings in the acute care setting often involve delivering bad news to patients and their families. A general roadmap for delivering bad news is summarized by the acronym SPIKES[33]:

- **Setting**—This represents the preparation before the meeting, such as arranging the meeting, identifying a location for the meeting, reviewing all pertinent information, and making sure there are enough chairs and that there is tissue in the room. Before the actual meeting starts, it is helpful to meet with the medical team (pre-briefing) to identify a meeting "leader" and the team's hopes and expectations for the meeting. Once everyone is present, it is important to make introductions.

- **Perception**—This is a way to assess the patient's understanding of the clinical situation and see if it matches the medical team's understanding. If there is any disagreement, it should be addressed at this time. What the patient says also gives insight into how he or she wants to *receive* information. For example, if the patient says, "I have widely metastatic lung cancer and my renal function is declining," then this is a hint to consider a more medically direct approach. Asking if the patient or family has experience in the healthcare profession may be helpful, as such experiences often strongly shape perception.

- **Invitation**—Invitation is a sign of respect. Asking permission to engage in conversation about a sensitive topic shows that the physicians are acknowledging the unique nature of the patient's narrative and that there is a time and a place for every conversation. It also serves as a warning statement and signals that a serious conversation is soon to follow. Sample invitations are: "Would it be all right if we talked about the results of the scan?" or "Would it be okay with you if we talked about something that has been worrying me?"

- **Knowledge**—This is the information the medical team wishes to convey: for example, "Your cancer has spread" or "Your loved one is dying." The key is to be concise and use simple language without medical jargon while allowing time for processing. Any questions that come up should be answered at that time.
- **Empathy**—Responding to emotion with empathy is where most healthcare professionals start feeling uncomfortable, but it is an area ripe for exploration. Helping a patients see through the fog of their own emotion makes underlying goals and expectations clearer and helps progress the plan of care. We discuss specific techniques for responding to emotion with empathy later in this chapter.
- **Strategy/Summary**—At the end of every family meeting, it is important to summarize what was discussed. Just as assessing perception at the beginning of a meeting provides valuable information, assessing perception at the end of a meeting helps identify any miscommunication or misunderstanding. A follow-up plan or a time to meet again in the near future should be established.

One of the most significant challenges in the acute care setting is the number of different medical services often consulted for care of a critically ill patient. With each physician entering the patient's room there is potential for the communication of a slightly different message. Arranging a family meeting with consultants, the primary team, social workers, the outpatient primary care physician, and family members helps minimize potential confusion and leads to more effective communication.[34,35]

One helpful tip for improving communication is to debrief with the medical team after the family meeting. This strategy allows time to reflect on the meeting, plan for the next steps, and discuss any perceived communication problems. Debriefing is another way to gauge the team's perception and to make sure that the primary and palliative care providers have the same perceptions of the patient's goals and expectations.[36]

Templates are often an effective means for contributing to communication efficiency through documentation. For instance, an electronic medical record (EMR) template for family conferences in the ICU might include elements regarding patient participation, decision-making capacity, surrogate information, participation from interdisciplinary team members, goals of care, prognosis, and areas of conflict.[37] Once clinicians acclimate to such a template, they may rapidly access information when needed after the conference has occurred. The template also acts as an educational tool, informing other providers about important palliative care considerations in family meetings. Furthermore, teams can track completion of each template item to assess the quality of conferences.

Establishing a strategy for conversing with patients is the first step in effective communication, but what of the actual conversation itself? The acute care setting is a high-stress environment, and there is often an expectation in family meetings for family members to make quick and life-changing decisions. The context of these conversations is often emotionally overwhelming. Responding to emotion with empathy is one of the more challenging aspects of the difficult conversation for many healthcare professionals. Physicians sometimes recognize an emotion but do not know how to respond; other times, they do not pick up on emotional cues at all.[38] After the family meeting is finished, nurses and social workers who check in often face a flood of emotion as family members begin to process information at their own pace. Responding with empathy to emotion is not only respectful and considerate; it also helps the patient better understand and cope with the situation.[38,39] Responding to emotion with empathy is summarized by the acronym NURSE[40,41]:

- **Name** the emotion—"It sounds like this has been overwhelming..."
- **Understand** the emotion—"I can't imagine how hard this must be for you."
- **Respect** the patient/family—"You are an amazing advocate for your father."
- **Support** the patient/family—"We will be here for you and your father."
- **Explore** the emotion—"What other things are you worried about?"

Potential uncertainty surrounding prognosis in the acute care setting often triggers intense emotion, and using the NURSE statements helps explore these reactions with empathy. Providing prognosis as a time frame (e.g., "weeks to months" instead of "14 days") helps set realistic expectations, while normalizing the uncertainty of prognosis leads to an honest and empathetic relationship with the patient.[42] Consider saying: "I wish I could give you a more certain time frame" or "I'm hearing you want more specific information on how much time is left. The truth is it's very hard to predict." Acknowledging the uncertainty of prognosis and the resulting emotional cues helps patients live in the moment rather than in constant fear of the unknown future.[43]

In addition to the these suggestions, the use of silence during family meetings is a very helpful tool, though many healthcare professionals find it uncomfortable. Giving the patient and family space to speak and allowing moments of silence often provides valuable insight into the emotional state, opens doors for further exploration and clarification, and leads to increased satisfaction and a decreased sense of conflict.[44] Filling silence with technical data often confuses and further overwhelms the situation, and it does not give the patient an opportunity to process things at his or her own pace.

Example of a Difficult Conversation

The following interaction illustrates communication in the acute care setting by modeling the SPIKES roadmap, a team approach, and NURSE statements as an empathic response to emotion.

Case Details

Mr. J is a 70-year-old man with stage IV lung cancer and chronic obstructive pulmonary disease. He was admitted five days prior for worsening dyspnea and was transferred to the ICU two days ago for oxygen desaturation and lethargy. He was intubated and is currently sedated and unresponsive. His renal function has started to decline, and his chest X-ray shows a new aspiration pneumonia. The senior resident in the medical intensive care unit (MICU) feels like a family meeting is appropriate to discuss goals of care and to address Mr. J's code status. He discusses the case with the

MICU social worker (LSW), who notices that Mr. J's daughter, Mrs. B, is the healthcare power of attorney. The social worker suggests consulting palliative care for assistance with the family meeting. A meeting is arranged with the social worker, Mr. J's nurse (RN), the palliative care physician (MD), the senior resident, and Mr. J's family, including his wife and daughter. Before starting the meeting, the palliative care physician finds a quiet meeting room, makes sure there is tissue, and discusses the plan with the team. The resident asks the palliative care physician to lead the meeting. The goal of the MICU and palliative care team is to explore Mr. J's goals and values, discuss his code status, and clarify end-of-life wishes.

The Conversation	Specific Strategies and Skills
MD: Thank you all for coming in and meeting us. My name is Dr. M, I was hoping we could all go around and introduce ourselves quickly (introductions made). Thank you. Our hope with this meeting is to provide you with a medical update to make sure that we're all on the same page and working together to make the best decisions for Mr. J. Is there anything else you would like us to address?	Introductions, and setting of expectations for the meeting. Assessing the family's agenda.
Mrs. J: No, thank you.	
MD: I can only imagine you've met a lot of providers here at the hospital and heard a lot of things that may be confusing. What is your understanding of what's going on right now with Mr. J?	Assessing perception (S**P**IKES) while expressing empathy for a potentially confusing and overwhelming situation.
Mrs. B: We know he has end-stage lung cancer, and there's no cure for it. We were told he has a bad pneumonia and needs to be on the breathing machine.	Perception matches perception of the medical team.
MD: Yes, that's right. (silence). Would it be okay if I gave you an update on how he's doing?	Using silence to allow processing, pausing for questions. Asking for an invitation (SPI**K**ES).
Mrs. B and Mrs. J: Yes, please.	
MD: Over the past two days his kidneys have started to shut down. With the pneumonia and his lung cancer, I'm worried that he won't recover from this.	Presentation of information (SPI**K**ES) without using technical medical terminology.
Mrs. B: So . . . he's not getting any better?	
MD: I wish he was. (silence)	Responding with empathy (SPIK**E**S), using silence.
Mrs. B: (crying) I knew it. I was afraid this would happen.	Fills silence with an emotional cue.
MD: Afraid that what would happen?	Exploring emotion: fear (**N**URSE).
Mrs. B: That he would be like this at the end, connected to machines. I don't want him to suffer. (Turning to his nurse) Is he in pain?	
RN: He seems very comfortable to me. We are using strong medicines for pain and anxiety. At the same time, I can't imagine how hard it must be to see him like this.	Providing reassurance, avoiding technical terminology, using an "understand" statement (N**U**RSE).
MD: Do you feel like he's suffering in some other way?	Exploring emotion and perception further (NURS**E**).
Mrs. B and Mrs. J: Yes . . .	
MD: Tell me more.	
Mrs. B: This just isn't him . . .	
MD: What would he say if he could sit here with us, and hear what we're saying, and see what's going on?	Assessing the patient's goals and values.
Mrs. J: He would hate it. This isn't like him, this isn't who he is.	Suggestion that this is an unacceptable state for Mr. J.
MD: Can you tell me a little bit more about who he is?	Assessing the patient's values.
Mrs. J: He was always very active, loved camping and playing sports. He was very independent, never wanted to be fussed over by anyone. He loves his grandchildren and loved spending time with them, holding them.	
Mrs. B: He would hate this, being like this, knowing that he wouldn't be able to get back to how he was.	
MD: It sounds to me like he is fiercely independent and loves being active and that this may not be an acceptable quality of life to him.	Identifying the patient's quality of life and his goals and values as it relates to his current condition.
Mrs. J: No, it wouldn't.	

Mrs. B: (*Turning to the social worker*) It's just so hard to make these decisions . . .	*Emotional cue: overwhelmed? guilt?*
LSW: I can't begin to imagine how devastating and overwhelming this is. We're here to provide guidance—we're not asking *you* to make decisions. We're asking you to tell us what Mr. J would say, so we can make sure he gets the treatments that match his values.	*Responding with empathy (SPIK**E**S). Naming the emotion, providing an understand statement, providing support (**NU**RSE).*
Mrs. B: Thank you. I know he wouldn't want any of this.	
Mrs. J: So . . . what do we do now?	*Asking for guidance? A recommendation?*
MD: Would it be helpful if I gave you my recommendation, based on everything you've said about Mr. J?	*Asking for an invitation (SP**I**KES) to offer guidance tailored specifically to who he is as a person.*
Mrs. B: Yes . . . please . . .	
MD: Based on everything you've said about how independent he is, and what he would say about his current condition, my suggestion is that we shift our energy to making him comfortable and not prolong a state of existence that he would find unacceptable. And that when he dies, we make sure he is comfortable and not try to bring him back.	*Offering a tailored plan that encompasses his goals and values without becoming overly technical, and without discussing the often overwhelming details of resuscitation.*
Mrs. B: Yes, that's what he would want.	
MD: Then to summarize briefly, we will focus now on making sure he is comfortable and not suffering in any way and stop things that may not be adding to his comfort.	*Strategy/summary statement (SPIKE**S**).*
Mrs. J: Yes, thank you.	

Barriers to Teamwork and Communication

Given the unique environment of the acute care setting, a number of communication barriers exist that reflect the complexity of team dynamics and hospital culture. Communication is more effective when it is one-on-one and concise[23] and often becomes more confusing as additional team members get involved. Acute care hospitals, particularly teaching academic hospitals, often have attending physicians, hospitalists, interprofessional healthcare students, and rotating learners coming on and off service at varying times. Identifying the appropriate chain of communication and making sure that the message is correctly conveyed is often challenging. Coordinating communication between multiple, different consulting services with different clinic and inpatient schedules is also difficult, particularly when arranging a family meeting. Additionally, there are logistical and monetary motivations from the acute care hospital administration to reduce lengths of stay,[45] and sometimes this translates into hurried communication and pressured planning.

With the extensive, and necessary, use of EMR, there is sometimes a lack of communication due to the assumption that all team members have read the documentation thoroughly and understand the plan clearly.[46] This is a dangerous assumption, and the palliative care team should make every effort to communicate directly with other healthcare providers. As previously mentioned, the acute care setting is a transition between long-term care environments, and as such communication between the acute care hospital and the discharge destination is important. If completed, POLST documents and advanced directives travel with patients on discharge, but these are often lost or not included in the EMR.[47] While such forms are effective tools for documenting end-of-life wishes, searching for them or completing a new form with each admission is frustrating for medical teams and families alike.

The sudden, emotionally charged, and often overwhelming nature of an acute hospitalization is another barrier to communication between patients, families,[48] and medical teams. Often there is the pressure to "fix" a situation or help someone consider the inner meaning of illness. Additionally, prognostic information is often unclear or poorly communicated.[49,50] Unforeseen family dynamics and psychosocial-spiritual factors also affect communication in the acute care setting, making the development of a positive and mutually attentive relationship challenging.

Ways to Improve Communication

A wide range of tools exist to improve the quality of communication. Communication skills training increases provider use of skills related to empathy and goal-setting, often involving role-play or simulation with feedback based on direct observation in the clinical setting. Protocols for communication may improve the timeliness and effectiveness of interdisciplinary communication, while templates improve efficiency and consistency of palliative care interventions as well as improve the availability of key information to other providers.

Conclusion

The acute care hospital setting is a vast and constantly evolving mix of healthcare professionals, patients, families, emotions, and expectations. As such, communication is critical in providing quality care centered on a patient's unique goals and values. While there are many differences between the ED, the general inpatient service, and the ICU, the skills and techniques for communication are applicable across all acute care settings. Respecting the complicated nature of the primary team–palliative care consultant relationship, utilizing conversational roadmaps such as SPIKES to help facilitate communication, and using NURSE skills to respond to emotion with empathy all help clarify patient goals and expectations. Acknowledging barriers to communication as they occur and taking steps to actively improve communication skills with reflection and constructive feedback helps to ensure that patients receive individualized care consistent with their goals and values and that communication is maintained across all levels of patient care.

References

1. Center to Advance Palliative Care. Growth of palliative care in U.S. Hospitals: A 2013 snapshot. http://www.capc.org/capc-growth-analysis-snapshot-2013.pdf. Published January 2013. Accessed June 21, 2014.
2. Temel JS, Greer JA, Muzikansky A, et al. Early palliative care for patients with metastatic non-small-cell lung cancer. *N Engl J Med.* 2010;363(8):733–742.
3. Morrison RS, Penrod JD, Cassel JB, et al. Cost savings associated with US hospital palliative care consultation programs. *Arch Intern Med.* 2008;168:1783–1789.
4. Smith AK, McCarthy E, Weber E, et al. Half of older Americans seen in emergency department in last month of life; most admitted to hospital, and many die there. *Health Aff.* 2012;31:1277–1285.
5. Bailey C, Murphy R, Porock D. Trajectories of end-of-life care in the emergency department. *Ann Emerg Med.* 2011;57:362–369.
6. Lamba S, Nagurka R, Murano T, Zalenski RJ, Compton S. Early identification of dying trajectories in emergency department patients: Potential impact on hospital care. *J Palliat Med.* 2012;15(4):392–395.
7. Lamba S, Nagurka R, Walther S, Murphy P. Emergency-department-initiated palliative care consults: A descriptive analysis. *J Palliat Med.* 2012;15(6):633–636.
8. Lamba S, Quest TE. Hospice care and the emergency department: rules, regulations and referrals. *Ann Emerg Med.* 2011;57:282–290.
9. Lamba S, Desandre PL, Todd KH et al. Integration of palliative care into emergency medicine: The Improving Palliative Care in Emergency Medicine (IPAL-EM) collaboration. *J Emer Med.* 2014;46(2):264–270.
10. Smith TJ, Coyne PJ, Cassel JB. Practical guidelines for developing new palliative care services: Resource management. *Ann Oncol.* 2012;23(Suppl 3):70–75.
11. Mosenthal AC, Murphy PA, Barker LK, Lavery R, Retano A, Livingston DH. Changing the culture around end-of-life care in the trauma intensive care unit. *J Trauma.* 2008;64:1587–1593.
12. Lautrette A, Darmon M, Megarbane B et al. A communication strategy and brochure for relatives of patients dying in the ICU. *N Engl J Med.* 2007;356(5):469–478.
13. Norton SA, Hogan LA, Holloway RG, et al. Proactive palliative care in the medical intensive care unit: Effects on length of stay for selected high-risk patients. *Crit Care Med.* 2007;35:1530–1535.
14. Shalowitz DI, Garrett-Mayer E, Wendler D. The accuracy of surrogate decision makers: A systematic review. *Arch Intern Med.* 2006;166(5):493–497.
15. Back AL, Arnold RM. Dealing with conflict in caring for the seriously ill. *JAMA.* 2005;293(11):1374–1381.
16. Youngwerth J, Twaddle M. Cultures of interdisciplinary teams: How to foster good dynamics. *J Palliat Med.* 2011;14(5):650–654.
17. Wittenberg-Lyles E, Oliver DP, Demiris G, Regehr K. Interdisciplinary collaboration in hospice team meetings. *J Interprof Care.* 2010;24:264–273.
18. Patterson K, Grenny J, McMillan R, Switzler A. *Crucial Conversations.* 2nd ed. New York, NY: McGraw-Hill; 2012.
19. Mellor MJ, Hyer K, Howe JL. The geriatric interdisciplinary team approach: Challenges and opportunities in educating trainees together from a variety of disciplines. *Educ Gerontol.* 2002;28:867–880.
20. Thomas JD, Arnold RM. Giving feedback. *J Palliat Med.* 2011;14(2):233–239.
21. Goldman L, Lee T, Rudd P. Ten commandments for effective consultations. *Arch Intern Med.* 1983;143(9):1753–1755.
22. Weissman DE. Consultation in palliative medicine. *Arch Intern Med.* 1997;157(7):733–737.
23. Salerno SM, Hurst FP, Halvorson S, Mercado DL. Principles of effective consultation: An update for the 21st-century consultant. *Arch Intern Med.* 2007;167(3):271–275.
24. Morrison RS, Meier DE. Palliative care. *N Engl J Med.* 2004;350(35):2582–2590.
25. Billings JA. The end-of-life family meeting in intensive care, Part 1: Indications, outcomes, and family needs. *J Palliat Med.* 2011;14(9):1042–1050.
26. Meier DE, Back AL, Morrison RS. The inner life of physicians and care of the seriously ill. *JAMA.* 2001;286(23):3007–3014.
27. Solet DJ, Norvell JM, Rutan GH, Frankel RM. Lost in translation: Challenges to physician communication during patient hand-offs. *Acad Med.* 2005;80:1094–1099.
28. Coleman EA, Berenson RA. Lost in transition: Challenges and opportunities for improving the quality of transitional care. *Ann Intern Med.* 2004;141(7):533–536.
29. Tolle SW, Tilden VP, Nelson CA, Dunn PM. A prospective study of the efficacy of the physician order form for life-sustaining treatment. *J Am Geriatr Soc.* 1998;46(9):1097–1102.
30. Silveira MJ, Kim SYH, Langa KM. Advance directives and outcomes of surrogate decision making before death. *N Engl J Med.* 2010;362(13):1211–1218.
31. Collins LG, Parks SM, Winter L. The state of advance care planning: One decade after SUPPORT. *Am J Hosp Pall Care.* 2006;23(5):378–384.
32. National Consensus Project for Quality Palliative Care: Clinical practice guidelines for quality palliative care, executive summary. *J Palliat Med.* 2004;7:611–627.
33. Baile WF, Buckman R, Lenzi R, Glober G, Beale EA, Kudelka AP. SPIKES—a six-step protocol for delivering bad news: Application to the patient with cancer. *Oncologist.* 2000;5(4):302–311.
34. Lilly CM, De Meo DL, Sonna LA, et al. An intensive communication intervention for the critically ill. *Am J Med.* 2000;109(6):469–475.
35. Mosenthal AC, Murphy PA, Barker LK, Lavery R, Retano A, Livingston DH. Changing the culture around end-of-life care in the trauma intensive care unit. *J Trauma.* 2008;64(6):1587–1593.
36. Back AL, Arnold RM, Tulsky JA. *Mastering Communication with Seriously Ill Patients: Balancing Honesty With Empathy and Hope.* New York, NY: Cambridge University Press; 2009.
37. Nelson JE, Walker AS, Luhrs CA, Cortez TB, Pronovost PJ. Family meetings made simpler: A toolkit for the intensive care unit. *J Crit Care.* 2009;24:626 e7–e14.
38. Butow PN, Brown RF, Cogar S, et al. Oncologist's reactions to cancer patients' verbal cues. *Psycho-Oncology.* 2002;11:47–58.
39. Butow PN, Kazemi JN, Beeney LJ, et al. When the diagnosis is cancer: Patient communication experiences and preferences. *Cancer.* 1996;77:2630–2637.
40. Fischer G, Tulsky JA, and Arnold RM. Communicating a poor prognosis. In: Portenoy R, Bruera E, eds. *Topics in Palliative Care.* 4th ed. New York, NY: Oxford University Press; 2000:75–94.
41. Tulsky, JA. Doctor-patient communication issues. In: Cassel C, Leipzig R, Cohen H, et al, eds. *Geriatric Medicine.* 4th ed. New York, NY: Springer; 2004.
42. Hagerty RG, Butow PN, Ellis PM, et al. Communicating with realism and hope: Incurable cancer patients' views of the disclosure of prognosis. *J Clin Oncol.* 2005;23:1278–1288.
43. Smith AK, White DB, Arnold RM. Uncertainty—the other side of prognosis. *N Engl J Med.* 2013;368(26):2448–2450.

44. McDonagh JR, Elliott TB, Engelberg RA, et al. Family satisfaction with family conferences about end-of-life care in the intensive care unit: Increased proportion of family speech is associated with increased satisfaction. *Crit Care Med.* 2004;32(7):1484-1488.
45. Carey K. Hospital length of stay and cost: A multilevel modeling analysis. *Health Serv Outcomes Res Methodol.* 2002;3:41-56.
46. Coiera E, Tombs V. Communication behaviours in a hospital setting: An observational study. *BMJ.* 1998;316(7132):673-676.
47. Danis M, Southerland LI, Garrett JM. A prospective study of advance directives for life-sustaining care. *N Engl J Med.* 1991;324:882-888.
48. Schenker Y, Crowley-Matoka M, Dohan D, Tiver GA, Arnold RM, White DB. I don't want to be the one saying "we should just let him die": Intrapersonal tensions experiences by surrogate decision makers in the ICU. *J Gen Intern Med.* 2012;27(12):1657-1665.
49. Yourman LC, Lee SJ, Schonberg MA, Widera EW, Smith AK. Prognostic indices for older adults: A systematic review. *JAMA.* 2012;307:182-192.
50. Campbell TC, Carey EC, Jackson VA, et al. Discussing prognosis: Balancing hope and realism. *Cancer J.* 2010;16(5):461-466.

CHAPTER 40

Team Communication in the Outpatient Care Setting

Jennifer Philip, Jenny Hynson, and Jennifer Weil

Introduction

Outpatient palliative care generally occurs in two settings: in the patient's home, where care is delivered according to the long-established hospice and palliative care models, or in the outpatient clinic, a newer model of palliative care delivery regarded as "a new frontier for palliative care."[1] An important third form of outpatient palliative care is the multidisciplinary cancer meeting. Of note, skilled nursing facilities and residential nursing facilities are also an increasing outpatient care setting for palliative care. These are not inpatient palliative care units or hospice units but places to go when people require a level of care beyond what can be achieved at home and may have a recoverable illness. Palliative care in the nursing home setting is discussed in another chapter in this volume. All models of care have been proven to provide benefits, and each present different communication challenges and opportunities.

Palliative care delivery settings are often thought about in isolation, but in reality, patients move between healthcare settings as their needs change. For example, the patient who prefers home care may need outpatient reviews, acute hospital admissions, and inpatient palliative care unit stays along the way. The system and the healthcare providers working within it must have the capacity to respond to these changing needs as patients move through their illness course: communication is key. Patient-centered care has been recognized as the ideal, with communication playing a vital role in achieving this optimal care.[2] After all, patient-defined values and goals direct palliative care therapy. In defining values and goals, the patient influences the composition of the healthcare team.

The multidisciplinary structure of the palliative care team will depend on the particular outpatient setting (e.g., clinic, palliative home care service, multidisciplinary cancer meeting) and the service itself. Disciplines represented in palliative home care services and, perhaps less so, hospital-based consultancy services vary considerably among even neighboring services and certainly internationally. Regardless of the particular disciplines involved, communication is clearly essential to providing optimal palliative care to patients and their families.

Communication with families deserves special mention, as care incorporating the family is one of the components that defines and distinguishes palliative care.[3] We know that families and/or caregivers frequently have information needs distinct from the patient,[4,5] and accommodating and responding appropriately to those needs in the outpatient setting can challenge healthcare providers. Indeed, the family's information needs and the healthcare provider response can, on occasion, conflict with the patient-centered paradigm of care.

The provision of outpatient palliative care in the home enables very ill patients to receive nursing and medical care, allied health support, and other assistance when they are too frail to leave their home to attend appointments. This care philosophy enables patients to remain in their own surroundings and community, living their remaining life in a manner that reflects their values, not subject to the medicalization and imperatives of an acutely oriented health system.[6] This form of care can be considered a component of hospice care, community palliative care, or palliative care home services. For purposes of clarity, this chapter uses the single term "palliative care home services."

The palliative care home services model varies significantly. In some settings, the patient is no longer receiving life-prolonging care such as chemotherapy to lengthen survival or supported ventilation for acute respiratory distress. In other settings, such therapies or access to such therapies may be delivered concurrently with palliative care home services. The care delivery model will profoundly affect the composition of the healthcare team and its communication. The benefits of palliative care home services have been long described and include a greater likelihood of death at home (the preferred option of most), improved satisfaction, reduced symptom burden, and reduced hospitalization and emergency department presentation, resulting in reduced cost.[7-12]

The palliative care outpatient clinic is designed to deliver palliative care to patients who are continuing to attend healthcare appointments and perhaps receive life-prolonging treatment. The clinic enables palliative care access earlier in an illness course. For example, in the United States, this ensures palliative care access to many patients not yet eligible for hospice care programs and represents an equitable palliative care delivery model. The palliative care outpatient clinic improves patient satisfaction with care and physicians while improving symptoms, quality of life, and psychological state. In addition, the outpatient clinic reduces the use of healthcare resources: fewer emergency department visits, hospitalizations, and primary care visits; less chemotherapy in the last 2 weeks of life; and overall healthcare cost reduction.[13-16]

Other benefits include providing follow-up for patients returning home from acute hospital admission or a palliative care inpatient unit; the ability to target special populations in need, such as those with advanced heart failure; the possibility of a deeper and emerging patient and family understanding of disease goals in an environment distant from the acute event; and recognition of the role of the family caregiver who has specific information needs.[1,17] Finally, the outpatient clinic is a relatively resource-friendly way to provide equivalent broad and equitable palliative care access. Of note, however, in the United States the configuration of clinics has been determined by reimbursement. For instance, Muir and colleagues embedded palliative care in an oncology practice but had only a physician and nurse practitioner on the team because those were the only reimbursed services.[18,19]

The third and final form of team-based care predominantly delivered to outpatients is the multidisciplinary cancer or tumor board meeting. In these meetings, surgical, medical and radiation oncologists, pathologists, and radiologists discuss cancer patients who are at some critical illness point, such as first diagnosis.[20] Palliative care providers, primary care physicians, nurses, and allied health practitioners may also attend and contribute to the formulation of management plans. In most instances, the patient does not attend the meeting.

Palliative Care Home Services

Much has been written about the provision and potential benefits of palliative care in the home. Many patients indicate a preference for dying at home, and most developed countries have services available to support this.[6,9,11] The home setting takes healthcare providers out of their usual environment and firmly places the patient and family in control. This significantly alters the flow and imperatives of the consultation. While this can be time-consuming and even unsettling for some providers, it is far more patient- and family-centered. Addressing family/caregiver specific concerns can occur easily in the home environment, with the patient's explicit consent. In more complex circumstances, opportunities for communication can be more readily affected (e.g., a family member who accompanies the healthcare provider outside the house ostensibly to bid farewell and imparts further information or concerns).

Team Composition of Palliative Care Home Services

In the home setting, the palliative care team composition is fluid. Healthcare providers, including physicians, nurses, social workers, allied health professionals, psychologists, pastoral care workers, and alternative therapists, often comprise the team. Volunteers associated with the palliative care home service or other community groups may also work alongside these paid professionals. The substantive work of caring is born by the patient's family and community, a vital unpaid and nonprofessional team component, who perform tasks as varied as cooking and cleaning to assisting with medications and complex care provision such as home dialysis.[21] The healthcare team must communicate effectively to achieve the best possible care and support for the patient.

The patient is considered a care recipient, an active participant, and a team member. The patient who actively shares his or her values, assists in goal-setting and reports on responses to therapies may be considered an active team participant. Even the patient who assigns his or her family or healthcare provider the task of decision-making must be considered a team member who engages, receives, trusts, and gives within the realm of care.

Communication Within the Palliative Care Home Services Team

Intrateam communication in the home setting involves many skills that are similar to those used in other outpatient settings. An important similarity is the necessity of assessing and documenting the healthcare team, both in the community and in the hospital(s), including formal and informal healthcare providers. It is essential for patients to feel that providers understand their individual care arrangements and demonstrate a willingness and ability to communicate and work effectively with their already established healthcare team both now and in the future. Often patients' awareness and understandings of the complexities and challenges that this can create, particularly across services and geographical locations, is limited. Recognizing and regularly communicating with this broad, patient-defined team is critical to good care and, in many cases, is essential to establishing a therapeutic relationship. Timeliness and selecting the appropriate mode of communication are important.

Communication Between Interdisciplinary Teams

Palliative care home services are often for referred patients who have strong connections with multiple, usually hospital-based providers. An oft-quoted example is the medical oncologist with whom a patient and family describe many years of a trusting relationship. As advanced disease progresses and the patient spends more time at home, he or she can feel abandoned by this very same physician and, indeed, by the entire hospital-based health service. Managing this "transition" to palliative care is a core communication task for palliative providers[22] and one balanced with another fundamental communication task: to re-establish frequently neglected community links, particularly with the patient's family physician. It is fairly common for the family physician not to have seen the patient during the anti-cancer treatment, with frequent hospital visits replacing community care. In extreme cases, some family physicians receive no communication at all from hospitals and may be entirely unaware of a patient's diagnosis until contacted by the palliative care home service. Understandably in such circumstances, requests for emergency responses or medication prescriptions from palliative care home services can engender an abrupt or even terse reaction.[23]

Model for Palliative Care Home Services

The ways in which palliative care home services interact with the healthcare system's other arms differ widely. The patient may be primarily managed by the palliative care team with input from both home- and hospital-based services simultaneously or, alternatively, by any combination of these. Even within the palliative care home service, models of care incorporating the multiple disciplines and multiple providers may differ. While some services may still adopt a primary nursing model, increasingly, services are employing a team-based approach whereby patients are allocated to all team members to encourage familiarization and shared knowledge. Regular team meetings involving case discussion and presentation and the maintenance of high-quality (often electronic and readily portable) medical records enable healthcare providers to care for large numbers of patients. Despite best intentions, however, a large team may be challenged by the need to be aware, at all times, of the rapidly changing status of a significant number of complex patients, each with particular nuances of their medical situations and family relationships.

Communication Opportunities in Palliative Care Home Services

Patient and provider interaction in the home care setting distinctly differs from the hospital setting and brings particular opportunities. Communication is much more than the words that are spoken. The very act of visiting a patient in his or her home has great meaning. It tells patients that the service is willing to come to them and this, in itself, can lay the foundation for meaningful communication. In addition, patients may feel more powerful and relaxed in the home setting and perhaps be more inclined to share their hopes and fears. Seeing a patient surrounded by his or her own possessions, family, and sometimes friends can provide a better sense of the person. This can be very helpful to the palliative care provider who, in seeking to enhance a patient's quality of life, must understand something of what that patient values and what challenges he or she faces. The home environment provides clues through the objects displayed, the people present, and the facilities available. There may also be an opportunity to speak to family members who have not been able to attend the hospital.

Challenges for the Palliative Care Home Service Team

Entering another person's world brings a responsibility to respect cultural and other practices and preserve privacy.[24] Some patients may be anxious and even ashamed about the state of their home and reluctant for strangers to visit. Healthcare providers have less control over who is present and how discussions unfold, and they are more vulnerable in the face of aggression and other extreme emotional reactions. Boundaries with patients and family can be less clear, and meticulous attention to these is essential.

A challenge common to many palliative care home services is a lack of available information both detailing what has gone before (the patient's full diagnostic, treatment, and prognostic information; outcomes of previous assessments; what information has previously been relayed to the patient and family) and issues that emerge over time. Working with patients in the home environment brings challenges in accessing diagnostic and other specialist input. The healthcare team frequently spends substantial amounts of time trying to collate these pieces to ensure consistent, accurate information and healthcare is delivered.

Case 1: William

William, aged 19, has metastatic osteosarcoma. News of disease progression comes after many years of treatment at a cancer center in a tertiary hospital. Although he has increasing pain and dyspnea, William has decided to go home where his parents will care for him.

The palliative care team visits William at home for the first time. When asked about their understanding of palliative care, he and his mother tell the team that it is "like hospital in the home" and he needs this because of pain and shortness of breath. Further inquiry highlights a mismatch between the family's understanding of the prognosis and the information contained in the referral from the inpatient unit. It is February, and while William is talking about plans for a holiday in December, the referral states that he has been discharged for "end-of-life care" and is expected to die within the month. As this conversation unfolds, William's mother looks through some written material provided by the palliative care home service team. She becomes agitated and concerned about some of the content and hurriedly finishes the meeting. The team leaves without a clear plan for follow-up. A call to the inpatient unit reveals that the oncologist did not actually tell William how long he might expect to live. He assumed the family understood the gravity of the situation, because they had chosen to go home and accept palliative care support.

In this case, the patient, family, and the home healthcare team have suffered the consequences of poor communication. William is now at home without a clear understanding of his illness and potentially without support. Verbal communication between the two services prior to the home visit may have highlighted the gap between William's expectations and those of his oncologist. The inpatient team could have then addressed this prior to discharge. Alternatively, if William had already been discharged, the home-based team could have tailored their approach and facilitated a process through which his understanding could have been improved (e.g., a return to the hospital for an outpatient review).

There are many ways in which poor communication between teams negatively affect care across the hospital-community interface. Other examples include:

- The role and availability of the palliative care home service is not adequately explained prior to discharge. When patients discover, for example, that there is limited support after hours, they may become angry and upset with the palliative care home services. Worse, their decision to go home may have been based on the belief that a nurse could visit after hours, and they now find themselves unable to manage.

- There is a lack of clarity around return to hospital, if this is required. Who should they or the palliative care home service team call?

- Details are missed and lead to adverse events (e.g., medication side effects, aggressive family members).

Hospital-based healthcare providers often have no experience working in the home and may not appreciate the challenges this setting brings. The equipment, medications, and support from colleagues that are so readily available in a hospital are not necessarily available in the community. Home-based healthcare providers understand this environment, and a conversation between the two can help ensure information is conveyed and other needs are met. Key elements of this conversation are highlighted in Box 40.1.

It is extremely helpful and reassuring for the patient to see evidence of teamwork.[24] There are a number of ways this can be demonstrated. A simple comment such as, "I've talked to your team in the hospital and, if it is okay, when we are finished today I'd like to let them know how things are going for you," provides a sense that healthcare providers are working together. In some cases, it is possible for a member of the inpatient team to visit the patient at home with the palliative care home service. A joint home visit of this kind has many advantages and should be encouraged whenever possible. It helps strengthen the working relationship

> **Box 40.1** Key Information and Questions to Consider Before Transfer From Hospital to Home
>
> - A general discussion of the patient's clinical and social history including key family members
> - Insights into the patient's personality, coping style, values, spiritual beliefs, hopes, and fears
> - Detailed exploration of the patient's understanding of his or her illness, prognosis, goals of care, ongoing treatment, and palliative care. What conversations have been had and with whom?
> - The inpatient team's expectations of the home-based service and how they have described the service to the patient
> - The home-based team's perspective on their role and availability
> - The inpatient team's ongoing role, if any, in the patient's care
> - Lines of communication should clinical advice or readmission be necessary
> - Practicalities including any medications, drug orders, documentation, or equipment that must be sent home with the patient

between the two healthcare teams, shows patients that they have not been abandoned by the inpatient unit, and builds trust.

In advanced illness, circumstances change, sometimes dramatically, and patients may seek support from emergency services, hospitals, and family physicians sometimes without calling the palliative care home service. Anticipating and planning for possible scenarios is a key skill for the palliative care provider and involves discussion within the healthcare team.

Palliative Care Outpatient Clinic

The outpatient clinic setting conforms to the usual medical model, and so communication with the patient proceeds, with the main constraint being time and appropriate prioritization of tasks. Addressing the often disparate information needs of patient, family, and/or other providers is an important palliative care communication task; however, it is not easily addressed in the outpatient clinic environment.[4] The main barriers to this are time and privacy concerns, though the latter are readily addressed by seeking the patient's consent.

Team Composition of Palliative Care Outpatient Clinic

In the palliative care outpatient clinic, the healthcare team is frequently modeled on the traditional mode of care delivery in acute facilities, reflecting the positioning and development of the majority of clinics. Palliative care outpatient clinics are predominantly part of the larger health system such as an acute hospital or cancer center. Most commonly, they are staffed by physicians, advance practice nurses or nurse practitioners, nurses, and/or social workers.[25] The reasons for referring patients to these clinics are reflective of this staffing profile and site of care, predominantly for pain and symptom management and for determining the goals of care.[25] Which patients are referred depends on the referral parameters of that center as well as funding models of the clinic. For example, a clinic funded by provider billings will usually require a medical referral for the patient to attend the clinic. Therefore, the characteristics of the patient population attending such a clinic will depend on the referring physicians' recognizing a palliative care need, which tends to occur only if symptoms are present. In contrast, nurses may more readily refer patients to palliative care for psychosocial concerns.[26]

Communication Within the Palliative Care Outpatient Team

Most often, palliative care outpatient clinics, unlike other models of palliative care service delivery, are staffed by a sole healthcare provider, which can complicate rather than simplify the communication tasks. Within the consultation's limited time frame, the healthcare provider needs to establish clearly which providers comprise the patient's "healthcare team," within and outside the hospital, to ensure that all providers are included in communication about the consultation, decision-making, and ongoing follow-up and treatment, if necessary. Given the time required to address issues arising from complex diagnoses as well as other patient needs, thought must be given to the most appropriate mode of communication.

Communication Between Interdisciplinary Teams, Beyond Palliative Care

Outpatient palliative care is largely a consultative specialty and, as such, relies on a referral base. The maintenance of this referral base requires good relationships and trust.[27]

It is rare for patients seen in a palliative care outpatient clinic not to have other medical providers involved in their care, and, indeed, there are often several. As discussed, establishing who is involved and communicating with them about the consultation is essential. A challenge may arise when a patient presents with a new problem and the decision must be made regarding which healthcare provider is responsible and should act on it and, in the case of those patients managed across different institutions, where the management should take place. Obviously, if good working relationships exist between the different healthcare providers, this can be straightforward; however, in some instances, the palliative care referral has been implied (e.g., at a multidisciplinary team meeting) or occurred via an alternate provider (e.g., the radiation oncologist referred for symptom management without explicit discussion with the treating medical oncologist). So, at times, changing management must be delicately and carefully negotiated, mindful of colleagues' sensitivities but nevertheless advocating for patient needs.

Model for Palliative Care Outpatient Clinic

The palliative care outpatient clinic model may entail handing over patient management to the palliative care team. In a more consultative service model, the referring provider remains the primary healthcare provider with the palliative care team supplementing or complementing this care. Once again, the healthcare team for such palliative care outpatient clinics will depend on these models of care. The team may include one or two palliative care providers, the referring physician, and an attendant team of healthcare professionals who continue to be involved in care such as restoring health and rehabilitation programs, as well as family caregivers.

The responsibilities of the healthcare providers in the palliative care outpatient clinic are built around communication tasks, with addressing symptoms and facilitating coping the mainstay of consultations.[28] In one study detailing the "anatomy" of outpatient visits, the early visits were spent elucidating patient and family understanding of the illness and prognosis and building relationships. Subsequent visits focused on treatment preferences and approaches to care, including inpatient care.[28] Other studies have specifically examined the time spent on various tasks, noting the average consultation is a median of 55 minutes, with a predominant focus on symptom management, followed by family coping, illness understanding, and education.[29]

Communication Opportunities in the Palliative Care Outpatient Clinic

The palliative care outpatient clinic offers many communication opportunities for the healthcare team involved in patient and family care. As noted, one such important possibility is the early engagement with palliative care services for patients who may not regard themselves as near the end of life.[1] This form of care has been demonstrated, in a cohort of patients with metastatic non-small cell lung cancer who had early palliative care input through clinic attendance, to improve quality of life, reduce depression, lessen aggressive end-of-life care, and improve survival.[30] Others have similarly documented less aggressive care at the end of life for those patients seen in a palliative care outpatient clinic, suggesting important communication tasks occur within these encounters.[15] Some groups have embedded palliative care providers in the broader outpatient clinic (e.g., a lung cancer treatment clinic) and have demonstrated that such a model also assists early engagement with palliative care. The relationships and trust that the embedded palliative care provider engenders overcomes patient, family, and referring physician hesitations about palliative care referral.[31]

Challenges in the Palliative Care Outpatient Clinic

Communication with multiple providers both within the palliative care team and with the broader healthcare team requires considerable time and effort. Electronic medical records have been helpful in addressing this communication burden and allow real-time documentation of clearly legible medical information. However, the electronic medical record information is available only within the institution employing the technology and to the healthcare providers working within the institution, rather than for the broader patient-defined healthcare team that usually crosses services and institutions. While universally accessible electronic medical records have long been advocated as a solution to information-sharing problems, particularly for emergency departments, privacy concerns and logistical issues continue to confound any real progress.[32,33] So while an electronic medical record may address the communication requirements of the acute hospital, its palliative care service, and emergency department, it does not negate the need to communicate directly with community-based teams or nonaffiliated units at other healthcare facilities. Equally, a courtesy call to the other healthcare providers involved in the patient's care is often required when a significant change occurs, perhaps not even because it will alter management but because respect for the patient's relationships with other healthcare providers, etiquette, safeguarding future referrals, and maintaining positive working relationships demand it.[27,34]

Case 2: John

John is a 58-year-old brick-layer, still working in the family business with his sons. He was diagnosed with lung cancer when he developed scapular and chest pain earlier in the year. Initially thought to be operable, curative resection was abandoned when a thoracotomy showed John had scattered small pleural nodules, which were biopsy-proven positive for metastatic disease. John had radiotherapy but without improvement of pain despite having very small volume disease, and he refused chemotherapy. His cardiothoracic surgeon referred him to the palliative care outpatient clinic for his ongoing management.

The outpatient clinic is frequently the first point of contact with palliative care, and multiple tasks must be simultaneously undertaken:

- Assembling all information about current cancer status and other intercurrent illnesses, with consideration given to ensure these are optimally managed
- Understanding the patient's perceptions and expectations of his or her illness and of palliative care
- Establishing a sense of the patient's responses to hardship and previous stresses
- Developing rapport with the patient and attending family members and determining patient support network
- Considering symptoms and appropriate responses
- Considering support needs (e.g., psychological, practical aids, and appropriate responses)
- Developing a management plan that incorporates all of these variables with appropriate follow-up
- In some outpatient clinics, undertaking clinical trials, in which case the healthcare provider may be considering if the patient or family is eligible for clinical research.

John arrives at the clinic alone, in his work clothes and smelling of alcohol. He is apparently anxious and states he is unsure why he is here but just needs some help with the pain. When asked about his health and how things have unfolded leading up to this appointment, he relates his disappointment at surgery not being possible and discusses his bewilderment and frustration that he continues to have pain despite all this. He is not troubled by his surgeon's suggesting ongoing care in palliative care, just "so long as you can help me." While he skirts around his understanding of the stage of his cancer and deliberately changes the direction of the conversation, his tearfulness at this time suggests at least some recognition of its incurability. His most recent CT scan is 2 months old and does not provide correlation between the known sites of disease and the pain complaint, so uncertainty of the pain mechanism exists.

Discussion with the surgeon must occur to determine his views on the pain mechanism based on operative findings, as well as his views on healthcare oversight: John's only symptom is pain and he is self-caring and working—thus not a "usual" patient managed solely by palliative care providers. Radiological review needs to be undertaken to determine if other sites of disease are present that may explain the pain, such as neurological invasion. Furthermore, communication with his family physician must take place to provide information about John's significant anxiety and apparent alcohol intake despite doing heavy, and potentially dangerous, manual labor.

In this case, the pain control need has ensured (relatively early) palliative care referral of a man who is otherwise fit and working a physically demanding job. The pain relief goal is overriding for John, and he is willing to move his care wholly to palliative care oversight if analgesia can be achieved. The coordination of his ongoing care, however, requires careful discussion with the broader team of healthcare providers: his surgeon, radiologist, family physician, and palliative care physician. John may need any one of these doctors in the near future, as his disease course unfolds, and all must be kept abreast of new information.

The clinic affords the opportunity for relationships to develop and therapeutic tasks to unfold over time. Trust around the successful relief of a symptom may enable discussion of seemingly tabooed subjects such as prognosis in a manner not possible earlier.

Multidisciplinary Cancer or Tumor Board Meetings

The prototype of the cancer or tumor board meetings is discussed in this section. In cancer care, these meetings are increasingly seen as an essential healthcare component, as reflected by guidelines and supported by a small but growing evidence base.[35-38] They are usually held in large tertiary-referral centers and involve an interdisciplinary specialists group presenting and discussing individual patients, frequently outpatients, to provide a consensus plan for their management and treatment. The patient and family are not usually present, although most will have clinic appointments to discuss the meeting outcome and the ongoing healthcare plan. A meeting sponsor (a healthcare provider who has reviewed the patient) usually presents the case, then a specialist pathologist and radiologist review their relevant pathology and imaging findings, respectively.[20] The subsequent discussion and final consensus care plan is documented in the (often) electronic medical record, ideally using a systematized pro forma.

Palliative care has, in some centers, been a relatively late addition to these meetings, and in many instances team members are still forming relationships and developing a voice. Despite the name, the multiple healthcare providers referred to in these meetings are largely medical, with surgeons, medical, and radiation oncologists the main protagonists. This strong medical viewpoint, alongside the treatment-focused rationale, challenge the palliative care role and can particularly intimidate the inclusion of nonmedical palliative care providers as well as other nonmedical multidisciplinary team members.[20] Palliative care participation in these multidisciplinary team meetings is desirable: to influence decision-making for those relevant patients, increase the likelihood of palliative care referral, encourage early referral as per best-practice guidelines,[30] develop relationships, and reflect a more accurate multidisciplinary composition. However, such participation needs to be balanced against the significant time commitment and the often low referral yield given the amount of healthcare provider time these meetings require.

Communication Within the Multidisciplinary Meeting

A key task for the palliative care provider attending a multidisciplinary cancer meeting is to report on known patients during the meeting and to communicate any referrals/salient information to the relevant palliative care providers at the meeting's conclusion. Both tasks may be complicated by the meeting organization and structure and the nuances of the different palliative care services, in addition to the systematic impediments to information flow between different services and institutions. For example, there may be no systematized way of knowing which of the patients scheduled for discussion at a multidisciplinary meeting are known to a palliative care home service or, indeed, the palliative care acute hospital consultancy services, beyond the single institution. Equally, the palliative care provider attending the meeting may not know the patient and/or his or her progress, despite their being well known to others in the service. Just establishing the correct services to contact prior to the meeting can be time consuming. Although it is preferable for a palliative care provider to liaise with other palliative care services, the palliative care provider attending the meeting has rarely met the patient, and so the quality of information shared is often diminished, along with perhaps even the message itself. Some formal structure around internal and external communication after multidisciplinary meetings is needed to ensure that the greatest value is extracted from the significant time required to attend. Privacy and logistical concerns have thus far confounded efforts to communicate this type of information electronically, such as through shared electronic medical records. Other tools, such as email, are more commonly used but are also increasingly seen as a potential privacy concern; the ideal tool to communicate multidisciplinary meeting outcomes to the broader team remains elusive.

The role of palliative care in multidisciplinary cancer meetings is relatively new. The treatment planning focus of the meeting often overrides symptom discussions, and, even in cases where symptoms are known to be present, healthcare providers rarely consider approaches to management outside disease-specific therapies. With such a focus, and compounded by limited patient information and the heavily medical (and in some cases surgical) perspective, establishing the role for palliative care may be challenging. Given that most patients discussed as a result of the meeting go on to meet with a surgeon, oncologist, and radiation oncologist at a minimum, to suggest another review, no matter how appropriate, can seem excessive. Some centers have included palliative care in the subsequent clinic reviews, creating a true multidisciplinary clinic after the meeting (a "mega clinic" where patients can see all their care providers).[31] In a well-integrated meeting a palliative care healthcare provider can suggest symptom-control measures to be delivered in parallel or as an alternative to disease-directed therapy. For those patients with incurable disease, the importance of quality of life domains, advance care planning (ACP), and the role of community and family support can be highlighted either as the primary focus of care or to supplement disease-directed therapies.

Model for Multidisciplinary Meetings

Because the multidisciplinary meeting has traditionally focused on diagnostic and tumor-specific management, healthcare providers frequently fail to consider psychosocial information. Suggestions to better incorporate such information have been made, despite the concerns and constraints of time and privacy.[20] Similarly, there have been efforts to include allied healthcare providers in the meetings and decision-making. Devitt and colleagues conclude, "It is only through the active engagement and incorporation of the views of all those involved in cancer care decisions that multidisciplinary meetings will function most effectively."[20(pe20)] While a universal solution to this problem remains elusive, for now, most would agree that participation, though imperfect, is best.

Since patients and families are not usually present for multidisciplinary team meetings, communication of the agreed-on management plans is usually done by a healthcare provider already known to the patient and family in a subsequent outpatient clinic.

Communication Opportunities in Multidisciplinary Meetings

These meetings provide a series of opportunities as a result of the greater trust, ease, and familiarity that develops within the relationships of the broader healthcare team. It is within the context of these enhanced relationships that earlier palliative care referrals may eventuate, as well as the opportunity to influence the discourse and decision-making around patients with advance disease or advanced comorbid disease when they are discussed at time of diagnosis. The palliative care provider can refocus the discussion from survival outcomes to quality of life, symptom relief, and best care in a place of patient's choice. These are all worthy contributions.

Challenges in Multidisciplinary Meetings

Some multidisciplinary cancer meetings have an atmosphere whereby healthcare providers give credibility only to disease-modifying therapies. This can be intimidating and make it difficult to raise and sustain meaningful discussion in the areas outlined previously. Palliative care involvement at such meetings should be viewed as a long-term project. With time, perceived responsiveness, and palliative care utility, particularly in the care of seemingly challenging or key patients and families, trust will develop on all sides. Through relationships forged within the multidisciplinary cancer meeting, the palliative care provider can educate other providers about the benefits and services palliative care may offer cancer patients.

Case 3: Barry

Barry is an elderly man with chronic obstructive airways disease, bronchiectasis, asbestosis, and an ongoing smoker. He presents with mild chest pain and is diagnosed with metastatic non-small cell lung cancer with a pleural based mass and extensive hilar lymphadenopathy. He is deemed to have incurable disease at the multidisciplinary cancer meeting. He lives with his wife who has advanced dementia, and he is her main healthcare provider. At the meeting, the option of radiotherapy, which is to be delivered over 10 days, is offered with the intention of disease control and pain relief. On specific inquiry by the palliative care provider about the patient's social circumstances, the lung cancer nurse offers that Barry is very worried about his wife. Since bringing her home from a high-level care facility, he has provided all her care. It is difficult for him to leave her alone and attending treatment will likely create some complexity.

It is agreed that radiotherapy will be put "on hold," and Barry will be seen in the palliative care outpatient clinic. When seen, Barry is very clear that his main goal is to be with his wife. Providing her care is arduous, but he is fully committed to the task and wants to care for her until he is no longer able to do so. He does not wish to leave her in the care of strangers; this makes attending treatments and even clinic appointments difficult. His pain is mild to moderate but responds readily to pharmacological management, and radiotherapy is postponed. The palliative care home service is engaged and offers community support to Barry, minimizing his clinic attendances. They also mobilize appropriate community aged-care support to facilitate more assistance for Barry's wife at home, as well as volunteers of the same cultural background to enable some socialization and short outings for Barry, while they stay with his wife.

In this case, the inquiry made by the palliative care provider at the multidisciplinary cancer meeting prompted the tabling of substantial social information, which had a significant impact on the treatment decision. It also facilitated an alternative approach to symptom relief, using medication, which better matched the patient's goals than that provided by disease-directed therapy.

Barry remains stable over the next 2 months but then develops a new pain over the contralateral chest wall. When sent back to clinic by the palliative care home service, the palliative care physician organizes imaging, and his case is subsequently reviewed at the multidisciplinary cancer meeting where the bone scan reveals a new rib metastasis. Barry is treated with a single fraction of radiotherapy to the painful rib with good symptom relief. Barry remains at home, caring for his wife until 1 week before death, when both are admitted to a local community aged care facility, as organized by both the palliative care home service and community aged care services. Barry dies soon after, and his wife continues her care in the facility.

The engagement of the palliative care provider in the multidisciplinary cancer meeting and subsequent communication with the team facilitated pain treatment at diagnosis in a manner that was both successful and more commensurate with his goal of staying home. Radiotherapy was subsequently sought as new disease-related problems developed, with targeted short therapy, again consistent with Barry's goals. Finally, through the multidisciplinary cancer meeting engagement with palliative care, Barry (and his wife) received enhanced and coordinated support for this final phase of life.

Tools and Innovations to Assist Communication In the Outpatient Setting

A number of authors have developed tools to assist communication tasks in the outpatient setting. The varying patient and family caregiver information needs at particular time points of an illness trajectory, rather than only and exclusively at time of diagnosis, have been reported.[4,39] In response, one approach has been to use the illness trajectory as a prompt to offer additional information.[4,39] Instituting a proactive model of care is another approach. Healthcare providers detect problems early through formalized screening in the outpatient setting, then plan and provide responses, rather than responding only once such problems are present and emergency department presentation and hospitalization are likely.[4]

To respond effectively to patient and family concerns during outpatient appointments, a prompt list of questions for patients to bring to appointments has been developed.[40] Using such prompts empowers patients to raise and articulate concerns at clinic appointments. Individuals are able to seek information in a way appropriate to their particular style of information engagement (e.g., seeking more or less); additionally, patients have some control in the consultation as it unfolds, with a focus on issues important to them.[41] A randomized controlled trial of advanced cancer patients attending outpatient clinics revealed that those who had the prompt list asked more questions of their healthcare providers, covered more issues, were more likely to seek prognostic information, and were more likely to discuss end-of-life concerns than control patients. Furthermore, those with the prompt list had fewer unmet information needs than those in the control group. The levels of anxiety between the prompt and control groups did not differ.[42] Box 40.2 provides sample questions from the question prompt list booklet used in the development of this research.

The degree to which such tools can be used in different settings and patient groups, including different cultural groups, is less well determined. Preliminary work suggests some differences in nuances of prompt sheets are required between Australian and US populations, as both patients and healthcare providers approach end-of-life issues and prognosis with slightly different emphases.[42] These differences are apparent between two cultures that may be broadly seen as similar in many ways, suggesting limits to the universal application of such instruments.

The reluctance of some patients to consider palliative care and referral to palliative care, either real or perceived by their healthcare providers, has meant that a number of patients are not referred in a timely manner.[4,5] The difficulty physicians have in engaging in these conversations often means they are avoided.[4,5] In this manner, communication by other disciplines who make up the broader team caring for outpatients requiring or receiving palliative care is constrained. In a bid to address this, Fairview Health System in Minnesota developed a script for family physicians and primary providers to introduce the concept of palliative care to patients.[1] The script explains palliative care tasks; for example, "The palliative care clinic works with me, your primary doctor, to better manage your pain, shortness of breath . . . They are specialists/experts in looking at this holistically and make a comprehensive plan for how best to relieve your symptom."[1] Other portions of the script answer questions about the future, confirm the treatment plan, or provide support and coping aids. In addition, the script suggests responses to patient questions. For example, for the patient who asks, "Why do I need this?" a suggested response may include, "As you know, you have XXX disease, and this appointment will help you know what to expect and make sure our care plan is in line with your goals and values." Further suggested phrases include suggestion of additional information and services and reassurance of nonabandonment by the primary care physician.[1] By providing the primary care physician with information and explanations, he or she has suggested language to negotiate these potentially difficult conversations when palliative care referral care is broached.

The outpatient clinic and home-based care afford the opportunity, when the patient is not acutely unwell, to discuss the patient's future goals and values and, within that discussion, consider how medical care best matches these goals. Discussing preferences for future care or ACP is an important task and one that is usually addressed over a number of consultations as the relationship within the consultation unfolds.[28] Furthermore, the discussion may be revisited and, indeed, preferences modified, as illness and its complications unfold or other factors emerge. Since the discussion is a dynamic one, the appropriate documentation assumes multiple challenges. The entire healthcare team must be aware of the patient's preferences as new illness complications develop. For example, emergency physicians report frustration at having to make decisions in the event of an acute emergency department presentation without access to the outcomes of ACP discussions.[32,43] A study in the United States has determined that the documentation of ACP discussions was not well recorded in electronic medical records, with just 34% of those who had actually held an ACP discussion having it recorded in a form that was legally valid (i.e., had been signed by the relevant parties). Furthermore these valid, as well as the invalid, documents were stored throughout the electronic medical record and were neither easy to find nor consistently filed, even within the same institution.[44] The authors concluded that a standardized documentation location is necessary so that the documentation can be located under any circumstances and in a timely manner.

Information Technology

Information technology is being increasingly utilized in healthcare; it includes the use of electronic records, medical imaging technology, videoconferencing, and telemedicine.[45] The use of these technologies in palliative care is evolving but has not yet been well studied.[46] Technologies such as videoconferencing allow providers in tertiary or other healthcare settings to interact with patients or other healthcare providers in homes or remote healthcare facilities. Although small in scale, there are studies that highlight the potential of videoconferencing and telemedicine to improve patient outcomes

---

Box 40.2 Sample Questions From the Question Prompt List Booklet, *Asking Questions Can Help: An Aid for People Seeing the Palliative Care Team*

♦ **Questions to Ask About the Palliative Care Service and Team**

- Who are the members of the palliative care team and what do they do?
- How do I access the services offered by the palliative care team?
- What does the palliative care team offer that is different to the services provided by the other doctors/nurses whom I see?
- How can I contact the palliative care team?
- Does the palliative care team speak to or write to my GP and other specialists about my care?

Source: ©Dr. Josephine Clayton, Prof. Phyllis Butow, and Prof. Martin Tattersall, Medical Psychology Research Unit, University of Sydney, 2002. All rights reserved. Printed in Australia. http://www.palliativecare.org.au/portals/46/resources/askingquestionscanhelp.pdf

and reduce palliative care costs. For example, in pediatric palliative care where the necessary expertise may be available only in a tertiary center distant from the patient's home, case reports describe how telemedicine can improve access to this specialist care.[47]

Technology has the potential to enhance communication, reduce costs, and improve efficiency. It may be possible, for example, for a nurse to be present in the home with the patient while the family physician video- or teleconferences with both. Along with huge opportunities, new technologies bring challenges. The provision of palliative care is very dependent on the relationship between healthcare provider and patient, and some healthcare providers have expressed concern that technologies may affect this relationship. It can be difficult for the healthcare provider to attend to nonverbal cues when teleconferencing, for example, and such interaction can feel less personal. There is little doubt that information technology will become a major part of modern healthcare. The question for the palliative care sector regards which patient encounters are best managed in person and which are satisfactorily managed through the use of technologies. For now, it is probably best considered a complementary tool.[48]

Electronic media holds other challenges and opportunities for palliative care services in patient and family care. The patients' ability to access healthcare provider email addresses, either with consent or from websites, and to use these to contact providers and seek advice and information requires reflection. In effect, the patient request and the healthcare provider response take the form of "giving advice," and this, along with subsequent electronic conversations, form a parallel medical record. Important parameters must be established around this form of patient communication and must be understood by all parties. For example, the healthcare provider may access emails infrequently, in which case patients need to be aware that the request may not be immediately seen or acted on. The electronic conversation forms a medical record that must be saved and possibly shared with the healthcare team. Furthermore, privacy issues with regard to the electronic information transfer need to be explicitly discussed. These parameters apply to other electronic forms of information transfer as well.

The use of a broader and somewhat depersonalized team has emerged in the development of online second medical opinions. Palliative care patients commonly seek second opinions to ensure current treatment approaches are appropriate to their circumstances, for reassurance, for improved information transfer, and to ensure "no stone is left unturned."[49] The Internet offers patients an opportunity to seek second medical opinions online whereby, for a cost, information is provided to a healthcare provider who, after review, offers an opinion on management.[50] This online treatment relationship raises challenges for the healthcare providers involved in the patient's care on the ground, as there is no real opportunity for interteam communication, and the risk of inconsistent information and, in turn, inconsistent goals, emerges.

Conclusion

The benefits of patients outside the hospital accessing palliative care and advice through palliative care home services, outpatient clinics, and multidisciplinary cancer meetings or via electronic media are dependent on consistent, sensitive, and compassionate communication. In order to ensure this type of communication, and its potential benefits are realized, palliative care providers must work hard within the healthcare team—both within their own team and within the wider healthcare network, as dictated by the patient goals and needs. This is an often arduous and time-consuming task but is always worthwhile. Only if done effectively will patient and family goals be achieved within their nominated team of healthcare providers.

References

1. Meier DE, Beresford L. Outpatient clinics are a new frontier for palliative care. *J Palliat Med.* 2008;11(6):823–828.
2. Bauman AE, Fardy HJ, Harris PG. Getting it right: Why bother with patient-centred care? *Med J Austral.* 2003;179(5):253–256.
3. World Health Organization. National cancer control programmes: Policies and managerial guidelines. 2nd ed. Geneva: World Health Organization, 2002. http://www.who.int/cancer/media/en/408.pdf.
4. Collins A, Lethborg C, Brand C, et al. The challenges and suffering of caring for people with primary malignant glioma: Qualitative perspectives on improving current supportive and palliative care practices. *BMJ Support Palliat Care.* 2014;4:68–76.
5. Philip J, Gold M, Brand C, Miller B, Douglass J, Sundararajan V. Facilitating change and adaptation: The experiences of current and bereaved carers of patients with severe chronic obstructive pulmonary disease. *J Palliat Med.* 2014;17(4):421–427.
6. Higginson IJ, Sen-Gupta G. Place of care in advanced cancer: A qualitative systematic literature review of patient preferences. *J Palliat Med.* 2000;3(3):287–300.
7. Hongoro C, Dinat N. A cost analysis of a hospital-based palliative care outreach program: Implications for expanding public sector palliative care in South Africa. *J Pain Symptom Manage.* 2011;41(6):1015–1024.
8. Brumley R, Enguidanos S, Jamison P, et al. Increased satisfaction with care and lower costs: Results of a randomized trial of in-home palliative care. *J Am Geriatr Soc.* 2007;55(7):993–1000.
9. Gomes B, Calanzani N, Curiale V, McCrone P, Higginson IJ. Effectiveness and cost-effectiveness of home palliative care services for adults with advanced illness and their caregivers. *Cochrane Database Syst Rev.* 2013;6(6):CD007760.
10. Luckett T, Davidson PM, Lam L, Phillips J, Currow DC, Agar M. Do community specialist palliative care services that provide home nursing increase rates of home death for people with life-limiting illnesses? A systematic review and meta-analysis of comparative studies. *J Pain Symptom Manage.* 2013;45(2):279–297.
11. Riolfi M, Buja A, Zanardo C, Marangon CF, Manno P, Baldo V. Effectiveness of palliative home-care services in reducing hospital admissions and determinants of hospitalization for terminally ill patients followed up by a palliative home-care team: A retrospective cohort study. *Palliat Med.* 2014;28(5):403–411.
12. McNamara B, Rosenwax L. Factors affecting place of death in Western Australia. *Health & Place.* 2007;13(2):356–367.
13. Rabow MW, Dibble SL, Pantilat SZ, McPhee SJ. The comprehensive care team: A controlled trial of outpatient palliative medicine consultation. *Arch Intern Med.* 2004;164(1):83–91.
14. Rabow M, Kvale E, Barbour L, et al. Moving upstream: A review of the evidence of the impact of outpatient palliative care. *J Palliat Med.* 2013;16(12):1540–1549.
15. Hui D, Kim SH, Roquemore J, Dev R, Chisholm G, Bruera E. Impact of timing and setting of palliative care referral on quality of end-of-life care in cancer patients. *Cancer.* 2014;120(11):1743–1749.
16. Yennurajalingam S, Atkinson B, Masterson J, et al. The impact of an outpatient palliative care consultation on symptom burden in advanced prostate cancer patients. *J Palliat Med.* 2012;15(1):20–24.
17. Rabow MW, Schanche K, Petersen J, Dibble SL, McPhee SJ. Patient perceptions of an outpatient palliative care intervention": It had been

on my mind before, but I did not know how to start talking about death..." *J Pain Symptom Manage.* 2003;26(5):1010–1015.
18. Muir JC, Daly F, Davis MS, Weinberg R, Heintz JS, Paivanas TA, Beveridge R. Integrating palliative care into the outpatient private practice oncology setting. *J Pain Symptom Manage.* July 2010;40(1):126–135.
19. Alesi ER, Fletcher D, Muir C, Beveridge R, Smith TJ. Palliative care and oncology partnerships in real practice. *Oncology.* November 30, 2011;25(13):1287–1290, 1292–1293.
20. Devitt B, Philip J, McLachlan S-A. Team dynamics, decision making, and attitudes toward multidisciplinary cancer meetings: Health professionals' perspectives. *J Oncol. Pract.* 2010;6(6):e17–e20.
21. Rabow MW, Hauser JM, Adams J. Supporting family caregivers at the end of life: They don't know what they don't know. *JAMA.* 2004;291(4):483–491.
22. Broom A, Kirby E, Good P, Wootton J, Adams J. The troubles of telling: Managing communication about the end of life. *Qual Health Res.* 2014;24(2):151–162.
23. Aubin M., Vezina L, Verreault EA, et al. 2011. Family physician involvement in cancer care and lung cancer patient emotional distress and quality of life. *Support Care Cancer.* 19(11):1719–27.
24. Holmberg L. Communication in action between family caregivers and a palliative home care team. *Journal Hospice Palliat Nurs.* 2006;8(5):276–287.
25. Smith AK, Thai JN, Bakitas MA, et al. The diverse landscape of palliative care clinics. *J Palliat Med.* 2013;16(6):661–668.
26. Hanratty B, Hibbert D, Mair F, et al. Doctors' perception of palliative care for heart failure: Focus group study. *BMJ.* 2002;325(7364):581–585.
27. Meier DE, Beresford L. Consultation etiquette challenges palliative care to be on its best behavior. *J Palliat Med.* 2007;10(1):7–11.
28. Yoong J, Park ER, Greer JA, et al. Early palliative care in advanced lung cancer: A qualitative study. *JAMA.* 2013;173(4):283–290.
29. Jacobsen J, Jackson V, Dahlin C, et al. Components of early outpatient palliative care consultation in patients with metastatic nonsmall cell lung cancer. *J Palliat Med.* 2011;14(4):459–464.
30. Temel JS, Greer JA, Muzikansky A, et al. Early palliative care for patients with metastatic non–small-cell lung cancer. *N Engl J Med.* 2010;363(8):733–742.
31. Le BH, Mileshkin L, Doan K, et al. Acceptability of early integration of palliative care in patients with incurable lung cancer. *J Palliat Med.* 2014;17(5):553–558.
32. Jelinek GA, Marck CH, Weiland TJ, et al. Caught in the middle: Tensions around the emergency department care of people with advanced cancer. *Emerg Med Australas.* 2013;25(2):154–160.
33. Neame R. Effective sharing of health records, maintaining privacy: A practical schema. *Online J Public Health Informat.* 2013;5(2):217.
34. von Gunten CF, Weissman DE. Consultation etiquette in palliative care # 266. *J Palliat Med.* 2013;16(5):578–579.
35. Boxer MM, Vinod SK, Shafiq J, Duggan KJ. Do multidisciplinary team meetings make a difference in the management of lung cancer? *Cancer.* 2011;117(22):5112–5120.
36. Kesson EM, Allardice GM, George WD, Burns HJ, Morrison DS. Effects of multidisciplinary team working on breast cancer survival: Retrospective, comparative, interventional cohort study of 13 722 women. *BMJ.* 2012;344:e2718.
37. Wright F, De Vito C, Langer B, Hunter A. Multidisciplinary cancer conferences: A systematic review and development of practice standards. *Eur J Cancer.* 2007;43(6):1002–1010.
38. Ruiz-Casado A, Ortega MJ, Soria A, Cebolla H. Clinical audit of multidisciplinary care at a medium-sized hospital in Spain. *World J Surg Oncol.* 2014;12(1):53.
39. Philip J, Collins A, Brand CA, Moore G, Lethborg C, Sundararajan V, Murphy MA, Lethborg C, Gold M. "I'm just waiting..." An exploration of the experience of people living and dying with primary malignant glioma. *Support Care Cancer.* 2014: 22(2):389–397.
40. Clayton J, Butow P, Tattersall M, et al. Asking questions can help: Development and preliminary evaluation of a question prompt list for palliative care patients. *Br J Cancer.* 2003;89(11):2069–2077.
41. Clayton JM, Butow PN, Tattersall MH, et al. Randomized controlled trial of a prompt list to help advanced cancer patients and their caregivers to ask questions about prognosis and end-of-life care. *J Clin Oncol.* 2007;25(6):715–723.
42. Walczak A, Mazer B, Butow PN, et al. A question prompt list for patients with advanced cancer in the final year of life: Development and cross-cultural evaluation. *Palliat Med.* 2013;27(8):779–788.
43. Marck C, Weil J, Lane H, et al. Care of the dying cancer patient in the emergency department: Findings from a national survey of Australian emergency department clinicians. *Inter Med J.* 2014;44(4):362–368.
44. Wilson CJ, Newman J, Tapper S, et al. Multiple locations of advance care planning documentation in an electronic health record: Are they easy to find? *J Palliat Med.* 2013;16(9):1089–1094.
45. Lindberg B, Nilsson C, Zotterman D, Söderberg S, Skär L. Using information and communication technology in home care for communication between patients, family members, and healthcare professionals: A systematic review. *Int J Telemed Appl.* 2013;2013:461829.
46. Demiris G, Parker Oliver D, Wittenberg-Lyles E. Technologies to support end-of-life care. *Semin Oncol Nurs.* 2011;27(3):211–217.
47. Bradford N, Herbert A, Walker R, Pedersen L, Hallahan A, Irving H, Bensink ME, Armfield NR, Smith AC. Home telemedicine for paediatric palliative care. *Stud Health Technol Informat.* 2010;161:10–19.
48. Bradford N, Armfield NR, Young J, Smith AC. The case for home based telehealth in pediatric palliative care: A systematic review. *BMC Palliat Care.* 2013;12(1):4.
49. Philip J, Gold M, Schwarz M, Komesaroff P. Second medical opinions: The views of oncology patients and their physicians. *Support Care Cancer.* 2010;18(9):1199–1205.
50. Tattersall M. Can a second medical opinion in a patient with cancer be truly independent? *Asia-Pacific J Clin Oncol.* 2011;7(1):1–3.

CHAPTER 41

Team Communication in the Hospice Setting

Anne Arber

Introduction

Living with a serious or terminal illness affects all aspects of life, creating enormous challenges for patients and their families. It is therefore unlikely that one healthcare professional could meet all of a patient's and family's complex needs. By integrating psychological, physical, social, and spiritual aspects of the patient and family into care planning, hospice and palliative care uniquely provide a "total care" approach through team-based care.[1] The patient and family are at the center of the team, including children as part of the family, enabling person-centered and family-centered care through the combined skills of an interdisciplinary team of professionals.[2] Cicely Saunders, founder of the modern hospice movement in the United Kingdom, believed that a total care approach was dependent upon a division of labor among team members.[3] Saunders' vision encapsulated a nonhierarchical, egalitarian approach to all aspects of interdisciplinary work among healthcare providers, patients, families, and volunteers. Team communication and coordination are integral to achieving shared decision-making, facilitating access to team resources, and providing quality hospice care.

The World Health Organization's definition of palliative care[4] states:

> Palliative care is an approach that improves the quality of life of patients and their families facing the problems associated with life-threatening illness, through the prevention and relief of suffering by means of early identification and impeccable assessment and treatment of pain and other problems, physical, psychosocial and spiritual.

Although this is a globally accepted definition of palliative care, this definition does not include how the team should work together or who should be members of the team. The ways that teams practice, the different roles team members play, and the overlap or blurring of roles differ across different service models and nations. Different models of teamwork exist and practices in the United Kingdom may differ from those in other parts of the world. In the United States, for example, federal requirements define hospice team composition to include physicians, nurses, social workers, and spiritual care providers. Given these variances, the terms "hospice team" and "palliative care team" are used interchangeably in this chapter.

Although several definitions of hospice care exist (depending on the country of origin), the European definition[5] emphasizes teamwork to meet the patient's holistic needs:

> Hospice care is for the whole person, aiming to meet all needs—physical, emotional, social and spiritual. At home, in day care and in the hospice, they are for the person who is facing the end of life and for those who love them. Staff and volunteers work on interprofessional teams to provide care based on individual need and personal choice, striving to offer freedom from pain, dignity, peace and calm.

In this definition of hospice care, staff and volunteers act as important team members working together to meet patient and family needs, enable patient and family choice in care decision-making, strive for care plans that prioritize patient dignity, and focus on pain and symptom management. In the United Kingdom, palliative care and hospice care refer to any setting where palliative care is practiced such as the hospital, the community, and the inpatient hospice. Nevertheless, wherever hospice and palliative care is practiced, the concept of teamwork is identified as central to such practice, as single disciplines cannot meet the integrated care needs of patients and families.[6]

Purpose and Function of the Hospice Team

Early in the development of the hospice and palliative care movement, a team approach was utilized and face-to-face team meetings were the model developed to facilitate communication, planning, and support. The case manager, often the nurse, coordinated the care of the patient's and the family's complex needs at the end of life by reporting on the patient during team meetings. Person-centered care was enabled through the teamwork of a variety of disciplinary team members who worked across professional boundaries. The goal of the team meeting is to improve communication among the different disciplinary team members, enabling a diversity of professional expertise to be available to manage complex problems. Teamwork contributes to accurate assessment and integrated medical and social care, with frequent and open communication among all involved;[7] it has been found to improve communication about end of life decisions, including advance directives and do not resuscitate orders in the intensive care unit.[8]

Traditionally, a hospice team consists of a core team of physicians, nurses, psychologists, social workers, physiotherapists, and chaplains. Other staff who may also be core team members include bereavement support workers, administrative support workers, speech and language therapists, occupational therapists, dieticians, pharmacists, complementary therapists, and librarians. Sometimes, however, these disciplines work in a liaison structure with the core hospice team.[9] The core team usually meets face to face to discuss their patients once weekly, sometimes more regularly.[10] The team may consist of a relatively small number of people depending on the context in which they practice, and the core (specialist) professionals differ according to the setting of the service. In the United Kingdom, physicians tend to have joint appointments with inpatient hospices and acute hospital settings in the community. However, specialist hospice and palliative care nurses generally work either at inpatient hospices or in specialist roles within a hospital setting or in the community. Therefore, hospice physicians attend team meetings in different hospital, inpatient hospice, and community settings, while other palliative care specialists such as chaplains, social workers, and nurses are usually employed in one setting. In one flagship service in the United Kingdom, a palliative care unit situated in the community identifies the clinical nurse specialist as the care coordinator. This coordinator integrates care within the hospice team and the wider network of general palliative care providers and has rapid access to specialist skills and care provision, enabling home-based, end-of-life care.[11]

The team meeting offers the opportunity for healthcare providers to communicate openly with each other, enabling them to tell the story of their patient encounters and to hear about other's encounters.[12] Highly experienced palliative care nurses report the importance of facilitating the patient story; these nurses are skilled at communicating the patient/family story in the team meeting.[13] Increasingly, the family is the focus of care, particularly at the end of life, and the conceptualization of dying begins to emerge and focus on the patient as part of the family.[14] This relational approach to care enables the family needs to be addressed as part of patient- and family-centered care.

Of course team communication does not take place only in the formal setting of the team meeting; much communication may be informal and backstage, during breaks or in corridors. This communication is called "embedded teamwork."[15] Embedded practices were found by Ellingson[15] to be flexible ways for blurring disciplinary boundaries and working around hierarchical structures and boundaries, enabling micro-negotiations to take place away from the formal team meeting. The hospice team may also be a "virtual team," a wider team supporting the patient and family. The virtual team consists of other general palliative care providers such as the general practitioner (GP), district nurse, pharmacist, and school support staff, for example. In the United Kingdom, there is recognition of the wider team offering general palliative care team in primary care.[16] The general palliative care professionals have training in the palliative care approach and can draw on the hospice team for support.[17]

Use of e-Technology in Hospice Teams

Increasingly, innovative approaches use telemedicine within hospice work, and the concept of the e-hospice and the virtual hospice has emerged. Within the virtual hospice, video conference software and Skype can facilitate virtual visits by interdisciplinary team members to patients at home. The use of e-technologies can facilitate communication at a distance and enable the patient and family to contribute to hospice team meetings. One such innovation is ACTIVE (Assessing Caregivers for Team Intervention via Video Encounters) that enables patient and family presence and involvement in hospice team meetings.[18] The ACTIVE intervention was found to increase caregiver's confidence and trust in the team.[19] Use of e-hospice initiatives provides an inclusive approach to patient and family participation in decision-making and helps overcome geographic barriers to patients' and caregivers' active involvement.

Barriers to Teamwork and Team Communication

While the goal of the team is to work together and collaboratively develop holistic care plans for patients and families, several barriers to teamwork can impede the team's process. First, some team members may be protective of their area of expertise and reluctant to work in an interdisciplinary way, resulting in professional rivalries and conflict.[20] In one study, a lack of cooperation was identified as "different perspectives on prognosis and objectives" for a patient; it was also reported that there were strong views on what should and should not be discussed in team meetings.[21] Second, teamwork can be eroded when team members are critical of hard-to-help patients and forego professionalism with colleagues.[22] However, for collaboration to emerge from the team meeting format, team members must take a neutral position when presenting and discussing patients[23] and have the confidence to challenge others' negative presentations of the patient.[24] Specialist nurses who take a neutral position when presenting patients in team meetings have been found highly effective in solving complex family problems.[25]

The portrayal of patients and families in hospice team meetings can affect patient and family outcomes as well as decision-making. Opie cites an example of a team that lacked generosity and imagination, where the patient was characterized as greedy and demanding; that characterization, left unchallenged, could have had negative effects for the patient.[26] Taking a neutral position in team meetings and "thinking jointly" together is a marker of teamwork. Skilled communication strategies enable the team to move beyond a focus on biomedical information to sharing knowledge of the patient (and the family) as a person with emotional, psychosocial, physical, and spiritual concerns, thus enabling person-centered, holistic care.

Finally, ethical and moral dilemmas among team members can impede teamwork and team communication. For example, team decisions about the use of palliative sedation or discussions about best placement for patient care can reveal differences of opinion among team members and cause conflict. Teams that are interdisciplinary in scope and focus on emotional and spiritual concerns as well as the physical and medical aspects of care are able to more effectively navigate ethical dilemmas related to care plan decision-making.[27] When dilemmas arise, threats to interdisciplinary teamwork can emerge from overly strong medical or nursing direction with unequal regard for psychological and spiritual care planning. More training is needed so that team members from psychosocial disciplines (such as social work and chaplaincy) develop the communication skills necessary to competently and confidently speak up during difficult decision-making.[28]

Studying Team Talk

Talk among colleagues in team meetings, known as team talk, is one way that team members demonstrate professional knowledge and skill of practice to colleagues.[29] Hospice team members perform and display their disciplinary expertise and skills by giving a credible account of their patient practice. Team members communicate and display their professional identity and manage their credibility with other team members by demonstrating attention to total care and symptom management.[30] Case presentation sets the tone for team talk within the team meeting, and the specialist nurse can influence the direction of the team's discussion.

This section provides naturally occurring data taken from an audio-recorded hospice team meeting. Box 41.1 shows the audio-recording transcript of a hospice team meeting as part of my 2004 research. The aim of the research was to understand how the hospice team carried out interdisciplinary teamwork in practice, and the focus was on the everyday accomplishment of hospice team meetings. The study was situated as ethnography of institutional discourse, and the tools of discourse analysis were applied to the data to enable an in-depth analysis of team talk.

Present at the meeting were two community palliative care nurses (CPCN), a social worker, and two physicians. A CPCN describes a distressing situation that emerged when she visited a confused, upset patient and her distressed daughter in a local care home. Telling a story is one way to command the attention of other team members; stories told in medical settings have different genres such as puzzle, mystery, or atrocity story.[31] Here, the CPCN tells a mystery story concerning patient P, a former ballet dancer, who has dementia and is in pain. The CPCN reports on the distressing situation that has occurred with the daughter in the care home. As the CPCN presents the case, she crosses a number of disciplinary boundaries, including the boundary with the physician and the social worker, to sort out the troubles presented within the care home.

The CPCN describes how the daughter has gone to see her mother in the care home and found her very distressed and agitated (line 26). The CPCN presents the situation from the daughter's and the nursing home's point of view. She presents the daughter's distress as linked to the mother's distress. She tells the story objectively without criticizing the daughter, despite the daughter's reported criticisms of the care home's failing to manage her mother's pain. The CPCN understands the nursing home's dismay, especially as the daughter was trying to contact the GP. The story is told as a dramatic incident with a breakdown of relationships within the nursing home and possibly with the GP. However, the CPCN is cautious; she does not attribute blame for this situation and tells the story carefully, keeping a neutral footing that enables her to eventually sort out the situation. The daughter's criticism threatens the care home staff and their inability to act appropriately and relieve her mother's pain.

The CPCN, by using interactional caution, minimizes the conflict and team disagreement. The CPCN works to maximize agreement among team members by distancing herself from the situation in the care home; her objectivity promotes consideration of the problem and active problem-solving through discussion.

Box 41.1 Transcript From an Audio Recording of a Hospice Team Meeting, Part 1

1	CPCN	We're doing psychological yeah psychosocial.
2		I've been to sort out one of Estelle's patients at lunchtime
3		that's why I'm late. Do you remember, doctor, a little lady
4		called P who is now 88? Ah who is in a ()
5		nursing home one of [nurse E] and she's she was
6		referred to us I think by St Paul's and she's hmm got
7		metastatic squamous carcinoma of the skin and possibly bone
8		and hmm
9	Dr	Yeah
10	CPCN	And hmm when she was referred, Louise from
11		St. Paul's, had put her on a fentanyl patch because she felt
12		she had some some pain hmm. She has also got quite severe
13		dementia. She's the ex-ballet dancer does anyone (ring any
14		bells) her?
15	Dr	Did she come in?
16	CPCN	No. Estelle's just done, I think, either one or two
17		visits.
18	Dr	I seem to remember Estelle talking about it, about her
19		being a ballet dancer.
20	CPCN	Estelle went on the 24th and had various phone
21		calls and was planning to meet the daughter on the 4th so
22		that's where it is up to. Anyway ah in the message book, that
23		the deputy had written, various phone calls, yesterday, from the
24		daughter who has got herself quite distressed, because she had
25		gone to see her mother in the nursing home and her mother
26		was very distressed and agitated and she felt she had
27		significant pain and she didn't think the fentanyl 25
28		micrograms was touching her. This lady does get distressed
29		when she's not in pain apparently ah because of her dementia
30		and then she can be, you know, very agitated and striking out
31		at people and things like that. But with the daughter yesterday
32		she wasn't doing that she was just, according to the daughter,
33		in a lot of pain and she couldn't get the nursing home to do
34		anything constructive about the pain, and so the daughter was
35		sort of looking through the notes and trying to ring the GP,
36		and all that, which of course upset the nursing home as well.
37		You can imagine. So hmm

Note: CPCN = community palliative care nurse.

This approach, called professional neutralism, has also been found in studies of family mediation.[32] A neutralistic footing allows mediators, in this case the nurse, to constitute their relationship in professional terms and discourages team members from heightening the emotional intensity implicit in disputes within interactions. The CPCN speaks to the patient's daughter and offers her further support, and she also sorts out P's medication so her pain can be managed more effectively. The CPCN proceeds with caution and tact with regard to the daughter, the nursing home, and the team. By objectively presenting the evidence and the solution, the CPCN diffuses the explosive situation in the care home. Her neutral positioning enables team members to see her as a professional, able to solve a difficult situation.

Box 41.2 shows the continuation of this conversation. The CPCN believes that P could benefit from some Oramorph, to which the doctor replies, "Liquid. Absolutely" (line 38). Also, the daughter believes her mother is able to take a liquid on a teaspoon (line 40). This action is agreeable to the doctor and to the daughter; the CPCN has spoken to the GP, who presumably also agrees with this. Following the sorting out of the pain problem with oral medication, the CPCN launches into a "psychosocial reading" of the case by identifying the daughter's need for support, the daughter leading a very busy life traveling with a lot on her mind. The CPCN identifies her knowledge of supportive care for the caregiver: "I think [she] could do with psychological support" (lines 42–48). The CPCN understands the daughter's difficult circumstances. The CPCN suggests that the daughter's distress is, in some part, caused by her lack of psychosocial support. The CPCN's interpretation is bolstered by reports that the daughter is eager to accept psychosocial support when it is offered. The daughter responds: "yes please" (line 48). In this shift, the CPCN accomplishes what the mystery is and the cause of the troubles, namely a lack of support for the patient's daughter. The CPCN is now acting as an intermediary for P's daughter and in her reading of the daughter's need for support.

The CPCN, by interpreting and acting on the problems in the nursing home, undertakes "rectification work."[33] By spending time talking with various people and maintaining a neutral footing, the CPCN begins to stabilize the disruption caused by the daughter's criticism of the staff's competence. However, if the CPCN had chosen to frame the story as an "atrocity story," the case presentation would have highlighted the insensitive behavior of the nursing home staff. Instead, the CPCN focuses on problem-solving and establishes her professional strengths with team members. With this approach, she is able to organize her report in a way that makes her look professionally competent.[34]

The case presentation enables team members to work together to resolve a difficult situation in a mutually acceptable way. The CPCN achieves "definitional privilege,"[35] an approach that conveys neutrality and defines the case as "not just about pain." She leads the team to focus on the psychosocial interpretation of the problem. This supports White's contention that the case is, in part, constituted through the telling, and in telling cases, healthcare providers are not only engaged in using knowledge but also in making knowledge.[35] The CPCN makes this case of psychosocial support the business of the team. During her discussion of the support needs of P's daughter, the doctors remain silent. The CPCN successfully shapes the patient's case as inclusive of pain and psychosocial distress, thereby achieving definitional privilege.

Box 41.2 Transcript From an Audio Recording of a Hospice Team Meeting, Part 2

38	Dr	Liquid. Absolutely.
39	CPCN	Because the daughter thought she would take a
40		liquid. She thought she would take a teaspoon if it had been
41		available to give her. So I rang Dr. Jordan regarding that but
42		also what I did do was hmm I talked a long time to the
43		daughter about if she thinks she could benefit from some
44		support because this daughter is travelling to and from
45		America and you know she's got a lot on her mind and you
46		know she's lost all her control since the mother's at the
47		nursing home and she's I think could do with psychological
48		support. When she said, "yes, please." So hmm I was going to
49		do a referral to you, but I don't know if your inundated? I'm
50		quite happy to take her on because I've got some space so I'll
51		do a referral and hmm hmm you can
52	Social Worker	Well, we are both quite busy at the moment we
53		had quite a lot of referrals.
54	CPCN	Okay.
55	Social Worker	Ahm.
56	CPCN	I don't mind whichever way you want to play it,
57		but I really think, you know, that she would you know, she's
58		beginning to see, difficult to see the wood from the trees,
59		really but I think you know she's actually asking for support,
60		and I think from the commotion that happened yesterday.
61		You know, the fact that she rang here and was saying, "what is
62		the hospice about," you know, because it didn't come out. So,
63		you know, I think she's reached sort of fever pitch and I think
64		she really needs
65	Social worker	And yeah, you've obviously have met the daughter.
66	CPCN	And because Estelle will be coming back to work
67		with the mother, I'm quite happy to take her on because I
68		won't probably be involved with her again. Well shall I just do it then?

Note: CPCN = community palliative care nurse.

The power of this interaction is best explained by White as a "not just medical" case presentation.[35] In a study of healthcare providers' talk in child health settings, White concluded that there are three types of case presentations: medical, psychosocial, and "not just medical." The "not just medical" is a mixture of medical and psychosocial case formulations; "powerful definitional privilege" involves the ability to determine whether a problem was medical, psychosocial, or a combination of both. The "not just medical stories" requires complex storytelling that includes rigorous attention to detail and the cross-checking of accounts. Negotiating the "not just medical," however, seems to be dependent on the competencies that the individual provider brings to the meeting, not just clinical and psychosocial skills but the ability to give a credible account of one's work with patients and families. To render a credible account, the evidence presented "must be seen to appear that way to anyone."[36] Thus, when producing a credible account, one device is to draw attention away from the person producing the account toward the facts and evidence being reported.[37]

In this case, the CPCN goes on to make a claim to provide psychosocial support for the patient's daughter and then addresses the social worker (lines 47–48). The CPCN indicates that she could provide the support to the daughter, if the social worker is in agreement. The CPCN presents her request in a way that defers to the social worker, "so I'll do a referral and hmm hmm you can" (lines 50–51). The CPCN is again being cautious; she avoids overstepping the mark by taking on a role that is usually the prerogative of the social worker. However, at lines 85–86, she leaves the decision to the social worker, who appears happy for the CPCN to assume this role. The CPCN has competently sorted out the care home commotion by persuading the social worker that she can give the daughter the support needed. The CPCN functions as a specialist practitioner, competent in both pain work and psychosocial support. She successfully negotiates across both the doctor and social worker boundary. This example supports the contention that functions usually considered part of the medical domain may be modified in practice and disciplinary boundaries blurred and negotiated in hospice team meetings. The hospice team is an important space for the construction and sharing of expert knowledge about the patient and for displaying one's expertise and reputation as an effective team member. In the data presented here, hospice team members together construct their reputation and expertise through team talk that successfully solves the upset in the care home. The collegial positioning of team members enables the practitioners to shape patient and caregiver identity when they present cases. They have considerable influence on how the medical and psychosocial aspects of the patient experience are framed. The ability to listen to patient and caregiver stories, solve problems, and reach decisions in team settings involves a high degree of emotional labor that may, however, be difficult for hard-pressed staff with large caseloads.

Techniques for Improving Team Communication

Team communication can be improved by examining the discourses that shape the information presented in team meetings and the representations of patients, families, and other healthcare providers to colleagues.[38] Care-planning decisions that focus on autonomy, loss, change, grief, and dependence are different from care-planning discussions that focus primarily on physical care needs. Transcripts from team meetings can be used as a basis of discussion to heighten awareness of team communication and decision-making.

Improving team communication involves taking the time to reflect on team processes and team communication. Thinking and working jointly, the process by which team members think about their work process, includes acknowledging the inevitability of differential power relations between patients and healthcare providers and the ways that communication can be used to minimize these differences. Other aspects of review that can improve team communication are feedback on performance from an outside evaluator and identification of mechanisms that foster appreciation between team members. It should also be noted that team outcomes and goals need to be part of team reflection; this can be done by reviewing patient deaths and patient preferences for goals of care to see if care planning objectives were met. Reflection on the process of collaboration, plans of care, discharges, and review following a patient's death are important processes for reviewing team effectiveness and support.

Reflexivity allows team members to focus on their work together, how team values emerge and influence team decision-making, and how these values reflect care planning decisions.[39] Moral deliberation, a pause to reflect on decisions and to make prudent decisions,[40] is suggested as a way for team members to transcend their disciplinary backgrounds and take into account other team member's perspectives.[41] For newly formed teams, it is important to be aware of the process of building a team and the need to reflect on the challenges and conflicts as they arise.

Future Research

There is still much to study to improve patient- and family-centered care. Future research is needed on the effectiveness of hospice team communication and patient outcomes, the advantages of the various hospice models, the role of informal and embedded teamwork in teamwork processes and patient outcomes, and patient and family participation in team meetings and how their participation affects patient outcomes. Innovative research has shown that when family caregivers are included in team meetings, more psychosocial information is shared and patient-centered goals become more central within care plans.[42] The impact of patient and family involvement in team decision-making in hospice has yet to be known.

There is some evidence, however, to suggest effectiveness of the hospice team in relation to facilitating home care and patient-centered care at the end of life.[43] More research is needed to explore patient and family participation in team meetings, how this impacts case presentation and patient outcomes, and the ways that this approach can inform the use of technology as well as serve as a resource for team education.

Conclusion

Interdisciplinary teamwork and communication are central to patient and family centred care. Team communication strategies used by healthcare providers during interdisciplinary team meetings were described in this chapter. These strategies include use of interactional caution to minimize conflict, professional neutralism to enable mediation on behalf of patients and caregivers, problem-solving across professional boundaries by focusing on physical as well as psychosocial issues for patients and caregivers, and negotiation of resources on behalf of patients to enable patient and family focused care. Barriers to communication can cause team conflict including issues of power as well as a lack of integration of physical and psychosocial issues by an overlying biomedical approach. However, ways to improve team collaboration and teamwork are considered and practical approaches to development are suggested through focused reflection, moral deliberation on decisions taken, and team building activities supported by education and research.

References

1. Saunders C. The evolution of palliative care. *Patient Educ Couns.* 2000;41:7–13.
2. Saunders C. *Selected Writings 1958-2004.* Buckingham, UK: Open University Press; 2006.
3. Clark D. "Total pain," disciplinary power and the body in the work of Cicely Saunders, 1958–1967. *Soc Sci Med.* 1999;49:727–736.
4. World Health Organization. Palliative care. http://www.who.int/cancer/palliative/definition/en/. Accessed September 19, 2014.
5. Help the Hospices. Hospice care. www.helpthehospices.org.uk/about-hospice-care/what-is-hospice-care/. Accessed September 19, 2014.
6. Radburch L, Payne S. White paper on standards and norms for hospice and palliative care in Europe: Part 1. *J Pain Symptom Control.* 2009;16:150–168.
7. Haugen DF, Neuck F, Caraceni A. The core team and the extended team. In: Hank G, Cherney NI, Christakis WA, eds. *Oxford Textbook of Palliative Medicine.* Oxford: Oxford University Press; 2010:167–176.
8. O'Mahony S, McHenry J, Blank AE, et al Preliminary report on the integration of a palliative care team into an intensive care unit. *Palliat Med.* 2010;24:154–165.
9. Radburch L, Payne S. White paper on standards and norms for hospice and palliative care in Europe: Part 2. *J Pain Symptom Control.* 2009;17:22–33.
10. Arber A. Building reputation: The significance of pain talk in hospice and palliative care team meetings. PhD thesis. Goldsmiths College, University of London; 2004.
11. Thiel V, Sonola L, Goodwin N, Kodner DL. *Midhurst Macmillan Community Specialist Palliative Care Service: Delivering End-of-Life Care in the Community.* London, UK. The Kings Fund, 2013.
12. Maddocks I. Communication: An essential tool for team hygiene. In: Speck P, ed. *Teamwork in Palliative Care.* Oxford: Oxford University Press; 2006:137–152.
13. Gamlen E, Arber A. First assessments by specialist cancer nurses in the community: An ethnography. *Eur J Oncol Nurs.* December 2013;17(6):797–801.
14. Broom A, Kirby E. The end of life and the family: Hospice patients' views on dying as relational. *Sociol Health Illn.* 2013;35:499–513.
15. Ellingson LL. Interdisciplinary health care teamwork in the clinic backstage. *J Appl Commun Res.* 2003;31:93–117.
16. Edwards S M. District nurses lived experiences of planning care for patients at the end of life. Unpublished MSc diss. University of Surrey, Guidlford, UK; 2014.
17. Council of Europe. Recommendation Rec (2003) 24 of the Committee of Ministers to member states on the organisation of palliative care. www.coe.int/t/dg3/health/Source/Rec(2003)24_en.pdf. Published November 12, 2003. Accessed September 13, 2014.
18. Parker Oliver D. The use of videophones for patient and family participation in hospice interdisciplinary team meetings: A promising approach *Eur J Cancer Care.* 2010;19:729–735.
19. Parker Oliver D, Alvright DL, Kruse RL, Wittenberg-Lyles E, Washington K, Demris G, Caregiver evaluation of the ACTIVE intervention. *Am J Hosp Palliat Med.* 2014;31:444–453.
20. Wittenberg-Lyles E, Goldsmith J, Ferrell B, Ragan SL. *Communication in Palliative Nursing.* New York, NY: Oxford University Press; 2013.
21. Junger S, Pestinger M, Elsner F, Krumm N, Radbruch L. Criteria for successful multiprofessional cooperation in palliative care teams. *Palliat Med.* 2007;21:347–354.
22. Li S. Symbiotic niceness: A study of psychosocial care in palliative care settings. Unpublished PhD thesis. Goldsmiths College, University of London; 2002.
23. Arber A, Gallagher A. Generosity and the moral imagination in the practice of teamwork. *Nurs Ethics.* 2009;16:775–785.
24. Crepeau EB. Reconstructing Gloria: A narrative analysis of team meetings. *Qualit Health Res.* 2000;10:766–787.
25. Arber A. "Pain talk" in hospice and palliative care team meetings. *Int J Nurs Stud.* 2007;44:916–926.
26. Opie A. Thinking teams, thinking clients: Issues of discourse and representation in the work of health care teams. *Soc Health Illn.* 1997;19:259–280.
27. O'Connor M, Fisher C, Guilfoyle A. Interdisciplinary teams in palliative care: A critical reflection *Int J Palliat Nurs.* 2006;12:132–137.
28. Piers RD, van Eechoud IJ, van Camp S, Grypdonck M. et al Advance care planning in terminally ill and frail older persons. *Patient Educ Couns.* 2013;90:323–329.
29. Arber A. Team meetings in specialist palliative care: Asking questions as a strategy within interprofessional interaction. *Qual Health Res.* 2008;18;1323–1335.
30. Hibbert D, Hanratty B, May C, Mair F, Litva A, Capewell S. Negotiating palliative care expertise in the medical world. *Soc Sci Med.* 2003;57:277–288.
31. Atkinson P. *Medical Talk and Medical Work.* London: SAGE; 1995.
32. Greatbatch D, Dingwall R. Professional neutralism in family mediation. In Sarangi S, Roberts C, eds. *Talk, Work and Institutional Order.* New York, de Gruyter; 1999:271–292.
33. Strauss A, Fagerhaugh S, Suczek B, Wiener C. Sentimental work in the technologised hospital *Soc Health Illn.* 1982;4:254–278.
34. Erickson F. Appropriation of voice and presentation of self as a fellow physician: Aspects of a discourse of apprenticeship in medicine In: Sarangi S, Roberts C, eds. *Talk, Work and Institutional Order.* New York: de Gruyter; 1999:109–143.
35. White S. Accomplishing "the case" in paediatrics and child health: Medicine and morality in inter-professional talk. *Soc Health Illn.* 2002;24(4):409–435.
36. Smith DE. K is mentally ill: The anatomy of a factual account. *Sociology.* 1978;12:23–53.
37. Erickson F. Appropriation of voice and presentation of self as a fellow physician: Aspects of a discourse of apprenticeship in medicine In: Sarangi S, Roberts C, eds. *Talk, Work and Institutional Order.* New York: de Gruyter; 1999:109–143.
38. Li S, Arber A. The construction of troubled and credible patients: A study of emotion talk in palliative care settings. *Qualit Health Res.* 2006;16:27–45.
39. Gracia D. From conviction to responsibility in palliative care ethics. In: Ten Have H, Clark D, eds. *The Ethics of Palliative Care: European Perspectives.* Buckingham, UK: Open University Press; 2002:87–105.
40. Gracia D. Moral deliberation: The role of methodologies in clinical ethics. *Med Health Care Philos.* 2001;4:223–232.
41. Hermensen MA, Ten Have H. Palliative care teams: Effective through moral reflection. *J Interprof Care.* 2005;19:561–568.
42. Wittenberg-Lyles E, Oliver DP, Demiris G, Burt S, Regehr K. Inviting the absent members: Examining how caregivers' participation affects hospice team communication. *Palliat Med.* 2010;24:192–195.
43. Higginson IJ, Finlay IG, Goodwin DM, Hood K, Edwards AGK, Cooke A, Douglas H-R, Normand CE. Is there evidence that palliative care teams alter end-of-life experiences of patients and their caregivers? *J Pain Symptom Manage.* 2003;25:150–168.

CHAPTER 42

Team Communication in the Nursing Home Setting

Carol O. Long

Introduction

Long-term care refers to a broad range of medical and social services provided in community settings for individuals who need assistance ranging from personal care through the end of life. Community-based settings that are classified as long-term care consist of adult day care, home healthcare, assisted living, hospice, and nursing homes.[1] Professional and paraprofessional healthcare services may be provided in a person's own home or in institutional settings, such as the nursing home or assisted living/residential care homes. The focus and purpose of this chapter is to describe nursing homes, nursing home residents, current efforts to integrate palliative care, and the essence of interdisciplinary teamwork and communication as a necessary intervention for promoting quality of care in the final years, months, and days of life. Two exemplars of team communication in nursing homes are also provided.

Historically, nursing homes in the United States emerged in the mid-18th century to meet the needs of the sick and poor and were located mostly in large cities.[2] Over time, these settings became homes for the aged and spread widely throughout the United States. With the Social Security Act of 1935 and later healthcare insurance through Medicare and Medicaid, federal and state assistance for nursing home care became more available. Nursing homes are now a mainstay in the continuum of care, largely due to the limited ability or time of family members to care for their aged or infirmed parent and increasing life expectancy of older adults. People living in nursing homes are generally referred to as residents. Today, nursing home settings are designed to meet the ongoing short or long-term care needs of residents, young and old, who cannot routinely manage personal or medical care services in their own home.

As of 2011, there were 15,683 nursing homes with over 1.7 million beds across urban and rural areas in the United States.[3] Approximately 1,000 nursing homes are classified as care continuing care retirement communities that offer the continuum of care from independent living to assisted living and skilled nursing. Presently, nursing homes are mostly for-profit status (71%) with the remaining designated as nonprofit (23%) and government-owned (6%). Nursing homes can be stand-alone, independent, or part of a corporate entity or chain. Roughly 84% of nursing homes have 199 beds or less, and the national occupancy rate is 82%.[4]

Today, close to 1.4 million residents live in nursing homes.[5] Over 63% of the residents are female and 82% are over the age of 65. Most are white (68%) followed by black (21%), and the remaining are Hispanic, Asian, Native American, or of two races/ethnicities.[3] The percentage of adults living in a nursing home increases dramatically with age.[6] Among Medicare beneficiaries in nursing homes, 49% are covered by Medicaid.[6] Additional ongoing care needs may be paid for by privately or through long-term care insurance.[7] While it is expected that there will be tremendous growth in the number of aging adults in the years to come, the number of nursing homes and occupancy rate has dropped over the past decade. Resident acuity and segmentation of care has increased in the nursing home setting as individuals with more complex needs and comorbidities require higher intensity of care, placing greater strain on this industry and healthcare personnel providing care.[8] Still, the projected scope, quantity, and locations of nursing homes needed to meet the demands of an aging population is not known, and the financial support needed to sustain long-term care settings has not been calculated.

State and federal nursing home regulations guide everyday practice and safety. The Omnibus Budget Reconciliation Act of 1987 is the federal law that was signed into law by President Ronald Reagan and included nursing home reform. The Centers for Medicare and Medicaid Service have federal jurisdiction over nursing homes that participate in the Medicare or Medicaid program. Nursing homes are licensed in each state and are deemed certified if they meet the federal conditions of participation. Over 95% of nursing homes are dual-certified by state and federal entities. Quality measures for each facility are publicly reported on the government website Nursing Home Compare.[9] External federal and state government and private entities, such as state and regional quality improvement organizations, the Administration on Aging Long-Term Ombudsman Programs, and Advancing Excellence in Nursing Homes support and monitor the quality of nursing home care.

Nursing homes are largely staffed by professional and paraprofessional nursing personnel. Professional nurse and certified nursing assistant (CNA) staffing remains a challenge in nursing homes.[5] Reports indicate an annual turnover rate of 66% or greater for CNAs.[10] Maintaining continuity of staff in nursing homes is often a challenge to quality care, and significant turnover of staff may lead to decreased understanding of the residents' wishes or needs.

Supportive healthcare includes an array of contracted or in-house licensed or registered staff that are similar to acute care settings, such as dietary, pharmacy, therapy, and social services. An activities or therapeutic recreation department also organizes leisure activities for residents. Medical care is delivered by an individual or a group of physicians or nurse practitioners of a resident's own choosing or through a contract with the nursing home. A medical director is responsible for the oversight of medical management in the nursing home.

Individuals residing in nursing homes generally require supportive care due to deficits in executing activities of daily living; in fact over 80% of residents have impairments with one or more activities of daily living. Half of nursing home residents are over the age of 85[6] and 68% are cognitively impaired.[11] Some residents reside in a nursing home for an abbreviated time. Typically referred to as "short stay," these individuals are typically admitted for skilled or rehabilitative care following an acute care or hospital stay. Skilled care in the nursing home is a Medicare benefit. Residents using the skilled benefit are not eligible to use the Medicare Hospice Benefit at the same time.[12] "Long-stay" residents are those who reside in the facility for longer than 100 days, require continuing or intermediate care, and typically do not return to the community or their home. While some residents may wish to return home, many are unable to do so. Oftentimes these individuals live out their final days in the nursing home setting. There is limited national data on the causes of deaths in nursing homes, and it is considered largely inaccurate. Among decedents 65 years of age and older, non-Hispanic white females are mostly likely to die in nursing homes.[13] Those receiving formal end-of-life care are more likely to have at least one advance directive (AD).[14]

The nursing home industry has changed and evolved over the years, responding to external regulatory forces or a self-identified need to improve care. A recent thrust in the nursing homes is "culture change," or the paradigm shift to reform care and improve satisfaction and quality of life for residents.[15,16] Nursing homes are adopting person-centered care as part of the culture change movement. An emerging evidence base and grassroots effort support positive resident, staff, and facility outcomes related to this initiative.[17] Thus resident choices are solicited, documented, and honored.

Another movement in long-term care is for residents to "age in place," whereby individuals live at home until their death. More recently this term has been applied and expanded to include long-term care settings, such as nursing homes. Aging in place refers to a model of care where a full range of services is provided in one setting to address different levels of care.[1,18] However, limited staffing, clinical knowledge, and skills expertise are barriers to providing end-of-life care to nursing home residents.

Currently there is a national initiative to reduce readmissions of all hospital discharged patients, including residents who were hospitalized within the past 30 days.[19] Likewise, there is increased attention aimed at reducing the number of Medicare nursing home residents admitted to hospitals, as some medical conditions may be cared for in the nursing home. In a recent government report, medical conditions such as septicemia (13.4%), pneumonia (7.0%), and heart failure (5.8%), which account for an estimated 6% of admission diagnoses, could be largely managed in a nursing home setting.[20] Thus the cost of expensive and yet sometimes futile hospital care has provided momentum to ensure that residents receive quality care in the most appropriate setting.

Palliative Care in Nursing Homes

Palliative care spans the continuum of care and is a necessary component in all healthcare settings, including the nursing home. Palliative care moves end-of-life care principles upstream in the trajectory of care, occurring long before the last 6 months of life, and includes hospice in the continuum of care. Considering that almost one-quarter of residents die in nursing homes each year, it is imperative that palliative care is a standard service and philosophy of care in these settings. In an analysis of Medicare claims, the proportion of nursing home decedents who received hospice care was 33.1% in 2006; most were female (67%), white (90%), and older than age 85 (55%).[20] Accordingly, 18.3% of hospice recipients received end-of-life care in a nursing facility in 2011.[21] Unfortunately, the Medicare Hospice Benefit cannot be provided when the resident is receiving the Medicare skilled nursing facility benefit; therefore, the resident may forgo expert end-of-life care services if palliative care is not an integral part of the nursing home structure.[12,22]

However, recent Centers for Medicare and Medicaid Service regulations in nursing homes include key elements of palliative care. There are three federal and state licensure and certification requirements specific to end-of-life care in nursing homes. First, when a resident is enrolled in hospice while residing in the nursing home, hospice staff, the nursing home team, and the resident or representative must be actively engaged in the plan of care, which includes methods to manage pain and symptoms.[23] The hospice team and nursing home staff must communicate with each other when changes are indicated to the plan of care, and each party must remain aware of his or her role in providing palliative care. Second, the interdisciplinary team (IDT), with support and guidance from the physician, is responsible for the review, evaluation, indications for, potential risks, and benefits associated with feeding tube placement.[24] This includes having a discussion about feeding tube placement or discontinuation with the resident or responsible party. The third requirement is related to ADs, which is specified in F-tag 155.[25] Buoyed by the 1991 Patient Self-Determination Act, residents in nursing homes must be told of their right to execute an AD. Results from the 2004 National Nursing Home Survey and 2007 National Home and Hospice Care Survey indicated that 65% of nursing home residents had completed at least one AD, most commonly consisting of living wills and "do not resuscitate" healthcare orders. Residents over age 85 and white were more likely to have an AD. Research shows that AD selection is largely determined by "individual attitudes, cultural beliefs, health conditions, and trust in healthcare professionals."[26(p1)]

Compliance with these regulations stipulates that policies and procedures should be in place regarding the right of residents to formulate ADs and to decline treatment and other related interventions. It further specifies that residents need to be informed and educated about these rights with the opportunity to develop an AD with the assistance of long-term care staff. Advance care planning is the process by which individuals identify their life plan for the future when they are no longer able to make those decisions. It includes clarifications of values, preferences, and specifications of care. A documented AD allows people to communicate their healthcare preferences and designate a medical care proxy. Furthermore, the nursing home must determine a resident's capacity to understand information and make treatment decisions and then monitor care and services to ensure consistency with his or her documented choices and goals. The nursing home IDT, along with the medical provider, is responsible for the execution and ongoing commitment to the completion of ADs and following residents' expressed wishes.

Even with these regulations, several barriers to the implementation of palliative care in nursing homes exist, including limited financial resources for nursing homes and residents, less than satisfactory coordination and communication of care between the palliative care team and nursing home staff, inadequate pain and symptom management, and a lack of palliative care education for staff and staffing inadequacies, to name a few. Additionally, hospice is not widely used in nursing homes due to financial disincentives related to Medicare payment mechanisms, and the services and benefits may not be well understood.[27] Nursing homes may feel threatened when the resident is "shared" with a hospice agency.[28] Advance care planning is often limited and not specified, and, when this happens, there is a greater chance for burdensome and futile care. Overall, the shift to palliative care is incongruent with federal and state standards.[29]

Geropalliative care is an emerging concept in palliative care that describes quality of care for older adults and families in the last years of life.[30] Geropalliative care includes management of multimorbid conditions, recognizing the complexity of care for older adults.[31,32] Geropalliative care is not setting or disease specific; rather it transcends these elements and illuminates broader care needs applicable in the nursing home setting. Differing health illness trajectories, burdensome treatments at the end of life, and lack of adequate advance care planning supports a holistic model of geropalliative care in nursing homes.

Burdensome transitions, treatments, interventions, and the prevalence of clinical patterns and symptoms in older adults reveal the need for palliative care in nursing homes. Health–illness trajectories depict progressive decline and have wide applicability for residents in nursing homes, characterized by a short period of evident decline, prolonged dwindling, and long-term limitations with intermittent serious episodes.[33,34] These trajectories, and their implications for different medical conditions, are useful in guiding practice and the work of the nursing home IDTs, particularly when a resident experiences a significant obvious change in condition (e.g., hip fracture, stroke, myocardial infarction) or one that is less obvious (e.g., weight loss, pain, falls, incontinence, repeated infections). The high incidence of pain, prevalence of feeding tubes, restraint use, pressure ulcers, multiple hospitalizations, time spent in the intensive care unit, lack of hospice care, and unexpected weight loss are described as discomfort and identified by poorer quality of care, particularly for those with advanced cognitive impairment.[35–37]

General knowledge about palliative care is essential but also lacking for staff in nursing homes.[38] Targeted palliative care education is necessary for direct care workers, support staff, and management. The End-of-life Nursing Education Consortium geriatric curriculum provides fundamental principles in palliative care practice.[39,40] Following a person-centered approach, staff need to know what residents want and how to create a culture of comfort.

They also need to be able to recognize geriatric syndromes, uncomfortable symptoms, pain, and the primary causes of death for older adults so that targeted comfort approaches can be instituted early on in the care trajectory. Content and concepts related to loss, grief and bereavement, quality of life, spirituality, and culture are essential skills. Topics on communication with residents and other team members are necessary for the nursing home staff and members of the IDT.

Thus while current palliative care guidelines and government regulations emphasize the principles of palliative care, formal palliative or "comfort" care has yet to become adopted or widely available in nursing homes.[41] A palliative care approach affirms life and maximizes quality of life in the end-of-life journey and needs to be widely available for residents in nursing homes. A model of palliative care in nursing homes must include an identifiable IDT structure with a working knowledge of geropalliative care principles to augment best practices.

Models of Palliative Care in the Long-Term Care Setting

The World Health Organization defines a team as two or more people working interdependently toward a common goal.[42,43] IDTs, which are composed of people from more than one discipline, rely on the synergy and expertise of team members to actively communicate, collaborate, and share information to work toward a common goal.[43] Both palliative care and long-term care settings rely on team-based structures. The lack of a defined team and turnover of staff can lead to inconsistent care and not "knowing the person." While models of teamwork and communication methods and tools require specificity, various palliative care models are evident for some nursing home settings and nonexistent in others.

In the nursing home setting, Medicare requirements stipulate that interdisciplinary care conferences be held on admission, quarterly, and as the medical condition of the resident changes. A registered nurse must conduct and coordinate each assessment with the appropriate participation of healthcare professionals. These meetings are attended by other IDT members, and comprehensive care plans are reviewed and needs addressed upon completion of the comprehensive assessment that includes the physician and other appropriate staff, the resident (if able), and resident's family or legal representative.

To integrate palliative care into the nursing home setting, and to enable the palliative care and nursing home IDTs to work together, Meier proposes using one of the following models: palliative care consultation services, hospital-based palliative care consultation service, or nursing home services–integrated palliative care and hospice care.[44,45] More recently three other models for palliative care in nursing homes have been suggested. These include nursing home–hospice partnerships, external palliative care consultative teams, and in-house teams or specialized palliative care units.[46] Table 42.1 lists three of the prevalent palliative care models that interface with nursing homes.

Nursing Home Teams and Communication Education

Often related to size and the organizational mission, different team structures exist in nursing homes. These may include

Table 42.1 Comparison of Nursing Home Palliative Care Models

Model	Description	Team Interface
Nursing Home—Hospice Partnerships	Under the Medicare Hospice Benefit or commercial insurer, hospice care is provided to the resident in the nursing home usually under contract. The nursing home provides room, board, medications, and the usual services but is paid for by hospice.	Hospice oversees the plan of care and supplements nursing home services. Joint team meetings between hospice and the nursing home guide the plan of care. Hospice brings expertise in pain and symptom management.
External Palliative Care Consultation Teams	These community-based teams are based in medical provider office practices, hospices, or hospital palliative care services. Medical consultation is paid for by existing Medicare or commercial payors directly and not through the nursing home or hospice.	Resident-specific consultations focusing on palliative care management are conducted in the nursing home. No formal communication or team model is known.
Internal Team or Specialized Palliative Care Units	In this model, the nursing home has built-in capacity to provide palliative care to residents through specialized programs or in palliative care units (see exemplars in text). Hospice is still provided to residents.	The nursing home in-house team is the palliative care team, managing care and advance care planning as an integral part of the nursing home structure. Usual nursing home team communication is followed.

administrative teams, ad hoc teams, care teams, IDTs, and others. Regarding palliative care, nursing homes interface with external teams, such as hospice or hospital/community-based palliative care teams, and others may create their own palliative care team. Regardless of the team structure, a core palliative care skillset is necessary, and team members participating in a palliative care or any other IDT should include skilled nursing staff, the CNA, medical providers, and social service, dietary, and activity staff, at a minimum. A team model is essential, and communication structure and flow must be defined. Palliative care IDTs can significantly improve the lives and reduce negative outcomes in the residents who live in nursing homes.[14,43,47]

Although not tested in nursing home settings, the COMFORT™℠ curriculum provides seven principles for patient and family care and includes modules on Communication, Orientation and Opportunity, Mindful presence, Family, Openings, Relating, and Team.[48,49] As a model of interprofessional communication, members of the nursing home IDT would benefit from instruction on COMFORT™℠, as the curriculum includes attention to self-awareness, collaborative practice, and person-centered communication. The COMFORT™℠ curriculum incorporates principles of team cohesion, consistency, and managing conflict. Overall, it supports team camaraderie, a necessary component of any effective nursing home setting structure.

Two additional evidence-based team models and educational approaches have been developed for use in nursing home settings: Team Strategies and Tools to Enhance Performance and Patient Safety (TeamSTEPPS™) and the Geriatric Interdisciplinary Team Training (GITT). While originally targeted toward patient safety initiatives, TeamSTEPPS™ focuses on four competency areas: team leadership, situation monitoring, mutual support, and communication. TeamSTEPPS™ Long-Term Care has been adapted to include long-term care settings such as nursing homes, assisted living, and care continuing care retirement communities. The standards of effective communication are completeness, clarity, brevity, and timelines. The TeamSTEPPS™: Long Term Care Version coaches staff in nursing home settings to use tools to communicate efficiently.[50]

The GITT training is a Hartford Institute for Geriatric Nursing resource created in 1995 and is currently being updated for the training of IDTs who care for older adults.[51] While the curriculum does not specifically address palliative care, the manual and training includes topics about the team, teamwork roles and responsibilities, communication and conflict resolution, care planning, multiculturalism, ethical care, and teamwork. GITT is a standard resource for geriatric team training.

Several methods of training that accentuate the team approach and communication have been developed that are specific to palliative care or geriatric IDTs; however, none address the unique context of nursing home settings. Elements to consider in nursing home IDTs include structural or foundational features, process components, and measureable outcomes. Necessary structural components may include an identifiable palliative care IDT and clear designation or roles of team members with specified interface with the nursing home organization. Process components focus on interprofessional education in palliative care, collaborative and coordinated approaches to care, and communication channels. Outcomes for residents could range from specific problem areas, such as incompletion of Ads, to targeted palliative care for residents who are high risk using geropalliative care principles.

Palliative Care Communication in the Nursing Home

Good communication is at the heart of the nursing home service delivery model, and it is an essential competency for all staff. Various communication tools and measures have been propagated in nursing homes, although none are specific to palliative care. While a curriculum in palliative care communication is necessary, several tools and methods are presently available and used in nursing home IDTs to improve communication and augment resident-focused practice. Many can be used or adapted by the internal nursing unit team, palliative care team, or external palliative care team or hospice staff who come to the nursing home to care for a resident. A summary of communication strategies are briefly outlined next.

Briefs or Huddles

Briefs or huddles are short- or long-term quick staff meetings to share and problem-solve issues "on the spot."[52] Huddles can occur at the start or end of a shift or target quality improvement topics related to clinical care and may or may not include the entire IDT. Huddles provide an effective way to foster ongoing communication at the time the need is more pressing, such as evolving critical issues. All staff hears the information at the same time with the meetings lasting no more than 5 to 15 minutes. Plans, outcome, and contingency plans are discussed. With a focus on quality of life and palliative care, specific targeted areas should include pain and symptom management, grief and family support, and general comfort needs. Perhaps residents are complaining about unanswered call lights when requesting pain medications. Staff may meet once to identify the problem and agree on the need to explore further. Future targeted meetings focus on possible causes and remediation with an objective to resolve the complaint.

Debriefs

Debriefs are short, informal, information-exchange and feedback meetings held after an event or end of a shift. Debriefs hone in on teamwork skills while examining targeted outcomes with efforts for future improvement. Debriefs could be used after a problem on the nursing unit. An example of a debrief may be the difficulty staff members have after the death of a resident. Staff members routinely meet in the lunch room to debrief by sharing stories about the resident and meaningful times spent together as a way to cope with the loss.

Daily Stand-Up Meetings

These meetings are similar to huddles but occur at the start of each day with similar goals: to help start the day well, to support improvement, to reinforce focus on the right things, to reinforce the sense of team, and to communicate what is going on. This team-building skill focuses on communication and teamwork and fosters self-management and empowerment and reinforces open communication that allows staff to raise questions and offer solutions within the team. Everyone attends. While staff members still receive individual reports from the shift leaving the unit, this method captures team spirit and affirms the focus on resident care and comfort. For example, daily stand-up meetings are useful to discuss residents new to hospice and current trends from the Minimum Data Set 3.0 reports on problem areas related to pressure ulcers, pain, or other measures that necessitate palliative care intervention.

Situation–Background–Assessment–Recommendation

SBAR is a standardized format for communicating to other team members about a resident's condition and is known to be used across a variety of clinical settings. For example, SBAR can be used by the registered nurses to "hand off" or communicate to the physician about a resident's need for pain medication. In this communication, both the medical prescriber and staff member dialogue about the presenting issues and joint recommendations are reached.

Check-Backs and Call-Outs

A check-back validates information exchanged, confirming that the message was communicated and the sender verified receipt of the message. A call-out communicates critical information about a resident during an emergency. An example of a call-out situation may be an unexpected hemorrhage at the end of life. An example of a check-back is when both the message sender and receiver verify the information received, repeating it back to the sender.

In this situation, both parties may agree on clinical interventions that support the resident and the family, such as rapid sedation and possible environmental changes that promote comfort.

Handoffs

Sometimes called "handovers," handoffs are the effective sharing of pertinent information to other team members. Handoffs can be used at the end of shifts or intermittently when new care team members need to be apprised or updated about a resident's condition. Handoff information typically includes the residents' diagnosis, recent changes in their condition, treatment and services, the plan or goals of care, and any recent or anticipated changes. During the handoff, authority and responsibility is transferred to the other team member. An example of a handoff may be a CNA who is leaving the nursing unit for lunch and is communicating to a fellow CNA and nurse about the terminal condition of a resident. During the handoff, both CNAs and the nurse may visit the bedside of the resident.

Resident Rounds

As noted, as people age, they are likely to be institutionalized in a nursing home and are most likely to die there. At-risk rounds help to target residents who may trigger for an emergency department transfer event, geriatric syndromes, progressive medical condition or disease trajectories, and unrelieved chronic pain.[53] Bedside rounds conducted at regular intervals focus specifically on goals of care; an example would be the daily evaluation of residents for fall risk or those new to pain medications.

Practice Tools

The Interventions to Reduce Acute Care Transfers (INTERACT) Version 3.0 program focuses on the means and tools to equip nursing homes to reduce transfers to the hospital and has numerous tools that augment palliative care.[54] INTERACT includes advance care planning tools; decision-support tools for change in condition, such as a review of acute care transfers and numerous care paths; and quality improvement and communication tools to facilitate information-sharing between the nursing home and hospital. When used routinely, these tools guide practice and are known to reduce admissions to acute care settings.

While current communication approaches tools target teamwork, it is important to note that the resident's family members are an integral part of the team. Family members may become isolated and feel like visitors while their loved one is in a nursing home. It is not uncommon for family members to feel tremendous guilt related to the resident's nursing home placement. Especially at the end of life, family members need the opportunity to advocate for their dying relative, as they can feel misinformed and excluded from care planning.[55] The palliative care IDT can work with nursing home staff to ensure that family members understand the dying process.[56] Family conferences are one communication tool that can be used to strengthen relationships among the care team, family, and resident. The care conference is best suited when the setting is right, the entire interdisciplinary care team is present, and a structure or agenda is in place.[57] The palliative care team can help provide family support by offering assistance with finances and finding community resources. The palliative care team is also able to help nursing home staff facilitate family conferences aimed at making care decisions congruent with resident and family goals of care and engaging family members in emotion work by recounting the resident's life and wishes. A main component of these conversations include education about palliative care, hospice, and quality of life.

Team Communication in a Nursing Home

Understanding teams and implementing communication best practices in nursing homes has been largely understudied and palliative care communication not well described in the literature. The best way to illuminate practice is to provide two exemplars featuring varying methods of teamwork and team communication.

Exemplar 1: Beatitudes Campus in Phoenix, Arizona

Beatitudes Campus, a nonprofit, faith-based, continuing care retirement community, serves 700 older adults and thousands of families in Phoenix, Arizona. The campus employs approximately 450 staff members who work around the clock in a variety of roles from many different departments. The Health Care Center is a 72-bed nursing home comprised of two Neighborhoods that serve residents with long-term care, rehabilitation, and dementia care needs. Staff communication has always been highly valued, yet one area that has proven to be particularly challenging is communication across departments and shifts as it relates to caring for people living with dementia. Stressful situations range from a team of painters interrupting a much-loved musician who only plays once a week to family communication challenges about care decisions when a resident's condition changes. To meet these challenges, the staff at Beatitudes Campus were required to complete a standardized communication plan for all departments and shifts, giving structure to a team-based model of communication.

A team meeting approach was developed to facilitate dialogue across departments and shifts in the Health Care Center. Formal meetings, called Neighborhood and Core meetings, were created to collect and disseminate information among providers. Facilitated by a trusted, nonbiased staff member, each team meeting is held weekly on the same day and time for 30 minutes. Members of each team are encouraged to discuss barriers and concerns regarding implementation of palliative care, and team members are required to provide a reasonable solution to the concern. Using this team-based approach for care planning empowers staff to work as a team and develop a culture that promotes comfortable and successful experiences for everyone.

Neighborhood meetings are attended by staff working in a particular area or Neighborhood in the Health Care Center. Each member of the team is encouraged to participate in the meeting and has an equal voice regardless of his or her position or department. The purpose of the Neighborhood meeting is to create comfort and eliminate distress by exchanging information about residents and families. The meeting focuses on getting to know each person in depth and sharing strategies that would maximize individual comfort and minimize distress. Staff learn from each other what strategies worked best for "Mrs. Jones" or "Mr. Green," and the exchange brings them closer together as team.

The second team meeting, known as Core meetings, represent all Beatitudes Campus departments but does not include every staff member from the Neighborhood. Again, each member of the Core team has an equal voice and is responsible for bringing concerns of people with dementia to the meeting. The purpose of this meeting is to review all healthcare systems and implement changes toward dementia-friendly practices. Because Core meeting members represent the larger Neighborhood staff, they are obligated to promote the well-being of everyone.

Still, team communication challenges remain. Initially, some staff members believed they had all of the answers and that other people's opinions or decisions did not matter. Other staff were reluctant to speak up and share information or engage in decision-making activities. Managers had concerns that either the Neighborhood or Core meeting would result in staff arguments, would decrease morale, or that team members would go outside their scope and ability by attempting to create changes that were not appropriate. In these situations, open communication was thwarted. Each of these challenges was eliminated by ensuring total transparency in the communication process. Meeting minutes are taken and available for every staff member to read. When warranted, staff were coached individually on how to embrace differing opinions of peers from other shifts or departments or how to speak up and or participate in decision-making activities during meetings. Finally managers, with the help of both the Neighborhood and Core members, drafted parameters for what could and could not be done within the scope of the meetings.

The process of developing and implementing team communication plan took approximately 6 months. Once in place, the Neighborhood and Core meetings were successful across all departments and shifts. The teams have experienced continuous success as staff members see their work come to life. As a result, the Neighborhood has developed and implemented a strong pain management program, reduced rejection of care, and limited use of antipsychotics or anxiolytics; in addition, families are satisfied with this shift toward palliative care. Staff from all departments have benefitted greatly as well, with improved morale and job retention.[58]

Exemplar 2: Donald Coburn Centre in Sydney, Australia

The Donald Coburn Centre is a 180-bed nursing home located in Sydney, Australia. It is one of 17 residential aged care facilities administered by Anglican Retirement Villages (ARV), a not-for-profit Christian organization and large aged care provider caring for over 6,000 residents and clients across the diocese of Sydney. Care is provided in both residential care homes and within the community. The nursing home is in a growing area of Sydney, and the majority of residents come from a middle-class Anglo-Australian background, although the resident demographic is becoming increasingly multicultural. Residents require high-level nursing assistance, and most are older adults who are physically frail and living with multiple comorbidities. Forty-five of the nursing home beds are contained within a dementia-specific unit. People residing in this area are those who have been found to have more challenging behavior, ranging in age from 50 to 100 years old.

The nursing home has access to the organization's palliative care nurse specialists, who provide a system of referral for those residents whose end-of-life needs are complex. The palliative care nurse team offers support, advice, and education to residents, families, staff, and general practitioners. The palliative care nurse specialists have close working relationships with specialist palliative care community teams for further support when required.

Recognizing that many of the residents entering the nursing home are in the latter stages of their lives, a family conference is called with the resident present (if appropriate) and the family (or responsible party) within the first 28 days of admission to the facility. Attendance at this meeting is open to any staff member who is involved in the resident's care, including but not limited to the registered nurse, physiotherapist, lifestyle leader, chaplain or pastoral care worker, care staff, and supervisor of food services. The senior registered nurse is responsible for organizing this meeting and leading a discussion of care needs and reviewing any family concerns or problems.

At the first family conference, emphasis is placed on opening discussion around future care wishes, especially when there is a decline in the health of the resident. Senior registered nurses at the center have been coached in conducting these sensitive conversations, allowing the family and the resident to consider medical interventions that would or would not be acceptable. To further support these conversations, a brochure is available to explain advance care planning procedures and topics. The meeting includes the palliative care nurse specialist if it is perceived that the resident or family is in discord or struggling with decisions. Information acquired and outcomes of the meeting are documented within the resident's computerized notes by the staff member who led the meeting. If and when completed, an advance care plan is placed at the front of the hard-copy notes so that it is visible to team members and can be countersigned by the general practitioner. All documentation is accessible by team members through the computer system.

Team members working in the nursing home setting come from many diverse backgrounds, countries, and cultures. This represents unique challenges to palliative care communication and end-of-life care situated in a first-world country. In order to practice cultural humility (see chapter 11), team members who are identified as having an interest in palliative care are given the opportunity to undertake a palliative care course delivered by ARV's palliative care nurse specialists. Upon completion, team members are recognized as palliative care specialists with the capacity to coach other care staff on the principles of end-of-life care.

Communication between the ARV palliative care nurse specialist team and nursing home staff is achieved by building relationships among all disciplinary team members, including the management team. Prompt response to referrals, being easily accessible to assist staff with concerns when delivering end-of-life care, bedside coaching of evidence-based practice, and the development of tools to enhance bedside care ensure the success of this model of palliative care in the long-term care setting.[59]

Conclusion

In conclusion, nursing homes are undergoing significant transformative change, yet more is needed. It is expected that older adults will continue to reside and die in nursing homes, many without the benefit of a geropalliative care skill set from an IDT. It is speculated that without defined patterns and methods of communication, positive resident outcomes may not be achieved and burdensome treatment may persist. Regulatory mandates are reinforcing the need for progressive change that supports a culture of palliative care; however, palliative care in these care settings require clarity on team structure and collaborative communication channels and methods. Two quite different exemplars of teamwork and communication were offered to provide insight into the ways palliative care can be delivered in long-term care settings. Formalized approaches and research supporting new and improved palliative care approaches that endorse the interdisciplinary care model of collaborative practice in nursing homes is still needed.

References

1. Miller CA. *Nursing for Wellness in Older Adults*. 6th ed. Philadelphia, PA: Wolters Kluwer/Lippincott Williams & Wilkins; 2012.
2. Long Term Care Education.com. Types of long-term care. http://www.ltce.com/learn/typesofcare.php. Published 2014. Accessed March 2, 2014.
3. Centers for Medicare and Medicaid Services. CMS Nursing Home Data Compendium. http://www.aanac.org/docs/reference-documents/nursinghomedatacompendium_508.pdf%7B?%7Dsfvrsn=2 Published 2012. Accessed March 20, 2014.
4. National Center for Health Statistics. Table 109: Nursing homes, beds, residents and occupancy rates by state: US selected years 1995–2011. In: *Health, United States, 2012: With Special Feature on Emergency Care*. Hyattsville, MD: US Department of Health & Human Services; 2013:317–318. http://www.cdc.gov/nchs/data/hus/hus12.pdf. Accessed May 16, 2014.
5. US Department of Health & Human Services. A profile of older Americans: 2013. http://www.aoa.gov/Aging_Statistics/Profile/2013/docs/2013_Profile.pdf. Accessed March 23, 2014.
6. Harris-Kojetin L, Sengupta M, Park-Lee E, Valverde R. *Long-Term Care Services in the United States: 2013 Overview*. Hyattsville, MD: National Center for Health Statistics; 2013. http://www.cdc.gov/nchs/data/nsltcp/long_term_care_services_2013.pdf. Accessed April 14, 2014.
7. Kaye HS, Harrington C, LaPlante MP. Long-term care: Who gets it, who provides it, who pays, and how much? *Health Aff*. 2010;29(1):11–21.
8. Mor V, Caswell C, Littlehale S, Nieme J, Fogel B. Changes in the quality of nursing homes in the US: A review and data update. http://www.ahcancal.org/research_data/quality/Documents/ChangesinNursingHomeQuality.pdf. Published August 15, 2009. Accessed April 29, 2014.
9. Medicare.gov. Nursing home compare. http://www.medicare.gov/nursinghomecompare/search.html. Accessed July 31, 2014.
10. Mukamel DB, Spector WD, Limcangco R, Wang Y, Feng Z, Mor V. The cost of turnover in nursing homes. *Med Care*. 2009;47(10):1039–1045.
11. Alzheimer's Association. 2013 Alzheimer's disease facts and figures. *Alzheimers Dement*. 2013;9:208–245.
12. Aragon K, Covinsky K, Miao Y, Boscardin WJ, Flint L, Smith AK. Use of the Medicare posthospitalization skilled nursing benefit in the last 6 months of life. *Arch Intern Med*. 2012;172(2):1573–1579.
13. Kelly A, Conell-Price J, Covinsky K, Cenzer IS, Chang A, Boscardin WJ, Smith AK. Length of stay for older adults residing in nursing homes at end of life. *J Am Geriatr Soc*. 2010;58(9):1701–1706.
14. Bercovitz A, Decker FH, Jones A, Remsburg RE. *End-of-life care in nursing homes: 2004 national nursing home survey*. National Health and Statistics Report 9. Hyattsville, MD: US Department of Health & Human Services; 2008.
15. Rahman AN, Schnelle JF. The nursing home culture-change movement: Recent past, present and future directions for research. *Gerontologist*. 2008;48:142–148.
16. Bowers B, Nolet K, Roberts T, Esmond S. Implementing change in long-term care. A practical guide to transformation. https://www.pioneernetwork.net/Data/Documents/Implementation_Manual_ChangeInLongTermCare%5B1%5D.pdf Accessed April 25, 2014.
17. Grabowski DC, O'Malley J, Afendulis CC, Caudry DF, Elliot A, Zimmerman S. Culture change and nursing home quality of care. *Gerontologist*. 2014;54(Suppl 1):S35–S45.

18. Shippee TP. "But I am not moving": Residents' perspectives on transitions within a continuing care retirement community. *Gerontologist.* 2009;49:418–427.
19. US Department of Health & Human Services, Centers for Medicare and Medicaid Services. Initiative to reduce avoidable hospitalizations among nursing facility residents. http://www.cms.gov/Medicare-Medicaid- Coordination/Medicare-and-Medicaid-Coordination/Medicare-Medicaid- Coordination-Office/Reducing Preventable Hospitalizations AmongNursing FacilityResidents.html. Published 2014. Accessed February 22, 2014.
20. US Department of Health & Human Services, Office of the Inspector General. Medicare nursing home resident hospitalization rate merits additional monitoring. https://oig.hhs.gov/oei/reports/oei-06-11-00040.pdf. Published November 2013. Accessed March 10, 2014.
21. National Hospice and Palliative Care Organization. *NHPCO's Facts and Figures: Hospice Care in America.* Washington, DC: National Hospice and Palliative Care Organization; 2013.
22. Huskamp HA, Stevenson DG, Grabowski DC, Brennan E, Keating NL. Long and short stay hospice stays among nursing home residents at the end of life. *J Palliat Med.* 2010;13(8):957–964.
23. US Department of Health and Human Services, Centers for Medicare/Medicare. Interpretive guidelines for long-term care, Facilities F tag 309 (quality of care): Advance copy. https://www.cms.gov/Medicare/Provider-Enrollment-and-Certification/SurveyCertificationGenInfo/Downloads/Survey-and-Cert-Letter-12-48.pdf. Published September 27, 2012. Accessed February 24, 2014.
24. US Department of Health & Human Services, Centers for Medicare/Medicare. Interpretive guidelines for long-term care : Facilities F tag 322 (feeding tube) : Advance copy. http://www.cms.gov/Medicare/Provider-Enrollment-and-Certification/SurveyCertificationGenInfo/Downloads/Survey-and-Cert-Letter-12-46.pdf. Published September 27, 2012. Accessed February 24, 2014.
25. US Department of Health & Human Services, Centers for Medicare/Medicare. F tag 155: Advance directives: Revised advance copy. https://www.cms.gov/Medicare/Provider-Enrollment-and-Certification/SurveyCertificationGenInfo/Downloads/Survey-and-Cert-Letter-13-16.pdf. Published March 8, 2013. Accessed February 24, 2014.
26. Jones AL, Moss AJ, Harris-Kojetin LD. *Use of Advance Directives in Long-Term Care Populations.* NCHS Data Brief 54. Hyattsville, MD: National Center for Health Statistics; 2011. http://www.cdc.gov/nchs/data/databriefs/db54.pdf Accessed May 16, 2014.
27. Miller SC. A model of successful nursing home-hospice partnership. *J Palliat Med.* 2010;13(5):525–533.
28. Long CO. Palliative care in nursing homes. In: Panke J, Coyne PJ, eds. *Conversations in Palliative Care.* 3rd ed. Pittsburgh, PA: Hospice and Palliative Nurses Association; 2011:255–264.
29. Forrest J, Long CO, Kuhn D, Alonzo TR, Frazier AL. Palliative care for advanced dementia: Regulatory friend or foe? *Ann Long-Term Care: Clin Care Aging.* 2012;20(1):17–20.
30. Lee SM, Coakley EE. Geropalliative care: A concept synthesis. *J Hospice Palliat Nurs.* 2011;13(4):242–248.
31. Arnold RM, Jaffe E. Why palliative care needs geriatrics. *J Palliat Med.* 2007;10(1):182–183.
32. Kapo J, Morrison LJ, Liao S. Palliative care for the older adult. *J Palliat Med.* 2007;10(1):185–209.
33. Lynn J, Adamson DM. *Living Well at the End of Life. Adapting Health Care to Serious Chronic Illness in Old Age.* Rand Health White Paper WP-137. Washington, DC: Washington Home Center for Palliative Care Studies; 2003.
34. Lunney JR, Lynn J, Foley DJ, Lipson S, Guralnik JM. Patterns of functional decline at the end of life. *JAMA.* 2003;289(18):2387–2392.
35. Gozalo P, Teno JM, Mitchell SL, Skinner J, Bynum J, Tyler D, Mor V. End-of-life transitions among nursing residents with cognitive issues. *N Engl J Med.* 2011;365:1212–1221.
36. Mukamel DB, Caprio T, Ahn R, Zheng N, Norton S, Quill T, Temkin-Greener H. End-of-life quality of care measures for nursing homes: Place of death and hospice. *J Palliat Med.* 2012;15(4):438–446.
37. Teno JM, Gozalo PL, Bynum JPW, Leland NEP, Miller SC, Morden NEMM, Scupp T, Goodman DC, Mor V. Change in end-of-life care for Medicare beneficiaries: Site of death, place of care, and health care transitions in 2000, 2005, and 2009. *JAMA.* 2013;309:470–477.
38. Grossman S. Educating RNs regarding palliative care in long-term care generates positive outcomes for patients with end-stage chronic illness. *J Hosp Palliat Nurs.* 2007;9(6):323–328.
39. End of Life Nursing Education Consortium. ELNEC fact sheet. www.aacn.nche.edu/elnec/factsheet.htm. Accessed March 1, 2014.
40. Kelly K, Ersek M, Virani R, Malloy P, Ferrell B. End-of-life nursing education consortium geriatric training program: Improving palliative care in community geriatric care settings. *J Gerontol Nurs.* 2008;34(5):28–35.
41. Meier DE, Lim B, Carlson MD. Raising the standard: Palliative care in nursing homes. *Health Aff.* 2010;29(1):136–140.
42. World Health Organization. Team building. http://www.who.int/cancer/modules/Team%20building.pdf. Published 2007. Accessed May 5, 2014
43. Youngwerth J, Twaddle M. Cultures of interdisciplinary teams: How to foster good dynamics. *J Palliat Med.* 2011;14(5):650–654.
44. Center to Advance Palliative Care. Improving palliative care in nursing homes. http://www.capc.org/support-from-capc/capc_publications/nursing_home_report.pdf. Published 2008. Accessed April 4, 2014.
45. Morrison RS. Suffering in silence: Addressing the needs of nursing home residents. *J Palliat Med.* 2009;12(8):671–672.
46. Ersek M, Carpenter, JG. Geriatric palliative care in long-term care settings with a focus on nursing homes. *J Palliat Med.* 2013;16(10):1180–1187.
47. Comart J, Mahler A, Schreiber R, Rockett C, Jones RN, Morris JN. Palliative care for long-term care residents: Effect on clinical outcomes. *Gerontologist.* 2012;53(5):874–880.
48. Wittenberg-Lyles E, Goldsmith J, Ragan SL. The COMFORT Initiative. Palliative nursing and the centrality of communication. *J Hosp Palliat Nurs.* 2010;12(5):282–292.
49. Wittenberg-Lyles E, Goldsmith J, Ferrell B, Ragan SL. *Communication in Palliative Nursing.* Oxford: Oxford University Press; 2013.
50. Agency for Healthcare Research and Quality. TeamSTEPPS: Long Term Care version. http://www.ahrq.gov/professionals/education/curriculum-tools/teamstepps/longtermcare/. Reviewed October 2012. Accessed June 14, 2014.
51. Hartford Institute for Geriatric Nursing Website. http://hartfordign.org/education/gitt/ Accessed July 31, 2014.
52. Pioneer Network. Huddles tip sheet. https://www.pioneernetwork.net/Providers/StarterToolkit/Step1/HuddlesTipSheet. Accessed February 22, 2014.
53. Caffery C. Potentially preventable emergency department visits by nursing home residents. NCHS Data Brief No. 33. http://www.cdc.gov/nchs/data/databriefs/db33.pdf. Published April 2010. Accessed April 26, 2014.
54. Ouslander JG, Bonner A, Herndon L, Shutes J. The Interventions to Reduce Acute Care Transfer (INTERACT) quality improvement program: An overview of medical directors and primary care clinicians in long term care. *J Amer Med Dir Assoc.* 2014;15:162–170.
55. Shield RR, Wetle T, Teno J, Miller SC, Welch LC. Vigilant at the end of life: Family advocacy in the nursing home. *J Palliat Med.* 2010;13(5):573–579.

56. Hanson LC, Ersek M. Meeting palliative care needs in post-acute settings: "To help them live until they die." *JAMA*. 2006;95(6):681–686.
57. Cohen Fienberg I, Kawashima M, Asch SM. Communication with families facing life-threatening illness: A research-based model for family conferences. *J Palliat Med*. 2011;14(4):421–427.
58. This exemplar was contributed by Tena Alonzo, MA, Director of Research, Beatitudes Campus, Phoenix, AZ.
59. This exemplar was contributed by Christine Lancaster RN, RM, MCN, Postgrad Cert Cancer Nursing, Postgrad Cert Palliative Care, Clinical Nurse Consultant Palliative Care, Anglican Retirement Villages, Sydney, Australia.

CHAPTER 43

Communication Education for Physicians

Jillian Gustin, Katie H. Stowers, and Charles F. von Gunten

Introduction

Communication is a critically important skill for all physicians to master in their clinical practice. The Accreditation Council for Graduate Medical Education (ACGME) requires all physicians to demonstrate competency in "interpersonal and communication skills that result in the effective exchange of information and collaboration with patients, their families, and other health professionals."[1] Much has already been written on the topic of teaching communication skills to physicians from a variety of perspectives and approaches. This chapter is not an exhaustive overview of those perspectives. Instead, it draws from a review of the literature and our own experience as seasoned clinical educators to present a "toolbox" of strategies for teaching communication skills, particularly related to teaching physicians new to the field of hospice and palliative medicine (HPM). This toolbox includes the following:

- A conceptual model for patient- and family-centered communication that can be used to help learners operationalize communication strategies and to demystify the "magic" in complex communication encounters that trainees often attribute to their attending physicians.
- An outline of various approaches to teaching communication skills such as simulated patient experiences, clinical bedside checklists, and so on.
- A discussion of the importance of and approaches to providing effective feedback as an integral part of teaching communication skills.
- A discussion of the importance of communication skills in common HPM clinical settings, such as family meetings and telemedicine.

Communication as an Essential Skill

Communication is a core skill essential to the daily practice of caring for patients and their families facing serious or advanced illness.[2] Consequently, ACGME-accredited HPM fellowships require graduating physicians to exhibit competence in the following communication skills[3]:

1. Initiate informed relationship-centered dialogues about care
2. Demonstrate empathy
3. Demonstrate ability to recognize and respond to own emotions and those of others
4. Demonstrate the ability to educate patients/families about the medical, social, and psychological issues associated with life-limiting illness
5. Use age-, gender-, and culturally appropriate concepts and language when communicating with families and patients
6. Demonstrate these skills in the following paradigmatic situations with patients or families and document an informative, sensitive note in the medical record (e.g., giving bad news, discussing transitions in care, introducing a palliative care consultation, etc.)
7. Organize and lead or cofacilitate a family meeting
8. Collaborate effectively with others as a member or leader of an interdisciplinary team
9. Develop effective relationships with referring physicians, consultant physicians, and other healthcare providers
10. Maintain comprehensive, timely, and legible medical records

Given the complexity inherent in demonstrating these competencies of HPM training, many physicians in our field assert that communication is HPM's core "procedure."

There are many benefits of quality communication. It improves patient and family satisfaction, decreases the psychological morbidity for patients and families, improves quality of life, fosters adherence to therapeutic regimens, avoids malpractice litigation, and supports bereavement adjustment for families.[4-7] Nonetheless, provider communication often fails to meet the needs of patients and families,[6, 8-11] and the outcomes of poor communication are dire. Adverse mental health sequalae, late hospice referrals, and more aggressive, unwanted life-prolonging care are all potential consequences of ineffective communication.[7]

Multiple barriers exist in communication with patients and their families. In part, ineffective communication can be related to the characteristics of the physician such as emotional stress, competing time demands, and fear of confronting illness and death.[12,13] Moreover, most physicians receive inadequate communication training and thus report discomfort with complex communication tasks.[14,15] Multiple studies have revealed that residents feel unprepared to provide end-of-life care and ill equipped to facilitate medical decision-making with patients and families.[14,15]

Communication education has made great advances over the past decade, with an increase in the implementation of communication curricula across the training spectrum (medical student, resident, fellow). Numerous studies have illustrated the valuable use of feedback, deliberate practice, simulation, communication roadmaps, and so on for honing communication skills particularly related to patients with serious or advanced illness. However, many of the training strategies have focused on discrete communication tasks such as breaking bad news, having a code discussion, and/or facilitating a family meeting. This has required learners to remember and employ separate communication rubrics for distinct situations, often making complex communication tasks feel even more complicated. To make teaching and learning communication less daunting, discrete communication tasks should be integrated into a comprehensive conceptual model for physician–patient–family communication. This schema allows the teacher and learner to move beyond a communication task approach and operationalize the elements and associated skills that foster communication in most contexts.

Patient- and Family-Centered Communication: The Five Elements and Their Associated Tools

This chapter's conceptual model builds on the concept of shared decision-making through patient- and family-centered communication. Communication in HPM often involves highly charged discussions and decisions related to breaking bad news, transitions in care plans, and advance care planning related to end-of-life care. Shared decision-making is often the crux of these discussions with five basic tenets[16] (see Table 43.1). Most simply, shared decision-making requires a patient-centered approach whereby healthcare providers engage in a partnership with patients and families to develop medically appropriate care plans that are consistent with patients' values and goals.

Although the evidence to support any particular communication practice is limited, multiple organizations such as the ACGME, the American College of Critical Care Medicine, and the National Cancer Institute, to name a few, all advocate the importance of patient- and family-centered communication. The National Cancer Institute[17] offers clear components of patient-centered communication that assure the core functions of communication[18] (see Table 43.1).

The following section integrates these concepts into a model that is grounded in a patient- and family-centered approach and centered on the concept of shared decision-making. It delineates the elements and skills of communication as a model from which to teach communication to physician learners. This model is comprised of the following five elements: assess patient perspective, exchange information, attend to emotion, manage uncertainty, and engage in shared decision-making. Most discussions between HPM physicians and patients/families involve shared decision-making with varying degrees of gravity (e.g., symptom management, resuscitation status, breaking bad news, advance care planning, and/or goals of care, etc.). Regardless of the type of discussion, the five elements of quality communication remain the same and can be employed for all types of discussions. Some discussions will require more of an emphasis on a particular element of the model (e.g., attending to emotion when breaking bad news). Nonetheless, all the skills are necessary to some greater or lesser degree for most HPM discussions. This conceptual model is not meant to be linear. Instead, it provides a cognitive framework, or scaffolding, on which to build and learn communication (Figure 43.1).

When visualizing this conceptual model, the top three circles are clearly part of patient- and family-centered communication and shared decision-making. We have added "managing uncertainty" as a crucial element to the model, related to common discussions in HPM. For many HPM patients and their families, prognostication and its inherent uncertainty are integral to the illness experience and decision-making.[19] Although there are no clear best practices for discussing uncertainty, managing

Table 43.1 Comparison of Shared Decision-Making, Patient-Centered Communication, and Core Functions of Communication

Shared Decision-Making[16]	Patient-Centered Communication[17]	Core functions of Effective Communication[18]
Discussing the nature of the decision to be made	Eliciting and understanding patient perspective (concerns, ideas, expectations, needs, feelings, and functioning)	Fostering the relationship
Exchanging relevant medical information and information about a patient's values	Understanding the patient within his or her unique psychosocial and cultural context	Gathering information
Checking for understanding of information for both the healthcare provider and the patient	Reaching a shared understanding of patient problems and its treatments	Providing information
Discussing preferred roles in decision-making	Helping a patient share power by offering him or her meaningful investment in choices related to his or her health	Decision-making
Achieving consensus about the treatment course most consistent with the patient's values and preferences		Enabling disease and treatment-related behaviors
		Responding to emotion

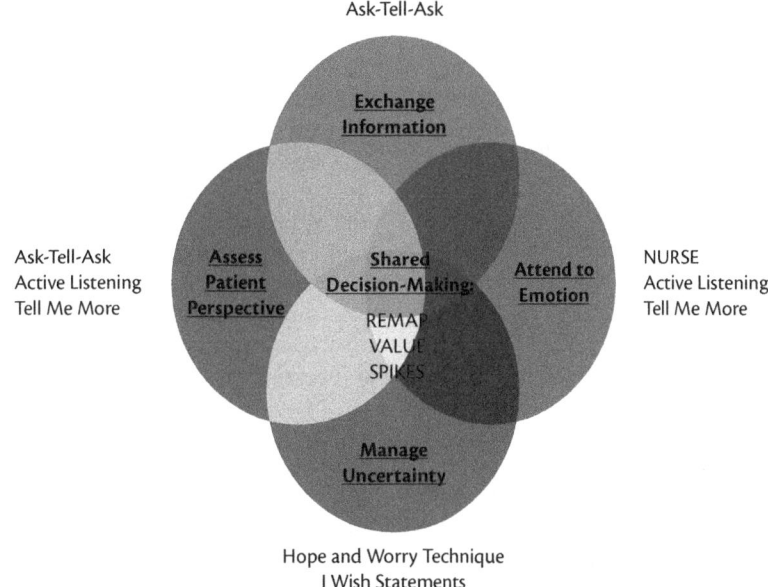

Figure 43.1 Patient- and family-centered communication: The five elements and associated tools

uncertainty while promoting prognostic awareness is an essential skill for HPM physicians, whose primary goal is to foster medical decision-making based on patients' values and realistic goals.[16]

This model transforms complex communication into a learnable skill by parsing it into essential elements and tools that can be taught and practiced. The elements are the "what" that constitutes quality communication and the tools are the "how" to employ the elements. These are not difficult skills, and many learners will have been introduced to some of them at some point during their training as roadmaps for specific types of discussions (e.g., SPIKES for breaking bad news,[20] VALUE for goals of care discussions in the intensive care unit [ICU][21], NURSE for addressing emotion[22]). When these roadmaps are deconstructed, they contain similar, if not identical, elements. This conceptual model takes these roadmaps and maps them onto the five elements central to patient- and family-centered communication for HPM physicians. The remainder of this section outlines each element, and its associated tools, with examples to guide the clinician educator in utilizing this conceptual model for teaching communication.

Assessing Patient Perspective and Exchanging Information

The goal of "assessing patient perspective" is to elicit how a patient and/or family understands and experiences the illness. It involves a biopsychosocial model of inquiry that assesses a patient's understanding of his or her illness from both a cognitive and emotional framework (i.e.: What does the patient know about his or her medical condition and what are his or her feelings related to the illness?). In addition, it includes an understanding of how a patient is being impacted by and making meaning out of his or her illness (i.e.: How does the illness affect functioning, relationships, self-perception, etc.?). The tools associated with this element of the conceptual model include Active Listening, Ask-Tell-Ask, and Tell Me More.

Active Listening

Active Listening involves paying attention to nonverbal cues, using reflective questions and statements, and practicing compassionate silence.[23] Quality communication often relies on close attention to nonverbal cues from both the patient and physician. Teaching communication to physician-learners requires an explicit discussion of the importance of nonverbal body language such as presenting an open body posture, encouraging patient input with nodding, sitting down or attempting to be at eye level with the patient, and maintaining eye contact. The setup of the room is another important feature to discuss with learners and includes such factors as minimizing distractions (i.e., silencing phones or pagers), finding a private place for a discussion (e.g., closing the door or curtain), sitting close to the patient, and so on.[12]

Reflective questions and statements show the patient that the physician is listening.[12] With this tool, learners reiterate and/or paraphrase what the patient has said to ensure that there is a mutual understanding of the patient's comments: "It sounds like you are saying that you are in a lot of pain. Do I understand you correctly?" Sometimes there is a buried question behind a patient's statement. A reflective question or statement that elucidates or interprets the buried question can often help move a conversation forward: "It sounds like you are saying that your pain is getting in the way of your ability to work."

In practicing compassionate silence, learners first need to practice allowing patients to talk without interruption. Once a learner has practiced this skill, the educator can introduce the application of compassionate silence. The literature underscores the importance of silence and allowing a patient and family to lead the conversation to areas important to them. Some silences can be invitational or expectant of a response from the patient. In contrast, the main objective of compassionate silence is to be present with the patient, without expectation, and is often helpful in times of high emotion. By employing compassionate silence, physicians create a sense of mutual understanding, caring, and compassion.

Compassionate silence can be a very difficult skill to master, thus teachers should normalize the challenges of employing this tool for learners.

Ask-Tell-Ask

The Ask-Tell-Ask[24] is used to explore patients' understanding of their disease, provide information to them as needed, and ensure that the information provided by the physician was received. The initial Ask is exploratory about the patient's and/or family's understanding of the illness:

> "What have the doctors told you so far?"
> "To make sure that we're on the same page, can you tell me what is your understanding of your illness?"

The first Ask should also explore how a patient wants to receive information; that is, who does the patient want involved in the discussion for support, such as a spouse or friend; how much information does he or she want to receive at a particular time; what is the best way to convey information in terms of level of detail versus general impressions?[25,26] Overall, the first ask is a strategy for eliciting what the patient already knows to provide the framework on which to build more knowledge and understanding.

As healthcare providers, we often need to deliver information to our patients about treatment options, results of testing, prognostic information, and so on. The "Tell" of "Ask-Tell-Ask" is the provision of information to the patient and/or family. Learners are encouraged to avoid medical jargon and give information in small, digestible chunks; receivers of information often cannot maintain attention for a prolonged period of time. The Tell requires completion of the initial ask, so that the physician can build on the knowledge of the patient without unnecessarily repeating what is already known. A Tell following the first Ask can also help the physician correct misinformation or misunderstanding of a patient's knowledge.

The second Ask is to ensure that the physician and patient have achieved a common understanding by asking for the patient's synopsis. In addition, the second Ask can include assessing what questions the patient may still have, after receiving the Tell:

> "I want to ensure that my explanation was effective. Will you tell me in your own words what you understand from what I have just said?"
> "What questions do you have about what we have just discussed?"

Tell Me More

Tell Me More[24] is a tool for helping learners drill deeper into their assessment of patient perspective. It is an invitation for patients to tell the physician more about whatever topic they have identified as important. Learners can use Tell Me More to uncover the hidden stories or questions in a patient's communication and to try to understand the full illness experience of the patient beyond just the physical changes to their health. It is a tool that can be used to explore a patient's cognitive and emotional perspective on their illness:

> "Tell me more about your understanding of your illness."
> "Tell me more about how you are feeling about your illness."
> "Tell me more about how you are making sense of all of this."
> "Tell me more how your illness is impacting your life."

Attending to Emotion

HPM discussions frequently focus on emotionally charged events such as giving serious news or considering advance care planning for one's impending death. An emotional reaction to difficult news is an expected response from patients and their families. Although physicians often purposefully try to remain emotionally neutral to provide accurate information, communication requires physicians to recognize the emotions of their patients and respond to them. Attending to emotion[12,27] can strengthen the patient–physician relationship by explicitly acknowledging and normalizing that emotions play a role in decision-making. If emotions are attended to, physicians can help decrease subsequent psychological morbidity in the future for patients and their families. In addition to Tell Me More and Active Listening, another tool associated with attending to emotion is NURSE statements—a helpful mnemonic of empathetic phrases made by the physician for the same purpose. These tools are used to attend to, explore, and support a patient when emotions have been expressed verbally and nonverbally.

NURSE Statements

In NURSE statements,[22,27,28] each letter stands for a particular aspect of the approach.

N = NAME. Learners begin by naming a patient's emotion to themselves as a way of noting what is happening in an encounter. By acknowledging the emotion silently, learners have a better understanding of where to focus the conversation. In some cases, it may be useful to name the emotion to the patient as a way of showing that the physician is attuned to what the patient is experiencing. By naming the emotion, the physician validates that emotion as expected and normal.

> A patient has just learned from recent imaging her disease is worse. Her head is bowed down, and she is visibly tearful. A Naming statement would be: "It seems that this is very upsetting to you"

U = UNDERSTAND. This type of statement shows an appreciation by the physician for the patient's predicament or feelings. It helps build rapport and focuses on what the patient is experiencing. An Understanding statement, at its most simple, is an empathic statement.

> A patient expresses the difficulty of managing work responsibilities with his chemotherapy regimen. An Understanding statement would be: "I can't imagine what it is like to balance your treatments with your work life."

R = RESPECT. Physicians show respect for their patients with nonverbal cues such as good eye contact, body posture, and so on. At the same time, a verbal statement that explicitly states that emotions are not only allowable but important is a helpful way of respecting a patient's emotions. Patients and their families often respond positively to validating statements of their coping in the face of a challenging road.

> A husband has been at his wife's bedside in the ICU daily for two weeks. A Respecting statement would be: "I have been so impressed by your ability to sit at the bedside every day to ensure that your wife is receiving the best care possible. I can't imagine how hard that must be."

S = SUPPORT. Patients are often fearful of being abandoned at the end of life by their physicians. A statement about a physician's willingness to help regardless of the outcome can alleviate a patient's fears of abandonment.[29,30] Ultimately, a Support statement is a verbal recognition of the physician-patient partnership, regardless of illness stage.

> A patient has shown no improvement after 2 weeks in the ICU. The patient's husband has agreed to transition the care plan for his

wife to intensive comfort measures. A Support statement would be: "You are not alone in this. We will continue to be here for you to help you and your family with the next steps."

E = EXPLORE. This tool may incorporate other skills such as Tell Me More to explore further the emotion of the patient and allow the patient and/or family to express the emotional areas most challenging to them.

> A terminally ill patient with young children has expressed profound sadness and guilt at not being able to parent her children as they grow up. An Explore statement would be: "I can only imagine how upsetting it must be to consider leaving your kids. Can you tell me more about your concerns?"

Managing Uncertainty

Many of the aforementioned skills such as Active Listening and Tell Me More can be used as tools to manage uncertainty for patients and their families. There are two additional tools that help learners incorporate assessing and promoting prognostic awareness while supporting their patients' coping: Hope and Worry and I Wish . . .

Hope and Worry

When using Hope and Worry, physician statements of nonabandonment help patients and their families cope with the uncertainty of their illness trajectory.[31,32] Many patients and their families often hope for outcomes that the healthcare provider feels may be unobtainable. Nonetheless, targeted questions that ask patients to identify hopes, and at the same time explore their concerns, often reveal a patient's clear understanding of the likely illness trajectory, despite the unrealistic wishes. To assess prognostic awareness, a healthcare provider may simply ask: "Putting together everything that we have talked about, what are you hoping for, and what are you worried about?"

This tool may also be used to promote prognostic awareness[32] and foster realistic expectations and goals, when a patient and/or family has difficulty expressing the likely, and oftentimes undesired, outcome. It is a way of reframing hope by encouraging a dual agenda: hoping for the best and preparing for the worst.[33] An important aspect of promoting prognostic awareness should include a discussion of possible trajectories: the best, the worst, and the most common, including not only mortality but also changes in function.[34] Example statements include: "Are there other hopes that you have? We have discussed what you are hoping for. May we talk about what if our hopes aren't realized?" "I am hoping with you that the treatment works, and I am worried that it may not. If it doesn't work as we would like, I will still continue to work with you to ensure that you are well taken care of."

I Wish . . .

This tool is a means to promote prognostic awareness while cultivating a partnership and alignment with the patient and/or family. I Wish[28,35] statements are an expression of empathy and an implied acknowledgment that the likely outcome is undesirable and emotionally difficult. I Wish statements also acknowledge implicitly that the healthcare provider is limited in his or her control of the outcome. This tool has the ability to temporarily suspend the physician from the medical expert role, so that the healthcare provider and patient can sit together in their sadness at the likely unwanted outcome. For example, "I wish I had more answers for you as to why your body is not responding to the treatment in the way we had hoped."

Shared Decision-Making

Many roadmaps capture the elements of shared decision-making and patient-centered communication. For some learners, mnemonics and roadmaps can be helpful tools for organizing discussions with patients, whether one on one or in a family meeting. For others, the tools associated with the other four elements of patient-centered communication will be sufficient to achieve shared decision-making. Certain mnemonics may be used as potential tools for achieving shared decision-making, including REMAP, VALUE, and SPIKES. REMAP is the mnemonic most focused on shared decision-making. The following examples illustrate its use. SPIKES and VALUE are other mnemonics that may be helpful to learners as guidelines for complex conversations.

REMAP is a mnemonic developed for addressing goals of care.[36,37] It consists of the following:

R = REFRAME. This is a statement that signals a disruption of the current clinical status, often following the delivery of serious news.

> "Given this news, it seems like a good time to talk about what to do now"
> "We are in a different place now."

E = EXPECT EMOTION AND EMPATHIZE. A learner can use the tools associated with Attending to Emotion at this point such as Active Listening, Tell Me More, and NURSE statements.

> "I can see how hard this is to hear. Is it ok for us to talk about what it means?"

M = MAP THE FUTURE. The physician may outline the different trajectories and elicit the patient's concerns, worries, and goals. This may be a place to use the skills in Managing Uncertainty to ensure a mutual understanding of the likely illness trajectory.

> "Given this situation, what is most important to you?"

A = ALIGN WITH THE PATIENT'S VALUES. This is an attempt to reconfigure a new orientation to living from the patient given his or her new and oftentimes undesired clinical context.

> "As I listen to you, it sounds like the most important things are being at home with your family and avoiding future hospitalizations."

P = PLAN MEDICAL TREATMENTS THAT MATCH PATIENT VALUES. A healthcare provider may offer possible directions that match the patient's articulated goals while underscoring continued involvement and nonabandonment.

> "Here's what I can do now that will help you do those important things. What do you think about that?"

VALUE is a mnemonic developed to improve communication between physicians and families of critically ill patients in the ICU.[21] VALUE stands for Value the comments made by the family, Acknowledge family emotions, Listen, Understand the patient as a person, and Elicit family questions. SPIKES is a mnemonic developed for delivering bad news. It can be applied to facilitating family meetings and goals of care discussions with some modifications.[20] SPIKES is a six-step protocol that includes Setting up the interview, assessing the patient's Perception, obtaining the patient's Invitation, giving Knowledge and information to the patient, addressing the patient's Emotion and empathic responses, and Summarizing.

Strategies for Teaching Communication Skills to Physicians

Interventions to promote communication skills development are largely successful in transferring new skills to learners.[38] Certain teaching strategies have proven more effective than others. Teaching strategies engaged in active learning, namely those involving practice (e.g., simulated patient experience), as well as teaching strategies that include feedback in response to skills training, have consistently demonstrated effectiveness at promoting skill development. On the other hand, those engaged in passive learning, namely training involving instruction (e.g., lectures), are most effective when used as supportive strategies.[38] Components of successful communication skills training programs include the following principals:

- Lecture-style methods alone are ineffective.
- Adult learning principles should be used.
- Teaching must include skills practice.
- Teaching must attend to learner attitudes and emotions.
- The learning environment should integrate knowledge, skills, and attitudes.
- Reenforcement is critical for the learning process.[39]

Communication skills training programs highlighted in the literature include the OncoTalk[39] and GeriTalk[40] programs that are comprised of multiday, small-group interventions. These skills training programs were designed around the aforementioned key educational principals and include a multimodal approach to skills training comprised of instruction, practice, and feedback.

Communication Instruction

Lectures and written handouts are useful teaching strategies when used as part of a multimodal training program. In our experience, the use of lectures and handouts provide an avenue to introduce the fundamental communication skills concepts that can be built on as more advanced teaching strategies are employed. For example, a training session to develop the communication skill of attending to emotion should begin with a lecture introducing the NURSE mnemonic tool and a handout with examples of NURSE statements, followed by an opportunity for the learner to practice these skills. The use of instructional teaching strategies increases the learner's knowledge of different communication skills and use in different contexts.[41]

Modeling is another form of communication instruction and refers to learning by watching and imitating others.[42] For communication training, modeling occurs when a expert performs a particular communication skill for the benefit of teaching learners a specific behavior. This can occur in a live or videotaped setting utilizing real or simulated patients.[42,43] For this strategy to be successful, it is imperative to identify the specific skill that is being modeled prior to initiating the interview. The learner should be instructed to observe not only what is said and how it is delivered but also the impact of the delivered skill on the patient—including both verbal and emotional responses. For example, when using modeling at the bedside that will likely include breaking bad news, the learner could be instructed to specifically observe for emotive statements used by the physician in response to patient distress.

After leaving the patient's room, the physician and learner should discuss the encounter, including the physician's actions, the patient's response, and suggestions for alternative approaches. The modeling teaching strategy, much like the other instructional techniques described here, has not proven effective when used in isolation but is successful in transferring skills to learners when combined with other techniques.[42]

Communication Practice

Practice teaching strategies are simulated scenarios in which participants act out situations to allow learners to practice specific communication skills.[42] Included in this category are simulated patient experience and role play.

The benefits of these strategies include providing a safe learning environment for learners to experiment with new skills, allowing opportunity for repetition, feedback, and replay.[41] For the palliative care learner, this safe learning environment is essential when developing skills to lead family meetings and goals of care discussion, as these conversations can be emotionally charged for both the patient and the learner. Additionally, these learning strategies provide exposure to multiple scenarios less frequently encountered during clinical practice, such as discussions regarding artificial nutrition and hydration and requests for hastened death. Successful role play and simulated patient encounters require facilitator training to provide a safe training environment and a culture of effective feedback.[41] Lack of learner engagement due to performance anxiety can be common with both approaches.[41,44]

Simulated patient experience refers to the use of a trained actor portraying a medical scenario conducted for purely educational purposes.[44] Simulated patients are different from standardized patients. Definitions vary in the literature, but, in general, a standardized patient provides consistent verbal, behavioral, and physical responses to the stimulus provided by the learner.[44] Standardized patients are best utilized for summative evaluation. Comparatively, simulated patients deliver a less structured performance, allowing variability of responses and behaviors in response to learner performance, thereby providing more flexibility during communication skills training.

In our experience, simulated patient training is best performed in a small-group setting, comprised of multiple learners, a trained facilitator, and a trained simulated patient. Learners should have the opportunity to familiarize themselves with the case and ask question prior to initiation of the simulated patient experience. The room should be organized such that learner and simulated patient can engage in a physician–patient type encounter (i.e., two chairs facing each other or a hospital bed and chair) with the observing learners and facilitator sitting within close range to see and hear the interaction. The observing learners and facilitator should be observing not only what is said but body language, facial expressions, and emotions. The facilitator can stop the simulation if the learner becomes "stuck" or at other opportune times to provide feedback and engage the observing learners in group discussion about what went well and alternate approaches to the simulation. This provides an opportunity to allow the learner to "retry" the simulation to incorporate the feedback.

A successful simulated patient experience hinges on creating a learning environment that feels authentic and fosters successes for learners, so they remain engaged and willing to participate. Learner resistance is common and is often due to performance anxiety. It can be alleviated by creating a safe learning environment, which includes a semiprivate, quiet setting without much distraction or observation from others outside the group.[41] The importance of the "time-out" cannot be underrated, as this not only provides security to the learner but also provides an opportunity for immediate feedback and group discussion. Finally, simulated patients need adequate training to foster success for learners. Simulated patient training can be a complex and time-consuming endeavor and often requires help from the leadership of a simulation center.

Role-play refers to the use of the learners as both patient and physician during a simulated scenario, alternating roles with other learners.[41] There are many similarities between role play and simulated patients. The same elements described previously that are pertinent for successful simulation apply to role play (excluding the training of the simulated patient). Additionally, the same setup and ground rules apply as well.

Compared to simulated patients, role play provides the benefit of allowing the learner to experience the perspective of the patient during the simulated encounter.[41] Without the constraint of the simulated patient cost and training, role play allows for more flexible and inexpensive skills education that can be beneficial to smaller or impromptu training sessions. However, learners often report that role play with other learners feels "unnatural," and success of this training strategy relies heavily on the learner's willingness to play the role of the patient authentically.[41]

Feedback

Feedback refers to providing learners with information describing their performance with the intent of guiding future performance.[45] Feedback is endorsed by all major medical education organizations (Liaison Committee on Medical Education, ACGME, Alliance for Clinical Education, American Medical Association) as essential to physician training. In general, it is an informed, nonevaluative, objective appraisal of performance intended to improve clinical skills, in this case communication.[45] Feedback helps learners identify areas of high performance and gaps between their performance and the standard. The literature on formative feedback in medical education shows that it enhances student satisfaction as well as improves clinical performance, patient satisfaction, and self-assessment accuracy.[46-50] In the absence of explicit feedback, learners "infer" about their abilities, often incorrectly.

Self-assessment is an important element of feedback particularly related to communication training. Self-assessment comprises learners' self-evaluation of their abilities against perceived norms. Although there are many challenges to self-assessment and little evidence that it changes clinical practice, it provides a window into a learner's insight and is more likely to generate learning goals than feedback provided by an observer.[51,52] Asking for learning goals requires students to think about their own developmental stage and to bring effort to deliberate improvement.[53] Finally, the opportunity for students to reflect on their experience and to enhance their self-assessment improves their ability for self-directed learning in the future.

The literature on feedback describes a mismatch in perceptions of its utility by students and teachers.[54-56] Both learners and faculty value feedback but are often ambivalent about receiving or giving it.[46,57,58] Faculty report feeling ill equipped to provide it due to lack of training, inadequate time, fear of retribution, and the underlying belief that feedback does not necessarily change behavior.[59,60]

Feedback becomes more challenging when the focus is on communication. All physicians come to training with ingrained habits related to communication from years of interacting with friends, family, and other professionals. Learners may perceive feedback as a personal attack on a communication style as opposed to a comment on a learned skill.[61] Moreover, learners who have integrated habits from watching previous role models may feel that feedback on their style denigrates the skills of a prior respected role model. Many learners and educators see communication skills as innate and immutable rather than as skills that can be identified and improved.

Despite its challenges, feedback regarding communication skills is a necessity for learners and an attainable skill for educators.[62,63] Much has been written on how to improve the efficacy of feedback. Here we highlight a few of the essential elements compiled from multiple sources:[45, 64-68]

Establish an Appropriate Climate

First, educators should find an appropriate location and time for providing feedback. A private, quiet space where the learner does not have competing responsibilities is preferable. An appropriate climate is one in which feedback is an intrinsic part of the supervisory role. The educator should explicitly inform learners that feedback is expected and clearly state its purpose, timing (preferably immediately following an encounter), and likely mode of delivery (e.g. checklist, verbal feedback, etc).

Set Specific Goals

Goals for the communication task should be specific enough that they are manageable in scope (ideally focusing on only one or two skills) and achievable. Moreover, goals should be learner-centered, such that the choice of a communication goal is negotiated and mutually agreed upon by the learner and teacher.

Utilize Learner Self-Assessment

Prior to an educational activity or encounter, educators should ask the learner to identify his or her likely communication challenges to help establish specific shared goals. After the encounter, educators again should ask the learner to identify his or her successes and challenges with achieving the desired goal. This will allow the educator to gain insight into the learner's self-perception and help guide further learning activities. Finally, the opportunity for students to reflect on their experience and to hear their self-assessment in juxtaposition with the comments of faculty can improve their ability to evaluate their own performance. For example, prior to a family meeting with discordant family members (mother and son) of a critically ill patient, a learner may reveal his discomfort with emotional conflict. The mutually agreed-upon goal for feedback could be attending to emotion. After the encounter, the learner reflects that he was able to name the son's frustration but did not know how to handle the mother's tears. The educator may consider a role-play in the future to practice attending to sadness.

Provide Targeted Feedback on Observed Behaviors

Feedback should be targeted to the behavior related to the specific learning goal that was identified before the encounter. It is helpful for the educator to convey how the learner's skill affected the interaction positively to (a) increase the learner's awareness of that specific skill and (b) increase the frequency with which the learner uses it. When a learner has achieved the identified learning goal of attending to emotion and the patient reengages eye contact, the feedback may be: "You listened to the patient and used an empathic statement, when she seemed sad. I noticed that after your empathic statement, the patient lifted her head and looked at you again."

The educator should also describe the gap between what was observed and what was expected, related to a specific learning goal that was not achieved during an encounter. For example, the learning goal may be to set up the room for a difficult conversation with a family of an ill patient. However, the conversation with the family was interrupted multiple times by the learner's phone ringing. The feedback may be: "I noticed your phone rang frequently and interrupted you when you were talking with the family. Please silence it when you are in a patient or family interview to minimize distractions and ensure that the family feels heard."

Offer Suggestions for Improvement

Feedback is not complete without an action plan to continue to improve performance. When possible, educators should build upon the skills that the learner employs competently with deliberate practice (i.e., repeated goal-setting, practice, feedback) and subsequent further practice while offering more challenges to the skill. For example, a learner received feedback that her empathic response helped to reengage a tearful patient after breaking bad news. An action plan may be to try empathic statements in other contexts, such as code discussions or goals of care discussions, with planned feedback on this learning goal for the rest of the week.

Be ready for a Learner's Emotional Reaction to Feedback

Learners may have strong emotional reactions to receiving feedback that is not aligned with their self-perceptions regarding their communication skills. Be ready. An empathic response from the teacher may help the learner absorb the need for more practice.

Strategies for Providing Formative Feedback at the Bedside

In the clinical setting, feedback is often overlooked and forgotten—partly due to time constraints and poor training in how to provide effective and efficient feedback.[64] Checklists are the preferred method for providing feedback in the clinical setting. Checklists are a frequently used and effective method of providing feedback during communication skills training. They consist of a list of specific communication skills or behaviors that allow an observer to record the presence or absence of the skill/behavior being performed.[69] A versatile tool, checklists can be used to provide feedback in a variety of settings, including direct observation of interactions with real patients or simulated patient encounters and videotaped real or simulated encounters.[70]

A variety of published checklists is available that are specific for communication skills training, including the Kalamazoo Consensus Statement,[71] Calgary-Cambridge Observation guide,[72] and SEGUE Framework.[73] The American Academy of Hospice and Palliative Medicine recommends the SECURE Framework as the tool of choice for assessing communication skills for HPM fellows.[74] This checklist was adapted from the SEGUE framework for use in HPM and highlights specific communication tasks and observable behaviors essential to a communication encounter (Table 43.2). While the SEGUE framework has been validated, the SECURE has not.[73,74]

While checklists can provide a useful tool for providing formative feedback at the bedside, there are also inherent challenges in their use. The efficacy of the checklist in promoting skills development largely depends on the users' (both observer and learner) engagement with the tool. Without adequate buy-in or proper training to utilize the tool, the benefits of using this tool may not be realized.[69] The SPIKES protocol for breaking bad news is another tool that can be used to guide the provision of feedback.[64] The elements of effective feedback listed here can be transposed onto the elements of SPIKES, as shown in Table 43.3.

Communication in Hospice and Palliative Medicine Practice

Family Meetings

Facilitations of family meetings are frequently required of HPM physicians and are often triggered by serious changes in a patient's clinical status. Family meetings provide an opportunity to share medical information, reach consensus on treatment plans, facilitate advance care planning, resolve conflict, clarify roles, and attend to anticipatory grief. The crux of any family meeting should be patient- and family-centered communication and eventually result in shared decision-making based on patient values. The tools necessary to facilitate a family meeting effectively are those already described in the proposed conceptual model and do not require new or different skills.

Facilitation of family meetings, however, can be a demanding context within which learners try to employ their communication techniques. The elements and skills described in the conceptual model need to be applied not just to the patient but to multiple family members who have their own reactions and perspectives. Educators should normalize the inherent challenges to facilitating family meetings so that learners do not feel overwhelmed by their complexity.

Table 43.2 SEGUE and SECURE Frameworks Compared

SEGUE Framework	SECURE—Palliative Care Framework
Set the Stage	Set the Stage
Elicit Information	Elicit Information
Give Information	Convey Information
Understand the Patient's Perspective	Understand Patient and Family Perspective
End Encounter	Respond to Emotions
	End Encounter

Table 43.3 SPIKES Protocol for Breaking Bad News, Adapted for Giving Feedback

Breaking Bad News	Giving Feedback
S = **Set** up the interview	Private, safe environment
P = assess **Perception**	Diagnose the learner, self-assessment
I = obtain **Invitation**	Warning shot: Can I give you some feedback on what I observed?
K = give **Knowledge** and information to the patient	Describe the behavior
E = address patients' **Emotions** with **Empathic** responses	Address emotions; use empathy
S = **Strategize** and **Summarize**	Make an action plan about what the learner will think about next time and follow-up

A few unique elements are integral to facilitating family meetings and are not explicitly stated in the conceptual model. First, family meetings often are for patients with complex medical issues that have required multiple consultants. A preparatory pre-meeting is essential and should determine who should be present at the meeting (e.g., whether the patient has medical decision-making capacity and, if not, who the legal decision-maker is; which family members would like to participate, which medical teams should be represented at the meeting, etc.) and confirm medical facts, including prognosis, with the other members of the medical team to ensure that accurate information is conveyed to the family.

Second, family members often have different understandings and perspectives of the clinical situation and perhaps even the patient's wishes and values, which sometimes may lead to conflict. Learners need to use various tools from such elements as "assessing patient perspective" and "attending to emotion" to clarify family members' differing interpretations, handle conflict, and build consensus. This is further complicated when patients fully lack decision-making capacity. The HPM physician needs to describe the goal of substituted decision-making (i.e., to speak on behalf of the patient by making choices that the patient would make if he or she could speak). Learners should be encouraged to use their toolbox of skills to elicit from each family member what they believe the patient would choose if he or she could speak in an effort to build consensus.

Occasionally, conflict exists between family members and the medical teams. Conflict can usually be attributed to misunderstandings of information or personal factors. The misunderstanding can be about the diagnosis, prognosis, underlying causes, or conversations that may have occurred. Personal factors of distrust, grief, guilt, or secondary gain may be at work. Occasionally, there is a genuine value conflict over either goals or the worth of a treatment. This may be couched in terms of religion, belief in miracles, or the value of life. In general, it is useful first to explicitly identify that there seems to be conflict and then seek to understand the various points of view. In this context, educators should help learners acknowledge that conflict negotiation between family members and between family members and medical teams is considered a higher level communication skill that will take practice.

Third, oftentimes, family members will ask the physician not to tell the patient the diagnosis or other important information. While it is the physician's legal obligation to obtain informed consent from the patient, a therapeutic relationship also requires a congenial alliance with the family. Rather than confronting their request with "I have to tell the patient," we recommend the learners assess the family perspective by asking them why they do not want you to tell the patient, what it is they are afraid will be said, and what their experience has been with medical information. Inquire whether there is a personal, cultural, or religious context to their concern. Learners may need practice in going to the patient with family members to ask how much the patient wants to know about his or her health and what questions he or she might have.

E-Health and Telemedicine

As technology changes, a new challenge is how best to foster good communication techniques when not physically present with the patient and family. E-health, defined as "health services and information delivered or enhanced through the Internet and related technologies"[75] and telemedicine, defined as the "the use of medical information exchanged from one site to another via electronic communication to improve a patient's clinical health status"[76] are two emerging means of providing palliative care. Although there is a paucity of data to provide direction for teaching communication skills in such settings, new technology does not necessarily require new communication skills. The same approaches used in face-to-face encounters can be used on the telephone, via text or email, or in a telemedicine unit with video capabilities. However, learners must be aware that the absence of nonverbal cues from the physician and the patient and/or family can lead to misunderstandings and miscommunication. Moreover, tools such as compassionate silence may feel more awkward when on the phone or via telemedicine. Verbal statements of empathy and compassion are likely to be more effective in this context. This is an area that deserves more research to determine specific communication strategies, as e-health and telemedicine become more prevalent in palliative medicine.

Conclusion

In this chapter, a conceptual model of patient- and family-centered communication has been detailed, as well as various approaches to teaching these skills to physician learners who provide care to patients with serious and advanced illness. As shared decision-making is often the crux of most discussions with such patients and their families, the elements and tools described here can be employed for all types of common HPM discussion (e.g., breaking bad news, goals of care discussions) in a variety of contexts (e.g., one-on-one patient encounters, family meetings, and e-health), with the understanding that certain discussions will require more of an emphasis on a particular element of the model than others. Communication skills education should include a multimodal approach comprised of instruction, practice, and effective feedback. Quality communication in HPM patient encounters is often complicated and emotionally charged, such that it may feel unattainable to learners. Thus it is important for teachers to normalize the challenges of acquiring new communication skills and help learners build upon their successes. For learners and educators, remember that quality patient-centered communication is a learnable skill with deliberate practice over time. We hope the tools described in this chapter are helpful in planning for and facilitating communication training for new HPM physicians.

References

1. Accreditation Council for Graduate Medical Education. ACGME Common Program Requirement. https://www.acgme.org/acgmeweb/Portals/0/PFAssets/ProgramRequirements/CPRs2013.pdf. Published July 2007. Updated July 2013. Accessed August 2014.
2. National Consensus Project for Quality Palliative Care. Clinical practice guidelines for quality palliative care. 2nd ed. http://www.nationalconsensusproject.org/guideline.pdf. Published 2009. Accessed August 1, 2014.
3. American Association of Hospice and Palliative Care. Hospice and palliative medicine core competencies. Version 2.3. http://aahpm.org/uploads/education/competencies/Competencies%20v.%202.3.pdf. Published September 2009. Accessed August 1, 2014.
4. Buckley J, Addrizzo-Harris D, Clay A, et al. Multisociety task force recommendations of competencies in pulmonary and critical care medicine. *Am J Respir Crit Care Med.* 2009;180(4):290–295.
5. Lautrette A, Darmon M, Megarbane B, et al. A communication strategy and brochure for relatives of patients dying in the ICU. *N Engl J Med.* 2007;356(5):469–478.
6. Levinson W, Roter D, Mullooly J, Dull V, Frankel R. Patient communication: The relationship with malpractice claims among primary care physicians and surgeons. *JAMA.* 1997;277(7):553–559.
7. Wright A, Zhang B, Ray A, et al. Associations between end-of-life discussions, patient mental health, medical care near death, and caregiver bereavement adjustment. *JAMA.* 2008;300(14):1665–1673.
8. Steinhauser K, Christakis N, Clipp Elizabeth, McNeilly M, McIntyre L, Tulsky J. Factors considered important at the end of life by patients, family, physicians, and other care providers. *JAMA.* 2000;284:2476–2482.
9. Abbott K, Sago J, Breen C, Abernethy A, Tulsky J. Looking back: One year after discussion of withdrawal or withholding of life sustaining support. *Crit Care Med.* 2001;29(1):197–201.
10. Azoulay E, Sprung C. Family-physician interactions in the intensive care unit. *Crit Care Med.* 2004;32:1832–1838.
11. Azoulay E. The end-of-life family conference: communication empowers. *Am J Respir Crit Care.* 2005;171:803–804.
12. Buckman R. *Breaking Bad News: A Guide for Health Care Professionals.* Baltimore, MD: Johns Hopkins University Press; 1992.
13. Gay E, Pronovost P, Bassett R, Nelson J. The intensive care unit family meeting: Making it happen. *J Crit Care.* 2009;24:629e1–629e12.
14. Gorman T, Ahern S, Wiseman J, et al. Residents' end-of-life decision making with adult hospitalized patients: A review of the literature. *Acad Med.* 2005;80(7):622–633.
15. Schwarz C, Goulet J, Gorski V, Selwyn P. Medical residents' perceptions of end-of-life care training in a large urban teaching hospital. *J Palliat Med.* 2004;6(1):37–44.
16. White D, Braddock C, Bereknyei S, Curtis R. Toward shared decision making at the end of life in intensive care units. *Arch Intern Med.* 2007;167:461.
17. Epstein R, Franks P, Fiscella K, et al. Measuring patient-centered communication in patient-physician consultations: Theoretical and practical issues. *Soc Sci Med.* 2005;61:1516–1528.
18. King A, Hoppe R. "Best practice" for patient-centered communication: A narrative review. *J Grad Med Educ.* 2013;5(3):385–393.
19. White D, Engelberg R, Wenrich M, Lo B, Curtis J. Prognostication during physician-family discussions about limiting life support in intensive care units. *Crit Care Med.* 2007;35:442–448.
20. Baile W, Buckman R, Lenzi R, Glober G, Beale E, Kudelka A. SPIKES—A six-step protocol for delivering bad news: Application to the patient with cancer. *Oncologist.* 2000;5:302–311.
21. Curtis J, Engelberg R, Wenrich M, Shannon S, Treece P, Rubenfeld G. Missed opportunities during family conferences about end-of-life care in the intensive care unit. *Am J Respir Crit Care Med.* 2005;171(8):844–849.
22. Fischer G, Tulsky J, Arnold R. Communicating a poor prognosis. In:Portenoy R, Bruera E, eds. *Topics in Palliative Care*, Vol. 4. New York, NY: Oxford University Press; 2000:75–94.
23. Back A, Bauer-Wu S, Rushton C, Halifax J. Compassionate silence in the patient-clinician encounter: a contemplative approach. *J Palliat Med.* 2009;12(12):1113–1117.
24. Oncotalk. Module 1: Fundamental Communication Skills. http://depts.washington.edu/oncotalk/learn/modules.html. Accessed August 2014.
25. Back A, Arnold R. Discussing prognosis: "How much information do you want to know?" Talking to patients who do not want information or are ambivalent. *J Clin Oncol.* 2006;24:4214–4217.
26. Back A, Arnold R. Discussing prognosis: "How much do you want to know?" Talking to patients who are prepared for explicit information. *J Clin Oncol.* 2006;24:4209–4213.
27. Back A, Arnold RM, Tulsky J. *Mastering Communication with Seriously Ill Patients: Balancing Honesty With Empathy and Hope.* New York, NY: Cambridge University Press; 2009.
28. VitalTalk. Nurse statements for articulating empathy. http://www.vitaltalk.org/quick-guides. Accessed August 2014.
29. van Vliet LM, van der Wall E, Plum NM, Bensing JM. Explicit prognostic information and reassurance about nonabandonment when entering palliative breast cancer care: Findings from a scripted video-vignette study. *J Clin Oncol.* 2013;31(26):3242–3249.
30. Cooper R, Ferguson A, Bodurtha J, Smith T. AMEN in challenging conversations: Bridging the gaps between faith, hope, and medicine. *J Oncol Pract.* 2014;10(4):e191–e195.
31. West H, Engelberg R, Wenrich M, Curtis J. Expressions of nonabandonment during the intensive care unit family conference. *J Palliat Med.* 2005;8(4):797–807.
32. Jackson V, Jacobsen J, Greer J, Pirl W, Temel J, Back A. The cultivation of prognostic awareness through the provision of early palliative care in the ambulatory setting: A communication guide. *J Palliat Med.* 2013;16(8):894–900.
33. Back A, Arnold R, Quill T. Hope for the best, and prepare for the worst. *Ann Intern Med.* 2003;138(5):439–443.
34. Douglas S, Daly B, Lipson A. Neglect of quality-of-life considerations in intensive care unit family meetings for long-stay intensive care patients. *Crit Care Med.* 2012;40(2):461–467.
35. Quill T, Arnold R, Platt F. I wish things were different: Expressing wishes in response to loss, futility, and unrealistic hopes. *Ann Intern Med.* 2001;135(7):551–555.
36. VitalTalk. Addressing goals of care: REMAP. http://www.vitaltalk.org/quick-guides. Accessed August 2014.
37. Back A, Trinidad S, Hopley E, Edwards K. Reframing the goals of care conversation: "We're in a different place." *J Palliat Med.* 2014;17(9):1019–1024.
38. Dwamena F, Holmes-Rovner M, Gaulden C, et al. Interventions for providers to promote a patient-centred approach in clinical consultations. *Cochrane Database Syst Rev.* 2012;12:CD003267.
39. Back A, Arnold R, Baile W, et al. Faculty development to change the paradigm of communication skills teaching in oncology. *J Clin Oncol.* 2009;27(7):1137–1141.
40. Kelley A, Back A, Arnold A, et al. Geritalk: Communication skills training for geriatric and palliative medicine fellows. *J Am Geriatr Soc.* 2012;60(2):332–337.
41. Lane C, Rollnick S. The use of simulate patients and role-play in communication skills training: A review of the literature to August 2005. *Patient Educ Couns.* 2007;67(1–2):13–20
42. Berkhof M, Rijssen J, Schellart A, Anema J, van der Beek A. Effective training strategies for teaching communication skills to physicians: An overview of systematic reviews. *Patient Educ Couns.* 2011;84(2):152–162.

43. Maguire P, Pitceathly C. Key communication skills and how to acquire them. *BMJ*. 2002;325:697–700.
44. Adamo G. Simulated and standardized patients in OSCEs: Achievements and challenges 1992–2003. *Med Teach*. 2003;23(3):262–270.
45. Ende J. Feedback in clinical medical education. *JAMA*. 1983;250(6):777–781.
46. Torre D, Simpson D, Sebastian J, Elnicki D. Learning/feedback activities and high-quality teaching: Perceptions of third-year medical students during an inpatient rotation. *Acad Med*. 2005;80:950–954.
47. Veloski J, Boex J, Grasberger J, Wolfson D. Systematic reviw of the literature on assessment, feedback and physicians' clinical performance: BEME Guide No. 7. *Med Teach*. 2006;28:117–128.
48. Hattie J, Timperley H. The power of feedback. *Rev Educ Res*. 2007;77(1):81–112.
49. Srinivasan M, Hauer K, Der-Martirosian C, Wikkes M, Gesundheit N. Does feedback matter? Practice-based learning for medical students after a multi-institutional clinical performance examination. *Med Educ*. 2007;41(9);857–865.
50. Cope D, Linn L, Leake B, Barrett P. Modification of residents' behavior by preceptor feedback of patient satisfaction. *J Gen Intern Med*. 1986;1(6):394–398.
51. Davis D, Mazmanian P, Fordis M, Harrison R, Thorpe K, Perrier L. Accuracy of physician self-assessment compared with observed measures of competence: A systematic review. *JAMA*. 2006;296(9):1094–1102.
52. Colthart I, Bagnall G, Evans A, et al. The effectiveness of self-assessment on the identification of learner needs, learner activity, and impact on clinical practice: BEME Guide No. 10. *Med Teach*. 2008;30:124–145.
53. Eva K, Munoz J, Hanson M, Walsh A, Wakefield J. Which factors, personal or external most influence students'generation of learning goals? *Acad Med*. 2010;85(10):S102–S105.
54. Gil D, Heins M, Jones P. Perceptions of medical school faculty members and students on clinical clerkship feedback. *J Med Educ*. 1984;59:856–864.
55. Liberman A, Liberman M, Steinert Y, McLeod P, Meterissian S. Surgery residents and attending surgeons have different perceptions of feedback. *Med Teach*. 2005;27:470–472.
56. Sostok M, Coverly L, Rouan G. Feedback process between faculty and students. *Acad Med*. 2002;77(3):276.
57. Wolverton S, Bosworth M. A survey of resident perceptions of effective teaching behaviors. *Fam Med*. 1985;17:106–108.
58. Chur-Hansen A, Koopowitz L. Formative feedback in undergraduate psychiatry. *Acad Psychiatry*. 2005;29:66–68.
59. Barratt M, Moyer V. Effect of a teaching skills program on faculty skills and confidence. *Acad Pediatr*. 2004;4(1):117–120.
60. Vorvick L, Avnon T, Emmett R, Robins L. Improving teaching by teaching feedback. *Med Educ*. 2008;42:540–541.
61. Bing-You R, Trowbridge R. Why medical educators may be failing at feedback. *JAMA*. 2009;302:1330–1331.
62. Salerno S, O'Malley P, Pangaro L, Wheeler G, Moores L, Jackson J. Faculty development seminars based on the one-minute preceptor improve feedback in the ambulatory seeting. *J Gen Intern Med*. 2002;17:779–787.
63. Holmboe E, Fieback N, Galaty L, Huot S. Effectivenss of a focused educational internvention on resident evaluations from faculty. *J Gen Intern Med*. 2001;16:427–434.
64. Thomas J, Arnold R. Giving feedback. *J Palliat Med*. 2011;14(2):233–239.
65. Shute V. Focus on formative feedback. *Rev Educ Res*. 2008;78(1):153–189.
66. Locke E, Latham G. New directions in goal-setting theory. *Curr Dir Psyhcol Sci*. 2006;15(5):265–268.
67. Archer J. State of the science in health professional education: Effective feedback. *Med Educ*. 2010;44(1):101–108.
68. O'Neill L, Back A. What do palliative care clinicians need to know about teaching communication? In: Goldstein N, Morrison R, eds. *Evidence-Based Practice of Palliative Medicine*. Philadephia, PA: Elsevier Saunders; 2013:251–257.
69. Hales B, Terblanche M, Fowler R, Sibbald W. Development of medical checklists for improved quality of patient care. *Int J Qual Health Care*. 2008;20(1):22–30.
70. Duffy F, Gordon G, Whelan G, Cole-Kelly K, Frankel R. Assessing competence in communication and interpersonal skills: The Kalamazoo II report. *Acad Med*. 2004;79(6):495–507.
71. Makoul G. Essential elements of communication in medical encounters: The Kalamazoo consensus statement. *Acad Med*. 2001;76(4):390–393.
72. Kurtz S, Silverman J, Benson J, Draper J. Marrying content and process in clinical method teaching: Enhancing the Calgary–Cambridge guides. *Acad Med*. 2003;78(8):802–809.
73. Makoul G. The SEGUE Framework for teaching and assessing communication skills. *Patient Educ Couns*. 2001;45(1):23–34.
74. Hospice and Palliative Medicine Competencies Phase 3 Workgroup. Hospice and Palliative Medicine Competencies Project: Toolkit of Assessment Methods. http://aahpm.org/uploads/education/competencies/Toolkit%20Intro%202014.pdf. Published 2010. Accessed August 2014.
75. Eysenbach, G. What is e-health?. *J Med Internet Res*. 2001;3(2):e20.
76. American Telemedicine Association. What is telemedicine? http://www.americantelemed.org/. Published 2012. Accessed August 2014

CHAPTER 44

Communication Education for Nurses

Pam Malloy

Introduction

Excellent communication, the most valuable skill a nurse can possess, is important for helping patients formulate their goals of care, assessing families' fears and concerns, and reporting vital aspects of assessment and management to the interprofessional team. On the other hand, poor interpersonal communication skills result in ineffective relationships between patients, their families, and the healthcare team, as well as an increase in complaints/dissatisfaction, malpractice claims, and negative outcomes.[1] Hence it is vital that nursing students, as well as practicing nurses, have opportunities to use creative ways to practice good communication skills and that faculty and professional development educators extend didactic methods to include scenarios for various simulation-type experiences.

Nurses are in key positions to ask the right questions, listen, be present and bear witness with patients, their families, and other members of the interprofessional team. No other healthcare professional spends more time at the bedside or out in the community assessing and managing patients than the nurse. For the past 11 years, 85% of respondents to a Gallup poll have ranked nurses as the number one most trusted, honest, and ethical profession in the United States, followed by pharmacists (75%) and physicians (70%).[2] This honor is given to nurses because the profession is committed to exceptional care, collaboration, advocacy, and open and honest communication.

Excellent communication skills are vital in providing the best care possible to the patient and his or her family. The conversations in the middle of the night with patients who are frightened about their future, or those encounters with the family after the patient has left for surgery, belong uniquely to nurses. Their observations and assessments are essential as an interprofessional plan of care is developed and all attempts are made to clearly articulate benefits versus burden when talking about potential treatment and the prevention of suffering.

Patients and families appreciate opportunities to talk with nurses and have great need for communication with their nurse. Studies have shown specific behaviors that are valued by patients and their families. They all revolve around communication. These include[3-5]

- Being present, silent, "bearing witness"
- Being willing to be "in the moment"
- Knowing and being comfortable with oneself
- Having a connection with the patient and his or her family
- Affirming and valuing them
- Acknowledging that this is a vulnerable time for them all
- Empathizing and being willing to be vulnerable as a healthcare provider
- Utilizing intuition
- Providing and promoting serenity and silence, when needed

Stop and Practice: Role-play a nurse entering a room where a patient and his wife received "bad news" an hour ago. The nurse has known this patient for 2 weeks, as he has been going through tests and surgery. Spend 5 minutes listening and talking about this news and its meaning to the patient and his wife. Then consider: Which of the previously listed behaviors that are valued were displayed between the nurse, the patient, and his wife? What went well? What could have been improved?

Those teaching student and practicing nurses must know that people can be taught to communicate better.[1] This can be done through practice, feedback, and mentoring.

Clinical Practice Guidelines for Quality Palliative Care Provides Points of Emphasis in Teaching Communication

The National Consensus Project for Quality Palliative Care has created clinical practice guidelines in an effort to provide direction in improving palliative care. Embedded throughout the foundation of all eight of the domains within the National Consensus Project's document titled *Clinical Practice Guidelines for Quality Palliative Care* lies the importance of collaborating and providing consistent, high-quality care across all patient care. This document reinforces the important role communication has in defining and orchestrating the work of palliative care. For example:[6]

- Domain 1: Structure and Processes of Care—Emphasizes the importance of the interprofessional team in coordinating palliative care. It stresses "engagement and collaboration" between the team, patient, and family.
- Domain 2: Physical Aspects of Care—Promotes proactive assessment and management of physical symptoms. Attention to these symptoms requires excellent communication skills,

and the care will be superior only if the entire team is contributing their expertise.

- Domain 3: Psychological and Psychiatric Aspects—Stresses the significance of collaborative assessment and including patients and their families in these discussions so their goals of care can be articulated and honored.
- Domain 4: Social Aspects of Care—Highlights the importance of interprofessional engagement and "collaboration with patients and families to identify, support, and capitalize on patient and family strengths."[6(p10)]
- Domain 5: Spiritual, Religious, and Existential Aspects of Care—Capitalizes on the significance of the interprofessional team, especially those in chaplaincy service, to assess and coordinate spiritual care, honoring spiritual/religious rituals and practices.
- Domain 6: Cultural Aspects of Care—Communication can only occur if the healthcare team understands and honors the culture, including linguistic competence, and promotes services that align with each patient's unique cultural background.
- Domain 7: Care of the Patient at the End of Life—Highlights interprofessional communication and documentation of the signs and symptoms of impending death. Of particular importance is guiding family in knowing what to expect in the death and post-death processes.
- Domain 8: Ethical and Legal Aspects of Care—Promotes advance care planning, including ongoing discussions about goals of care.

Each of these eight domains requires excellent nurse communication in order to be fully implemented.

Using Simulation in Nursing Education to Promote Excellent Communication Skills

One way to provide student and practicing nurses with educational opportunities in communication is through various types of simulation. Simulation has been used in nursing education to address high-risk assessment and management needs, similar to what has been used in aviation, nuclear power agencies, and the military.[7] Simulation, whether it be high-fidelity, standardized patients (SPs), role plays, and so on, is defined as a "technique, not a technology, to replace or amplify real experiences with guided experiences, often immersive in nature, that evoke or replicate substantial aspects of the real world in a fully interactive fashion."[8(p2)] Using simulation in nursing education allows students to practice skills in a safe environment and permits errors and professional growth without a "live" patient being at risk.[7] Simulation also offers the opportunity to provide interprofessional standardized cases; promotes critical thinking, decision-making, and psychomotor skills; provides instant feedback from faculty to participants; integrates knowledge and skills; and provides opportunities for faculty to debrief with the participants about their feelings.[9]

There are both advantages and disadvantages to simulation. Advantages include (a) students can witness and be involved in a crisis situation before experiencing it in the clinical arena; (b) there are opportunities to evaluate and reflect on the activity in a safe environment; and (c) simulation opportunities can be provided in spite of overcrowded, hard-to-obtain clinical sites.[10] While these advantages address important issues, there are also some disadvantages to simulation as well as a need for more evidence-based research supporting simulation. A tremendous amount of time is spent in writing/creating scenarios and preparing the lab, and stellar clinical faculty must be available to assess the quality of the simulation.[10] In addition, simulation labs are costly.

Due to the high costs of setting up a simulation lab, some nursing education institutions use a form of simulation that includes the use of SPs, which has been reported to be innovative, creative, and promising.[11,12] SPs can be simulated or actual patients who are trained to portray a clinical scenario. Research studies provide a plethora of data showing that SP pedagogy provides learners with opportunities to interact in a variety of scenarios and to repeat and practice various skills. It also increases knowledge about specific clinical scenarios; improves communication and interviewing skills; and increases satisfaction for both faculty and students.[1,12,13]

Peer role play is another low-cost way to practice good communication, allowing students to exercise a wide variety of roles with their peers (e.g., playing the role of patient, caregiver, physician, nurse, chaplain, etc.). This method allows participants to "be in" various roles and promotes excellent and immediate feedback from faculty. Immediate feedback from faculty who are well educated in communication techniques can reinforce good interactions, as well as point out ways to improve the conversation when needed. Learners need to feel that they are in a safe place to practice these skills. In addition, faculty must prepare ahead of time for these learning opportunities. For example, they need to develop/choose realistic roles, make sure the role aligns with the participant's level of practice, and give feedback that will be helpful and memorable. Studies have shown that practicing communication skills with peers can be successful and that it improves communication more than just providing didactic content.[14,15] For examples of scenarios that could be used in simulation, see Box 44.1.

Practicing Difficult Areas of Communication: Team and Family Meetings

Unfortunately, there is no prescriptive script that students and practicing nurses can memorize in order to communicate with patients and families, as each situation is unique. Especially in difficult and tragic circumstances, it is critical that nurses actively listen, be present, and bear witness.[16] Nurses have shared that the areas in which they struggle most when communicating is discussing bad news, talking with physicians about palliative care issues, discussing spiritual concerns, and talking with patients/families from different cultures.[17] Many times, nurses may just need key phrases/words to get the conversation started (Table 44.1).

Team and family meetings are frequent occurrences for nurses. Collaboration and respect are key when working with the interprofessional team, as it promotes quality and safe care.[18,19] Team and family meeting scenarios can be acted out in the simulation lab or through role plays. This allows the student a safe place to witness one of these meetings. The purpose of a family meeting can be varied. For example, it can be focused on sharing information about treatment options, benefits and burdens of care, goals

Box 44.1 Examples of Role-Plays/Vignettes That Can Be Used in Simulation

Scenario: Neonatal

Premature infant, Sydney, was born with multiple cardiac and respiratory anomalies. Neonatologists have spoken with the family, stating that the child will not survive more than 3 to 4 days. The nurse comes in to talk to the mother and father about this conversation. The mother states, "I can't wait for my baby to get through this crisis so we can take him home." How should the nurse respond?

A 26-year-old mother goes into a diabetic coma, giving birth prematurely. Unfortunately, both the mother and baby die. The father, the mother's parents, and two young children (ages 4 and 6 years) are in the waiting room. The obstetrician/gynecological advanced practice nurse asks the family to come into a private office to give this bad news. How should she begin giving this news? Should the children be present? If not, where should they be?

Scenario: Pediatric

Timmy, age 8 years, was hit by a car on his way to school this morning. His single mom arrives in the emergency department and sits alone in the waiting room. After numerous resuscitation attempts, Timmy dies. The nurse and physician go to the waiting room to tell Timmy's mother that Timmy has died. The physician returns to the emergency department and the nurse stays to comfort the mother. What do you say? What do you do? Should Timmy's mother drive home?

Ashley is 5 years old and had an allogeneic bone marrow transplant 8 weeks ago. She has been battling graft-versus-host disease for the past 3 weeks. Her father is very concerned and asks, "Is my daughter going to die?" How should you respond?

Scenario: Adult

Sandra is 42 years old and has stage 4 breast cancer with metastasis to the bones and brain. She is married and has three children (ages 6, 10, and 12 years). She tells you that she is afraid she will die before her children grow up. She states that she hopes her children will always remember how much she loves them. Describe how you would communicate ways she could leave a legacy for her children.

Mark is 56 years old and has amyotrophic lateral sclerosis. He is considering being placed on a ventilator to improve his respiratory status. He asks you, as his home health nurse, if this is something to consider. He admits, "I am tired, and really want nature to take its course. But, I feel I should show my family I am willing to fight this." How should you respond?

Margaret is 38 years old and suffers from heart failure, type 1 diabetes, and hypertension. She is 5'4" and weighs 378 pounds. She is currently hospitalized because she had a stroke last week that left her with some cognitive and muscular-skeletal deficits. She asks you if she is going to die soon. How would you respond? Role-play the nurse with other members of the interprofessional team talking to Margaret about her goals of care.

Robert is 60 years old and has been undergoing chemotherapy for stage 4 pancreatic cancer over the past 3 months. He was admitted to the hospital last night because of dehydration, failure to thrive, and pneumonia. He confides in you that he doesn't think he can continue with the chemotherapy. "I am done with all of this," he says. You notice that no one has asked Robert what his goals of care are. How would you begin a conversation, asking about his goals?

Later, Robert confides that he does not want to continue with chemotherapy. He has recently read information on the Internet that his stage 4 pancreatic cancer is terminal. He is angry that his oncologist has not told him this when he was first diagnosed. "I would have rather spent time at home with my family than spending time at the infusion center getting chemotherapy." You speak with the oncologist about this conversation later in the day, and the oncologist tells you, "He would be dead by now if we had not given him chemotherapy." How would you respond to this physician?

Role-play a conversation with a physician who refuses to include the palliative care team on a 50-year-old patient with end-stage renal failure and multiple symptoms (i.e., anxiety, anorexia, fatigue, depression, etc.).

Eric is 36 years old and was in the Iraqi/Afghanistan War 15 years ago. He has a rare form of bone cancer and states his pain scores range between 8 and 10 (on a zero to 10 pain scale). When you explore what he takes for the pain, he states, "I don't take anything. I know what it is like to be addicted." He confides in you that he had a gunshot wound in his shoulder while in the war. "I got addicted to those pain medications and I don't want to ever take them again." Also, he states, "Sometimes you just have to be stoic and bear the pain." How would you respond? What misconceptions does he have about pain medication? What role does being a veteran play in his self-proclaimed "stoicism"?

Michelle is 32 years old and was diagnosed with advanced cervical cancer 2 months ago, with metastasis to the liver and lungs. While at the clinic, she confides in you that she feels guilty about having this disease and believes that God is punishing her. How would you respond?

Scenario: Older Adults

Miriam is 82 years old. She has lived in a nursing home for the past 20 years due to multiple illnesses. Three months ago, she was diagnosed with late-stage colon cancer. She has one daughter who lives 100 miles away and visits her mother once a year. This year, when the daughter arrives at the nursing home, she is shocked that her mother has lost so much weight. The nurse explains that her mother has eaten poorly since her colon surgery. Even though dietary services have been involved, she continues to lose weight, as she just does not want to eat. The daughter demands that a feeding tube be inserted. How would you interact with the daughter? What other team

(continued)

Box 44.1 (Continued)

members should be included in this conversation? Role-play what a conversation would look like with the advanced practice geriatric nurse, the dietician, and the primary nurse caring for Miriam.

Sally is 76 years old and has been in a head-on car accident. Her partner, Deborah, is waiting in the emergency room. The doctors state that her head injuries are very serious and that she is unable to breathe on her own. Sally does not have an advanced directive. Role-play the conversation needed between the physician, chaplain, nurse, and Sally's partner.

Edward is 92 years old and is a veteran of World War II. You are his home care nurse, and you make visits twice a week, monitoring his dementia, diabetes, and hypertension. You have been caring for Edward for the past 18 months. He recently had a left below-the-knee amputation due to complications of diabetes. Today when you visit, his two sons tell you, "Everything must be done to prolong our father's life for as long as possible. We need his veteran's pay." Edward has an advanced directive and has made it clear that he wants "no heroics." The children inform you they plan to contest that. How would you speak with the sons? How would you advocate for Edward?

---

of care, and advance care planning.[4,5] The goal of a family meeting is to improve communication regarding all issues dealing with palliative care and decision-making.[5]

Preparing to attend a family meeting takes time, preparation, and organization. With little time and resources, the healthcare team must be prepared not only to provide information but to listen to concerns of the patient/family, answer difficult questions honestly, and "be present." Components of a family meeting include preparing for the meeting; opening the meeting; making sure the family understands the current health status and available treatments; honoring patient and family values, preferences, and beliefs; addressing decisions that need to be made; closing the meeting; following up; and giving feedback to appropriate healthcare colleagues.[4]

◆ **Stop and Practice:** Role playing, using the eight components listed earlier for holding a family meeting, can give students and practicing nurses opportunities to rehearse these important skills. The following is an example of a role play with key concepts to promote the exchanges.

Situation: Kent is 46 years old and was diagnosed with stage 4 small cell lung cancer 8 months ago. His dyspnea is increasing, along with his fatigue and anxiety. He has lost 12 pounds in the last month (currently he weighs 138 pounds and is 6 feet tall).

Kent was born in Vietnam but came to the United States with his parents when he was 2 years old. He was employed as an electrician prior to his illness, has been divorced for 20 years with no significant other during that time, lives alone, has no children, and continues to smoke two packs of cigarettes per day. His parents and one sister live nearby. Kent is not affiliated with any religion but states he is "spiritual." He does not have an advanced directive.

Kent was admitted to the hospital yesterday, suffering a broken right arm and hip due to a fall at home. The orthopedic surgeon is concerned about operating on Kent due to his compromised condition. The oncologist schedules a meeting with Kent and invites the advanced practice nurse from the palliative care team to join them. Role play this scenario following the guidelines listed.[4,20] Actors for the role play include Kent's parents, the oncologist, and an advanced practice nurse.

◆ **Prepare for the meeting**
  - Review current medical issues, medical history, and social history.
  - Determine which healthcare team members will attend and who will lead the meeting.
  - Decide the purpose of the meeting. What will the goal(s) of the meeting be? What information do you want to be sure is conveyed?
  - Decide if the patient will attend as well as which family members.
  - Arrange to be in a quiet and private room, with ample seating.
  - Decide if arrangements should be made for those living long-distance to attend the conference via telephone or other electronic medium.
  - Turn off pagers, call phones to prevent any distraction.

◆ **Open the meeting**
  - Be sure everyone in the room is introduced and that patient and family understand the role of each healthcare professional.
  - Ensure each healthcare professional understands the caregiving role(s) of any of the family or friends attending the meeting.
  - Describe the purpose and goal(s) of the meeting. This needs to be clearly articulated at the beginning. Examples of ways to state the purpose include
  - *"The purpose of this meeting is to make sure everyone understands how Kent is doing. We also want to be available to answer any questions you might have."*
  - *"We've called this meeting because Kent's health is declining quickly and we need to consider future care."*
  - *"Kent's health is rapidly declining, and we need to make some decisions. Because there is no advanced directive, we must address these issues today.:*
  - Be flexible. The goals of the meeting may change, due to needs or concerns of the patient/family.

◆ **Determine the family understanding about what is happening to Kent.**
  - Have each family member state his or her understanding of Kent's condition.
  - An example to start this conversation may include

Table 44.1 Phrases to Consider When Speaking With Patients and Their Families

Appropriate Phrases to Begin a Conversation	Phrases to Avoid When Beginning a Conversation
Bad News	
"I am very sorry to hear that you received some difficult news today. I wish the news you received today had been better. Tell me what you understand about your diagnosis."	"I am sorry to hear about your bad news. I know how you feel." **Problem:** While the listener may be empathetic to the bad news, no one knows how someone else feels.
Quality of Life Assessment[31]	
"Please tell me how your disease has interfered with your daily activities." "How has it affected your family, friends? your work?" "Do you find yourself feeling worried or sad about your illness?" "What are the symptoms that bother you the most? What concerns you the most?" "Have your religious/spiritual beliefs been affected by your illness? If so, please explain?" "Many of my patients wonder about the meaning of their illness—do you?"	"Has your illness interfered with your daily activities, family, friends, work?" "Do you worry a lot or find yourself being sad? If so, that's okay." "Do you have pain, fatigue, dyspnea, or other symptoms?" "Are you seeing a clergy/chaplain about any religious/spiritual or existential problems?" **Problem:** Questions can be answered with "yes or no." None of these questions are open-ended.
Family Meeting	
"The purpose of this family meeting is to get to know each of you and to focus on your father's current health status. We recognize that you have known him longer than we have. We value any information you may have that would assist us in caring for him. Can you share your understanding of your father's illness?"	"The purpose of this family meeting is to share with you our goals of care for your father." **Problem:** The purpose of this meeting is to provide information, to clarify the patient's goals (not the healthcare team's), address problems, support the family, and provide resources to them as needed.
"Before we start the meeting, I would like to share with you that it is such a privilege to provide care to your father. Over these next few minutes, we would like to give you an update on the tests that were completed yesterday and to hear your thoughts on how we should proceed."	"Our team is busy and we have six other patients to see. We only have 10 minutes for this meeting." **Problem:** This attitude sets the tone for those attending. The patient/family knows that you are busy, and this statement does not promote an environment of compassion, listening, or being present.
Setting Goals	
"We have talked about the limited time you have left and you shared with me last week that you have a list of goals that you would like to accomplish before you die. What are your goals for these last few days/months of your life?"	**"We need you to make a decision right now."** **Problem:** Questions about goal-setting are rarely asked. By asking this question, you place value on the patient—their goals and dreams give you a window into their thoughts.
Artificial Feeding/Hydration[31]	
"Tell me what you know about artificial ways to provide food and drink to your loved one." "One of the body's signals that death is close is that patients lose interest in eating. This can occur days to weeks before death." "Your loved one will not die from dehydration or starvation. It will not promote suffering. It will be the disease that causes his death."	"Do you know anything about tube feedings?" "You don't want your loved one to starve to death. That's a terrible way to die." **Problem:** The question is not open-ended. Speaking about issues that have no data to support them is unprofessional and unethical.
Discussing Palliative Care With Physicians	
"Dr. Jones, you have taken excellent care of Mr. K. over the past 10 years with his various illnesses. Now with his new diagnosis, already-compromised physical state, and multiple health issues with his wife who is the caregiver, what are your thoughts about us contacting the palliative care team to work with us in addressing some of these issues?"	"Dr. Jones, can we have a palliative consult on Mr. K.?" **Problem:** Again, this is not an open-ended question. Where do you go after the physician says "No"? What information have you given the physician to even think a palliative care consult should occur?
Discussing Palliative Care With Patients/Families	
"Mrs. T., you have done a beautiful job of sharing with us what your goals of care are. You want to be as pain-free as possible, you would still like to enjoy some food, and you would like to talk to a spiritual advisor about some existential angst you are experiencing. It would be good to have someone from the palliative care team come and talk with you and make a plan for addressing each of these issues. I am very familiar with this team and they have worked with many of our patients to improve their quality of life for the time they have left. They are specially trained in assessing and managing your symptoms. In addition, they can also work with your husband and children as they deal with many changes in their lives since your illness. What are your thoughts about having the palliative care team come and talk with you today?"	"Mrs. T., your doctor and I talked today about having palliative care come and see you. Are you okay with that?" **Problem:** This is not an open-ended question. Patients may be confused about what palliative care is. This question does not provide necessary information for Mrs. T. to make a decision.

- *"What has the team told you about Kent's illness? What is your understanding of his condition?"*
- Speak clearly about the seriousness of the illness and how it is affecting Kent.
- After each family member has had an opportunity to speak, it is helpful to state, *"Is there anything that is not clear that you would like further information about?"*

♦ **Address patient and family values, preferences, and beliefs**
- Elicit goals of all family members present. Be prepared for multiple perspectives.
- Use open-ended questions.
  - *"Given that Kent has fallen and his lung cancer is getting worse, what do you hope for him?"*
  - *"Seeing a particular family member or friend can be an important goal for some patients. Are you aware of anyone that Kent would want to see at this time?"*
- Commit to exploring and understanding ethnic and cultural preferences and influences on communication, family relationships, medical treatments, and end-of-life care.
  - *"We really want to understand and respect Kent's cultural beliefs and practices so that we as a team can take the best possible care of him."*
- Keep the focus on the decisions made from the patient's perspective. Many times, this provides relief to family members and prevents guilt from making certain decisions.
  - *"Did Kent ever tell you what he wanted for himself if he became this ill? If so, please share what he requested."*
  - *"Did Kent ever have a family member or friend who was very ill and state that he would want that same type of care? If yes, please explain."*
  - *"Have you experienced a similar situation of having someone close to you being very ill? If so, how did you cope and react to the situation?"*
  - *"Please help me understand what I need to know about Kent's cultural beliefs in order to best care for him."*

♦ **Deal with decisions that need to be made**
- Be sure everyone has a common understanding of each issue.
- Begin with statements about the current assessment of Kent and talk about options for interventions.
- Provide clear recommendations that are based on patient and family goals.
  - *"Given our understanding of this latest health crisis and what you have told us about what you would want for Kent, I would recommend that we not obtain another orthopedic consult."*
- Consider coming to an agreement about a healthcare team recommendation, rather than details of a specific intervention.
  - *"We would like to focus on Kent's comfort and not do any invasive procedures that might cause or prolong suffering. What are your thoughts on that goal of care?"*
- Make sure everyone in the room understands the decisions that have been made.
  - *"I would like to make sure that everyone understands that we have decided to . . ."*

♦ **Close the meeting**
- Provide a short summary of the meeting.
- Ask if there any further questions or concerns.
- State your appreciation and respect for the family.
  - *"We thank you for meeting with us today and for giving us a better picture of Kent. We can only imagine how difficult this must be for each of you. We respect you for trying to do the right thing for Kent and for helping to make some challenging decisions."*
- Follow up. When is the next family meeting? Make sure family members know how to contact you.

♦ **Follow up on the meeting**
- Document the meeting in the patient's chart.
- Follow up with any plans that were made and any reassessment agreed upon.
  - *"At our last meeting, you were going to talk to your daughter about what we discussed two days ago. How did that conversation go?"*

♦ **Give feedback/follow-up to healthcare colleagues**
- This is a very important step—do not neglect it.
- Ask any of the healthcare professionals how the meeting went.
- Consider positives as well as potential areas for further evaluation.
- Provide feedback to colleagues about the meeting.

Nurses Witness Various Emotions When Holding Difficult Conversations

Many conversations regarding palliative care are full of emotions—it is the nature of the work. For example, patients hearing that their disease is progressing despite aggressive treatment, families receiving news that their loved one has only a few days of life remaining, or a parent who is shocked to hear that their child is in critical condition following an accident on the football field—all of these conversations are laden with difficult and heart-breaking emotions. This is a sacred moment, and students and practicing nurses must understand the privilege and opportunity they possess to be with patients and families during these vulnerable times.

♦ **Stop and Practice:** Mrs. Smith is 78 years old with heart and renal failure. She is the sole caregiver for her 84-year-old husband, who has Parkinson's disease. The home care nurse is visiting Mrs. Smith today at her home. This case will show the importance of how to respond to emotion by[21]

- Reflecting thoughts, emotions, or behaviors
- Affirming and respecting

- Summarizing/paraphrasing
- Making a plan

Nurse: "Hello, Mrs. Jones. Tell me about these tears." *(reflecting emotion)*

Mrs. Jones: "Things are happening so fast. My kidney status is failing and the dialysis is not working as it used to. I'm having trouble adjusting my heart and diabetic medicines. I have lost most of my doctors because they are not in my new insurance network, so I have had to look for new ones. Do you know how much energy that takes? Who is going to take care of my husband when I die? Because he has Parkinson's he can't be left alone. Medical bills are piling up. I just can't handle all of this. When will it stop?"

Nurse: "Mrs. Jones, you have a tremendous amount of stress on you. I am glad you could share these fears and concerns with me. Though I can't personally assist you with all of these issues, I do work with a wonderful team and together we can work with you to find solutions. It is so important that you communicate with us about how you feel—physically, psychologically, socially, spiritually. Together, we as a team can work with you to address these. Today, what is the most stressful thing you are dealing with? What can I work on right now to get you some relief?" *(affirmation and respect)*

Mrs. Jones: "At this point, my doctors say there is not much else left for me. My heart is slowly weakening. My kidneys are shot. I always knew this day would come. But I really need to focus on what I can control. Right now, my biggest concern is getting help for my husband. I believe that in a few short days/weeks, I will no longer be able to care for him."

Nurse: "Mrs. Jones, you have shared many concerns with me today. I am so impressed with the way you have taken such good care of your husband, despite your own problems. It is obvious you love him very much *(acknowledges her role, emotions)*. You have shared with me that your physical status is declining rapidly, you are concerned about financial issues, and you need to seek some new doctors. However, your biggest concern now is how to get help for your husband who is so dependent on you. Do I understand what is causing you the most angst at this time?" *(summarizing/paraphrasing)*

Mrs. Jones: "Yes, you are correct. My husband is requiring much more attention than I have the energy to provide. I don't know where to turn at this point."

Nurse: "Mrs. Jones, I am going to contact our social worker, so he can get right on this today. He will be able to connect you with several services in our community that can assist you and your husband. We will work to get the very best service here to work with you. This is an urgent situation and we want to take care of it immediately. While we will work with you to get your husband some care, we also need to talk more about you and your future *(address one concern, move to next)*. I will call your doctor today to see if there are any medication adjustments we should be making. I will be back tomorrow afternoon and together we can review options for providing care for your husband. I would also like to discuss having palliative care come and see you both in the next few days. We spoke about this last week and I left some pamphlets for you to read. Is it okay to discuss this further tomorrow, as well as some of the financial concerns you have?" *(make a plan)*

Mrs. Jones: "Yes. I know I am going to need to make some adjustments. I have read the palliative care pamphlets and I have some questions."

Emotional conversations, such as this one, happen every day. Nurses need to be prepared for them. They need to practice these types of encounters. It is easy to become overwhelmed with the numerous and complicated needs of patients, but nurses must stay focused, listen, and be present in order to respond to the emotion by reflecting, affirming/respecting, and summarizing/paraphrasing. Each of these actions are critical in helping the patient and family develop a plan of care. Further resources are available to assist in teaching and practicing patient- and family-centered communication (Table 44.2).

Telehealth: Excellent Communication Skills Are Vital

The world is changing rapidly, and the need to provide quality and value-based healthcare is a tremendous challenge. Almost 20% of Americans live in rural areas (59,492,276, 19.3%),[22] representing 80% of all land in the United States.[23] Many who live in rural areas are poor, older, and have chronic illness(es), and they have little or no access to healthcare. It is difficult to

Table 44.2 Educational Resources to Promote Communication in Palliative Nursing

Resource: Websites	Overview
BREAKS Protocol for Delivering Bad News http://www.ncbi.nlm.nih.gov/pmc/articles/PMC3144432/	A six-step protocol to provide communication strategies for breaking bad news.
Center to Advance Palliative Care http://www.capc.org/ipal/ipal-icu/improvement-and-clinical-tools	Provides assessment tools regarding family conferencing, language to use, etc.
Palliative Care Communication Institute http://www.pccinstitute.com	Provides teaching tools for nurses and other members of the interprofessional team, as well as research opportunities and an iOS app.
End-of-Life Nursing Education Consortium Core, Pediatric Palliative Care, Geriatric, Critical Care www.aacn.nche.edu/ELNEC	National education project dedicated to educate nurses in palliative care. One of the modules in each of these curricula is devoted entirely to communication.
End of Life/Palliative Education Resource Center Fast Facts http://www.eperc.mcw.edu/EPERC/FastFactsandConcepts (On right-hand screen, click "Communication")	A compilation of over 60 "fast facts" about a wide variety of communication scenarios, such as giving bad news, setting up a family meeting, how to inform a family member about their loved one's death, etc.
Silver Hour http://silverhour.info/teaching-resources	Provides numerous examples of simulations dealing with palliative care issues.

entice healthcare professionals to practice in rural areas.[23] As the traditional fee-for-service system begins to shrink and new models of care are implemented (e.g., accountable care organizations, patient-centered medical homes), telehealth will continue to play an important role in healthcare, especially as outcomes are sought and measured.[23] In addition, the cost of telehealth technologies are dropping; it is becoming easier to use, more prevalent in the marketplace, and more accessible.[23] Videoconferencing via two-way interactive video, the Internet, email, fax, telephone, store-and-forward imaging, streaming media, and terrestrial and wireless communications are examples of various telehealth technologies that nurses use to promote healthcare.

Along with increasing changes in telehealth technology, chronic illnesses are also on the rise. Chronic illnesses are the leading cause of disability and death in the United States.[24] Since 2012, approximately half of all adults in the United States (117 million people) have one or more chronic diseases, and 25% of US adults have two or more chronic health conditions.[25] Heart disease and cancer account for almost 48% of all deaths.[26] Obesity continues to be a tremendous healthcare challenge, as more than one-third of all adults (~78 million) and nearly one-fifth of children ages 2 to 19 years are considered obese.[27] Kidney failure, lower limb amputations, and new cases of blindness are caused primarily by diabetes in adults.[28] With these various chronic diseases, it is becoming more essential that patients and their families be better informed and more empowered to participate in self-management activities. Students and practicing nurses must be familiar with this technology, as they are generally on the front line caring for those in rural and other areas where telehealth is used.

Thus there is a need to be familiar with the technology, to be comfortable in educating and communicating via this technology, and to collaborate with other interprofessional team members in planning for future care While these telehealth technologies have the potential to increase and enhance access, availability, quality, and cost-effectiveness of services related to healthcare, it is extremely important that healthcare providers have the communication skills to maximize care and improve the delivery of services.[29] A study published in 2014 supported the use of video conferencing among a sample of hospice end users, including both interprofessional team members and caregivers, and demonstrated that meaningful conversation can occur.[30] With the rise in medical costs and decrease in practitioners, the demand for telehealth will only increase. Nursing faculty, continuing education providers, and staff development educators must stress the important role that nurses have in designing and implementing e-health tools and provide opportunities to access and provide excellent communication via these various telehealth options.

Conclusion

Communication is a nonnegotiable skill that every nurse must have. Research and theory associated with meaningful and purposeful communication must be taught, role-played, and assessed. Immediate feedback must be given and opportunities provided to promote mentorship in developing excellent communication. Student and practicing nurses need to understand and value the important role and privilege they have in caring for patients and their families during their most vulnerable time(s). It is an honor to be trusted, to have late-night conversations, to advocate, to share assessments with other members of the interprofessional team, to pay attention to words and actions, and to assist in scripting goals of care. All of these opportunities require excellent patient- and family-centered communication. For those who teach, mentor, and role-model communication, the opportunity to inspire others is tandem to this work we call education.

References

1. Lin ECL, Chen SL, Chao SY, Chen YC. Using standardized patient with immediate feedback and group discussion to teach interpersonal and communication skills to advanced practice nursing students. *Nurs Educ Today*. 2012;33:677–683.
2. Laidman J. Nurses remain nation's most trusted professionals. Medscape Medical News. http://www.medscape.com/viewarticle/775758 Published December 6, 2012. Accessed August 22, 2014.
3. Boreale K, Richardson B. Communication. In: Panke J, Coyne P, eds. *Conversations in Palliative Care*. 3rd ed. Pittsburgh, PA: Hospice and Palliative Nurses Association; 2011:33–44.
4. Dahlin C, Wittenberg-Lyles E. Communication in palliative care: An essential competency for nurses. In: Ferrell BR, Coyle N, Paice, J, eds. *Oxford Textbook of Palliative Nursing*. 4th ed. New York, NY: Oxford University Press; 2015.
5. Wittenberg-Lyles E, Goldsmith J, Ferrell B, Ragan S. *Communication in Palliative Nursing*. New York, NY: Oxford University Press; 2012.
6. National Consensus Project for Quality Palliative Care. Clinical practice guidelines for quality palliative care. www.nationalconsensusproject.org. Published 2013. Accessed August 22, 2014.
7. Galloway SJ. Simulation techniques to bridge the gap between novice and competent healthcare professionals. *Online J Issues Nurs*. 2009;14(2). http://www.nursingworld.org/MainMenuCategories/ANAMarketplace/ANAPeriodicals/OJIN/TableofContents/Vol142009/No2May09/Simulation-Techniques.aspx Accessed August 22, 2014.
8. Gaba D. The future vision of simulation in healthcare. *Qual Saf Health Care*. 2004;13(Suppl 1):2–10.
9. Fowler C, Alden KR. Enhancing patient safety in nursing education through patient simulation. *Patient Safety and Quality: An Evidence-Based Handbook for Nurses*. Rockville, MD: Agency for Healthcare Research and Quality; 2008. http://www.ncbi.nlm.nih.gov/books/NBK2628/ Accessed August 22, 2014.
10. Sanford PG. Simulation in nursing education: A review of the research. *Qual Rep*. 2010;(15)4:1006–1011.
11. Luctkar-Flude M, Wilson-Keates B, Larocque M. Evaluating high-fidelity human simulators and standardized patients in an undergraduate nursing health assessment course. *Nurs Educ Today*. 2012;32(4):448–452.
12. Shawler C. Palliative and end-of-life care: Using a standardized patient family for gerontological nurse practitioner students. *Nurs Educ Perspect*. 2011;32(3):168–171.
13. Lee CA, Chang A, Chou CL, Boscardin C, Hauer KE. Standardized patient-narrated Web-based learning modules improve students' communication skills on a high-stakes clinical skills examination. *J Gen Intern Med*. 2011;26(11):1374–1377.
14. Bosse HM, Schultz JH, Nickel M, et al. The effect of using standardized patients or peer role play on ratings of undergraduate communication training: A randomized controlled trial. *Patient Educ Couns*. 2011;87:300–306.
15. Lane C, Rollnick S. The use of simulated patients and role-play in communication skills training: A review of the literature to August 2005. *Patient Educ Couns*. 2007;67:13–20.
16. Ladd C, Grimley K, Hickman C, Touchy TA. Teaching end-of-life nursing using simulation. *J Hosp Palliat Nurs*. 2012;15(1):41–51.

17. Malloy P, Virani R, Kelly K, Munevar C. Beyond bad news: Communication skills of nurses in palliative care. *J Hosp Palliat Nurs*. 2010;12(3):166–174.
18. American Association of Critical Care Nurses. ACCN standards for establishing and sustaining healthy work environments—a journey to excellence. www.aacn.org/WD/HWE/Docs/HWEStandards.pdf Accessed August 22, 2014.
19. Freise C, Manojlovich M. Nurse-physician relationships in ambulatory oncology settings. *J Nurs Scholarsh*. 2012;44(3):258–365.
20. End-of-Life Nursing Education Consortium Website. http://www.aacn.nche.edu/elnec. Accessed August 22, 2014.
21. Center to Advance Palliative Care. Critical care communication. http://www.capc.org/palliative-care-professional-development/Training/c3-module-ipal-icu.pdf Accessed August 22, 2014.
22. US Census Bureau. Frequently asked questions. https://ask.census.gov/faq.php?id=5000&faqId=5971. Accessed August 22, 2014.
23. Institute of Medicine. The role of telehealth in an evolving healthcare environment. http://www.hrsa.gov/ruralhealth/about/telehealth/. Accessed August 22, 2014.
24. Centers for Disease Control and Prevention. Chronic diseases and health promotion. http://www.cdc.gov/chronicdisease/overview/index.htm?s_cid=ostltsdyk_govd_203. Accessed August 22, 2014.
25. Ward BW, Schiller JS, Goodman RA. Multiple chronic conditions among US adults: A 2012 update. *Prev Chronic Dis*. 2014;11:130389. http://dx.doi.org/10.5888/pcd11.130389. Accessed August 22, 2014.
26. Centers for Disease Control and Prevention. Death and mortality. http://www.cdc.gov/nchs/fastats/deaths.htm. Accessed August 22, 2014.
27. Centers for Disease Control and Prevention. NCHS obesity data. http://www.cdc.gov/nchs/data/factsheets/factsheet_obesity.htm. Accessed August 22, 2014.
28. Centers for Disease Control and Prevention. National diabetes fact sheet. http://www.cdc.gov/diabetes/pubs/pdf/ndfs_2011.pdf Accessed August 22, 2014.
29. Wakefield BJ, Bylund C, Holman JE, et al. Nurse and patient communication profiles in a home-based telehealth intervention for heart failure management. *Patient Educ Counsel*. 2007;71:285–292.
30. Wittenberg-Lyles E, Oliver DP, Kruse RL, Demiris G, Gage LA, Wagner K. Family caregiver participation in hospice interdisciplinary team meetings: How does it affect the nature and content of communication? *Health Commun*. 2013;(28)2:110–118.
31. Improving Palliative Care-Intensive Care Unit. Responding to emotion: Communication phrases in palliative care. http://www.capc.org/ipal/ipal-icu/improvement-and-clinical-tools. Accessed August 22, 2014.

CHAPTER 45

Communication Education for Social Workers

John G. Cagle and Kaila Williams

Introduction

Palliative care is a model of care that strives to address the multidimensional needs of patients and their families. These needs include an individual's physical, social, cognitive/emotional, and spiritual dimensions. Although there is substantial role overlap between palliative care disciplines, social workers are often charged with handling the social and emotional dimensions of care. Social workers must ensure open and clear communication between patients, families, and providers in the potentially difficult discussions about coping resources, care planning and advance directives, death and dying, and financial matters. Furthermore, social workers are frequently involved in crisis situations—for example, mediating family conflict, assisting with urgent decision-making, or intervening to allay heightened patient/family distress. This chapter provides an overview of communication education for social workers as well as a critical description of related curriculum standards in social work education and innovative modes of communication education.

Communication Education and Training in Social Work

Communication is an integral part of social work education at both the graduate and undergraduate level. Graduates from accredited programs can expect fundamental communication training, knowledge, and skills. The Council on Social Work Education (CSWE), the sole accrediting body for schools of social work in the United States, lists communication skills as a priority for social work education in multiple policy statements. Specifically, the CSWE has endorsed curricula that focus on the development of professional communication, competency, and critical thinking when interacting with clients and organizations and articulating the importance and impact of diversity in their clients' lives.[1] International social work organizations such as the British Association of Social Workers and the International Federation of Social Work have a similar emphasis on the development of communication skills.

In 2009 the CSWE issued a white paper titled "Palliative Care with Older Adults," which includes a description of the role of social work in palliative care.[2] This document highlights the strengths, skills, and perspective that social workers bring to the interprofessional palliative care team. Notably, the authors argue that social workers are needed because of their communication expertise. Social workers use their communication skills to understand the client's unique experiences, which in turn guides interactions between the healthcare team and the client. The CSWE also identifies social workers' distinctive ability to communicate between patients, families, the healthcare team, and the community at large. Thus social workers may serve as the linchpin that connects and galvanizes healthcare members. In short, the CSWE prioritizes communication education and training for generalist social workers—and especially for those with specialized palliative care training.[1,2]

NASW Standards for Social Work Practice in Palliative and End-of-Life Care

In 2004, the National Association of Social Workers (NASW) published standards for social work practice in palliative and end-of-life care.[3] These standards, meant to establish common expectations for practice, include a number of communication-related domains, such as the ability to recognize patterns of communication and decision-making in the family; facilitate communication among clients, family members, and members of the healthcare team; communicate the client's and family's psychosocial needs to the interdisciplinary team; and communicate and work collaboratively as an interdisciplinary team member to achieve care goals. The tenets of these guidelines have been echoed elsewhere in the social work literature,[4,5] and, when coupled with the CSWE's emphasis on the importance of cultivating strong communication skills in social work, the clarion call is clear—palliative care social workers *must* be equipped with knowledge of communication dynamics and the ability to facilitate difficult discussions in the clinical context.

Essentials in Communication Education for Palliative Social Work

Building from fundamental social work communication skills such as empathy, rapport-building, and client advocacy (see chapter 6), essential palliative care education includes a strong foundation of relevant theory and careful attention to language, culture, and clinical presence.

Social work is known for embracing a strengths-oriented focus to practice, a focus that is congruent with the principles and ethics of palliative care. Solution-focused communication is a way of framing problems from the perspective of the patient/family and empowering them to utilize their coping skills and resources to find ways to achieve what is most important. Ideally, communication education for palliative social workers should be grounded in a critical review of prevailing theories about serious illness, dying, and loss. Appraisals of the conceptual work advanced by Kübler-Ross, Worden, Pearlin, Lazurus and Folkman, Stoebe and Stroebe, Rando, Glasser and Strauss, and Corr, for example, provide social workers with the theoretical context they need to understand coping with life-threatening illness, the stressors of providing care, and loss. These frameworks inform palliative care communication during assessment and intervention.

Comprehensive communication education for palliative social workers should include careful attention to the use of language—and in particular, the use of metaphors, hyperbole, and hidden meanings—as well as nonverbal communication. Communication is much more than just the words that are spoken during a conversation. The meaning of a given statement is defined by numerous contextual factors, including the speaker's tone of voice, body posture, and the external circumstances surrounding the discussion. Social workers should be aware of how their own appearance can shape the meaning of an interaction. For example, leaning forward, raising eyebrows, and making eye contact can indicate that a listener is receptive to a speaker. On the other hand, crossed arms may suggest defensiveness, feeling threatened, or a desire to end the conversation. Leaning back or fidgeting with objects may also signify that you are nervous, disinterested, or bored. It is also important to acknowledge that nonverbal cues are culturally determined and that different gestures, facial expressions, or physical positions may mean different things to different people.

Individual perceptions about serious and life-threatening illness are shaped, in large part, by one's unique history and cultural background. These perceptions include theories about how and why illness develops, taboos against truth-telling, and beliefs about healing. The centrality of the patient/family-centered approach in palliative care resonates with many immigrant cultures, but true family-centered advance care planning, efforts to understand the patient's culture, and involvement of trained interpreters take time, which may clash with administrative challenges such as large caseloads and short medical appointments. Some cultures hold fatalistic beliefs that discussing potentially negative events may contribute to their eventual occurrence.[6] This belief can complicate prognostication and advance care planning. Conventional (i.e., Western-based) practice concepts and approaches may not be applicable to diverse populations.

To enhance cultural awareness and patient/family-centeredness, palliative social workers should be taught how to be clinically present. Clinical presence involves attentive behavior and active listening skills. In the context of palliative care, being present means starting where the patient/family are and communicating in a manner that makes them feel heard and not alone. Presence is demonstrated by a relaxed body posture and the judicious use of therapeutic silence—that is, deliberate pauses in conversations that allow patients and families the opportunity to contemplate what is being said and formulate well-reasoned questions and/or responses.

One way to practice clinical presence is to engage in reflection. Reflection is a basic communication skill and a central component of active listening. It involves rephrasing and summarizing what is heard during a conversation. The social worker demonstrates that he or she is listening and understands what the speaker is saying. Reflection also provides the speaker the opportunity to correct the listener's interpretation of what was said. Rephrasing what is said lets patients know that they were heard and provides an opportunity to avoid ambiguity or correct misinterpretation. Reflection can also be used to summarize the main points of a lengthy conversation or to clarify next steps for action.

Comprehensive Psychosocial Assessment

The psychosocial assessment provides palliative care social workers with a framework of topics considered important to patients and families dealing with serious illness. These assessment topics are often communication starters or launching points for in-depth discussions about the family's experiences, needs, hopes, and fears. During the assessment encounter, social workers are often simultaneously trying to establish trust and rapport with families while also evaluating risks, support needs, and patient/family priorities. Assessment questions can seem impersonal, awkward, or intrusive (e.g., regarding financial matters or how the illness is affecting intimate relationships). However, responses to such questions inform the care plan and allow the social worker to better understand the patient/family perspectives and context. With practice and training, healthcare providers can seamlessly integrate their assessment inquiry into an introductory conversation with the patient and family.

Team Communication

Interprofessional cooperation within a palliative care team requires close communication, a foundation of mutual trust, worker autonomy, a supportive work environment, role clarity, and belief in the team-based philosophy of care.[7] Palliative social workers should feel comfortable assertively articulating their clinical judgment in team meetings, care planning activities, and the implementation of psychosocial interventions. In particular, social workers should remain a staunch and vocal advocate for patient and family needs and preferences. Furthermore, social workers should become conversant with common medical terminology and the professional terms so they can understand, advise, and translate during team-based communication. Some medical systems may still have strongly entrenched professional hierarchies, and thus social workers should be attuned to the existing dynamics within their own team—and educate themselves on how to diplomatically negotiate these dynamics to facilitate a more "flattened" and equitable team structure.

An important aspect of professional communication is being able to succinctly articulate one's role and responsibilities to others. Palliative care social workers should be able to clearly and concisely explain their role to patients, families, and fellow team members. This may be challenging, as both palliative care providers and social workers have struggled to operationalize their professional positions within a large and constantly evolving, hierarchically layered, profit-conscious health system. Social workers may define their role differently depending on their specific job responsibilities, but the role typically includes, among other things, connecting families to needed resources, facilitating decision-making, and bolstering patient/family coping skills. This role can be especially demanding, both physically and emotionally. Thus it is important to note that palliative care professionals are susceptible to compassion fatigue, the affective toll of compound losses, and the stressors of a high-demand job. Social workers should also be able to succinctly articulate their own coping needs and manage these needs through supervision, peer support from fellow team members, mindfulness, and other self-care activities.

Facilitating Goals of Care Discussions

Social workers are often involved in patient/family conversations about treatment decisions and goals of care. Thus comprehensive communication training is needed to equip them with the necessary skills and knowledge to lead and facilitate such discussions. The increased use of documented treatment instructions (e.g., Medical Orders for Life Sustaining Treatment [MOLST]), for example, require in-depth discussions about patient priorities and preferences. Thus a comprehensive training program for palliative care social workers should also include the review and application of strategies for initiating such discussions.

One widely endorsed communication framework is the shared decision-making approach: (a) reviewing decisions that need to be made; (b) sharing information about the patient's values, current medical situation, and risks and benefits of treatment; (c) ensuring that all parties involved comprehend the information that is being provided; (d) discussing preferred roles in decision-making; and (e) reaching an agreement about a treatment approach that is consistent with the patient's values and preferences. Shared decision-making also ensures that all relevant care preferences and decisions are documented in advance directives and honored by healthcare providers. When initiating discussions about advance care planning, it may be helpful for social workers to begin by exploring the patient's priorities in terms of comfort, longevity, or functionality. Because goals and preferences change over time, such discussions should be considered part of an ongoing conversation, with advance directives updated when appropriate.

Helping to Manage Uncertainty

Although patients and family members may desire diagnostic clarity and clinical certainty, such precision is rarely available. Palliative care professionals must acknowledge this and feel comfortable saying "I don't know."[8] Discussions may need to include a frank conversation about "what is known" and "what is knowable," including the challenges of establishing prognosis.[8,9] Further complicating the issue is family members often "don't know what they don't know."[10] Patients and families may benefit more from a facilitated discussion about their questions, uncertainties, and concerns related to a life-limiting diagnosis, as opposed to simply providing information about possible outcomes. When practitioners invite families to discuss uncertainties regarding prognosis, it allows social workers to openly address related frustrations and anxieties.

Convening Family Meetings

Family meetings may generate consensus, profound emotional release, or heated debate. In this latter regard, these meetings may require the application of mediation skills (i.e., basic conflict resolution) to ensure that all parties have the opportunity to be heard, the various opinions are understood and acknowledged, and all parties feel respected. Hudson et al. published guidelines for conducting family meetings in palliative care, calling for them to be offered early in the clinical encounter (ideally at admission); proactive rather than crisis-driven; and facilitated by the team member (or members) with appropriate skills in palliative care, group dynamics, and clinical communication.[11] The family meeting is an ideal forum during which the social worker can take the lead by scheduling the meeting, preparing an agenda, facilitating discussion, taking notes, advocating for patients and caregivers, documenting decisions, and ensuring adequate follow-up.[12,13]

Education and Training Activities

Table 45.1 summarizes selected communication training activities that can be employed with interprofessional learners, including social workers. These include traditional educational modalities such as clinical rotations, didactic sessions, and self-study modules—as well as nontraditional methods such as standardized patients and families, reflective writing, palliative care vignettes, case-solving, and capstone projects. Forrest and Derrick described interprofessional case simulations with volunteer actors that emphasized the application of communication skills.[14] Student participants included representatives from social work, nursing, and chaplaincy. Significant improvement was demonstrated in self-rated skills and competency. Although patient simulation appears to be a promising model for communication training, the impact of these training approaches on the real-world patients and families requires further research. For example, a randomized trial of simulation training for physicians and nurse practitioners did *not* improve their perceived quality of communication.[15]

Standardized patients, role playing, and modeling are popular because they provide avenues for students to interact with a "trained" patient and seasoned healthcare providers. However, these activities take time to prepare and can be difficult to assess because of variability in responses. Reflective writing, classroom didactics, and case vignettes are more commonly used because they take less time to prepare and can outline a large amount of educational content within a short period of time. These latter educational activities, however, typically do not require learners to demonstrate their acquired knowledge and skills in an interactive situation.

Models for Sharing Life-Altering News

Because palliative care patients are often coping with debilitating and/or life-threatening conditions, it is essential that social workers prepare themselves to broach these difficult topics. Sharing life-altering news, such as the diagnosis of a terminal disease or the lack of effective treatment options, can be challenging for even seasoned practitioners. When communicating serious information, it may be helpful to use an existing communication framework to provide structure and guide the conversation. Palliative care educators may find the use of communication models particularly useful for novice learners with limited experience who are interacting with patients and families. Table 45.2 displays selected models for communicating life-altering news to patients

Table 45.1 Modes of Communication Education and Training for Palliative Care Social Work

Activity	Description	Pros	Cons
Standardized patient(s)	Trained actor(s) simulate a healthcare scenario through an interactive role play with learners	♦ Requires interactive application of knowledge/skills	♦ Expense ♦ Time training actors
Reflective writing	Diaries or other narrative writing exercises that encourage self-assessment of personal values, beliefs, and biases	♦ Self-review is considered an integral first step to effective palliative care practice	♦ Lack of applied interaction
Didactics	Lecture-based instruction involving dissemination of best-practice strategies	♦ Structured ♦ Time-tested training approach	♦ Lack of applied interaction
Self-directed activities	Semistructured learning assignments that allow learners to apply knowledge and skills to a population and/or setting of their choosing	♦ Allows learners to pursue unique interests ♦ Fosters creativity	♦ Lack of standardization ♦ Difficult to assess outcomes
Case vignettes	The presentation of clinically complex scenarios that involve common ethical dilemmas and communication challenges	♦ Allows for brainstorming with other learners	♦ Lack of real-time communication dynamics
Role-play	An interactive learning activity during which learners are tasked with assuming the role of the client or healthcare provider	♦ Allows learners to work through complex situations at their own pace	♦ Difficult to assess because of variability
Modeling	Demonstration of exemplary communication approaches by instructor(s)/expert(s)	♦ Structured and real-life examples	♦ May appear scripted/contrived

and families. While distinctly different, these models include a number of shared elements, including (a) preparation of self, the setting, and the patient/family; (b) building trust and rapport and being present; (c) exploring what the patient/family already knows and what they want to know; (d) providing clear, jargon-free information about the situation; (e) allowing space for emotional expressions and denial; (f) supporting and empathizing; and (g) summarizing and discussing next steps. Discussions involving life-altering news may also demand extensive flexibility, the reiteration of important information, and a review of hospice services. Educators and practitioners should also be aware of the limitations of using a formulaic communication approach. A dynamic, evolving approach—one that is responsive to the needs and reactions of the family—is usually preferred over a scripted "cookie-cutter" approach.[8,16]

In addition to sharing life-altering news such as a poor prognosis, unresponsive treatments, or death, palliative care social workers must also be willing to broach potentially taboo subjects such as family finances; the presence of mental illness; and issues related to sexuality, potential abuse/neglect, and spirituality.[3,17,18] These topics are essential components of a comprehensive psychosocial assessment, and yet exploring these issues can be perceived as rude or intrusive. Social workers in training can practice addressing these challenging subjects in a respectful manner by explaining the rationale behind the questions and asking permission to bring them up.

Advances in Communication Technology

Technological innovations have provided palliative care professionals with a growing number of useful communication tools. Live video streaming, mobile phones and messaging, email, and electronic documentation can facilitate efficient practice, overcome barriers to care and continuity, and reduce errors. Telemedicine, in particular, has strong potential for use in palliative care. For example, Parker-Oliver and colleagues demonstrated that use of a live video interface by hospice providers can improve outreach and support for rural-dwelling families and allow family caregivers greater opportunity to participate in team-based communication.[19] Palliative care educators and practitioners should stay abreast of the latest developments in communication technology and assess their potential to improve processes and outcomes in clinical practice. In many cases, however, the ever-evolving changes in communication technology are outpacing formal education and professional training. Furthermore, along with the advances in communication technology come questions about the effectiveness of such tools, as well as the ethical and legal implications of incorporating them into routine clinical practice. The blurring of professional boundaries, the potential for breach of protected health information, questions about data integrity, and worries about depersonalizing patient/family–provider interactions are a few of the many concerns noted by social work scholars and technology adopters. Moreover, some scholars have expressed concern about vulnerable populations (e.g., poor, elderly, rural dwellers) who may have limited access to the latest technology. Thus educators and practitioners should be mindful of how innovative communication tools may contribute to disparities—or be used to address them. For community-based palliative care providers, electronic documentation can allow for important medical chart information to be relayed to clinical team members in real time, regardless of their location. Additionally, the use of electronic documentation in hospice settings has been

Table 45.2 Selected Models for Communicating Difficult News Relevant to Palliative Care Providers

Model	Brief Description	Patient Populations and Settings	Evidence of Use by Social Work	Reference(s)
ABCDE	A = Advance preparation B = Build therapeutic environment C = Communicate well D = Deal w/patient/family reactions E = Encourage and validate emotions	None specified	Yes	Rabow and McPhee[21]
BREAKS	B = Background R = Rapport E = Explore patient's knowledge A = Announce a warning K = Kindling (i.e., space for emotions) S = Summarize	None specified	None identified	Narayanan et al.[24]
COMFORT™℠	C = Communication O = Orientation and opportunity M = Mindful presence F = Family caregiver communication O = Openings R = Relating T = Team	Setting(s): Home, nursing home, hospital, palliative care	Yes	Wittenberg-Lyles et al.[22]
Kaye 10-Step Approach	1. Preparation 2. What does the patient know? 3. Is more information wanted? 4. Give a "warning shot" 5. Allow denial 6. Explain (if requested) 7. Listen to concerns 8. Encourage ventilation of feelings 9. Summary and plan 10. Offer availability	None specified	None identified	Kaye[25]
SPIKES	S = Setup P = Perception I = Invitation K = Knowledge E = Empathize S = Summarize and Strategize	Population(s): cancer patients Setting(s): hospital, clinical settings	Yes	Baile et al.[26]

linked to greater attention to key palliative care quality domains, including advanced care planning, cultural needs, and the dying experience.[20]

Training Environments for Palliative Care Social Workers

Palliative care social workers can advance their communication-based knowledge and skills in a variety of educational environments. Possible settings include the traditional "brick-and-mortar" classroom, postgraduate training, online learning, continuing education seminars, and on-the-job training. Regardless of the setting, social workers looking to increase their palliative care communication skills may need direct client interaction in order to fully understand and apply these skills in a real-life setting. Classroom training, however, is often considered a necessary first step to equip trainees with essential information about relevant theory and evidence-informed practice approaches in social work communication. Many schools of social work now provide elective courses in death and dying, bereavement, managing chronic diseases, and working with families. Ideally, palliative care communication should be infused into classroom education to promote baseline knowledge, teach specific communication strategies, and ground social work practice in theory. Once social workers finish their in-class coursework, learning continues. In fact, the profession is charged with staying current about best practices, and thus postgraduate training and continuing education opportunities are essential to maintain practitioner competency and quality.

Postgraduate Training Opportunities

Certification Opportunities for Hospice and Palliative Care Social Workers

The NASW, in partnership with the National Hospice and Palliative Care Organization, offers two credentialing opportunities for hospice and palliative care social workers. Bachelor's-level social workers can pursue becoming a Certified Hospice and Palliative Social Worker (CHP-SW), and master's level practitioners can work to obtain the Advanced Certified Hospice and Palliative Social Worker (ACHP-SW) designation. The development of practitioner communication skills is a central component of these programs. For example, competencies for certification include the following:

- Communicates effectively and compassionately with patients, families, healthcare team, and community members about hospice and palliative care issues.
- Accurately documents and verbally communicates assessment information, treatment plans, and client system interactions as required by the organizational setting.
- Communicates and collaborates effectively as a member of the interdisciplinary team to develop the plan of care and facilitate ongoing revisions to address the biopsychosocial needs and goals of the patient family/caregiver.

Postgraduate Fellowships and Internships

Fellowships and internships provide advanced, intensive, hands-on, mentored training for an extended period (usually between 1 month and 2 years). The goals, focus, and structure of fellowships vary widely, and training may be clinically oriented, research focused, or a combination of both. The development of communication skills is usually a core component of training, particularly in clinically oriented settings. Fellowships and internships are often funded, and thus trainees may receive a modest stipend. However, a small number of fellowships are known to charge tuition, although tuition assistance is frequently available for participants who need financial help. Many fellowships involve a competitive application process. Thus interested candidates should inquire about the availability of positions, selection criteria, and requirements in advance. The Department of Pain Medicine and Palliative Care at Mount Sinai Beth Israel in New York has offered a recurring year-long social work fellowship in palliative and end-of-life care. New York University's Silver School of Social Work sponsors a 16-month leadership program in palliative and end-of-life care through the Zelda Foster Studies Program. A number of Veterans Administration hospitals also offer paid interprofessional and/or social work fellowships in palliative care.

Online Communication Training

Although the number of online offerings is increasing, some scholars have raised concerns about the effectiveness of using Web-based training to develop interpersonal and interprofessional communication skills. The concern is that online forums may not adequately allow for the development of the dynamic social skills needed to initiate and facilitate in-person discussions about challenging topics. That said, one potentially effective online training tool for palliative care social workers is the COMFORT communication curriculum developed by Wittenberg-Lyles and colleagues.[21] This course has been designed for a diverse audience of healthcare professionals to improve palliative care communication, ease transitions in care, and facilitate conversations about patient/family psychosocial needs. The course creators successfully implemented the Web-based learning modules with a sample of nurses, physicians, social workers, pharmacists, and other interprofessional learners. The approach is team oriented and includes adaptive communication strategies to match communication style to patient/family preferences and needs. More specifically, the COMFORT™™ curriculum consists of the following seven elements:[22]

C—communication (a narrative approach to clinical practice)

O—orientation and opportunity (assessment of health literacy)

M—mindful presence (attentive behavior, attention to nonverbal language, and self-care)

F—family caregiver communication (with key members of the patient's social sphere)

O—openings (opportunities for emotional expression)

R—relating (family denial and acceptance)

T—team (collaboration and patient/family advocacy in team meetings)

Another reputable online communication training curriculum is CancerPEN, developed by the Stanford University School of Medicine. The Web-based content features expert video presentations, case studies, and discussion forums on giving bad news, clarifying goals of care, managing family conflict, delivering information about resuscitation attempts, and more. Social workers who enroll can earn continuing education credits for course modules.

Other Continuing Education Forums

Social workers can obtain additional training in communication at the postgraduate level through continuing education in various formats. For example, one advanced continuing education and training program is the Communication Skills Training program offered at Memorial Sloan-Kettering Cancer Center.[23] The program teaches patient-centered communication skills through classroom teaching, video-recorded training, and interaction with trained actors. Communication is highlighted across eight core modules and includes verbal and nonverbal skills training with feedback and reflection. Topics include life-altering news, responding to patient anger, communicating through interpreters, discussing prognosis and goals of care, and conducting family meetings. Participants come from the fields of medicine, nursing, and social work.

Conclusion

Communication is a dynamic process that requires healthcare providers to quickly assess, interpret, and respond to verbal and nonverbal communication as well as implicit and explicit information. Social workers are core members of the palliative care team, who come equipped with a strong foundation of communication training and skills. As experts in family dynamics and communication skills, social workers can assume a primary role in facilitating difficult discussions about prognosis, expected disease progression, limitations of treatment, and advance care planning. It is incumbent, however, on social work practitioners and educators to stay current on the fast-paced innovations in palliative care communication approaches and training. By doing so, they can sharpen their communications skills to truly hear the rich histories and unique needs of their patients/families—and then advocate as needed on their behalf.

References

1. Council on Social Work Education. Education policy and accreditation standards. http://www.cswe.org/File.aspx?id=13780. Published March 27, 2010. Updated August 2012. Accessed September 27, 2014.
2. Christ G, Blacker S. Palliative care with older adults: Section 2: Social work role in palliative care. Council on Social Work Education. http://www.cswe.org/CentersInitiatives/CurriculumResources/MAC/Reviews/Health/22739/22741.aspx. Published September 11, 2009.
3. Bailey, G. *NASW Standards for Social Work Practice in Palliative and End of Life Care.* Washington, DC: National Academy of Social Workers; 2004.
4. Quinn K, Hudson P, Ashby M, Thomas K. "Palliative care: The essentials": Evaluation of a multidisciplinary education program *J Palliat Med.* 2008;11(8):1122–1129.
5. Otis-Green S, Sidhu, RK, Del Ferraro C, Ferrell, B. Integrating social work into palliative care for lung cancer patients and families: A multidimensional approach. *J Psychosoc Oncol.* 2014;32(4):431–446.
6. Braun KL, Tanji VM, Heck R. Support for physician-assisted suicide: Exploring the impact of ethnicity and attitudes toward planning for death. *Gerontologist*, 2001;41(1):51–60.
7. Jünger S, Pestinger M, Elsner F, Krumm N, Radbruch L. Criteria for successful multiprofessional cooperation in palliative care teams. *Palliat Med.* 2007;21(4):347–354.
8. Cagle JG, Kovacs PJ. Education: A complex and empowering intervention at the end of life. *Health Soc Work.* 2009;34(1):17–27.
9. Bern-Klug M, Gessert C, Forbes S. The need to revise assumptions about the end of life: Implications for social work practice. *Health Soc Work.* 2001;26(1):38–48.
10. Rabow MW, Hauser, JM, Adams, J. Supporting family caregivers at the end of life: "They don't know what they don't know." *JAMA.* 2004;291(4):483–491.
11. Hudson P, Quinn K, O'Hanlon B, Aranda S. Family meetings in palliative care: Multidisciplinary clinical practice guidelines. *BMC Palliat Care.* 2008;7(1):12.
12. Yennurajalingam S, Dev R, Lockey M, Pace E, Zhang T, Palmer JL, Bruera E. Characteristics of family conferences in a palliative care unit at a comprehensive cancer center. *J Palliat Med.* 2008;11(9):1208–1211.
13. Fineberg IC, Kawashima M, Asch SM. Communication with families facing life-threatening illness: A research-based model for family conferences. *J Palliat Med.* 2011;14(4):421–427.
14. Forrest C, Derrick C. Interdisciplinary education in end-of-life care: Creating new opportunities for social work, nursing, and clinical pastoral education students. *J Soc Work End Life Palliat Care.* 2010;6(1–2):91–116.
15. Curtis JR, Back AL Ford DW et al. Effect of communication skills training for residents and nurse practitioners on quality of communication with patients with serious illness: A randomized trial. *JAMA.* 2013;310 (21):2271–2281.
16. Wittenberg-Lyles EM, Goldsmith J, Sanchez-Reilly S et al. Communicating a terminal prognosis in a palliative care setting: Deficiencies in current communication training protocols. *Soc Sci Med.* 2008;66(11):2356–2365.
17. Cagle JG, Bolte S. Sexuality and life-threatening illness: Implications for social work and palliative care. *Health Soc Work.* 2009;34(3):223–233.
18. Cagle JG, Kovacs PJ. Informal caregivers of cancer patients: Perceptions of preparedness and the need for support during hospice care. *J Gerontol Soc Work.* 2011;54:92–115.
19. Parker-Oliver D, Demiris G, Wittenberg-Lyles E, Porock D. The use of videophones for patient and family participation in hospice interdisciplinary team meetings: A promising approach. *Eur J Cancer Care.* 2010;19(6):729–735.
20. Cagle JG, Durham DD, Rokoske FS, Schenck AP, Spence C, Hanson LC. Use of electronic documentation for quality improvement in hospice care. *Am J Med Qual.* 2012;27(4):282–290.
21. Rabow MW, McPhee SJ. Beyond breaking bad news: How to help patients who suffer. *West J Med.* 1999;171(4):260–263.
22. Wittenberg-Lyles E, Goldsmith J, Ferrell B, Burchett M. Assessment of an interprofessional online curriculum for palliative care communication training. *J Palliat Med.* 2014;17(4):400–406.
23. Kissane DW, Bylund CL, Banerjee SC, et al. Communication skills training for oncology professionals. *J Clin Oncol.* 2012;30(11):1242–1247.
24. Narayanan V, Bista B, Koshy C. "BREAKS" protocol for breaking bad news. *J Palliat Med.* 2014;17(4):400–406.
25. Kaye P. *Breaking Bad News: A 10 Step Approach.* Northampton, CT: EPL Publications; 1996.
26. Baile WF, Buckman R, Lenzi R, Glober G, Beale EA, Kudelka AP. SPIKES—a six-step protocol for delivering bad news: Application to the patient with cancer. *Oncologist.* 2000;5(4):302–311.

CHAPTER 46

Communication Education for Chaplains

Angelika A. Zollfrank and Catherine F. Garlid

Introduction

Chaplaincy in palliative care requires specialized knowledge in the spiritual aspects of a patient's pain, including spiritual distress, poor quality of spiritual and relational life, and/or a lack of meaning during chronic and life-threatening illness. There are many valid approaches to the communication education of chaplains that vary in academic and practical methodology. Recommendations for interdisciplinary spiritual care models that help all members of the healthcare team to identify spiritual issues and concerns have also guided the development of specialized communication education for chaplains in palliative care.[1] In the United States, the credentialing available through Clinical Pastoral Education (CPE) for board certification of several professional organizations equips chaplains to serve alongside other credentialed members of the palliative care team. In this chapter the primary focus is on CPE methods as a distinct pathway to communication competency in palliative care chaplaincy.

The main goal of the palliative care chaplain is to support patients, families, and staff in their religious and/or spiritual practice, coping, and development. CPE prepares healthcare chaplains for this task. In CPE healthcare chaplains and spiritual leaders learn to:

1. develop a spiritual plan of care that honors the patient's religious/spiritual background and development during chronic and life-threatening illness;

2. support and intervene toward positive coping through conversation, prayer, meditation, guided imagery, sacred text, ritual and worship;

3. collaborate with religious and spiritual communities and their leaders;

4. offer education and function as a broker among involved stakeholders regarding religious and spiritual principles and healthcare; and

5. contribute expertise concerning the ways that religion and spirituality influence patient and family treatment decisions and support clinical ethics consultation processes.[2(p430)]

Chaplaincy education is at its core communication education, which includes spiritual literacy in a wide variety of meaning-making and belief systems. Communication education also equips chaplains with the translational skills necessary to competently receive and transfer religious/spiritual information[3] on multiple levels, including physical, emotional, cultural, spiritual, religious, philosophical, and ethical aspects of care. Over the course of its development, communication education in chaplaincy has evolved in content and method. This chapter is organized into four parts: a representative case, a summary of the background of chaplaincy communication education, educational practices, and future opportunities.

Patti,[4] a 71-year-old Caucasian woman and former Roman Catholic, had identified her religious affiliation as "none." A passenger in a high-speed accident in her late teens, Patti became a paraplegic. Two years later, after multiple surgeries, Patti met the love of her life, Ron, also a paraplegic, in a rehabilitation hospital, and they married. Through intense determination and a zest for life, they achieved satisfying and productive work lives, designing their own home to fully accommodate their disabilities and wheelchair use. The palliative care chaplain met Patti in the intensive care unit. Intubated following major surgery for malignant colon cancer, Patti was fully alert when the chaplain met her and she wrote, "No religion! Spiritual." The chaplain's response was, "Works for me. Does it for you?" The chaplain attended a meeting with Patti, her husband, her primary care physician, and the palliative care nurse practitioner. The team spoke to Patti and shared that they did not expect her to be able to leave the hospital and presented several options for discontinuing aspects of her acute medical care and shifting to comfort measures. Patti needed time to think things over. As she came off the respirator, Patti shared with the chaplain that her goal was to regain her strength, get to a rehabilitation hospital, and then go home. The chaplain was in regular communication with the palliative care nurse practitioner. Patti told the chaplain about the generations of chipmunks that she and Ron had watched, fed, and tamed from their porch at the edge of a rural pasture. For Patti, her home with Ron provided her spiritual grounding, a sanctuary, and a source of hope.

The chaplain followed Patti until her discharge from rehabilitation and did not hear from her until 11 months later, when Patti was again hospitalized. For 9 months, Patti had enjoyed her life at home before her cancer came back and her symptoms became unmanageable. When she heard that the surgeon could operate but that it would "kill her," Patti called the chaplain, expressing her distress that the team had come once again to tell her she would die.

She was, however, grateful that the nurse had set her up with a morphine pump. "I can't stand the pain anymore." The next day, Patti, who was with Ron, asked to see the chaplain again, saying, "It's not good and I am having trouble letting go." After a long silence and warm eye contact, the chaplain said, "Maybe you could think of it not as letting go but as letting be."

The chaplain facilitated open sharing of Patti's fears about how Ron would manage after she died, about funeral plans, and about Patti's recent experience of being overmedicated, a sense of "fading away" that was not frightening, and about whether she, still a full code, would want to go back to the intensive care unit. Ron's comment was, "It would depend on the circumstances." However, 3 hours later, the nurse found Patti without a pulse and a code blue was called. Over the telephone in the midst of the code response, Ron said, "Let her go." The chaplain and the nurse practitioner were satisfied with how they helped Patti manage a difficult transition. Close team communication, recognition of the uniqueness of each patient's story, and effective use of the different clinical roles were key to compassionate care.

Background of Chaplaincy Communication Education

The Clinical Case Method as Primary Teaching Tool

The foundational method for teaching communication in chaplaincy has been the clinical case method. The method includes the clinical case study and the verbatim, a later adaptation of the clinical case study. Two of the founders of CPE, Anton Boisen, a Protestant minister and Richard Cabot, MD, encouraged student chaplains to focus on a particular patient and collect concrete observable data as opposed to having him or her accumulate knowledge from a distance later to be superimposed on the subject/object.[5] Cabot taught the skills of close observation, recall, and reporting of patient behavior and experience.

Having used clinical case studies while working with Cabot at Harvard Medical School, Boisen began studying religious experience through his own mental illness. Having suffered recurring psychotic episodes, he first used himself as primary case material in a thorough study of "the living human document." Boisen then bridged the academic education of clergy, ancient Judeo-Christian understandings, and the world of Western medical practice[2] using case study methodology. In an unpublished memo to Cabot, Boisen wrote,

> I wish to express in the first place my very great appreciation of the method of teaching ... this is the most satisfactory from the pedagogical standpoint in that it supplies concrete material on which to work [and] it places the stress on what the student does [experiential learning] rather than upon what the teacher says. The problems presented are of fundamental interest and importance, and the principles involved are so clearly brought out and summed up as we go along.[5(p86)]

Russell Dicks, a Methodist minister, was hired by Cabot as the first chaplain in a general hospital. Dicks pioneered the use of the verbatim, instead of the clinical case study, believing it was a tool better suited to shorter visits in a general hospital. The close recollection of the actual conversation was used to examine whether the communication between the patient and the chaplain was effective, appropriate, and congruent with the person's crisis or pain.[6(p124)] "Discussion and analysis of case studies should make use of, but also *transcend*, behavioral science perspectives in order to prepare the chaplain not as a psychotherapist but as a spiritual care giver with finely tuned communication skills."[6(pp125-126)] Table 46.1 specifies the main characteristics of the clinical case method, comparing verbatim and clinical case study, the primary tools for teaching communication in clinical pastoral education.

Over time, educators in CPE have continued to develop verbatim formats and seminars to suit differing objectives for communication education. Curricula often include the critical incident report, addressing end-of-life situations, or healthcare decision-making. The critical incident report captures an encounter with several individuals in a context that represents a crisis or opportunity for the learner. The report includes aspects of the environment that influenced the communication, such as internal and external mood, the general climate, responses, and results. For example, student chaplains might use a critical incident report to explore their role and communication in a team or family meeting.

In the 1970s David Duncombe, CPE supervisor and chaplain to Yale Medical School, used the verbatim in an interprofessional education experiment. He trained law, medical, nursing, and graduate-level theological students in a course titled "The Seminar on the Chronically Ill," for which he recruited patients with advanced chronic illness as "teachers." The students presented their work in small interdisciplinary groups using the verbatim as the primary teaching tool.[7] CPE today continues to emphasize the value of interprofessional contexts for learning.

Beginning in the 1980s, the demand for systematic skill building began to grow, influenced by the greater reach of secular counseling and psychology. Psychologist Egan introduced the basic skills required to build an alliance and rapport: the use of nonverbal behaviors such as eye contact and posture, the use of open questions and the avoidance of "why" questions, the use of gestures and "minimal prompters," "verbal following," paraphrasing of content and feeling, and summarization.[8] Hemenway wrote, "[CPE] is a direct response to the need 'to learn how to do it'[9(p195)] ... Human behavior in a given situation can be self-chosen, observable, measured, and changed."[9(p196)] She emphasized praxis and the movement between action and theory, empathy and detachment. She also stressed the need for the student chaplain's awareness of the clinical context while assessing communication.[9(p196)]

Responding to managed care in the 1990s, Hilsman stressed the importance of adapting chaplaincy communication education to the rapidly changing healthcare paradigm, emphasizing the importance of spiritual assessment and the articulation of a theory of healing.[10] In addition to teaching student chaplains to engage patients without a theological, spiritual, or emotional agenda, CPE also began to focus on the art of semistructured interviewing and spiritual assessment.[11,12] Later, in 2004, Wilson argued for the use of formalized role plays using volunteer actors. Using research to validate the effectiveness of his methods, Wilson videotaped the encounters, and the student chaplains received immediate critique from the volunteer and an observing peer, a technique similar to the current use of standardized patients in simulation centers.[13] Student chaplains were evaluated for their ability to join with the volunteer, listen actively, assess the volunteer's theological concerns, and intervene.[14]

Table 46.1 Comparison of Communication Teaching Tools in Current Chaplain Education

	Verbatim	Clinical Case Study
Goal(s)	a. To examine driving forces and barriers toward effective spiritual care provision b. To reveal learning areas in the student chaplain's practice c. To provide a record and tool for supervision and group learning	a. To track a chaplain/patient relationship *over time* (may include portions of several pastoral/spiritual conversations) b. To provide a record and tool for professional supervision, group, and interprofessional education c. To contribute to the published pool of cases in specific practice areas. d. To develop research questions regarding the effectiveness of religious/spiritual care
Method	a. To give a written account of a single conversation or encounter between a student chaplain and a patient/family for analysis	a. To provide a detailed written account of the patient's background including his or her medical, social, familial, psychological, cultural, and religious/spiritual context b. To examine the effectiveness of multiple encounters between chaplain/patient
Content	a. Context of the encounter b. Preliminary data including (to the extent known) patient's age, gender, marital or other lifestyle status, number of children, religion, race, ethnicity, medical diagnosis, date of admission, occupation, prior pastoral/spiritual care c. Record from memory of the dialogue between student chaplain and a patient/family/other d. Analysis including spiritual assessment, interpersonal, socioeconomic, spiritual/religious dynamics; evaluation of spiritual care provided; ethical questions; religious/spiritual care plan; documentation; and theological reflection	a. An overall narrative that includes the institutional context, detailed information about both patient and family or other significant relationships, medical course, demographics, social, familial, psychological, cultural, and religious/spiritual characteristics b. Primary focus is on chaplain/patient relationship in the clinical context c. A detailed spiritual assessment, including the patient's spiritual/religious practices, spiritual history, sense of vocation and purpose, ability to face life challenges, spiritual/religious coping, relationship to religious/spiritual authority or guidance, community, and experience and meaning d. An evaluative summary of the spiritual care provided to address patient's needs

Chaplaincy education today is grounded in teaching specific skills through observable data and includes practical exercises. The word "clinical" in CPE refers both to the context for learning and to the process of reflective practice both in the moment and later, through writing and group discussion. In order to develop the art of reflective practice, additional methods were added to chaplain education.

Process Notes

In addition to the verbatim as a written tool for reflection and assessment of communication skills, student chaplains are required to submit a weekly reflection report, known also as process notes. Student chaplains need to be able to consider their own role in communication and communicate their inner thoughts, conflicts, and areas for growth. Process notes may have an assigned outline, such as relationships, patient care, interdisciplinary communication, organizational and institutional systems, core beliefs, theological concepts, attitudes, spiritual practices, or satisfactions, learning, and identification of learning needs.

The material for reflection by the student chaplain and supervisor will include previously unconscious material, which comes to consciousness through the educational process. Engaging the suffering of a palliative care patient, whether physical or existential, might bring up personal memories and experiences in the student chaplain that will either be an asset or a liability in providing spiritual care. For example, student chaplain Jane discovered upon reflection that she repeatedly changed the subject when her dying patient, Helen, attempted to explore her grief about leaving her young children motherless. Jane discovered that her inability to attend to Helen's grief was related to the loss of a grandmother who lived with Jane's family when she was a child. This discovery helped Jane to listen and respond to Helen going forth.

Process Group

The process group, an experiential seminar, meets regularly throughout the program. Student chaplains are expected to participate actively in the group process with their peers and CPE supervisor(s). The group offers student chaplains a laboratory in which to improve listening skills, explore communication styles and effectiveness, both verbal and nonverbal, contribute effectively to the goals of a group, and balance interpersonal boundaries with empathy. Student chaplains also learn how group membership may yield cognitive and emotional experiences that affect one's ability to engage in intentional communication behaviors. Additionally, the process group offers an educational context for student chaplains to confront and engage mortality and suffering, which are at the core of all human life. As one child psychotherapist writes, "The amount of suffering in the world is not something added on; it is integral to the world, of a piece with our life in nature."[15(p10)]

For many palliative care patients and families, the chaplain represents the liminal space between the profane and sacred, life and death, the known and unknown, the concrete world and the imagined world. The student chaplain's communication role thus involves closing and bridging these gaps. The healthcare environment communicates implicitly to the patient, "You are part of nature, and nature takes its course. You are of the material world."

Spiritual and chaplaincy care communicates implicitly, "You are significant. You have ultimate worth, dignity, and belonging beyond your disease progression." Compassionate communication in palliative care chaplaincy represents these implicit values to the patient, his or her family, and the team.

Current Educational Practices

Current CPE has developed specific methods and content without compromising the values of emotional, spiritual self-awareness, and personal, professional formation. Today's professional healthcare chaplains are board certified after completing at least 400 educational hours and at least 1,200 clinical hours in CPE. Additionally, board certification requires demonstrating the ability to meet the standards of healthcare chaplaincy in writing and in a committee appearance. Online professional continuing education is available to advance board-certified chaplains toward palliative care subspecialty certification.[16] Nationally certified instructors leading CPE, as well as board-certified chaplains, must be endorsed by a faith tradition. However, by and large, chaplains work across religious/spiritual affiliations, beliefs, or spiritual paths, supporting patients, families, and staff of all faith traditions or no faith tradition.[3(p48)] Student chaplains come from a wide variety of religious, spiritual, cultural, and educational backgrounds, with different faith groups emphasizing different educational models and outcomes in the professional formation of their leaders.

The overall goal of palliative care chaplains' communication is the religious/spiritual accompaniment of the patient and his or her loved ones in the process of meaning-making and achieving peace independent of the healthcare outcome. Communication education in palliative care chaplaincy emphasizes the outcome orientation of religious/spiritual care. Box 46.1 offers questions useful in assessing the efficacy of religious/spiritual care interventions.

Screening Protocols

Palliative care programs vary in the use of screening protocols and determining whether healthcare providers or chaplains are responsible for spiritual screening.[17] Validation of several screening tools through rigorous research is underway,[18,19] and palliative care chaplains should recommend the most appropriate spiritual screening tool for their clinical context. Box 46.2 shows several spiritual screening tools that can be used in a variety of clinical settings.[20-22] Familiarity with different screening tools is essential as there is "a growing body of evidence (that) points to the negative impact of religious/spiritual struggle on quality of life and emotional adjustment to illness."[21(p2)] Specific screening for religious/spiritual struggles, which patients may not openly convey, is important.[21(p2),23(p300)] Box 46.2 summarizes different screening tools.

Framing the Spiritual Care Contact

By framing the spiritual care contact, mindful of nonverbal communication, eye contact, and energy, student chaplains learn to greet all persons present, if possible, by name. Introduction to the role of the chaplain may be adjusted depending on the clinical area or the patient's religious/spiritual background. Communication in the initial spiritual care contact includes explaining the visit's purpose and asking permission to enter. Creating the space and

---

Box 46.1 Guiding Questions for Assessing the Efficacy of Spiritual/Religious Care Interventions

Will the religious/spiritual care intervention help patients and their loved ones to:

- sustain and develop positive religious/spiritual coping skills?
- draw creatively on ancient and/or individually tailored religious/spiritual resources?
- elicit and connect with transcendent sources of meaning?
- access support during times of chronic illness, caregiving, and grieving?
- claim their underlying motivations, values, and beliefs?
- make medical decisions consistent with religious/spiritual beliefs and goals of care?
- address any religious/spiritual struggles?
- express emotional and spiritual concerns in team–family meetings?
- engage religious/spiritual aspects of a life that has a legacy and unique meaning?
- adjust to changing clinical realities while maintaining realistic hopes?
- utilize relationships and beliefs to prepare for death and enter into grieving?
- plan and engage transitional religious/spiritual rituals (i.e., wedding, renewal of vows, farewell rituals, or a funeral)?
- heal and continue relationships with those left behind?
- deal with broken relationships, regrets, or unresolved questions of meaning?
- handle practical, spiritually, culturally sensitive matters postmortem?
- continue to live well spiritually?

Box 46.2 Screening Tools for Spiritual Care

Screening Question	Reference
"Are you at peace?"	Steinhauser et al.[20]
"Are there any spiritual beliefs that you want to have discussed in your care with us here?"	Fitchett and Risk[21]
"How important is religion and spirituality in your coping?"	Puchalski[22(p204)]
"Is religion or spirituality important to you as you cope with your illness?" **If "yes,"** "How much strength/comfort do you get from your religion/spirituality right now?" **If "no,"** "Has there ever been a time that religion/spirituality was important to you?"	Fitchett[23(p300)]

narrating the purpose of one's care enhances rapport. A key learning for new student chaplains is not to take rejection personally and to work with patients' assumptions related to the chaplain's presence. Many palliative care patients and families bring a complex positive or negative history to interactions with spiritual/religious leaders. Other patients and families may equate the chaplain's visit with bad news or with forecasting of the patient's death. Yet others may be able to be comforted by the chaplain in ways that other care providers cannot. The chaplain's accompaniment in the patient's illness journey may lead to a sense of hope that transcends the presence.[24] Communication education equips student chaplains to work with such projections and assumptions when framing the spiritual care contact. Student chaplains learn to leave contact information, connect patients and loved ones with community religious/spiritual caregivers, and not make promises they cannot keep.

Cultural and Religious/Spiritual Humility Practices

Chaplaincy education in palliative care emphasizes cultural and religious/spiritual sensitivity. Knowledge of religious/spiritual beliefs and practices during illness, suffering, and at the end of life is just as necessary as knowledge of medical ethics related to specific faith traditions. Expanding such knowledge and competency is a lifelong process and includes knowledge of one's own cultural locations. Based on relational-cultural theory, communication education in spiritual communication across racial, ethnic, cultural, religious/spiritual, socioeconomic, and other differences aims to help student chaplains grow in relational competence. The following assumptions adopted from relational-cultural theory are useful:[25]

- Persons grow through, toward, and within relationships until they die.
- Healing encounters are characterized by a movement toward mutuality.
- Spiritual and emotional growth is expressed in an increasing ability to participate in complex and diversified relationships.
- Healing relationships foster mutual empathy and mutual empowerment.
- Authenticity is necessary for real engagement in healing relationships.

Dynamics of racial, ethnic, cultural, religious/spiritual, and socioeconomic differences are examined in detail in analyzing clinical interactions using verbatims. Particularly in clinical decision-making in palliative care, different understandings of autonomy and community, power and surrender, passivity and agency, illness and death come into play. Religious/spiritual aspects and core values may be culturally determined and need to be negotiated in caring communication in team–family relationships. Chaplains are trained to develop the ability to observe self and others, to adjust assumptions as necessary, and to foster mutually healing relationships. In genogram seminars student chaplains present their own and/or a palliative care family's spiritual and cultural family tree. The goal of this method is to foster greater awareness of diversity, cultural, and spiritual intergenerational family patterns, conflicts, or changes during times of crisis.[26] In cultural awareness seminars student chaplains also engage in exercises to identify their multicultural identities. Among a variety of models we found the RESPECTFUL Model[27(p58)] useful.

Empathic Responding Practice

Student chaplains learn to authentically communicate empathy and to effectively use their emotional and spiritual self to explore and respond to patients' and loved ones' emotional, spiritual, religious, ethical, and cultural experiences, perspectives, beliefs, and values. In highly charged conversations, student chaplains learn to engage in an increasingly wide range of emotional and spiritual experiences while staying nonanxious, centered, mindful, and nonjudgmental. For example, Mrs. Bogota felt unable to redirect her husband's care. Staff grew impatient as Mr. Bogota, who had stage 4 decubitus ulcers, was on antibiotics and a C-PAP machine and was unresponsive and somnolent. Healthcare providers felt they were hindering the patient's greater sense of peace during his dying process. The chaplain eased her way into the room, slowly and carefully building trust. Married for 52 years, Mrs. Bogota was focused on her husband. "Honey, I know you can get better, if you try. You must try, honey, okay?" Pain and separation anxiety were palpable. Mrs. Bogota manipulated the C-PAP equipment, attempted to prop the patient up, and forcefully opened her husband eyes. The chaplain stated tenderly and repeatedly, "You love him so much . . . You are heartbroken . . . You love him so much . . . You miss him already. You cannot bear losing your love." Two hours later, when the physician suggested again, "I think he would be more comfortable without the mask," Mrs. Bogota cried, "Sweetheart, I love you. I love you so much, my love . . . my life. I must let go . . . ." The chaplain supported her throughout her husband's death and in the immediate time afterward.

"Existential suffering and deep personal anguish at the end of life are some of the most debilitating conditions that occur in patients who are dying, and yet the way such suffering is treated in the last days is not well understood."[28(p604)] Existential suffering is a kind of suffering that cannot be borne. Spiritual care aims to authentically reach persons in those places of suffering. Student chaplains learn that palliative communication in chaplaincy involves relating without judgment to any human experience and developing the skills necessary to accompany others empathically using their own emotional experiences. Therapeutic use of self[29(p128)] requires self-awareness and the ability to distinguish between projecting one's life experience onto the patient versus using one's life experience to service the patient. For example, a Chinese American chaplain student visited the family of a dying Chinese man. The family was visibly upset, wanting their father, a devout Muslim, to be able to face Mecca. They insisted that the bed be turned toward the West. Although Christian himself, the student chaplain understood the family's culture and religion: in China the patient had prayed toward Mecca, which was in the West. Although Mecca is east of the United States, the family felt reassured by the chaplain's collaboration with nursing, which led to the patient's bed being turned toward the West.

In communication education, student chaplains learn to use emotional or biographical information to lend support without extensive self-disclosure. They learn to expand their range of emotional, spiritual, religious, ethical, and cultural experiences in order to meet the emotional, spiritual, religious, ethical, and cultural expressions of their patients. Such an ability to encounter another includes an exquisite ability to empathically relate to and enter into the world of the other. Based on McCluskey's work, empathy involves resonance, the process of accessing similar emotions to those expressed by the patient inside oneself, and then communicating to the patient that one has heard, felt, and seen what the patient has expressed.[30(pp49-50)] "Empathy can be understood as our capacity to move away from ourselves as the locus of our reference for understanding emotion and sensation and see these phenomena as they might be experienced by another person, given *their* context and the information coming to them from their senses and cognition."[30(p50)] Therefore, spiritual care communication involves emotional reasoning, associational linking, and clinical empathy.[31] Responses need to match the patient's or family member's affect, energy level, cadence, and rhythm. Such well-matched responses can be useful communication tools in working empathically toward conflict resolution in team–family meetings. For example, in response to the physician's summary of her husband's medical condition, the wife of a dying patient barely speaks in an audible tone, "I can't believe this is happening." Sitting next to the wife, the chaplain builds a communication bridge between the physician and the wife, stating in a gentle, equally low tone of voice, making eye contact and mirroring the wife's nonverbal behavior: "There is a lot of new medical information [pause] ... and a part of you just can't believe that this is what is happening now." Relating in this way can create a sense of closeness that can counterbalance power dynamics in relation to healthcare providers and can ameliorate separation anxiety in relation to the patient.

In CPE mirroring emotional tone, paraphrasing content, and responding empathically are clinical skills that are practiced with the "Capturing the Heart" exercise. The goal of this practice is "to experience the differences between listening—reflecting the heart of another's message—and interpreting or parroting it."[32] Box 46.3 details the Capturing the Heart exercise.

Narrating Observations

CPE student chaplains learn the skill of narrating observations, which can turn nonverbal communication into verbal behavior.[33] To practice this skill, student chaplains work in pairs. The first person uses his or her observations of the other, including any emotional observations. For example, "You appear fidgety. Is there anything unsettling to you?" Or "You are sitting on the opposite side of the room today." Or "You say that you are very sad and you are also smiling." The directive is for the second person to engage in whatever way he or she wishes to, while the first person keeps empathically narrating observations of the other.

Semistructured Interviewing

In communication education for palliative care chaplaincy, general communication education[33-35] and basic spiritual communication skills are combined with in-depth spiritual assessment skills. Student chaplains learn to assess patients' relationships as well as their orientation to meaning and purpose.[36] Several spiritual assessment models are taught and practiced. For its theoretical foundation and depth we have selected and summarized the 7×7 spiritual assessment.[11] The 7×7 model for spiritual assessment (summarized in Table 46.2) includes holistic assessment (seven dimensions of a person's life) and spiritual assessment (seven dimensions of a person's spiritual life). This is a functional approach to spiritual assessment aimed at drawing out people's spiritual stories in their own words. In role play and group education, student chaplains practice the art of semistructured interviewing as a way to elicit and evaluate the information necessary to complete a meaningful spiritual assessment. Box 46.4 provides a summary of useful semistructured interview questions.

Use of Prayer and Other Spiritual and Religious Practices

The goal of these specifically religious/spiritual interventional forms of communication is to ameliorate spiritual pain and contribute to positive life transformations in the face of life-threatening illness. Use of prayer and other spiritual and religious practices have several goals: (a) spontaneous prayer summarizes the patient's

---

Box 46.3 Capturing the Heart Exercise

In a role-play, Jennifer takes up the role of the chaplain. Bob role plays the brother of a terminally ill patient. Bob talks to Jennifer. Jennifer listens.

BOB: If only I could have said good-bye to my brother before he became unconscious.

Jennifer then paraphrases Bob's message.

JENNIFER: You regret not having said all of what you wanted to say and it makes you sad.

If Bob feels that Jennifer's paraphrase fit his message, then (and only then), Bob says to Jennifer, "that's exactly it."

If Bob feels that Jennifer's paraphrase does not reflect his message, then Bob repeats the part of the message he felt was either left out or misinterpreted. For example:

BOB: Actually I am not feeling sad as much as that I am feeling frustrated that I did not get here sooner.

Jennifer then tries again.

JENNIFER: Yes, you really feel some frustration over not having gotten here sooner.

BOB: Exactly. I just wish I could speak to him.

This continues until Bob feels truly understood.
After a while, Bob and Jennifer switch roles.

Table 46.2 The 7 × 7 Model for Spiritual Assessment

Holistic Assessment	Spiritual Assessment
Medical (Biological) Dimension	Beliefs and Meaning
Psychological Dimension	Vocation and Obligations
Family Systems Dimension	Experience and Emotions
Psycho-Social Dimension	Courage and Growth
Ethnic, Racial, Cultural Dimension	Rituals and Practice
Social Issues Dimension	Community
Spiritual Dimension	Authority and Guidance

Source: Fitchett G. *Assessing Spiritual Needs*. Lima, OH: Academic Renewal Press; 2002.

> **Box 46.4** Semistructured Interview Questions
>
> - If you were to die sooner rather than later, what would be left undone?
> - How is your family handling your illness?
> - What is the hardest part for you/your loved ones?
> - Any code or motto you have been living by? anything worth dying for?
> - What do you believe will happen after you die?
> - How would you like to be remembered?
> - How would your loved ones describe you? Anything you would add?
> - What will help you feel that you have lived up to your own ideals in the way you've dealt with your illness/your death?
> - What still puts a smile on your face?
> - What does a good day look like for you?
> - What are some of the ways you have found yourself growing or changing in this phase of your life?
> - Are there moments when you feel discouraged or heartbroken as you are facing this illness/your death?
> - Do you feel that God/the Divine/the Universe cares about you?
> - What are the religious/spiritual practices and beliefs that can help you through this?
> - Are there any relationships in your life, including the past, that need healing?
> - Do you believe God/Higher Power is with you?
> - What do you think God is thinking about all of this?
> - Are there moments of awe that you remember?
> - What, if anything, would you have done differently?
> - What, if anything, is hard for you to forgive?
> - Do you have a prayer or meditation practice? How is it going for you?
> - Do the important people in your life know what they mean to you?
> - Are there ways in which I can help you and your family to prepare for and deal with your death?
> - How would you like to say good-bye to the most important people in your life?
> - Is there anything else you would like to talk about?

concerns; (b) guided imagery can help a patient relax or find peace; (c) sacred text can assist patients in describing their own narrative of suffering in the meta-story of an ancient, sacred narrative; (d) chanting can offer a sense of collecting oneself, while also detaching from suffering; and (e) familiar prayers or spiritual rituals offer the solace of entering into what is known and finding comfort. All these goals of spiritual communication offer patients and loved ones an opportunity to gain greater perspective. In shifting perspective, meaning-making is enhanced and patients and family members may feel held in a friendlier universe or by a loving divine being.

Reframing

Since chaplains translate between the language of medicine and the language of religion/spirituality, reframing is a crucial clinical skill. For example, families who want "everything done" may be encouraged to reflect on what they want to do for their loved one. Student chaplains learn to reframe the language of "comfort measures only" to "intensive comfort measures," with the chaplain coaching loved ones to do what only they can do to enhance comfort. They may speak of redirecting care focusing on the comfort and dignity of a unique person. Student chaplains learn to explore sources of hope beyond medical interventions, bodily life, and life-altering health news. They learn to engage the patient/family's understanding of an afterlife, legacies, or values modeled by the patient that might be adopted by loved ones. Permission may be given and relief may be acknowledged in the process of letting go and letting be.

Conclusion

As palliative care has developed as a specialty, chaplains have been increasingly valued as core members of the interdisciplinary team. Some professional chaplaincy organizations have adopted a model for certifying specialized palliative care chaplains. The early methodology used for educating student chaplains is being applied to educate chaplains specializing in palliative care, focused on the use of the clinical case study and the rigorous, detailed observation, documentation, and interpretation of "the living human document." Arguably, the experiential focus of chaplaincy communication education leads to student chaplains learning from the least rather than the most experienced in the field. However, valuable methods for teaching reflective religious/spiritual care practice, such as verbatims, process notes and groups, specific communication skills, spiritual assessment, and interprofessional education are part of the rich pedagogy of chaplaincy communication education. Still, chaplain educators need to develop validated tools for assessing the effectiveness of chaplaincy communication education. The early focus on the clinical case method has been rediscovered with the recognition that a published body of cases will direct outcome-oriented chaplaincy, evidence-based practice, and research. Going forward, research should focus on tracking and analyzing the communication practices and skills exhibited by palliative care chaplains that are reported within case studies. While educational objectives, outcomes, and standards for professional chaplaincy are consistent throughout the United States, these may need to be compared and competencies for communication developed.

References

1. Puchalski C, Ferrell B, Virani R, et al. Improving the quality of spiritual care as a dimension of palliative care: The Report of the Consensus Conference. *J Palliat Med.* October 2009;12(10):885–904.
2. Zollfrank AA, Garlid CF. Curriculum development, courses, and CPE: Part II: Clinical pastoral education. In: Cobb M, Puchalski CM, Rumbold B, eds. *Oxford Textbook of Spirituality in Healthcare.* Oxford: Oxford University Press; 2012:429–433.

3. Cadge W. *Paging God: Religion in the Halls of Medicine*. Chicago, IL: University of Chicago Press; 2012.
4. Used with permission from the patient's husband.
5. Asquith G. The case study method of Anton T. Boisen. *J Past Care*. 1980;34(2):84–94.
6. Asquith G. The case study. In: Hunter RJ, ed. *Dictionary of Pastoral Care and Counseling*. Nashville, TN, Abingdon Press; 1990:123–126.
7. Duncombe DC. Five years at Yale: "The Seminar on the Chronically Ill." *J Pastoral Care Counsel*. 1974;28(3):152–162.
8. Egan G. *The Skilled Helper*. 2nd ed. Monterey, CA. Brooks/Cole; 1982
9. Hemenway JE. Position paper on CPE supervision. *J Pastoral Care*. 1982;36(3):194–202.
10. Hilsman GJ. Crafting clinical pastoral education: Teaching competencies for the new spiritual care work. *J Pastoral Care*. 1997;51(1):3–12.
11. Fitchett G. *Assessing Spiritual Needs: A Guide for Caregivers*. Lima, OH: Academic Renewal Press; 2002.
12. Lucas A, VandeCreek L. *The Discipline for Pastoral Care Giving: Foundations for Outcome Oriented Chaplaincy*. Binghamton, NY: Haworth Pastoral Press; 2001.
13. Tartaglia A, Dodd-McCue D. Enhancing objectivity in pastoral education: Use of standardized patients in video simulation. *J Past Care Counsel* 2010;64(2):2.1–10.
14. Wilson DR. Virtual visiting seminar replaces verbatim seminar in clinical pastoral education. *J Past Care Counsel*. 2004;58 (1–2):95–100.
15. Phillips A. *Darwin's Worms: On Life Stories and Death Stories*. New York, NY: Basic Books; 2000.
16. HealthcareChaplaincy Network Website. http://www.healthcarechaplaincy.org/professional-continuing-education.html. Accessed June 28, 2014.
17. Derrickson PE. Screening patients for pastoral care: A preliminary report. *Caregiver J*. 1995:11(2):14–18.
18. Grossoehme D, Fitchett G. Testing the validity of a protocol to screen for spiritual struggle among parents of children with cystic fibrosis. In: Piedmont RL, Village A, eds. *Research in the Social Scientific Study of Religion*. Leiden, Boston, MA: Brill; 2013:282–308.
19. King SDW, Fitchett G, Berry DL. Screening for religious/spiritual struggle in blood and marrow transplant patients. *Support Care Cancer*. 2013;21:991–1001.
20. Steinhauser KE, Voils CI, Clipp EC, Bosworth HB, Christakis, NA, Tulsky JA. "Are you at peace?" One item to probe spiritual concerns at the end of life. *Arch Intern Med*. 2006;166:101–105.
21. Fitchett G, Risk JL. Screening for spiritual struggle. *J Past Care Counsel*. 2009;63(1–2):1–12.
22. Puchalski CM. Restorative medicine. In: Cobb M, Puchalski CM, Rumbold B, eds. *Oxford Textbook of Spirituality in Healthcare*. New York, NY: Oxford University Press; 2012:197–210.
23. Fitchett G. Next steps for spiritual assessment in healthcare. In: Cobb M, Puchalski CM, Rumbold B, ed. *Oxford Textbook of Spirituality in Healthcare*. New York, NY: Oxford University Press; 2012:299–308.
24. Nolan S. *Spiritual Care at the End of Life. The Chaplain as "Hopeful Presence."* London, Philadelphia, PA: Jessica Kingsley; 2012.
25. Comstock DL, Hammer TR, Strentzsch J, Cannon K, Jacqueline Parsons J, Salazar G. Relational-cultural theory: A framework for bridging relational, multicultural, and social justice competencies. *J Couns Dev*. 2008;86:279–280.
26. Anderson RG. Spiritual/cultural competencies: Methods in diversity education. *J Pastoral Care Counsel*. 2012;66(4):1–11.
27. Ivey AE, Ivey MB, Zalaquett CP. *Intentional Interviewing and Counseling: Facilitating Client Development in a Multicultural Society*. 7th ed. Belmont, CA: Brooks/Cole; 2010.
28. Boston P, Bruce A, Schreiber R. Existential suffering in the palliative care setting: An integrated literature review. *J Pain Symptom Manage*. March 2011;41(3):604–618.
29. Cooper-White P. *Shared Wisdom: Use of the Self in Pastoral Care and Counseling*. Minneapolis, MN: Augsburg Fortress. 2004.
30. McClusky U. *To Be Met as a Person: The Dynamics of Attachment in Professional Encounters*. London, New York, NY: Karnac; 2005.
31. Halpern J. *From Detached Concern to Empathy*. Oxford, New York, NY: Oxford University Press; 2001.
32. Systems-Centered Training Website. http://www.sctri.com/en-us/training.aspx. Accessed June 28, 2014.
33. SAVI Communications Website. http://www.savicommunications.com/about.html. Accessed June 29, 2014.
34. Kidd RA. Foundational listening and responding skills. In Roberts S, ed. *Professional Spiritual and Pastoral Care. A Practical Clergy and Chaplain's Handbook*. Woodstock, VT: SkyLight Paths; 2013:92–105.
35. Benjamin B, Yaeger A. *Conversation Transformation: Recognize and Overcome the 6 Most Destructive Communication Patterns*. New York, NY: McGraw-Hill; 2012.
36. Donavan DW. Assessments. In: Roberts SB, ed., *Professional Spiritual and Pastoral Care: A Practical Clergy and Chaplain's Handbook*. Woodstock, VT, SkyLight Paths; 2013:42–60.

CHAPTER 47

Interprofessional Education

Barbara Anderson Head and Tara J. Schapmire

Introduction

According to the World Health Organization, interprofessional education (IPE) occurs when students from two or more professions learn about, from, and with each other in order to enable effective collaboration and improve health outcomes.[1] The Education Task Force of the American Association of Colleges of Pharmacy developed a more comprehensive definition of IPE:

> IPE involves educators and learners from two or more health professions and their foundational disciplines who jointly create and foster a collaborative learning environment. The goal of these efforts is to develop knowledge, skills, and attitudes that result in interprofessional team behaviors and competence. Ideally, IPE is incorporated throughout the entire curriculum in a vertically and horizontally integrated fashion.[2(p2)]

The Interprofessional Education Collaboration (IPEC) states the goal of such education is to prepare all health profession students for deliberatively working together with the common goal of building a safer and better patient-centered and community/population-oriented healthcare system. At the core of IPE is the unifying concept of interprofessionality:

> the process by which professionals reflect on and develop ways of practicing that provide an integrated and cohesive answer to the needs of the client/family/population ... Interprofessionality requires a paradigm shift, since interprofessional practice has unique characteristics in terms of values, codes of conduct, and ways of working.[3(p9)]

It is not enough to simply have learners from different backgrounds in the same room; "shared learning" wherein learners actively participate to achieve learning goals that enhance their personal development and improve the care of patients must occur.[4] Improved communication with and understanding of individuals from other disciplines should be an outcome of all interprofessional learning activities. In this chapter, we explore the mandates and competencies currently influencing IPE and team practice. Recent initiatives and research efforts related to interprofessional communication training in palliative care is described, including those directed toward students, continuing education of healthcare professionals, and the development of existing teams.

The Current Mandate for Interprofessional Education

In the past 5 years, there have been numerous studies and legislative/policy mandates for IPE of healthcare professionals, but such recommendations by authoritative bodies have a history of over 40 years. In 1972 the Institute of Medicine issued the report *Educating for the Health Team*, in which it encouraged academic health centers to conduct IPE and provide team-based clinical experiences. The report also suggested that a national clearinghouse be developed for the sharing of instructional and practice models.[5] From the issuing of this report through the early 1990s, scattered programs developed with the help of external funding by the Health Resources and Services Administration and various foundations. These programs were usually elective and targeted small numbers of students, and such efforts failed to mainstream IPE.

In the early years of the 21st century, the concern with healthcare quality and safety fueled recommendations for team-based care and related education. Three Institute of Medicine Reports[6-8] called for the development of effective teams by equipping the workforce with new skills and related competencies taught via IPE.

In 2009 IPEC was formed by the American Association of Colleges of Nursing, the American Association of Colleges of Pharmacy, the American Association of Colleges of Osteopathic Medicine, the American Dental Education Association, the Association of Schools of Public Health, and the Association of American Medical Colleges. The goal of this organization is to "advance substantive interprofessional learning experiences to help prepare future clinicians for team-based care of patients."[9(p6)] IPEC's first initiative was the development of core competencies for interprofessional collaborative practice[10] to guide curricula development in health professions. IPEC developed four competency domains for interprofessional collaborative practice: Values/Ethics for Interprofessional Practice, Roles and Responsibilities, Interprofessional Communication, and Teams and Teamwork. The General Competency Statement and specific competencies for the domain of interprofessional communication are detailed in Box 47.1. Although not specific to communication in palliative care, these competencies are inclusive of the skills necessary for communication in team-based practice, regardless of specialty.

Also applicable to palliative care is the 2010 Patient Protection and Affordable Care Act that promotes team-based care as a strategy for meeting patient demands and reducing the costs of healthcare. The 2010 World Health Organization report *Framework for Action on Interprofessional Education and Collaborative Practice* also claimed that interprofessional practice was an important means to bolster the global health workforce and address the shortage of health workers.[1] New models encouraged by the Affordable Care Act, such as medical homes, accountable care

> **Box 47.1** Interprofessional Education Collaboration's Communication Competencies for Interprofessional Collaborative Practice
>
> **Interprofessional Communication Domain of the Core Competencies for Interprofessional Collaborative Practice**
>
> **General Competency Statement:** communicate with patients, families, communities, and other health professionals in a responsive and responsible manner that supports a team approach to the maintenance of health and treatment of disease.
>
> CC1—Choose effective communication tools and techniques, including information systems and communication technologies, to facilitate discussions and interactions that enhance team function.
>
> CC2—Organize and communicate information with patients, families, and healthcare team members in a form that is understandable, avoiding discipline-specific terminology when possible.
>
> CC3—Express one's knowledge and opinions to team members involved in patient care with confidence, clarity, and respect, working to ensure common understanding of information and treatment and care decisions.
>
> CC4—Listen actively, and encourage ideas and opinions of other team members.
>
> CC5—Give timely, sensitive, instructive feedback to others about their performance on the team, responding respectfully as a team member to feedback from others.
>
> CC6—Use respectful language appropriate for a given difficult situation, crucial conversation, or interprofessional conflict.
>
> CC7—Recognize how one's own uniqueness, including experience level, expertise, culture, power, and hierarchy within the healthcare team, contributes to effective communication, conflict resolution, and positive interprofessional working relationships.
>
> CC8—Communicate consistently the importance of teamwork in patient-centered and community-focused care.
>
> Interprofessional Education Collaborative Expert Panel. *Core Competencies for Interprofessional Collaborative Practice: Report of an Expert Panel*. Washington, DC: Interprofessional Education Collaborative; 2011.

organizations, and home-based primary care, expanded the roles of many healthcare providers previously peripheral to the physician-dominant delivery models.[11] These newer delivery models emphasize teamwork, and healthcare providers must be taught the skills and master the competencies of interprofessional care in order to effectively practice in this new paradigm. Interprofessional team-based practice has become an established approach in palliative care, geriatrics, hospice, rehabilitation, and mental health but is rarely found in other areas of health delivery. Therefore, those specialties experienced in team practice have the expertise to lead the movement to make team-based care the norm for healthcare provision.

The Institute of Medicine report, *Redesigning Continuing Education in the Health Professions*[12] and the World Health Organization report[1] both pointed to IPE as the means for preparing the workforce of the future. In recent years, the Josiah Macy Jr. Foundation has funded model programs and scholars focusing on IPE. The foundation seeks "to foster innovation in health professional education and to align the education of health professionals with contemporary health needs and a changing health care system."[13]

In 2012 the National Center for Interprofessional Practice and Education was formed as a private–public partnership through a cooperative agreement with the Health Resources and Services Administration and four private foundations: the Josiah Macy Jr. Foundation, the Robert Wood Johnson Foundation, the Gordon and Betty Moore Foundation, and the John A. Hartford Foundation. Located at the University of Minnesota, the center leads, coordinates, and studies the advancement of collaborative, team-based health professions' education and patient care as an efficient model for improving quality, outcomes, and cost.[14] It serves as a clearinghouse for ideas and resources and allows for networking among those creating, implementing, and evaluating IPE initiatives.

IPE and Palliative Care—A Natural Partnership

As recognized in the *Clinical Guidelines for Quality Palliative Care*, teamwork is essential for the provision of palliative care. The structure and delivery of palliative care requires attention to IPE to meet patient and family needs. A growing body of recognition and recommendations for addressing the supportive care needs of patients with serious illness across the illness continuum exists.[15–17] Professional groups and associations, such as the American Society for Clinical Oncology,[18] the American Heart Association,[19] the Coalition for Supportive Care in Kidney Disease,[20] and the National Comprehensive Cancer Network,[21] have called for palliative care integration throughout the disease continuum, making it essential that all healthcare providers working with chronic and serious illness have basic palliative care skills. Providers must be able to communicate not only with patients and families but also with fellow team members and institutions where teams interface with patients and families (i.e., family meetings, goals of care discussions, joint home visits, team meetings). The most effective venues for teaching and practicing such skills involve interdisciplinary learners and teaching faculty that represent a variety of disciplines.

Graduate and Postgraduate Education

While interprofessional learning opportunities and the teaching of palliative care knowledge and skills (including communication skills) is not the norm in the majority of healthcare professional education programs, more programs are incorporating such content into the core curriculum or offering elective courses and seminars. A variety of approaches and teaching techniques have been described in the literature.

The most common approach is to offer a course or workshop (required or elective) that includes students from a variety of disciplines who come together to learn palliative care principles and skills. Such courses usually include some didactic teaching, coupled with interactional activities in which communication skills may be practiced or evaluated. Most often, students are assigned to interdisciplinary learning teams (ILTs) for learning activities and experiential practice.

The University of Utah provides such a course for nursing, social work, and pharmacy students: Interdisciplinary Approaches to End of Life and Palliative Care teaches the skills essential for ILT collaboration; dealing with family dynamics and communication challenges; and management of pain, suffering, and other symptoms. Interprofessional students observe a case presentation by an actual hospice ILT and work in ILTs to collaborate on a progressive case study. Evaluation of the students' online discussion boards and focus-group feedback indicated the students developed a better understanding of and respect for other roles on the team as well as methods for communicating and collaborating with other professionals.[22,23]

A 6-credit hour course offered at the University of British Columbia also assigned students from pharmacy, nursing, social work, and medicine to ILTs. The teams worked together in clinical settings and did presentations together. Individually, the students completed a reflective journal and analyzed a film's portrayal of palliative care concepts. In the course evaluation, students validated learning of joint planning and decision-making skills and improved interprofessional knowledge and skills.[24]

Likewise, students of medicine, nursing, pharmacy, social work, and chaplaincy participated in a 5-week Interdisciplinary Palliative Care Seminar at the University of South Dakota. Case studies, role playing, film, journaling, and assigned readings were used in the seminar; additionally, the students completed home visits with one member of another discipline and shared these experiences in small groups of 8 to 10. Students showed significant improvements in their understanding of all disciplines, confidence regarding their role on the team and conflict resolution, and comfort in expressing views in meetings.[25] A shorter course focused on teaching spiritual assessment included second-year medical students, masters of social work students, and chaplain interns and residents. Interdisciplinary small groups worked together to explore their own spiritual perspectives and reflect on cases. The most frequently cited benefit of the course was that the students developed the ability to interact with peers from other professions.[26]

In London, a multiprofessional masters of science in palliative care is offered by King's College and St. Christopher's Hospice. Participants must have a degree in medicine, nursing, dentistry, life sciences, or social sciences, and all disciplines learn alongside each other. While communication skill development is not a singular focus of the courses offered, students completing the program state they learned to work effectively and efficiently with other professions, developed confidence in articulating their views, and improved their communication and teamwork skills.[27]

Teaching Approaches

The most common approach to IPE uses simulated patients (SPs), also referred to as standardized patients, sample patients, or patient instructors, who are individuals trained to act as "real" patients for the purpose of presenting symptoms or problems to be addressed by learners. Many teaching institutions have SP programs. SPs may be local amateur or professional actors, graduate students, retired healthcare providers, or actual patients. SPs receive training and may be expected to provide feedback to students about content and communication approaches. The SP presents the "gestalt" of the patient, including patient history and physical findings, body language, personality, and emotional state.[28,29] The SP is given some clinical information, but the focus is more on the personal characteristics of the character he or she is playing. This characterization enriches the SP's performance and increases the sense of reality as opposed to presenting stereotyped or assumed behavior.[29]

Instructors determine the learning experience objectives and instruct the SP to illustrate specific situations and clinical interactions. Interactions with SPs can be filmed to use as teaching tools, and they can be used for longitudinal encounters allowing students to follow a patient over time. The use of SPs allows students to practice and improve specific clinical and communication skills in a safe, controlled learning environment. Effective evaluation of the enacted scenario is essential to the students' learning. Structured constructive feedback is best given immediately after the interaction and should include successful elements and suggestions for alternative approaches.[29]

Work done at the University of Pennsylvania School of Nursing and the Perelman School of Medicine illustrates the use of SPs to teach multidisciplinary students important palliative care skills.[28] Objective Structured Clinical Examinations (known as OSCEs in medical education) were created to teach advanced practice nursing students and fellows in geriatrics, oncology, or palliative medicine the following skills: goals of care discussion, breaking bad news, and delirium assessment. The involved SPs received 4 hours of training in which they reviewed the learning goals, practiced the scenarios, learned how to complete evaluative checklists reflecting best practices and interpersonal skills demonstrated by the students, and considered how to give feedback to the students. Students rotated through the three stations, were debriefed afterward, and evaluated the learning experience. In a similar project, a group of educators in Ontario, Canada, adapted the traditional OSCE to create Team Observed Structured Clinical Encounters to assess student teams interacting at three stations.[30] At each station, the team was given an instruction sheet describing the encounter and then had to assign roles, decide what type of team was needed (acute care, homecare), and embark on an interview with SP(s) or a team meeting depending on the scenario. Two faculty observers (one from nursing, one from medicine) used score sheets as a basis for their feedback to participants. This format was found to be acceptable and feasible, and students stated it promoted a team attitude toward problem management.

SPs were used to allow nurse practitioners, internal medicine residents, and subspecialty fellows to practice communication skills during an interprofessional communication skills training course.[31] In this elective course, students received 32 hours of skills training, including building rapport, giving bad news, goals of care, advance directive and do-not-resuscitate discussions, dealing with interdisciplinary conflict, facilitating transition to hospice, and provision of bereavement support. Scenarios were constructed based on two patient stories, which unfolded longitudinally from diagnosis until death. SPs were trained to behave in a standardized way as either a patient or a family member and evaluated the student's skill. At training completion, evaluations showed student improvement in giving bad news and expressing sympathy when compared to students who had not received the training.

Educators in Manchester, UK conducted a short (8-hour) course in breaking bad news for medical students in their final year and third-year nursing students.[32] Students in physician–nurse dyads interacted with SPs and then received feedback from the SP, their peers who were observing the scenario, and the course facilitators. Qualitative analysis of student-completed questionnaires, focus groups, and field notes revealed three themes (challenging professional misconceptions, development of teamwork skills, and maintaining professional identity), indicating that interprofessional learning was as significant as the learning of a particular skill.

These efforts, while not all targeted at communication skill development per se, required students to practice and hone their communication skills as part of the learning activities. Overall, project evaluations demonstrated the value of using SPs as a teaching resource, but further evaluation of interprofessional simulation-based education is needed.[33]

Given the cost and/or absence of a SP program, many instructors use students or instructors as the "actors" to role-play scenarios. Role play is a less costly alternative and requires less time.[34] When using either role play or student interactions with SP scenarios, the instructor must address student anxiety and concerns about participation. Students should be reassured that it is only a rehearsal, and perfection is not expected. There should be a clear purpose and learning objectives for the role play, and it must be a realistic, challenging scenario. Using techniques such as setting ground rules related to confidentiality, allowing participants to seek help from other learners, allowing for time-outs, and setting time limits can make the learners more comfortable.[35–37] Evaluation and discussion of the role play is an essential part of the learning process. Role play not only facilitates the practice of clinical skills but also sensitizes students to the feelings and experiences of those receiving care. See Box 47.2 for suggestions for using role play and SP scenarios to teach interprofessional communication skills.

Using role play in IPE can be done in a variety of ways. Rao and Stupans developed a typology of role-playing learning opportunities, in which they described three types of role play: the "role switch", in which the student plays an unfamiliar role in order to understand the actions of others involved in a scenario; the "acting" model, which focuses on developing particular practice skills; and the "almost real-life category," where students participate in a role play that is as close to real experience as possible.[38] All three types are useful in teaching interdisciplinary communication skills. Demonstration role play can also be used by instructors or facilitators to illustrate specific skills or scenarios.[31,32] Such demonstrations can be set up to show either positive or negative interactions for the students to evaluate. Beginning a session with instructor/facilitator role play can help put learners at ease before expecting them to participate. A study of the use of scripted role play in teaching interdisciplinary palliative care communication skills demonstrated the value of this approach, as the participants showed significant improvements in comforting families, collaborating with other disciplines, and understanding professional roles.[34]

The use of patient simulators is also common in IPE. A patient simulator (or high-fidelity patient simulator) is a computer-controlled mannequin that can be programmed for physiologic responses. The simulator can receive and react to medical procedures and may be used to teach the use of medical equipment and medications. Although simulation has become an accepted strategy for teaching and evaluating student competencies in both nursing and medicine, there are few studies that compare simulation to other methods of teaching/learning and a few studies that evaluate the impact of simulation on communication skill development.[39] Reising et al. involved nursing and medical students working on teams in a mock code scenario using a patient simulator and found that it promoted interprofessional communication skill development and a sense of one's role on a team.[39] When compared to students learning in a roundtable discussion of the same patient scenario, those learning in the simulator scenario experienced a better sense of timing and realism. While the literature does not describe the use of such simulators in palliative care, they could be used to teach responses to patient death with or without the presence of family members or appropriate use of medications to control symptoms at the end of life and related team communication.

Students can benefit from observing and reflecting on the communication skills of experienced healthcare providers and from direct interactions with patients and colleagues in the clinical setting. A group of educators in England developed a program in which multidisciplinary teams of 12 students provided hands-on, around-the-clock care for a selected group of patients on an in-patient palliative care unit. Students were prepared for the placement during a 2-day induction program and were supervised by professional staff. Daily reflective sessions were held related to communication skills, and students reported that they learned how to be open and honest with patients, break bad news, and console patients. They also learned to appreciate the roles of other disciplines and support team members in tough patient communication scenarios.[40]

Even a brief observational clinical experience in palliative care can result in significant learning for students. Nurses and medical students in a palliative care course at a large academic medical center spent approximately 8 to 12 hours attending interdisciplinary team meetings, rounding with a team, or observing patient visits. Students' reflective narratives of their observation experience revealed important learning related to communication issues with patients and families, how to speak with patients and families, and communication within the interdisciplinary team.[41]

Finally, online education has emerged as a convenient, accessible way of providing IPE. Today's learners are becoming more comfortable with online learning, and advances in technology have enabled opportunities for interactive, multidisciplinary communication skills learning and practice in an online environment. Audiovisual materials such as clips from movies or television, recordings of actual patient/family encounters, self-directed tutorials, interactive case studies, and quizzes are commonly used online education approaches.[42] Advances in technology also enable Internet conferencing, both synchronous and asynchronous, allowing student-to-student and student-to-teacher communication about course material. Online learning allows students to participate at a convenient time, and access is unrestricted by location or time of day. Instruction can be tailored to meet the

> **Box 47.2** Tips for Successful Use of Role-Plays and Simulated Patient Scenarios in Interdisciplinary Palliative Care Communication Skills Training
>
> - Determine your teaching objectives and design the exercise according to your learning goals.
> - Use relevant, challenging cases. Actual case scenarios are the best sources.
> - Allow plenty of time.
> - Ensure that adequate representation of the disciplines involved are present. If not, learners can be assigned to "play" another profession as an alternative learning experience.
> - Allow adequate time for setting the stage, the actual role-play, and debriefing/feedback.
> - Provide content (didactic or reading) that will enable students to formulate their approach to the scenario before or at the beginning of the session. For instance, guidelines for giving bad news or conducting family meetings would be helpful to students practicing such skills. Role-plays are for practicing, not learning, new techniques or approaches.
> - Create a "safe" environment for the learners. Normalize student anxiety and discuss the ground rules. Allow students to discuss their discomfort. Let them know that perfection is not expected—this is a time to "rehearse" new skills.
> - Establish the importance of the skill to be taught (i.e., goals of care discussion, family meeting). Allow students to share past experiences related to such encounters.
> - Set the stage for the interaction. Be sure that students acting as patient or family member or standardized patients know their role. It may help to give them a written description (script) for their role. Use nametags or props to identify the players as appropriate.
> - Involve all students. Those not playing a role can be observers or they can serve as coaches for those in the role.
> - Establish mechanisms that foster group investment in the success of the activity. For instance, students can ask for help from other learners, call a time-out for feedback, or coach each other during the role play.
> - Faculty role-plays can be used as examples (good or bad) and are a means of putting the students at ease prior to their participation.
> - Monitor the role play. Set a time limit. Intervene with "time-outs" should the students get stuck or experience obvious discomfort.
> - Begin debriefing by having students evaluate their own performance (What did you do well? poorly? How did it feel for you?). Students will often point out their deficiencies/mistakes without the instructor's or observers' feedback.
> - Include the students playing patient or family member in the debriefing as this will provide valuable insight as to how the interaction "felt" for the recipient of care.
> - Discuss with the group alternative approaches to the scenario.
> - Focus the debriefing/feedback on the intended learning goal. Focus on positives; reframe criticisms as opportunities for improvement.
> - Encourage reflection. Ask open-ended questions that encourage deep thinking about the scenario and how it played out.
> - Have fun! Role-play can be an enjoyable experience for everyone involved.

needs of the learners who control the pace of the course. A 2008 meta-analysis of Internet-based learning in the healthcare professions found that such learning is associated with positive effects compared to no intervention; when compared with non-Internet instructional methods, effects are mixed and generally small, suggesting that the effectiveness of such learning is similar to more traditional methods.[43] Online education has the ability to reach large numbers of learners from multiple disciplines who might not otherwise receive training in palliative care communication and thus has significant potential in the education of both healthcare students and providers.

In IPE, online learning is often a component of a blended curriculum, using a variety of teaching modalities. Interprofessional students (medical, nursing, chaplaincy, and social work) were taught the spiritual and cultural aspects of palliative care in a blended course at Yale University. The course consisted of an online interactive case-based module and a live simulation workshop, in which the students observed a team-meeting simulation and then worked together to develop an interdisciplinary plan of care.[44] Although not focused on the teaching of communication skills per se, students overwhelmingly noted that the course was helpful in learning interprofessional communication skills and gaining a better sense of their role on the team. A similar program at the University of Louisville blended four teaching modalities: online didactic case-based modules; a clinical rotation in palliative care; a reflective writing experience coupled with interdisciplinary group sharing; and a face-to-face interdisciplinary experience in which students observed videos of SP scenarios, evaluated the interactions, and worked together to develop a plan of care.[45] Outcomes for this mandatory curriculum for nursing, medical, chaplaincy residents, and graduate social workers showed a significant difference when pre-and posttest scores on the End-of-Life Professional Caregiver Survey[46] were compared.

A relatively new form of online education involves the creation of the virtual patient (VP). A VP is an interactive computer simulation of a clinical scenario used for the training, education, and/or assessment of students. Students react to scenarios and are able to explore the consequences of their treatment decisions and healthcare interventions. Similar to the recreational role plays done in online gaming, avatars or self-created digital characters are used for the simulation. Interaction and communication can occur either synchronously or asynchronously through text-based mediums. Used by some educators to create virtual learning environments, Second Life[47] offers the technology to create three-dimensional virtual worlds where avatars can interact. Vokis™, online speaking avatars, can be customized and given voice-using software readily available online. Instructors can use Vokis™ to present content or scenarios, and Vokis™ offers a classroom management function.[48]

Educators in the Department of Family Medicine at the University of Alberta developed and implemented an online VP clinical case in palliative care. Students rated the VP realism as good to excellent, and their comfort with end-of-life patient management increased significantly as a result of the experience.[49] Group work has been successfully taught in a virtual environment using an asynchronous online role play, demonstrating the ability of online learning approaches to teach interactive skills.[50] The downside of such virtual entities and communities is the inability to incorporate realistic facial expressions, speech intonation, and body language, which are important aspects of communication. However, VPs can instruct and allow for the teaching of communication content.

Continuing Education of Interdisciplinary Healthcare Professionals

In 2010 the Macy Foundation funded a study of continuing education for healthcare providers that recommended that continuing education efforts be interdisciplinary in nature to allow for the development of interprofessional patient-centered[12] skills.

Several continuing education initiatives have focused on development of communication skills in palliative care. COMFORT represents the seven basic principles to be taught and implemented in early palliative care communication: Communication, Orientation and Opportunity, Mindful presence, Family, Openings, Relating, and Team. Each module consists of a didactic portion introducing core concepts and skills, video clips of interactions between teams and family caregivers, and roundtable discussion conducted by faculty. An evaluation of four of the communication modules found that participants' perceptions of the learning were positive and that the learning objectives were achieved.[51] The COMFORT communication curriculum is offered through an online platform with the goal of teaching palliative care communication. In Australia, a 7.5-hour online course in palliative oncology was developed to reach providers in rural and remote areas.[52] Based on the needs assessment, the course included communication training with particular emphasis on treatment decision-making.

A similar course designed to teach psychosocial cancer management included the use of discussion boards, email, and a "virtual classroom" to teach breaking bad news.[53] Attrition and final assessment performance rates were compatible with a face-to-face learning program. The Advocating for Clinical Excellence Project involved psycho-oncology professionals (psychologists, social workers, and spiritual care professionals) in an intensive advocacy and leadership training program. This program targeted skills in leadership, team-building, communication, collaboration, and palliative care, and participants reported substantial improvement in all five areas.[54]

Educators at the Royal Liverpool and Broadgreen University Hospital Trust in Liverpool, UK developed a 4-day program for practicing nurses and other allied healthcare providers.[29] SPs were used in the experiential training, which began with participants observing interactions between the SP and a course facilitator. After the scenario was played out, the facilitator and SP stayed in their roles so that students could interact and clarify certain points, ask questions, and recreate new role plays for the SPs and facilitator to "re-run." This approach was successful in overcoming student discomfort with role play and receiving feedback on their communication skills.

In Australia, a nine-session, 2-day program included sessions on communication with patients, families, colleagues, and a multidisciplinary team.[55] Evaluation revealed that communication skills showed the most improvement related to interest, knowledge, and confidence. In Scotland, a 3-day experiential interprofessional course focused on communication and relationship skills for palliative care found that learning was sustained and increasingly transferred into practice if the workplace was supportive,[56] and another course teaching physicians and nurses communication skills identified that increased self-efficacy was maintained over time.[56]

Ongoing Interdisciplinary Team Communication Training and Development

Due to the nature and intensity of palliative care practice and as mandated by the *Clinical Practice Guidelines for Quality Palliative Care*,[57] practicing teams should also have ongoing opportunities for team-building and communication skills development. Communication, both formal and informal, is the dominant factor influencing team success.[58] A breakdown in communication leads to ineffective teamwork and can directly affect patient care and outcomes. Despite its importance, interdisciplinary team functioning, including communication, has been neglected in palliative care research and education.[59]

The Medicare Hospice Benefit requires hospice agencies to conduct regular team meetings. In a survey of 145 hospice agencies, 61% of the agencies reported that team training does occur, with 33% stating that training included team-building. Over half reported that their teams need ongoing training in conflict resolution, communication/relationships, and teamwork. The training offered was limited to new employee orientation sessions, which did not occur in team environments. This study recommended that communication and team-building skills be taught to entire teams and that there be time devoted for such trainings separate from care planning duties.[60]

In his book *Teamwork in Palliative Care*, Peter Speck discusses multiple factors that come into play when team members communicate, including past experiences, coping styles, and conscious and unconscious processes that can contribute to their communication with the team.[61] Speck posited that a team, "like the individuals within it, will develop defenses against any emotions which may be perceived as too difficult or too painful to acknowledge, and may have a variety of ways of avoiding any real engagement."[61(p96)] Influences on team emotional responses can include events outside the organization (e.g., governmental policy changes or sources of conflict within the organization) such as competition between departments for scarce resources. Teams must also navigate team, department, and organization dynamics as well as the effects of the work itself (grief responses, transference and countertransference, and team-member attrition and change).

This emotional load—generated outside and inside the team—calls for supports such as clinical supervision, staff support groups, and debriefing in order to manage stress and conflict and facilitate effective communication and collaboration. In staff support groups, Speck pointed out that the focus—when clearly defined as work-related and supportive for team-building and communication—can have therapeutic benefit for the attendees. Debriefing time can be created separately or allocated during normal team meetings to allow team members to process events, stressors, or team dynamics. During the course of any of these activities, the need may emerge for personal supervision or support for individual team members, and teams should understand that such support must be sought separately from the team environment.[61]

Team-building is important for development among practicing palliative care teams. Malcom Payne wrote that palliative care raises three main issues for team-building: it is holistic (addresses physical, psychological, social, and spiritual aspects), multiprofessional (involves coordination of professionals to respond to human complexity), and specialist (integrates its work with a range of non-specialized aspects of social and healthcare). Therefore palliative care teams should focus on team-building wherever and however possible in everything they do.[62] This author suggested that while team-building based on psychological theories of group forming and relations—often organized outside of everyday work in teams, usually by external consultants—may sometimes be necessary, a more helpful approach is knowledge management.

This approach to team-building focuses on how palliative care team members deal with disciplinary knowledge in a constant, everyday way. Focusing on knowledge management prioritizes doing a good job in the task that the team is formed to do. The palliative care task defines the team members' identities. While interpersonal issues may arise, knowledge management argues that teams are united by the task and can put interpersonal issues to the side. Knowledge management allows palliative care team members to come together and reveal the various aspects of knowledge and skill that they bring together in the care of those affected by serious illness. "The task of leadership in the team is to allow different aspects of knowledge to come forward, be expressed and used collectively"[62 (p122)]

Important aspects of everyday team-building include developing and following rules about how to raise difficult issues, different types of knowledge, and how these interact with patient and family needs. By developing regular review of teamwork and joint activities, maintaining interpersonal support and an appropriate social climate, and responding to individual development needs, the palliative care team provides a context to enable everyday team-building to take place.[62]

While the necessity of team-building, including activities that improve communication and collaboration, is well established, there is little research on how teams communicate or optimally function and few published studies in the area of team-building and ongoing training. One study of a team-building workshop provided to a palliative care team reported that staff found it to be helpful in promoting understanding of roles and developing good working relationships; the study concluded that providing the opportunity for staff to share in team development exercises in a neutral environment appears to be of value.[63] The content of the workshop was not shared in the article. Arber analyzed the language used in the interactions of a palliative care team and found that the strategic use of questions enabled palliative care nurses to influence and manage interprofessional interactions in a polite, diplomatic manner. As a result, she suggested that teams reflect on how meetings are conducted and that review of transcripts might help develop insights into how the team works together, leading to interactional competencies to guide team practice and education.[64]

One notable effort to establish and develop teams is TeamSTEPPS®, a national program developed and implemented by the Agency for Healthcare Research and Quality and the Department of Defense.[65] This evidenced-based teamwork system aims to improve communication and teamwork skills among healthcare professionals. Six regional training centers offer training to develop a national network of master trainers who then train front-line healthcare workers. Support and guidance is provided to all using the model via Web conferences, discussion forums, and a national website. The curriculum provides a customized training plan to develop teamwork skills. Short case studies and videos illustrating teamwork opportunities and successes are shared. While not directed at palliative care and hospice teams, some teams in these areas have found the tools and training useful, especially when a new team is formed.

It has been hypothesized, but not proven, that teams would benefit from team-building and communication skills training. Such efforts might include using an outside "coach" or consultant to evaluate and improve team interactions, using communication and/or coping style evaluation instruments to develop a better understanding of how to relate and communicate with fellow team members, or holding retreats that allow for team sharing and getting to know each other. Just as in the educational efforts described earlier in this chapter, existing teams could benefit from role playing, including "rehearsals" of family meetings or other interactions anticipated as being difficult, use of SPs to practice communication and alternative approaches to situations, and exploration of cases entailing team challenges. The results of such efforts should be rigorously evaluated so that a body of evidence can be built to justify the value of such activities.

Interprofessional communication training is necessary if providers are to be prepared for essential palliative care skills such as team communication and collaboration, team meetings, goals of care discussions, family meetings, communication with colleagues outside the team, and team-based care. Multiple obstacles to IPE efforts include lack of funding, unbalanced representation of the disciplines, educational isolation of the disciplines, integration of such efforts into already overloaded curricula, logistical challenges, and lack of advocates for such efforts.[45] While IPE is becoming more prevalent in undergraduate and graduate education of healthcare providers, more rigorous evaluation of such endeavors is needed to create a body of evidence as to how to best plan, overcome the obstacles, orchestrate, and incorporate such offerings into existing curricula.

Ongoing team development and team-building should be mandatory for practicing palliative care teams, and attention to the evaluation of team-enhancing activities would contribute to development of models for the field. Comprehensive evaluation, including measurement of the longitudinal impact of both student and practitioner training, is necessary; such evidence can guide those initiating such efforts and establish standards for IPE on palliative care communication.

References

1. World Health Organization. *Framework for Action on Interprofessional Education and Collaborative Practice.* Geneva: World Health Organization Department of Human Resources for Health; 2010.
2. Buring SM, Bhushan A, Broeseker A, et al. Interprofessional education: Definitions, student competencies, and guidelines for implementation. *Am J Pharm Educ.* July 10, 2009;73(4):59.
3. D'Amour D, Oandasan I. Interprofessionality as the field of interprofessional practice and interprofessional education: An emerging concept. *J Interprof Care.* May 2005;19(Suppl 1):8–20.
4. Lawrie I, Lloyd-Williams M. Training in the interdisciplinary environment. In: Speck P, ed. *Teamwork in Palliative Care: Fulfilling or Frustrating?* New York, NY: Oxford Univeristy Press; 2006:153–165.
5. Institute of Medicine. *Educating for the Health Team.* Washington, DC: National Academies of Science; 1972.
6. Committee on Quality of Health Care in America. *To Err is Human: Building a Safer Heatlh System.* Washington, DC: Institute of Medicine; 1999.
7. Committee on Quality of Health Care in America. *Crossing the Qualtiy Chasm: A New Health system for the 21st Century.* Washington, DC: Institute of Medicine; 2001.
8. National Research Council. *Health Professions Education: A Bridge to Quality.* Washington, DC: Institute of Medicine; 2003.
9. Interprofessional Education Collaborative. Team-based competencies: Building a shared foundation for education and clinical practice. Paper presented at: Team-Based Competencies, Washington, DC; 2011.
10. Interprofessional Education Collaborative Expert Panel. *Core Competencies for Interprofessional Collaborative Practice: Report of an Expert Panel.* Washington, DC: Interprofessional Education Collaborative; 2011.
11. National Academies of Practice. *Toward Interdisciplinary Team Development: A Policy Paper of the National Academies of Practice.* Cleveland, OH: Center for Community Solutions; 2011.
12. Committee on Planning a Continuing Health Professional Education Institute. *Redesigning Continuing Education in the Health Professions.* Washington, DC: Institute of Medicine; 2010.
13. Josiah Macy Jr. Foundation. Organizational priorities. http://macyfoundation.org/priorities/c/interprofessional-education-and-teamwork. Accessed June 24, 2014.
14. National Center for Interprofessional Practice and Education. About us. https://nexusipe.org/about. Accessed June 24, 2014.
15. Nelson JE, Hope AA. Integration of palliative care in chronic critical illness management. *Respir Care.* June 1, 2012;57(6):1004–1013.
16. Levy MH, Adolph MD, Back A, et al. Palliative Care. *J Natl Compr Canc Netw.* October 1, 2012;10(10):1284–1309.
17. Morrison RS, Meier DE. *America's Care of Serious Illness: A State-by-State Report Card on Access to Palliative Care in Our Nation's Hospitals.* New York, NY: Center to Advance Palliative Care; 2011. http://reportcard.capc.org/pdf/state-by-state-report-card.pdf. Accessed June 4, 2014.
18. American Society of Clinical Oncology. ASCO recommends palliative care as a part of cancer treatment. http://www.cancer.net/research-and-advocacy/asco-care-and-treatment-recommendations-patients/asco-recommends-palliative-care-part-cancer-treatment. Accessed June 30, 2014.
19. American Heart Association Website. http://www.heart.org/HEARTORG/Conditions/HeartFailure/Planning-Ahead-Advanced-Heart-Failure_UCM_441935_Article.jsp. Accessed June 30, 2014.
20. Coalition for Supportive Care for Kidney Patients Website. http://www.kidneysupportivecare.org/Home.aspx. Accessed June 30, 2014.
21. National Comprehensive Cancer Network. Palliative Care Clinical Practice Guidelines. Clinical practice guidelines for oncology. http://www.nccn.org/professionals/physician_gls/pdf/palliative.pdf. Accessed June 30, 2014.
22. Supiano KP, Berry PH. Developing interdisciplinary skills and professional confidence in palliative care social work students. *J Soc Work Educ.* 2013;49:387–396.
23. Supiano KP. Weaving interdispclinary and discipline-specific content into palliative care education: One successful model for teaching end-of-life care. *Omega.* 2013;67(1–2):201–206.
24. Cadell S, Bosma H, Johnston M, et al. Practising interprofessional teamwork from the first day of class: A model for an interprofessional palliative care course. *J Palliat Care.* 2007;23(4):273–279.
25. Shrader S, McRae L, King WMt, Kern D. A simulated interprofessional rounding experience in a clinical assessment course. *Am J Pharm Educ.* May 10, 2011;75(4):61.
26. Lennon-Dearing R, Florence JA, Halvorson H, Pollard JT. An interprofessional educational approach to teaching spiritual assessment. *J Health Care Chaplain.* 2012;18:121–132.
27. Koffman J, Higginson IJ. Assessing the effectiveness and acceptability of interprofessional palliative care education. *J Palliat Care.* 2005;21(4):262–269.
28. Corcoran AM, Lysaght S, LaMarra D, Ersek M. Pilot test of a three-station palliative care observed structured clinical examination for multidisciplinary trainees. *J Nurs Educ.* 2013;52(5):294–298.
29. Donovan T, Hutchison T, Kelly A. Using simulated patients in a multiprofessional communications skills programme: Reflections from the programme facilitators. *Eur J Cancer Care.* 2003;12(2):123–128.
30. Hall P, Marshall D, Weaver L, Boyle A, Taniguchi A. A method to enhance student teams in palliative care: Piloting the McMaster-Ottawa Team Observed Structured Clinical Encounter. *J Palliat Med.* 2011;14(6):744–750.
31. Bays AM, Engelberg RA, Back AL, et al. Interprofessional communication skills training for serious illness: Evaluation of a small-group, simulated patient intervention. *J Palliat Med.* 2014;17(2):159–166.
32. Cooke S, Chew-Graham C, Boggis C, Wakefield A. "I never realised that doctors were into feelings too": Changing student perceptions through interprofessional education. *Learn Health Social Care.* 2003;2(3):137–146.
33. Gough S, Hellaby M, Jones N, MacKinnon R. A review of undergraduate interprofessional simulation-based education (IPSE). *Collegian.* 2012;19(3):153–170.
34. Spear ML, Guillen U, Elliott DJ, Roettger L, Zukowsky K. The use of role play for interdisciplinary teaching of palliative care communication skills. *J Palliat Med.* 2013;16(8):825.
35. Joyner B, Young L. Teaching medical students using role play: Twelve tips for successful role plays. *Med Teach.* 2006;28(3):225–229.
36. End-of-Life Nursing Education Consortium. Tips for using role play exercises. In: ELNEC Core Curriculum. Washington, DC: American Association of Colleges of Nursing; 2013:M6-55–M56-57.
37. Jackson VA, Back AL. Teaching communication skills using role-play: An experience-based guide for educators. *J Palliat Med.* 2011;14(6):775–780.
38. Rao D, Stupans I. Exploring the potential of role play in higher education: Development of a typology and teacher guidelines. *Innov Educ Teach Int.* 2012;49(4):427–436.

39. Reisling DL, Carr DE, Shea RA, King JM. Comparison of communication outcomes in traditional versus simulation strategies in nursing and medical students. *Nurs Educ Perspect.* 2011;32(5):323–327.
40. Dando N, d'Avray L, Colman J, Hoy A, Todd J. Evaluation of an interprofessional practice placement in a UK in-patient palliative care unit. *Palliat Med.* 2012;26(2):178–184.
41. Phillips M, Breakwell S, Kim M, Faut-Callahan M. Clinical observation reflections from students in an interdisciplinary palliative care course. *J Hospice Palliat Nurs.* 2012;14(4):274–282.
42. Pulsford D, Jackson G, O'Brien T, Yates S, Duxbury J. Classroom-based and distance learning education and training courses in end-of-life care for health and social care staff: A systematic review. *Palliat Med.* 2013;27(3):221–235.
43. Cook DA, Levinson AJ, Garside S, Dupras DM, Erwin PJ, Montori VM. Internet-based learning in the health professions: A meta-analysis. *JAMA.* 2008;300(10):1181–1196.
44. Ellman MS, Schulman-Green D, Blatt L, et al. Using online learning and interactive simulation to teach spiritual and cultural aspects of palliative care to interprofessional students. *J Palliat Med.* 2012;15(11):1240–1247.
45. Head BA, Schapmire T, Hermann C, et al. The Interdisciplinary Curriculum for Onology Palliative Education (iCOPE): Meeting the challenge of interprofessional education. *J Palliat Med.* 2014;17(10):1107–1114.
46. Lazenby M, Ercolano E, Schulman-Green D, McCorkle R. Validity of the End-of-Life Professional Caregiver Survey to assess for multidisciplinary educational needs. *J Palliat Med.* 2012;15(4):472–431.
47. What is Second Life? http://secondlife.com/whatis/. Accessed June 27, 2014.
48. About Voki. http://www.voki.com/about_voki.php. Accessed June 26, 2014.
49. Tan A, Ross SP, Duerksen K. Death is not always a failure: Outcomes from implementing an online virtual patient clinical case in palliative care for family medicine clerkship. *Med Educ Online.* 2013;18(22711).
50. Levine J. Teaching groupwork at a distance using an asynchronous online role-play. *Groupwork.* 2013;23(1):56–72.
51. Wittenberg-Lyles E, Goldsmith J, Ferrell B, Burchett M. Assessment of an interprofessional online curriculum for palliative care communication training. *J Palliat Med.* 2014;17(4):400–406.
52. Koczwara B, Francis K, Marine F, Goldstein D, Underhill C, Olver I. Reaching further with online education? The development of an effective online program in palliative oncology. *J Cancer Educ.* 2010;25(3):317–323.
53. Kinghorn S. Delivering multiprofessional Web-based psychosocial education: The lessons learnt. *Int J Palliat Nurs.* 2005;11(8):432–437.
54. Otis-Green S, Ferrell B, Spolum M, et al. An overview of the ACE Project—Advocating for clinical excellence: Transdisciplinary palliative care education. *J Cancer Educ.* 2009;24:120–126.
55. Quinn K, Hudson P, Ashby M, Thomas K. "Palliative care: The essentials": Evaluation of a multidisciplinary education program. *J Palliat Med.* 2008;11(8):1122–1129.
56. Andrew J, Taylor C. Follow-up evaluation of a course to develop effective communication and relationship skills for palliative care. *Int J Palliat Nurs.* 2012;18(9):457–463.
57. National Consensus Project. *Clinical Practice Guidelines for Quality Palliative Care.* Pittsburgh, PA: Hospice and Palliative Nurse's Association; 2013.
58. Youngwerth J, Twaddle M. Cultures of interdisciplinary teams: How to foster good dynamics. *J Palliat Med.* 2011;14(5):650–654.
59. O'Connor M, Fisher C. Exploring the dynamics of interdisciplinary palliative care teams in providing psychosocial care: "Everybody thinks that everybody can do it and they can't." *J Palliat Med.* 2011;14(2):191–196.
60. Baldwin PK, Wittenberg-Lyles E, Oliver DP, Demiris G. An evaluation of interdisciplinary team training in hospice care. *J Hospice Palliat Nurs.* 2011;13(3):172–182.
61. Speck P. Maintaining a healthy team. In: Speck P, ed. *Teamwork in Palliative Care.* New York: Oxford University Press; 2006:95–115.
62. Payne M. Team building: How, why and where? In: Speck P, ed. *Teamwork in Palliative Care.* New York: Oxford University Press; 2006:117–135.
63. Donaghy K, Devlin B. An evaluation of teamwork within a specialist palliative care unit. *Int J Palliat Nurs.* 2002;8(11):518–525.
64. Arber A. Team meetings in specialist palliative care: Asking questions as a strategy within interprofessional interaction. *Qual Health Res.* 2008;18(10):1323–1335.
65. Agency for Healthcare Research and Quality. TeamSTEPPS®.. http://teamstepps.ahrq.gov/about-2cl_3.htm. Accessed June 27, 2014.

CHAPTER 48

Qualitative Communication Research

Patrick J. Dillon and Lori A. Roscoe

Introduction

> In daily life, we ground our ideas about people and experiences in data that are constantly presented to us. Researchers build upon that discovery process by imposing a rigor that overcomes many of the conceptual biases that tempt social actors ... [Qualitative] research perspectives reflect the intuitive ways that we seek knowledge, and they prod us to go a little further. (p. 542)[1]

Qualitative research is a field of inquiry in its own right; it has its own history, subdivisions, and controversies.[2-4] Although these broader issues may be of interest to some readers, the focus in this chapter is to explore qualitative communication research as a broadly defined set of assumptions and techniques that can be used to understand and represent the various ways human beings understand and participate in social reality. More specifically, our aim is to describe the ways qualitative researchers investigate communication phenomena--such as family relationship patterns, cultural expectations, situated meanings, institutional policies/procedures, and personal histories--in palliative care contexts. The chapter also emphasizes qualitative research that is oriented toward improving palliative care practice and, ultimately, promoting better outcomes for patients and their loved ones. Thus this chapter focuses on applied communication research, which is defined as the study of real-world communication concerns, issues, and problems.[5]

Clinicians have traditionally been trained to think logically and inferentially and to draw upon pathophysiologic rationales and deductive reasoning in their medical practice; this orientation is reflected in the biomedical research literature, which tends to emphasizes deductive quantitative epidemiological studies and clinical trials.[6] In providing answers to questions that ask "whether" (e.g., whether taking a particular medication reduces patients' A1c count) or "how much" (e.g., how much a low platelet count predisposes a cancer patient receiving chemotherapy to febrile neutropenia), quantitative studies are necessary in order to provide appropriate, evidence-based medical care.[6] Contemporary healthcare practice, however, is more than a biomedical, quantitative science; it is also an interactive, communicative "process in which both the [provider] and patient, with all their experiences and expectations, are active agents in co-creating and co-interpreting what occurs" during healthcare encounters (p. 532).[1] Crandall and Marion note, for example,

> Clinicians who will thrive in their work will have the capacity for being able to toggle back and forth between objectivity and receptivity. In essence, effective clinicians attend to the patients' whole story in tandem with clinical reasoning, which leads to a mutually satisfactory process and outcome. (p. 1175)[7]

This balance between what some have described as the mechanistic science and interpretive art of medicine requires more than answers to "whether" and "how much"; it also requires answers to the "what," "how," and "why" of health, illness, and medical care.[6,8,9] The need for such answers is evident in palliative care, because patients are dealing not only with serious physical illness but also with the larger questions of quality of life, mortality, and the limits of medical science. Attending to patients' and their families' physical, intellectual, emotional, social, and spiritual needs requires clinicians who understand the complex perspectives and factors that influence their patients' illness experiences, including their health beliefs/literacy, cultural/religious preferences, living environment, relational considerations, and treatment preferences.[10,11] For example, how do a patient's spiritual beliefs influence his or her willingness to discontinue aggressive medical care in order to begin receiving hospice services? Or why is one adult child supportive of increasing her mother's morphine dosage while her sibling is not? Answers to questions such as these are essential to understand in order to provide high-quality, patient/family-centered palliative care and are best approached using qualitative methods.

Quantitative and qualitative communication research display some general similarities. For example, both types of research allow scholars and providers to better understand how communicative actions shape the social world, and both require training in data collection, analysis, and presentation.[4,12] There are also, however, clear differences between them. Quantitative research is, as noted, most often oriented toward answering "whether" and "how much" questions.[6] It involves isolating discrete variables, identifying relationships among various factors, operationalizing theoretical relations, measuring and quantifying phenomena, and attempting to generalize findings to large populations.[12,13]

Although quantitative research can capture important behavioral trends and demonstrate statistical relationships, it is ill suited to provide in-depth, nuanced insight into the relational, emotional, and experiential aspects of everyday life. In contrast, qualitative research provides systematic, inductive methods for engaging the "what," "why," and "how" of social action and, in so doing, engages the messiness of local, contextually situated knowledge and practices.[2,12,13] Additionally, as Warren and Karner[11] note, while quantitative studies produce "experientially distant" numerical summaries of human interaction, qualitative studies are what Clifford Geertz[14] calls "experience near" the people, relationships, and social settings they investigate. Both quantitative and qualitative research methods are invaluable tools for generating knowledge about palliative care practice; there are, however, many aspects of communication in palliative care settings that can best be illuminated by qualitative inquiry.[4,6,11]

As an example, consider hospice enrollment. Quantitative studies demonstrate that of the more than 1.5 million patients who receive end-of-life services through hospice each year, nearly 35% are enrolled for 7 or fewer days,[15] and more than 50% die within the first 30 days.[16] Further, a quantitative analysis of the Family Evaluation of Hospice Care data repository revealed substantial variation in patients' family members' perceptions of whether their loved one was referred "too late,"[17] which was not statistically correlated with hospice organization characteristics or the market where services were provided.[18] To better understand this issue, Teno and colleagues[19] conducted a qualitative study that included narrative interviews with 100 family members of patients referred to hospice care in the last 7 days of life. The interviews focused on two questions: (a) Why are persons referred to hospice in the last 7 days of life? and (b) Why do family members believe a referral to hospice within 7 days of death was either "at the right time" or "too late"?

Of the 100 participants who took part in narrative interviews, 41% of respondents stated that their family member was referred "too late," and 58% stated hospice referral was "at the right time" (one respondent did not respond to this question). When families stated that referral was "at the right time," their perceptions were based on the patient's having refused earlier referral, a rapid decline in the patient's condition that resulted in the late referral, or a belief in all things coming together as they were meant to be. When families stated that referral was "too late," their reasons centered on concerns with the healthcare providers' role in decision-making, with concerns being inadequate physician communication, not recognizing the patient was dying, or problematic hospice delays in referral from the nursing home or home health agency. Teno and colleagues'[19] qualitative research approach provided important insights that would not have been discovered in a quantitative study; likewise, qualitative communication research, in general, is an invaluable tool for understanding and improving palliative care practice. It is through this lens that the rest of this chapter is written, with the intent of providing an overview of various procedures and tools that are used to collect and analyze qualitative data in a systematic and transparent manner.

We continue with a description of the ontological and epistemological paradigms that inform qualitative research in the communication discipline and then briefly describe the process of generating qualitative research data through fieldwork and in-depth interviews. Next, the analytic procedures that are associated with some of the prevailing traditions in qualitative communication research—grounded theory, ethnography, phenomenology, meta-ethnography, and mixed methods research—all of which have applications in palliative care settings, are discussed. Finally, we conclude by discussing how issues such as generalizability, validity, and reliability apply to qualitative inquiry.

Ontological and Epistemological Perspectives

As noted in the introduction, qualitative communication researchers study how human beings understand and participate in social reality; thus the way one defines what research is and how it should be done is intimately connected to one's philosophical beliefs about the nature of that reality (ontology) and how it may be known or studied (epistemology).[4,19] Conducting qualitative research, then, proceeds from particular ontological and epistemological perspectives. The paradigmatic underpinnings of various approaches to qualitative communication research are complex.[2,4,19] While a thorough review of these perspectives is beyond the scope of this chapter, we provide a brief overview. Two of the most commonly referred to ontological/epistemological perspectives are (a) positivism/postpositivism and (b) interpretivism.[4,12,19] Although positivism/postpositivism is often associated with quantitative research and interpretivism with qualitative inquiry, we note that qualitative studies may proceed from each of these viewpoints.[2,4,6,12,19]

Positivism, as a research paradigm envisioned by Comte,[20] assumes that a singular, objective reality exists apart from the "knower" or observer. From this perspective, the concepts and methods of the natural sciences (e.g., detachment, objectivity, experimentation, variable manipulation, and control) offer viable approaches to document this essential reality.[4,19,20] Through the continual refinement and systemization of research methods, the ultimate goal of positivist social science research is to identify and explain the cause-and-effect relationships that determine human behavior.[4] Although its influence is still widespread across social science disciplines, few contemporary communication scholars, particularly those who conduct qualitative research, align themselves with rigid or essentialist positivism.[4,19,21] Instead, those who are committed to scientific approaches to studying communication largely identify with the postpositivist paradigm. Similar to positivism, postpositivists adopt a "realist" ontology, which assumes that physical and social reality exist outside of human perception. At the same time, however, postpositivists acknowledge that gaining an objective picture of reality in "a phenomenologically messy and methodologically imperfect world" is difficult (p. 93). Thus, although obtaining an objective understanding of communicative phenomena through rigorous, scientifically informed research methods remains the goal, most postpositivists admit that their findings reflect a reasonable approximation of reality that is consistent with what was observed or recorded during the research process.[4,19]

The interpretive paradigm draws from several 19th- and 20th-century intellectual traditions, including German idealist philosophy, phenomenology, hermeneutic philosophy, and American pragmatism.[4] Although there are many ways to describe the interpretive perspective, we--like Guest and colleagues[19]-- prefer the definition offered by Walsham:

> Interpretive methods of research start from the position that our knowledge of reality, including the domain of human action, is a social construction by human actors and that this applies equally to researchers. Thus there is no objective reality which can be discovered by researchers and replicated by others, in contrast to the assumptions of positivist science. (p. 5)[23]

As this definition implies, interpretive researchers assume that conceptions of reality are unique, pluralistic, and contextual.[4] From this perspective, reality does not exist "out there"; it is instead continually (re)created through communicative expressions and interpretations.[4,24] Interpretive research is often associated with the theoretical framework of social constructionism.[12] Social constructionism assumes that generating knowledge about social life requires researchers to identify the meaning that participants assign to their lived experiences while simultaneously acknowledging the ways the researchers' own perspectives influence the research process.[12] Consistent with this perspective, interpretive communication research proceeds from the notion that, rather than seeking to capture one objective reality, qualitative methods can and should provide important insights into the multiple realities that are continually (re)created and experienced through human interaction.[4,12,19,24] Interpretive researchers seek to achieve deep understanding of the actions, motives, and feelings that constitute people's perceptions of reality while acknowledging that their knowledge claims are inevitably partial.[4,24] Rather than attempting to maintain objective distance from the study setting or research participants, interpretive scholars frequently acknowledge, emphasize, and even celebrate the ways their own experiences, biases, and theoretical and methodological commitments influence the research process.[2,24]

As noted, qualitative communication research in palliative care settings may proceed from either of the paradigms discussed here (as well as several others). The appropriateness of one set of foundational assumptions over another depends upon the researcher's training and ideological commitments, as well as what is most appropriate and useful for the research questions at hand. Each of these ontological/epistemological perspectives (and the qualitative research that draws from them) can provide useful ways of understanding, talking about, and improving palliative care. In the next section, the various types of qualitative research data are discussed.

Generating Qualitative Research Data

Regardless of the paradigmatic underpinnings or goals of a particular study, qualitative researchers generally draw upon the same data types. At a very basic level, qualitative research data may include anything that does not indicate ordinal values.[19,25] As this description implies, qualitative data can take a wide variety of forms. At one end of the spectrum, a researcher may collect one-word responses to an open-ended question (e.g., "What is the name of your primary care doctor?"). Another researcher, however, may produce audio-recordings of first-person narratives that recount each research participant's experience with palliative care, which could be several hours long. Yet another qualitative researcher may choose to collect naturally occurring conversations by observing medical interviews or family meetings. Ryan and Bernard's[26] typology of qualitative research organizes qualitative data into its three main forms—text, images, and sounds. They further divide textual data into two primary components—text as an object of analysis (e.g., conversations, narratives, etc.) and text as a proxy for experience (e.g., participants' recollections and perceptions of past events).[19,26] Although communication research in palliative care contexts may incorporate a wide range of qualitative data, including visual images, recorded (spontaneous) conversations, and personal/organizational documents, it generally involves analyzing textual data collected through fieldwork and/or interviews; the generation of these types of qualitative data is the focus of this section.

Fieldwork

Fieldwork, or participant observation, involves present-time, face-to-face interaction with people in a particular setting (i.e., the field), which may include anything from a family's home to an intensive care unit.[4,12] Fieldwork is the process of watching and learning about a setting and the people who inhabit it while participating in the daily realities that characterize the study environment.[27,28] A researcher's level of participation during fieldwork may range from nonparticipant (observer only) to complete participation.[29] For example, in her study of hospice volunteers, Elissa Foster was a complete participant in the volunteer process.[30] She went through volunteer training and visited Dorothy--her assigned hospice patient--and Dorothy's family for more than a year. A researcher's participation level during fieldwork is largely dependent on the research topic and how easy/difficult it is to gain access to the study site[29] and has implications for how the results of the study are developed. Immersing one's self in the field, in the way Foster did, generally leads to results that include personal reflections about one's experience, as well as how the researcher may have influenced the events that transpired.

Whatever the degree of participation, conducting fieldwork is designed to produce detailed knowledge of communicative actions in the study setting that are based on researchers' observations and reflections on their (potential) meanings.[4] In order to document and analyze communication in a chosen setting, field researchers must document their observations and reflections. While this process may involve video/audio-recording certain events and conversations and/or taking photographs, it has traditionally been associated with producing handwritten, textual artifacts known as field notes.[4,12] In communication research, field notes focus on "describing and interpreting the symbolic (i.e., textual) qualities of communication as social action" (p. 155).[4] Ultimately, field notes (and other forms of documentation) provide the evidentiary material that field researchers use to develop and support their claims.

Interviews

Interviews are purposeful conversations between two or more people that explore topic(s) of interest through the asking and answering of questions.[31] Interviewing is a qualitative research method that is popular in health communication and other social science disciplines. One of the benefits of using interviews as a research method is that they can be adapted for a variety of settings and purposes. Qualitative research interviews may include face-to-face interaction, telephone contact, or Internet-mediated communication.[12] Interview topics may focus on recounting and assigning meanings to past or present experiences; in some cases, they may focus on projections toward the future. The most common form of interview is a dyad (i.e., one interviewer and one respondent), but research interviews may also be triadic (e.g., one researcher may simultaneously interview a palliative care patient and his or her designated caregiver).[12] Focus groups, which typically involve one or more researchers and a group of respondents, are an additional research interview format.[12] Scholars interested in palliative care may use interviews to gain insight into the health experiences of patients, providers, and family members and/or develop health communication theory.[31] In particular, interviews can be a valuable tool for learning about participants' experiences with sensitive topics without encroaching on these deeply personal events. For example, Wittenberg-Lyles and colleagues[32] used qualitative interviews to gain insight into the challenges that caregivers face after a loved one begins receiving hospice (discussed in more detail later in this chapter).

Research interviews may take a variety of forms, but they generally fall into one of three categories: (a) highly structured interviews, (b) semistructured interviews, or (c) unstructured interviews.[31] Highly structured interviews include a specific set of questions that are asked of participants in the same way with no follow-up questions. Semistructured interviews involve a set of specific questions but also include spontaneous questions that may ask for more information or clarification. Unstructured interviews may include a list of topics, but questions are phrased spontaneously to stimulate conversation. Each of these interview styles has benefits and drawbacks, and it is important that scholars consider the setting and purpose of their research before choosing an interview format.[4,12,31] Whatever the style, format, or topic(s) of qualitative research interviews, they are typically audio- or video-recorded and then transcribed to serve as the data for analysis.[4,12,31]

Qualitative Communication Research Approaches

In this section, we briefly describe and provide examples of a few of the more common approaches to collecting and analyzing qualitative communication data in palliative care contexts. This is not comprehensive, and other important approaches--including ethnomethodologic,[33,34] photovoice,[35,36] and material culture research—are not discussed here.[4,12] Additionally, although we distinguish between various approaches in this section, these distinctions are not always evident in qualitative research practice, as there is substantial overlap among them.[1,4,12,19]

Grounded Theory

Grounded theory was originally developed by sociologists Barney Glaser and Anselm Strauss during the 1960s.[37] Grounded theory is a specific form of inductive thematic analysis, a general term used to describe qualitative analysis that involves identifying themes in collected data, coding those themes, and then interpreting the structure and content of the themes.[37,38] Inductive thematic analysis more generally and grounded theory in particular is likely the most common qualitative data analysis in the social, behavioral, and health sciences.[19] Charmaz, who updated grounded theory to better align with the social constructionist perspective, defines it as a set "of systematic, yet flexible guidelines for collecting and analyzing qualitative data to construct theories 'grounded' in the data themselves." (p. 2)[39] Consistent with this description, grounded theory is an iterative process for identifying recurring thematic categories that appear within qualitative data and then organizing the categories into formal theoretical models.[39,40] The process involves reviewing units of text (e.g., words, sentences, paragraphs, stories) to first capture and code emerging themes. The relationships between the themes are noted, and as more data are analyzed, the thematic codes are continually reexamined and redefined through the constant comparison method, which involves comparing and contrasting all textual units with each other.[19,39,40] Research teams often begin by individually coding their data and then coming together to compare interpretations and refine their analytic framework.[19,39,40] As researchers engage in this process, the primary objective is to present the data in a plausible, coherent way.

Wittenberg-Lyles and colleagues[32] provide an example of using grounded theory in qualitative communication research in their exploration of how family communication patterns influence caregivers' concerns after their loved ones started hospice care. Their data included audio-recorded interviews with 89 caregivers that ranged from 35 minutes to an 1.5 hours in duration. Data analysis began with two members of the research team listening to the interview recordings and transcribing all segments of talk that mentioned "family." The research team members next engaged in a series of individual readings of the transcripts, using a Family Communication Patterns Theory[41] as a sensitizing concept, and coded caregiver talk into one of the following mutually exclusive codes: family hierarchy, preservation of family authority, minimal talk with family but with sustained contact, explicit talk of assumed family roles, reference to open discussion among family members, the absence of an authoritarian family member, little interaction among family, or emotional detachment from family.

Next, the research team grouped these codes together by family patterns: family hierarchy and preservation of family authority (*consensual* family communication pattern), minimal talk with family but with sustained contact and explicit talk of assumed family roles (*protective* family communication pattern), reference to open discussion among family members and the absence of an authoritarian family member (*pluralistic* family communication pattern), and little interaction among family and emotional detachment from family (*laissez-faire* family communication pattern). The team members addressed coding disagreements by collectively returning to the transcripts and discussing differing interpretations until they reached consensus. Finally, the data grouped by family communication pattern was then thematically analyzed using a constant comparison method, where individual team members coded the data and then came together to refine the initial codings into a thematic typology of family caregiver types: (a) Manager, (b) Carrier, (c) Partner, and (d) Loner. As Wittenberg-Lyles and colleagues noted,[32] identifying family caregiver types can help clinicians better understand and address their needs. Thus, in this case, the iterative, grounded theory process of individually and collectively analyzing interview transcripts helped identify recurring patterns of behavior.

Ethnography

As a qualitative research approach, ethnography rests on the premise that culture and human behavior are complicated phenomena that are composed of, and influenced by, a multitude of factors, which might include history, physical contexts, institutional structures, and other symbolic influences (e.g., language, rituals).[1,19] An ethnographic perspective further assumes that cultural meanings, assumptions, and values are evident in the ways people interact with each other.[1,42] Ethnography typically involves immersing one's self in a cultural setting, community, or organization in order to learn, through direct observation, participation, and interaction, about the environment and the people who inhabit it.[1,4] Thus while ethnography does not technically refer to a specific data collection method,[4] it most often is associated with fieldwork[1,19,42] and frequently includes formal and informal interviews with key informants.[4] One of the key features of ethnography is that it takes place in "natural settings"; that is, researchers typically observe people's behaviors and interactions in settings that are part of their everyday lives.[1,4,19,42] This is one of the strengths of ethnography, as it provides insights that other research methods cannot.[19] In disciplines such as anthropology, ethnography has historically relied on long-term research studies, which often last a year or longer.[19] Contemporary ethnographic research is generally much shorter in duration, but producing a detailed, insightful ethnographic analysis does require considerable time and effort.[1,19] Although some ethnographers, like others who practice fieldwork, may try to remain unobtrusive by observing at a distance, many ethnographies include researchers' direct participation in the study setting.[1,4]

Pesut et al.[43] used ethnography to explore rural palliative care, with a particular focus on the responsibilities that support good palliative care from rural participants' perspectives. The researchers began their study by identifying four rural communities in Western Canada to include in their study. The communities were considered rural because they had populations of fewer than 10,000 residents and were located at least a 3-hour traveling distance from a palliative care treatment center.[43] All four communities had one or two designated palliative beds in acute medical units and/or residential care centers; however, these beds were also used for general patients and were not always available for palliative care patients.

Pesut and colleagues' ethnographic data collection took place over a 15-month period.[43] Data sources for their study were collected more than 51 days of fieldwork, which included more than 74 hours of direct participant observation. These observations were conducted by following nurses who provided palliative care in patients' homes and acute care settings. The observations were documented using field notes. The researchers also conducted 95 interviews with key informants, including family caregivers, volunteers, nurses, physicians, social workers, and healthcare administrators.[43] Interviews lasted between 30 and 90 minutes, were audio-recorded, and were transcribed verbatim. The research team analyzed the collected data (i.e., field notes and transcripts) jointly using inductive thematic analysis (see previous discussion). Although previous studies indicated that palliative care quality deteriorated as distance from urban centers increased,[44] Pesut and colleagues found that palliative care services in the rural communities they studied were not uninformed or substandard; they did discover, however, that the fluidity of palliative care roles and organizational policies (e.g., hiring providers outside the community, limiting inpatient palliative care beds) had a negative impact on palliative care practice in these rural communities.[43] They also found that palliative care responsibilities were often negotiated through fluid, informal communication processes between healthcare providers, patients, and lay caregivers.[43]

Phenomenology

Within the communication discipline, phenomenology refers to the qualitative study of people's perceptions, feelings, and lived experiences.[1,19] There is, thus, little emphasis on physical and/or social characteristics of reality apart from the meaning people assign to them.[1] In this way, the focus of phenomenological research is to understand how people constitute experiences through consciousness.[1,19] Edmund Husserl--a German philosopher--is widely regarded as the founder of the phenomenological perspective.[1] He described a phenomenological method called eidetic reduction or bracketing.[45] According to du Pré and Crandall:

> [When] following such a process, a person seeks to imagine a thing or concept and "bracket" out all nonessential elements of it. The objective is to arrive at its essential properties, those that ultimately define it as being different from other phenomena. (p. 538)[1]

While Husserl[45] argued that human beings regularly engage in this activity in their everyday life, qualitative communication researchers attempt to guide study participants through a similar process, usually through open-ended, in-depth interviews.[1,19] Specific to palliative care, researchers may explore the meanings people assign to notions such as "health," "illness," "suffering," "terminal," or "compassion." Interestingly, those who practice qualitative research of various types have adopted many characteristics of phenomenology; many qualitative research approaches are, to some extent, phenomenological, as they attempt to document people's "lived experiences and the behavioral, emotive, and social meanings that these experiences have for them." (p. 11)[19]

Erichsen et al.[46] conducted a phenomenological study of nurses' understanding of "honesty" in palliative care. The research team recruited participants from two different hospitals in a county of approximately 400,000 residents in southeast Sweden. The study sample included 16 female palliative care nurses. Data collection involved audio-recorded, open-ended interviews with each nurse. In order to encourage informants to focus on the concept, all the interviews commenced with the question: "Do you think honesty is important?" Consistent with the phenomenological approach, Erichsen and colleagues[46] described the analysis process as consisting of four steps. They began by reading interview transcriptions to familiarize themselves with the data. Next, they identified the statements that were most relevant to the concept of honesty. These statements were then compared to each other in order to identify sources of variation and agreement. Finally, they focused on the structure of participants' experiences in order to synthesize the data into an overarching framework that described the lived experience of honesty.

The study results indicated that while the nurses had some difficulty defining honesty, they considered it a basic need for all human beings and an essential component of providing patient- and family-centered palliative care. Consistent with the principles of virtue ethics, the nurses' reasons for being honest were that honesty was expected from them as professionals, that a lie would be exposed anyway, and that they wanted to provide good care of high quality. The nurses also reported moral conflicts related to honesty, such as when family members asked them to withhold certain information from patients or when they were forced to describe the potential benefits of a certain treatment when patients were unlikely to experience them.[46] Ultimately, the researchers called for greater emphasis on patient autonomy and a commitment to being honest in palliative care contexts while recognizing that honesty can also create uncertainty and ethical conflict.[46]

Meta-Ethnography

A qualitative meta-analysis is a structured study that analyzes the findings of other qualitative studies linked by the same topic area.[47] Although various approaches have been used to guide the synthesis of qualitative research,[48] meta-ethnography is the most developed method for such analysis.[49] Meta-ethnography provides a systematic framework for evaluating previous research and developing a coherent analysis of what can be learned from a body of evidence.[50] Noblit and Hare[47] originally developed meta-ethnography as an inductive process for identifying and connecting themes and concepts identified in interpretive studies. Although the authors firmly positioned meta-ethnography within the interpretive paradigm, researchers have extended the meta-ethnographic process to synthesize various types of qualitative studies.[51] Meta-ethnography generally involves seven distinct steps:[52] (1) developing a suitable research question, (2) identifying/evaluating existing studies, (3) reading the individual studies, (4) determining how the studies are related, (5) translating the studies into an emerging theoretical framework, (6) finalizing the analytic framework, and (7) presenting the results.

Dillon et al.[50] conducted a meta-ethnographic synthesis of qualitative studies in order to identify factors that influenced African Americans' decisions about hospice care. Hospice enrollment disparities among this population have been well documented by quantitative studies, and a number of qualitative studies have sought to understand how African American patients and their loved ones make the decisions they do about hospice. As the authors argued, however, these studies were often interpreted in isolation without productive links to previous inquiry.[50] Meta-ethnography was used as a starting point to develop culturally targeted health messages[53] about hospice care. The study began by conducting a systematic literature search in order to identify topically relevant, peer-reviewed studies published from 2000 to 2010. The initial search generated a total of 788 abstracts for review, which was then narrowed to 96 articles by eliminating those that did not focus on hospice decisions by African Americans in the United States. The synthesis sample was further narrowed to 12 articles by asking two specific questions: (a) "Does this paper report on findings from research that involved qualitative methods of data collection and analysis?" and (b) "Is this research relevant to the synthesis topic?" The research team then appraised the quality of each article and decided that all 12 should be included in their analysis. Finally, using the synthesis articles' findings and interpretations as primary data, the researchers used a grounded theory approach to develop a coherent thematic framework that identified three primary factors that influenced African Americans' hospice decisions: (a) necessary knowledge about hospice care (e.g., available services, quality of care, financial information, etc.), (b) family members' needs and preferences, and (c) religious/spiritual considerations. Building from these identified factors, the authors emphasized the need for health messages designed to promote hospice enrollment among African Americans to emphasize the role of family caregivers and position hospice as a "partnership" between healthcare providers and patients' loved ones. The study also highlighted the importance of incorporating the narratives of actual African American hospice patients in hospice promotion messages, which was validated by another recent study.[54]

Mixed-Methods Research

Given the differing goals and findings associated with quantitative and qualitative research, researchers are increasingly combining both methodologies to generate insights that would not emerge from using either approach alone.[19] Although there is not consensus on this issue, some have argued that using a mixed-methods approach strengthens the overall research design (by offsetting the strengths and weaknesses of the other), encourages interdisciplinary research, and encourages the integration of multiple ontological/epistemological paradigms.[19,55] Although there are multiple ways of integrating qualitative and quantitative approaches, the concurrent design appears to be most helpful. In a concurrent design, data are integrated into the analysis at the same time.[19,55] The advantage of this design is that, rather than using one method to inform the analysis of the other, it allows researchers to simultaneously compare quantitative and qualitative data in order to identify areas of convergences, divergence, and contradiction.[19,55]

Roscoe et al.[56] used a concurrent mixed-methods design to explore competing definitions of effective communication in head and neck cancer care at the end of life. The research team recruited 14 head and neck cancer patients from a local cancer center to participate in the study. Eligibility criteria limited patient participants to those with head and neck cancer for which conventional treatments (surgery, radiation therapy, combined chemotherapy/radiation therapy) were not recommended and who had been told by their oncologist that their prognosis was terminal (i.e., that death was likely to occur within 6 months, if the disease took its usual course). Consistent with the mixed-methods approach, patients participated in semistructured interviews and also completed two quantitative measures: the McGill Quality of Life Questionnaire–Cardiff Short Form[57] and the University of Washington School of Medicine Quality of Communication Questionnaire.[58] The quantitative survey results were reported using descriptive statistics, and interview data was analyzed using grounded theory.

This quantitative and qualitative data revealed that patients rated their physicians highly in terms of their general communication skills as well as their comfort in discussing end-of-life issues, as revealed through statistical analysis of responses to the quality of communication questionnaire. Patient interview data suggested that they considered their oncologists straightforward communicators who were willing and able to answer questions. There were, however, some alarming trends that were identified as part of the qualitative analysis of interview data. The research team found that a number of patients could not rate their physicians' end-of-life communication skills because they had not been told of their terminal diagnosis—despite a documented terminal diagnosis being an inclusion criterion for patients. The interview data shed some light on these inconsistencies. As Roscoe and colleagues explained,

> Patients indicated their physicians were willing to answer questions, and physicians and other clinical health professionals in this study reported a willingness to answer questions. However, this

question-and-answer approach assumes patients know what questions to ask and feel comfortable doing so. (p. 189)[56]

These findings suggest that discussions about terminal diagnosis and/or end-of-life care may not occur unless patients and their loved ones explicitly inquire about these issues, which many patients/family members may be unwilling or unable to do; patients and their loved ones may also be unsure about the appropriateness of such concerns. Roscoe and colleagues'[56] study demonstrates the value of mixed-methods research; even though the quantitative data suggested that patients rated their physicians' communication skills highly, the qualitative data was able to identify potential shortcomings of communicating terminal diagnoses and end-of-life options in head and neck cancer care.

Generalizability, Validity, and Reliability

Quantitative social science research has long been concerned with issues of generalizability, validity, and reliability.[2,4,12] This section provides a brief discussion of how these considerations apply to qualitative communication research. The purpose of quantitative (often positivist or postpositivist) research is frequently to generalize from a study sample to the larger population from which participants are drawn; for example, a researcher who distributes the Quality of Communication Questionnaire to 600 palliative care patients in Memphis, Tennessee, may hope to generalize his or her findings to the city's entire palliative care population. The generalizability of the sample would be made possible through random-sampling techniques, just as the random assignment of participants to experimental or control groups is meant to facilitate generalizability in experimental studies.[4,12] Qualitative communication researchers are generally less concerned with generalizability in the traditional sense, because qualitative epistemologies typically assume that social reality is emergent and contextual.[4,12] This is not to suggest that qualitative research findings do not have value or are not applicable outside of the study setting. Communication challenges (e.g., discussing prognosis and end-of-life options[56]) and patterns of interaction (e.g., family communication patterns[32]) identified in a single study are often relevant to other contexts. Thus the degree to which qualitative communication research is generalizable (and qualitative scholars rarely use that term) is dependent on others' ability to identify with a study's findings and not its statistical relationship to a greater population.[12]

In quantitative studies, such as clinical trials, the term "validity" refers to the truthful correspondence between study results and an objective reality.[6] Qualitative research offers empirical insights into personal and social experiences, which are, of course, more subjective than biomedical phenomena.[4,6,12] Qualitative researchers often use words such as "credibility" or "plausibility" to describe a conceptually similar yet distinct idea.[6,12] To this end, Altheide and Johnson suggest that qualitative researchers who seek to demonstrate credibility or plausibility must "provide an account that communicates with the reader the truth of the setting or situation as the [researcher] has come to know about it." (p. 496)[59] Similarly, qualitative and quantitative researchers often have different conceptions of reliability. In quantitative studies, "reliability" refers to the idea that different researchers would reach the same conclusions if they analyzed identical data.[12] Since (almost) all qualitative data can be interpreted in multiple ways, this notion of reliability is not applicable to qualitative inquiry; however, qualitative researchers do often attempt to demonstrate that there is a level of consistency between their findings and the meanings that participants assign to study phenomena.[4,12]

While quantitative researchers employ statistical tests to assess reliability and validity, qualitative communication researchers may attempt to assess the validity and reliability of their results through procedures such as "triangulation" and "member checking."[4,12,19] Triangulation refers to the practice of incorporating different data types and analytic procedures into the research; the implicit assumption behind this practice is that if more than one data collection/analysis procedure points toward the same conclusion, validity is enhanced.[4] Member checking (or validation) means taking findings back to study participants in order to determine whether they recognize them as accurate or plausible.[4,12] This is, of course, a tricky process, as study participants (like researchers) may have different understandings of what constitutes an accurate conclusion and may have various reasons for supporting and/or critiquing particular findings.[12]

Quantitative notions and tests of generalizability, validity, and reliability are rarely applicable to qualitative research, but the concerns that underlie these concepts are frequently addressed in different ways. There are no easy answers when it comes to supporting and evaluating qualitative analysis and interpretation. Often, the best thing that qualitative scholars can do is avoid manipulating data collection and analysis in ways that distort field settings and/or participants' experiences while being forthright about the methods they used to reach their conclusions.[4]

Conclusion

Qualitative communication research is a broadly defined set of assumptions and techniques that are useful in attempting to understand and represent the various ways human beings understand and participate in social reality. This chapter has offered an overview of qualitative methods used to study palliative care communication.

References

1. du Pré A, Crandall SJ. Qualitative methods: Bridging the gap between research and daily practice. In: Thompson TL, Parrott R, Nussbaum JF, eds. *The Routledge Handbook of Health Communication*. 3rd ed. New York, NY: Routledge; 2011:532–545.
2. Denzin NK, Lincoln YS. *The Landscape of Qualitative Research*. Los Angeles, CA: SAGE; 2008.
3. Bochner AP. *Coming to Narrative: A Personal History of Paradigm Change in the Human Sciences*. Walnut Creek, CA: Left Coast Press; 2014.
4. Lindlof TR, Taylor, BC. *Qualitative Communication Research Methods*. 3rd ed. Thousand Oaks, CA: SAGE; 2011.
5. Frey LR, Cissna KN. *Routledge Handbook of Applied Communication Research*. New York, NY: Routledge; 2009.
6. Giacomini MK, Cook DJ. Users' guides to the medical literature: XXIII. Qualitative research in health care A: Are the results of the study valid? *JAMA*. 2000;284(3):357–362.
7. Crandall SJ, Marion GS. Commentary: Identifying attitudes towards empathy: An essential feature of professionalism. *Acad Med*. 2009;84(9):1174–1176.

8. Battista RN, Hodge MJ, Vineis P. Medicine, practice and guidelines: The uneasy juncture of science and art. *J Clin Epidemiol.* 1995;48(7):875–880.
9. Charon R. *Narrative Medicine: Honoring the Stories of Illness.* Oxford: Oxford University Press; 2006.
10. National Consensus Project for Quality Palliative Care. *Clinical Practice Guidelines for Quality Palliative Care.* 3rd ed. Pittsburgh, PA: National Consensus Project for Quality Palliative Care; 2013.
11. Connor, SR. *Hospice and Palliative Care: The Essential Guide.* New York, NY: Routledge; 2009.
12. Warren CAB, Karner TX. *Discovering Qualitative Methods: Field Research, Interviews, and Analysis.* New York, NY: Oxford University Press; 2010.
13. Flick U. *An Introduction to Qualitative Research.* 2nd ed. London: SAGE; 2002.
14. Geertz C. *Interpretation of Cultures.* New York, NY: Basic Books; 1973.
15. National Hospice and Palliative Care Organization. NHPCO facts and figures: Hospice care in America. http://www.nhpco.org/sites/default/files/public/Statistics_Research/2014_Facts_Figures.pdf. Accessed October 15, 2014.
16. Waldrop DP, Rinfrette ES. Making the transition to hospice: Exploring hospice professionals' perspectives. *Death Stud.* 2009;33:557–580.
17. Teno JM, Shu JE, Casarett D, et al. Timing of referral to hospice and quality of care: Length of stay and bereaved family members' perceptions of the timing of hospice referral. *J Pain Symptom Manage.* 2007;34:120–125.
18. Farrell TGP, Casarett D, Connor S, et al. It's too late: Examining the role of hospice and market factors in late hospice referrals. *J Am Geriatri Soc.* 2008;56:S1–S2.
19. Guest G, Namey EE, Mitchell, ML. *Collecting Qualitative Data: A Field Manual for Applied Researchers.* Thousand Oaks, CA: SAGE; 2013.
20. Comte A. *A General View of Positivism.* New York, NY: R. Speller; 1957.
21. Corman SR. Postpositivism. In: May S, Mumby DK, eds. *Engaging Organizational Communication Theory & Research: Multiple Perspectives.* Thousand Oaks, CA: SAGE; 2005:15–34.
22. Patton M. *Qualitative Research and Evaluation Methods.* 3rd ed. Thousand Oaks, CA: SAGE; 2002.
23. Walsham G. *Interpreting Information Systems in Organizations.* Chichester, UK: Wiley; 1993.
24. Bochner AP. Perspectives on inquiry III: The moral of stories. In: Knapp ML, Daly JA, eds. *Handbook of Interpersonal Communication.* 3rd ed. Thousand Oaks, CA: SAGE; 2002:73–101.
25. Nkwi PN, Nyamongo IK, Ryan GW. *Field Research into Socio-Cultural Issues: Methodological Guidelines.* Yaoundé, Cameroon: International Center for Applied Social Sciences, Research, and Training; 2001.
26. Ryan G. Bernard R. Data management and analysis methods. In: Denzin NK, Lincoln YS, eds. *Handbook of Qualitative Research.* Thousand Oaks, CA: SAGE; 2000:769–802.
27. Lofland J, Lofland, LH. *Analyzing Social Settings: A Guide to Qualitative Observation and Analysis.* 3rd ed. Belmont, CA: Wadsworth; 1995.
28. Spradley JP. *Participant Observation.* New York, NY: Holt, Rinehart & Winston; 1980.
29. Merrigan G, Huston CL. *Communication Research Methods.* 2nd ed. New York, NY: Oxford University Press; 2009.
30. Foster E. *Communicating at the End of Life: Finding Magic in the Mundane.* Mahwah, NJ: Lawrence Erlbaum Associates; 2006.
31. Dillon PJ. Interviewing in the health care context. In: Thompson TL, ed. *Encyclopedia of Health Communication.* Thousand Oaks, CA: SAGE; 2014:752–754.
32. Wittenberg-Lyles, E, Goldsmith, J, Demiris, G, Oliver, DP, Stone, J. The impact of family communication patterns on hospice family caregivers. *J Hosp Palliat Nurs.* 2012;14(1):25–33.
33. Garfinkel H. *Studies in Ethnomethodology.* Cambridge, MA: Polity/Basil Blackwell; 1967.
34. Heritage J. *Garfinkel and Ethnomethodology.* Cambridge, MA: Polity; 1984.
35. Wang CC. Photovoice: A participatory action research strategy applied to women's health. *J Womens Health.* 1999;8(2):185–192.
36. Angelo J, Egan, R. Family caregivers voice their needs: A photovoice study. *Palliat Support Care.* 2014;13(3):701–712.
37. Glaser BG, Strauss AL. *The Discovery of Grounded Theory: Strategies for Qualitative Research.* Chicago, IL: Aldine; 1967.
38. Guest G, MacQueen KM, Namey EE. *Applied Thematic Analysis.* Los Angeles, CA: SAGE; 2012.
39. Charmaz K. *Constructing Grounded Theory: A Practical Guide Through Qualitative Analysis.* London: SAGE; 2006.
40. Corbin, JM, Strauss, AL. *Basics of Qualitative Research: Techniques and Procedures for Developing Grounded Theory.* Los Angeles, CA: SAGE; 2008.
41. Koerner AF, Fitzpatrick MA. Toward a theory of family communication. *Commun Theory.* 2002;12(1):70–91.
42. Atkinson P, Hammersley M. Ethnography and participant observation. In: Denzin NK, Lincoln YS, eds. *Handbook of Qualitative Research.* Thousand Oaks, CA: SAGE; 1994:248–261.
43. Pesut B, Robinson CA, Bottorff, JL Among neighbors: An ethnographic account of responsibilities in rural palliative care. *Palliat Support Care.* 2014;12(2):127–138.
44. Schuurman N, Crooks VA, Amram O. A protocol for determining differences in consistency and depth of palliative care service provision across community sites. *Health Soc Care Community.* 2010;18(5):537–548.
45. Husserl, E. *The crisis of European Sciences and Transcendental Phenomenology: An Introduction to Phenomenological Philosophy.* Evanston, IL: Northwestern University Press; 1970.
46. Erichsen E, Danielsson EH, Friedrichsen M. A phenomenological study of nurses' understanding of honesty in palliative care. *Nurs Ethics.* 2010;17(1):39–50.
47. Noblit, GW, Hare, RD. *Meta-Ethnography: Synthesizing Qualitative Studies.* Newbury Park, CA: Sage Publications; 1988.
48. Bosma H, Apland L, Kazanjian A. Review: Cultural conceptualizations of hospice palliative care: more similarities than differences. *Palliat Med.* 2010;24(5):510–522.
49. Campbell R, Pound P, Pope C, et al. Evaluating meta-ethnography: A synthesis of qualitative research on lay experiences of diabetes and diabetes care. *Soc Sci Med.* 2003;56(4):671–684.
50. Dillon PJ, Roscoe LA, Jenkins JJ. African Americans and decisions about hospice care: Implications for health message design. *Howard J Commun.* 2012;23(2):175–193.
51. Dillon PJ, Basu A. HIV/AIDS and minority men who have sex with men: A meta-ethnographic synthesis of qualitative research. *Health Commun.* 2014;29(2):182–192.
52. Atkins S, Lewin S, Smith H, et al. Conducting a meta-ethnography of qualitative literature: Lessons learnt. *BMC Med Res Method.* 2008;8(1):21.
53. Kreuter MW, Wray RJ. Tailored and targeted health communication: Strategies for enhancing information relevance. *Am J Health Behav.* 2003;27(1):227–232.
54. Enguidanos S, Kogan AC, Lorenz K, Taylor G. Use of role model stories to overcome barriers to hospice among African Americans. *J Palliat Med.* 2011;14(2):161–168.
55. Creswell JW, Plano Clark V. *Designing and Conducting Mixed Methods Research.* Thousand Oaks, CA: SAGE; 2007.
56. Roscoe LA, Tullis JA, Reich RR, Mccaffrey JC. Beyond good intentions and patient perceptions: Competing definitions of effective

communication in head and neck cancer care at the end of life. *Health Commun.* 2013;28(2):183–192.
57. Cohen SR, Mount BM, Strobel MG, Bui F. The McGill Quality of Life Questionnaire: A measure of quality of life appropriate for people with advanced disease: A preliminary study of validity and acceptability. *Palliat Med.* 1995;9(3):207–219.
58. Curtis JR, Wenrich MD, Carline JD, Shannon SE, Ambrozy DM, Ramsey PG. Patients' perspectives on physician skill in end-of-life care: Differences between patients with COPD, cancer, and AIDS. *Chest.* 2002;122(1):356–362.
59. Altheide DL, Johnson JM. Criteria for assessing interpretive validity in qualitative research. In: Denzin NK, Lincoln YS, eds. *Handbook of Qualitative Research.* Thousand Oaks, CA: SAGE; 1994:485–499.

CHAPTER 49

Quantitative Communication Research

Melinda M. Villagran and Brenda L. MacArthur

Introduction

We learn about the influence of communication in health and palliative care through research. As research evolves and patterns begin to form, our collective knowledge about the relationships between communication and health grows. Communication shapes our understanding of health, our beliefs about what is healthy, and our decisions regarding health promotion and prevention behaviors. When research findings are made public, patients and providers can use the new evidence to make informed healthcare decisions for themselves and their patients. If knowledge brings power, then reliable and valid research findings provide powerful information enabling us take control of our lives. But what determines whether research findings are *good evidence* to use in making future decisions? How can the measurement of communication provide evidence to describe, explain, predict, or control future health events?

Quantitative communication research is the use of numerical measurement to answer questions through the application of scientific and systematic procedures. It is considered *empirical* because it is based on observations or experiences of communication.[1] Quantitative communication research is often used in studies examining the effects of messages disseminated through health campaigns. It is, however, more challenging in palliative care research due to health, logistical, and ethical concerns about conducting research with seriously ill patients. Only in recent years have palliative and end-of-life care begun to integrate research with clinical practice.[2] Recently, there have been calls for more rigorous clinical trials to build the body of evidence about communication and palliative care, but these types of studies hinge on researchers' ability to recruit research participants and properly utilize measurement and statistical testing to draw conclusions.[3] Unfortunately, challenges exist that may limit the number of scientifically rigorous studies on communication in palliative care due to a lack of access to palliative care patients and a lack of behavioral research experience among some healthcare providers. Palliative care patients often have variable and short periods of survival, have multiple health issues and comorbidities, and are often too ill to complete surveys or participate in interviews.[4] Palliative care providers may lack sufficient experience with communication research design and measurement, may be put off by an addition to their workload,[2] or may simply have too few patients at one time to conduct rigorous quantitative studies with sufficient sample sizes.[4] Together, these challenges have limited the number of randomized controlled trials using quantitative methods conducted to build the palliative care evidence base.[3]

Despite these challenges, quantitative communication research offers many unique benefits. First, it allows researchers to target and compare specific communication interventions (e.g., completing an advance directive or participating in a family meeting) and adds to the body of evidence regarding the effects of such interventions on patients' health outcomes.[5] Second, quantitative methods typically result in strong evidence about the effectiveness of interventions across settings because of their high level of precision and objectivity in the research design.[1,5] Even when the replication of results from a nonexperimental intervention produces consistent results across multiple settings, critics may question whether the intervention provides definitive evidence to support large, system-wide change. For researchers seeking to bring about individual or system-wide changes to provide greater access and use of palliative care, randomized controlled trials using quantitative research methods are considered more scientifically rigorous because key variables are controlled and systematically measured.[5] In general, study findings resulting from scientifically rigorous quantitative methods are viewed as the most credible evidence on which to make healthcare decisions.[5]

This chapter explores some of the benefits associated with quantitative research and explains common practices and methods used by quantitative researchers in the palliative care context. Before considering the processes associated with quantitative research, it is important to understand what quantitative research is and what it offers for those studying palliative care communication.

What Is Quantitative Research?

In its most basic form, quantitative research is the use of numbers to provide statistical support for claims based on theory. The use of quantitative methodology helps to ensure researchers report accurate results that are statistically supported and replicable. In order to conduct this type of research, communication phenomena are measured based on the amounts, frequencies, degrees, values, or intensity of the occurrence.[1] The degree to which a patient experiences a change in health outcome can be reported as a percentage. For example, if Patient A experiences a 10% change in a specified health outcome, a second study should result in statistically similar results for Patient B, if the studies were conducted using random assignment of participants, similar control and treatment conditions, and systematically controlled measurement techniques.

Quantitative research is based on deductive reasoning. In this form of research, the hypotheses are rooted in evidence from an existing theory or similar studies, and the goal for quantitative research is ultimately to include or exclude alternative explanations for measured changes in the variables of interest. In other words, a researcher may examine general literature to find a theory, set of concepts, definitions, or similar studies that present a systematic view of a given communication phenomena[1] and then apply that general information to a specific palliative care issue. The most useful theories for examining communication in palliative care focus on the unique needs of seriously or terminally ill patients and the crucial roles that their providers, caregivers, and/or family members play in their care. Table 49.1 presents a summary of theories often used in quantitative communication research and applicable to palliative care communication.

In the field of communication, quantitative research provides a number of benefits for examining and reporting data. Unlike qualitative research that relies on researcher interpretation of subjective data, quantitative research employs techniques to measure statistically significant outcomes. Quantitative researchers do not typically seek to uncover emergent patterns in data unless the pattern was hypothesized at the beginning of the study. By moving from a general claim or idea (e.g., provider communication can be improved through communication training) to a more specific issue that is measured (e.g. measuring learner communication confidence following exposure to a one-time communication training course), quantitative researchers ably confirm or disconfirm their hypotheses based on manifest content of measured variables (e.g., the learner's ability to apply new communication skills). Quantifying the level of change that occurs as a result of a controlled intervention also allows researchers to use meaningful comparison to calculate the statistically significant outcomes of the study.

An example of quantitative research is a study that examined how a tailored pain management coaching intervention could contribute to better cancer pain control among advanced cancer patients.[6] In this study, the researchers used quantitative methods to analyze data on patients' pain severity, active communication with their physician about pain, and changes in medication. By statistically analyzing this data, the researchers were able to conclude that increased patient communication about pain with their physicians led to changes in physicians' prescribing of medication. Because this hypothesis was statistically supported, statements such as "cancer patients with poorly controlled pain could prompt changes in their pain medication by more actively communicating their questions, concerns, needs, and preferences" reveal new knowledge created through the research. This statement now carries more weight in research and in practice and can be used to guide future healthcare decisions for patients and providers.

Comparison

Using numbers to represent communication phenomena (such as how many times a question was asked or how satisfied a patient is with a provider's communication) allows for *comparison* between and among communication variables. Patient A's rating of an experience can be compared to the experience of Patient B's rating of the same experience to more precisely assess differences in health outcomes. For example, if one patient reports a pain level of 3 while another describes his or her pain closer to a 9, the researcher can compare the two participants to see if communication-related factors such as level of patient's disclosure of information, perceived satisfaction with care, or perceptions of patient-centered communication accounts for this difference. An entire data set can also be represented as a whole by averaging the individual scores to obtain one mean score for pain. The mean score can then be compared to other variables based on disease type or patient characteristics. Comparing data helps researchers explain why results were either expected or unexpected and allows them to isolate results based on criteria such as participants' existing attitudes or beliefs, interventions, or demographic features.

Credibility

The use of numbers to represent communication variables ensures *credibility* or truthfulness when reporting results. Credibility refers to the researchers' capacity to remain objective.[1] Statistical tests ensure that there is a 95% or greater chance that the results did not happen by chance alone. In order to achieve this small level of error, quantitative research is bound by *reliability* and *validity*. Reliability ensures that if a study is replicated, the same result can also be replicated over time. Validity ensures that the researchers measured the constructs they claimed to measure.[1] Threats to validity can occur through misinterpretation of meaning, such that there is a lack of uniformity between what the researcher is studying and what is actually being measured by the selected measurement techniques. For example, the difference between a patient's reporting of satisfaction with his or her healthcare provider and satisfaction with his or her ability to communicate with the healthcare provider is an important distinction that can skew results, leading to the reporting of inaccurate information. A study about prostate cancer patients' information-seeking behaviors and its relationship to satisfaction examined the latter.[7] The study focused on patients' satisfaction with their own abilities. However, if a participant misunderstood the question as

Table 49.1 Health Communication Theories

Theory	Palliative Care Context
Communication Privacy Management[24]	Managing privacy boundaries for patients and providers regarding the disclosure of personal information
Relational Dialectics[25]	Patients must manage the tensions experienced in personal relationships throughout the palliative care experience
Expectancy Violations Theory[26]	Patient expectations regarding accuracy and sensitivity of provider interactions
Sensemaking[27]	Patients and caregivers manage the palliative care experience through interactions
Transactional Model of Stress and Coping[28]	Stressors experienced in the palliative care environment require action to restore balance
Theory of Reasoned Action[29]	Behavioral intention to adopt specific palliative care protocol

asking about his satisfaction with his provider, the participant's incorrect response could detrimentally affect the entire data set.

Measuring Communication

Information deduced from quantitative communication research can have powerful implications for patients, families, and providers. However, in order to obtain such results, the consistent and accurate measurement of communication phenomena is essential. When using quantitative methods, it is especially important that the study is properly designed in a way that ensures reliability and validity. This requires careful consideration of how the data will be analyzed, which will in turn guide decisions about how the data will be collected. This section focuses on the use of surveys to collect data, the measurement of variables, and the use of health interventions to examine changes in health outcomes.

Surveys

The use of surveys or questionnaires is perhaps the most common technique researchers use to obtain quantitative data about human communication across disciplines.[1] Quantitative communication researchers often employ survey research techniques to gather data about patients' attitudes, beliefs, experiences, satisfaction, or knowledge of a topic. This type of information is not typically collected as part of routine charting, so surveys often provide a viable alternative for collection of such information from patients and caregivers. For example, one study examined affection deprivation or the longing for more affectionate touch (hugging, hand-holding, kissing) as a factor related to specific health outcomes.[8] This study found that when patients perceive affection deprivation, they are more likely to experience a host of deficits related to their general well-being, social health, mental health, and physical health. Specifically, patients who perceived more affection deprivation were more likely to experience stress, depression, mood and anxiety disorders, and secondary immune system disorders.[8] Such studies highlight the importance of communication variables such as affection in significantly contributing to patients' health outcomes.

Surveys are often used because they can obtain information about participants' experiences or characteristics quickly, efficiently, and often without interfering in the patients' treatment protocol or family members' grieving process. A survey of bereaved family members illustrates how online surveys can be used to unobtrusively collect data without interrupting participants during the grieving process.[9] The study measured family members' satisfaction with their deceased loved ones' hospice services prior to death. Because the researchers collected data from participants who had recently experienced the loss of a loved one and were interested in the family members' satisfaction with specific healthcare providers, a survey design provided participants with convenience and an added layer of privacy during this difficult time. With the use of technology, surveys can also be distributed to a large number of participants regardless of geographic location through multiple channels with the click of a button. Participants can be recruited to complete surveys via email, websites, or social media channels. The delivery of surveys using online channels allows participants to access the content at a time and location that is convenient for them. A recent multinational online survey measured the percentages of volunteers in four countries involved in palliative care who engaged in emotional care of patients and families and who completed a variety of tasks as part of patients' care.[10]

Sometimes, online surveys afford participants a level of anonymity when researchers seek information about stigmatized issues that may be considered controversial or embarrassing. For instance, researchers examined the unmet supportive needs of men with prostate cancer.[11] An online survey was used to obtain information about patients' perceptions of unmet needs relating to psychological issues, sexuality, pain or discomfort, and depression. In this case, an online survey ensured participants a level of anonymity to encourage them to share personal information honestly, without the risk of having to reveal their identities to researchers face to face. As demonstrated by this study, the anonymity afforded by online surveys is especially important for researchers interested in collecting personal or embarrassing health-related information if participants would be less likely to share information in the presence of researchers. Examples of stigmatized health-related information may include information about sexual health, drug use, addictive behaviors, or mental health.

Variables and Measurement

The use of surveys is efficient because a single survey may contain multiple measures of different communication variables that may reveal additional information to explain results. Rarely do researchers include just one measure in a survey. Instead, they typically include a set of scales that collectively measure variables for a study. Variables that may be of specific interest to researchers examining communication in the palliative care context are summarized in Table 49.2. Table 49.3 provides examples of communication measures for quantitative research.

To conduct quantitative communication research, individual scales are developed and validated based on analysis of scale responses across various participant types, association with previously validated scales; feedback from patient, caregivers, and providers; or feedback from experts who examine the scale items for validity.[12] For example, researchers utilized quantitative measures to gather data regarding provider and family satisfaction

Table 49.2 Examples of Communication Variables Used in Quantitative Research

Communication Variable	Example
Utterances	Phrases or sentences (e.g., see Box 49.1)
Nonverbal cues	Eye contact, head nodding, touch, space
Source cues	Credibility associated with the communication source, (e.g., provider, institution, website, organization)
Mode of delivery	Face-to-face, written (email, letter, text messaging) via technology (e.g., video conference)
Message content	Topic (such as delivering a poor prognosis, goals of care); communication education script or protocol; educational materials
Message response	Emotional reactions to messages
Message valence	Negative or positive psychological value associated with message

Table 49.3 Example Communication Measures for Quantitative Research

Communication Construct	Scale/Measure	Reliability and Validity	Source
To measure any kind of belief	Generalized Belief Measure	Alpha reliability estimate above .90.	McCroskey JC, Richmond VP. *Fundamentals of Human Communication: An Interpersonal Perspective*. Prospect Heights, IL: Waveland Press; 1996
To obtain information concerning how competent people feel when they are in a variety of communication contexts and with a variety of people	Self-Perceived Communication Competence Scale	This measure has generated good alpha reliability estimates (above .85) and had strong face validity. It also has been found to have substantial predictive validity.	McCroskey JC, McCroskey LL. Self-report as an approach to measuring communication competence. *Commun Res Rep.* 1988;5:108–113
To measure individual ethnocentrism	Ethnocentrism Scale	Alpha reliability estimate in the range of .80 to .90 in most cases. For validity information on this scale see: Neuliep, JW. Assessing the reliability and validity of the Generalized Ethnocentrism Scale. *J Intercult Commun Res.* 2002;31:201–215	Neuliep JW, McCroskey JC. The development of a U.S. and generalized ethnocentrism scale. *Commun Res Rep.* 1997;14:385–398
To measure the feeling of fear when communicating with a physician	Fear of Physician	Alpha reliability estimates for this instrument should be near .90.	Richmond VP, Smith RS, Heisel AM, McCroskey JC. The impact of communication apprehension and fear of talking with a physician and perceived medical outcomes. *Commun Res Rep.* 1998;15:344–353
To measure a member's perception of his or her organization's orientations toward change	Perceived Organizational Innovativeness Scale	Highly reliable (alpha above .90) and very good predictive validity.	Hurt HT, Teigen CW. The development of a measure of perceived organizational innovativeness. In: Ruben, BR, ed. *Communication Yearbook I*. New Brunswick, NJ: Transaction Books; 1977:377–385
To measure nonverbal immediacy as an other- or observer-report	Nonverbal Immediacy Scale-Observer Report	Alpha reliability estimates around .90 should be expected. This measure also has more face validity than previous instruments because it has more diverse items. Its predictive validity is also excellent.	Richmond VP, McCroskey JC, Johnson AE. Development of the Nonverbal Immediacy Scale (NIS): Measures of self- and other-perceived nonverbal immediacy. *Commun Q.* 2003;51:502–515
To provide a simple, general measure of patients' overall quality of received medical care	Perceived Quality of Medical Care	Alpha reliability estimates should be expected to be above .90.	Richmond VP, Smith RS, Heisel AM, McCroskey JC. The impact of communication apprehension and fear of talking with a physician and perceived medical outcomes. *Commun Res Rep.* 1998;15:344–353
To measure communication apprehension in the intercultural context	Personal Report of Intercultural Communication Apprehension	Alpha reliability estimates should be expected to be above .90 when completed by native English speakers.	Neuliep JW, McCroskey JC. The development of intercultural and interethnic communication apprehension scales. *Commun Res Rep.* 1997;14:385–398
To provide a simple, general measure of patients' satisfaction with their physician	Satisfaction With Physician	Alpha reliability estimates should be expected to be above .90.	Richmond, VP, Smith RS, Heisel AM, McCroskey JC. The impact of communication apprehension and fear of talking with a physician and perceived medical outcomes. *Commun Res Rep.* 1998;15:344–353
To measure state communication apprehension in any context	Situational Communication Apprehension Measure (SCAM)	Alpha reliability estimates of .85 to .90.	Richmond VP. The relationship between trait and state communication apprehension and interpersonal perception during acquaintance stages. *Hum Commun Res.* 1978;4:338–349
To measure a person's willingness to initiate communication	Willingness to Communicate)	Alpha reliability estimates for this instrument have ranged from .85 to well above .90.	McCroskey JC, Richmond VP. Willingness to communicate. In: McCroskey JC, Daly JA, eds. *Personality and Interpersonal Communication*. Newbury Park, CA: SAGE; 1987:119–131
To measure patient and provider beliefs regarding patient-centeredness	Patient-Practitioner Orientation Scale	Has been efficaciously validated and used in a variety of medical contexts as well as adapted for traditionally non-Western cultures.	Trapp S, Stern M. *Critical Synthesis Package: Patient-Practitioner Orientation Scale (PPOS)*. Washington, DC: MedEdPORTAL Publications; 2013
To measure an organization's health literacy level to develop a strategy for the clear communication of medical information	Communication Climate Assessment Toolkit		Wynia MK, Johnson M, McCoy TP, Griffin LP, Osborn CY. Validation of an organizational communication climate assessment toolkit. *Am J Med Qual.* 2010;25(6):436–443

with end-of-life care for patients who recently died in an academic medical center.[13] In this study, the research team created a survey that included scales to measure satisfaction with care. Participants rated their satisfaction with the following aspects of the end-of-life care: symptom management, providers' level of communication with the patient and family, expectations of the illness, emotional care, and spiritual care. Two groups of participants completed the survey: (a) providers categorized as attending physicians, house staff, and nurses, and (b) families of patients. By obtaining numerical data from both groups of individuals, the researchers were able to compare providers' satisfaction with the end-of-life care they provided to the patient and the families' satisfaction with the care their loved one received. The researchers also compared different providers' satisfaction with the care they provided. Because numerical data was collected, the researchers were able to compare different types of providers, revealing that intern and resident physicians reported lower satisfaction than attending physicians.[13]

To reliably measure satisfaction using quantitative methods, the construct was assessed on a 1 to 4 Likert-type scale where 1 = not very satisfied, 2 = moderately satisfied, 3 = very satisfied, 4 = completely satisfied. Likert-type scales use numbers to help participants categorize the degree of their feelings. Other studies use semantic differentials that use word pairs as bipolar adjectives anchored on a numeric scale (e.g., happy–sad, quick–slow, easy–hard).[1] For these measurement tools, participants select a value on a 7-point rating scale between the two adjectives. Semantic differential scales allow researchers to measure both directionality and intensity of a participant's rating of a particular phenomena.[1]

Interventions

Palliative care communication interventions typically exhibit four general characteristics: experimental or quasi-experimental research designs; statistically significant positive health outcomes for the target population; publication of results in a peer-reviewed journal or other professional publication; and high-quality intervention materials, training and support resources, and quality assurance procedures.[14] Although some qualitative studies employ research designs that are similar to quantitative studies, the numerical data produced by quantitative studies allows researchers to more meaningfully compare results across groups. For example, if a study finds there is a 10% change in health outcomes for patients who receive a certain health intervention, it is possible to assess whether a second population receiving the same intervention has the same results. Unlike qualitative data that provides more descriptive information about a single group or intervention, quantitative data provides a level of certainty that a result can be replicated over time through a number of studies. One of the major benefits of conducting quantitative research is the ability to meaningfully compare results across studies and over time. Narrative data from qualitative studies provides a deeper description of the conditions in a single study, but quantitative data from a controlled experimental study allows researchers to predict the potential success of a health intervention and measure the outcome of the study in a way that has universal meaning based on the numerical results.

Experimental Research Design

Studies that employ an experimental design use random assignment of participants to a treatment or control group. Those in the treatment group take part in the intervention being tested, while those in the control group do not typically take part in the intervention. Quantitative data from participants allows for meaningful comparison of results at the end of the study to determine whether the intervention produced statistically significant results different from those who took part versus those who did not take part in the treatment intervention. In addition, pre- and posttest assessments of each group allow researchers to assess whether the intervention resulted in a significant change after the intervention when compared to a baseline measure of the specific variables.

An experimental research design was used in a study aimed at examining the effects of a patient participation-based dietary intervention on health outcomes for patients diagnosed with stomach cancer.[15] Patients were randomly placed into a treatment group that received the intervention or a control group that did not. For those in the treatment group, nurses coached and empowered patients through education, while patients in the control group received usual care. Patients completed a pretest on the day before hospital discharge following a gastrectomy and posttests at 2 weeks and 12 weeks post-op. The researchers were able to report that patients in the treatment group demonstrated significant improvements in overall functioning, adherence to dietary guidelines, and satisfaction over those in the control group. The use of treatment and control groups, combined with statistical analyses, enables researchers not only to test the effects of an intervention but also to support differences found between groups. In this case, participants' scores for overall functioning in the treatment group increased by 22 points from the pretest to the second posttest, where patients' scores in the control group increased by only 14 points. Because this difference was statistically significant, the researchers could conclude that this change was likely a result of the intervention (nurse-facilitated communication and education on diet).

Quasi-Experimental Research Design

Studies that employ quasi-experimental research designs do not use random assignment of participants to a treatment condition. These types of interventions still use a control group for comparison to the treatment group who receive the intervention and typically also include a pre- and posttest assessment of the effectiveness of the intervention.

Successful interventions are typically those that result in outcomes consistent with the hypotheses. Most often, the target group will respond in an expected manner based on their exposure to some form of intervention, and their outcome will be significantly different from members of the control group who do not participate in the intervention. When the intervention has an intended effect on members of the target group, there will usually be statistically significant behavioral outcomes that yield a p value of less than or equal to .05. For example, imagine that a group of 50 physicians use a new communication protocol with patients, and a separate group of 50 physicians do not use the new protocol in communication with patients. Examples of communication intervention protocols include various types of messages, various modes of message delivery, and patient and family coaching to help improve understanding and shared decision-making. The intervention would be the new communication protocol, and the hypothesized outcome might be greater communication satisfaction and quality of life based on information presented by the physicians to their patients. A successful intervention such as providing communication coaching for patients and families might result in statistically significant higher communication satisfaction scores and statistically significant more quality of life among the patients who engaged in the new communication protocol. Replication of these results over a number of studies adds to the validity of the intervention for use in populations where the results were established.

Publication of Results

Sharing the results of successful quantitative interventions through peer-reviewed publications allows researchers to replicate intervention methods across different patient populations. If a study is published in a peer-reviewed publication, it means a group of scholars who are experts in the topic have critically analyzed the manuscript and support the claims and results of the study based on the information provided in it. The peer-review process provides an additional level of confidence for providers when selecting an intervention for their patient. Unfortunately, few interventions are 100% reliable 100% of the time. In fact, results of an intervention method vary from study to study, but, over time, successful interventions gain acceptance as standard treatment protocols when they repeatedly produce statistically significant results. The peer-review process allows researchers and providers to gain a greater level of confidence in published studies that have a strong history of predicable results. Although a lot of health communication research is published in communication-specific publications such as *Health Communication, Journal of Health Communication,* or *Communication and Medicine,* it is important to note that a great majority of these studies are also published in the health sciences. In these publications, palliative care is often emphasized in clinical communication. Such publications include *Patient Education and Counseling* and *Journal of General Internal Medicine.*

Providers are more likely to use interventions they believe will be effective for their patients, and the best way to assess what might be effective is to use established protocols from previously successful interventions that have been published in peer-reviewed journals or documented in comprehensive evaluation reports. The controlled environment of an experimental study, and the quantitative data it produces, allow providers to gauge exactly how well the intervention might improve health outcomes for their own patients who share similar personal or health characteristics with the target population who previously had success with the same intervention methods.

Assessing the Quality of Interventions

When providers elect to use quantitative interventions in patient care, there are six general characteristics to be considered: (a) the needs of the patient given his or her health situation, such as the patient's prognosis; (b) the fit or match of existing protocols with the patient's personal and health characteristics (e.g., disease, age, racial or ethnic group affiliations); (c) the resources available to implement and measure the effectiveness of the intervention (e.g., the ability to measure provider, patient, and family interactions); (d) existing evidence about the potential value of the treatment intervention for the patient or family such as matching appropriate messages and channels with patient needs; (e) the availability of resources to understand, apply, and measure the success of the intervention, as demonstrated by the communication health literacy of the patient and caregivers, and (f) the capacity of the patient, caregivers, and providers to successfully deliver the intervention based on the patient's needs, such as the patient's perceived communication competence of the providers and family members involved, given the goals of the intervention.[16]

All evidence derived from research is not the same. A recent report from the Agency on Healthcare Research and Quality on evidence-based practices for improving healthcare among seriously ill patients rated published studies from low to high quality based on the "strength" of the evidence presented in the study.[17] The authors operationalized the strength of evidence based on the types of research designs used in each study. The quantitative assessments of interventions included in the report allowed for stronger comparisons across the studies due to more consistent reporting of effect sizes and confidence intervals for reported outcomes. For researchers seeking to replicate existing results, the quantitative measurements in these studies provide a great deal of information about the magnitude of the change in health outcomes among patients in the treatment group. For communication researchers, the ability to replicate a study is essential, because it is through this replication and consistent results that communication theories are formed and expanded. Continued theoretical development is essential, because theory allows researchers to describe, explain, and predict communication phenomena related to health. As a result, those theories are indicative of behavior change, which in turn have the ability to affect health outcomes.

Quantitizing Talk

Quantitizing refers to a process of content analysis in which researchers gather relevant communication data using qualitative methods and then convert that qualitative information into quantitative data that allows for meaningful comparison of information from one participant to another.[18] For example, sometimes qualitative data such as recordings from provider–patient interactions can be converted into quantitative data to more accurately assess the data based on objective criteria. Quantitizing allows researchers to transform verbal or visual data (e.g., from interviews, videotaped clinical interactions, or clinic notes) into constructs or variables that can be represented numerically and are, therefore, more easily used in comparison across groups.

The result includes numerically represented variables that can be statistically analyzed and compared to other variables because the original dialogue has been transformed into a numerical dataset. These numbers represent the presence or absence of a specific type of information or behavior during the interaction.

Analyzing Audio-Recording Content

For a number of reasons, researchers may use audio-recording devices to obtain data. In certain instances, it may not be appropriate for the researchers to be physically present during an interaction. In other circumstances, researchers may interview participants and record the conversation to preserve the naturalness of the environment and capture the exact context of a given utterance. In order to statistically analyze such data, those recordings must be transcribed and coded into quantifiable data. An example of a study that converted audio recordings into quantitative data examined prognosis communication during palliative care consultations with seriously ill, hospitalized patients.[19] In this study, the researchers audio-recorded patient consultations with physicians. In order to preserve the real situation, digital recorders were placed in unobtrusive locations in patients' hospital rooms. All participants gave written consent for the use of recorders during the interaction.

The use of digital recorders provides many benefits for researchers. First, audio-recordings provide word-for-word accounts of the interaction. Researchers are able to understand the context of specific utterances and are also able to take note of crucial instances of pausing, hesitation, or utterances such as "um" or "uh." Second, the use of digital recorders allows researchers to obtain more genuine data without actually being present in the room during the interaction. Using devices in discrete locations are not as distracting as the presence of the researchers themselves. In addition, the presence of researchers may cause participants to alter their communication behaviors in order to please the researchers.

In this particular study, once the interactions were recorded, the conversations were coded or broken down into quantifiable data. The audio transmissions were coded for speaker (patient, family member, or member of the palliative care team), topic of the prognosis communication (patient's length of life vs. patient's quality of life), focus of the prognosis communication (expectations for population vs. expectations for the individual patient), and affective framing (pessimistic cues [things said or behavior that reflected pessimistic attitudes] vs. optimistic cues). Coding requires multiple trained coders who are able to code transcripts nearly identically. To achieve this, a codebook that provided specific instructions for coding each topic and precise definitions was utilized. Box 49.1 provides an example of such a codebook, and Box 49.2 provides an example of how the coding would be recorded as numerical data.

Based on the significance of statistical tests, the researchers identified key differences between physicians and patients when communicating about a patient's prognosis in palliative care. The researchers were able to report significant findings that providers communicated about prognosis information more frequently than their patients. Information about such differences was uncovered because of quantitative analytical methods. The researchers were able to provide detailed information about this result because of the numbers, which provided statistically significant support for their conclusions.

Analyzing Video-Recording Content

Videotaped clinical interactions can also be quantified by using existing typologies or other coding schemes. Videotaped interactions that employ a standardized patient, someone recruited by the research team to play a patient or family role, can be examined to assess the quality of a training protocol for healthcare students. Standardized patients, primarily used in communication education in nursing and medicine, are provided a script, which allows educators and researchers to maintain consistency across interactions. This quantitative research approach was taken in a research study examining an interaction-based approach to breaking bad news.[20] In this study, medical students were videotaped delivering bad news (regarding a terminal illness) to a standardized patient after completing an instructional unit on a commonly used breaking bad news protocol. Coders watched the video-recorded interactions and coded for each step of the breaking bad news protocol performed by students. To analyze the data, researchers examined the frequency of each step of the protocol employed by students, revealing that several steps of the protocol were not utilized.

E-Health Interventions

The central role of communication in palliative care makes e-health interventions a potentially attractive option for researchers seeking

---

Box 49.1 Sample Code Book for Active Patient Participation Behaviors

Instructions to the coder: Please mark 1 (present) or 2 (not present) on your coding sheet when reviewing the video recordings.

1. **Asking Questions:** Utterances in interrogative form intended to seek information and clarification. Examples:

   What does that medicine do?

   Why does it hurt when I lift my arm?

   When should I get my next checkup?

2. **Expressions of Concern:** Utterances in which the patient expresses worry, anxiety, fear, anger, frustration, and other forms of negative affect or emotions. Examples:

   I'm worried about cancer given my family history.

   I'm afraid this might be something serious.

   I'm so tired of this hurting all the time!

   I didn't like the way that other doctor treated me.

3. **Assertive Responses:** Utterances in which the patient expresses his or her rights, beliefs, interests, and desires as in offering an opinion, making recommendations, making a request, disagreeing, or interrupting. Examples:

   I would like to see if it gets any worse before I think about surgery.

   Could I have a note for my employer?

   Before I go, there's one other thing I want to talk about.

   That's not what I want to do. I'd rather just get a refill of my prescription.

Box 49.2 Sample Data for Code Book in Box 49.1

Study ID Number: _____

Study Variable: Active Patient Participation Behaviors

Use "1" for present and "2" for not present.

1. Asking Questions: _____
2. Expressions of Concern: _____
3. Assertive Responses: _____

to conduct measurements, enhance communication, or increase the availability of palliative care resources and services to patients, caregivers, and healthcare teams in geographically separate locations. E-health has been defined as health services and information that are delivered or enhanced through the Internet and related technologies.[21] A recent review of e-health interventions in palliative care examined studies using integrated technology to deliver patient care.[22] Regarding the effectiveness of e-health, the review found that these interventions in palliative care had results ranging from improved quality of care and improved communication to reduced documentation effort and reduced costs.[22] Quantitative outcomes for system-wide palliative care interventions included data reporting a decrease in the number of hospital admissions by 66%, the number of emergency room visits by 19%, and the number of bed days by 77% after introducing the text messaging and videophone devices to patients in the study.[23]

Conclusion

Quantitative communication research is becoming more prevalent across academic disciplines, across professional roles, and across various types of patient populations. Box 49.3 summarizes journal outlets for publishing health communication research. The popularity of health communication is driven, in part, by the increased realization that communication matters. No matter how many treatment protocols and technological advances are available for treating patients, there is no escaping the essential role of communication in healthcare. As long as patients, family members, and providers need to interact together in the care process, research will be needed on how to maximize communication.

References

1. Keyton J. *Communication Research: Asking Questions, Finding Answers*. New York: McGraw-Hill; 2011.
2. Bullen T, Maher K, Rosenberg JP, Smith B. Establishing research in a palliative care clinical setting: Perceived barriers and implemented strategies. *Appl Nurs Res*. 2014;27:78–83.
3. LeBlanc TW, Lodato JE, Currow DC, Abernethy AP. Overcoming recruitment challenges in palliative care clinical trials. *J Oncol Pract*. 2013;9: 277–282.
4. National Palliative Care Research Center Website. http://www.npcrc.org/ Published 2014.
5. Chan RJ, Phillips J, Currow D. Do palliative care health professionals settle for low-level evidence? *Palliat Med*. 2014;28:8–9.
6. Street R, Tancredi D, Kravitz R, et al. A pathway linking patient participation in cancer consultations to pain control. *Psycho-Oncology*. 2014;23:1111–1117.
7. Cegala D, Bahnson R, Pohar K, et al. Information seeking and satisfaction with physician-patient communication among prostate cancer survivors. *Health Commun*. 2008;23:62–69.
8. Floyd K. Relational and health correlates of affection deprivation. *West J Commun*. 2014;78:383–403.
9. Rhodes RL, Mitchell SL, Miller, SC, Connor SR, Teno JM. Bereaved family members' evaluation of hospice care: What factors influence overall satisfaction with services? *J Pain Symptom Manage*. 2008;35:365–371.
10. Burbeck R, Low J, Sampson E, et al. Volunteers in specialist palliative care: A survey of adult services in the United Kingdom. *J Palliat Med*. 2014;17:568–574.
11. Cockle-Hearne J, Charnay-Sonnek F, Faithfull S, et al. The impact of supportive nursing care on the needs of men with prostate cancer: A study across seven European countries. *Br J Cancer*. 2013;109:2121–2130.
12. Purusothaman V, Ryther RC, Bertrand M. et al. Developing the pediatric refractory epilepsy questionnaire: A pilot study. *Epilepsy Behav*. 2014;37:26–31.
13. Galanos AN, Morris DA, Pieper CF, Poppe-Ries AM, Steinhauser KE. End-of-life care at an academic medical center: Are attending physicians, house staff, nurses, and bereaved family members equally satisfied? Implications for palliative care. *Am J Hosp Palliat Med*. 2012;29:47–52.
14. National Registry of Evidence-Based Programs and Practices Website. http://www.nrepp.samhsa.gov/Index.aspx. Accessed October 21, 2014.
15. Kim H, Suh EE, Lee H, Yang H. The effects of patient participation-based dietary intervention on nutritional and functional status for patients with gastrectomy: A randomized controlled trial. *Cancer Nurs*. 2014;37:E10–E20.
16. Blasé K, Kiser L, Van Dyke M. *The Hexagon Tool: Exploring Context*. Chapel Hill, NC: National Implementation Research Network, FPG Child Development Institute, University of North Carolina at Chapel Hill; 2013.
17. Dy SM, Aslakson R, Wilson RF, et al. *Improving Health Care and Palliative Care for Advanced and Serious Illness. Closing the Quality Gap: Revisiting the State of the Science*. AHRQ Publication No. 12(13)-E014-EF. Rockville, MD: Agency for Healthcare Research and Quality; 2012.
18. Sandelowski M. Combining qualitative and quantitative sampling, data collection, and analysis techniques in mixed-method studies. *Res Nurs Health*. 2000;23:246–255.

Box 49.3 Journal Outlets for Publishing Research in Health Communication

American Journal of Health Behavior
American Journal of Hospice and Palliative Medicine
American Journal of Public Health
Communication and Critical/Cultural Studies
Communication Education
Communication Monographs
Health Communication
Health Education & Behavior
Health Promotion Practice
Human Communication Research
Journal of Applied Communication Research
Journal of Cancer Education
Journal of Clinical Oncology
Journal of Communication in Healthcare
Journal of Health Communication
Journal of Hospice and Palliative Nursing
Journal of International and Intercultural Communication
Journal of Interprofessional Care
Journal of Palliative Medicine
Journal of Psychosocial Oncology
Journal of Research in Interprofessional Practice and Education
Medical Informatics and Decision Making
OMEGA—Journal of Death and Dying
Patient Education and Counseling
Psycho-Oncology
Qualitative Health Research
Qualitative Inquiry
Review of Communication
Seminars in Oncology Nursing
Social Science and Medicine

19. Gramling R, Norton SA, Ladwig S. et al. Direct observation of prognosis communication in palliative care: A descriptive study. *J Pain Symptom Manage.* 2013;45:202–212.
20. Villagran M, Goldsmith J, Wittenberg-Lyles E, Baldwin P. Creating COMFORT: A communication-based model for breaking bad news. *Commun Educ.* 2010;59:220–234.
21. Eysenbach G. What is e-health? *J Med Internet Res.* 2001;3:E20.
22. Capurro D, Ganzinger M, Perez-Lu J, Knaup P. Effectiveness of e-health interventions and information needs in palliative care: A systematic literature review. *J Med Internet Res.* 2014;16:e72.
23. Maudlin J, Keene J, Kobb R. A road map for the last journey: Home telehealth for holistic end-of-life care. *Am J Hosp Palliat Med.* 2006;23:399–403.
24. Petronio S. Communication boundary management: A theoretical model of managing disclosure of private information between marital couples. *Commun Theory.* 1991;1:311–335.
25. Baxter LA, Montgomery BM. *Relating: Dialogues & Dialectics.* New York, NY: Guilford Press; 1996.
26. Burgoon JK., Hale JL. Nonverbal expectancy violations: Model elaboration and application to immediacy behaviors. *Commun Monogr.* 1988;55:58–79.
27. Weick KE. *Sensemaking in Organizations.* Thousand Oaks, CA: SAGE; 1995.
28. Antonovsky A. *Health, Stress, and Coping.* San Francisco, CA: Jossey-Bass; 1979.
29. Fishbein M. A theory of reasoned action: Some applications and implications. *Nebr Symp Motiv.* 1979;27:65–116.

CHAPTER 50

The State of the Science on Palliative Care Communication

Elaine Wittenberg

Introduction

The chapters in this volume summarize the barriers to and benefits of palliative care communication across a variety of contexts, patient and family populations, care settings, diseases, and trajectories. The full range of interdisciplinary authors contributing to this volume all conclude that communication transcends patient and family healthcare experiences. With 60% of Americans aged 67 and older having three or more chronic diseases,[1] palliative care communication is vital to providing quality healthcare. Hospital-based palliative care programs have become a permanent fixture across healthcare settings, and outpatient palliative care continues to expand. Still, limited knowledge about palliative care among patients, families, providers, and the public remains one of the field's biggest challenges.[2,3] Perhaps the most challenging misperception of palliative care is that it is synonymous with end-of-life care and hospice, that it is only for dying patients, and that it is synonymous with a reduction in care services.[4]

Palliative care's "identity problem"[5] directly impacts consumer access and, as pointed out in chapter 4, there is a need for a public education campaign.[4] In part, the difficulty in understanding the meaning of palliative care services is due to the use of inconsistent language and terms such as "supportive care" and "comfort care."[6] Defining the palliative care patient population also causes ambiguity, with terms such as "serious illness" or "advanced illness" often creating further confusion.[7] These linguistic differences only highlight the importance of palliative care communication and the provider's ability to describe, define, and explain the difference between palliative care and hospice to patients, families, colleagues, and consumers.[5,8]

Palliative care providers are often considered communication experts by their colleagues, and there are high expectations for quality communication when a palliative care provider is consulted for a patient and family. There has always been a deep connection between communication and palliative care, as detailed in chapter 2, and the unique emphasis on communication skills has long separated palliative care providers from other healthcare professionals. This reputation and expectation for communication expertise, coupled with findings in this volume depicting the burgeoning area of palliative care communication, suggest that palliative care's identity problem may soon be fully articulated in healthcare. For palliative care and its practitioners, this is a period of reflection, analysis, and exploration in order to define and practice excellence in palliative communication.[9,10] Palliative care is recognized as a leader in clinical communication, and it is now time to establish delivery structures and communication content to further shape the field.

Of primary concern to hospital administrators and policymakers is research on the effectiveness of palliative care demonstrating better patient and caregiver outcomes; it is vital that this research account for core communication variables in the delivery of palliative care. An overview of randomized controlled trials (RCT) on palliative care (Table 50.1), comprising the evidence base for palliative care concurrent with standard care, demonstrates the incongruity of communication structures and practices between studies. Notably, not all RCTs included an interdisciplinary palliative care team,[11] with interventions varying from counseling to a nursing education intervention. Variance in the palliative care communication interventions among these studies includes a lack of details about the disciplines represented, the role and involvement of family caregivers, the scope of topics discussed, and the provision of written materials in addition to oral, face-to-face sessions. As this volume demonstrates, palliative care communication is broad and includes language (chapter 4), culture (chapter 11), relationships (chapter 3), and variety of platforms/channels for communication, including one on one and one to many (chapter 13).

In order to promote effectiveness research on palliative care teams, studies need to include the structures and processes of team-based care and identify standards for such structures and processes. This research is especially important since interdisciplinary teams vary radically in performance.[12] Comparisons to usual care are inconclusive if we cannot account for structural and procedural factors contributing to team performance in a communication intervention.[13] While the effectiveness of palliative care services can be demonstrated, the specific communication characteristics (e.g., communication interventions, timing of the intervention, topics discussed, placement in care trajectory, team composite, interpersonal approaches, etc.) remain

Table 50.1 Overview of RCTs on Palliative Care and Communication

RCT Study on Palliative Care	Palliative Care Communication in the Intervention
Temel et al[33]	♦ Palliative care team comprised of six physicians and one nurse ♦ Average initial consultation (averaging 55 minutes) by one member of the team ♦ Initial consultation addressed patient and family coping (averaging 15 minutes) and education about illness (averaging 10 minutes)
Pantilat et al[34]	♦ Provided by single MD
Rabow et al[35]	♦ Comprised of seven components, including assessment and referral for quality of life domains, advance care planning ♦ Physicians rarely directly interviewed or examined the patient ♦ Psychological care provided via telephone by social worker ♦ Family caregiver training and support provided by nurse ♦ Support groups offered and facilitated
Brumley et al[36]	♦ Goals of care conversations ♦ Provided by physician, nurse, social worker team, with chaplain services referred to as needed ♦ Advance care planning provided
Gade et al[37]	♦ Delivered by palliative care team comprised of all four core disciplines ♦ Patients only ♦ Goals of care conversations, included advance directive forms ♦ If appropriate, patient/family meetings were part of consultation
Bakitas et al[38]	♦ Intervention delivered by advanced practice nurses ♦ Four weekly educational sessions (averaging 41–30 minutes) with patients and at least monthly telephone follow-up ♦ Patients and caregivers could attend shared medical appointments with physician and nurse practitioner
Meyers et al[39]	♦ Intervention delivered by trained educators (discipline unknown) ♦ Patient and caregiver dyads participated in intervention ♦ Intervention consisted of face-to-face sessions plus written booklet as resource
Zimmerman et al[11]	♦ Physician and nurse consultation ♦ Patient only ♦ Routine telephone contact follow-up by nurse ♦ Monthly outpatient follow-up (average 20–50 minutes)

Note: RCT = randomized controlled trial.

unknown. The goal of this final chapter of the volume is to provide a summary and analysis of palliative care communication, explore the state of the science, and offer future direction for moving the field forward.

Measuring Effectiveness

One of the primary goals of palliative care communication research is to demonstrate the effectiveness of communication interventions (e.g., family meetings, consultations about goals of care, transitions in care conversation, and shared decision-making). The Institute of Medicine prioritizes the need to establish standards for palliative care communication that are measurable, actionable, and evidence based.[2] However, effectiveness measurement in the field of palliative care has been challenging, with inconsistencies existing in quality measurement and communication viewed as a palliative care domain that is difficult to measure.[14]

Considered an aspect of quality care, communication is primarily measured as satisfaction with the care experience.[13] In a values-based program, approximately 30% of a hospital's incentive payment is based on the patient care experience, assessed through the Hospital Consumer Assessment of Healthcare Providers and Systems. Four of the eight dimensions of the Patient Experience of Care domain measure communication: communication with physicians, communication with nurses, communication about medication, and discharge information. Within the values-based program, communication with nurses can account for up to 15% of values-based program payments.[15]

The National Quality Forum has recommended 14 measures for palliative and end-of-life care. Two of the 14 measures aim to assess communication. Namely, the Family Evaluation of Hospice Care and Consumer Assessments and Reports of End of Life Care assess the perception of the quality of care and rating for quality of care.[16] While the survey items do assess family information needs and wants, primarily related to physical care, the measures are mortality follow-back surveys intended to assess information provision at the end of life. This approach excludes any assessment of hospital-based or community-based outpatient palliative care and upstream communication needs and preferences during decision-making, prognosis, treatment, and disease trajectories that may include survivorship. In essence, survey items do not provide an accurate measure of the quality of communication in palliative care.

Cancer patients and families report that questions written specifically for the assessment of communication experiences cover content that is not routinely included in satisfaction surveys.[17] In fact, patient satisfaction measures do not include assessment of the process, purpose, or goal of communication. Questions are typically stated as: How do you rate the hospital overall? How do you rate your overall satisfaction? How do you rate your satisfaction with care? Chapter 29 offers a more detailed way of examining patient-centered communication with specific measurable behaviors. Communication preferences and needs can vary among and between patients and families, as detailed in chapters 16, 17, and 18, pointing to the need to explore communication-based outcomes of both patients and family members.

Having established the benefit and satisfaction of palliative care services, it is time for researchers to develop a standardized measure of patient/family satisfaction that is grounded in communication. Figure 50.1 provides an excellent example of how to measure the core functions of patient-centered communication as part of patient satisfaction assessment.[17] Communication strategies and interventions should be designed to include these behaviors rather than measuring perception of quality of care or satisfaction with care.[14] Research should aim to validate and document the benefits

Please mark the extent to which the following statements accurately describe *your* experience with *members of the palliative care team* who talked with you about *your* care				
Members of the Palliative Care Team...	To A Great Extent	Somewhat	Very Little	Not At All
...helped me understand my treatment choices.	○	○	○	○
...listened to my views on what was most important to me in my cancer treatment.	○	○	○	○
...encouraged me to express my views about my treatment.	○	○	○	○
...took my views into account in recommending my cancer treatment.	○	○	○	○
...treated me with sensitivity and respect.	○	○	○	○
...gave me the information that I needed at that time.	○	○	○	○

*Items based on the six core functions of patient-centered communication
*Adapted from: Mazor KM, Gaglio B, Nekhlyudov L, et al. Assessing patient-centered communication in cancer care: stakeholder perspectives. *J Oncol Pract*. Sep 2013;9(5): e186–193.a

Figure 50.1 Sample patient satisfaction assessment measuring communication

of palliative communication[18] and include an operationalization of communication variables (e.g., people, messages, channels, context) as part of data collection and analysis. This could include such things as testing the relationship between the number of family meetings and goals of care conversations and patient/family level of anxiety; physician-nurse delivery of life-altering information and physician-only delivery of information on patient/family understanding; use of responsive listening behaviors with team members and impact on perception of teamwork; impact of family mediation on family comprehension of level of care; association between how a patient communicates with his or her support network and providers and utilization of supportive care services; gender differences on treatment preferences and information preferences; patient/family perception of feedback topics when participating in a healthcare team meeting; or patterns of communication within disease-specific populations. Chapters 27, 31, and 38 reveal that no interventions or assessments can be accurate without recognizing and including the pivotal role of family members in palliative care communication.

Communication Education

With the introduction of palliative care into mainstream hospital systems over the past decade, there also has been an increase in attention to communication education for healthcare professionals.[19] Approaches to communication education have included clinical observation of mentors and real-time practice in order to learn skills,[20] with more recent development of formal curriculum. Chapters 6 through 10 summarize the pivotal communication roles and responsibilities of key palliative care providers and offer a first step toward outlining standards for training. Collectively, chapters 43 to 46 reveal that patient simulation and interprofessional education have emerged in healthcare programs to teach palliative care communication. Simulated-based communication training in one study was found to improve learners' communication skills, knowledge, confidence, and overall performance; however, when learners engaged patients and families following training, no significant changes to patient- and family-reported outcomes of quality of communication or quality of end-of-life care were found.[21] Furthermore, the study found no improvement in patient outcomes. This demonstrates the remaining knowledge gap between better training and the impact of training on patient and family outcomes. Specifically, chapter 47 suggests that interprofessional education is the key to better training. All of the chapters in this volume highlight the need for communication education to include self-reflection of biases (see chapters 28, 36, and 37), the ways that experiences influence approach or avoidance, and the ways that these perspectives impact communication skills performance.

New models of palliative care education and training are needed to advance the field.[4] Six of the eight recommendations for training and career developing in palliative care[22] involve communication: offer communication workshops to develop core curricula, promote institutional communication training to increase knowledge about palliative care, teach fellows how to conduct communication research, collaborate with communication researchers, mentor outside the discipline and include social sciences and humanities, and identify key communication research needs. Importantly, given that team-based care is foundational to palliative care, professional education and development should include all healthcare profession students in order to expand awareness of palliative care and increase knowledge among all providers.[2] Chapters on team communication presented in this volume (chapters 39–42) highlight how setting influences team processes.

While the philosophical underpinnings of palliative care position all team members to be competent in their ability to engage patient/family in any type of communication intervention—ranging from goals of care conversations to providing spiritual support—communication education has been predominantly physician-focused. The American Academy of Hospice and Palliative Medicine has established hospice and palliative medicine competencies for physicians that include interpersonal and communication skills to be assessed by the attending physician, peer assessment, and self-assessment.[23] These advances in medical education are very encouraging. A recent study aimed at developing generalist-level palliative care competencies for medical students and residents placed communication skills among the most critical domains of proposed palliative care competencies.[8] Specific attention to using patient-centered techniques when giving bad news, exploring patient and family understanding of illness, and engaging in shared decision-making were identified as most important for medical students and residents.

The majority of curricular work in palliative care communication has similarly come from medicine, which implicitly suggests that the physician is primarily responsible for all communication tasks ranging from sharing life-altering news to handling family meetings to discussing transitions in care. Remaining team members in nursing, social work, and chaplaincy are often not mentioned or are depicted only in supporting communication roles. While improving physician communication is undoubtedly of utmost importance, real progress depends on enhanced communication for all disciplines. The fields of nursing, social work, and chaplaincy have not established communication competencies for their palliative communication roles, and they have little or sporadic exposure to communication education in their professional preparation. Available curriculum is often limited to a few topics such as how to give information; this volume expands palliative care communication by summarizing challenging discussions about psychological issues (chapter 9), social issues (chapters 25 and 33), and spiritual issues (chapters 31 and 37). Healthcare profession educators have received minimal preparation or resources to teach communication—the goal of this volume is to serve as a pioneering text for explicating communication processes and to serve as a clinical guide in teaching palliative communication.

Communication education should include development and testing of a standardized communication curriculum, development and assessment of core communication competencies for all core disciplines, established communication practice standards for palliative care teams, formalized preparation for health profession educators to teach communication, extended pedagogical approaches beyond didactic teaching, and an intentional effort to address the culture of care so that communication skills are valued.[4] To prepare the future workforce, palliative communication education needs to be interdisciplinary in scope and include methodologically rigorous research to build an evidence base for quality practice.[22] We have included chapters on qualitative communication research (chapter 48) and quantitative communication research (chapter 49) to facilitate development of these skills. Infrastructure to promote quality communication education to address difficult-to-reach populations and disparities in palliative care as well as research methods to conduct studies on communication interventions, decision-making, and advance care planning are needed. While it has been noted that there are few programs to train junior investigators in palliative care research,[22] programs are also needed that provide mentoring for educators, clinicians, and researchers of palliative care communication.

Designing Communication Interventions

Specific attention to the design of communication interventions thus far has focused on advance care planning and family meetings. These two areas of practice are prime targets for the field to model improved care. This volume includes two chapters devoted to advance care planning (chapters 24 and 35). Research shows there is room for improvement in both of these areas of practice. Family conferences, while shown to be effective and beneficial to families in the intensive care unit setting, have not demonstrated an impact in oncology/palliative medicine settings.[24] Advance care planning, a component of palliative care closely linked to communication, was assessed in five of the RCT studies (Table 50.1), with two studies finding no difference, two reporting an increase in documentation, and one with nonsignificant results. One reason for these study results has been the focus on care structure and the logistical arrangements and documentation of the communication.

To move the field forward, we need to focus on quality communication strategies and processes within these and other communication interventions. How do we ensure that advance care planning material is written in a manner that is easy to read, understand, and access? How can we change delivery structures so that family meetings include the presence and participation of all palliative care team members? To what extent can we provide visual and audio communication support to assist in patient and family decision-making? What steps can be taken to help providers use plain language and simple terms when explaining diagnosis, treatment, or the dying process to patients and families? How can the explanation of palliative care occur early in the course of a disease process instead of later?

Quality communication interventions are dependent upon practice and payment incentives, as providers continue to be concerned with the time it takes to have clinical conversations and current billing systems have minimal channels to account for this.[4] Advances in communication technology will likely impact the design of future communication interventions. For example, a recent study on Medigram, a HIPAA-compliant application for smartphones that facilitates group messaging, found group messaging more effective than one-way pagers for team communication and integration into workflow during rounds and patient discharge.[20] Incentive changes are necessary to promote learning communication strategies and the use of interactive tools for decision-support and team communication.

Likewise, the design and evaluation of a specific communication intervention (such as a question prompt list for patient use prior to a clinical visit, use of a pamphlet or video to aid family decision-making, or structured protocol for sharing information) should address communication function and anticipated functional outcomes of communication. Communication functions, related skills, and functional outcomes have been outlined by Street and De Haes[25] in accordance with the patient-centered communication framework and provide an evidence-based guide for the design of communication research in palliative care.

Communicating With Tomorrow's Patient

Increasing cancer prevalence, rising numbers of cancer survivors, and newly insured patients entering the healthcare system[26] intensify the demand for palliative care. There are more than 170 Food and Drug Administration–approved anti-cancer drugs, whereas 50 years ago there were only a handful of hard-to-tolerate cancer treatment options.[26] Advances over the next 20 years are expected to be more rapid than those of the past five decades, with incentives for treatment and novel therapies causing an increase in costs and resulting in more complex cancer care.[26] As healthcare becomes individualized and personalized, there will be a need for more data, more tools, and new technology. In-home care settings will become commonplace, mobile clinician communication will be standardized, oral administration of new medicines will be prioritized, and there will be new challenges in educating and communicating with family caregivers about treatment adherence and side effects. Similar advances have occurred in cardiac, pulmonary, and renal disease, in which treatments have become more complex and care far more prolonged. For palliative care, this also means expanding communication intervention development to include communicate protocols for communicating life support and artificial hydration (chapter 34) and addressing the unique needs of the homeless and mentally ill (chapter 25) as well as veteran populations (chapter 26).

The 2014 Institute of Medicine report on end-of-life care emphasizes that improvement is needed in engaging patients and families in shared decision-making and advance care planning.[2] Four of the 10 recommendations for improved quality care include communication:

♦ Provide patients and their families with understandable information about cancer prognosis, treatment benefits and harms, psychosocial support, and costs.

♦ Provide patients with end-of-life care that meets their needs, values, and preferences.

♦ Ensure coordinated and comprehensive patient-centered care.

♦ Ensure that all individuals caring for cancer patients have appropriate core competencies.

Within the past 5 years, patient priorities have shifted from "promptness in responding to the call button" to effective communication, empathy, and relationship-building as the top three inpatient concerns.[27] Healthcare reform has prompted changes toward value-based payment models, including a provision for children to receive hospice and curative care simultaneously. The Joint Commission initiated an Advanced Certification Program in Palliative Care in 2011 emphasizing "processes which support the coordination of care and communication among all care settings and providers."[28] The focus is now clearly on the quality and cost of care;[6] the challenge for palliative care is to provide quality communication interventions that result in lower healthcare costs.

Integrated Palliative Care Communication

The integration of palliative care across the continuum of care has been emphasized by the World Health Organization[3] and the Institute of Medicine.[2] The integrated care model of palliative care posits that communication should take place incrementally, with conversations about this care occurring over the trajectory of a disease process, allowing patients and family members to explore the meaning of illness and its impact, as well as psychologically manage the diagnosis and prognosis. Engaging in these conversations early, prior to high symptom burden and management, also prioritizes the caregiver's role and quality of life in the palliative care trajectory.[29] Open and continuous communication should occur through frequent conversations with patient and family and should begin at any age or state of health.[2]

Currently, family meetings, breaking bad news (which I prefer phrased as "sharing life-altering information"[30]), goals of care, and transition in care conversations are the recognized palliative care communication interventions, with communication education detailing approaches to initiate these conversations. However, not all communication skills taught in a curriculum are applicable for every patient/family visit.[31] Placement in the

Table 50.2 Integrated Palliative Care Communication

Disease Trajectory	Communication Objective	Patient/Family Decision Point[a]
Diagnosis	♦ Explain the diagnosis ♦ Explain treatment options (including the option of no treatment) ♦ Discuss advance care planning	Selecting a surrogate and other advance care planning decisions
Treatment	♦ Address and assess quality of life domains ♦ Address and assess patient/family values and needs ♦ Address caregiver needs for home care	Treatment choices when cure is not possible Whether to be admitted to ICU and receive life-prolonging treatments or to focus on comfort care
Survivorship	♦ Address and assess quality of life domains ♦ Address and assess patient values and needs ♦ Address psychosocial care such as sexuality	Selecting a surrogate and other advance care planning decisions
End-of Life-Care	♦ Explain the diagnosis, if applicable ♦ Address and assess quality of life domains ♦ Explain dying process and natural death ♦ Inquire about cultural beliefs and rituals	Selecting a surrogate and other advance care planning decisions Where to receive end-of-life care

[a] Bakitas M, Kryworuchko J, Matlock DD, Volandes AE. Palliative medicine and decision science: The critical need for a shared agenda to foster informed patient choice in serious illness. J Palliat Med. 2011;14(10):1–8.

> **Box 50.1** Development and Assessment of Palliative Care Communication Interventions
>
> - What are the components of the palliative care communication intervention?
> - How does the intervention address the needs of the family/caregiver?
> - What is the purpose of the communication in the intervention?
> - What are the expected communication outcomes of the interaction?
> - Are written materials included?
> - Is the intervention tailored to meet individual needs?
> - When is the intervention implemented?
> - Is there follow-up or reinforcement of the intervention?
> - Are visual aids used?
> - Does the intervention go beyond basic decisions (e.g., advance directives) to address psychosocial or spiritual concerns?
> - How are various disciplines included?

> **Box 50.2** Opportunities for Advancing Palliative Care Communication
>
> - Outline the tenets of palliative care communication
> - Define the characteristics of palliative care communication across the disease trajectory
> - Draft utilization guidelines and detail who should adopt these guidelines and why
> - Write policies to establish structure and financing for palliative care communication
> - Create communication education guidelines for healthcare providers practicing palliative care
> - Develop and offer communication training for volunteers
> - Establish research networks to share effective models for the delivery of communication interventions
> - Publish details on communication education curricula, details on protocols for communication interventions, and effectiveness of decision support aids

disease trajectory influences communication approaches within conversations, the framing of the conversation, and emphasis on different communication objectives. Palliative settings vary in degree and scope, with different trajectories of disease, diagnosis, and prognosis and different demands on decision-making. Patients and family members report that any assessment of communication experiences should include the type of cancer, treatment, and prognosis, as it impacts experiences.[17] Moreover, the relational dimensions of provider–patient–family caregiver communication dramatically influences communication quality and content.[19]

Frequent conversations are needed across the disease trajectory, as patients and families engage in a variety of decision points.[2,32] As Table 50.1 depicts, integrated palliative care communication requires attention to the patient's placement in the disease trajectory, articulation of specific communication objectives provided using patient-centered communication strategies, and identification of specific decision points as communication outcomes. Longitudinal discussions of prognosis should begin in the outpatient setting as well.[29] Box 50.1 offers several questions to guide development and assessment of communication interventions across the disease trajectory. Patients, families, and clinicians all agree that measuring communication is important.[17] Box 50.2 summarizes opportunities for advancing palliative care communication.

Conclusion

As recognized experts in communication within healthcare systems, palliative care providers are positioned to define quality communication in healthcare. Future work is needed to outline objectives and competency guidelines for palliative care communication across different settings and disease-specific trajectories. Organizations such as the American Academy of Hospice and Palliative Medicine, Healthcare Chaplaincy, Hospice and Palliative Nurse Association, and the Social Work Palliative Network could offer a powerfully supportive voice in this effort. The editors and authors of this text represent an international cadre of professionals deeply committed to advancing communication as an essential element of quality palliative care. The intent of this first *Textbook of Palliative Care Communication* is to provide a roadmap for the journey ahead.

References

1. DuGoff EH, Canudas-Romo V, Buttorff C, Leff B, Anderson GF. Multiple chronic conditions and life expectancy: A life table analysis. *Med Care*. August 2014;52(8):688–694.
2. Institute of Medicine. *Dying in America: Improving Quality and Honoring Individual Preferences Near the End of Life*. Washington, DC: Institute of Medicine of the National Academies; 2014.
3. World Health Organization. Strengthening of palliative care as a component of integrated treatment throughout the life course. *J Pain Palliat Care Pharmacother*. Jun 2014;28(2):130–134.
4. Hutchinson C. The state of palliative care in the US. *Clin Oncol News*. June 2014;9(6). Accessed June 16, 2015, http://www.clinicaloncology.com/ViewArticle.aspx?d=Current+Practice&d_id=155&i=June+2014&i_id=1070&a_id=27639
5. Parikh RB, Kirch RA, Smith TJ, Temel JS. Early specialty palliative care—translating data in oncology into practice. *N Engl J Med*. December 12, 2013;369(24):2347–2351.
6. Fletcher DS, Panke JT. Improving value in healthcare: Opportunities and challenges for palliative care professionals in the age of health reform. *J Hosp Palliat Nurs*. 2012;14(7):452–461.
7. Sinclair C. Increasing palliative care awareness: The 2011 CAPC public opinion research. http://www.pallimed.org/2011/06/increasing-palliative-care-awareness.html. Published June 29, 2011. Access date: June 16, 2015.
8. Schaefer KG, Chittenden EH, Sullivan AM, et al. Raising the bar for the care of seriously ill patients: Results of a national survey to define essential palliative care competencies for medical students and residents. *Acad Med*. July 2014;89(7):1024–1031.
9. Erikson EH. *Childhood and Society*. New York, NY: W.W. Norton; 1993 (Orignally published 1950)

10. Erikson EH. *Identity: Youth and Crisis.* New York, NY: W.W. Norton; 1968.
11. Zimmermann C, Swami N, Krzyzanowska M, et al. Early palliative care for patients with advanced cancer: A cluster-randomised controlled trial. *Lancet.* 2014;383(9930):1721–1730.
12. Fine P, Davis M, Muir J. An evaluation of time and cost variability in hospice interdisciplinary group meetings and comparative clinical quality outcomes. *J Hosp Palliat Nurs.* 2014;16(7):414–419.
13. Wen J, Schulman KA. Can team-based care improve patient satisfaction? A systematic review of randomized controlled trials. *PLoS One.* 2014;9(7):e100603.
14. Dy S. Measuring the quality of palliative care and supportive oncology: Principles and practice. *J Support Oncol.* 2013;11:160–164.
15. Press Ganey Associates. *The Rising Tide Measure: Communication With Nurses.* Boston: Press Ganey; 2013.
16. National Quality Forum. Endorsement summary: Palliative care and end-of-life care measures. http://www.qualityforum.org/projects/palliative_care_and_end-of-life_care.aspx. Published February 2012.
17. Mazor KM, Gaglio B, Nekhlyudov L, et al. Assessing patient-centered communication in cancer care: Stakeholder perspectives. *J Oncol.* September 2013;9(5):e186–e193.
18. El-Jawahri A, Greer JA, Temel JS. Does palliative care improve outcomes for patients with incurable illness? A review of the evidence. *J Support Oncol.* May-June 2011;9(3):87–94.
19. De Vries AM, de Roten Y, Meystre C, Passchier J, Despland JN, Stiefel F. Clinician characteristics, communication, and patient outcome in oncology: A systematic review. *Psycho-Oncology.* April 2014;23(4):375–381.
20. Przybylo JA, Wang A, Loftus P, Evans KH, Chu I, Shieh L. Smarter hospital communication: Secure smartphone text messaging improves provider satisfaction and perception of efficacy, workflow. *J Hospital Med.* September 2014;9(9):573–578.
21. Curtis JR, Back AL, Ford DW, et al. Effect of communication skills training for residents and nurse practitioners on quality of communication with patients with serious illness: A randomized trial. *JAMA.* 2013;310(21):2271–2281.
22. Aziz NM, Grady PA, Curtis JR. Training and career development in palliative care and end-of-life research: Opportunities for development in the U.S. *J Pain Symptom Manage.* December 2013;46(6):938–946.
23. Sanchez-Reilly S, Ross JS. Hospice and palliative medicine: Curriculum evaluation and learner assessment in medical education. *J Palliat Med.* January 2012;15(1):116–122.
24. Powazki R, Walsh D, Hauser K, Davis MP. Communication in palliative medicine: A clinical review of family conferences. *J Palliat Med.* 2014;17(10):1167–1677.
25. Street RL Jr, De Haes HC. Designing a curriculum for communication skills training from a theory and evidence-based perspective. *Patient Educ Couns.* October 2013;93(1):27–33.
26. American Society of Clinical Oncology. The state of cancer care in America, 2014. http://jop.ascopubs.org/content/early/2014/03/10/JOP.2014.001386. Published 2014.
27. Press Ganey Associates. *Hospital Pulse Report 2009: Patient Perspectives on American Health Care.* Boston: Press Ganey; 2009.
28. Joint Commission. Advanced Certification Program for Palliative Care. http://www.jointcommission.org/certification/palliative_care.aspx.
29. Ritchie CS. Ushering in an era of community-based palliative care. *J Palliat Med.* August 2013;16(8):818–819.
30. Wolfe AD, Frierdich SA, Wish J, Kilgore-Carlin J, Plotkin JA, Hoover-Regan M. Sharing life-altering information: Development of pediatric hospital guidelines and team training. *J Palliat Med.* September 2014;17(9):1011–1018.
31. Fettig L. Dismiss simulation for palliative medicine communication training? Not so fast. http://www.pallimed.org/2013/12/dismiss-simulation-for-palliative.html. Published December 23, 2013.
32. Bakitas M, Kryworuchko J, Matlock DD, Volandes AE. Palliative medicine and decision science: The critical need for a shared agenda to foster informed patient choice in serious illness. *J Palliat Med.* October 2011;14(10):1109–1116.
33. Temel JS, Greer JA, Muzikansky A, et al. Early palliative care for patients with metastatic non-small-cell lung cancer. *N Engl J Med.* August 19, 2010;363(8):733–742.
34. Pantilat SZ, O'Riordan DL, Dibble SL, Landefeld CS. Hospital-based palliative medicine consultation: A randomized controlled trial. *Arch Intern Med.* December 13, 2010;170(22):2038–2040.
35. Rabow MW, Dibble SL, Pantilat SZ, McPhee SJ. The comprehensive care team: A controlled trial of outpatient palliative medicine consultation. *Arch Intern Med.* January 12, 2004;164(1):83–91.
36. Brumley R, Enguidanos S, Jamison P, et al. Increased satisfaction with care and lower costs: Results of a randomized trial of in-home palliative care. *J Am Geriatr Soc.* July 2007;55(7):993–1000.
37. Gade G, Venohr I, Conner D, et al. Impact of an inpatient palliative care team: A randomized control trial. *J Palliat Med.* 2008;11(2):180–190.
38. Bakitas M, Lyons KD, Hegel MT, et al. Effects of a palliative care intervention on clinical outcomes in patients with advanced cancer: The Project ENABLE II randomized controlled trial. *JAMA.* 2009;302(7):741–749.
39. Meyers FJ, Carducci M, Loscalzo MJ, Linder J, Greasby T, Beckett LA. Effects of a problem-solving intervention (COPE) on quality of life for patients with advanced cancer on clinical trials and their caregivers: Simultaneous care educational intervention (SCEI): linking palliation and clinical trials. *J Palliat Med.* April 2011;14(4):465–473.

Index

Page numbers followed by "b," "f," and "t" indicate boxes, figures, and tables.

ABCDE model, 379t
Absent grief, 312
Access, 91, 96, 156
Accreditation Council for Graduate Medical Education (ACGME), 355
Acculturation, 156
ACHP-SW. *See* Advanced Certified Hospice and Palliative Social Worker
ACP. *See* Advance care planning
Acting model of role-play, 393
Activation, 243
ACTIVE intervention, 341
Active listening, 64, 357–358
Acute care team communication
 barriers to, 327
 families, patients and, 324–326
 improving, 327
 overview of, 321–322, 327–328
 strategies for, 322–324
AD. *See* Advance directives
Adaptive responses, 217
Addiction, 265–266, 267t. *See also* Drug-addicted patients
Administration on Aging Long-Term Ombudsman Programs, 346
Adolescents, 223, 226. *See also* Pediatric palliative care communication
Advance care planning (ACP)
 adolescents and, 201
 barriers and enablers to effective discussions, 290–292
 conversation through process of, 285–286
 decision-maker appointment and, 286
 decision-support tools for, 289, 290b
 discussion points for, 286–289, 288–289t
 HIV/AIDS and, 197, 202b
 interpersonal communication theories and, 197–198
 lesbian, gay, bisexual, and transgender individuals and, 230–231
 nurses and, 58–59
 outpatient care setting and, 337
 overview of, 285, 292
 social work and, 36, 40
 strategies for communication, 286, 287–289t
 written plans and, 286
Advance Care Planning Australia, 287t
Advanced Certification Program in Palliative Care, 421

Advanced Certified Hospice and Palliative Social Worker (ACHP-SW), 380
Advance directives (AD)
 disparities in use of, 113
 health literacy and, 91, 93
 Jehovah's Witnesses and, 259
 lesbian, gay, bisexual, and transgender individuals and, 230–231
 nursing communication and, 58
 nursing homes and, 347–348
"Advance Directives" (Project Grace), 58
Advancing Effective Communication, Cultural Competence, and patient- and Family-Centered Care- A Roadmap for Hospitals (TJC), 101
Advancing Excellence in Nursing Homes, 346
Affect, 17
Affirmation, 224
Affordable Care Act, 139, 246, 390–391
Afghanistan War veterans, 215–216, 217
Agency, 28
Agent Orange, 215
Aging in place, 347
Aging with Dignity, 58
AHRQ Health Literacy Universal Precautions Toolkit, 101
AIDS. *See* HIV/AIDS, people living with
Albom, Mitch, 17
Alcohol abuse, 208t. *See also* Drug-addicted patients
"Allow-Natural-Death (AND) and Other Orders" (Schlairet and Cohen), 283
Allow natural death orders, 58
Almost real-life category of role-play, 393
ALS. *See* Amyotrophic lateral sclerosis
Alternative medicine, 271–274
AMEN model, 68, 256, 259b
American Academy of Hospice and Palliative Medicine, 24t, 87, 420
American Cancer Society, 24t, 25, 123t
American Cancer Society Action Network, 24t, 25f, 26f
American Childhood Cancer Organization, 24t
American Heart Association, 26f
American Liver Foundation, 122t
American Medical Association, 101
American Nurses Association, 54
American Society of Addiction Medicine, 265

American Society of Clinical Oncology, 24t, 122t
American Stroke Association, 26f
Amitrityline, 268t
Amyotrophic lateral sclerosis (ALS), 215
Ancestry, 155t. *See also* Cultural considerations
Anglican Retirement Villages, 351
Anticipatory grief, 313, 314, 316–319
Anticipatory guidance, 224
Antonovsky, Aaron, 130
APPEAL tool, 201
Artificial intelligence, 124
Artificial nutrition and hydration
 building end-of-life plans and, 281, 282t
 decision-making burden and, 281–282
 fundamental science of, 276–277
 holistic approach to care and, 278–279
 illness prognosis and, 277, 277t
 overview of, 276, 283
 previous provider experiences and, 282–283
 provider-driven vs. patient-directed healthcare and, 279–281
 removal of, 278
 signs and symptoms and, 277–278
 social work and, 41
Asbestos exposure, 214
Asking Questions Can Help, 337b
Ask-Tell-Ask tool, 173–174, 175t, 176, 177, 178, 358
Assessment
 clinical psychologists and, 72–73
 family caregiving and, 139, 140t
 spirituality and, 304t, 305
Assurance Wireless, 209
Atomic bombs, 214
Atrocity stories, 343
Attentive listening, 31
ATTUNE acronym, 280, 281b
Audio technology, 93, 413–414. *See also* Technology
Auditory learning, 57
Autonomy, 28–29, 277

Backstage communication, 19
Bar graphs, 94
BATHE model, 17
Battlemind, 216
Bearing, Vivian, 17

Beatitudes Campus, 351
Beavin, Janet, 15
Beneficence, 28–29
Bereavement. *See also* Grief reactions
 anticipatory grief, 314, 316–319
 classification of, 313
 complicated, 314–315
 depression and, 315
 disenfranchised grief and, 315
 framework for understanding, 311–313, 312b
 loss and, 313–314
 noncomplicated, 314
 overview of, 311
 palliative social work and, 40
 plans of care and, 316–319
 self-awareness and, 315–316
Bias, 115
Biomedical model of medicine, 238
Biopsychosocial model of medicine, 238
The Birth of the Clinic (Foucault), 129
Bisexual individuals. *See* Lesbian, gay, bisexual and transgender individuals
BMT. *See* Bone marrow transplantation
BODE Index, 179, 179t
Body mapping, 296
Boisen, Anton, 383
Bone marrow transplantation (BMT), 193–194
Bowker, John, 63
BPI. *See* Brief Pain Inventory
Bracketing, 403
BREAKS protocol, 372t, 379t
Bridging the Gap curriculum, 85b
Brief Pain Inventory (BPI), 264
Briefs, 349–350
Broyard, Anatole, 128–129
Burnout, 76–77

Cabot, Richard, 383
Calgary-Cambridge Observational Guide, 362
California State University Institute for Palliative Care, 77
Call-outs, 350
CAM. *See* Complementary and alternative medicine
Cambia Health Foundation, 3
CAM-Cancer, 273t
Canadian Hospice Palliative Care Association, 287t
Canadian Virtual Hospital, 287t
Cancer. *See* Oncology
Cancer board meetings, 335–336
CancerPEN, 380
Cancer Survivorship and Agency Model (CSAM), 28
Cancer Terms Pro, 151t
Can't We Talk About Something More Pleasant? (Chast), 1, 2f
"Capturing the Heart" exercise, 387, 387b
Cardiac transplantation, 191–192
Care conferences, 225
Caregiver Competence Scale (CCS), 140t
Caregivers. *See also* Family caregiving
 anticipatory grief in, 314
 health literacy and, 92–93
 impacts of caregiving on, 137–138
 types of, 148–150, 148t
Caregiver support, 92
"Caregiving in the U.S." (NAC), 137
CareSearch, 50t
CareZone, 151t

CaringBridge, 151t
Carrier caregivers, 148, 148f, 148t
Case managers, transitions in care and, 249t
Case vignettes, 378t
CCS. *See* Caregiver Competence Scale
Cell phones, 209
Centers for Disease Control and Prevention, 100
Center to Advance Palliative Care, 23, 23b, 24t, 154, 212, 372t
Center to Advance Palliative Care 2011 Public Opinion Research on Palliative Care, 23, 23b
Centrifugal force, 19
Centripetal force, 19
Certified Hospice and Palliative Social Worker (CHP-SW), 380
Change agents, nurses as, 60
Chaplaincy care, 66f, 66t
Chaplaincy communication
 background of education for, 383–385
 current educational practices for, 385–388
 definition problem and, 65–66, 66t
 emergence of chaplaincy as profession and, 65
 emerging best practice and, 67–68
 hope, denial and, 258
 interdisciplinary teams and, 68
 overview of, 63, 68, 382–383, 388
 pain management and, 269
 scope problem and, 66–67
 spirituality/religion and, 64–65
Charon, Rita, 16
Chast, Roz, 1, 2f
Check-backs, 350
Chemo Brain Doc Notes, 151t
Child life specialists, 248t
Children, 223. *See also* Pediatric palliative care communication
Chochinov's Dignity Therapy, 305
Chodren, Pema, 283
CHP-SW. *See* Certified Hospice and Palliative Social Worker
Chronic fatigue syndrome, 216
Chronic obstructive pulmonary disease and heart failure
 advanced treatments and technologies for, 177–180
 communication challenges in patients with, 173f
 communication strategies for patients with, 174–175, 175t, 176t
 future of, 180
 overview of, 173, 174t, 180
 palliative care needs of, 173
 REMAP tool and, 176–177, 177t
 transplantation and, 192–193
City of Hope National Medical Center, 246, 251–253, 252f
CLAS. *See* National Standards for Culturally and Linguistically Appropriate Services
Clergy confidentiality, 67
Clinical case studies, 383–384, 384t
Clinical Communication Collaborative, 372t
Clinical deliberation, 31
Clinical gaze, 129, 129t
Clinical intimacy, 31
Clinical Pastoral Education (CPE)
 background of, 65, 383–385
 current practices, 385–388

 overview of, 382–383, 388
Clinical Practice Guidelines, 287t
Clinical Practice Guidelines for Quality Palliative Care (NCP), 85b, 144
Clinical presence, 17–18, 64, 376
Clinical psychology, communication in
 assessment services provision and, 72–73
 challenges and future directions of, 77
 family systems involvement and, 75–76
 interdisciplinary teams and, 71, 74–75, 76–77
 overview of, 71–72
 training, competencies and, 77
 treatment services provision and, 73–75
Clinical rotations, cultural humility and, 85b
Clinical sensitivity, 31–32
Clinical Trial Seek, 151t
Coburn Centre, 351–352
Cognitive behavioral therapy, 74
Cognitive impairments, health literacy and, 100
Cohen, Richard, 283
Coherence, 129t, 130
Collaboration, 382. *See also* Coordination; Interdisciplinary teams
Comfort care orders, 58
Comfort measures
 building end-of-life plans and, 281, 282t
 decision-making burden and, 281–282
 fundamental science of, 276–277
 holistic approach to care and, 278–279
 illness prognosis and, 277, 277t
 overview of, 276, 283
 previous provider experiences and, 282–283
 provider-driven vs. patient-directed healthcare and, 279–281
 removal of, 278
 signs and symptoms and, 277–278
COMFORT model
 homeless, drug-addicted, mentally ill patients and, 205, 211
 interprofessional education and, 395
 nursing homes and, 349
 overview of, 5, 6–7, 6b, 48, 50t
 social workers and, 379t, 380
Communicating at the End of Life (Foster), 17
Communication and Medicine, 413, 415b
Communication brokers, 222
Communication Climate Assessment Toolkit, 411t
Communication privacy management, 5, 409t
Community, health literacy tools for, 95
Comparison, 409
Compassionate presence, 304t, 305–306
Compassionate silence, 357–358
Competencies. *See also* Specific competencies
 clinical psychologists and, 77
 future of education and, 420
 for interprofessional education, 390, 391b
 nursing communication and, 55b
 patient-centered communication and, 243–244
Complementary and alternative medicine (CAM), 271–274
Complicated grief, 313, 314–315
Comskil training program, 5, 50t
Confidentiality, 32–33, 67
Conflicts, 68, 323–324, 363
Consent, 41, 221
Consultants, 248t

Consultation teams, 349t
Consumer Assessments and Reports of End of Life Care, 418
Consumers
  lack of understanding of palliative care by, 23–25, 23b
  overview of issue, 22, 25–26
  Patient Quality of Life Coalition and, 25
  quality of life, quality of living and, 22–23
  resources for communicating with, 24t
Content meaning, 198
Content skills, 231
Continuing education, 380, 395
Continuity, pediatric palliative care and, 225
Conversation analysis, 5
Conversation Project, 287t, 290
Conversations. *See* Family conversations
Coordination
  City of Hope National Medical Center and, 251–253, 252f
  nursing homes and, 349
  overview of, 246, 253
  palliative social work and, 36–37
  provider communication and, 246–247, 247–250t
COPD. *See* Chronic obstructive pulmonary disease and heart failure
COPD patient decision aid, 180
Coping and Communication Support, 141t
Coping Skills Training, 141t
Core Competencies for Interprofessional Collaborative Practice, 391b
Council on Social Work Education (CSWE), 375
Counseling the Culturally Diverse (Sue and Sue), 80
Couples counseling, 76
Courageous Parents Network, 24t
CPE. *See* Clinical Pastoral Education
Credibility, 405, 409–411
CRIES scale. *See* Crying, Requiring oxygen, Increased vital signs, Expression, Sleepless scale
Critical incident reports, 383
"Crossing the Quality Chasm" (IOM), 238
Crying, Requiring oxygen, Increased vital signs, Expression, Sleepless (CRIES) scale, 263–264
CSAM. *See* Cancer Survivorship and Agency Model
CSWE. *See* Council on Social Work Education
Cues, transactional communication and, 15
Cultural awareness, 80t
Cultural brokering, 80t
Cultural change, 347
"Cultural Competence in the Social Work Profession," 80
Cultural competency, 39, 80–81, 80t, 81t
Cultural considerations
  advance care planning and, 286, 291–292
  advances in palliative care and, 154
  artificial nutrition and hydration and, 277
  case study, 157–158, 158t
  clinical psychologists and, 73
  comfort measures and, 278
  culture and palliative care and, 154–155
  disparities in palliative care and, 113–114, 153, 155
  faith, hope, miracles and, 258–259
  overview of, 153–154, 155t, 159

pain communication and management and, 264–265
practice implications of, 158–159
seriously-ill veterans and, 216–217
social determinants of palliative care, 156–158
social worker communication and, 38–39, 376
symptom management and, 267–268
transactional communication and, 15
transplantation and organ donation and, 189
Cultural Formulation Interview, 85b
Cultural humility
  barriers to training and awareness, 83–85
  cultural competency and, 80–81
  historical background of, 79–80, 80b
  overview of, 79, 87
  self-awareness perspective and, 82–83
  training tools for, 81–82, 81t, 82t, 84t, 85–86b
Cultural meaning systems, 155t
Cultural safety, 80t
Cultural sensitivity, 80t, 201, 202b
Culture, 155t. *See also* Cultural considerations
Culture brokers, 68
CURE Magazine, 151t
Current Opioid Misuse Measure, 265
Cystectomy patients, 246, 251–253, 252f

Daily stand-up meetings, 350
Debriefs, 350
de Bronkert, Dave, 105
Decision-making. *See also* Healthcare proxies; Shared decision-making
  appointment of proxy, 286
  burden of, 281–282
  chaplaincy communication and, 383
  patient-centered communication and, 242–243
  pediatric palliative care and, 221, 223–224
  providers' previous experiences and, 282–283
Decision-Making Tools, 224
Deductive reasoning, 409
Defibrillators, 177
Definitional privilege, 343
Delegitimization, 129t, 131
Deliberative decision-making, 31
Delivery mode, 410t
Demonstration role-play, 393
Denial, 257–258, 291
Depression, bereavement and, 315
Depression and Bipolar Support Alliance, 122t
Derek (Gervais), 17
Detachment, 14
Dexamethasone, 268t
Diagnosis, 35, 200, 200b. *See also* Prognostication
Diagnosis, Intractability, Risk, Efficacy score, 265
Dialectic tensions, 19
Dialogue, spirituality and, 304t, 306–307
Diazepam, 268t
Dicks, Russell, 383
Didactics, 378t
Dietitians, 269
Dignity, 306
Dignity therapy, 40, 132–133, 305, 306
Dioxin, 215

Direct communication, 81t
Discharge, 324
Discrimination, 115
Disease-Specific Advance Care Planning Interview, 199t
Disenfranchised grief, 315
Disenfranchisement, 231, 315
Disenrollment from hospice, 112
Disparities
  contributing factors, 113–115, 113f
  future research and interventions to address, 115–116, 116t
  lesbian, gay, bisexual, and transgender individuals and, 230
  overview of, 111, 116
  in palliative care use, 113, 153, 155
  trust, hope, miracles and, 258–259
Distrust, 30, 232
Diversity, 18. *See also* Cultural considerations
Docusate sodium, 268t
Donald Coburn Centre, 351–352
Drive theory of sexuality, 294
Drug-addicted patients
  communication characteristics and, 209
  description of, 206–207
  families and, 210–211, 210f
  future research and, 211–212
  interdisciplinary care teams and, 211
  overview of, 205, 211–212
  recommendations for, 211
  theoretical framework for, 205–206, 206t
  trust and, 207–208
Drugs.com, 123t
Dual Process Model, 312
Duncombe, David, 383
Dying in America report, 54

Economic concerns, 37, 113
ED. *See* Emergency departments
Educating Future Physicians in Palliative and End-of-Life Care, 287t
Education. *See also* Health literacy; Interprofessional education
  bereavement and, 316–317, 318
  clinical case methods and, 383–384
  clinical practice guidelines for quality care and, 366–367
  clinical psychologists and, 76
  communication as essential skill and, 355–356
  cultural humility and, 80, 81–82, 81t, 82t, 83, 84t, 85–86b
  empathic response and, 386–387
  family caregiving and, 150
  framing and, 385–386
  health literacy and, 94
  models for, 377–378, 379t
  narrating observations and, 387
  nurses as change agents and, 60
  oncology patients and families and, 187
  overview of for chaplains, 382–383
  overview of for nurses, 366, 372–373
  overview of for physicians, 355–356, 363–364
  overview of for social workers, 36, 375–377
  physician communication and, 360–362
  process groups and, 384–385
  process notes and, 384
  screening protocols and, 385
  semistructured interviewing and, 387, 388b

Education (*Cont.*)
    simulations and, 360–361, 367
    state of science and, 419–420
    strategies for forative feedback at bedside and, 362
    team and family meetings and, 367–371
    team communication and, 376–377
    technological advances, 378–379
    training activities for social workers, 377
    training environments and, 379–380
    transitions in care and, 249t
Education for Phsicians of End-of-Life Care project, 276
Education in Palliative and End-of-Life Care, 50t, 77, 321
Effectiveness measures, 418–419
Eidetic reduction, 403
Elder Guru, 287t
ELNEC. *See* End-of-Life Nursing Education Consortium
Email communication, 103–104, 107t
Embedded model of understanding, 19
Embedded teamwork, 341
Emergency departments (ED), 321. *See also* Acute care setting
Emotional enabling, 64
Emotional intelligence, 57
Emotional resilience, 129t
Emotional support, 316–317, 318, 396
Emotions
    comfort measures and, 278–279
    communication instruction and, 362
    nursing communication and, 371–372
    patient-centered communication and, 241–242, 358
    transactional communication and, 16
Empathic listening, 35, 64
Empathic opportunities, 16
Empathic opportunity continuers, 16
Empathic opportunity terminators, 16
Empathic responses, 16–17, 386–387
Empathic witness, 129t, 131, 132–133
Empathy, 16–17, 325
Empathy and Relational Science Program (MG) study, 279
Empowerment, 106–107
End-of-Life Nursing Education Consortium (ELNEC), 50t, 60, 321, 348, 372t
End-of-Life/Palliative Education Resource Center, 372t
End-of-life plans, 281, 282t
End-of-life psychotherapy, 74
Environmental factors, 15
Epstein, Ronald, 244
Ethics
    chaplaincy communication and, 68
    communication between healthcare providers and, 29–31
    communication with the patient and, 31–33
    in framework for palliative care communication, 27–29
    hospice teams and, 341
    overview of, 27, 33
    palliative social work and, 40–41
    pediatric palliative care and, 221
    therapeutic communication as core obligation and, 28–29
Ethnicity, 155t, 157t, 190. *See also* Cultural considerations
Ethnocentrism Scale, 411t

Ethnography, 5, 129–131, 129t, 402–403
Existential issues, 38
Existential psychotherapy, 74
Expectancy Violations Theory, 409t
Explanatory models of illness, 155t
Ex-PLISSIT, 296
Exploratory models, 129t
Expressive touch, 295
External palliative care consultation teams, 349t

Face, Legs, Activity, Cry, Consolability (FLACC) scale, 263–264
FACE-HIV model and intervention, 198–200, 199t, 201b
FACES. *See* Family Assessment Collaboration to Enhance End of Life Support
FACES-revised, 263
Fairview Health System, 337
False hope, 257–258
Families. *See also* Family caregiving; Patient- and family-centered communication
    advance care planning and, 291
    clinical psychologists and, 75–76
    confidentiality and, 33
    homeless, drug-addicted, mentally ill patients and, 210–211, 210f
    lesbian, gay, bisexual, and transgender individuals and, 231
    pain management and, 267–268
    patient-centered communication and, 239–241, 239f, 240–241
    pediatric palliative care and, 221–222, 226
    relationships with nurses, 58
    symptoms and, 119–120, 122–123
    team communication and, 324–326
Families of choice, 231
Family and Medical Leave Act, 139, 140
Family Assessment Collaboration to Enhance End of Life Support (FACES), 140t, 263
Family Caregiver Communication Tool (FCCT), 150
Family caregiving
    assessment tools and, 139, 140t
    changing relationships and roles, 136–137
    COMFORT model and, 6b, 7
    communication patterns and, 147–148
    communication types and, 148–150, 148t
    evidence-based interventions for, 140, 141t
    family communication in, 145–146
    future of, 140
    hematopoietic stem cell/bone marrow transplantation and, 193
    impacts of, 137–138
    multiple goals and, 146
    overview of, 135, 144–145, 150
    positive responses and benefit finding, 138
    pre-illness relationship and, 135–136
    privacy and, 146–147
    resources for, 150, 151t
    situational factors impacting, 138–139
Family-centered care, 30, 198
Family communication patterns theory, 4–5
Family conversations, 161–168, 169t
Family Evaluation of Hospice Care, 400, 418
Family meetings
    nurses and, 59
    nursing communication and, 367–371
    palliative social work and, 37, 38f
    physician facilitation of, 362–363
    social worker communication and, 377

FCCT. *See* Family Caregiver Communication Tool
Fear of Physician measure, 411t
Federal legislation, 25
Feedback, 344, 361–362, 363t
Fee-for-service model, 95
Fellowships, 380
Fence-sitting, 11
Ferrell, Betty, 3
Fibromyalgia, 216
FICA tool, 305, 305b
Fieldwork, 401
Financial strain, 37
Finger writing, 298
Five Wishes, 58, 199, 199t, 290b
Fluoxetine, 268t
Focus groups, 169, 401–402
FOCUS program, 141t
Forums, 105–106, 107t. *See also* Support groups
Foster, Elissa, 401
Foucault, Michael, 129
4x7 Model for Spiritual Assessment, 387t
Framework for Action on Interprofessional Education and Collaborative Practice (WHO), 390
Framing, 94, 385–386
Frank, Arthur W., 133
Frankl, Viktor, 306
Frequency, percentage vs., 94
Freud, Sigmund, 294
Frontstage communication, 19
Functional Assessment of Chronic Illness Therapy- Spiritual Well Being Inner Peace Factor, 306
Funding, health literacy and, 95

Gawande, Atul, 3, 97
Gay individuals. *See* Lesbian, gay, bisexual, and transgender individuals
Geertz, Clifford, 400
Generalizability, 405
Generalized Belief Measure, 411t
Genograms, 210–211, 210f, 386
Gen Silent, 229
Geriatric Interdisciplinary Team Training (GITT), 349
GeriTalk, 180, 360
Geropalliative care, 348
Gervais, Ricky, 17
Gilda's club, 42b
GITT. *See* Geriatric Interdisciplinary Team Training
Glaser, Barney, 402
Globalization, 154
Global meaning, 63
Goals, 73–74, 146, 377
Gordon and Betty Moore Foundation, 391
Gottman, John, 280
Graphs, health literacy and, 94
Grayness, 11
Grief reactions. *See also* Bereavement
    anticipatory grief, 314, 316–319
    classification of, 313
    disenfranchised grief and, 315
    framework for understanding, 311–313, 312b
    loss and, 313–314
    overview of, 310, 311
    plans of care and, 316–319
    self-awareness and, 315–316

Grief work, 312
Grounded theory, 402
Gulf War veterans, 215–216, 217
Gunderson Health System, 58, 287t

Haloperidol, 268t
Handoffs/handovers, 350
Hartford Institute for Geriatric Nursing, 349
Hays, Ross, 224
Hazelton, Sue, 20
Healthcare durable power of attorney, 58–59, 200b, 285, 286
Healthcare proxies, 58–59, 200b, 285, 286
Health Care Reform Act, 157
Health Communication, 413, 415b
"Health Communication" resource, 24
Health.gov, 100
Health literacy
   clinical psychologists and, 72
   considerations for special populations, 99–100
   disparities in use of palliative care and, 114
   introduction to, 90
   key resources for, 100–101
   lessons from recent experiences, 97
   overview of, 97
   research and practice priorities, 95–97
   role of, 90–92
   strategies and tools for, 92–95
   written communication and, 103
Health Literacy: A Prescription to End Confusion (IOM), 100
Health Literacy Interventions and Outcomes: A Updated Systemic Review (AHRQ), 100
Health Literacy Online, 101
Health Resources and Services Administration, 101
Heart disease. *See* Cardiac transplantation; Chronic obstructive pulmonary disease and heart failure
Heedful interrelating, 18–19
HeLa cell line, 259
Hematopoietic stem cell transplantation (HSCT), 193–194
Heuristic devices, 224
Hierarchies, 31, 147
History of palliative care communication
   barriers and, 11–12, 13t
   evolving focus on communication in, 10, 11t
   future and, 12–13
   honest and open communication and, 11
   hope and, 11
   introduction to, 10
   pediatric, 12
   technology and, 12
HIV/AIDS, people living with
   adolescents and, 201
   comorbidities, aging, and need for new paradigms, 201–202
   cultural and religious sensitivity and, 201, 202b
   diagnosis disclosure and, 200, 200b
   FACE-HIV model and intervention, 198–200, 199t, 201b
   lesbian, gay, bisexual, and transgender individuals and, 230, 231
   overview of, 197, 202

   patient-family provider communication models for, 201
   person- and family-centered approach to, 198
Holistic approach to care, 278–279
Homeless patients
   communication characteristics and, 208–209
   description of, 206
   families and, 210–211, 210f
   future research and, 211–212
   interdisciplinary care teams and, 211
   overview of, 205, 211–212
   recommendations for, 211
   theoretical framework for, 205–206, 206t
   trust and, 207–208
Home services. *See* Outpatient care setting, communication in
Honesty, 11
Hope
   addressing chronic obstructive pulmonary disease and heart failure and, 175t
   African Americans and, 258–259
   AMEN model and, 259–261, 259b
   communicating, 11
   conversation framed by, 261
   dialect of, 307
   miracles and, 257–258
   overview of, 255–256, 261–262
Hope and Worry tool, 359
"Hope for the best, prepare for the worst" framework, 175
Hope Project, 261
Hospice, 10, 40
Hospice and Palliative Nursing Association (HPNA), 55, 55b
Hospice Mazatlan, 287t
Hospice teams
   barriers to teamwork and, 341–342
   etechnology and, 341
   future of, 344
   overview of, 337, 340, 344–345
   purpose and function of, 340–341
   team talk and, 342–344, 342b, 343b
Hospital Consumer Assessment of Healthcare Providers and Systems, 418
HPNA. *See* Hospice and Palliative Nursing Association
HSCT. *See* Hematopoietic stem cell transplantation
Huddles, 349–350
Human nature, 154
Humility. *See* Cultural humility; Narrative humility
Husserl, Edmund, 403
Hydration, artificial. *See* Artificial nutrition and hydration
Hyoscine butylbromide, 268t
Hyperbole, 376

I*CARE program, 50t
Iatrogenic suffering, 305
Ibuprofen, 268t
ICD. *See* Implantable cardioverter defibrillators
Icon arrays, 94
ICU. *See* Intensive care units
Identity problem, 417
Illness as Metaphor (Sontag), 129
Image matrices, 94

Immigrants, 38
Implantable cardioverter defibrillators (ICD), 177
Incarcerated individuals, 99
Indian Health Service, 95
Indirect communication, 81t
Information
   delivery of, 4
   palliative social work and, 36
   patient-centered communication and, 241
   pediatric palliative care and, 224, 225
   transactional model of communication and, 4
Informed consent, 41
Initiative for Pediatric Palliative Care, 86b
Initiative on Methods, Measurement, and Pain Assessment in Clinical Trials, 264
Inpatient setting, 321, 322. *See also* Acute care setting
Inspire Cancer Treatment, 123t
Institutional constancy, 81
Insurance coverage, 113
Intangibles, 14
Integrated palliative care communication, 421–422, 421t
Integrating Cultural Competency and Humility Training into Clinical Clerkships, 86b
Intensive care units (ICU), 321, 322. *See also* Acute care setting
INTERACT. *See* Intervention to Reduce Acute Care Transfers
Interaction details, micro-analysis of, 5
Interagency Registry for Mechanically Assisted Circulatory Support (INTERMACS), 178
Intercultural communication, 155t
Interdisciplinary Approaches to End of Life and Palliative Care (UU), 392
Interdisciplinary Palliative Care Seminar (USD), 392
Interdisciplinary teams (IDT). *See also* Team communication
   chaplaincy communication and, 68
   clinical care psychologists and, 71, 74–75, 76–77
   future of palliative care communication and, 12
   home care services and, 331
   nursing communication and, 59
   nursing homes and, 347, 348
   pain management and, 268
   pediatric palliative care and, 226
   physician communication and, 48
Interfaith chaplains, 64
INTERMACS. *See* Interagency Registry for Mechanically Assisted Circulatory Support
International Palliative Care Family Career Research Collaboration, 140
Internet
   communication and, 103–104, 105–106, 107t
   health literacy and, 96
   hospice teams and, 341
   interprofessional education and, 393–395
   outpatient care setting and, 337–338
   physician education and, 363
   qualitative research and, 401
   quantitative research and, 410, 414–415
   social worker training and, 380
   symptom management and, 123, 124

Internships, social work and, 380
Interpersonal communication, 3, 197–198
Interpretivism, 400–401
Interprofessional Communication competency, 390
Interprofessional education (IPE)
  continuing education, 395
  current mandate for, 390–391
  graduate and postgraduate education and, 391–392
  ongoing training and development, 395–397
  overview of, 390
  palliative care and, 391
  teaching approaches for, 392–395
Interprofessional Education Collaboration (IPEC), 390
Interruptions, 14
Intervention to Reduce Acute Care Transfers (INTERACT), 350–351
Interviewing, 401–402
Invitation, 324
IPE. See Interprofessional Education
IPEC. See Interprofessional Education Collaboration
iPharmacy, 151t
Iraq War veterans, 215–216, 217
"I-Thou" connectedness, 229
I Wish. tool, 359

Jackson, Don, 15
Jehovah's Witnesses, 259
John A. Hartford Foundation, 391
Josiah Macy Jr. Foundation, 391
Journal of General Internal Medicine, 413, 415b
Journal of Health Communication, 413, 415b
Journals, 413, 415b. *See also Specific journals*
Journey metaphor, 313–314

Kalamazoo Consensus Statement, 362
Kaleidoscope metaphor, 128
Kaye 10-Step Approach, 379t
Kidney disease, 190
Kinesthetic learning, 57
Kings College, 392
Kleinman, Arthur, 128, 129–131, 132b
Knowledge, 290, 325
Korean War veterans, 215, 217
Kreps' model of communication and symptom management, 121–122, 121f
Kusher, Harold, 63

Lacks, Henrietta, 259
Language. *See* Vocabulary
Larkin, Philip, 14
Lavender families, 231
Law of double protection, 75
Leadership, 202b
Leaflets, end-of-life, 104–105, 107t
Learning styles, 57
Leeds Assessment of Neuropathic Symptoms and Signs, 264
Left ventricular assist devices (LVAD), 178
Legislation, 25, 95, 140. *See also Specific legislation*
LEP. *See* Limited English proficiency
Lesbian, gay, bisexual, and transgender individuals
  challenges of communication, 231–232
  future and, 234–235
  overview of, 229–230, 235–236
  palliative care needs of, 230–231
  strategies for communication, 232–234, 233–234t, 235t
Leukemia, 189–190, 193
LGBT individuals. *See* Lesbian, gay, bisexual, and transgender individuals
Life expectancy. *See* Prognostication
Life-prolonging measures, 277
Life review, 40
Life support
  building end-of-life plans and, 281, 282t
  decision-making burden and, 281–282
  fundamental science of, 276–277
  holistic approach to care and, 278–279
  illness prognosis and, 277, 277t
  overview of, 276, 283
  previous provider experiences and, 282–283
  provider-driven vs. patient-directed healthcare and, 279–281
  removal of, 278
  signs and symptoms and, 277–278
Liminal space, 17
Limited English proficiency (LEP), 99
Line graphs, 94
Literacy. *See* Health literacy
Liver transplantation, 191–192, 191t
Living wills, 58
Lone caregivers, 148f, 148t, 149
Long-stay nursing homes, 347
Loperamide, 268t
Lorazepam, 268t
Loss, 216, 313–314. *See also* Grief reactions
Lou Gehrig's disease, 215
Lung transplantation, 192
LVAD. *See* Left ventricular assist devices
Lyon Family Centered Advance Care Planning Survey, 199, 199t

Macy Foundation, 391
Maddux, Stu, 229
"Making Choices" document, 58
Making your Wishes Known: Planning Your Medical Future, 290b
Maladaptive responses, 217
Management continuity, 225
Manager caregivers, 148–149, 148f, 148t
Massachusetts General Hospital Pain center, 264
Mayo Clinic, 101
McGill Pain Questionnaire, 264
McGill Quality of Life Existential subscale, 307
McGill Quality of Life Questionnaire, 302, 404
Meaning, 4, 198, 306–307
Meaning-based therapy, 132
Meaning-making, 63
Measures, comfort. *See* Comfort measures
Mechanical ventilation, 178–179
Medical gaze, 129, 129t
Medical homes, 390
Medical Orders for Life Sustaining Treatment (MOLST), 36, 377
Medicare and Medicaid, 346, 347, 395
Medication administration, 163
Medigram, 420
Meier, Diane, 1–2
Member checking, 405
Memorial Pain Assessment Card, 264
Memorial Sloan-Kettering Cancer Center, 380
Mentally ill patients
  communication characteristics and, 209–210
  description of, 207
  families and, 210–211, 210f
  future research and, 211–212
  interdisciplinary care teams and, 211
  overview of, 205, 211–212
  recommendations for, 211
  theoretical framework for, 205–206, 206t
  trust and, 207–208
Merck Manual of Diagnosis and Therapy, 80
Meta-ethnology, 404
Metaphors, 128, 129, 133, 272, 313–314, 376
MetLife Mature Market Institute, 139
Metoclopramide, 268t
Micro-analysis of interaction details, 5
Microsoft HealthVault, 151t
Mindful communication, 6b, 7
Mindfulness, 18–19
Miracles
  African Americans and, 258–259
  AMEN model and, 259–261, 259b
  chaplaincy communication and, 68
  hope, denial and, 257–258
  overview of, 255–256, 261–262
Mistrust, 115, 258–259
Misunderstandings, 277, 277t, 279
Mixed-methods research, 404–405
Modeling, 360, 378t
MOLST. *See* Medical Orders for Life Sustaining Treatment
Moral agency, 28
Moral deliberation, 344
Moral injury, 216–217
Moral practice, palliative care as, 27–28
Morphine, 268t
Mothers Against Drunk Driving, 212
Mount Sinai Beth Israel, 380
Multidisciplinary meetings, 335–336
Multifaith chaplains, 64
Multiple goals theory, 146
Multiple Sclerosis Foundation, 122t
Mutual assessment, 57
Mutual respect, 18–19
My Cancer Manager, 151t
My Pillbox, 151t
My Voice Planning Ahead, 290b

NAFC-C. *See* Needs Assessment of Family Caregivers- Cancer
Narrative, 131, 133, 387
Narrative humility, 129, 129t
Narrative inquiry, 5, 6
Narrative medicine, 6
Narrative theory, 4–5
National Action Plan to Improve Health Literacy (USDHHS), 100
National Advance Care Planning Cooperative, 288t
National Alliance for Caregiving, 139
National Alliance for the Mentally Ill, 212
National Association of Social Workers (NASW), 80, 86b, 375, 380
National Cancer Institute, 122t
National Center for Complementary and Alternative Medicine, 273t
National Center for Interprofessional Practice and Education, 391
National Comprehensive Cancer Network (NCCN), 66, 251

National Consensus Development Conference for Caregiver Assessment, 135
National Consensus Project for Quality Palliative Care, 10, 11t, 56, 71, 154, 301
National Council for Palliative Care, 288t
National Family Caregivers Association, 135
National Family Caregiver Support Program, 139
National Gold Standards Framework, 288t
"National Healthcare Disparities Report," 80
National Health Care for the Homeless Commission, 211
National Home and Hospice Care Survey, 347
National Hospice and Palliative Care Organization, 77, 269, 273t
National Hospice Foundation, 20
National Institute on Drug Addiction, 212
National Institutes of Health, 24t
National Nursing Home Survey, 347
National Quality Forum Clinical Practice Guidelines, 55t, 154, 418
National Resource Center on LGBT Aging, 234
National Standards for Culturally and Linguistically Appropriate Services (CLAS), 80
A Natural History of Family Cancer (Beach), 161
Navigators, 93, 96, 248t
Needs Assessment of Family Caregivers-Cancer (NAFC-C), 140t
Negative effects. *See* Symptom management
Neighborhood and Core meetings, 351
Neonatal Infant Pain Scale (NIPS), 263-264
Neonatal intensive care units (NICU), 225
Neonatal palliative care, 200, 225. *See also* Pediatric palliative care
Nephrotalk, 180
Neuropathic pain, 263
Neuropathic Pain Questionnaire, 264
Neuropathic Pain Scale, 264
Neutrality, 342-343
Newest Vital Sign (NVS), 91, 101
NHS Choices, 273t
NICU. *See* Neonatal intensive care units
NIPS scale. *See* Neonatal Infant Pain Scale
Noise, 15
Nolan, Steve, 258
Nonabandonment, 260
Noncomplicated bereavement, 314
Nonheterosexual individuals. *See* Lesbian, gay, bisexual, and transgender individuals
Noninvasive positive pressure ventilation (NPPV), 179
Nonmaleficence, 28-29
Nonverbal communication
  chaplaincy communication and, 383
  clinical sensitivity and, 32
  cultural competency training and, 81t
  grief and, 313
  nursing and, 56
  quantitative research and, 410t
  social workers and, 376
Nonverbal Immediacy Scale-Observer Report, 411t
NPPV. *See* Noninvasive positive pressure ventilation
NURSE statements, 325, 357, 358-359, 360
"Nursing Care and Do-Not Resuscitate and Allow Natural Death Decisions" position statement, 54

Nursing communication. *See also* Providers
  barriers to, 59-60
  change agents and, 60
  clinical practice guidelines for quality care and, 366-367
  common conversations and, 58-59
  cultural humility and, 85b
  emotions and, 371-372
  interdisciplinary teams and, 59
  interprofessional education and, 392
  introduction to, 54-56, 55b, 55t
  overview of, 56-57, 60
  overview of education for, 366
  relationship with family and, 58
  relationship with patient and, 57-58, 57t
  simulations and, 367, 368-369b
  team and family meetings and, 367-371
  telehealth and, 372-373
  transitions in care and, 247-248t
  When Cancer Calls and, 168, 169t
Nursing Home Compare, 346
Nursing home team communication
  education and, 348-349
  exemplars of, 351-352
  models for, 348, 349t
  overview of, 346-347
  palliative care and, 347-348
Nutrition, artificial. *See* Artificial nutrition and hydration
NVS. *See* Newest Vital Sign

Objective Structured Clinical Examinations (OSCE), 392
Observing gaze, 129, 129t
Ohio State University Medical Center, 101
Omnibus Budget Reconciliation Act of 1987, 346
Oncology
  challenges of communication, 184
  multidisciplinary cancer or tumor board meetings and, 335-336
  overview of, 183, 184t, 188
  palliative care needs of patients and families, 183-184
  pediatric palliative care and, 220
  provider education and, 187
  recommendations for communication, 185-188
  shared decision-making and, 246, 249t, 250-253, 252f
  tomorrow's patient and, 420-421
OncoTalk, 180, 360
Online learning. *See* Internet
Open questions, 383
Open Society Institute, 10
Opioid Risk Took, 265
Organ donation. *See* Transplantation and organ donation
Origin, 155t. *See also* Cultural considerations
OSCE. *See* Objective Structured Clinical Examinations
Osler, William, 244
Ottawa Hospital Research Institute, 180
Oucher, 263
Outcome-Oriented Chaplaincy, 67
Out of Hospital DNR form, 324
Outpatient care setting, communication in
  in home care setting, 36-37, 331-333, 333b
  information technology and, 337-338

multidisciplinary cancer or tumor board meetings and, 335-336
  in outpatient clinic setting, 333-335
  overview of, 330-331, 338
  tools to assist, 336-337
Outpatient clinics, 333-335

Paasche-Orlow and Wolf's health literacy framework, 91-92
Pain Care, 151t
Pain management
  in absence of patient communication, 267-268
  assessment in special populations and, 263-264
  chronic pain assessment scales and, 264
  complications of, 265-266
  cultural considerations of, 264-265
  disparities in, 112
  at end of life, 266-267
  hematopoietic stem cell/bone marrow transplantation and, 193
  interdisciplinary teams and, 268
  oncology patients and families and, 185
  overview of, 263, 268
  pain histories and, 263
  palliative social work and, 36
  treatment goals, therapeutic responses and, 265
PAIN Report It, 123
Palliative Care and Hospice Education Training Act, 25
Palliative Care Australia, 287t
Palliative Care Communication Institute, 24, 24t
Palliative Care Leadership Centers, 212
Palliative Care Victoria, 122t
"Palliative Care with Older Adults" (CSWE), 375
Palliative medicine communication course, 50t
Palliative Nursing: Scope and Standards of Practice (HPNA), 55, 55b
Partner caregivers, 148f, 148t, 149-150
Pastoral care, 66f, 66t
Patient 2.0 Empowerment, 106-107
Patient- and Family-Centered Care Core Principles, 220
Patient- and family-centered communication, physician education and, 356-359, 357f
Patient-centered checklists, 3
Patient-centered communication. *See also* Written communication
  comfort measures and, 279
  competence and, 243-244
  decision-making and, 242-243
  emotions and, 241-242
  functions of, 239-240, 240f
  information provision and receipt and, 241
  overview of, 2-3, 238-239, 239f, 244
  patient- and family-centered communication and, 356t
  patient/family-provider relationship and, 240-241
  physician education and, 356-359, 357f
  self-management and, 243
  uncertainty and, 242
Patient Centered Quality Care for Life Act, 25
Patient decision aids (PtDA), 93
Patient Dignity Inventory (PDI), 306

Patient Education and Counseling, 413, 415b
Patient empowerment, 106–107
Patient Experience of Care measures, 418
Patient experience of illness
　challenge of metaphor and, 128–129
　empathic witness and, 132–133
　kaleidoscope as metaphor for, 128
　mini-ethnography of, 129–131
　overview of, 127–128, 133–134
　reciprocity of experience and, 128
　theoretical framework for, 131–132, 132b, 132t
Patient instructors. *See* Simulations
Patient navigators, 93, 96, 248t
Patient-Practitioner Orientation Scale, 411t
Patient Protection and Affordable Care Act. *See* Affordable Care Act
Patient Quality of Life Coalition, 25
Patients
　assessing perspective of, 357–359
　disparities in use of palliative care and, 114–115
　ethical communication with, 31
　relationships with nurses, 57–58, 57t
　spirituality and, 302–303
　symptoms and, 119–120
　team communication and, 324–326
　tools for health literacy and, 92–93
　virtual, 394–395
　When Cancer Calls and, 168, 169t
Patient Self-Determination Act, 36, 347
Patient simulators, 393. *See also* Simulations
Patriarchal model, 221
Payment systems, health literacy and, 95
Payne, Malcom, 396
PCS. *See* Preparedness of Caregiving Scale
Pediatric palliative care communication
　adult palliative care needs vs., 221
　assessment and intervention implementation, 224–225
　clinical psychologists and, 76
　conversation involvement and, 222–223, 223t
　cultural humility and, 86b
　disparities in, 112
　history of, 12
　improvement needs, 226
　managing logistical efforts, 225
　needs of, 221–222
　overview of, 220, 226
　pain management and, 263–264
　population description, 220–221
　problem-solving, decision-making and, 221, 223–224
　specific populations and needs, 225–226
Peer role-play, 367
Peplau, Hildegard, 205
Perceived Organizational Innovativeness Scale, 411t
Perceived Quality of Medical Care, 411t
Percentage, frequency vs., 94
Perception, 231, 324
Perinatal palliative care, 225. *See also* Pediatric palliative care communication
Persistent complex bereavement, 313, 314–315
Personal Health Records (PHR), 218
Personal Report of Intercultural Communication Apprehension, 411t
Person-centered care, 15–18, 198, 347
Perspective, assessing, 357–359

Pharmacy personnel, 249t
Phase I trials, 255
Phenomenology, 403–404
PHR. *See* Personal Health Records
Physical losses, 313
Physical pain. *See* Pain management
Physician assistants, 248t
Physician communication. *See also* Providers
　barriers to, 46, 47t, 48t
　family meetings and, 362–363
　interdisciplinary team approach to, 48
　learning, unlearning, relearning and, 48–49
　need for improved, 45–46, 46t
　overview of, 44–45, 49–51
　overview of education for, 355–356, 363–364
　patient-and family-centered communication and, 356–359
　prognostication and, 46–48, 48t
　strategies for formative feedback at bedside and, 362
　strategies for teaching, 360–362
　transitions in care and, 248t
　When Cancer Calls and, 168, 169t
Physician Data Query, 273t
Physicians Orders for Life-Sustaining Treatment (POLST), 287t, 324, 327
Pictographs, 94
The Place of Suffering in the Religions of the World (Bowker), 63
Plain Language Planner for Palliative Care, 267, 268t
Planning, advance care. *See* Advance care planning
Plans of care, 35, 316–319, 382
Plausibility, 405
Policy. *See* Legislation
Pollock, Lois, 14
POLST. *See* Physicians Orders for Life-Sustaining Treatment
Positivism, 400
Postpositivism, 400
Posttraumatic stress disorder (PTSD), 214, 217
Power
　chaplaincy communication and, 65
　communication models and, 14, 15
　cultural humility and, 81, 82, 82t
　trust, hope and, 257, 258–259
Practice tools, 350–351
The Pragmatics of Human Communication (Watzlawick et al.), 15
Preexisting conditions, trust as, 256–257
Premorbid functioning, 72
Preparatory grief, 313, 314, 316–319
Preparedness of Caregiving Scale (PCS), 140t
Preparedness Plan (Swetz et al.), 178
PREPARE website, 24, 24t, 290b
Presence, 17–18, 64, 376
Prior events
　distrust based on, 30, 232
　negative touch associations and, 298
　provider decision-making and, 282–283
Prison, 99
Privacy, 146–147
Privacy management theory, 5, 6
Problematic integration theory, 4–5, 6
Problem solving, 74
Procedural touch, 295
Process groups, 384–385
Process notes, 384
Process skills, 231

Prognostication
　addressing chronic obstructive pulmonary disease and heart failure and, 178–179
　comfort measures and, 277
　nurses and, 59
　oncology patients and families and, 185–186, 186t
　patient-centered communication and, 242
　physician communication and, 46–48, 48t
Project Grace, 58
Prolonged grief disorder, 313, 314–315
Proselytizing, 64
Providers. *See also* Nursing communication; Physician communication
　advance care planning and, 290–291
　bereavement and, 315–316
　care coordination and, 246–247, 247–250t
　comfort measures and, 279
　disparities in use of palliative care and, 115, 116
　ethical communication and, 29–31
　health literacy and, 91–92, 93–95
　oncology patients and families and, 188
　patient-centered communication and, 240–241
　spirituality and, 303
　transitions in care and, 247–250t
Proxies, 58–59, 285, 286
Psychology. *See* Clinical psychology
Psychosocial assessment, 376
Psychosocial distress, 37
Psychosocial losses, 313
Psychosocial support, 343–344
Psychotherapy, 74
PtDA. *See* Patient decision aids
PTSD. *See* Posttraumatic stress disorder
Public messaging. *See* Consumers
Public Opinion Research on Palliative Care (2011), 23, 23b

Qualitative research
　data generation, 401–402
　ethnography and, 402–403
　generalizability, validity, and reliability of, 405
　grounded theory and, 402
　meta-ethnology and, 404
　mixed-methods research and, 404–405
　ontological and epistemological perspectives, 400–401
　overview of, 5, 399–400, 405
　phenomenology and, 403–404
　quantitative research vs., 399–400
Quality of Communication Questionnaire, 404, 405
Quality of life, 22–23
Quality of living, 22–23
Quantitative research
　assessing quality of, 413
　comparison and, 409
　credibility and, 409–411
　e-health interventions for, 414–415
　experimental design and, 412
　interventions and, 412
　measures of, 410–413, 410t, 411t
　overview of, 408–409
　publication of results from, 413, 415b
　qualitative research vs., 399–400
　quantitizing talk and, 413–414

quasi-experimental research design and, 412–413
surveys and, 401
variables, measurement and, 401, 401t
Quantitizing talk, 413–414

Race, 190. *See also* Cultural considerations
Radiating pain, 263
Rahner, Karl, 302
Randomized controlled trials (RCT), 417, 418t
Rapid Estimate of Adult Literacy in Medicine (REALM), 91, 103
Rapid Estimate of Adult Literacy in Medicine-Short Form, 101
RCCM. *See* Relationship-Centered Care Model
RCS. *See* Rewards of Caregiving Scale
Reach Out Wireless, 209
ReACT. *See* Respect a Caregiver's Time
Reagan, Ronald, 346
REALM. *See* Rapid Estimate of Adult Literacy in Medicine
Reasoned action, 409t
Rebranding, 96
Receivers, 4
Receptivity, 31
Reciprocity, 18, 128
"Recommended Care Core Curriculum Guidelines on Culturally Sensitive and Competent Health Care," 80
Redesigning Continuing Education in the Health Professions (IOM), 391
Referrals, 304t, 306, 317, 318
Reflection, 376
Reflection reports, 384
Reflective questions and statements, 357
Reflective writing, 378t
Reflexivity, 344
Reframing, 388
"Registered Nurses' Roles and Responsibilities in Providing Expert Care and Counseling at the End of Life" position statement, 54–55
Relating, 6b, 7
Relational communication, 15–16, 57
Relational continuity, 225
Relational-cultural theory, 386
Relational dialectic theory, 5, 19, 409t
Relationship-Centered Care Model (RCCM), 18, 19
Relationship-centered interaction skills, 234, 235r
Relationship meaning, 198
Relationships, 4. *See also* Transactional communication
Reliability, 405, 409, 411t
Religion. *See also* Hope; Miracles
advance care planning and, 286
chaplaincy communication and, 64–65, 66f, 66t, 386
cultural considerations and, 157t
disparities in use of palliative care and, 114
health literacy and, 95
HIV/AIDS and, 201, 202b
pain management and, 264–265
palliative social work and, 38
spirituality and, 301–302
symptom management and, 267–268
REMAP tool, 176–177, 177t, 180, 359
REMATCH trial, 178
Remoralization, 129t

Rephrasing, 376
Resident rounds, 350
The Resilient Clinician (Wicks), 16
Respect, mutual, 18–19
Respect a Caregiver's Time (ReACT), 139
Respectful Death Model of Care, 74
RESPECTFUL model, 386
Respecting Choices model, 198, 202b
Respecting Choices Next Steps ACP Interview, 199
Respecting Patient Choices, 287t
Rewards of Caregiving Scale (RCS), 140t
Risk communication, 94
Robert Wood Johnson Foundation, 10, 391
Rockers in Recovery, 212
Role ambiguity, 60
Role-play
chaplaincy communication and, 383
interprofessional education and, 393, 394b, 396
nursing communication and, 366, 367, 368–369b
physician education and, 361
social worker communication and, 379t
Roles and Responsibilities competency, 390
Role switches, 393
Ross, Elizabeth Kubler, 10
Roter's Interactional Analysis System, 5
Rounding, 225
Royal Liverpool and Broadgreen University Hospital Trust, 395
Royal Marsden, 273t
Ryan White Care Act Programs, 95

SACR-D mnemonic, 302, 303t
SafeZone Programs, 234
Safran, Dana, 18
SAGE. *See* Services and Advocacy for Gay, Lesbian, Bisexual, & Transgender Elders
Sample patients. *See* Simulations
Satisfaction with Physician measure, 411t
Saunders, Cicely, 1, 6, 32, 340
SBAR. *See* Situation-Background-Assessment-Recommendation
SCAM. *See* Situational Communication Apprehension Measure
Schema-based interventions, 132–133
Schlairet, Maura, 283
Schwartz, Morrie, 17
Scope, chaplaincy communication and, 66–67
Scope and Standards of Practice (ANA), 54
Screener and Opioid Assessment for Patients with Pain-Revised, 265
SDM. *See* Shared decision-making
Seattle Heart Failure Model (SHFM), 179
Second Life, 395
SECURE framework, 362, 362t
SEGUE framework, 5, 362, 362t
Self-activation, 243
Self-assessment, 361–362
Self-awareness
bereavement and, 315–316
cultural humility and, 82–83
spirituality and, 303–305, 304t
trust, hope, miracles and, 256–257
Self-care, 76–77, 92
Self-determination, 40
Self-image, 30
Self-management, 243

Self-Perceived Communication Competence Scale, 411t
Self-reflection, 81, 82, 82t, 85b
Semistructured interviewing, 383, 387, 387t, 388b, 402
Senders, 4. *See also* Transmission model of communication
Senna, 268t
Sensemaking theory, 409t
Sense of coherence, 129t, 130
Sensitivity, 31–32
Sensuality, 294–295
Services and Advocacy for Gay, Lesbian, Bisexual, & Transgender Elders (SAGE), 232
Setting, acute care team communication and, 324
Settling, 138
Severe and persistent mental illness. *See* Mentally ill patients
Sexuality, 298–299. *See also* Lesbian, gay, bisexual, and transgender individuals; Touch
Shame, 91
Shared decision-making (SDM)
care coordination and, 246–247, 247–250t
City of Hope National Medical Center and, 246, 251–253, 252f
comfort measures and, 282
overview of, 359
patient-centered communication and core functions of communication vs., 356t
provider communication and, 246–247, 247–250t, 359
social worker communication and, 377
transitions from acute care hospitals and, 250–251, 250t
Shared meaning, 198
SHARE model, 48
SHFM. *See* Seattle Heart Failure Model
Short-stay homes, 347
Side effects. *See* Symptom management
Silence
assessing patient perspective and, 357–358
communicative value of, 4
cultural competency training and, 81t
history of palliative care communication and, 10
transactional communication and, 15
Silver Hour, 372t
Simply Put (CDC), 100–101
Simulations
future of education and, 419
interprofessional education and, 392–393, 394b
nursing communication and, 367, 368–369b
physician communication and, 360–361
social worker communication and, 377, 378t
Situational Communication Apprehension Measure (SCAM), 411t
Situational meaning, 63
Situation-Background-Assessment-Recommendation (SBAR), 350
Skilled communicators, 244
Skype, 12
Sliding door moments, 280
Social dying, 17
Social factors, 15
Social media, 60, 96, 123

Social work, communication in
  care of imminently dying patient and, 40
  case study, 41–42b
  cultural considerations and, 38–39, 157–158
  education and training for, 375, 377, 378t
  essentials in education for, 375–377
  ethical and legal aspects of care and, 40–41
  models for sharing life-altering news, 377–378, 379t
  NASW standards and, 375
  overview of, 35, 41, 375, 380–381
  physical aspects of care and, 36–37
  psychosocial and psychiatric aspects of care and, 37
  social aspects of care and, 37–38
  spiritual, religious, and existential aspects of care and, 38
  structure and process of care and, 35–36
  technological advances, 378–379
  training environments and, 379–380
  transitions in care and, 248t
Society of Critical care Medicine Palliative Noninvasive Positive Pressure Ventilation Task Force, 179
Society of Teachers of Family Medicine, 80
Sojourner Award in palliative care, 3
Solid organ donation, 190
Solution-focused communication, 376
Somatic pain, 263
Sontag, Susan, 128, 129
Source cues, 410t
Space, chaplaincy communication and, 65
Specialized palliative care units, 349t
Speck, Peter, 395–396
SPIKES protocol, 48, 49f, 324–325, 359, 363t, 379t
SPIRIT intervention, 201
Spiritual assessment, 66f, 66t, 383, 387
Spiritual care, 66f, 66t, 306
Spirituality
  advance care planning and, 286
  assessment and, 304t, 305
  chaplaincy communication and, 64–65, 66f, 66t, 67, 386
  compassionate presence and, 304t, 305–306
  cultural considerations and, 157t
  dialogue and, 304t, 306–307
  disparities in use of palliative care and, 114
  end-of-life leaflets and, 105
  impact of addressing issues of, 302–303
  overview of, 301–302, 307
  palliative social work and, 38
  patient-patient forums and, 106
  patient preferences and, 303
  providers and, 303
  refer to additional spiritual supporters and, 304t, 306
  religion and, 301–302
  self-awareness and, 303–305, 304t
Staffing patterns, 30–31, 113
Standardized patients. See Simulations
Standards, 80, 86b, 375. See also Specific standards
Standards for Cultural Competence in Social Work Practice (NASW), 80
State of science
  education and, 419–420
  effectiveness measures and, 418–419
  future patients and, 420–421

  integrated communication and, 421–422, 421t
  intervention design and, 420
  overview of, 417–418, 422
Status-based power, 257
St. Christopher's Hospice, 392
Stereotyping, 79, 155
Storytelling, 133, 342–343
Strand, Jacob, 15
"Strategies for Culturally Effective End-of-Life Care" (Crawley et al.), 82
Strategy/summary, 325
Strauss, Anselm, 402
Strengths-oriented practice, 376
Struggling, caregiving and, 138
Study to Understand Prognoses and Preferences for Outcomes and Risks of Treatment (SUPPORT) study, 173
Substance abuse. See Drug-addicted patients
Substance Abuse and Mental Health Services Agency, 212
Suffering, 138, 153
Suggestion, 362
Support groups, 123, 123t. See also Forums
Supportive care, 96, 347
SupportScreen, 251
SUPPORT study, 44
Surrogate decision-makers, 58–59, 200b, 285, 286
Surveys, 401, 418
Symbolic losses, 313
Symptom management. See also Pain management
  advance care planning and, 291
  communication and delivery of palliative care and, 121–122, 121f
  culture, religion and, 267–268
  future of, 123
  negative effects on, 119–120
  oncology patients and families and, 185
  overview of, 119, 124
  palliative social work and, 36
  patient response to negative effects on, 120–121
  resources for, 122t, 123t
  strategic communication and, 122–123, 122t

Taboos, 157t
Tailored Caregiver Assessment and Referral, 141t
Taking the Leap (Chodren), 283
Talkback sessions, 169
Targeted communication patterns, 81t
Task communication, 57
Teach-back method, 94, 241
Team-building, 396
Team communication. See also Interdisciplinary teams; Specific teams
  acute care setting and, 321–322
  barriers to, 327, 341–342
  COMFORT model and, 6b, 7
  education and, 347–348
  exemplars of, 351–352
  families, patients and, 324–326
  future of, 344
  in home care setting, 331–333, 333b
  improving, 327, 344
  information technology and, 337–338
  models of, 347, 348t

  multidisciplinary cancer or tumor board meetings and, 335–336
  in outpatient care setting, 330–331, 333–335
  overview of, 321, 327–328, 330, 338, 340–341, 344–345, 346–347, 352
  social worker communication and, 376–377
  strategies for, 322–324, 348–351
  team talk and, 342–344, 342b, 343b
  tools to assist in outpatient care setting, 336–337
Team meetings, 367–371
Team Observed Structured Clinical Encounters, 392
Team rotation, 30–31
Teams and Teamwork competency, 390
Team Strategies and Tools to Enhance Performance and Patient Safety (TeamSTEPPS), 349, 396
Team talk, 342–344, 342b, 343b
Teamwork, 18–19
Teamwork in Palliative Care (Speck), 395–396
Technology. See also Internet; Telemedicine
  addressing chronic obstructive pulmonary disease and heart failure and, 177–180
  health literacy and, 92, 95, 96
  history of palliative care communication and, 12
  hospice teams and, 341
  interprofessional education and, 393–394
  nursing communication and, 372–373
  outpatient care setting and, 337–338
  physician education and, 363
  quantitative research and, 413–415
  social worker communication and, 378–379
  symptom management and, 124
Telehealth information systems, 123, 372–373
Telemedicine, 363, 378
Tell Me More tool, 358
Temel study, 187, 187t
Terminology. See Vocabulary
Test of Functional Health Literacy in Adults (TOFHLA), 91, 101, 103
Theory of Reasoned Action, 409t
The Science of Trust (Gottman), 280
"Thinking Ahead" Gold Standard Framework Advance Care Planning Discussion, 290b
TOFHLA. See Test of Functional Health Literacy in Adults
Toolkit for Making Written Material Clear and Effective (CMMS), 101
Touch
  assessment of patient experiences, 296–298
  chaplaincy communication and, 65
  continuum of, 294, 295f
  expressive and procedural touch, 295–296
  overview of, 294, 299
  professional barriers and obstacles, 298
  sensuality of, 294–295
  sex affirmative healthcare environments and, 298–299
  unlearning negative associations, 298
Touch Continuum, 294, 295f
TOUCH intervention, 296–297, 296b
Tough Talk: Helping Doctors Approach Difficult Conversations, 50t
Towards Cultural Competency in End-of-Life Communication Training, 85b
Training. See Education
Transactional communication

advance care planning and, 198
overview of, 15, 19–20
person-centered care and, 15–18
teamwork and, 18–19
transmission model of communication vs., 3–5
Transactional Model of Stress and Coping, 409t
Transcultural Concepts in Nursing Care (Andrews and Boyle), 81
Transcultural Nursing: Assessment & Intervention, 85b
Transgender individuals. *See* Lesbian, gay, bisexual, and transgender individuals
Transition coaches, 251
Transitions. *See also* Coordination
from acute care hospital, decision-making and, 250–251, 250t
communicating, 247–249
from curative to palliative, 3
overview of, 246, 253
Transmission model of communication, 3–5, 14–15
Transplantation and organ donation
cardiac transplantation, 192–193
hematopoietic stem cell/bone marrow transplantation, 193–194
kidney disease and, 190–191
liver transplantation, 191–192, 191t
lung transplantation, 192
non-solid transplantation, 189–190
overview of, 188, 194
palliative care and, 189–190
solid organ, 190
Triangulation, 405
Trust
African Americans and, 258–259
comfort measures and, 279–281
homeless, mentally ill, and drug-addicted patients and, 207–208
overview of, 255–256, 261–262
power and, 257
as preexisting condition, 256–257
Truthfulness, 32
Truth-telling, 41
Tuesdays with Morrie (Albom), 17
Tumor board meetings, 335–336
Turn-taking, 81t
Twelve Tips for Teaching Diversity and Embedding it in the Medical Curriculum, 86b

UK General Medicine Council, 288t
Uncertainty
patient-and family-centered communication and, 356–357, 357f, 359
patient-centered communication and, 242
social worker communication and, 377
Unequal Treatment (IOM), 155
University of Alberta, 395
University of British Columbia, 392
University of California San Francisco, 24t, 122t
University of Louisville, 394
University of South Dakota, 392
University of Utah, 392
University of Washington Center for Palliative Care Education, 77
University of Washington School of Medicine Quality of Communication Questionnaire, 404, 405
Unstructured interviewing, 402
Utilization, 90, 156
Utterances, 410t

Valence, 410t
Validation, 405
Validity, 405, 409, 411t
VALUE acronym, 357, 359
Value-based medicine, 278
Values, 175t
Values/Ethics for Interprofessional Practice competency, 390
Variables, 401, 401t
Ventilation, 177–178
Verbal following, 383
Verbatims, 383, 384t
Veterans, seriously ill
communication challenges for, 217–218, 217b
Gulf War, Afghanistan, and Iraq War, 215–216
interventions for, 218, 218b
Korean War, 215
overview of, 214, 218b
palliative care needs of, 216
unique stresses experienced by, 216–217
Vietnam War, 215
World War II, 214
Video technology, 12, 93, 378, 414. *See also* Technology
Vietnam War veterans, 215, 217
Vignettes, 378t

Virtual patients, 394–395
Visual learning, 57
VITAL talk, 180
Vitaltalk, 24t
Vocabulary
challenges of communication and, 417
grief and, 313
lesbian, gay, bisexual, and transgender individuals and, 232–234
nursing communication and, 370t
pain management and, 264–265, 267–268, 268t
public messaging and, 23–25
social worker communication and, 376
spirituality and, 306
Vokis, 395

Warehousing, 162–163
Warrior culture, 216–217
Watzlawick, Paul, 15
WBFPRS. *See* Wong Baker Faces Pain Radiating Scale
We Are MacMillan Cancer Support, 273t
WebMD, 122t, 123t
Weisman, Avery, 258
When Cancer Calls, 162, 168–170, 169t
Wicks, Robert, 16
Willingness to Communicate measure, 411t
Winfrey, Oprah, 261
Wong Baker Faces Pain Radiating Scale (WBFPRS), 263
Work, 133, 239
Worldviews, 154
World War II veterans, 214, 217
Written communication, patient- and family-centered
advance care planning and, 285, 286
cultural humility and, 85b
email, 103–104, 107t
end-of-life leaflets, 104–105, 107t
health literacy and, 103, 107t
importance of, 102–103, 107t
online patient-patient forums, 105–106, 107t
overview of, 102, 106–108, 107t
text types for, 103

Yale University, 394
Young, Jeffrey, 132–133
Your Life, Your Choices, 290b

Zitter, Jessica, 2–3